DISEASES of METABOLISM

DETAILED METHODS OF DIAGNOSIS AND TREATMENT

A Text for the Practitioner

Edited by

GARFIELD G. DUNCAN, M. D.

Chief of Medical Service "B," Pennsylvania Hospital; Clinical
Professor of Medicine, Jefferson Medical College,
Philadelphia, Pennsylvania

CONTRIBUTORS

WALTER BAUER

ABRAHAM CANTAROW

GARFIELD GEORGE DUNCAN

FERDINAND FETTER

CYRIL NORMAN HUGH LONG

LOUIS HARRY NEWBURGH

TOM D. SPIES

HUGH R. BUTT

TRACY DONALD CUTTLE

FRANK ALEXANDER EVANS

FRIEDRICH KLEMPERER

EDWARD HALTON MASON

JOHN PUNNETT PETERS

LEANDRO MAUÉS TOCANTINS

ABRAHAM WHITE

FULLY ILLUSTRATED
INCLUDING 7 PLATES IN COLOR

PHILADELPHIA AND LONDON

W. B. SAUNDERS COMPANY

1942

"DURING the past few decades the clinician and the laboratory worker have been drawn closer together, to the mutual benefit of each. This symbiosis has stimulated research. There has been an increasing flow of new facts. These facts have led to a better understanding of both the normal and the abnormal. There are few branches of medical science in which sound knowledge has advanced so rapidly as has been the case in the field of the diseases of metabolism.

"Metabolism can be treated as an entity in a laboratory but, in dealing with diseases of metabolism, it is found necessary to invade the fields of nutrition, endocrinology and even hematology. The purpose of this book is to present the fundamental knowledge of metabolism, to apply this knowledge to the explanation of diseases of metabolism and to outline a rational basis for the treatment of these diseases.

"To present to the physician, the teacher and the student of medicine the true picture, as it is today, of the diseases of metabolism is a great responsibility. The editor has wisely chosen a group of outstanding authorities to assist him in this task. It is hoped that this book will fill the need for ready information on a subject which is so important in all fields of medical science."

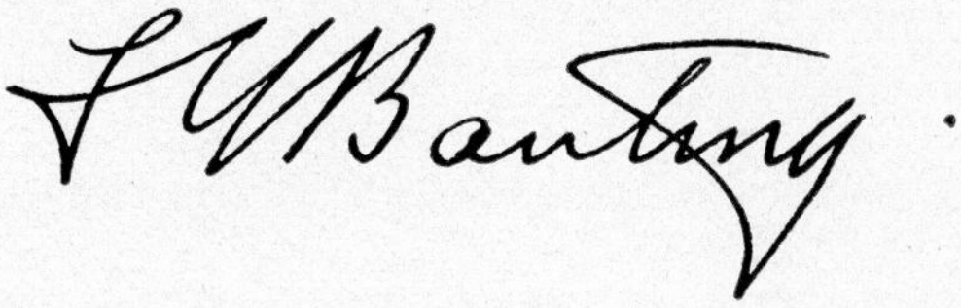

F W Banting

iii

CONTRIBUTORS

WALTER BAUER, M.D.

Associate Professor in Medicine, Harvard Medical School; Physician in Medicine, Massachusetts General Hospital; Director, Robert W. Lovett Memorial.

HUGH R. BUTT, M.D.

Consultant, Division of Medicine, the Mayo Clinic; Instructor in Medicine, the Mayo Foundation, Graduate School of the University of Minnesota.

ABRAHAM CANTAROW, M.D.

Associate Professor of Medicine, Jefferson Medical College; Assistant Physician, Jefferson Hospital; Biochemist, Jefferson Hospital.

TRACY DONALD CUTTLE, M.D.

Demonstrator in Medicine, Jefferson Medical College; Assistant Physician to the Pennsylvania Hospital; Chief of Out-patient Clinic, Medical Service B, and Clinical Assistant of Diabetic Clinic, Jefferson Hospital.

GARFIELD GEORGE DUNCAN, M.D.

Chief of Medical Service "B," Pennsylvania Hospital and Associate Professor of Medicine, Jefferson Medical College, Philadelphia.

FRANK ALEXANDER EVANS, M.D.

Chief of Medical Division, Western Pennsylvania Hospital, Pittsburgh.

FERDINAND FETTER, M.D.

Associate in Medicine, School of Medicine, University of Pennsylvania; Assistant Physician, the Pennsylvania Hospital; Associate Physician, Presbyterian Hospital, Philadelphia.

FRIEDRICH KLEMPERER, M.D.

Assistant in Medicine, Harvard Medical School; Graduate Assistant in Medicine, Massachusetts General Hospital.

CYRIL NORMAN HUGH LONG, M.D.

Sterling Professor of Physiological Chemistry, Yale University School of Medicine.

EDWARD HALTON MASON, M.D.

Associate Professor of Medicine, McGill University; Physician, Royal Victoria Hospital, Montreal.

LOUIS HARRY NEWBURGH, M.D.

Professor of Clinical Investigation, the Medical School, University of Michigan.

JOHN PUNNETT PETERS, M.D.

John Slade Ely Professor of Medicine, Yale University; Associate Physician, New Haven Hospital and New Haven Dispensary.

TOM D. SPIES, M.D.

Associate Professor of Medicine, University of Cincinnati College of Medicine.

LEANDRO MAUÉS TOCANTINS, M.D.

Associate Professor of Medicine, Jefferson Medical College; Physician, the Pennsylvania Hospital; Assistant Physician, Jefferson Hospital, Philadelphia.

ABRAHAM WHITE, Ph.D.

Assistant Professor of Physiological Chemistry, Yale University School of Medicine.

PREFACE

THE abiding aim in the writing of this book has been to provide for the physician a practical basis for the understanding, diagnosis and treatment of the various metabolic disorders. A practical consideration of the physiology of metabolism, the pathological physiology as observed in the various diseases of metabolism, and the methods of detecting and of treating these disturbances is presented. The fundamentals are reviewed and are interpreted in the light of recent investigative work. The gap is bridged between the investigator employing chemical and physiological methods and the physician who applies the results of laboratory investigation in the identification and treatment of disease.

Metabolism, be it normal or abnormal, offers a complicated problem. The authors have simplified their respective phases of the subject as much as is possible to do, and yet they have made their presentations sufficiently comprehensive and sufficiently enlightening to give the reader a working knowledge of the disorders under discussion. Subjects about which much controversy exists have been for the most part omitted, as have the advanced scientific considerations which have little or no practical application at the present time.

Clinical considerations are presented in detail. Laboratory data are important in most diseases of metabolism. They are considered here in the light of being aids in understanding, aids to diagnosis and aids in the conduct of treatment of these diseases.

No attempt has been made to present a complete bibliography. References have been restricted to works which, in the opinion of the authors, are the most important and comprehensive.

The presentation of a comprehensive work on the subject of metabolism is fraught with certain difficulties. It is difficult to know how far the fields of nutrition and endocrinology should be invaded to have in the end a complete book on metabolism. The subjects of nutrition and nutritional or deficiency diseases are inseparably linked with the subject of metabolism. Hence they have been included. The vitamins of known clinical value are dealt with in detail.

Reason defeats tradition when the anemias due to a deficiency either of the maturation factors or of iron are discussed with the other deficiency diseases. Objectively the problems relating to these diseases are largely hematological, but etiologically and therapeutically they are problems of nutrition and metabolism.

Endocrine disturbances have been included only when they are directly related to disorders generally recognized as metabolic diseases. Obesity associated with endocrine disturbances, and the disturbances in calcium metabolism in diseases of the parathyroid gland are examples. Diseases of the thyroid gland which cause nutritional and metabolic disturbances are discussed. There has been no attempt to include endocrinology as a whole.

I am exceedingly grateful to the late Sir Frederick Banting for his encouragement in this undertaking. In a letter received from Sir Frederick early in the course of the preparation of this volume, he said: "I have been forced to travel a great deal on pressing business and have had little time to think of what to say or how to say it." The Foreword was received but a few days before Sir Frederick's untimely death, which occurred in the conduct of that "pressing business." Humanity's indebtedness to this great man is inestimable.

My thanks are due Dr. Frederick M. Allen, to whom I owe my early interest in diseases of metabolism, and to him I am indebted for a happy and profitable two years spent as his first assistant; and to my predecessor at the Pennsylvania Hospital, the late Professor Thomas McCrae, whose clinical training and tutelage during an association which lasted eight years did much to encourage clinical interpretations of medical problems.

I wish to express my gratitude to the co-authors, who by their cooperation and promptness have made it possible to have a composite book, authoritatively presented, available in a remarkably short time.

I am grateful also to Professors Walter E. Lee, John B. Flick, Thomas A. Shallow and George P. Muller for permission to observe and report on patients under their care. Acknowledgment and thanks for giving me the benefit of their knowledge on many points are due many of my friends and associates, especially to Drs. F. Fetter, A. Cantarow, J. T. Durkin, L. S. Carey, L. Tocantins, J. T. Bauer, W. A. Wolff, T. D. Cuttle, C. W. Wirts, L. W. Parkhurst and colleagues at the Pennsylvania and Jefferson Hospitals too numerous to mention.

For the painstaking secretarial efforts I am indebted to Miss Mary Smyth, Miss Eleanor Roulston and especially to Dorthea E. Duncan. I am grateful also to the nurses and dietitians, especially Miss Mary Harding, Miss Martha Tarbox and Miss Martha Alderman, who have labored in behalf of my diabetic patients. My appreciation is also due the publishers, W. B. Saunders Company, for their cooperation and counsel. For permission to reproduce in part previous publications, I am indebted to Lea & Febiger Company and to the publishers of the International Clinics, the Medical Clinics of North America, and the Bulletin of the Ayer Clinical Laboratory, Pennsylvania Hospital.

GARFIELD G. DUNCAN.

January, 1942.

CONTENTS

ix

CHAPTER IV

CHAPTER V

CHAPTER VIII

CHAPTER IX

CHAPTER X

CHAPTER XI

XANTHOMATOSES, GLYCOGEN DISEASE, AND DISTURBANCES OF INTER-
MEDIARY METABOLISM 592

BY EDWARD MASON

CHAPTER XII

GOUT 609

BY WALTER BAUER AND FRIEDRICH KLEMPERER

CHAPTER XIII

HYPERINSULINISM 655

BY GARFIELD G. DUNCAN

CHAPTER XIV

CHAPTER XV

CHAPTER XVI

BY GARFIELD G. DUNCAN

DISEASES OF METABOLISM

CHAPTER I

INTRODUCTORY CONSIDERATIONS

By Garfield G. Duncan

*Hast thou marked nature's diligence? The body of everything
that takes nourishment dies and is constantly reborn.*
—LEONARDO DE VINCI

METABOLISM

Definitions.—*Metabolism* is the sum total of tissue activity as considered in terms of physicochemical changes associated with and regulated by the availability, utilization and disposal of protein, fat, carbohydrate, vitamins, minerals, water, and the influences which the endocrines exert on these processes. These processes have to do with growth, tissue repair, the regulation of the body temperature, energy production for muscular activity, and the maintenance of vital functions.

Anabolism is a term, not freely used in clinical circles, employed to denote the assimilative processes of metabolism relating to tissue growth, maintenance, and repair. *Catabolism* constitutes those changes which involve the breaking down of tissue into simple constituents in which form they are readily excreted under normal conditions.

Alterations from these normal metabolic processes as recognized by clinical and chemical examinations constitute *diseases of metabolism.*

Nutritional Requirements of Man.—There is, in normal individuals, a beautifully balanced mechanism which, by automatically adjusting the desire for food and its repletion, maintains a normal body weight. A normal appetite gauges the amount and kind of food necessary to maintain the total metabolism with extraordinary exactness. It is altered in direct proportion to increases and decreases in the total metabolism. In this manner under normal conditions, three demands comprising the *total* energy metabolism are satisfied and loss of weight is prevented. These demands are: (1) the specific dynamic action of food (S.D.A.), (2) the energy expenditure for the execution of physical work, and (3) the basal metabolism or the minimal caloric needs which for the normal adult approximates 25 calories per Kg. of body weight.

The Specific Dynamic Action of Food (S.D.A.).—The raising of the metabolism above the basal rate caused by the metabolism of food is known as the *specific dynamic action of food.* This effect, commencing within one hour after the ingestion of food, increases gradually, reaching the peak about the third hour, where it is maintained for several hours. The increases

1

above the basal metabolism brought about by the respective foods are as follows:

Protein.. 30 per cent
Carbohydrate.. 6 per cent
Fat... 4 per cent

A meal with a high protein content dissipates more energy than a meal containing liberal amounts of carbohydrate and fat with a small allowance of protein.

The specific dynamic action (S.D.A.) of protein is believed by Best to be dependent on the stimulating effect which amino acids have on the tissue cells. The liver is essential for this reaction, there being no such action in hepatectomized dogs. The *S.D.A.* of carbohydrate is believed to represent the energy liberated in the conversion of glucose to glycogen and in the case of fat to the speeding up of the oxidation of fat, which follows the ingestion of this food substance.

Energy Expenditure for Physical Work.—The expenditure of energy by physical exertion also increases metabolic activity. *Light muscular effort,* such as sitting, standing, dressing, undressing, etc., raises the metabolism 25 to 60 per cent above the basal level. *Moderate exercise,* such as walking, swimming, housework, carpentry, raises it 100 to 200 per cent; and strenuous exercise, such as competitive sports, heavy labor, sawing wood, etc., may increase it from 8 to 15 times the basal level.

TABLE 1

EXTRA CALORIES* OF METABOLISM PER HOUR ATTRIBUTABLE TO OCCUPATION—LUSK[1]

Occupations of Men	Extra calories per hour
Tailor...	44
Bookbinder..	81
Shoemaker...	90
Metal worker, filing and hammering....................	141
Painter of furniture..................................	145
Carpenter making a table.............................	164
Stone mason chiselling a stone.......................	300
Man sawing wood......................................	378
Occupations of Women	
Seamstress, needlework...............................	6
Typist—50 words per minute...........................	24
Seamstress using a sewing machine....................	57
Bookbinder..	63
Housemaid (moderate work)............................	81
Laundress (moderate work)............................	124
Housemaid (hard work)................................	157
Laundress (hard work)................................	214

* The calories referred to are those required in excess of the basal needs by the various occupations.

Mental effort, in contrast to physical effort, causes negligible increases above the basal rate.

BASAL METABOLISM

The minimum heat production of the body, measured directly or indirectly, is the *basal metabolism,* also referred to as the standard metabolism. It is usually determined by measuring the oxygen consumption or the carbon dioxide production of the patient under standard conditions, *i.e.*, in the postabsorptive state and with the subject at complete physical and mental rest (correction is made for the temperature and barometric pressure). A slightly lower oxygen consumption and hence a lower heat production is obtained during sleep, but studies of the gaseous exchange under these conditions are not practical clinically. The most widely employed method of determining the basal metabolism is by measuring the oxygen consumption per minute over a given period, usually six or eight minutes. In this manner it is a simple matter to calculate the heat (Calories) production per square meter of body surface per hour. The figure representing the oxygen consumption obtained after a correction for temperature and barometric pressure is recorded in percentage of the standard normal heat production (Calories) per square meter of body surface and is known as the *basal metabolic rate* (B.M.R.), a term introduced by Plummer and Boothby. The normal standards with which comparisons are made are presented in table 4 (p. 12).

The normal basal metabolic oxygen requirement per square meter of body surface is remarkably constant for individuals of the same height, weight, age and sex. Instances of exact physiological regulation are not confined to oxygen utilization. Such constancy is also observed in the regulation of body temperature, the number of red blood cells per cu. mm. of blood and the blood sugar concentration.

Lavoisier, toward the end of the eighteenth century, demonstrated that animal heat was the result of oxidation of carbon in the body. Oxygen was consumed and CO_2 was produced. A parallelism between the amount of heat generated in this process and the quantity of CO_2 liberated was established. Prior to Lavoisier's observation, Crawford observed a parallelism between the amount of oxygen used and the heat produced. The two *indirect methods* of determining the basal metabolic rates, clinically, are based upon these principles: carbon dioxide production is calculated when the Tissot apparatus or when the Douglas bag is used; oxygen consumption is measured when the Benedict-Roth, Sanborn, Jones, McKesson, and Krogh machines are employed. The method employed when any one of the latter machines is used avoids the error so common in the interpretation of the CO_2 production, namely, the *Auspumpung* or excessive elimination or washing out of CO_2 due to hyperventilation. The Knipping apparatus allows the combined analyses of oxygen consumption and the carbon dioxide production. The *direct* method of determining the basal metabolic rate entails placing the patient in a calorimeter and actually measuring the heat produced per unit of time. It is apparent from the principles of the three methods of determining the basal metabolic rate as outlined above that the basal metabolism may be expressed in three terms, *i.e.*, oxygen consumed, carbon dioxide liberated, and heat produced. Each indicates the heat (Calories) production per unit of time.

The basal metabolic rate, as demonstrated by Magnus-Levy, is especially valuable in confirming the clinical diagnosis of hyper- and hypothyroidism. It may be correlated with an excess or impairment of thyroid activity. Repeated tests give an opportunity to observe changes under treatment, *i.e.*, rest, iodine, roentgen ray therapy, and after surgical intervention and thyroid therapy for hyperthyroidism. The test is especially valuable as a guide in regulating thyroid therapy in cretinism and myxedema. It is an aid in uncovering hyperthyroidism masked by other diseases. Recently I have seen two patients suffering from heart disease with tachycardia. In neither was the pulse rate reduced following appropriate treatment and apparent improvement of the cardiac disorder. In one the basal metabolic rate was plus 75 per cent, and in the other plus 54 per cent. Neither patient exhibited the classical signs of hyperthyroidism. Indeed, the disorder was not suspected in one and in the other it was suggested by a medical student as a cause of the unexplained persistent tachycardia. In each instance a marked reduction of the basal metabolic rate and pulse rate followed the administration of iodides in preparation for a subtotal thyroidectomy.

I can do no better than present the conclusions which Means[2] has made regarding the value of determinations of the basal metabolism:

1. "Patients with an outspoken clinical picture of hyperthyroidism invariably show increased metabolism, and those with definite clinical pictures of hypothyroidism invariably show decreased metabolism. Those with goiters, but no signs or symptoms of abnormal function for the most part show normal metabolism.

2. "Patients with atypical or incomplete clinical evidence of abnormal thyroid function may show normal or abnormal metabolism. The majority show normal metabolism.

3. "By inference from the indirect evidence we believe that in these borderline thyroid cases, provided that in the first place a true basal rate is secured, and, provided that certain well recognized causes for increased metabolism, such as fever, acromegaly, leukemia and severe anemia are excluded, the finding of an increased basal metabolic rate is strong presumptive evidence of hyperthyroidism. In a similar way, provided that such conditions as starvation, hypopituitarism, and hyposuprarenalism are excluded, a low metabolic rate is strong presumptive evidence of hypothyroidism.

4. "To that extent, then, the metabolism test is distinctly useful in differential diagnosis. Like all other laboratory tests it should be interpreted only with due regard to all other clinical and laboratory findings, and with due regard for its limitations and pitfalls."

There are two indirect methods of determining the basal metabolic rate: (1) the closed or spirometric method—this method is extensively used in this country because of its accuracy, ease of operation, and because it does not entail chemical analyses; (2) the open or gasometric method—this method is not widely used because of the gas analyses involved.

The preparation for the test by either method is the same. The patient is instructed to retire early the night before the test. No food is to be taken after 8 P.M. and the test is conducted on the following morning from twelve to sixteen hours after the ingestion of food. The patient is kept quiet and not allowed to walk about before the test. If the apparatus for determining the basal metabolism is at some distant part of the hospital the patient is taken on a stretcher or wheel chair and allowed to lie motionless for twenty or thirty minutes before the test is made. The error introduced by exercise and emotional disturbance is greater in hyper- than in hypothyroidism.

It is more satisfactory, but not essential to have ambulatory patients admitted to the hospital over night and have the test done in a quiet room before breakfast. Records are made of the patient's height, weight, age, sex, pulse rate and body temperature. The temperature of the air in the spirometer and the barometric pressure are also recorded.

Closed or Spirometric Method.—The patient, when prepared for the preliminary test, breathes through a closely fitting soft rubber mouth piece. The nasal passages are shut off by an adjustable rubber clamp. The "system" is closed, the inspired air being drawn from the oxygen reservoir or spirometer chamber, passing through a rubber flutter valve which permits passage of air in one direction only. The expired air proceeds by another passage

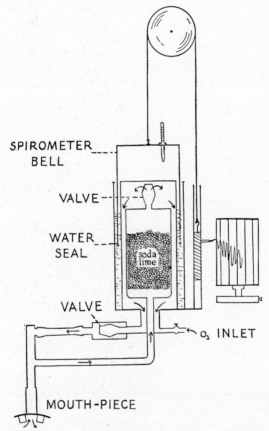

Fig. 1.—Sectional view of Benedict-Roth closed circuit respiration apparatus.

to a chamber containing soda lime, which removes the CO_2, thence via another one-way rubber flutter valve into the spirometer chamber, thus completing the circuit. The amount of air in the spirometer chamber, filled with oxygen before the test is begun, increases and decreases with expiration and inspiration respectively. This is facilitated by the sensitive balancing of the spirometer bell which rises, without noticeable effort to the patient, during expiration and falls during inspiration. Loss of oxygen and the entrance of outside air into the system are prevented by a water seal between the spirometer chamber and the external casing. The changing levels of the spirometer bell are permanently recorded on a drum which is uniformly revolved by a clock device. The level of the spirometer lowers in direct proportion to the rate of oxygen consumption. The volume of oxygen utilized over a given period is determined by simple calculation. A diagram of the apparatus is presented in figure 1.

TABLE 2*

THE SURFACE AREA OF THE BODY IS INDICATED IN SQUARE METERS, WHERE THE HORIZONTAL LINE DRAWN AT THE LEVEL OF THE PATIENT'S WEIGHT CROSSES A VERTICAL LINE DRAWN FROM THE PATIENT'S HEIGHT. ILLUSTRATION: PATIENT'S WEIGHT, 176 POUNDS AND HEIGHT 68.9 INCHES HAS A SURFACE AREA OF 1.96 SQ. METERS.

HEIGHT-CENTIMETERS

WEIGHT-KILOGRAMS	140	141	142	143	144	145	146	147	148	149	150	151	152	153	154	155	156	157	158	159	160	161	162	163	164
40	1.24	1.25	1.25	1.26	1.27	1.27	1.28	1.28	1.29	1.30	1.30	1.31	1.32	1.32	1.33	1.33	1.34	1.35	1.35	1.36	1.37	1.37	1.38	1.38	1.39
41	1.25	1.26	1.27	1.27	1.28	1.29	1.29	1.30	1.30	1.31	1.32	1.33	1.33	1.34	1.34	1.35	1.36	1.36	1.37	1.37	1.38	1.39	1.39	1.40	1.41
42	1.27	1.27	1.28	1.29	1.29	1.30	1.30	1.31	1.32	1.32	1.33	1.34	1.34	1.35	1.36	1.36	1.37	1.38	1.38	1.39	1.39	1.40	1.41	1.41	1.42
43	1.28	1.29	1.29	1.30	1.30	1.31	1.32	1.32	1.33	1.34	1.34	1.35	1.36	1.36	1.37	1.38	1.38	1.39	1.40	1.40	1.41	1.41	1.42	1.43	1.43
44	1.29	1.30	1.30	1.31	1.32	1.32	1.33	1.34	1.34	1.35	1.36	1.36	1.37	1.38	1.38	1.39	1.40	1.40	1.41	1.42	1.42	1.43	1.44	1.44	1.45
45	1.30	1.31	1.32	1.32	1.33	1.34	1.34	1.35	1.36	1.36	1.37	1.38	1.38	1.39	1.40	1.40	1.41	1.42	1.42	1.43	1.44	1.44	1.45	1.46	1.46
46	1.32	1.32	1.33	1.34	1.34	1.35	1.36	1.36	1.37	1.38	1.38	1.39	1.40	1.40	1.41	1.42	1.42	1.43	1.44	1.44	1.45	1.46	1.46	1.47	1.48
47	1.33	1.33	1.34	1.35	1.36	1.37	1.37	1.38	1.38	1.39	1.40	1.40	1.41	1.42	1.42	1.43	1.44	1.44	1.45	1.46	1.46	1.47	1.48	1.48	1.49
48	1.34	1.35	1.35	1.36	1.37	1.37	1.38	1.39	1.39	1.40	1.41	1.42	1.42	1.43	1.44	1.44	1.45	1.46	1.46	1.47	1.48	1.48	1.49	1.50	1.50
49	1.35	1.36	1.37	1.37	1.38	1.39	1.39	1.40	1.41	1.41	1.42	1.43	1.43	1.44	1.45	1.45	1.46	1.47	1.48	1.48	1.49	1.50	1.50	1.51	1.52
50	1.36	1.37	1.38	1.38	1.39	1.40	1.41	1.41	1.42	1.43	1.43	1.44	1.45	1.45	1.46	1.47	1.47	1.48	1.49	1.49	1.50	1.51	1.52	1.52	1.53
51	1.37	1.38	1.39	1.40	1.40	1.41	1.42	1.42	1.43	1.44	1.45	1.45	1.46	1.47	1.47	1.48	1.49	1.49	1.50	1.51	1.51	1.52	1.53	1.53	1.54
52	1.39	1.39	1.40	1.41	1.41	1.42	1.43	1.44	1.44	1.45	1.46	1.46	1.47	1.48	1.49	1.49	1.50	1.51	1.51	1.52	1.53	1.53	1.54	1.55	1.55
53	1.40	1.40	1.41	1.42	1.43	1.43	1.44	1.45	1.45	1.46	1.47	1.48	1.48	1.49	1.50	1.50	1.51	1.52	1.53	1.53	1.54	1.55	1.55	1.56	1.57
54	1.41	1.42	1.42	1.43	1.44	1.44	1.45	1.46	1.47	1.47	1.48	1.49	1.49	1.50	1.51	1.52	1.52	1.53	1.54	1.54	1.55	1.56	1.57	1.57	1.58
55	1.42	1.43	1.43	1.44	1.45	1.46	1.46	1.47	1.48	1.49	1.49	1.50	1.51	1.52	1.52	1.53	1.54	1.54	1.55	1.56	1.56	1.57	1.58	1.58	1.59
56	1.43	1.44	1.45	1.45	1.46	1.47	1.47	1.48	1.49	1.50	1.50	1.51	1.52	1.53	1.53	1.54	1.55	1.55	1.56	1.57	1.58	1.58	1.59	1.60	1.60
57	1.44	1.45	1.46	1.46	1.47	1.48	1.49	1.49	1.50	1.51	1.52	1.52	1.53	1.54	1.54	1.55	1.56	1.57	1.57	1.58	1.59	1.59	1.60	1.61	1.62
58	1.45	1.46	1.47	1.47	1.48	1.49	1.50	1.50	1.51	1.52	1.53	1.53	1.54	1.55	1.56	1.56	1.57	1.58	1.58	1.59	1.60	1.61	1.61	1.62	1.63
59	1.46	1.47	1.48	1.49	1.49	1.50	1.51	1.52	1.52	1.53	1.54	1.54	1.55	1.56	1.57	1.57	1.58	1.59	1.60	1.60	1.61	1.62	1.63	1.63	1.64
60	1.47	1.48	1.49	1.50	1.50	1.51	1.52	1.53	1.53	1.54	1.55	1.56	1.56	1.57	1.58	1.59	1.59	1.60	1.61	1.62	1.62	1.63	1.64	1.64	1.65
61	1.48	1.49	1.50	1.51	1.51	1.52	1.53	1.54	1.54	1.55	1.56	1.57	1.57	1.58	1.59	1.60	1.60	1.61	1.62	1.63	1.63	1.64	1.65	1.66	1.66
62	1.49	1.50	1.51	1.52	1.52	1.53	1.54	1.55	1.55	1.56	1.57	1.58	1.59	1.59	1.60	1.60	1.61	1.62	1.63	1.64	1.65	1.65	1.66	1.67	1.68
63	1.50	1.51	1.52	1.53	1.53	1.54	1.55	1.56	1.57	1.57	1.58	1.59	1.60	1.60	1.61	1.62	1.63	1.63	1.64	1.65	1.66	1.66	1.67	1.68	1.69
64	1.51	1.52	1.53	1.54	1.55	1.55	1.56	1.57	1.58	1.58	1.59	1.60	1.61	1.61	1.62	1.63	1.64	1.65	1.66	1.66	1.67	1.68	1.68	1.69	1.70
65	1.52	1.53	1.54	1.55	1.56	1.56	1.57	1.58	1.59	1.59	1.60	1.61	1.62	1.63	1.63	1.64	1.65	1.66	1.66	1.67	1.68	1.69	1.69	1.70	1.71
66	1.53	1.54	1.55	1.56	1.57	1.57	1.58	1.59	1.60	1.60	1.61	1.62	1.63	1.64	1.64	1.65	1.66	1.67	1.67	1.68	1.69	1.70	1.70	1.71	1.72
67	1.54	1.55	1.56	1.57	1.58	1.58	1.59	1.60	1.61	1.61	1.62	1.63	1.64	1.65	1.65	1.66	1.67	1.68	1.69	1.69	1.70	1.71	1.72	1.72	1.73
68	1.55	1.56	1.57	1.58	1.59	1.59	1.60	1.61	1.62	1.63	1.63	1.64	1.65	1.66	1.66	1.67	1.68	1.69	1.70	1.70	1.71	1.72	1.73	1.73	1.74
69	1.56	1.57	1.58	1.59	1.60	1.60	1.61	1.61	1.62	1.63	1.64	1.65	1.66	1.67	1.67	1.68	1.69	1.70	1.71	1.71	1.72	1.73	1.74	1.75	1.75
70	1.57	1.58	1.59	1.60	1.61	1.61	1.62	1.63	1.64	1.65	1.65	1.66	1.67	1.68	1.69	1.69	1.70	1.71	1.72	1.72	1.73	1.74	1.75	1.76	1.76
71	1.58	1.59	1.60	1.61	1.61	1.62	1.63	1.64	1.65	1.66	1.66	1.67	1.68	1.69	1.70	1.70	1.71	1.72	1.73	1.74	1.74	1.75	1.76	1.77	1.77
72	1.59	1.60	1.61	1.62	1.62	1.63	1.64	1.65	1.66	1.67	1.67	1.68	1.69	1.70	1.71	1.71	1.72	1.73	1.74	1.75	1.75	1.76	1.77	1.78	1.78
73	1.60	1.61	1.62	1.63	1.63	1.64	1.65	1.66	1.67	1.67	1.68	1.69	1.69	1.70	1.71	1.72	1.73	1.74	1.75	1.76	1.76	1.77	1.78	1.79	1.80
74	1.61	1.62	1.63	1.64	1.64	1.65	1.66	1.67	1.68	1.68	1.69	1.70	1.71	1.72	1.73	1.73	1.74	1.75	1.76	1.77	1.77	1.78	1.79	1.80	1.81
75	1.62	1.63	1.64	1.64	1.65	1.66	1.67	1.68	1.69	1.69	1.70	1.71	1.72	1.73	1.74	1.74	1.75	1.76	1.77	1.78	1.78	1.79	1.80	1.81	1.82
76	1.63	1.64	1.65	1.65	1.66	1.67	1.68	1.69	1.70	1.70	1.71	1.72	1.73	1.74	1.74	1.75	1.76	1.77	1.78	1.79	1.79	1.80	1.81	1.82	1.83
77	1.64	1.65	1.65	1.66	1.67	1.68	1.69	1.70	1.70	1.71	1.72	1.73	1.74	1.75	1.75	1.76	1.77	1.78	1.79	1.80	1.80	1.81	1.82	1.83	1.84
78	1.65	1.66	1.66	1.67	1.68	1.69	1.70	1.71	1.71	1.72	1.73	1.74	1.75	1.76	1.77	1.77	1.78	1.79	1.80	1.81	1.81	1.82	1.83	1.84	1.85
79	1.66	1.66	1.67	1.68	1.69	1.70	1.71	1.72	1.72	1.73	1.74	1.75	1.76	1.77	1.77	1.78	1.79	1.80	1.81	1.82	1.82	1.83	1.84	1.85	1.86
80	1.66	1.67	1.68	1.69	1.70	1.71	1.72	1.73	1.73	1.74	1.75	1.76	1.77	1.78	1.78	1.79	1.80	1.81	1.82	1.83	1.83	1.84	1.85	1.86	1.87
81	1.67	1.68	1.69	1.70	1.71	1.72	1.72	1.73	1.74	1.75	1.76	1.77	1.78	1.78	1.79	1.80	1.81	1.82	1.83	1.83	1.84	1.85	1.86	1.87	1.88
82	1.68	1.69	1.70	1.71	1.72	1.73	1.73	1.74	1.75	1.76	1.77	1.78	1.79	1.79	1.80	1.81	1.82	1.83	1.84	1.84	1.85	1.86	1.87	1.88	1.89
83	1.69	1.70	1.71	1.72	1.73	1.73	1.74	1.75	1.76	1.77	1.78	1.79	1.79	1.80	1.81	1.82	1.83	1.84	1.85	1.85	1.86	1.87	1.88	1.89	1.90
84	1.70	1.71	1.72	1.73	1.73	1.74	1.75	1.76	1.77	1.78	1.79	1.80	1.80	1.81	1.82	1.83	1.84	1.85	1.85	1.86	1.87	1.88	1.89	1.90	1.91
85	1.71	1.72	1.73	1.73	1.74	1.75	1.76	1.77	1.78	1.79	1.80	1.80	1.81	1.82	1.83	1.84	1.85	1.86	1.86	1.87	1.88	1.89	1.90	1.91	1.92
86	1.72	1.73	1.73	1.74	1.75	1.76	1.77	1.78	1.79	1.80	1.80	1.81	1.82	1.83	1.84	1.85	1.86	1.86	1.87	1.88	1.89	1.90	1.91	1.92	1.92
87	1.72	1.73	1.74	1.75	1.76	1.77	1.78	1.79	1.80	1.80	1.81	1.82	1.83	1.84	1.85	1.86	1.87	1.87	1.88	1.89	1.90	1.91	1.92	1.93	1.94
88	1.73	1.74	1.75	1.76	1.77	1.78	1.79	1.80	1.80	1.81	1.82	1.83	1.84	1.84	1.86	1.87	1.87	1.88	1.89	1.90	1.91	1.92	1.93	1.94	1.94
89	1.74	1.75	1.76	1.77	1.78	1.79	1.80	1.80	1.81	1.82	1.83	1.84	1.85	1.86	1.87	1.87	1.88	1.88	1.90	1.91	1.92	1.93	1.94	1.94	1.95
90	1.75	1.76	1.77	1.78	1.79	1.79	1.80	1.81	1.82	1.83	1.84	1.85	1.86	1.87	1.87	1.88	1.89	1.90	1.91	1.92	1.93	1.94	1.95	1.95	1.96
91	1.76	1.77	1.78	1.79	1.79	1.80	1.81	1.82	1.83	1.84	1.85	1.86	1.87	1.88	1.88	1.89	1.90	1.91	1.92	1.93	1.94	1.95	1.95	1.96	1.97
92	1.77	1.78	1.78	1.79	1.80	1.81	1.82	1.83	1.84	1.85	1.86	1.87	1.87	1.88	1.89	1.90	1.91	1.92	1.93	1.94	1.95	1.95	1.96	1.97	1.98
93	1.77	1.78	1.79	1.80	1.81	1.82	1.83	1.84	1.85	1.86	1.87	1.87	1.88	1.89	1.90	1.91	1.92	1.93	1.94	1.95	1.95	1.96	1.97	1.98	1.99
94	1.78	1.79	1.80	1.81	1.82	1.83	1.84	1.85	1.86	1.86	1.87	1.88	1.89	1.90	1.91	1.92	1.93	1.94	1.95	1.95	1.96	1.97	1.98	1.99	2.00
95	1.79	1.80	1.81	1.82	1.83	1.84	1.85	1.85	1.86	1.87	1.88	1.89	1.90	1.91	1.92	1.93	1.94	1.95	1.95	1.96	1.97	1.98	1.99	2.00	2.01
96	1.80	1.81	1.82	1.83	1.84	1.84	1.85	1.86	1.87	1.88	1.89	1.90	1.91	1.92	1.93	1.94	1.95	1.95	1.96	1.97	1.98	1.99	2.00	2.01	2.02
97	1.81	1.82	1.83	1.83	1.84	1.85	1.86	1.87	1.88	1.89	1.90	1.91	1.92	1.93	1.94	1.94	1.95	1.96	1.97	1.98	1.99	2.00	2.01	2.02	2.03
98	1.81	1.82	1.83	1.84	1.85	1.86	1.87	1.88	1.89	1.90	1.91	1.92	1.93	1.94	1.94	1.95	1.96	1.97	1.98	1.99	2.00	2.01	2.02	2.03	2.03
99	1.82	1.83	1.84	1.85	1.86	1.87	1.88	1.89	1.90	1.91	1.92	1.92	1.93	1.94	1.95	1.96	1.97	1.98	1.99	2.00	2.01	2.02	2.03	2.03	2.04
100	1.83	1.84	1.85	1.86	1.87	1.88	1.89	1.90	1.91	1.91	1.92	1.93	1.94	1.95	1.96	1.97	1.98	1.99	2.00	2.01	2.02	2.03	2.04	2.05	2.05
101	1.84	1.85	1.86	1.87	1.88	1.89	1.89	1.90	1.91	1.92	1.93	1.94	1.95	1.96	1.97	1.98	1.99	2.00	2.01	2.02	2.02	2.03	2.04	2.05	2.05
102	1.85	1.85	1.86	1.87	1.88	1.89	1.90	1.91	1.92	1.93	1.94	1.95	1.96	1.97	1.98	1.99	2.00	2.01	2.01	2.02	2.03	2.04	2.05	2.06	2.07
103	1.85	1.86	1.87	1.88	1.89	1.90	1.91	1.92	1.93	1.94	1.95	1.96	1.97	1.98	1.99	1.99	2.00	2.01	2.02	2.03	2.04	2.05	2.06	2.07	2.08
104	1.86	1.87	1.88	1.89	1.90	1.91	1.92	1.93	1.94	1.95	1.96	1.97	1.97	1.98	1.99	2.00	2.01	2.02	2.03	2.04	2.05	2.06	2.06	2.08	2.09
105	1.87	1.88	1.89	1.90	1.91	1.92	1.93	1.94	1.95	1.95	1.96	1.97	1.98	1.99	2.00	2.01	2.02	2.03	2.04	2.05	2.06	2.07	2.08	2.09	2.10
106	1.88	1.89	1.90	1.90	1.91	1.92	1.93	1.94	1.95	1.96	1.97	1.98	1.99	2.00	2.01	2.02	2.03	2.04	2.05	2.06	2.07	2.08	2.09	2.09	2.10
107	1.88	1.89	1.90	1.91	1.92	1.93	1.94	1.95	1.96	1.97	1.98	1.99	2.00	2.01	2.02	2.03	2.04	2.05	2.06	2.07	2.07	2.08	2.09	2.10	2.11
108	1.89	1.90	1.91	1.92	1.93	1.94	1.95	1.96	1.97	1.98	1.99	2.00	2.01	2.02	2.03	2.04	2.04	2.05	2.06	2.07	2.08	2.09	2.10	2.11	2.12
109	1.90	1.91	1.92	1.93	1.94	1.95	1.96	1.97	1.98	1.99	2.00	2.01	2.01	2.02	2.03	2.04	2.05	2.06	2.07	2.08	2.09	2.10	2.11	2.12	2.13
110	1.91	1.92	1.93	1.94	1.95	1.95	1.96	1.97	1.98	1.99	2.00	2.01	2.02	2.03	2.04	2.05	2.06	2.07	2.08	2.09	2.10	2.11	2.12	2.13	2.14
	55.1	55.5	55.9	56.3	56.7	57.1	57.5	57.9	58.3	58.7	59.1	59.5	59.8	60.2	60.6	61.0	61.4	61.8	62.2	62.6	63.0	63.4	63.8	64.2	64.6

* DuBois body surface chart from height and weight as modified by Boothby and Sandiford.

By an accessory valve, the patient breathes room air through the machine for a minute or two to gain confidence and allay fear. The marker records rate, regularity, and depth of respirations, but of most importance, the rate at which the spirometer bell is lowered (see Fig. 2). From this record the oxygen consumed per minute and the corresponding calories utilized per hour are calculated. A straight line touching the bottom of the greatest number of recorded respiration waves indicates the level of the spirometer bell at the beginning and end of the six-minute test. The amount of oxygen consumed in terms of Calories per hour is the difference between

165	166	167	168	169	170	171	172	173	174	175	176	177	178	179	180	181	182	183	184	185	186	187	188	189	WEIGHT-POUNDS
1.40	1.40	1.41	1.41	1.42	1.43	1.43	1.44	1.45	1.45	1.46	1.46	1.47	1.48	1.48	1.49	1.49	1.50	1.51	1.51	1.52	1.52	1.53	1.54	1.54	88
1.41	1.42	1.42	1.43	1.44	1.44	1.45	1.45	1.46	1.47	1.47	1.48	1.49	1.49	1.50	1.50	1.51	1.52	1.52	1.53	1.53	1.54	1.55	1.55	1.56	90
1.43	1.43	1.44	1.44	1.45	1.46	1.46	1.47	1.48	1.48	1.49	1.49	1.50	1.51	1.51	1.52	1.52	1.53	1.54	1.54	1.55	1.56	1.56	1.57	1.57	93
1.44	1.45	1.45	1.46	1.47	1.47	1.48	1.48	1.49	1.50	1.50	1.51	1.52	1.52	1.53	1.53	1.54	1.55	1.55	1.56	1.56	1.57	1.58	1.58	1.59	95
1.45	1.46	1.47	1.47	1.48	1.49	1.49	1.50	1.51	1.51	1.52	1.52	1.53	1.54	1.54	1.55	1.56	1.56	1.57	1.57	1.58	1.59	1.59	1.60	1.60	97
1.47	1.47	1.48	1.49	1.49	1.50	1.51	1.51	1.52	1.53	1.53	1.54	1.54	1.55	1.56	1.56	1.57	1.57	1.58	1.59	1.60	1.60	1.61	1.61	1.62	99
1.48	1.49	1.50	1.50	1.51	1.51	1.52	1.53	1.53	1.54	1.55	1.55	1.56	1.57	1.57	1.58	1.58	1.59	1.60	1.60	1.61	1.62	1.62	1.63	1.64	101
1.50	1.50	1.51	1.52	1.52	1.53	1.53	1.54	1.55	1.55	1.56	1.57	1.57	1.58	1.59	1.59	1.60	1.61	1.61	1.62	1.62	1.63	1.64	1.64	1.65	104
1.51	1.52	1.52	1.53	1.54	1.54	1.55	1.56	1.56	1.57	1.57	1.58	1.59	1.59	1.60	1.61	1.61	1.62	1.63	1.63	1.64	1.65	1.65	1.66	1.67	106
1.52	1.53	1.54	1.54	1.55	1.56	1.56	1.56	1.58	1.58	1.59	1.60	1.60	1.61	1.61	1.62	1.63	1.63	1.64	1.65	1.65	1.66	1.67	1.67	1.68	108
1.54	1.54	1.55	1.56	1.56	1.57	1.58	1.58	1.59	1.60	1.60	1.61	1.62	1.62	1.63	1.64	1.64	1.65	1.66	1.66	1.67	1.67	1.68	1.69	1.69	110
1.55	1.56	1.56	1.57	1.58	1.58	1.59	1.60	1.60	1.61	1.62	1.62	1.63	1.64	1.64	1.65	1.66	1.66	1.67	1.68	1.68	1.69	1.70	1.70	1.71	112
1.56	1.57	1.58	1.58	1.59	1.60	1.60	1.61	1.62	1.62	1.63	1.64	1.64	1.65	1.66	1.66	1.67	1.68	1.68	1.69	1.70	1.70	1.71	1.72	1.72	115
1.57	1.58	1.59	1.60	1.60	1.61	1.62	1.62	1.63	1.64	1.64	1.65	1.66	1.66	1.67	1.68	1.68	1.69	1.70	1.70	1.71	1.72	1.72	1.73	1.74	117
1.59	1.59	1.60	1.61	1.61	1.62	1.63	1.64	1.64	1.65	1.66	1.66	1.67	1.68	1.68	1.69	1.70	1.70	1.71	1.72	1.72	1.73	1.74	1.74	1.75	119
1.60	1.61	1.61	1.62	1.63	1.63	1.64	1.65	1.65	1.66	1.67	1.68	1.68	1.69	1.70	1.70	1.71	1.72	1.72	1.73	1.74	1.74	1.75	1.76	1.76	121
1.61	1.62	1.63	1.63	1.64	1.64	1.65	1.66	1.67	1.67	1.68	1.69	1.70	1.70	1.71	1.72	1.72	1.73	1.74	1.74	1.75	1.76	1.76	1.77	1.78	123
1.62	1.63	1.64	1.64	1.65	1.66	1.67	1.67	1.68	1.69	1.69	1.70	1.71	1.72	1.72	1.73	1.74	1.74	1.75	1.76	1.76	1.77	1.78	1.78	1.79	126
1.64	1.64	1.65	1.66	1.66	1.67	1.68	1.69	1.69	1.70	1.71	1.71	1.72	1.73	1.73	1.74	1.75	1.76	1.76	1.77	1.78	1.78	1.79	1.80	1.80	128
1.65	1.66	1.67	1.68	1.68	1.68	1.69	1.70	1.70	1.71	1.72	1.73	1.74	1.74	1.75	1.75	1.76	1.77	1.78	1.78	1.79	1.80	1.80	1.81	1.82	130
1.66	1.67	1.67	1.68	1.69	1.70	1.70	1.71	1.72	1.72	1.73	1.74	1.75	1.75	1.76	1.77	1.77	1.78	1.79	1.80	1.80	1.81	1.82	1.82	1.83	132
1.67	1.68	1.69	1.69	1.70	1.71	1.71	1.72	1.73	1.74	1.74	1.75	1.76	1.77	1.77	1.78	1.79	1.79	1.80	1.81	1.82	1.82	1.83	1.84	1.84	134
1.68	1.69	1.70	1.70	1.71	1.72	1.73	1.73	1.74	1.75	1.76	1.76	1.77	1.78	1.78	1.79	1.80	1.81	1.81	1.82	1.83	1.84	1.84	1.85	1.86	137
1.69	1.70	1.71	1.72	1.72	1.73	1.74	1.75	1.75	1.76	1.77	1.78	1.78	1.79	1.80	1.80	1.81	1.82	1.83	1.83	1.84	1.85	1.85	1.86	1.87	139
1.71	1.71	1.72	1.73	1.74	1.74	1.75	1.76	1.76	1.77	1.78	1.79	1.79	1.80	1.81	1.82	1.82	1.83	1.84	1.85	1.85	1.86	1.87	1.87	1.88	141
1.72	1.72	1.73	1.74	1.75	1.75	1.76	1.77	1.78	1.78	1.79	1.80	1.81	1.81	1.82	1.83	1.84	1.84	1.85	1.86	1.86	1.87	1.88	1.89	1.89	143
1.73	1.74	1.74	1.75	1.76	1.77	1.77	1.78	1.79	1.80	1.80	1.81	1.82	1.83	1.83	1.84	1.85	1.85	1.86	1.87	1.88	1.88	1.89	1.90	1.91	146
1.74	1.75	1.75	1.76	1.77	1.78	1.78	1.79	1.80	1.81	1.81	1.82	1.83	1.84	1.84	1.85	1.86	1.87	1.87	1.88	1.89	1.90	1.90	1.91	1.92	148
1.75	1.76	1.77	1.77	1.78	1.79	1.80	1.80	1.81	1.82	1.83	1.83	1.84	1.85	1.86	1.86	1.87	1.88	1.89	1.89	1.90	1.91	1.92	1.92	1.93	150
1.76	1.77	1.78	1.78	1.79	1.80	1.81	1.81	1.82	1.83	1.84	1.85	1.85	1.86	1.87	1.88	1.88	1.89	1.90	1.91	1.91	1.92	1.92	1.93	1.94	152
1.77	1.78	1.79	1.79	1.80	1.81	1.82	1.83	1.83	1.84	1.85	1.86	1.86	1.87	1.88	1.89	1.89	1.90	1.91	1.92	1.92	1.93	1.94	1.95	1.95	154
1.78	1.79	1.80	1.81	1.81	1.82	1.83	1.84	1.84	1.85	1.86	1.87	1.88	1.88	1.89	1.90	1.91	1.91	1.92	1.93	1.94	1.94	1.95	1.96	1.97	157
1.79	1.80	1.81	1.82	1.82	1.83	1.84	1.85	1.85	1.86	1.87	1.88	1.89	1.89	1.90	1.91	1.92	1.93	1.93	1.94	1.95	1.96	1.96	1.97	1.98	159
1.80	1.81	1.82	1.83	1.83	1.84	1.85	1.86	1.86	1.87	1.88	1.89	1.90	1.91	1.91	1.92	1.93	1.94	1.94	1.95	1.96	1.97	1.97	1.98	1.99	161
1.81	1.82	1.83	1.84	1.85	1.85	1.86	1.87	1.88	1.88	1.89	1.90	1.91	1.92	1.92	1.93	1.94	1.95	1.96	1.96	1.97	1.98	1.99	1.99	2.00	163
1.82	1.83	1.84	1.85	1.86	1.86	1.87	1.88	1.89	1.90	1.90	1.91	1.92	1.93	1.94	1.94	1.95	1.96	1.97	1.97	1.98	1.99	2.00	2.01	2.01	165
1.83	1.84	1.85	1.86	1.87	1.87	1.88	1.89	1.90	1.91	1.91	1.92	1.93	1.94	1.95	1.95	1.96	1.97	1.98	1.99	1.99	2.00	2.01	2.02	2.02	168
1.84	1.85	1.86	1.87	1.88	1.88	1.89	1.90	1.91	1.92	1.93	1.93	1.94	1.95	1.96	1.96	1.97	1.98	1.99	2.00	2.00	2.01	2.02	2.03	2.04	170
1.85	1.86	1.87	1.88	1.89	1.90	1.90	1.91	1.92	1.93	1.94	1.94	1.95	1.96	1.97	1.98	1.98	1.99	2.00	2.01	2.02	2.02	2.03	2.04	2.05	172
1.86	1.87	1.88	1.89	1.90	1.91	1.92	1.92	1.93	1.94	1.95	1.95	1.96	1.97	1.98	1.99	1.99	2.00	2.01	2.02	2.03	2.03	2.04	2.05	2.06	174
1.87	1.88	1.89	1.90	1.91	1.92	1.92	1.93	1.94	1.95	1.96	1.96	1.97	1.98	1.99	2.00	2.00	2.01	2.02	2.03	2.04	2.04	2.05	2.06	2.07	176
1.88	1.89	1.90	1.91	1.92	1.92	1.93	1.94	1.95	1.96	1.97	1.97	1.98	1.99	2.00	2.01	2.02	2.03	2.03	2.04	2.05	2.06	2.06	2.07	2.08	179
1.89	1.90	1.91	1.92	1.93	1.94	1.94	1.95	1.96	1.97	1.98	1.99	1.99	2.00	2.01	2.02	2.03	2.03	2.04	2.05	2.06	2.07	2.07	2.08	2.09	181
1.90	1.91	1.92	1.93	1.94	1.95	1.95	1.96	1.97	1.98	1.99	2.00	2.00	2.01	2.02	2.03	2.04	2.04	2.05	2.06	2.07	2.08	2.09	2.09	2.10	183
1.91	1.92	1.93	1.94	1.95	1.96	1.96	1.97	1.99	1.99	2.00	2.01	2.00	2.03	2.04	2.04	2.05	2.05	2.06	2.07	2.08	2.09	2.10	2.10	2.11	185
1.92	1.93	1.94	1.95	1.96	1.97	1.97	1.98	1.99	2.00	2.01	2.02	2.02	2.03	2.04	2.05	2.06	2.07	2.07	2.08	2.09	2.10	2.11	2.11	2.12	187
1.93	1.94	1.95	1.96	1.97	1.98	1.98	1.99	2.00	2.01	2.02	2.03	2.03	2.04	2.05	2.06	2.07	2.08	2.08	2.09	2.10	2.11	2.12	2.13	2.13	190
1.94	1.95	1.96	1.97	1.98	1.99	1.99	2.00	2.01	2.02	2.03	2.04	2.04	2.05	2.06	2.07	2.08	2.09	2.09	2.10	2.11	2.12	2.13	2.14	2.14	192
1.95	1.96	1.97	1.98	1.99	2.00	2.00	2.01	2.02	2.03	2.04	2.05	2.05	2.06	2.07	2.08	2.09	2.10	2.10	2.11	2.12	2.13	2.14	2.15	2.15	194
1.96	1.97	1.98	1.99	2.00	2.00	2.01	2.02	2.03	2.04	2.05	2.06	2.06	2.07	2.08	2.09	2.10	2.11	2.11	2.12	2.13	2.14	2.15	2.16	2.16	196
1.97	1.98	1.99	2.00	2.01	2.01	2.02	2.03	2.04	2.05	2.06	2.07	2.07	2.08	2.09	2.10	2.11	2.12	2.12	2.13	2.14	2.15	2.16	2.17	2.17	198
1.98	1.99	2.00	2.01	2.02	2.02	2.03	2.04	2.05	2.06	2.07	2.00	2.08	2.09	2.10	2.11	2.12	2.13	2.13	2.14	2.15	2.16	2.17	2.18	2.19	201
1.99	2.00	2.01	2.02	2.02	2.03	2.04	2.05	2.06	2.07	2.08	2.08	2.09	2.10	2.11	2.12	2.13	2.14	2.14	2.15	2.16	2.17	2.18	2.19	2.20	203
2.00	2.01	2.02	2.03	2.03	2.04	2.05	2.06	2.07	2.08	2.09	2.09	2.10	2.11	2.12	2.13	2.14	2.15	2.15	2.16	2.17	2.18	2.19	2.20	2.21	205
2.01	2.02	2.03	2.03	2.04	2.05	2.06	2.07	2.08	2.09	2.10	2.10	2.11	2.12	2.13	2.14	2.15	2.16	2.16	2.17	2.18	2.19	2.20	2.21	2.22	207
2.02	2.03	2.03	2.04	2.05	2.06	2.07	2.08	2.09	2.10	2.10	2.11	2.12	2.13	2.14	2.15	2.16	2.17	2.17	2.18	2.19	2.20	2.21	2.22	2.23	209
2.02	2.03	2.04	2.05	2.06	2.07	2.08	2.09	2.10	2.11	2.11	2.12	2.13	2.14	2.15	2.16	2.17	2.18	2.18	2.19	2.20	2.21	2.22	2.23	2.24	212
2.03	2.04	2.05	2.06	2.07	2.08	2.09	2.10	2.11	2.11	2.12	2.13	2.14	2.15	2.16	2.17	2.18	2.18	2.19	2.20	2.21	2.22	2.23	2.24	2.25	214
2.04	2.05	2.06	2.07	2.08	2.09	2.10	2.11	2.12	2.12	2.13	2.14	2.15	2.16	2.17	2.18	2.18	2.19	2.20	2.21	2.22	2.23	2.24	2.25	2.26	216
2.05	2.06	2.07	2.08	2.09	2.10	2.11	2.12	2.12	2.13	2.14	2.15	2.16	2.17	2.18	2.19	2.20	2.20	2.21	2.22	2.23	2.24	2.25	2.26	2.26	218
2.06	2.07	2.08	2.09	2.10	2.11	2.12	2.12	2.13	2.14	2.15	2.16	2.17	2.18	2.19	2.20	2.20	2.21	2.22	2.23	2.24	2.25	2.26	2.27	2.27	220
2.07	2.08	2.09	2.10	2.11	2.12	2.12	2.13	2.14	2.15	2.16	2.17	2.18	2.19	2.20	2.20	2.21	2.22	2.23	2.24	2.25	2.26	2.27	2.28	2.28	223
2.08	2.09	2.10	2.11	2.12	2.12	2.13	2.14	2.15	2.16	2.17	2.18	2.19	2.20	2.21	2.21	2.22	2.23	2.24	2.25	2.26	2.27	2.28	2.28	2.29	225
2.09	2.10	2.11	2.11	2.12	2.13	2.14	2.15	2.16	2.17	2.18	2.19	2.20	2.21	2.21	2.22	2.23	2.23	2.24	2.25	2.26	2.27	2.28	2.29	2.30	227
2.10	2.11	2.11	2.12	2.13	2.14	2.15	2.16	2.17	2.18	2.19	2.20	2.21	2.21	2.22	2.23	2.24	2.25	2.26	2.27	2.28	2.29	2.30	2.30	2.31	229
2.10	2.11	2.12	2.13	2.14	2.15	2.16	2.17	2.10	2.19	2.20	2.21	2.21	2.22	2.23	2.24	2.25	2.26	2.27	2.28	2.29	2.30	2.30	2.31	2.32	231
2.11	2.12	2.13	2.14	2.15	2.16	2.17	2.18	2.19	2.20	2.21	2.21	2.22	2.23	2.24	2.25	2.26	2.27	2.28	2.29	2.30	2.30	2.31	2.32	2.33	234
2.12	2.13	2.14	2.15	2.16	2.17	2.18	2.19	2.20	2.20	2.21	2.22	2.23	2.24	2.25	2.26	2.27	2.28	2.29	2.30	2.30	2.31	2.32	2.33	2.34	236
2.13	2.14	2.15	2.16	2.17	2.18	2.19	2.20	2.20	2.21	2.22	2.23	2.24	2.25	2.26	2.27	2.28	2.29	2.30	2.30	2.31	2.32	2.33	2.34	2.35	238
2.14	2.15	2.16	2.17	2.18	2.19	2.19	2.20	2.21	2.22	2.23	2.24	2.25	2.26	2.27	2.28	2.29	2.30	2.30	2.31	2.32	2.33	2.34	2.35	2.35	240
2.15	2.16	2.17	2.17	2.18	2.19	2.20	2.21	2.22	2.23	2.24	2.25	2.26	2.27	2.28	2.29	2.30	2.30	2.31	2.32	2.33	2.34	2.35	2.36	2.37	243
65.0	65.4	65.7	66.1	66.5	66.9	67.3	67.7	68.1	68.5	68.9	69.3	69.7	70.1	70.5	70.9	71.3	71.7	72.0	72.4	72.8	73.2	73.6	74.0	74.4	

HEIGHT-INCHES

these two levels. Should the respirations be irregular or uneven or should
the patient have been restless during the test it should be repeated. It is

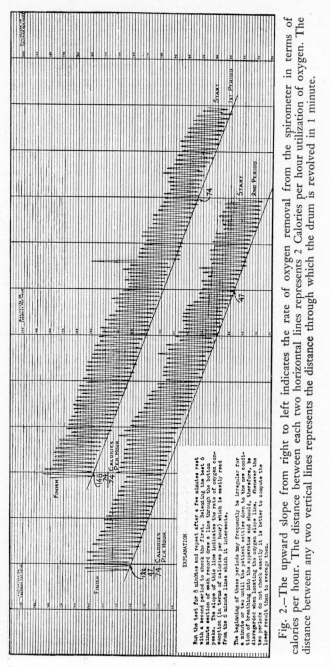

Fig. 2.—The upward slope from right to left indicates the rate of oxygen removal from the spirometer in terms of calories per hour. The distance between each two horizontal lines represents 2 Calories per hour utilization of oxygen. The distance between any two vertical lines represents the distance through which the drum is revolved in 1 minute.

well in any case to secure at least two six-minute graphs. They afford a
good check as to uniformity and the better tracing may be selected upon

which to base calculations. Tests for leaks in the apparatus are important. A small weight placed on the spirometer bell will alter the trend of the marker on the kymograph if a leak is present.

The oxygen consumption is proportionate to the surface area of the patient's body. The surface area is readily calculated for adults when the height and weight are known by using the DuBois Body Surface Chart, table 2.

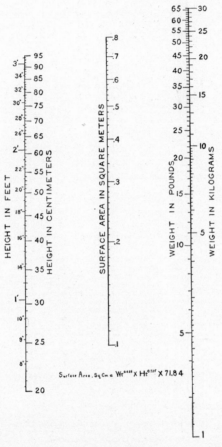

Fig. 3.—Nomogram devised by R. R. Hannon from the formula of DuBois and DuBois for the estimation of surface areas of children. The surface area is indicated when a straight line which connects the height and weight levels intersects the surface area column.

The surface areas of children are obtained by using the nomogram (Fig. 3) devised by Hannon from the formula of DuBois and DuBois.

The oxygen consumption is corrected for temperature and barometric pressure, table 3, and is compared with the modification by Boothby and Sandiford of the DuBois normal standard according to age and sex, table 4 (p. 12).

The final reading is given as plus or minus values in percentage above or below the normal standard oxygen utilization. Basal metabolic rates which are within 10 per cent above (+ 10 per cent) or 10 per cent below (— 10 per cent) that of the normal standard are considered to be within normal limits. In fact little credence should be placed in values which are not more than 15 per cent from the normal standard. Basal metabolic rates which exceed normal usually do so to a greater degree than rates which are below normal—*e.g.*, a B.M.R. of + 75 per cent is not uncommon, while rates below —30 per cent are rare.

Illustration of the Calculation of the Basal Metabolic Rate.—Female, aged 49 years, height 64 inches (160 cm.), weight 108 lb. (49 Kg.). Blood pressure 110/80. Pulse rate 72. Temperature of spirometer 20° C. Barometric

TABLE 3

TABLE FOR AND ILLUSTRATION OF THE CORRECTION FOR TEMPERATURE AND BAROMETRIC PRESSURE IN DELIVERING THE BASAL METABOLIC RATE (SEE TEXT)

Temperature in degrees Centigrade

mm	15	16	17	18	19	20	21	22	23	24	25	26	27	28	29	30	31	32	33	34	35
600	.735	.732	.728	.725	.721	.718	.715	.712	.708	.704	.701	.697	.693	.689	.685	.681	.677	.673	.669	.665	.661
605	.742	.739	.735	.731	.727	.724	.721	.718	.714	.710	.707	.703	.699	.695	.691	.687	.683	.679	.675	.671	.667
610	.748	.745	.741	.737	.733	.730	.727	.724	.720	.716	.713	.709	.705	.701	.697	.693	.689	.685	.680	.676	.672
615	.754	.751	.747	.744	.740	.737	.734	.730	.726	.722	.719	.715	.711	.707	.703	.699	.695	.691	.686	.682	.678
620	.760	.757	.753	.750	.746	.743	.740	.737	.733	.729	.725	.721	.717	.713	.709	.705	.701	.696	.692	.688	.684
625	.767	.764	.760	.756	.752	.749	.746	.743	.739	.735	.731	.727	.723	.719	.715	.711	.707	.702	.698	.694	.690
630	.773	.770	.766	.762	.758	.755	.752	.749	.745	.741	.737	.733	.729	.725	.721	.717	.713	.708	.704	.700	.696
635	.779	.776	.772	.768	.764	.761	.758	.755	.751	.747	.743	.739	.735	.731	.727	.723	.719	.714	.710	.706	.702
640	.785	.782	.778	.774	.770	.767	.764	.761	.757	.753	.749	.745	.741	.737	.733	.729	.725	.720	.716	.711	.707
645	.792	.788	.784	.781	.777	.773	.770	.767	.763	.759	.755	.751	.747	.743	.739	.735	.731	.726	.722	.717	.713
650	.798	.794	.791	.787	.784	.780	.777	.773	.769	.765	.761	.757	.752	.748	.744	.740	.736	.732	.727	.723	.719
655	.804	.800	.797	.793	.790	.786	.783	.779	.775	.771	.767	.763	.758	.754	.750	.746	.742	.738	.733	.729	.724
660	.810	.806	.803	.799	.796	.792	.789	.785	.781	.777	.773	.769	.764	.760	.756	.752	.748	.744	.739	.735	.730
665	.816	.812	.809	.805	.802	.798	.795	.791	.787	.783	.779	.775	.770	.766	.762	.758	.754	.749	.745	.741	.736
670	.822	.819	.816	.812	.809	.805	.801	.797	.793	.789	.785	.781	.776	.772	.768	.764	.760	.755	.751	.746	.742
675	.828	.825	.821	.818	.815	.811	.807	.803	.799	.795	.791	.787	.782	.778	.774	.770	.766	.761	.757	.752	.740
680	.834	.831	.827	.824	.821	.817	.813	.809	.805	.801	.797	.793	.788	.784	.780	.776	.771	.767	.763	.758	.754
685	.841	.837	.833	.830	.827	.823	.819	.815	.811	.807	.803	.799	.794	.790	.786	.782	.777	.773	.769	.764	.760
690	.848	.844	.841	.837	.833	.829	.825	.821	.817	.813	.809	.805	.800	.796	.792	.788	.783	.779	.775	.770	.765
695	.854	.850	.847	.843	.839	.835	.831	.827	.823	.819	.815	.811	.806	.802	.798	.794	.789	.785	.780	.776	.771
700	.860	.856	.853	.849	.845	.841	.837	.833	.829	.825	.821	.817	.812	.808	.804	.800	.795	.791	.786	.781	.777
705	.866	.862	.859	.855	.851	.847	.843	.939	.835	.831	.827	.823	.818	.814	.810	.806	.801	.796	.792	.787	.783
710	.872	.868	.865	.861	.857	.853	.849	.845	.841	.837	.833	.829	.824	.820	.816	.812	.807	.802	.798	.793	.788
715	.878	.874	.871	.867	.863	.859	.855	.851	.847	.843	.839	.835	.830	.826	.822	.818	.813	.808	.804	.799	.794
720	.885	.881	.877	.873	.869	.865	.861	.857	.853	.849	.845	.841	.836	.832	.823	.824	.819	.814	.810	.805	.800
725	.891	.887	.883	.879	.876	.872	.867	.863	.859	.855	.851	.847	.842	.838	.834	.830	.825	.820	.816	.811	.806
730	.897	.894	.890	.886	.882	.878	.874	.869	.865	.861	.857	.853	.848	.844	.840	.836	.831	.826	.822	.817	.812
735	.904	.900	.896	.892	.888	.884	.880	.875	.871	.867	.863	.859	.854	.850	.846	.842	.837	.832	.827	.822	.817
740	.910	.906	.902	.898	.894	.890	.886	.881	.877	.873	.869	.865	.860	.856	.852	.848	.843	.838	.833	.828	.823
745	.916	.912	.908	.904	.900	.896	.892	.887	.883	.879	.875	.871	.866	.862	.857	.853	.848	.844	.839	.834	.829
750	.922	.918	.914	.910	.906	.902	.898	.893	.889	.885	.881	.877	.872	.868	.863	.859	.854	.849	.845	.840	.835
755	.928	.924	.920	.916	.912	.908	.904	.899	.895	.891	.887	.883	.878	.874	.869	.865	.860	.855	.851	.846	.841
760	.934	.930	.926	.922	.918	.914	.910	.905	.901	.897	.893	.889	.884	.860	.875	.871	.866	.861	.857	.852	.847
765	.941	.936	.932	.928	.924	.920	.916	.911	.907	.903	.899	.895	.890	.886	.881	.877	.872	.867	.863	.857	.852
770	.947	.943	.939	.935	.930	.926	.922	.917	.913	.909	.905	.901	.896	.892	.887	.883	.878	.873	.869	.863	.858
775	.954	.949	.945	.941	.936	.932	.928	.923	.919	.915	.911	.907	.902	.898	.893	.889	.884	.879	.875	.869	.864
780	.960	.956	.952	.948	.943	.939	.935	.930	.926	.921	.917	.913	.908	.904	.899	.895	.890	.885	.880	.875	.870

pressure .750 mm. of Hg. Surface area of patient 1.5 sq. meter (Table 2). Actual oxygen consumption equals 74 Calories per hour (see Fig. 2). Correction for temperature and barometric pressure (Table 3): $74 \times .902 = 66.74$ Cals. per hour. Normal value (DuBois normal standard, table 4): 35.0 Cals. per square meter of body surface per hour and for actual surface area, $1.5 \times 35 = 52.5$ calories per hour.

Deduction: 52.5 calories are average per hour for a person of this age, sex, height and weight, whereas the actual consumption for this patient is 66.74 calories per hour. Excess of normal: $66.74 — 52.5 = 14.24$ calories per hour. 52.5 calories per hour = 100 per cent of normal. 14.24 calories per hour $= \dfrac{100}{52.5} \times 14.24 = 27$ per cent. Basal metabolic rate $= + 27$ per cent.

Some of the newer models of metabolism testing machines have an oxygen container with a rubber bellows substituted for the water chamber and spirometer bell. This has the advantage of lighter weight and greater portability. A fan for circulating the oxygen can also be used on these machines. The graph obtained is similar to that described, and from it is calculated the amount of oxygen (in cc. per minute) utilized by the patient. Correction for temperature and barometric pressure may be automatically made by introducing a measured amount of oxygen into the chamber.

The basal metabolic rate is easily computed when the oxygen consumption has been determined. After a correction for age and sex, the result is compared to the average figure (obtained from the tables) for the given height and weight, to determine whether the result is above or below the normal. If preferred, the whole computation can be made on a specially constructed slide rule on which the basal metabolic rate is read directly. This eliminates the use of the tables but of course there is still opportunity for numerical errors in the calculations.

Knowing the height and weight of the patient, one can obtain the surface area by referring to the tables based upon the height-weight formula of DuBois. The oxygen consumption per square meter of body surface is then compared with that of the normal standard.

Emotional Influences.—Undue importance attached to the test in conversation with the patient is certain to lead to error. Niederwiesser (1932) has warned against remarking to the patient, "The basal metabolism test will tell whether or not an operation is necessary." Needless to say a reliable result could not be expected under these circumstances. Emotional reactions, apprehension and discomfort increase the metabolism. Aub[4] believes the increased metabolism resulting from emotional imbalance is due to an increase in the secretion of epinephrine. The kindly thoughtfulness and efficiency of the technician are of no little importance in relieving apprehension or actual fear. No doubt some B.M.R. readings reflect the mood of the person who makes the examination.

There are, then, many possibilities of error in making this test, but under ideal conditions the results are of great value. It will be of greater value to the consultant if the following information is recorded on the laboratory report: Patient's name, temperature by mouth, pulse rate, blood pressure, height, weight, age and sex. It should be stated also if this was the first test to which this patient had been subjected and if the machine was checked for leaks and with normal controls. Restlessness, fatigue or apprehension on the part of the patient should be recorded and a note should be made of the length of the rest period before test. In borderline cases in which the results may be $- 10$ to $- 15$ or $+ 10$ to $+ 15$ per cent of normal, the test should be repeated. A series of tests is of much greater value than a single test.

CONDITIONS WHICH ALTER THE BASAL METABOLIC RATE

Physiologic Conditions.—Physiological variations in the basal metabolic rates are subject to age and sex, race and climate, occupation, body mass, pregnancy, diet, and the administration of certain drugs. It was not, therefore, until normal standards, which incorporated these fluctuations, were evolved that it was possible to make deductible evaluations of changes in the rate of oxygen consumption.

Age and Sex.—The heat production and hence the basal metabolic rate of the newborn infant is low (approximately 25 calories per square meter of body surface), but within a few weeks the rate has doubled. The rate continues to increase until the age of five years. A decline in the rate ensues from five to ten years of age, with a modest increase at puberty. A further decline occurs between puberty and twenty years of age, but from this age to old age the decrease is extremely gradual. These changes are depicted in figure 4, which presents the "Sage" or Aub and DuBois standards.

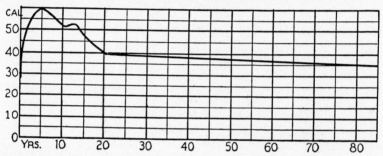

Fig. 4.—Curve depicting the levels of the basal metabolism, expressed in terms of calories per hour per square meter of surface area, at different ages. (After Aub and DuBois.)

The basal metabolic rates of females are from 6 to 10 per cent lower than those of males of the same age group. These differences as presented in table 4 are allowed for in the routine calculation of basal metabolic rates.

TABLE 4

CALORIES PER SQUARE METER OF BODY SURFACE PER HOUR
(HEIGHT-WEIGHT FORMULA OF AUB AND DUBOIS)

Age, Years	Males	Females
14–16	46.0	43.0
16–18	43.0	40.0
18–20	41.0	38.0
20–30	39.5	37.0
30–40	39.5	36.5
40–50	38.5	36.0
50–60	37.5	35.0
60–70	36.5	34.0
70–80	35.5	33.0

Race and Climate.—American subjects have been used in compiling the normal standards quoted in this book. Differences in race and climate explain, in part at least, the disparity in standards in different countries and, indeed, in one country, such as the United States, where there are great differences in climate. It has been amply verified that the basal metabolic rate is reduced in hot climates. Even so, the greatest difference found in rates between extremes of heat and cold were only 12 per cent.

The sensation of chilliness is accompanied by an increase in the metabolic rate. This may increase two or four times above the basal level if shivering occurs. Warm temperatures, on the other hand, have a less marked effect on the basal rate. The important feature for accurate testing is that the patient should be comfortable before and during the test period if misleading results are to be avoided. DuBois quotes Durig and Zuntz and others to the effect that altitude or reduced barometric pressure causes but small variations in the basal metabolism.

DuBois[6] summarizes the effect of race as follows, ". . . there are distinct racial differences in metabolism apart from the effects of climate. Native Australians show a low metabolism, Chinese slightly low, Japanese close to the American figures. Natives of certain parts of India and Syria are distinctly low, perhaps partly on account of differences in diet and muscular activity. The white inhabitants of Central and South America seem to show no racial divergencies, but perhaps a slight lowering due to the warm climate. On the other hand the Maya Indians and Araucanians are well above the averages for whites in North America."

Occupation.—The basal metabolic rate is generally 1 to 5 per cent higher than the average standard in individuals who are accustomed to heavy manual labor or athletics, and 1 to 6 per cent lower in those who do light work, such as barbers and school teachers. During sleep the basal metabolism decreases from 7 to 12 per cent.

Diet.—The diet taken for several days preceding the test affects the metabolism little if any. No significant differences have been observed between the rates of vegetarians and nonvegetarians.

Pregnancy.—Of thirty cases of pregnancy observed by Boothby, 80 per cent had metabolic rates between − 15 per cent and + 15 per cent, three patients had rates between + 16 and + 20 per cent, and three exceeded the + 20 per cent rate. When the rate of metabolism is altered by pregnancy it does so on the plus side, there being a slow increase in the rate in the last three months with a prompt reduction after the termination of pregnancy.

Drugs.—Caffeine causes an increase of 3 to 10 per cent in the basal metabolic rate in the first hour, and epinephrine increases the rate up to 10 per cent in the course of two hours after administration. Dinitrophenol, taken orally, increases the metabolism abruptly from 20 to 30 per cent within the first hour.[7] Unfortunately, the side effects (skin reactions, liver damage, cataracts and agranulocytosis) caused by this drug prohibit the clinical use of what might otherwise be a valuable remedy in the management of obese patients. Of the sedatives, morphine, heroin, chloral hydrate, barbital, ipral, neonal, and phanodorn tend to reduce the oxygen consumption slightly. Low metabolism values have been observed in children treated with nirvanol (phenylethylhydantoin).

Potassium iodide causes no alteration in normal metabolism in contrast to the great reduction in the rate which ensues when it is administered to patients suffering from hyperthyroidism.

Pathologic Conditions.—The basal metabolic rate is below normal in starvation, anorexia nervosa, undernutrition, shock, cretinism, myxedema, thyroiditis (Riedel's struma), Addison's disease, lipoid nephrosis and obesity, resulting from pituitary dysfunction or hypothalamic disorders, and Simmond's disease (hypophyseal cachexia). It is above normal in hyperthyroidism, toxic adenomata, and malignancy of the thyroid gland, diabetes insipidus, fever, cardiorenal disease with dyspnea, severe anemias, diabetic

pseudodwarfism, leukemia, and polycythemia. Metabolism may be elevated
in basophilic adenomata of the hypophysis and adrenal cortical tumors.

Undernutrition.—Undernutrition may be voluntary, such as that observed in professional fasters. It may be due to disease or to design in the
treatment of disease, as in obesity, diabetes, and heart disease. The reduction
in metabolism which results from starvation is proportionately greater than
the reduction in body mass. The phenomena underlying this apparently
protective reaction are not understood. A case report by Magnus-Levy was
that of a barber whose metabolic rate was reduced by undernutrition to
— 33 per cent. His metabolism was restored to normal by improving his
nutrition. Undernourished diabetic patients in the Allen era had low metabolic rates, being from 15 to 20 per cent below the normal average.

TABLE 5

ALTERATIONS IN BASAL METABOLISM IN DISEASE

Increased B.M.R.	Decreased B.M.R.
Hyperthyroidism	Myxedema
Toxic adenomata of thyroid gland	Cretinism
Malignancy of thyroid gland	Thyroiditis (Riedel's struma)
Polycythemia	Nephrosis
Severe anemia	Hypopituitarism
Leukemia	Simmonds' disease
Diabetes insipidus	Addison's disease
Advanced cardiac decompensation	Undernutrition (starvation, anorexia nervosa)
Drug poisoning	Shock
(*a*) thyroid	
(*b*) dinitrophenol	
Diabetic pseudodwarfism	

Similar values are encountered in patients suffering from anorexia nervosa.
Master[8] has applied the principle of the reduction of metabolism by means
of undernutrition, in the treatment of congestive heart failure, angina
pectoris, and thrombosis of the coronary arteries.

Thyroid.—MYXEDEMA AND CRETINISM.—The basal metabolism in these
two diseases is reduced below the normal average in proportion to the reduction in the secretion of thyroxin. Rates between 20 and 30 per cent
below normal are not unusual and in the occasional extreme cases the rate
may be — 40. The rate is restored and maintained within a normal range by
the proper and continued administration of thyroid substance. Low metabolic values associated with destruction of the anterior lobe of the hypophysis may be mistaken for myxedema. These patients are so extremely sensitive to even small doses of thyroid, that fatalities have occurred following
the administration of amounts of thyroid which ordinarily would be inadequate to control myxedema.

Thyroxin (1 mg.) when given intravenously to a myxedematous patient
causes an average increase of 2.8 per cent in the basal metabolic rate. The
amount necessary to achieve a desired result is closely predictable.

A large dose of thyroxin given intravenously is followed by a rise in the
basal metabolism after a latent period of twenty-four hours. The rise increases steadily, reaching its peak between the third and tenth days. A gradual reduction then occurs, the rate reaching subnormal levels about the fifty-
second day. It has been estimated that thyroxin is destroyed at the rate of 0.2

to 0.4 mg. daily in the myxedematous patient. As a therapeutic agent thyroxin has no advantages over dried thyroid; it is more expensive and given orally it is less effective. It is not necessary to keep the basal metabolic rate up to normal if the patient is free from symptoms with the rate at a lower level.

It is well to emphasize (1) that the potency of various thyroid preparations varies greatly (page 238), hence the different products available commercially are not interchangeable without due consideration of this fact, and, (2) that the maximum increase in the basal metabolic rate does not occur immediately but develops gradually over a period of seven to ten days and that after withdrawal of the drug a diminishing effect remains for several weeks.

HYPERTHYROIDISM, TOXIC ADENOMATA, AND MALIGNANCY OF THE THYROID GLAND.—The basal metabolism is increased in toxic goiters, *i.e.*, in hyperthyroidism, toxic adenomata, and malignancy of the thyroid gland.

In hyperthyroidism, also referred to as Graves' disease, and exophthalmic goiter, the highest metabolic rates are found. They vary from + 30 to + 75 and even higher, according to the severity of the disease. The metabolism is reduced temporarily by administering iodides (Chap. V). It also usually decreases after roentgen ray therapy to the gland. The most effective measure for restoring metabolism to normal, however, is subtotal thyroidectomy, done after preliminary treatment with iodides.

In cases of toxic adenomas the average metabolic increase reaches + 30 per cent. The response to iodine is not so marked as in Graves' disease but surgical removal of the adenomas restores normal metabolic rates. Malignancy of the thyroid also increases the metabolic activity but to a less degree.

Addison's Disease.—A lowering of the metabolism is common in Addison's disease. Values of − 15 to + 30 per cent are obtained. One cannot say to what extent this reduction is due to the reduced adrenal secretion and the resulting influence on the thyroid gland. The reader is referred to works of Koehler[9] and of Boothby and Sandiford[10] for more detailed discussions on this subject.

Pituitary.—Hyperpituitarism, in general, tends to increase and hypopituitarism to decrease metabolism. The changes are not nearly so striking as in diseases of the thyroid gland, however. Of Boothby and Sandiford's 58 cases of hypopituitarism all but a third were within 15 per cent of normal, but in this one-third the metabolism was depressed below − 15 per cent of normal.

Reports of the metabolism in pituitary disease are confusing. This is doubtless due to the fact that the transitory phase of hyperpituitarism due to increased chromophilic activity gives way to hypopituitarism. Hence, decreased metabolic activity occurs in some acromegalic patients.

Forty-nine of Cushing and Davidoff's[11] seventy-two acromegalic patients had basal metabolic rates varying from + 2 to + 61 per cent. In six, the rates were below − 10 per cent. The metabolism decreased following the administration of Lugol's solution, or after thyroidectomy. In 107 patients with hypopituitarism the average basal metabolic rate was − 14 per cent with fluctuations between − 10 and − 36. The administration of pituitary extracts usually does not affect the rate of metabolism but when it does the change is that of an increase.

Lipoid Nephrosis.—Moderate depression of the metabolic activity occurs in lipoid nephrosis. Epstein[12] noted metabolic rates varying from 8 to 18 below normal. These observations have been amply confirmed. An error is likely to be overlooked if allowance is not made for the increased weight due to inert fluid which accumulates in the tissues and serous cavities of patients suffering from this disease. Normal rates of metabolic activity are restored when adequate amounts of thyroid are given.

Obesity.—Overweight directly attributable to too much food or too little exercise, or both, causes no appreciable change in metabolic activity. Values slightly below the normal level should be discounted because of error introduced by the masses of inert fat, the metabolic activity of which must be extremely small. Of ninety-four cases of obesity studied by Boothby and Sandiford[10] 95 per cent had metabolic rates within the accepted normal range, between + 15 and − 15 per cent. It can be definitely stated that, contrary to a too prevalent belief, the basal caloric needs are not altered by exogenous obesity.

Accumulation of water in the tissues of obese patients may mislead. Newburgh and Johnston[13] pointed out that a patient on an undernutrition regimen may actually gain in weight temporarily from water retention, but the body weight will eventually be reduced according to prediction. These authors emphasize that metabolism of the obese is normal. The basal requirement is usually not changed, even in the most severe cases.

Obesity due to hypothyroidism, castration, or hypopituitarism—the so-called endogenous obesity—is another matter and is dealt with under the corresponding headings.

Fever.—Fever increases the basal oxygen requirement. In most febrile disturbances, tuberculosis excepted, this is remarkably uniform, the average increase being 13 per cent for each degree C. rise above the normal temperature (7.2 per cent increase for each degree F.).[14] In pulmonary tuberculosis the rise in metabolic activity is considerably less than in febrile reactions of other diseases. The small degree of toxemia and lower protein breakdown in this disease is offered as an explanation of this disparity.

Cognizance of the effect of fever on metabolism is important if a positive nutritional balance is to be maintained in prolonged fevers, such as typhoid fever.

Diabetes Insipidus.—The ingestion of large quantities of water, the temperature of which is below that of the patient's body, causes readjustment of the heat-regulating mechanism. Increases in the basal rates as high as 20 to 40 per cent have been observed in patients suffering from diabetes insipidus. Excessive renal activity has been suggested as a cause of this change. Metabolism is restored to normal when the disorder is controlled by appropriate hormonal therapy.

Leukemia.—Increases in the metabolic rate in myelogenous and lymphatic leukemia reach levels as high as are observed in hyperthyroidism. Fourteen of Boothby and Sandiford's sixteen patients suffering from leukemia exceeded the normal metabolic rate by more than 20 per cent.

The increased metabolism has an apparent direct relationship with the increased total white blood cell count and the percentage of immature leukocytes.

Polycythemia.—The subject dealing with the increased metabolism in polycythemia vera has been reviewed by Minot and Buckman.[15] It has been suggested that this change, usually a moderate one, is caused by the blood-forming organs or immature red cells, or the rate of uric acid production going hand in hand with the destruction of nuclear material. Actually the cause or causes of the changes in metabolic activity in this disease are obscure.

Diseases of the Heart.—The effect of heart disease on metabolism is in direct relation to the degree of dyspnea present. In the absence of dyspnea the metabolism is normal but as the dyspnea appears and becomes progressively worse the metabolic rate rises. Hence, changes in metabolism are directly related to the presence and degree of cardiac decompensation. It may be assumed that the dyspneic patient is not being studied under strictly basal conditions. If it were possible to correct for energy expended in the effort of difficult breathing it is quite likely that the basal rates would be normal in all patients with uncomplicated cardiac decompensation. As one might expect, the metabolic activity is found to rise as the vital capacity of the lungs decreases, and vice versa.

Total ablation of the thyroid gland in individuals with a normal metabolism as a means of reducing the basal and total metabolism below normal has been advocated[16] as a treatment for selected cases of congestive heart failure and angina pectoris. If all the benefit secured is attributable to the reduced metabolism, this surgical measure in many instances can be replaced by a regimen of undernutrition. By this means Master[8] secured a reduction in metabolic rate quite as great (— 20 to — 30 per cent) as that obtained by total thyroidectomy. This is not the place to deal with the treatment of disease of the heart, but it is not out of place to stress the benefit which accrues to these patients from reduced metabolism and to point out that undernutrition is a suitable means of securing this change in selected cases.

Miscellaneous disorders which cause clinically unimportant changes in the basal metabolism are diabetes, nephritis, arterial hypertension, disturbance of the sex glands, anemia, and arthritis. Allen and DuBois[17] found insignificant increases in metabolism in diabetes and observed the lowering effect which the undernutrition treatment had on the metabolic rate. DuBois agrees with Grafe's conclusion that a total absence or diminished function of the sex glands only exceptionally diminishes the metabolic processes. In primary anemia a moderate rise in the basal metabolism occurs in the majority of cases. In nephritis the altered metabolic rate appears to depend upon the process of decompensated cardiac lesions with dyspnea, or upon a renal acidosis.

BIBLIOGRAPHY

1. Lusk, G., J.A.M.A., **70:** 821, 824, 1918.
2. Means, J. H. and Burgess, H. W., Arch. Int. Med., **30:** 507, 1922.
3. Boothby, W. M. and Sandiford, I., Am. J. Physiol., **90:** 290, 1929.
4. Aub, J. C., J.A.M.A., **79:** 95, 1922.
5. DuBois, E., Basal Metabolism in Health and Disease, Lea & Febiger, Philadelphia, 1936, p. 151.
6. Ibid., p. 200.
7. Cutting, W. C., Mehrtens, H. G., Tainter, M. L., J.A.M.A., **101:** 193, 1933; ibid., **101:** 1472, 1933.
8. Master, A. M., J.A.M.A., **105:** 337, 1935; also Am. Heart J., **12:** 549, 1936.
9. Koehler, A. E., J.A.M.A., **91:** 1457, 1928.

10. Boothby, W. M. and Sandiford, I., Physiol. Rev., **4:** 69, 1924; also J. Biol. Chem., **54:** 783, 1922.
11. Cushing, H. and Davidoff, L. M., Arch. Int. Med., **39:** 673, 1927.
12. Epstein, A. A., J.A.M.A., **87:** 913, 1926.
13. Newburgh, L. H. and Johnston, M. W., Ann. Intern. Med., **3:** 815, 1930; also J. Clin. Invest., **8:** 197, 1930.
14. DuBois, E., Basal Metabolism in Health and Disease, Lea & Febiger, Philadelphia, 1936, p. 432.
15. Minot, G. R., Buckman, T. E., Amer. J. Med. Sci., **166:** 469, 1923.
16. Blumgart, H. L., Levine, S. A., Berlin, D. A., Arch. Intern. Med., **51:** 866, 1933.
17. Allen, F. M., DuBois, E., Arch. Intern. Med., **17:** 1010, 1916.

CHAPTER II

CARBOHYDRATE METABOLISM

By C. N. H. Long

CARBOHYDRATES OF BIOLOGICAL IMPORTANCE

A large number of carbohydrates are present in both the food and tissues of animals. Some of these are found in the free state while others form a part of more elaborate molecules. The appended table gives an indication of the character and distribution of these substances. The most important dietary carbohydrates are the *monosaccharides* glucose and fructose, the *disaccharides* sucrose, lactose, and maltose, and the *polysaccharide*, starch. The *pentoses*, although important constituents of nucleic acids, and certain of the intracellular co-enzymes are not found in the body in a free state except in the condition of the pentosuria. In herbivora the bacterial digestion of the polysaccharide cellulose serves to liberate soluble sugars that are utilized as a source of energy. Since this does not occur in man, this widely distributed carbohydrate is of no nutritive value although its inclusion in the diet is credited with certain beneficial effects on the motility of the intestinal tract.

A discussion of the chemistry of carbohydrates is not included here but may be found in text books of organic and biochemistry.

DIGESTION OF CARBOHYDRATES

While the main function of saliva is to moisten the food and facilitate its swallowing, it also contains, at least in man, an enzyme known as **ptyalin** which exerts a powerful effect upon boiled starch. Under its influence starch is rapidly broken down by successive stages into dextrins of various molecular sizes and finally into maltose. This conversion may be followed by the change in the color given by starch with an iodine solution until a point is reached (achroodextrins) at which no further color is produced on addition of the reagent.

Although the time usually spent by starches in the mouth is not sufficient to allow any considerable degree of hydrolysis to occur, the food swallowed is thoroughly mixed with saliva and accumulates in the upper portions of the stomach. Here the ptyalin continues to act until the hydrochloric acid of the stomach has penetrated the mass and reduced its alkaline reaction to a point where the action of this enzyme is inhibited (around pH 4). Since this often takes a considerable time a large portion of the ingested starch may be hydrolyzed by this enzyme.

The simpler carbohydrates are not attacked by ptyalin nor by any other constituent of the saliva. Indeed, salivary digestion of starch is not essential since the saliva of many animals does not possess diastatic activity.

19

TABLE 1

CARBOHYDRATES OF BIOLOGICAL IMPORTANCE

Carbohydrate	Sources	Chemical Form
I. *Monosaccharides*		
(a) Trioses:		
Glycerose	Muscle	Combined with phosphoric acid
Dihydroxyacetone		
(b) Pentoses:		
l-Arabinose	Fruits, gums	As polymer araban
d-Ribose	Yeast	Nucleic acids and derivatives
d-2-Desoxyribose	Animal tissues	Riboflavin phosphate (Vitamin B₂)
d-xyloketose	Urine of pentosuric patients	Free
(c) Hexoses:		
d-Glucose	Fruit, vegetables and animal tissues	Free, combined and polymerized forms
d-Fructose	Fruit, vegetables and animal tissues	Free and combined forms
d-Galactose	Milk	Combined form
II. *Disaccharides*		
Maltose	Starches	Glucose + Glucose
Lactose	Milk	Glucose + Galactose
Cellobiose	Cellulose	Glucose + Glucose
Melibiose	Trisaccharide Raffinose	Glucose + Galactose
Sucrose	Fruits, beet, cane	Glucose + Glucose
III. *Trisaccharides*		
Raffinose	Sugar beet, molasses	Galactose + Glucose + Fructose
IV. *Polysaccharides*		
(a) Pentosans:		
Arabans	Vegetable gums	Polymers of pentoses
Xylans		
(b) Hexosans:		
Cellulose	Structural elements of plants	Polymer of glucose
Starch	Vegetable foodstuffs	Polymer of glucose
Glycogen	Animal tissues	Polymer of glucose
Inulin	Jerusalem artichoke	Polymer of fructose
V. *Other Carbohydrate Containing Substances*		
Pectins	Fruit and plants	Arabinose, galactose and pectic acid
Mucopolysac- charides	Mucin, cartilage, chitin, bacterial polysaccharides, heparin	Amino sugar and uronic sulfate
Glycoproteins		
Albumins	Carbohydrate combined with protein	
Gonadotropic hormones		

VI. *Other Carbohydrate Derivatives of Biological Importance*
Vitamin C, Lactic Acid ,Pyruvic Acid, Glycuronic Acid

It should be noted that unboiled starch is only very slowly attacked both by ptyalin and by the diastatic enzymes of the pancreatic juice and, indeed, if large amounts of it are ingested, a considerable portion will ultimately appear unchanged in the feces.

While the acidity of the gastric juice brings to an end the activity of ptyalin it also contributes to carbohydrate digestion by commencing the hydrolysis of the disaccharides, particularly sucrose. At one time it was thought that this inversion of cane sugar was due to a special enzyme, invertase, but this view is unnecessary since inulin, a polysaccharide that yields fructose on hydrolysis, is also attacked by gastric juice and thus can serve as a source of dietary carbohydrate.

Fluids Affecting Carbohydrate Digestion.—The most important digestive fluids affecting carbohydrates are those of the pancreas and intestine. The pancreatic juice contains an enzyme, *amylase*, that completes the hydrolysis of starches to maltose. At this point, the digestion is completed by a second enzyme, *maltase*, that converts this disaccharide into glucose. The pancreatic juice does not attack any other disaccharide.

On the other hand, the intestinal secretions contain three enzymes that hydrolyze the disaccharides. First of these is a *maltase* that converts maltose into glucose. The second is a *lactase* that splits lactose or milk sugar into glucose and galactose. Finally, there is present an *invertase* that hydrolyzes sucrose or cane sugar into glucose and fructose.

Thus on the completion of intestinal digestion all the major disaccharides and polysaccharides of the diet have been converted into hexoses, mainly glucose, but also fructose and galactose. It is in this form that they are absorbed and it is noteworthy that these three monosaccharides together with *mannose** are probably the only sugars that are directly assimilable by higher animals.

THE ABSORPTION OF CARBOHYDRATES

Under normal circumstances the absorption of carbohydrates occurs in the small intestine and by the time the products of digestion have reached the ileocecal valve all assimilable carbohydrates have been removed. The capacity of the stomach to absorb glucose is a limited one except when this sugar is introduced in very high concentrations. Under such circumstances Morrison, Shay, Ravdin and Cahoon have shown that a considerable portion of a 40 per cent solution may disappear within an hour. Since such concentrations of glucose are rarely ingested, it may be reasonably concluded that the stomach plays an insignificant rôle in this regard.

The same conclusion has been reached regarding the ability of the large intestine and rectum to absorb glucose. As has just been pointed out, little, if any, of the hexoses ever reach the large intestine in the normal individual, and the problem of large intestinal absorption arises only when glucose solutions are introduced for therapeutic reasons into the lower bowel. Even when 10 per cent solutions are used little significant absorption occurs,[1] unless hypoglycemia is present. Furthermore, study of the blood glucose curve indicates that practically no absorption takes place.[2]

The problem of the absorption of carbohydrates is largely that of the absorption of hexoses and occasionally pentoses, since in the ordinary course of digestion all the carbohydrates of the diet (except cellulose) are absorbed in either of these two forms. Before discussing this, however, a little may be said regarding the utilization of disaccharides. While these form a notable proportion of dietary carbohydrates since they are absorbed as the constituent monosaccharides, it is noteworthy that in their original form they are not assimilated by the organism. Thus, the intravenous or parenteral injection of sucrose and lactose is followed by their complete excretion in the urine. Since the blood apparently contains a maltase, injection of maltose is followed by a certain proportion of its utilization as glucose. Thus, even though the disaccharides are freely soluble in water and are diffusible, any quantity that passes in an unchanged form through the intestinal wall

* Mannose is, however, such a rare constituent of the diet that it plays no practical part in animal metabolism

and enters the blood stream is rejected by the organism. The appearance of lactose in the urine during pregnancy and lactation is an example of its resistance to hydrolysis once it has entered the blood.

Absorption of the Dietary Hexoses.—It may be categorically stated that the absorption of the dietary hexoses is not entirely governed by the ordinary laws of diffusion and consequently the intestinal mucus membrane must participate in this process. The evidence for this is as follows:

1. In the intact intestine, glucose will pass from within out but not in the reverse direction. The existence of one-sided permeability is in itself not conclusive evidence of selective absorption since other complex but non-living membranes may exhibit the same property.

2. The absorption of glucose is to a large extent independent of the blood glucose concentration.[3] This is also true for the pentose and xylose.

3. The hexoses (glucose, fructose, galactose and mannose) pass through the intestinal wall at a more rapid rate than the pentoses (xylose and arabinose). This is the reverse of what might be expected from the laws of diffusion,[4, 5] since the latter are of smaller molecular size. When injected intraperitoneally the absorption rates are the same.[6]

4. The work of Cori is of particular importance. He showed that not only were the hexoses absorbed at a different rate than the pentoses but also the absorption rate of the hexoses themselves differed widely. Thus, if the absorption rate of glucose is taken as 100, the rates for the other sugars are as follows: d-galactose 110, d-glucose 100, d-fructose 43, d-mannose 19, l-xylose 15, l-arabinose 9. Furthermore, the rate of absorption of these sugars is independent of the concentration in which they are given (by stomach tube) and of the amount administered. Thus, the intestinal membrane to a large extent guards the organism against sudden and large influxes of sugar and must be regarded as an important factor in the regulation of carbohydrate metabolism.

Cori points out, as evidence of the remarkable selectivity of this membrane, that relatively slight changes in the structure of the sugar molecule markedly affect their absorption rate. Thus, the keto-sugar fructose is absorbed at half the rate of the aldo-sugar glucose, while mannose, a stereo-isomer of glucose, is absorbed at one-fifth the rate.

The actual mechanisms involved in this selective absorption are not yet clearly understood. In the first place the majority, if not all, of the sugars enters the blood after passing through the intestinal wall and little, if any, enters the lymphatics. Earlier workers were of the opinion that in transit from the intestinal wall glucose was converted into some other substance, one of those suggested being glycogen. Such a transformation would also assist absorption by increasing the diffusion gradient but so far there has been but little evidence to indicate that the glycogen content of the mucosa is altered during glucose absorption.

Phosphorylation.—The most attractive hypothesis is that processes involving phosphorylation are concerned. It has been well established, as will be seen later, that the intermediary metabolism of glycogen and glucose in the tissues involves a series of chain reactions in which phosphorylation and dephosphorylation play an essential rôle. Furthermore, it is probably safe to assume that the absorption processes require the expenditure of energy by the cells of the mucosa. The analysis of the mechanisms involved requires a study not only of the manner in which the sugars are transferred across the membrane but also of the processes within the cells affecting this transfer. In neither of these phases of the problem has a satisfactory answer been obtained.

However, in a series of experiments,[7] it has been concluded that phosphorylation is an essential part of the absorption process. Following the analogy of the effect of mono-iodoacetic acid in inhibiting lactic acid formation in skeletal muscle, Verzár and his colleagues claim to have demonstrated that the injection of this substance into rats reduces the absorption rate of glucose to that of xylose, the absorption of the latter remaining unchanged. Similar results were found with galactose and fructose. Since it is assumed that the pentoses are not phosphorylated during absorption, it would appear from these results that iodoacetic acid has inhibited such a process, thus reducing the absorption rate to that effected by simple diffusion. Another series of experiments using phloridzin, a substance that is also claimed to inhibit phosphorylation, gave comparable results.

Other workers have, however, failed to confirm these results. Klinghoffer[8] found that while iodoacetic acid did reduce the rate of glucose absorption that of xylose was also affected. Furthermore, the absorption of sodium chloride was also reduced and this investigator attributed the results to the general toxicity of the drug rather than to any specific effect on phosphorylation.

The measurement of absorption by giving single sugars is not a strictly physiological procedure for during normal digestion a mixture of carbohydrates together with the products of protein and fat digestion are being simultaneously absorbed. Experiment has shown that when two carbohydrates or a mixture of a carbohydrate and amino acid are being absorbed, there occurs a reduction in the rate of each. This has been termed "mutual inhibition of absorption." [9]

There are in addition other factors that influence the rate of absorption from the intestine. One of the most important is the general condition of the animal. Thus, prolonged starvation, vitamin deficiencies, infections and various intoxications will greatly reduce the absorption of all foodstuffs. This is a fact of considerable clinical importance particularly when the tolerance for carbohydrates is being tested by the oral administration of glucose.

Endocrine Factors.—Recently there has been advanced some evidence that certain endocrine factors directly influence carbohydrate absorption.

As has been pointed out above, Verzár and his colleagues believe that the selective absorption of glucose is due to its phosphorylation in the intestinal mucosa. They have found after adrenalectomy that the rate of glucose absorption is sharply reduced while that of xylose is not affected. The injection of cortical extract restored glucose absorption to normal. Verzár et al. conclude that the *cortical hormone* is concerned with phosphorylation processes not only in the intestine but elsewhere in the body, and that its absence interferes with glucose absorption by reason of the defects occurring in this process. These results have not been generally confirmed, for while most investigators will admit that adrenalectomized animals may show marked defects in absorption this is reported not to occur if the animals (rats) are adequately maintained by the administration of sodium salts[10] so that the secondary effects of adrenal cortical insufficiency are avoided.

The removal of the thyroid gland has been shown to exert a very definite retarding effect on glucose absorption which is alleviated by the administration of thyroxin.[11, 12] These findings have had an interesting sequel in the work of Russell,[13] who has shown that the diminished glucose absorption rate of hypophysectomized rats is due to the concomitant thyroid atrophy and that absorption may be returned to normal by thyroxin injections, although these do not correct any other abnormality of metabolism in these animals except the lowered basal metabolic rate.

CARBOHYDRATES OF THE BLOOD AND THE BLOOD GLUCOSE

Glucose is not the only carbohydrate found in the blood although it is present in by far the largest amount. Since the blood consists of cellular elements as well as plasma there are also found certain carbohydrates and their derivatives that are typical of the former. Thus, the leukocytes contain small quantities of glycogen, which is said to be increased in severe diabetes mellitus. Hexose phosphates are present in the red cells and traces of such sugars as mannose have also been reported in the plasma in combination with glucosamine and proteins. All these other carbohydrates, however, do not under normal circumstances constitute more than a few per cent of the total.

In certain conditions abnormal quantities of sugars other than glucose may be detected in the blood. The presence of maltose has been reported and during pregnancy and lactation small amounts of lactose may be found. The administration of galactose or fructose brings about a temporary increase in the quantity of these hexoses in the blood.

A clear distinction should be borne in mind between the actual quantities of *reducing* sugars (almost entirely glucose) in the blood and the values given by various methods based on the reduction of copper or iron salts. Some of these reagents are reduced by such noncarbohydrate substances as glutathione, and consequently give abnormally high values for the blood sugar. Others, particularly the more recent methods such as those of Benedict and Somogyi, are more insensitive to these substances and give values closely approximating those found by yeast fermentation of the blood filtrates. By the use of the yeast method combined with an appropriate reagent the presence of nonfermentable sugars of the type of pentoses and galactose may be detected.

In the discussions that follow it should be clearly understood that the level of blood glucose under any set of conditions is a resultant of the opposing forces of glucose utilization and production within the organism together with the operation of such factors as intestinal absorption and renal excretion. Consequently deductions based on the level of the blood glucose alone should be made with caution. Thus, both insulin and phloridzin injections produce hypoglycemia, but for very different reasons: the former produces it by increasing glucose utilization (and decreasing production); while the effect of the latter is due to its influence on the renal tubules and certainly not because of any favorable influence on glucose utilization.

In a normal individual under normal circumstances, the true glucose level of the blood plasma is held within rather narrow limits. During fasting it is approximately 80 mg. per cent (70–90 mg. per cent) and will be maintained at this level for long periods. Under these circumstances the concentration of glucose in the venous and arterial blood is approximately equal with a small difference in favor of the latter. It may be remarked at this point that free flowing capillary blood has the same glucose content as that drawn directly from an artery and is usually used in man for estimations of the arterial content.

The ingestion of a mixed diet is followed by moderate increases in the blood glucose level, the extent of which is largely governed by the quantity of preformed carbohydrate ingested. The difference between the arterial and venous blood becomes much exaggerated and for a short time after ingestion of food may reach between 50 and 100 mg. per cent. The return to normal levels takes place more rapidly in the veins than it does in the arteries, a fact of some importance in the interpretation of glucose tolerance curves (cf. below).

THE GLUCOSE TOLERANCE CURVE

The *major factors* that determine the response of the blood glucose to the ingestion of carbohydrates are:

(a) **The Method of Administration.**—The usual custom is to give glucose in solution by mouth in quantities of 50 to 100 grams or, better, 1 gram per kilo of body weight. When the carbohydrate is given in this manner the rate of intestinal absorption is an important factor and atypical responses may be obtained if the activity of this organ is impaired. In order to avoid this possibility it is necessary to give the sugar intravenously in quantities of about 1 gram per kilo of body weight. In animals the most accurate method is to give the glucose continuously by vein using for this purpose some type of infusion pump. Recently Exton and Rose[14] have advocated the two-dose (by mouth) test. The advantage claimed for this method is that it makes the diagnosis of mild diabetes easier, for, whereas in normal individuals the second dose does not produce so marked an elevation of blood glucose as the first (Staub-Traugott effect), in diabetes there occurs a greater degree of hyperglycemia.

(b) **The Diet of the Individual Prior to the Test.**—This is of great importance. It has been shown by Himsworth[15] and others that the composition of the diet prior to the test greatly influences the results obtained (Fig. 5). Thus, both in men and animals, a previous diet high in fat produces a much greater and more prolonged degree of hyperglycemia when glucose is given than does one rich in carbohydrate. Abstinence from food, when the metabolic mixture is largely protein and fat, also results in the "diabetic" type of tolerance curve. This effect was defined by Hofmeister in 1890 and has been termed *hunger diabetes*. As mentioned above the administration of a second quantity of carbohydrate produces a lessened degree of hyperglycemia and a third still less.

(c) **The Nutritive State.**—Malnutrition may be due to an actual lack of food or to an associated vitamin deficiency, either of which will alter the response of the individual. This is particularly true when the vitamin deficiency is due to a lack of the B complex.

(d) **Exercise.**—Increased muscular activity before or during the test will modify the response to glucose since it not only increases glucose production from liver glycogen but also increases utilization.

(e) **Age.**—In older individuals both the extent and duration of the hyperglycemia may be prolonged while infants are reported to require relatively larger quantities of glucose than adults to induce the same degree of hyperglycemia.

(f) **Alterations in Endocrine Function.**—Hypo- or hyperactivity of several members of the endocrine system are associated with marked alterations in carbohydrate metabolism. These are discussed below. Indeed, the glucose tolerance test is used chiefly to detect the impairment of carbohydrate metabolism associated with diabetes mellitus and other endocrine disorders.

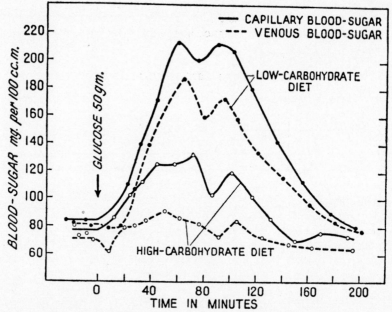

Fig. 5.—Two experiments in the same healthy subject, showing the rise of capillary blood-sugar and the rise of venous blood-sugar after ingestion of 50 gm. of glucose. Before one experiment the subject was taking a low-carbohydrate diet; before the other a high-carbohydrate diet. The area enclosed between the capillary and venous blood-sugar curves indicates the amount of sugar removed from the blood by the peripheral tissues. The areas are approximately equal in both experiments. (From Himsworth, H. P., Lancet, II: 1, **55**, 118, 117, 1939.)

The **normal curve** is illustrated in figure 6, which also shows the variations in both venous and capillary (arterial) blood. The following points are worthy of notice:

(*a*) The blood glucose in both venous and capillary blood reaches a maximum within the first hour after ingestion of glucose. The latter, however, increases to almost twice the level of the former.

(*b*) Following this peak there is a rapid decline so that in about an hour the venous blood has returned to the initial level, while the capillary blood although also falling sharply is still above its initial level.

(*c*) Within the next hour the venous blood declines below the initial level—*the hypoglycemic phase*, which in some individuals may be more marked than in others. The same tendency, but to a lessened degree, is also seen in the capillary blood. Since the contours of the blood glucose curves may be markedly different in different individuals, Himsworth[16] has suggested the use of the area circumscribed by the tolerance curve as a more reliable measurement of the state of the carbohydrate metabolism.

The Effect of Ingestion of Carbohydrates Other than Glucose.—The ingestion of an equivalent amount of boiled *starch* gives a curve that is identical with that following glucose. When *galactose* is given a much greater degree of hyperglycemia is encountered which persists for a much longer time. This is in accord with its poor capacity as a precursor of liver glyco-

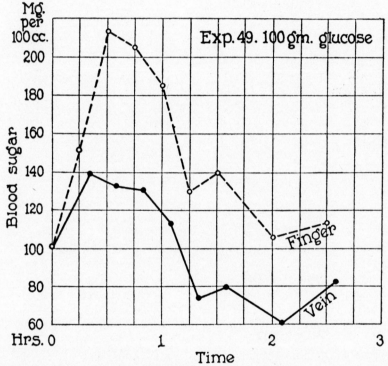

Fig. 6.—Sugar of venous and finger blood after ingestion of glucose. (From Foster, G. L., J. Biol. Chem., **55**: 291, 1923.)

gen[25] and the large proportion that is excreted in the urine (up to 60 per cent in rats).

The behavior of fructose is somewhat confusing. This sugar although absorbed at only half the rate of glucose has an equal capacity as a glycogen precursor. This may be due to the fact that fructose is apparently largely converted into glucose by passage through the intestinal wall.[17] The ingestion of this sugar yields a blood glucose curve that does not rise as markedly as with glucose and is also attended with a well defined increase in blood lactic acid.

GLUCOSE IN OTHER BODY FLUIDS

In general all the extracellular fluids such as the lymph and the spinal, synovial, and peritoneal fluids contain glucose in quantities approximating those of the plasma. Spinal fluid is often regarded as containing a smaller quantity than plasma but this may be due to the greater content of non-carbohydrate reducing substances in the latter. The presence of bacteria in any of these fluids leads to a great destruction of glucose.

GLUCOSE CONTENT OF THE TISSUES

The glucose content of the cells (*i.e.*, of the intracellular water) varies in different organs and tissues. Since the red blood cell is the most accessible it has been the one most frequently studied although it is by no means representative of all. In man the red cell is freely permeable to glucose so that its concentration in the water of the plasma and cell is the same.[18] In other animals, however, the glucose content of the red cells may be considerably less than in the plasma.

The glucose in the liver varies between wide limits according to the state of the carbohydrate metabolism, since it is a glucose forming organ. The free glucose of the muscles is much lower than that of the blood and this is probably true of all active organs. In comparisons of this kind it is important to remember that the calculations should be based on the glucose content per hundred parts of water of cell or plasma. Failure to do this may result in wide discrepancies between the "apparent" and "actual" ratios.

THE GLYCOSURIAS

Although the term *glycosuria* is usually used to denote the presence of glucose in the urine, other sugars are occasionally found and since their presence does not carry the clinical complications that the presence of glucose does it is well to bear in mind that they may be found from time to time.

It has already been pointed out that in the normal individual the venous blood sugar following glucose ingestion does not increase beyond 160 to 170 mg. per cent. Under these conditions, no excess of glucose appears in the urine. It is usually stated that the normal urine does not contain glucose, but examination by more refined methods than those usually employed reveals that small but nevertheless constant amounts are excreted by most individuals. These quantities, however, are insufficient to cause any reduction of Fehling's or Benedict's solution, and consequently, the presence of amounts of glucose that cause precipitation of these copper reagents are looked upon as abnormal.

It is now well established that when the venous blood sugar rises above 180 mg. per cent, the kidney allows some glucose to escape reabsorption and to appear in the urine. This level is termed the *renal threshold for glucose*, but it should be remembered that the level in the arterial blood at which glucosuria occurs is greater than that in the venous blood, and furthermore, the renal threshold for glucose is by no means fixed at a given level, even in the same individual. Thus, in long standing cases of diabetes, the renal threshold for glucose may gradually be elevated to such an extent that no sugar is present in the urine, although the glucose tolerance curve may reveal that well marked disturbances in carbohydrate tolerance are present.

Glucosuria may arise as a result of various circumstances and it is important to realize that although some of these are without ultimate detriment to the organism, others are of such a nature that their continuance constitutes a threat to the individual's well-being.

In consequence, it is of no little importance when confronted with a glycosuria to decide, first of all, what particular sugar is present and then, if this sugar is glucose, to determine the circumstances under which its excretion is occurring.

The methods employed to identify a reducing substance in the urine will be found in any of the more commonly used textbooks, but, in general, they consist of a differentiation between reducing sugars by their fermentation with yeast and the osazones which they form when treated with phenylhydrazine. (cf. Chap. XV, Melituria.)

Conditions Enhancing Glucosuria.—If glucose is identified in the urine, we have to consider the various conditions in which glucosuria may be present. These are:

(a) *Alimentary.*—In some normal individuals the ingestion of large quantities of carbohydrates is said to be followed by the excretion of small quantities of glucose.

(b) *Renal.*—As mentioned above, the renal threshold for glucose is not rigidly adjusted to one blood sugar level, and in some cases it is lowered to such an extent that glucosuria is present even when the blood sugar is within normal limits. These cases often offer a great deal of difficulty, inasmuch as they are likely to be mistaken for true diabetes. A study of glucose tolerance usually reveals no abnormalities and since this condition is harmless, it is of some importance to bring it to the attention of the individual.

(c) *Emotion and Asphyxia.*—It is known that conditions attended by strong emotional stress result in the discharge of increased amounts of epinephrine from the adrenal glands. This hormone will increase the blood sugar and will, at times, lead to glucosuria. In a similar manner, asphyxial conditions stimulate the discharge of epinephrine and glucosuria occurs. Glucosuria is not uncommon following injuries to the base of the brain; in such cases it may be presumed that the higher sympathetic centers have been stimulated by the lesion. These glucosurias disappear when the conditions exciting them are withdrawn.

(d) *Phloridzin.*—The glucoside phloridzin decreases the renal permeability to glucose, and extensive glucosuria follows. This condition, of course, is not encountered in man, but the use of this drug has been of great service in our knowledge of the intermediary metabolism of carbohydrate.

(e) *Endocrine Diseases.*—The commonest cause for the appearance of glucose in the urine is *diabetes mellitus*. A few years ago the presence of this disorder would have been considered as due to an insufficient supply of insulin, but today we are not at all sure that in all instances it is due to this cause. Nevertheless, it is apparent that dysfunction of several endocrine organs may result in an impairment of carbohydrate metabolism of such a degree that glucosuria occurs. Among the endocrine glands whose functional derangement may precipitate this occurrence is most certainly the *pancreas*, and it is still true that destruction of the islets of Langerhans beyond a certain degree will cause glucosuria.

On the other hand, it is equally well established that hyperfunction of the *anterior pituitary* gland, owing to either a secreting tumor or other

pathological condition, is accompanied by a decreased carbohydrate tolerance and glucosuria. Hyperthyroidism or certain tumors of the adrenal
cortex not infrequently give rise to glucosuria.

The interrelationship between these various endocrine glands in the
control of carbohydrate metabolism will be considered in a later section.
The continued presence of glucose in the urine after the ingestion of food
should always be taken as indicative of a gross disturbance in carbohydrate metabolism, particularly if it is accompanied by an abnormal blood
sugar curve.

Lactosuria.—The sugar other than glucose most frequently found in the
urine is lactose. This occurs during pregnancy and lactation and is not indicative of any disturbance in carbohydrate metabolism. However, since lactose is a reducing sugar, an unfortunate diagnosis may be made if care is not
taken to identify the reducing agent.

Pentosuria.—Although the pentoses are widely distributed in the plant
world, chiefly in the polymerized form of pentosans, they do not form a
major form of utilizable carbohydrate in animals. It is true that they are
metabolized since some of them are found in all animal tissues as constituents
of nucleic acids. Nevertheless, the ingestion of large quantities of certain
fruits and berries is followed by the appearance of pentoses in the urine.
This may be termed alimentary pentosuria to differentiate it from the far
rarer condition of "essential or familial pentosuria." These individuals continually excrete pentose regardless of their diet and the pentose found is
l-xyloketose. Pentoses in the urine may be identified by the Salkowski reaction, details of which are given in any text book of biochemistry.

Fructosuria.—The presence in the urine of fructose is usually regarded as
a rare anomaly yet Silver and Reiner[19] reported the finding of six cases
within a year. They regard fructosuria as probably an inborn error of metabolism since in their cases there was no evidence of a more generalized disturbance in carbohydrate metabolism. Earlier workers have, however,
claimed[20] that fructose is frequently present in diabetic urine. It is, however,
extremely doubtful if the analytical methods employed would stand modern
scrutiny.

Glycuronic Acid.—Although glycuronic acid is not a sugar, being the
uronic acid of glucose, it has in recent years come to be recognized as a
not uncommon constituent of urine. This substance is used by the organism
as a conjugating agent in detoxicating mechanisms. While it has been known
for some time that many foreign substances such as menthol are coupled
with glycuronic acid before excretion, the recent work of Cohen and Marrian[21] and of Venning[22] has shown that the hormones of the ovary (estrogens
and progesterone) are in the course of their metabolism united to glycuronic
acid and excreted as glycuronides. Since the glycuronides are much less active than the free hormones this may be an important method for the control of their activity. In pregnancy considerable quantities of glycuronic acid
are found in the urine combined both with the hormones themselves and
with the end products of their metabolism (*i.e.*, *pregnandiol*). Those who
are interested in the origin of glycuronic acid (probably from glucose)
should consult the papers of Quick.[23]

Urines containing glycuronides do not reduce the usual sugar reagents
unless previously boiled with acid.

THE INTERMEDIARY METABOLISM OF GLUCOSE

Following digestion the assimilable carbohydrates of the diet are converted almost entirely into fructose, glucose, and galactose. Fructose, on its passage through the intestinal wall, is converted to some extent into glucose, while galactose apparently passes through unchanged.

All three hexoses enter the portal blood and are carried to the liver where they act to a different degree as precursors of glycogen. Since this polysaccharide on hydrolysis yields glucose which again enters the blood it is convenient, although perhaps somewhat arbitrary, to describe the intermediary metabolism of carbohydrates in terms of this one sugar.

When the organism is presented with a given quantity of glucose it disposes of it in three main ways: (a) By deposition in the liver and muscles as glycogen, (b) by oxidation and (c) by transformation into fat. While a great deal is known of the first two mechanisms and the factors that control them, little knowledge is available concerning the third process although it is as Bodansky[24] remarks "an established fact and a matter of common knowledge and experience."

The Liver and Metabolism.—The liver plays an essential rôle in many phases of metabolism and is rightly regarded as the organ that is responsible for the supply to the tissues of practically all the metabolites upon which their function depends. While this is not the place to detail all the metabolic activities of the liver, it will be recalled that the following important metabolic functions are performed by it: (a) Deamination of amino acids, urea and uric acid formation, (b) Desaturation of depot fatty acids and acetone body formation, (c) Detoxication and conjugation of foreign substances and certain hormones, (d) Glycogen synthesis from various sources, (e) Protein synthesis including fibrinogen and probably other serum proteins and (f) Storage of certain vitamins and essential elements such as iron and copper. A detailed account of its influence on protein and fat metabolism will be found elsewhere.

Glycogen Formation in the Liver.—The glycogen content of the liver varies within wide limits, being greatest after the ingestion of considerable quantities of carbohydrate, less when a high proportion of fat is present in the meal and least when all food is withheld. It also undergoes rapid changes during exercise, conditions involving a marked emotional response and as a result of the action of certain hormones, particularly epinephrine and insulin.

The three major hexoses that result from the digestion of carbohydrate possess different capacities to form liver glycogen. Thus, Cori[25] found the following quantities of liver glycogen after feeding glucose, galactose and fructose (cf. Table 2).

It will be noted that when expressed as a percentage of the sugar absorbed, fructose is a better glycogen former than glucose while galactose is markedly inferior. This last observation is in keeping with the finding that a considerable proportion of this sugar is excreted unchanged in the urine. The pentoses do not form liver glycogen when fed in this manner.

One of the most important facts concerning the rôle of the liver in metabolism is the observation that proteins and certain of their amino acid constituents are capable of increasing the liver glycogen. Investigators in the last century clearly showed that the feeding of well washed meat to fasting

2

animals increased the liver glycogen. In more recent times the conversion of proteins into glucose (and liver glycogen) has been extensively studied both by direct observations on the ability of amino acids to form liver glycogen and indirectly by the use of animals injected with phloridzin. Since the latter procedure has proved to be a valuable method in the study of intermediary metabolism a brief description of its technic will be of future value.

Phloridzin is a glucoside (glucose combined with phloretin) found in the root bark of certain trees. When suspended in oil and injected subcutaneously into animals, it produces a profuse glycosuria which is apparently due to its effect on the renal tubules. Normally all the glucose in the glomerular filtrate is reabsorbed as it passes down the tubules provided that its

TABLE 2

LIVER GLYCOGEN FORMATION AFTER FEEDING VARIOUS SUBSTANCES TO FASTED RATS

Substance fed	Liver glycogen		Per cent excreted	Absorption coefficient (g/100 g/hour)
	Per cent	As per cent of amount absorbed		
None...................	0.21	....	.....	.....
Glucose[1]...............	3.68	16.8	0	0.176
Fructose[1]...............	3.95	39.4	0	0.081
Galactose[1]..............	1.16	4.9	60.5	0.186
d-Lactic acid (Sodium salt)[2]..	1.56	61.8	....	0.030
dl-Alanine[3]...............	0.63	....	....	0.071
Glycine[3]..................	0.20	....	....	0.042–0.055
Leucine[3].................	0.19	....	....	0.034–0.057
Glutamic acid[3]...........	0.33	....	....	0.053–0.074
Casein and butter[3].........	1.67	....	....	.....
Butter[4].................	0.29	....	....	.....
Propionic acid[5]...........	1.36	....	....	.....
Valeric acid[5].............	0.67	....	....	.....
Oleic acid[5]...............	0.20	....	....	.....
Glycerol[5]................	0.65	....	....	.....

[1] From C. F. Cori, J. Biol. Chem., **70:** 577, 1926.
[2] From C. F. Cori and G. T. Cori, J. Biol. Chem., **81:** 396, 1929.
[3] From R. H. Wilson and H. B. Lewis, J. Biol. Chem., **85:** 559, 1929–30.
[4] From M. G. Bodley, H. B. Lewis and J. F. Huber, J. Biol. Chem., **75:** 715, 1927.
[5] From H. J. Deuel, J. S. Butts, L. F. Hallman and C. H. Cutler, J. Biol. Chem., **112:** 15, 1935–36.

concentration does not exceed 180–200 mg. per cent (the renal threshold). It has been suggested by Lundsgaard that phloridzin inhibits a phosphorylation process upon which this reabsorption depends and consequently practically all the glucose in the glomerular fluid escapes into the urine. The interesting and important feature of phloridzin glycosuria is that the blood glucose is below normal and this in turn leads to a stimulation of glucose formation by the liver from noncarbohydrate sources and also an increased fatty acid catabolism to satisfy the energy requirements.

If a carbohydrate or any substance that is capable of forming glucose during the course of its metabolism is given to a phloridzinized animal then an almost equivalent quantity of glucose will appear in the urine due to the rapidity with which the affected kidneys remove glucose from the blood.

It is by the use of such preparations that it has been shown that proteins and certain amino acids form glucose, since their administration is followed by the appearance in the urine of an extra quantity of this carbohydrate. Not all the amino acids form glucose when given to phloridzinized animals, and investigation has shown that some of the latter group form acetone bodies when perfused through an isolated liver. A third group of amino acids does not form either glucose or acetone bodies.

The administration of fats produces only a slight augmentation of glucose excretion in phloridzinized animals and this is believed due to the glycerol portion of the molecule. It is a fact of importance in considering the question of the conversion of fatty acids with an even number of carbon atoms to glucose that these substances are without effect in either enhancing an existing glycosuria or increasing the liver glycogen.

In addition to the substances that are normal constituents of the diet, there are certain others that possess a marked ability to increase liver glycogen of normal animals or the glycosuria of phloridzinized animals. The chief of these are lactic and pyruvic acids, which are excellent glycogen formers (cf. Table 2) and, strikingly enough, the fatty acids with an odd number of carbon atoms such as propionic and valeric acids. Fatty acids of this type do not constitute a major part of natural fats.

The major sources of liver glycogen are the preformed carbohydrates and the proteins of the diet. It should be noted that even during fasting the liver is not completely devoid of glycogen and under such circumstances glycogen formation must have occurred from noncarbohydrate sources, of which only the tissue proteins are able to furnish any significant amount. The formation of glycogen (or glucose) from such noncarbohydrate sources is spoken of as *glyco-* or *gluconeogenesis*.

The Regulation of Blood Glucose by the Liver.—The liver is the predominant organ in the regulation of the blood glucose concentration since it is the only organ that (*a*) possesses a store of glycogen that can be rapidly converted into glucose and (*b*) is capable of forming glucose from noncarbohydrate sources.

The accuracy of this regulation is shown by the narrow limits within which the blood glucose is held in a normal individual in spite of the extreme variations in the quantity of carbohydrate in the diet. While no deleterious effects are known to be associated with blood glucose levels above the normal limits (provided of course there is no associated disorder of metabolism), a reduction in the blood glucose beyond the lower limit of normal is followed by serious consequences. Indeed, prolonged exposure to low blood glucose levels has a fatal outcome probably due to the apparent dependence of the central nervous system on this substance as its sole source of energy. The normal organism reacts vigorously to any measure that forces the blood glucose down towards critical levels and it is the liver that is the site of these corrective measures.

The symptoms of *hypoglycemia* vary somewhat in different species but follow the same general pattern in all. As the blood glucose declines, restlessness and anxiety for food are commonly seen followed by such signs of central nervous system involvement as hyperexcitability of the reflexes and (in man) mental aberrations of all kinds. With a still further decline in blood glucose excitability is followed by convulsive seizures and finally coma and death. The exact pattern of events accompanying hypoglycemia varies in different species: some, such as the sheep, goat and birds, show little change in behavior until convulsions suddenly appear. Others, and man in particular, show marked premonitory symptoms at higher blood glucose levels.

The key to the regulation of blood glucose by the liver is the fact, first recognized by Claude Bernard, that this organ can vary its glucose production in response to the needs of the organism. Furthermore, as indicated above, it is not dependent on a supply of preformed carbohydrate but can convert other metabolites into glucose for this purpose.

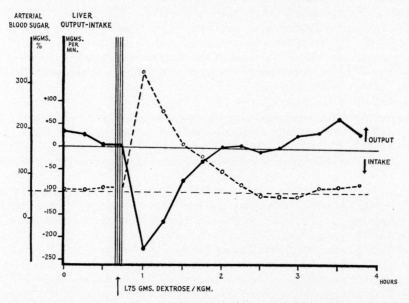

Fig. 7.—Effects of the intravenous injection of five minutes' duration, of 1.75 gm. dextrose per kilogram of body weight. Note particularly the period which follows the large retention of sugar by the liver. There is no intake of sugar and the liver does not immediately resume its output. During this period the level of sugar in the arterial blood falls below its original control value, and does not return to normal until after the liver has resumed its output. (From Soskin, S., Essex, H. E., Herrick, J. F. and Mann, F. C., Amer. J. Physiol., **124:** 558, 1938.)

EXPERIMENTAL EVIDENCE.—The evidence on which the above conclusion is based has been derived from a number of experimental procedures, the chief of which are the following:

(a) *Direct Measurement of Glucose Intake and Output.*—In this method blood samples are simultaneously withdrawn from the portal and hepatic blood vessels of anesthetized animals, and a sample of arterial blood is also taken. A more elegant method devised by London consists of inserting suitably designed cannulæ around the vessels at a previous operation, the open ends of which protrude through the abdominal wall. At a later period blood may be drawn from unanesthetized animals by passing needles down these cannulæ. Analysis gives the glucose content at the moment of withdrawal of the samples and to obtain a measure of the total intake and output the volume of blood traversing the liver must be known. In the above method this is determined on a separate series of animals and the average value obtained is used. Obviously, this may be a source of error since the blood flow through the liver can vary greatly under different conditions. To avoid this difficulty, Soskin and his colleagues[26] have measured the blood flow in the hepatic artery, and the portal and hepatic veins during the experiment by means of electrical flow recorders directly attached to the vessels. A typical experiment of these investigators is shown in figure 7. It will be observed that in the fasting state the liver is adding glucose to the blood but after the administration of glucose by vein there is a large retention by the liver which does not again begin to add glucose until the blood level has declined below its original value.

It has been emphasized by Soskin and his collaborators in a series of papers[27, 28, 29] that regulation of the blood glucose is in large part due to the *homeostatic* activity of the liver. Thus, when the blood glucose rises the liver responds by diminishing its glucose output and conversely a fall in blood glucose is counteracted by an increased hepatic output. The participation of certain endocrine glands in this mechanism will be discussed later.

(*b*) *The Hepatectomized Animal.*—Information of great significance has been derived from studies on hepatectomized animals not only concerning carbohydrate metabolism but other phases of metabolism as well. The technical difficulties involved in the removal of the liver from mammals are considerable and it was not until the work of Mann and his collaborators that a method was developed that yielded a preparation whose condition was such that some final conclusions could be drawn as to the normal activity of this organ. In brief, the method of Mann[30] (which has been modified and in some ways simplified by later investigators) consists of a three-stage operation. At the first operation the blood flow from the inferior vena cava was diverted into the portal system by anastomosing these vessels and ligating the vena cava above. The increased portal flow and pressure open up anastomotic channels between the systemic and portal circulations and at a second operation some weeks later the portal vein is ligated. As a result all the blood in the vena cava and portal vein is carried by the anastomotic channels and in this way is carried around the liver. Consequently, at the final operation of actual removal of the liver, the venous circulation is not acutely obstructed and rapid death from this cause does not occur.

Following hepatectomy and recovery from the anesthetic the animals (usually dogs) appear and behave in a normal manner for an hour or more. Gradually, however, the animal becomes lethargic and convulsions follow which unless relieved are soon followed by death. The lethargy and convulsions are now known to be associated with the progressive hypoglycemia (Fig. 8) that begins as soon as the liver is removed. They are immediately relieved by glucose injection but soon appear again unless the sugar is given continuously. By this means the life of the animals may be prolonged for many hours although ultimately death occurs from causes other than those associated with a low blood glucose level.

The failure of liverless animals to maintain a normal blood glucose level clearly indicates that this organ is the sole source of glucose in the organism. Although the muscles contain large quantities of glycogen it is quite evident that this cannot substitute for the liver glycogen. Furthermore, the animals still possess, in the form of tissue protein, quantities of a glucose precursor which in normal animals are adequate to maintain the blood glucose during many days of fasting but which in the absence of the liver are quite unusable for this purpose.

Consequently, the liver is the organ in which the conversion of amino acids to glucose must occur and this is borne out by the observation that urea formation also ceases after hepatectomy since under normal conditions the ammonia liberated by the deamination of amino acids is rapidly converted into urea. The production of amino acids from the tissue proteins

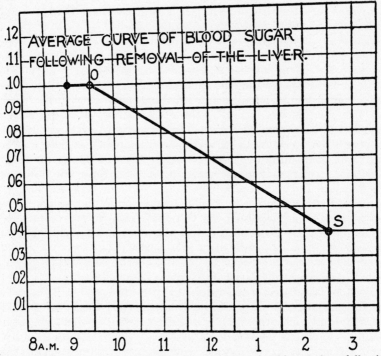

Fig. 8.—The average change in blood sugar noted in thirteen dogs following removal of the liver. O: Point at which the liver was removed. S: Point at which the animal became moribund. (From Mann, F. C. and Magath, T. B., Arch. Int. Med., **30**: 73, 1922.)

continues after hepatectomy as is shown by their steady increase in the blood and in some animals by their appearance in the urine.

The importance of glucose as the major carbohydrate of the circulating fluids is also shown by the fact that this sugar is far superior to any other in relieving either the hypoglycemia of hepatectomized animals or that produced by insulin in normal animals. Fructose, particularly if given intravenously, does prevent hypoglycemia but no other sugar except mannose is at all effective. Amino acids, lactic acid or pyruvic acid are also quite without effect.

The quantity of glucose required to maintain the glucose level of hepatectomized animals is approximately 0.2 gm. per kilo of body weight. This value has been taken as a measure of the glucose output of the liver that is necessary to maintain a normal blood glucose level. However, care should be exercised not to place too much emphasis on this value since glucose is not the only metabolite normally supplied to the tissues by the liver. It is now known for example that this organ is the sole source of the acetone bodies whose rôle as a source of energy in animals deprived of carbohydrate has only recently been fully appreciated. Consequently, in the hepatecto-mized animals the major source of substances providing the metabolic needs of the organism is suddenly withdrawn. Under such conditions the quan-tity of glucose necessary to maintain the normal blood glucose level may or may not be indicative of the requirement under normal circumstances.

One of the most surprising observations made on hepatectomized animals is that if they are *depancreatized* prior to the removal of the liver the blood glucose declines almost as rapidly as in animals that retain their pancreas and hypoglycemic convulsions appear that are relieved by glucose injection. Furthermore, the quantity of glucose necessary to maintain a normal blood glucose level in depancreatized and hepatectomized dogs is stated to be only slightly less than that required by animals from which the liver only is re-moved. The essential character of the liver as the sole source of glucose is emphasized by these experiments and the bearing of these findings upon the problem of the metabolism of the diabetic animals is evident.

The Liver and Gluconeogenesis.—The use of the term gluconeogenesis to signify the formation of glucose from noncarbohydrate sources has come into widespread use. It has been already pointed out that the liver is the site of those processes whereby amino acids and certain other substances such as glycerol and lactic acid are converted into liver glycogen. A dis-cussion of the hypothesis that fatty acids may also serve as a source of glu-cose will be found in the section on the interconversion of the foodstuffs but whatever may be the truth of this proposition its proponents are agreed that it is also in the liver that it occurs.

There appears to be a relationship between the quantity of preformed carbohydrate in the diet, the response of the blood glucose to the ingestion of a large quantity of carbohydrate, and the glycogen content of the liver.

It has already been pointed out that the smaller the proportion of pre-formed carbohydrate in the diet, the greater the hyperglycemia after glu-cose ingestion.

In a recent study[31] it was found that the glycogen content of the liver after a period of fasting was greater in rats that had previously received a high protein diet than in those to whom a carbohydrate rich diet had been given. In addition, exposure to cold or the injection of phloridzin did not deplete the glycogen reserves as rapidly in the protein fed group. In the fully fed condition the glycogen content of the liver of the carbohydrate fed rats was approximately four times as great as in those fed protein, so that the maintenance of the glycogen reserves in the latter could not be attributed to their higher initial content. The authors conclude that this phe-nomenon is related to the previous rate of gluconeogenesis. Since this is already going on at a high rate in the protein fed group, the withdrawal of food does not necessitate the abrupt alteration in the metabolic mixture that it does in the carbohydrate fed group. This view is supported by two further pieces of evidence, for it was found that by the third day of fasting the glycogen levels in the groups were approximately the same, indicating that in the carbohydrate fed group the processes of gluconeogenesis were now proceeding at a rate comparable to those of the protein fed rats. In addition, a study of the nitrogen excretion during fasting showed initially a very much greater quantity of protein catabolism in the group previously fed protein, but again by the third day the excretion of both groups had almost equalized. It is also of interest that *adrenalectomy* abolished this effect of protein feeding.

Experiments of a similar significance but using an entirely different technic have been reported by G. T. Evans.[20] This author exposed fasting rats to atmospheres containing 10.5 per cent oxygen for twenty-four hours and observed a striking increase in the liver glycogen content. That this procedure had stimulated the formation of glucose from protein was shown by the increased nitrogen excretion that accompanied it. This effect was also abolished by adrenalectomy or hypophysectomy.

Mechanism of Glucose and Glycogen Formation in the Liver.—The equation $(C_6H_{10}O_5)_n + n\,H_2O \rightleftharpoons n\,C_6H_{12}O_6$, while illustrating the reversibility of the glycogen-glucose relationship in the liver, does not reveal either the intermediate steps involved or the mechanism by which the transformation is effected. The conversion of liver glycogen to glucose can occur with great rapidity as is shown by the rapid elevation of the blood glucose following stimuli that excite the sympathetic nervous system and the adrenal medulla. It is also probable that glucose is polymerized into glycogen at an equally high rate.

For many years it was thought that a liver amylase was responsible for the hydrolysis of glycogen and there are many experiments on record which indicate that suitable liver extracts will hydrolyze glycogen. The recent work of Cori and Cori[33] has, however, shown that an amylase is not the enzyme concerned although the presence of this ferment in blood may complicate studies made on liver extracts. The work of these authors, together with that of Ostern, Herbert and Holmes,[34] has shown that the main pathway of liver glycogen breakdown is through phosphorylation with inorganic phosphate, the product of the reaction being glucose 1-phosphate, a substance first isolated from muscle by Cori, Colowick and Cori.[35]

$$\text{Glycogen} + H_3PO_4 \longrightarrow \text{Glucose 1-Phosphate}$$

This reaction is catalyzed by an enzyme known as a *phosphorylase* and, as very recently shown by the work of the Coris, the reaction can be reversed in vitro so that for the first time a synthesis of glycogen outside the animal body has been achieved.

The next step in the decomposition of glycogen is the splitting of the glucose phosphate by another enzyme—a phosphatase. This reaction yields glucose and regenerates inorganic phosphate which can again phosphorylate glycogen. The complete cycle of events in the liver is then:

$$
\begin{array}{l}
\text{Liver Glycogen} + H_3PO_4 \quad \longleftarrow \\
\qquad \uparrow \quad \downarrow \qquad\qquad \text{Phosphorylase} \\
\quad \text{Glucose 1-Phosphate} \\
\qquad \downarrow \quad \uparrow \qquad\qquad \text{Phosphatase} \\
\text{Blood} \rightleftarrows \text{Glucose} + H_3PO_4 \longleftarrow
\end{array}
$$

Since the reaction between liver glycogen and glucose is a reversible one and glucose 1-phosphate is converted into glycogen by the phosphorylase it appears that glycogen synthesis from glucose must also be achieved through a preliminary stage involving the addition of inorganic phosphate. This would depend on the reversibility of the phosphatase but the exact mechanism is not entirely known at present. The work of Ostern, Herbert and Holmes has shown that while liver slices synthesize glycogen from glucose with ease, this fails to occur after a preliminary maceration of the tissue. The process is an aerobic one and appears to require the presence of calcium. Sodium fluoride inhibits the synthesis and also the breakdown of glucose 1-phosphate to glucose.

As will be seen later the breakdown of muscle glycogen follows the same initial stages as the liver glycogen does, but the end products are quite different. The universality of phosphorylation in processes involving carbohydrate degradation and synthesis is shown by the fact that almost identical mechanisms are present in yeast [36] and in plants.[37]

CARBOHYDRATE METABOLISM IN THE TISSUES

I. **Glycogen Formation.**—While the liver is the organ responsible for the supply of glucose, it is the tissues—particularly the muscles—in which utilization occurs. The blood glucose level at any time merely indicates the balance between production and utilization.

The glycogen in the tissues is no longer available as a source of glucose except by an indirect series of changes which again involve the activity of the glycogenic mechanisms of the liver.

The glycogen content of the tissues, with the exception of the skeletal muscles and the heart, is quite low, being of the order of 0.2 gm. per cent. In the muscles the quantity varies according to the nutritive state and the species studied. In the white rat which has been extensively used in such work the skeletal muscle glycogen after a fast of twenty-four hours is about 0.5 gm. per cent and after glucose feeding about 0.8 gm. per cent. Fasting for periods as long as three days does not materially decrease the muscle glycogen below 0.5 gm. per cent and the tenacity with which this tissue retains its glycogen stores is in marked contrast to the behavior of the liver glycogen. Indeed, animals dying in diabetic coma will be found to possess considerable stores of muscle glycogen. The glycogen content of the cardiac muscle is of the same order as that in skeletal muscle and in this tissue pancreatectomy is claimed to bring about a striking increase.[38] Smooth muscle, on the other hand, has a low glycogen content 0.05 gm. per cent.[39]

It is extremely probable that the only source of muscle glycogen in the organism is the blood glucose. This does not exclude the participation of other metabolites, such as lactic acid, but these apparently undergo a preliminary transformation into glucose in the liver before they can be used for this purpose.

II. **Carbohydrate Balance Sheets.**—The manner in which an animal disposes of a known quantity of glucose (or any other carbohydrate) has proved one of the most valuable methods for the study of carbohydrate metabolism. The present most widely used technic is that introduced by the Coris.[40] Standard fasting white rats are fed a known amount of glucose by stomach tube, the quantity fed being in excess of that which can be absorbed during the period of observation. After feeding, the animals are placed in a respiration apparatus and the oxygen consumption and respiratory quotient over the period determined. They are then anesthetized and the following determinations are made: (a) the glucose remaining in the intestinal tract, (b) the blood glucose, (c) the muscle glycogen, and (d) the liver glycogen. From these quantities together with the respiratory data and comparison with non-fed animals it is possible to calculate what proportion of the glucose absorbed (a) was oxidized, (b) was deposited as liver glycogen, (c) was deposited as muscle glycogen, and (d) remained circulating in the body.

The results of such an experiment are given below in table 3.

It will be observed that for every 100 parts of glucose absorbed, 18 parts were accounted for as liver glycogen, 25 parts as muscle glycogen and 44

TABLE 3

DISPOSITION OF GLUCOSE IN A FASTED RAT*

	Grams	Per cent
Glucose absorbed (4-hour period).................	1.065	100
Increase in liver glycogen	0.192	18
Increase in body glycogen........................	0.263	25
Glucose oxidized	0.465	44
Total..	0.920	87

* From Cori, C. F. and Cori, G. T., J. Biol. Chem., **70**: 557, 1926.

parts by oxidation. The total recovery of 87 per cent is to be considered as excellent, particularly as small quantities of other carbohydrate intermediaries are not included in the estimations.

Under these circumstances glycogen formation in the liver and muscles is approximately equal to the glucose oxidized and the quantity of glucose deposited as muscle glycogen is greater than that retained by the liver.

Similar balance sheets have not been made in fed animals but in these it is probable that some transformation of the absorbed glucose into fat occurs. The extent of this in short term experiments has not been measured.

III. **Carbohydrate Metabolism in the Skeletal Muscles and Its Relation to the Contraction Process.**—Practically all our knowledge of carbohydrate utilization and oxidation in the tissues has been derived from the study of skeletal muscles. This is not only because these tissues constitute nearly half the body weight and hence are the seat of the major part of metabolism, but because muscular movements that place such a heavy demand on the energy supply of the body are carried out to a large degree by the breakdown and utilization of the muscle carbohydrates. Nor is it probable that the mechanisms involved in these phases of metabolism are unique to the skeletal muscles. Indeed, there is every reason to believe that carbohydrate utilization is carried out in all tissues by the same systems and for that matter even in such lowly organisms as yeast.

Lactic Acid in Muscle.—The appearance of lactic acid in muscles in rigor mortis had been observed for many years but that it had its source in muscle glycogen was not known until the work of Parnas and Wagner in 1914.[41] Prior to this, in a classical paper, Fletcher and Hopkins[42] had shown that lactic acid appeared in a stimulated muscle and disappeared again during recovery. They also made the important observation that much greater quantities of lactic acid appeared under anaerobic conditions and were not removed until oxygen was available. Since muscles will contract for considerable periods without oxygen the association of these phenomena was evident, but its real significance was not appreciated until the work of Meyerhof, whose first paper appeared in 1920.[43] In this paper Meyerhof showed that there was a relationship between the oxygen consumption, glycogen disappearance, and lactic acid formation of exercised muscles of frogs.

The figures showed that lactic acid appearance during stimulation of isolated muscles of frogs was equivalent to glycogen disappearance and that the oxygen consumption which took place during recovery accounted for only a part (one-fifth) of the lactic acid that disappeared during this period. The remaining quantity of lactic acid that was removed was accounted for by the resynthesis of glycogen. As a result of these experiments as well as the measurements of heat production during contraction and recovery by A. V. Hill,[44] it was thought that these reactions accounted for the energy production of muscle and that the carbohydrate cycle that occurred formed the basis of muscular contraction. The events taking place during activity could be then represented as follows:

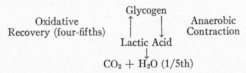

This simple scheme has, however, not entirely stood the test of further investigation although there is no doubt that muscle glycogen does not break down to glucose, as does the liver glycogen, but passes through a variety of other intermediates of which lactic acid is the one which accumulates in greatest quantity when the oxygen supply is deficient.

Even prior to the work of Meyerhof it was appreciated that glycogen did not form lactic acid directly. Embden in an extensive series of papers between 1914 and 1927 had shown that hexose phosphates, particularly glucose 6-phosphate, were formed in contracting muscle and that these substances then gave rise to lactic acid. At this point the analogy between carbohydrate breakdown in muscle and yeast became particularly striking.

Harden and Young had found in 1908 that the fermentation of glucose by yeast involved a preliminary phosphorylation and that alcohol and CO_2 production paralleled the formation of this ester. Furthermore, they showed that ester formation was catalyzed by a yeast enzyme, *hexokinase*. In muscle, lactic acid and CO_2 are the end products but, as Meyerhof showed, the yeast enzyme will also catalyze glucose breakdown in muscle extracts. Finally, it was shown that the muscle extracts contained not one enzyme but a whole series of catalysts which degrade glycogen in a stepwise manner.

The dissection of this chain of events has occupied the attention of a large number of investigators in recent years, and while the whole cycle is not yet complete, enough is known to indicate that the general pattern of carbohydrate breakdown in muscle and yeast is almost identical.

Before discussing this it is necessary to mention one other investigation which clearly indicated that the simple mechanism of Meyerhof and Hill was unsatisfactory as a full explanation of the chemical processes occurring in contracting muscle. In 1930 Lundsgaard[45] had found that if animals (rabbits or frogs) were injected with iodoacetic acid ($CH_2I.COOH$) and the muscles were stimulated, these muscles contracted for a while and then went into rigor. Examination of the muscles showed that although glycogen had decreased no lactic acid formation had occurred. Instead, considerable quantities of hexose phosphates had accumulated. Even more significant were the alterations in the creatine phosphate content of the tissue (see table 4).

TABLE 4

CHEMICAL CHANGES IN MUSCLES TREATED WITH IODOACETIC ACID*

	Lactic acid (mg. per cent)	Phosphate (mg. per cent)	Creatine phosphate (as PO_4) (mg. per cent)
Normal resting..........	25	21	61
Normal working........	84	29	46
Poisoned resting........	16	29	57
Poisoned working.......	15	28	0

* After Lundsgaard, Biochem. Zeitsch., **217**: 102, 1930.

Creatine Phosphate.—The presence of creatine phosphate in muscles had been discovered three years previously by both Eggleton and Eggleton[46] and Fiske and Subbarow.[47] Its formula is:

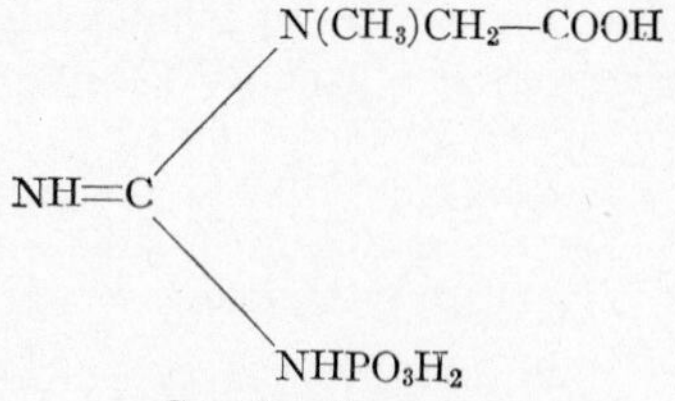

$$
\begin{array}{c}
N(CH_3)CH_2\!-\!COOH \\
/ \\
NH\!=\!C \\
\backslash \\
NHPO_3H_2
\end{array}
$$

Creatine Phosphate

These investigators had found that during muscular contraction this substance is split into creatine and phosphoric acid which renders phosphate available for combination with the muscle carbohydrate. Furthermore, during recovery creatine phosphate is resynthesized. Thus, not only is there a carbohydrate cycle in muscle but also one involving phosphate.

Adenylic Acid.—Creatine phosphate, however, is not the only phosphorus compound that undergoes decomposition during muscular contraction. Embden and Zimmerman in 1928[48] had isolated adenylic acid from muscle. Its formula is:.

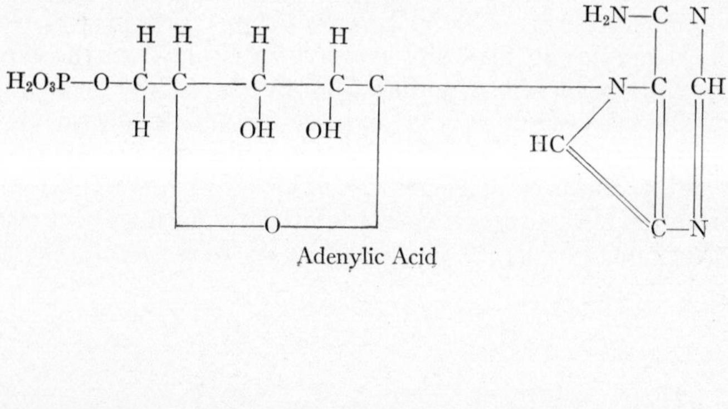

Adenylic Acid

This substance is a mono-nucleotide and contains in addition to the phosphate radical, a pentose, d-ribose, and a purine, adenine. Two years later Lohmann[49] isolated from muscle the pyrophosphate of this compound known as adenylic acid pyrophosphate or adenylpyrophosphate. This substance is a key compound in the processes involved in carbohydrate breakdown in muscle. It acts as a co-enzyme and during muscular contraction is broken down to adenylic acid yielding two molecules of phosphate which then phosphorylates the carbohydrate.

The relation of creatine phosphate to these changes is that the former apparently acts as a phosphate reserve from which adenylpyrophosphate is regenerated. A partial reconstitution of creatine phosphate under anaerobic conditions is made possible by the fact that the phosphate attached to the carbohydrate in the initial stages is later discarded and thus is again made available for further carbohydrate decomposition:

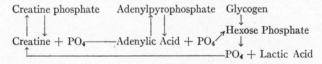

These changes it will be observed are all anaerobic and involve the transfer of phosphate first to the carbohydrate and then back to the adenylpyrophosphate via creatine phosphate.

Further study has shown that between the initial formation of hexose phosphate and lactic acid several other intermediaries are involved. The present conception of the chain reactions occurring is as follows but is subject to further modification as this active phase of investigation is pursued.

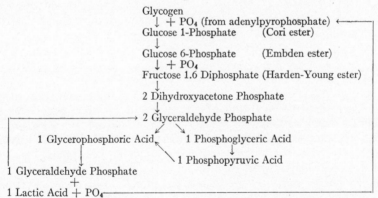

It will be observed that the initial stages of glycogen breakdown on muscle are similar to those in liver since glucose 1-phosphate is formed in both tissues. However, in liver this is immediately decomposed to glucose and phosphate. In muscle the addition of a second phosphate radical together with a reorientation of the carbohydrate molecule yields fructose diphosphate, whose metabolic pathway is then fixed so that lactic acid is in muscle the end product of glycogen breakdown.

Degradation and Regeneration of Glycogen.—There are still two important questions to be considered. The first of these is the manner in which the glycogen stores of muscle are replenished. It will be recalled that the original Meyerhof scheme (largely worked out on isolated frog muscles) postulated that four-fifths of the lactic acid formed was reconverted into glycogen, the oxidation of the remainder providing the necessary energy. However, in the intact mammal with its rapid circulation considerable quantities of the lactic acid formed during hard muscular exercise may escape into the blood stream and consequently become unavailable for such a process. Even more damaging, however, is the fact that lactic acid while a good precursor of liver glycogen apparently does not form muscle glycogen when infused into an animal.[50, 51] Furthermore, as Long and Grant[52] showed in fasted rats during recovery from exercise, lactic acid removal from both the muscle and the blood is comparatively rapid while muscle glycogen regeneration is slow but if glucose is given its regeneration soon occurs (C. N. H. Long and E. G. Fry—unpublished results).[53] Consequently, in the intact animal, muscle glycogen regeneration is largely dependent on the glucose brought to it by the blood stream. Furthermore, it is also entirely possible that the lactic acid that accumulates in muscles when the oxygen supply is deficient is largely removed by the blood and converted by the liver into glucose before it can again serve as a source of muscle glycogen.

The second question is of even greater importance. The conversion of glycogen to lactic acid yields only a small part of the energy of the glycogen available for work and is consequently a most uneconomical method for its utilization. Oxidation, on the other hand, yields all the available energy. It is certain that glycogen can be degraded to lactic acid under anaerobic conditions in muscle but it is not at all certain that this is the usual pathway except under conditions in which the oxygen supply is inadequate to meet the rate of work, *i.e.*, strenuous exercise. In any case the lactic acid formed must ultimately be oxidized and the question has been raised as to whether carbohydrate oxidation can occur in muscle without an intermediary formation of lactic acid by anaerobic processes.

Anaerobic and Aerobic Degeneration.—A clear distinction should be drawn between the anaerobic and aerobic degradation of carbohydrate. The former may well be an emergency mechanism allowing muscular activity to take place and repaying the oxygen at a later date during recovery —the oxygen debt. From the extensive studies of Hill, Long and Lupton,[54] it is known that all except the mildest forms of exercise are associated with an increased blood lactic acid and a period of extra oxygen consumption after the exercise is finished. Evidently some metabolites accumulate, particularly at high levels of work, which require oxidation before the organism returns to its pre-exercise condition. The dissociation of work from the necessity of a contemporary oxygen supply of sufficient magnitude is a distinct advantage since short violent efforts can be made at a level of energy expenditure far beyond that available to the muscles through their blood supply. Thus, a man can run a hundred yards in somewhat under ten seconds without drawing a breath, yet following this his tissues will consume in the next hour an extra ten liters of oxygen. Since the maximum oxygen supply that can be transported by the blood is about five liters a minute, the advantage in being able to accumulate a large oxygen debt is apparent, and not only from the point of view of athletic performance alone.

The mechanisms by which glycogen or lactic acid are oxidized in muscles have also been extensively studied in recent years. Although the oxidation of metabolites by tissues consists essentially of the union of oxygen atoms with their carbon, hydrogen, nitrogen or sulfur atoms, it is carried out by the operation of a complicated series of enzymes and catalysts, whose action is coordinated so that the degradation of the molecules proceeds in a step-like manner. Since only a certain proportion of the total energy of the metabolite is liberated by each step, a smooth delivery of this energy is afforded in a manner most advantageous to the cell. The rapid oxidation by cells of substances which outside the body are regarded as unusually stable compounds is a remarkable demonstration of the efficiency of these biological systems.

In order to understand our present knowledge of the oxidation of the carbohydrates and of their derivatives, it is first necessary to describe these enzyme systems in general terms.

In the first place the oxidation of an organic compound can take place (a) by the direct addition of oxygen, or (b) by the withdrawal of hydrogen. A moment's thought will show that dehydrogenation leaves the molecule in a more highly oxidized and more unstable condition and, furthermore, can occur in the absence of oxygen provided that some other compound is available to which the liberated hydrogen can be attached. Such a compound is termed a *hydrogen acceptor*. The hydrogen of the metabolite is loosened from its attachment in the parent molecule by the action of an enzyme known as a *dehydrogenase*. These are specific in their nature and are usually named after the substrate upon which they act, *i.e.*, lactic acid dehydrogenase.

The interaction between metabolite, dehydrogenase, and hydrogen acceptor may be featured as follows:

$$1. \text{ MH}_2 \xrightarrow{\text{Dehydrogenase}} \text{M} + \text{H}_2$$

$$2. \text{ H}_2 + \text{A (Hydrogen acceptor)} \rightarrow \text{AH}_2$$

Now, in order for this system to work continuously it must be reversible, which means that the reduced hydrogen acceptor must be oxidized and thus returned to its original state.

This is carried out by the interaction between the reduced hydrogen acceptor and an oxidizing enzyme (oxidase).

$$3. \text{ AH}_2 + \text{X}\tfrac{1}{2}(\text{O}) \longrightarrow \text{A} + \text{X} + \text{H}_2\text{O}$$

The now reduced oxidase is reoxidized by oxygen brought to the cell by the blood and the process starts over again. Summing these equations shows that as a result of the operation of this series of enzymes there has occurred an oxidation of the hydrogen of the metabolite to water. The union of hydrogen with oxygen yields the maximum quantity of energy. However, this union has not occurred immediately but over a series of steps at each one of which part of the energy of the hydrogen is released.

As to the actual enzymes involved there exists as indicated above a series of dehydrogenases which activate the hydrogen of the metabolite so that it can unite with the hydrogen acceptor. The most important hydrogen acceptors in muscle are the cytochromes, iron containing pigments related to haem and which like this respiratory pigment are combined with a protein.

Three such substances have been recognized in muscle and are termed cytochrome A, B and C. All participate in cellular respiration and they probably act in series.

CYTOCHROME OXIDATION AND REDUCTION.—The oxidation and reduction of the cytochromes consists in the alternate oxidation and reduction of the iron atom they contain, so that what actually occurs when the cytochrome accepts hydrogen from the substrate is the acceptance by the iron atom of an electron donated by the hydrogen.

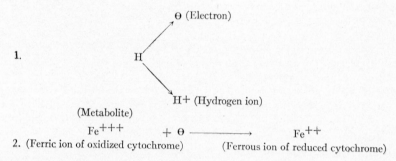

1.

Θ (Electron)

H

H+ (Hydrogen ion)

(Metabolite)

2. (Ferric ion of oxidized cytochrome) Fe^{+++} $+ \Theta \longrightarrow$ Fe^{++} (Ferrous ion of reduced cytochrome)

The further union of the hydrogen ion with oxygen and the reacceptance of the electron from reduced cytochrome is affected by another enzyme termed *cytochrome oxidase*. This enzyme is also known by the name of "Warburg's respiratory enzyme" (*Atmungsferment*). It also contains iron atoms in organic combination (probably a haem), which are united to a specific protein.

The oxygen carried to the cell unites with the cytochrome oxidase and oxidizes its iron atom which in turn accepts the electron from the cytochrome. The oxygen having donated a positive charge to the Fe^{++} atom becomes an oxygen ion. Two such ions will then unite with four hydrogen ions derived from the metabolite and form two molecules of water.

3. Fe^{++} $+$ $(+) \longrightarrow Fe^{+++}$
(Ferrous ion of cytochrome oxidase)   (From oxygen)

4. O_2 $2+$ $2O^=$

5. $2O^= + 4H^+ \longrightarrow 2H_2O$

6. Fe^{+++} $+$ $\Theta \longrightarrow Fe^{++}$
(Ferric ion of cytochrome oxidase)   (Θ from reduced cytochrome)   (Ferrous ion of cytochrome oxidase)

It should be noted that the rôle of oxygen is limited to the acceptance of an electron derived from hydrogen and the union of the ensuing oxygen ion with the hydrogen ions to form water. However, the transfer of hydrogen involves further enzymes and catalysts than those indicated above. It has been shown by Szent-Györgyi[55] that between the dehydrogenases and the cytochromes is inserted a series of catalysts which heretofore had been regarded merely as metabolites. These are the dicarboxylic acids, oxaloacetic, malic, fumaric and succinic acids. The discovery of their catalytic action in cellular respiration is based on the observation by Szent-Györgyi that the addition of minute traces of fumaric acid to minced and washed pigeon breast muscle would support the respiration, which soon declined in its absence. Further extensive investigation showed that these dicarboxylic acids acted as follows:

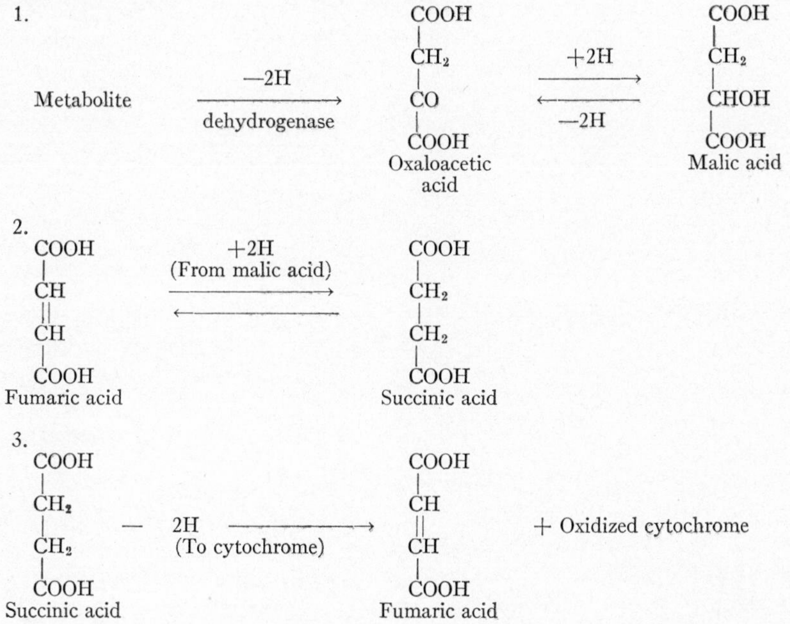

1.

$$
\text{Metabolite} \xrightarrow[\text{dehydrogenase}]{-2\text{H}}
\begin{array}{c}
\text{COOH} \\
| \\
\text{CH}_2 \\
| \\
\text{CO} \\
| \\
\text{COOH} \\
\text{Oxaloacetic} \\
\text{acid}
\end{array}
\begin{array}{c}
\xrightarrow{+2\text{H}} \\
\xleftarrow[-2\text{H}]{}
\end{array}
\begin{array}{c}
\text{COOH} \\
| \\
\text{CH}_2 \\
| \\
\text{CHOH} \\
| \\
\text{COOH} \\
\text{Malic acid}
\end{array}
$$

2.

$$
\begin{array}{c}
\text{COOH} \\
| \\
\text{CH} \\
|| \\
\text{CH} \\
| \\
\text{COOH} \\
\text{Fumaric acid}
\end{array}
\begin{array}{c}
\xrightarrow{\substack{+2\text{H} \\ (\text{From malic acid})}} \\
\xleftarrow{}
\end{array}
\begin{array}{c}
\text{COOH} \\
| \\
\text{CH}_2 \\
| \\
\text{CH}_2 \\
| \\
\text{COOH} \\
\text{Succinic acid}
\end{array}
$$

3.

$$
\begin{array}{c}
\text{COOH} \\
| \\
\text{CH}_2 \\
| \\
\text{CH}_2 \\
| \\
\text{COOH} \\
\text{Succinic acid}
\end{array}
\quad -\quad 2\text{H} \xrightarrow[(\text{To cytochrome})]{}
\begin{array}{c}
\text{COOH} \\
| \\
\text{CH} \\
|| \\
\text{CH} \\
| \\
\text{COOH} \\
\text{Fumaric acid}
\end{array}
\quad + \text{ Oxidized cytochrome}
$$

Two pairs of dicarboxylic acids are involved. In the first stage (1) the hydrogen of the metabolite reduces oxaloacetic acid to malic acid. This then yields by the action of a dehydrogenase two atoms of hydrogen to fumaric acid (2), thus regenerating oxaloacetic acid and reducing the fumaric acid to succinic acid. The action of another dehydrogenase (succinic acid dehydrogenase) then allows the passage of two hydrogen atoms to cytochrome (3) which then carries the hydrogen forward as already described, at the same time reducing the succinic acid back to fumaric acid.

The hydrogen of the metabolite is thus passed steadily over these two pairs of dicarboxylic acid liberating at each step a certain portion of its energy.

SOURCE OF CO_2 IN RESPIRATION.—One of the questions most frequently asked is the source of the CO_2 that appears during respiration, since the above scheme only postulates the oxidation of hydrogen to water. This problem has not yet been successfully solved but two views have been put forward. Szent-Györgyi believes that the respiratory CO_2 arises by processes independent of the oxidation of hydrogen. He postulates that at some stage following the dehydrogenation of the carbohydrate molecule pyruvic acid is formed which is then decarboxylated, yielding CO_2. Pyruvic acid is a highly reactive substance that can react under both aerobic and anaerobic conditions with a variety of substances. Thus, by direct decarboxylation such as occurs in yeast it yields CO_2 and alcohol. In brain it may follow several pathways (all of which, however, yield CO_2), or it may be both oxidized and decarboxylated to yield CO_2 and acetic acid. It is of exceeding interest that the co-enzyme of the decarboxylating system is the diphosphate of vitamin B_1.[56]

Krebs and Johnson[57] have put forward a scheme that accounts not only for the oxidation of hydrogen but for that of carbon as well. This is in a sense an extension of Szent-Györgyi's work but it involves the addition of other steps, particularly the formation of citric acid by the union of oxaloacetic and pyruvic acid. It is claimed that citric acid, like fumaric and succinic acids, catalyses the respiration of washed pigeon muscle, a point on which all investigators are not agreed.[58] In brief the "citric acid cycle" is:

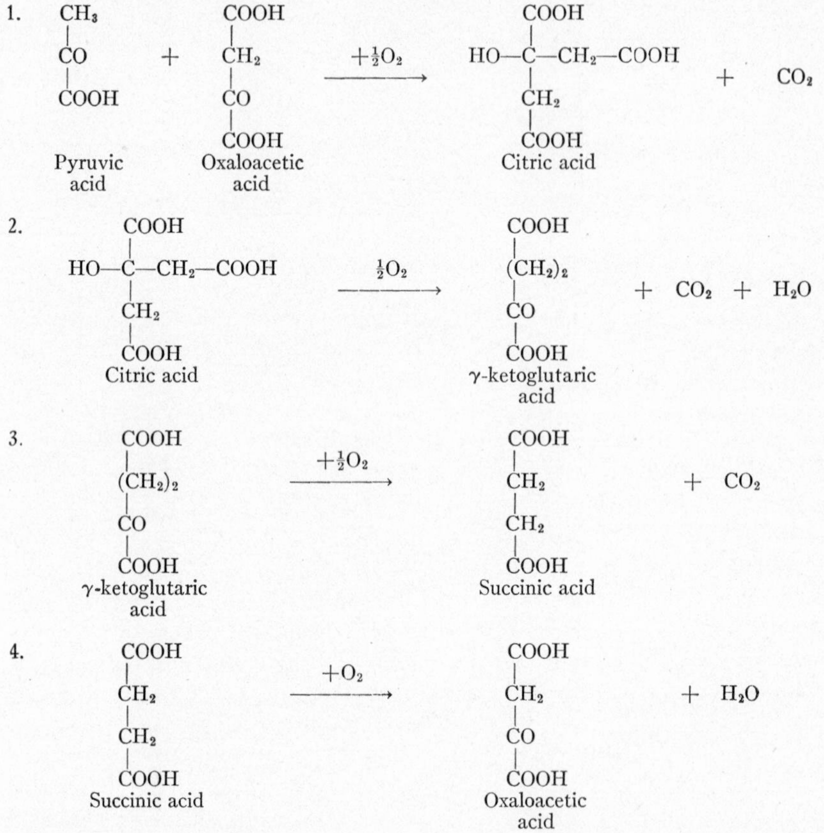

1.

$$\underset{\text{Pyruvic acid}}{\begin{array}{c}CH_3 \\ | \\ CO \\ | \\ COOH\end{array}} \quad + \quad \underset{\text{Oxaloacetic acid}}{\begin{array}{c}COOH \\ | \\ CH_2 \\ | \\ CO \\ | \\ COOH\end{array}} \quad \xrightarrow{+\frac{1}{2}O_2} \quad \underset{\text{Citric acid}}{\begin{array}{c}COOH \\ | \\ HO-C-CH_2-COOH \\ | \\ CH_2 \\ | \\ COOH\end{array}} \quad + \quad CO_2$$

2.

$$\underset{\text{Citric acid}}{\begin{array}{c}COOH \\ | \\ HO-C-CH_2-COOH \\ | \\ CH_2 \\ | \\ COOH\end{array}} \quad \xrightarrow{\frac{1}{2}O_2} \quad \underset{\gamma\text{-ketoglutaric acid}}{\begin{array}{c}COOH \\ | \\ (CH_2)_2 \\ | \\ CO \\ | \\ COOH\end{array}} \quad + \quad CO_2 \quad + \quad H_2O$$

3.

$$\underset{\gamma\text{-ketoglutaric acid}}{\begin{array}{c}COOH \\ | \\ (CH_2)_2 \\ | \\ CO \\ | \\ COOH\end{array}} \quad \xrightarrow{+\frac{1}{2}O_2} \quad \underset{\text{Succinic acid}}{\begin{array}{c}COOH \\ | \\ CH_2 \\ | \\ CH_2 \\ | \\ COOH\end{array}} \quad + \quad CO_2$$

4.

$$\underset{\text{Succinic acid}}{\begin{array}{c}COOH \\ | \\ CH_2 \\ | \\ CH_2 \\ | \\ COOH\end{array}} \quad \xrightarrow{+O_2} \quad \underset{\text{Oxaloacetic acid}}{\begin{array}{c}COOH \\ | \\ CH_2 \\ | \\ CO \\ | \\ COOH\end{array}} \quad + \quad H_2O$$

It will be observed that the net result of these reactions is the oxidation of one molecule of pyruvic acid to CO_2 and H_2O, *viz.*

$$C_3H_4O_3 + 2\tfrac{1}{2}O_2 \longrightarrow 3CO_2 + 2H_2O$$

The original molecule of oxaloacetic acid has been regenerated and is able to start the chain of reactions again by combining with another molecule of pyruvic acid (or another triose).

In a recent paper Colowick, Kalckar and Cori[104] have shown that in cell free extracts of heart muscle and kidney, the phosphorylation of glucose is coupled with the succinic-fumaric oxidative system and that the oxidation of one molecule of glucose is accompanied by the phosphorylation of five molecules of glucose. Since the oxidation of glucose follows the path of triose phosphate—phosphoglycerate—pyruvate—CO_2 + H_2O, these substances are apparently common intermediates in both the aerobic and anaerobic breakdown of glucose. In the absence of oxygen, pyruvic acid is transformed into lactic acid. These authors point out that while in these cell free systems the oxidative energy is used to phosphorylate glucose, in the intact cell this energy can be utilized for a variety of other cellular activities.

SUMMARY.—It is now possible to incorporate in a condensed scheme what is known concerning the anaerobic and aerobic breakdown of carbohydrate in muscle.

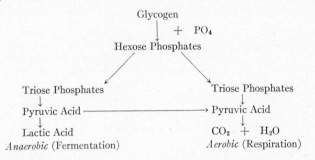

It should be emphasized that all the foregoing schemes are necessarily incomplete and in some cases are no more than approximations to the actual conditions existing in intact cells.

The muscles are not limited to the utilization of carbohydrates for their energy supply. It is known that they oxidize the acetone bodies with equal facility and can probably utilize amino acids and fatty acids as well. Consequently, it must be assumed that they possess equally efficient enzyme systems for these metabolites. Of these not a great deal is known at present. Glutamic acid dehydrogenase is present in muscle and by its action converts the amino acid into γ-ketoglutaric acid, an intermediary in the Krebs "citric acid cycle." Such a change suggests that many intermediary metabolites may be derived from all the major foodstuffs and hence may ultimately follow a common path. A conspicuous example of these is pyruvic acid, which is derived both from carbohydrates and protein (by the oxidative deamination of alanine). By condensation with acetic acid, beta-hydroxybutyric acid, a fatty acid intermediary, may also be formed.[59]

For an extensive discussion of biological oxidation the reader is referred to Szent-Györgyi's book (cf. above) or the recent monograph by Green.[60]

In summary, it may be said that carbohydrate utilization in muscles receiving an adequate oxygen supply may be entirely oxidative and not involve lactic acid formation. On the other hand, it seems clear that under circumstances where the oxygen supply is deficient lactic acid is formed by anaerobic processes and is then oxidized when oxygen becomes available. A third possibility is that the initial stages of carbohydrate breakdown are always anaerobic since the rapidity with which the oxygen requirement rises during muscular activity is far beyond the immediate capacity of the oxygen transporting mechanism. At a later date this may become adequate and the contraction process entirely oxidative, a view that is taken by Sacks.[61] Obviously, however, in severe exercise for short periods the energy requirements must be met by anaerobic breakdown of metabolites which are oxidized or otherwise removed after the effort.

The primary reaction in muscular contraction is unknown but it seems likely that one of the keys is adenylpyrophosphate; its decomposition initiates the glycolytic cycle and is also responsible for the preliminary phosphorylation of muscle glycogen, which may then follow either the aerobic or anaerobic path of metabolism.

IV. Carbohydrate Metabolism of the Heart.—The heart is the most important muscle in the body and operates under somewhat different circumstances from either voluntary or involuntary muscle. The cardiac muscle is in continuous activity and lacks the advantage which the other muscles have, of being able to rest for comparatively long periods. Consequently, it is not surprising to find that the cardiac muscle is exceedingly dependent on a contemporary supply of oxygen and possesses only a limited ability to go into oxygen debt[62] and to accumulate lactic acid. Nevertheless, the heart contains considerable quantities of glycogen which is apparently utilized and rebuilt in the same manner as in skeletal muscle. If an adequate oxygen supply is available, the carbohydrate content changes but little over a long period; but a reduction or complete withdrawal of the oxygen supply leads to rapid glycogen disappearance although the beat ceases long before this has proceeded to the point reached in skeletal muscle.[63] A prolongation of activity may be obtained in isolated hearts if they are perfused with fluids rich in glucose so it may be presumed that under anaerobic conditions glycogen breakdown forms a major source of energy. Cardiac muscle also contains phosphocreatine and adenylpyrophosphate and it is probable that these play a similar rôle to that of voluntary muscle.

Under aerobic conditions the heart is in no way dependent on carbohydrate alone for its energy requirements and can also, like voluntary muscle, oxidize protein and fat as well. According to Evans[64] the heart will also oxidize lactate directly and this may furnish nearly half the energy requirements under normal circumstances. Furthermore, it can also use beta-hydroxybutyric acid.[65]

The relation of an altered cardiac metabolism to disease is an important question but so far no important correlations have been made. It is known, however, that diphtheria toxin decreases the cardiac glycogen and that infarction of the heart muscle is followed by a reduction in both glycogen and phosphocreatine.

For a more detailed discussion of cardiac metabolism the reader is referred to the book by Clark[66] and the reviews by Evans[64] and Cruickshank.[67]

V. Carbohydrate Metabolism of the Nervous System.—The nervous tissue is unique in that its sole source of energy appears to be glucose or such related substances as lactate, pyruvate or succinate. This dependence is clearly shown by the behavior of brain slices in a respiration apparatus. Unless one of the above substances is added to the Ringer's solution in which the slices are suspended, the respiration soon fails but if these are present it is maintained for long periods.[68, 69] Himwich and Nahum studied the metabolism of the brain in situ and found that regardless of the quantity of carbohydrate that was being oxidized in the remainder of the body, the brain always oxidized carbohydrate. This was true even in totally depancreatized animals. The implications of these studies are highly interesting. In the first place, the nerve cells seem to require only two substances, oxygen and glucose, for their metabolic needs. Reduction of the latter by such measures as the administration of insulin provokes serious disturbances in the nervous system culminating in convulsions and death. Reduction of the oxygen supply, as is well known, also excites a violent response. Now, while limitation of the oxygen supply is ultimately fatal to all tissues, reduction of the glucose supply is without effect on any tissue except that of the nervous system. Thus, Himwich and Fazekas[70] have shown that as the blood glucose is decreased by insulin the oxygen consumption of the brain declines along with its glucose utilization, but the muscles of the same animal, while they also show a comparable reduction in carbohydrate utilization, do not diminish their oxygen consumption. This indicates, as pointed out before, that this tissue is able to draw on substances besides glucose for its energy requirements.

In recent years insulin and metrazol have been widely used in the treatment of various forms of nervous diseases of a functional nature. As Himwich, Bowman, Fazekas and Crenstein[71] have pointed out insulin depresses cerebral metabolism by withdrawing glucose while metrazol exerts its effects by decreasing the oxygen supply.

THE FORMATION OF FAT FROM CARBOHYDRATE

This is an important transformation of carbohydrate and probably occurs in all individuals that may be said to be well nourished. Nevertheless, the mechanism of this change is unknown although it was in 1883 that Meersl and Strohmer showed in the hog that during a two-day period over 300 grams of fat were formed from glucose. A little later an equally great deposition of fat from carbohydrate was shown to occur in the goose by Voit and Lehmann. Although the hog and the goose apparently deposit fat from carbohydrate at a high rate, this transformation has also been shown to occur in dogs and of course is a common procedure in the "fattening" of cattle.

Comparison of the formulae of glucose and a fatty acid such as palmitic acid indicates that the transformation involves not only a marked alteration in molecular structure but also the removal of oxygen and the fusion of several glucose molecules into one of the fatty acids.

$$n\ C_6N_{12}O_6 \longrightarrow CH_3\text{---}(CH_2)_{14}\text{---}COOH$$

Furthermore, energy is required for such a transformation since the resulting fatty acid yields a greater quantity of heat when oxidized than the parent substance yields. This might well be furnished by the oxidation of part of the glucose available which serves to convert some of the remainder into fatty acid. A simple equation of this type is:

$$6C_6H_{12}O_6\ +\ 13O_2 \longrightarrow 20CO_2\ +\ C_{16}H_{32}O_2\ +\ 2OH_2O$$

The respiratory quotient of such a process is 1.54 and values approaching this order were obtained by Wierzuchowski and Ling[72] in their studies on the respiratory metabolism of a young hog fed a mixture of starch and glucose. In this animal at the height of the process fat was being formed from carbohydrate at a rate of over 7 grams an hour.[73]

The exact chemical changes involved are at the present time entirely hypothetical. The usual scheme, suggested first by Magnus-Levy, is the successive condensation of acetaldehyde (which might be derived from pyruvic acid) into an hydroxy aldehyde which is finally converted into a fatty acid.

1. $CH_3—CO—COOH$ $\longrightarrow$ $CH_3—CHO + CO$
              Pyruvic acid   Acetaldehyde
              (from glucose)

2. $CH_3—CHO + CH_3—CHO$ $\longrightarrow$ $CH_3—CHOH—CH_2—CHO$
                   Acetaldehyde   Aldol

3. $CH_3—CHOH—CH_2—CHO$ $\longrightarrow$ $CH_3—CH_2—CH_2—COOH$
                   Aldol   Butyric acid

The equations above illustrate the formation of butyric acid by such a process. Repeated aldol condensation could lead in this manner to the formation of higher fatty acids.

It is likely that in the future much more work will be done on this transformation since it represents such an important metabolic pathway of glucose. In a recent paper Drury[74] has suggested that insulin catalyzes this process, a hypothesis which if confirmed is of great importance particularly as there have been rather persistent clinical claims that this hormone had a markedly beneficial effect in the treatment of underweight individuals.

The Conversion of Fatty Acids into Glucose.—This has been a controversial problem for a number of years, particularly because of the bearing that it has on the factors involved in the production of both experimental and clinical diabetes. (For a discussion of the latter the reader is referred to the section on the etiology of diabetes [see Chap. XVI] and the mechanism of insulin action.) Within the last year, however, the work of Stadie and his associates[75] would seem to have established that this transformation does not occur. However, since it is unlikely that the protagonists of this view will accept this work as final it is of value to briefly review the evidence both for and against it.

An equation illustrating the conversion would be:

$$2C_3H_5(C_{18}H_{33}O_2)_3 + 64O_2 \longrightarrow 16C_6H_{12}O_6 + 18CO_2 + 8H_2O$$
           Triolein   Glucose

The respiratory quotient of such a process is 0.28, a value that has never been observed in any mammal excepting perhaps the hibernating marmot. Since the respiratory quotient for the oxidation of triolein to CO_2 and H_2O is 0.71, any values significantly below this might well indicate that a certain proportion of fat was being transformed into glucose. While respiratory quotients below this level have been reported in certain diabetes with severe ketosis it must be remembered that in these abnormal circumstances the theoretical fat quotient of 0.71 would be modified [73] and may be as low as 0.67. Values even lower than this have been reported from time to time but are extremely rare.

It is probable that in the past too much emphasis has been placed on the level of the respiratory quotient as evidence that a certain process is or is not occurring. For instance, if fatty acids were converted into glucose and the glucose oxidized, then the overall respiratory quotient would be that of fat. More concrete and direct evidence must be sought and this so far has not been forthcoming.

The main arguments against the conversion are: (a) The respiratory quotient of totally depancreatized animals is not sufficiently depressed below the level indicating fat oxidation (cf. above). (b) The ratio of urine glucose to nitrogen in totally depancreatized or phloridzinized fasting animals is between 3.0 and 4.0 to 1. Such values indicate that the urinary glucose could be all derived from protein catabolism since any extensive glucose formation from fat would greatly increase this ratio. The validity of both these arguments depends on the assumption that totally depancreatized or phloridzinized animals are oxidizing only minimal quantities of glucose, a contention which has been challenged. (c) The feeding of fats or fatty acids does not increase the liver glycogen nor when fed to depancreatized animals do they increase the glycosuria beyond the quantity expected from the glycerol portion of the fat molecule. (d) The exposure of diabetic animals to conditions involving a large increase in fat catabolism does not increase the glucose excretion.

The evidence cited in favor of such a conversion is largely indirect and for its support requires the acceptance of the hypothesis that the glucose output in diabetic animals is not a true measure of glucose production in the organism. Thus, it is held that the glucose production by the liver is of such an order that it cannot have originated solely from protein or already formed carbohydrate. If this be allowed, then it must also be accepted that a considerable quantity of glucose formed is oxidized even in a totally diabetic animal.

As may well be imagined this last hypothesis has not gone unchallenged. The most convincing evidence would be a clearcut demonstrations that fatty acids or their intermediary metabolites were converted into glycogen or glucose. Such proof has not been forthcoming although recently Weil-Malherbe[76] has reported that kidney slices form glucose from acetoacetic acid, a claim that is denied by Stadie and his colleagues.[75]

The question would appear to be settled for the time being by the recent studies of Stadie, Zapp and Lukens.[75, 77] These investigators, using liver slices from diabetic animals, constructed a balance sheet relating the total oxygen consumption to that required for acetone body formation, oxidative deamination and CO_2 formation (see table 5).

The results are also of extreme importance regarding the mechanism of acetone body formation (cf. chapter on Lipid Metabolism), and for the present discussion indicate that when the oxygen required for acetone body formation, oxidative deamination, and CO_2 formation is subtracted from the total oxygen consumption none remains for glucose formation from fatty acids. Furthermore, in spite of the intense fat catabolism there was no direct evidence of glucose formation while the fatty acid disappearance was accounted for by acetone body formation.

Carbohydrate Formation from Protein.—This conversion has already been discussed and there is no doubt that proteins either ingested in the diet

TABLE 5*

The Oxidative Metabolism of Liver Slices from Totally Depancreatized Cats

Oxidative process	Mean oxygen uptake per gram of liver per hour (micromoles)
Deamination of amino acids	8.2 ± 1.2
Carbon dioxide formation	28.0 ± 5.0
Ketone body formation	63.0 ± 4.0
Sum of known oxidations	99.2 ± 6.5
Observed oxygen uptake	87.5 ± 4.0
Difference	-11.7 ± 7.6†

* Stadie, Zapp and Lukens, J. Biol. Chem., **132**: 423, 1940.
† Difference not significant.

or derived from the tissues themselves are the most important noncarbo-hydrate source of glucose. Not all the constituent amino acids are con-verted into glucose, however. There are also certain discrepancies regarding some of the amino acids according to the method employed for testing their glycogenic value. The two methods employed have been (a) administra-

TABLE 6

Glucose Formation from Amino Acids in Phloridzinized Animals and Liver Glycogen Formation in Normal Animals

Amino acid	Glucose formation in phloridzinized animal	Liver glycogen formation in normal animal
(A) *Mono-amino monocarboxylic acids*		
Glycine	+	+
d-Alanine	+	+
l-Serine	+	+
d-Threonine	+	+
d-Valine	−	?
Norleucine	?	?
l-Leucine	−	−
d-Isoleucine	−	−
(B) *Mono-amino dicarboxylic acids*		
l-Aspartic	+	+ (?)
d-Glutamic	+	+ (?)
(C) *Diamino monocarboxylic acids*		
d-Arginine	+	?
d-Lysine	−	−
(D) *Sulfur-containing acids*		
l-Cystine	+	−
l-Methionine	+	−
(E) *Aromatic amino acids*		
l-Phenylalanine	−	+
l-Tyrosine	−	−
(F) *Heterocyclic acids*		
l-Histidine	−	−
l-Proline	+	?
l-Hydroxyproline	+	?
l-Tryptophane	−	−

tion to phloridzinized animals and (b) feeding to normal animals and deter-mining the effect on the liver glycogen level. The following indicates the results obtained by these two methods (see table 6).

From the results obtained on phloridzinized dogs it can be calculated that proteins can form from 45 to 60 grams of glucose per 100 grams. If none of the glucose formed is oxidized, the urinary glucose-nitrogen ratio would be between 2.8 and 3.65.

THE ENDOCRINE CONTROL OF METABOLISM

General Principles.—Before discussing in detail the endocrine control of carbohydrate metabolism a few remarks on the general character of the humoral control of the processes of metabolism would seem appropriate.

The study of metabolism is the investigation of all the chemical processes occurring in living organisms. It is now recognized that life continues by virtue of the capacity of living cells to carry out an extraordinary variety of diverse and complicated chemical reactions. This study has been actively pursued since the fundamental observations of Lavoisier between the years 1780 and 1790, and as a result of a large volume of work since that time we have learned to appreciate that every vital phenomenon, whether it be in animal or plant cells, is associated with chemical changes in its substance.

Now, even to the casual observer, it is apparent that living creatures exhibit two fundamental characteristics. The *first* of these is a correlation between the various parts of the organism so that it reacts as a whole; this is particularly true in the higher forms where masses of cells are associated in organs, each with a special set of functions. The *second* is the adaptability of living things to a wide variety of internal and external circumstances so that the emphasis of existence may, at least for a time, be almost wholly diverted to a particular end.

In the most highly specialized forms, which include the mammals and birds, organ correlation and adaptability to external circumstances has reached such a high point of development that the internal environment of the body remains virtually constant throughout life in spite of the very large strains that may be imposed from time to time on its resources. Familiar examples of the constancy of the internal environment are to be seen in the narrow limits within which the body temperature and hydrogen ion concentration are maintained.

It was this recognition of the constancy of the internal environment that was one of the great achievements of Claude Bernard, and his concept has been extended and elaborated in our time by the work of Cannon, who has coined the term "homeostasis" to describe this phenomenon.

It is now recognized that the cells of the body are surrounded by a circulating body of fluid containing solutes. Some of these solutes pass freely in and out of the cells; others do not pass or pass only with difficulty. The fluid within the cells has a different composition from that without, although there is every reason to believe that the composition of this intracellular fluid is kept within as narrow a range as that of the extracellular fluid. Apart from the nervous system the only means of communication between cells and organs is through the extracellular fluid and the introduction of chemical agents into this fluid is the means by which the chemical processes within the cells may be profoundly modified. Such substances are often termed *humoral agents* and are not necessarily hormones. Alterations in the normal proportions of substances in the extracellular fluid may be produced in a variety of ways, many of them take place as a result of physiological processes, such as digestion, and indeed, as we shall see, the main function of the controlling mechanisms of the body is to keep these changes within the limits in which normal cellular function can continue.

It follows that in the simpler organisms where the extracellular fluid is not enclosed within the body itself the metabolism of the cells must, in large part, be determined by what occurs in the external environment since control of its composition by the organism is impossible. The advantages of placing the external environment of the cells within the control of the whole organism are enormous and undoubtedly made possible the development of the higher forms of life.

Apart from the fluctuations in chemical composition that result from the operation of physiological and pathological processes the extracellular fluid receives, either continuously or intermittently, the secretions of certain specialized groups of cells that are termed endocrine or ductless glands. In all there are eight well recognized organs of this character: (*a*) the anterior pituitary, (*b*) the posterior pituitary, (*c*) the thyroid, (*d*) the parathyroids, (*e*) the adrenal cortex, (*f*) the adrenal medulla, (*g*) the gonads, and (*h*) the pancreas. While in addition there are in association with the digestive system certain other groups of cells whose secretions influence this function.

The *secretions*, or hormones, of all these glands may influence the metabolism of the major number of cells in the body, or their effect may be limited to certain organs or tissues. An example of the first type is that of the thyroid hormone, which increases the basal oxygen consumption of all tissues, whereas the gonadal hormones, which exert their influence almost exclusively on the organs related to the reproductive function, is representative of the second.

In the broadest sense of the term all the hormones influence the metabolism or chemical processes occurring in cells. The acceleration of general body growth by the anterior pituitary hormones, the contraction or relaxation of smooth muscle by epinephrine, and the hypertrophy of the accessory genital organs produced by the gonadal hormones, all must divert the chemical processes within these various types of cells into channels that result in the observed effects.

The term "endocrine control of metabolism" is, however, used in a more limited sense. It is used to indicate the influence of certain endocrine glands upon the chemical changes undergone by the various substances which the cells use for the production of energy or for the formation of compounds not found in the foodstuffs ingested by the organism. Now, the object of digestion is to provide the cells of the body with the materials required for their activity and surprisingly enough, in view of the variety of foodstuffs ingested, the materials that ultimately reach the cells are in the form of a comparatively few types of compounds consisting in the main of glucose, a variety of amino acids, and fats. To these, of course, must be added some quantities of inorganic salts and certain essential substances known as "vitamins."

From this mixture of glucose, amino acids, fats, and accessory substances the organism forms all the compounds found in living tissues largely by the operation of synthetic processes of a diverse and complicated character. These processes require the provision of energy for their completion and to provide this and the other forms of energy necessary, a large proportion of the foodstuffs ingested is ultimately oxidized.

Metabolic Hormones.—While the limitation of the term "endocrine control of metabolism" to the influence of hormones on the metabolism of carbohydrate, fat and protein is entirely artificial and restricts the broad viewpoint of their function, it is convenient when we have to discuss the details of their operation. Thus, although we speak of "carbohydrate metabolism hormones" and "protein metabolism hormones," it should not be forgotten that no such isolation of the various phases of metabolism occurs in the body. The metabolic channels of fat, protein and carbohydrate are not shut off from each other. Carbohydrates are transformed into fats; amino acids follow the pathway of carbohydrate and fat, possessing as well a special metabolism of their own. This interlocking of the metabolism of the major foodstuffs has led to confusion regarding the number of metabolic hormones that exist, since an alteration in one phase of metabolism will induce secondary changes in the other types which may be and have been interpreted as evidence for the existence of several hormones, where in reality only one is present.

The endocrine glands do not operate as individual units whose functional level is independent of each other. They constitute a bodily system in the same sense as do the circulatory or digestive systems. Alterations in the function of one member is followed both by an unbalanced operation of others and by compensatory efforts on their part to readjust the normal state of equilibrium.

The imbalance or compensatory effects following a single endocrine hyper- or hypofunction is apt to produce, particularly if operative over a long period, a series of events that may completely obscure their original cause. This is particularly true of endocrine disorders in man and has led to great confusion in this field. Indeed, a great future lies in this field as soon as we can correctly interpret the symptomatology of human endocrine dysfunction.

The Anterior Pituitary and the Integration of the Endocrine System.— One of the most important discoveries of recent years is that the functional as well as the anatomical integrity of several endocrine glands is dependent on the secretions of the anterior pituitary. The work of a number of investigators, particularly P. E. Smith, has clearly demonstrated that removal of this organ is followed by marked atrophy of the gonads, thyroid, and adrenal cortex, and that conversely the injection of anterior pituitary extract into normal animals results in hypertrophy of these organs. There is now no doubt that through its "tropic" hormones the anterior pituitary acts as the dominant and controlling member of a large part of the endocrine system. With the exception of the adrenal medulla and posterior pituitary, the only major ductless gland upon which there is any doubt concerning the influence of the anterior pituitary is the islet tissue of the pancreas and even in this instance a clearly negative answer has not yet been found.

The control of the secretions of the adrenal medulla and posterior pituitary is now definitely known to be exerted by the nervous system, most probably by sympathetic centers in the hypothalamus and brain stem. Over these two organs there appears to be no tropic control by the anterior pituitary.

Another question that can only be briefly touched on, but yet is of exceeding importance, is the possibility that the anterior pituitary itself is also controlled by the nervous system. If this were so then the nervous system would, through its control of the tropic hormones of this gland, be in a position to integrate the whole endocrine system. Unfortunately, except in the case of the adrenal medulla and posterior pituitary, the present available evidence is somewhat scanty although interesting work on this subject has recently been published by Haterius, Brooks and Uotila.

We must therefore, for the time being, assume that the anterior pituitary is the major integrator of the endocrine system but must also recognize that this influence is not one sided since alterations in the functional level of such organs as the thyroid and the gonads will in time bring about alterations in the activity of the anterior pituitary.

Removal of the hypophysis or the injection of crude extracts of the anterior pituitary that contain all the hormones of this organ must in consequence produce a polyglandular syndrome and the dissection of this presents a complicated but nevertheless fascinating task for the experimenter.

The Anterior Pituitary and Growth.—Hypophysectomized animals do not grow even though every known element required is provided in their diet. On the other hand, the injection of suitable extracts of the anterior pituitary into such animals is immediately followed by the resumption of growth. Further, their injection into normal animals brings about an accelerated growth rate. Now, growth is a complicated process, involving both internal and external factors. Nevertheless, it requires above all else a capacity to synthesize and retain sufficient quantities of protein within the cells that are undergoing division. The mechanism governing synthesis of cellular protein is a problem in protein metabolism that has so far defied successful experimentation, yet as we shall see there are certain lines of evidence that definitely associate the growth-promoting action of the anterior pituitary with this phase of metabolism. Indeed, it may well be that this effect of the anterior pituitary is perhaps its most central significant action on metabolism since other phases of its activity are mediated by other endocrine glands.

It must, however, be admitted that the effects of this gland on carbohydrate and fat metabolism have not as yet been successfully integrated into a hypothesis in which its influence on protein metabolism can be shown to be the single determining factor. Nevertheless, it must be borne in mind that the growth principle has not yet been tested in a pure form and, as we shall see, the trophic effect of the anterior pituitary on other endocrine glands influencing metabolism introduces complications when crude extracts are used. There is, however, no doubt that the growth promoting principle is one that acts *directly* on the tissues and that its effects are not mediated by other endocrine glands even though the presence of their secretions may be essential for its action.

The Anterior Pituitary and Carbohydrate Metabolism.—The anterior pituitary has a widespread influence on carbohydrate metabolism both by its trophic effect on the thyroid and adrenal cortex and also by some principle that apparently acts directly on the tissues. A comprehensive review of the effect of the anterior pituitary on carbohydrate metabolism is that of Russell.[78]

(*a*) GLUCOSE ABSORPTION. It was shown by Phillips and Robb in 1934[79] that hypophysectomized rats have a much reduced intestinal absorption rate for glucose. Since Althausen[12] had shown that thyroxin increases the glucose absorption rate of rats, Russell[80] injected hypophysectomized rats with thyroxin and found the absorption rate to return to normal along with the basal metabolic rate although the other metabolic abnormalities of the animals were unaffected.

(*b*) CARBOHYDRATE LEVELS. It has been well established that fasted hypophysectomized animals rapidly deplete the carbohydrate levels of their blood, liver and muscles and are consequently extremely prone to hypoglycemic attacks that will have a fatal ending unless food is given. This rapid depletion of the carbohydrate levels is unique and is not found in any other endocrine deficiency. Furthermore, it has been found by Fisher and

TABLE 7

EFFECT OF HYPOPHYSECTOMY AND INJECTION OF ANTERIOR PITUITARY EXTRACT (A.P.E.) ON
THE DISPOSITION OF FED GLUCOSE IN RATS*
(All values expressed as milligrams per 100 grams of rat)

	Glucose absorbed	Non-protein R. Q.	Glucose oxidized	Glucose as liver glycogen	Glucose as muscle glycogen	Glucose in body fluids	Glucose recovered
Normal rats..............	854	0.862	453	122	120	30	724
Per cent of absorbed CH$_2$O.	....	....	53	14	14	4	86
Hypophysectomized rats...	568	0.925	420	28	85	11	544
Per cent of absorbed CH$_2$O.	....	....	74	5	15	2	96
Hypophysectomized rats + A.P.E.................	457	0.814	201	33	75	50	359
Per cent of absorbed CH$_2$O.	....	....	44	7	16	11	78
Normal rats + A.P.E......	789	0.782	243	104	158	40	545
Per cent of absorbed CH$_2$O.	....	....	31	13	20	5	70

* After J. A. Russell, Amer. J. Physiol., 121: 756, 1938.

Pencharz[81] and by Fisher, Russell and Cori[82] that not only are the glycogen stores of hypophysectomized rats lowered by a short fast but there is also a marked elevation of the respiratory quotient. It is evident that these animals are either failing to produce sufficient carbohydrate for their needs from noncarbohydrate sources or else are oxidizing their carbohydrate stores at an abnormally rapid rate. Since in normal fasting rats carbohydrate utilization is reduced to a minimum it may be tentatively concluded that an anterior pituitary factor is actively concerned either with (*a*) glucose production from noncarbohydrate sources, (*b*) an inhibiting effect on glucose utilization or (*c*) both glucose production and utilization.

Effect of Hypophysectomy and Injection of Anterior Pituitary Extract. Using the Cori technique of administering a known quantity of glucose by mouth and determining its disposition by oxidation and storage Russell has compared the behavior of (*a*) hypophysectomized rats (*b*) normal rats injected with anterior pituitary extract and (*c*) normal rats. The results are in table 7.

Less liver glycogen is stored in hypophysectomized rats; a larger proportion is oxidized. The injection of anterior pituitary extract reduces the proportion oxidized, while such injections into normal rats also reduce glucose oxidation and increase muscle glycogen storage. The ability of anterior

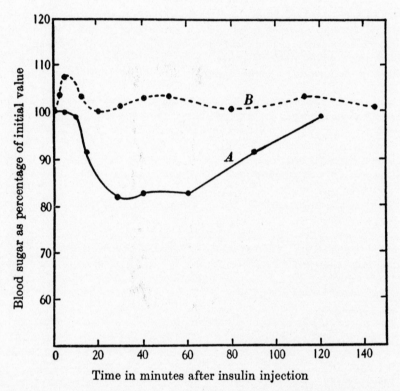

Fig. 9.—Blood sugar response to intravenously administered crystalline insulin, of rabbits receiving two preliminary injections of an anterior pituitary extract. Curve A. Average response to 0-1 unit of seven hypophysectomized rabbits, fasting 2½ hours, which received two pituitary injections equivalent to a total of about 13 Gm. of fresh anterior lobe tissue. Curve B. Typical response to 2 units of an intact rabbit which had received two pituitary injections equivalent to a total of about 4 Gm. of fresh anterior lobe tissue. Initial blood-sugar levels: A, 89 mg./100 c.c.; B, 103 mg./100 c.c. (From Newton, W. H. and Young, F. G., J. Physiol., **94:** 40 1938–39.)

pituitary extract to promote muscle glycogen storage or to prevent its loss in hypophysectomized animals has been termed by Russell "the glycostatic effect."

There is still some dispute as to whether the rapid exhaustion of the carbohydrate levels of hypophysectomized animals is due to a failure of glucose production or to an abnormal rate of glucose utilization. The former view is held by Soskin[83] while Russell[78] has advanced evidence that the peripheral rate of glucose utilization is increased to a point beyond the capacity of the organism to meet. This latter view does not necessarily deny that the capacity for glucose formation is unchanged after hypophysectomy.

(c) INSULIN SENSITIVITY. From what has been said above it might be anticipated that any agent which increases glucose utilization would more rapidly reduce the carbohydrate levels of hypophysectomized animals to the danger point. Such an agent is insulin and the demonstration of the marked sensitivity of these animals to this hormone was one of the major discoveries of Houssay and his colleagues.[84] A dose of insulin about one-tenth of that required to affect the blood glucose of a normal animal will cause severe hypoglycemia and convulsions in those deprived of the hypophysis. This sensitivity is abolished by the injection of anterior pituitary extract or, if this extract is given to normal animals a state of insulin insensitivity is produced (Fig. 9). Under such circumstances an injection of insulin will have practically no effect on the blood glucose level.

This effect of anterior pituitary extract is said to be due to a separate factor—the *glycotropic factor*.[85] It should be remembered, however, that if there exists a pituitary factor that inhibits carbohydrate utilization then such a result as a diminution of the response to insulin might be anticipated. Further chemical fractionation will be the only way in which the actual number of anterior pituitary hormones can be determined.

(d) THE DIABETOGENIC ACTION OF THE ANTERIOR PITUITARY. It was stated above that the injection of anterior pituitary extract into normal animals not only nullified the usual hypoglycemia of exogenous insulin but also reduced glucose utilization. Prior to these studies Houssay and his colleagues* had found that these crude extracts if injected into normal animals, particularly dogs, for a period of several days resulted not only in hyperglycemia but also a profuse glycosuria and acetonuria. There are also some interesting additional points about this effect that has been termed the "diabetogenic" action of the anterior pituitary: 1. It occurs only in fed animals. 2. It is most easily produced in those on a high carbohydrate diet, next on a high protein, while on high fat diets there is little if any glycosuria. 3. It does not depend on the presence of the pancreas. This is important since it shows that the effect is not produced by a mere neutralization of insulin. 4. The response varies markedly with the species of animal used; the dog is most susceptible, while only with the greatest difficulty is glycosuria produced in rats.

Houssay found in his original experiments that if the injections were prolonged the effect could no longer be elicited, this being due either to "antihormone" production or to a hypertrophy of the islets of Langerhans. More recently Young[87] has made the remarkable discovery that by continually increasing the quantity of anterior pituitary extract injected not only could the glycosuria and acetonuria be continued but, on cessation of the injections, a *permanent* diabetic state resulted. The important implications of these studies on the etiology of diabetes mellitus are discussed in Chapter XVI. It has been shown by Campbell and Best,[88] Richardson and Young.[89] and by Dohan and Lukens[90] that the islets of Langerhans are severely damaged by this treatment and it is this insulin deficiency that perpetuates the diabetic state. This sequence of events forms a remarkable example of

* A full account of the work of Houssay and his collaborators will be found in the New England Journal of Medicine, **214:** Nos. 19–23, 1936.[86]

the interplay between the various endocrine glands concerned with the regulation of metabolism.

The recognition that the anterior pituitary gland is concerned in the diabetic syndrome is due to the equally brilliant discovery of Houssay that removal of the pituitary gland from totally depancreatized animals is followed by an amelioration of the diabetic state. This work was first carried out on toads but was soon extended to mammals. The extent of the amelioration in dogs and cats may be judged from table 8 that is taken from the work of Houssay[86] and Long and Lukens.[91] The effects of total adrenalectomy are also included and their similarity to those of hypophysectomy will be noted.

TABLE 8

EFFECT OF HYPOPHYSECTOMY OR ADRENALECTOMY ON THE DIABETES OF TOTALLY DEPANCREATIZED DOGS AND CATS

Species	Condition	Survival (days)	Urine			G/N	Blood glucose mg. per cent
			Glucose *g/k/d	Nitrogen *g/k/d	Acetone *mg/k/d		
Dog....	Depancreatized	15	4.0	1.4	...	2.8	400
Dog....	Hypophysectomized-depancreatized	74	0.8	1.1	...	0.8	234
Cat.....	Depancreatized	5	3.2	1.3	116	2.7	347
Cat.....	Hypophysectomized-depancreatized	22	0.4	0.7	5	0.6	190
Cat.....	Adrenalectomized-depancreatized	14	0.6	0.6	13	1.0	186

* Signifies gm. or mg./kilo body weight/day.

Apart from the striking prolongation of life, which in some experiments was as long as a year, there is a virtual disappearance of the characteristic acidosis and ketosis as well as a marked decrease in the glucosuria and hyperglycemia. If fasted, these animals like those simply hypophysectomized will develop severe hypoglycemia requiring glucose for its relief. The problems posed by these "Houssay" animals are intricate ones touching as they do not only the question of glucose utilization in the absence of insulin, but also the nature of the effect of the anterior pituitary on carbohydrate metabolism.

The glucose tolerance of these animals while superior to that of depancreatized animals is, however, far from normal and the importance of insulin for a normal rate of utilization is not seriously questioned. The lesson to be learned from these experiments together with the results of anterior pituitary injection is that the utilization of glucose is both enhanced as well as depressed by hormonal factors. Insulin is the hormone that catalyzes the disposal of carbohydrate while the hormones of the anterior pituitary restrain its utilization and in addition through their influence on other endocrine glands (adrenal cortex and thyroid) increase glucose formation from noncarbohydrate sources. The result of this interplay is to endow the organism with a wide latitude in its ability to metabolize glucose. Not only can it dispose of large quantities ingested in the diet without markedly elevating the blood glucose, but it can conserve this substance when its supply is markedly reduced by reducing its utilization to a minimum.

This effect of the anterior pituitary would seem to offer an explanation of the variations produced in the glucose tolerance curve by the previous diet. During fasting or on diets low in carbohydrate and high in fat, the anterior pituitary hormones are present in the body fluids in increased quantity. The sudden influx of a large quantity of glucose requires adjustments in the hormonal balance that require a certain length of time. Until these are effected, the utilization of glucose remains at a low level with a consequent "high" type of tolerance curve. The administration of a second or third quantity of glucose finds the organism increasingly able to dispose of it with a consequent lowering of the tolerance curve.

The Pancreas and Carbohydrate Metabolism.—In earlier reviews of the endocrine control of carbohydrate metabolism, first place in the discussion would have been given to the influence of the islets of Langerhans. Important as this organ still is in the regulation of carbohydrate metabolism, it is now realized that it is only one member of the glandular system whose secretions participate in this control.

The essential rôle played by the internal secretion of the pancreas has been recognized since the fundamental discovery of Minkowski in 1893 that total pancreatectomy in several species of animals was followed by severe disturbances in carbohydrate metabolism which bore a striking resemblance to those found in diabetes mellitus in man. The characteristic changes observed in the metabolism of totally depancreatized dogs are as follows:

(*a*) There is pronounced glucosuria and hyperglycemia which does not disappear on fasting.

(*b*) There is disappearance of liver glycogen with some reduction of muscle glycogen, although the latter is maintained to a surprising degree.

(*c*) The ingestion of glucose is followed by its almost quantitative excretion in the urine. This is true only in the period soon after pancreatectomy. At a later date when severe emaciation is present a considerable portion of the glucose may be retained.[107]

(*d*) The respiratory quotient falls to the fat level (0.71) and is not elevated by glucose ingestion.

(*e*) In fasting animals or those on a meat diet, there is established a relative constancy between the nitrogen and glucose excreted in the urine. This $\frac{G}{N}$ ratio is in the neighborhood of 3.0 and indicates that a constant proportion of the protein derived from the diet or tissues is converted into glucose. Of equal importance is the increased level of nitrogen excretion in fasting animals which implies that the rate of tissue protein breakdown has been accelerated.

(*f*) Marked acetonuria develops which, according to the most modern view,[92] is due to the accelerated catabolism of fat.

(*g*) Finally, in totally depancreatized dogs and cats severe dehydration,

3

acidosis, and coma ensue, leading generally to death in four to fourteen days.

The injection of the pancreatic hormone—insulin—rapidly corrects all these metabolic disturbances and with appropriate dietary control totally depancreatized dogs have been kept in good health for years.

In partially depancreatized dogs and in many human diabetic patients the presence of variable quantities of pancreatic tissue modifies the disturbances produced. Thus, in the mildest state, the impaired carbohydrate metabolism may be detected only by placing a sudden load on the assimilatory capacity of the organism. This is usually done by the ingestion of a quantity of glucose. In the moderately severe forms glucosuria may be absent during fasting and present after meals; while the most severe types will approximate to the condition of the totally depancreatized dog in which glucosuria is always present.

The injection of insulin into normal fasting animals produces a rapid fall in blood glucose. If the insulin is given in sufficient quantity, severe hypoglycemic symptoms will occur which lead to convulsions and death if not relieved. No other carbohydrate is as effective as glucose, except those yielding considerable amounts of this substance, in relieving these symptoms.

If insulin is given to well-fed animals or its administration is accompanied by glucose ingestion or injection, the extent of the hypoglycemia is curtailed and it will be found that in addition to the marked increase in respiratory quotient considerable quantities of glycogen are deposited in the muscles. The behavior of the liver glycogen at first sight is paradoxical for with the exception of the young rabbit[93] the majority of investigations demonstrate that the hormone brings about a decrease. This would appear to be due to the fact that the liver glycogen is the reserve of carbohydrate which, under the influence of insulin, is either utilized or stored in the peripheral tissues at a rate greater than it is accumulated from the dietary carbohydrate or nonprotein sources. Furthermore, if as some believe, insulin also inhibits hepatic gluconeogenesis, then the combination of increased peripheral consumption plus decreased hepatic production of glucose must result in a lowering of the level of liver glycogen.

While there can be no dispute as to the consequences of pancreatectomy in the cat or dog or to the effects of insulin injection into animals or human diabetics, the exact manner by which insulin loss precipitates this chain of events or insulin injection corrects them is still not entirely clear.

The problem is one of utmost importance since its solution will have a profound effect on our understanding of the etiology of diabetes. It is apparent that this hormone greatly increases the capacity of the organism to assimilate glucose (and carbohydrates). Whether this is brought about by an accelerated oxidation in the peripheral tissues or by an inhibition of hepatic gluconeogenesis or both is perhaps still debatable, but the overall effect of the hormone indicates quite clearly its importance as a regulator of carbohydrate and, indirectly, of protein and fat metabolism.

The Adrenal Medulla and Carbohydrate Metabolism.—That the hormone of the adrenal medulla (*epinephrine, adrenin*) could bring about alterations in carbohydrate metabolism has been known since the work of Blum in 1901 who found that the injection of extracts of this gland into dogs was followed by hyperglycemia and glucosuria. This observation coming so soon after Minkowski's discovery of the effects of pancreatectomy excited much speculation as to the possible relationship between these two phenomena. From them arose the concept of Eppinger, Falta and others that carbohydrate metabolism was controlled by the interaction of several glands of internal secretion. The pancreatic hormone was regarded as antagonistic in its effects to that of the adrenal medulla so that when the pancreas was removed the unopposed action of the adrenal medulla drove up the glucose production to a point beyond the capacity of the organism to assimilate and glucosuria followed. The work of more recent years has, however, revealed further facts concerning this hormone that are not in harmony with the hypothesis that it is to be regarded as a diabetogenic agent.

In the first place, the hyperglycemic and glycosuric action of epinephrine is in large part, although not entirely, dependent on the presence of preformed liver glycogen. Under the influence of this hormone the liver glycogen is rapidly converted into glucose and the blood glucose level may in a few minutes be doubled or trebled if an adequate supply of glycogen is present.

It must also be recalled that epinephrine is unique inasmuch as the action of this hormone is identical with that produced by strong and widespread stimulation of the sympathetic nervous system. The relation of this part of the nervous system and the adrenal medulla to the "emergency" mechanisms of the body has been beautifully worked out by Cannon and his colleagues and their extensive papers and writings on this subject should be consulted for full details.

The work of Cori and Cori[94] has thrown further light on the mode of action of this hormone. While, as stated above, the most pronounced hyperglycemic action of epinephrine is seen in well-fed animals, it is also present to a lesser degree in rats that have been fasted until their liver glycogen was less than 0.5 gm. per cent. In these animals the injection of epinephrine produces a hyperglycemia that will persist for some hours and obviously cannot have been supported by such low initial liver glycogen levels. Furthermore, as these workers showed, the liver glycogen gradually *increases* during the period of epinephrine action (three to four hours after subcutaneous injection) while at the same time the muscle glycogen decreases. The link between these effects was shown by the increased lactic acid content of the blood during the period. The hormone evidently increases the rate of glycogen breakdown both in liver and muscle, liberating it in the former as glucose and in the latter as lactic acid, these being the normal carbohydrate intermediaries of these two tissues. The lactic acid derived from the muscle glycogen is transformed by the liver in glycogen which is again liberated as glucose, thus maintaining the hyperglycemia. Since, however, the muscles considered as an organ are at least ten times as large as the liver, the lactic acid supply is so large that the level of liver glycogen rises until a new equilibrium is established between the rate of formation and breakdown.

In well-fed animals a biphasic influence of epinephrine on liver glycogen is found. The first and immediate effect is a sharp decrease which is followed by secondary rise which may bring the level higher than the initial one.

Since it has also been clearly established that epinephrine does not increase protein breakdown, its effects on carbohydrate metabolism appear to be limited to the preformed carbohydrate stores of the liver and muscles. In both it increases the rate of glycogen breakdown and acts in this manner to redistribute the preformed stores. It does not stimulate glucose formation from noncarbohydrate sources and hence cannot be regarded as a "diabetogenic" agent in the ordinary sense of the term.

Nevertheless, epinephrine must be regarded as a hormone that enables considerable quantities of glucose to be rapidly liberated into the blood stream under conditions of violent effort or emotion, and consequently is rightly considered as a regulator of carbohydrate metabolism.

The Adrenal Cortex and Carbohydrate Metabolism.—A direct participation of the adrenal cortex in the hormonal control of carbohydrate metabolism has been the subject of vigorous debate for a number of years. The interest in this problem has centered not only in the interpretation of the alterations in carbohydrate metabolism that occur in adrenalectomized animals but also on their relation to the function of the adrenal cortex. This problem would appear to be capable of a simple solution were it not for the fact that other changes follow adrenalectomy which at first sight appear to be of greater significance than the disturbances in carbohydrate metabolism.

The most important of these other changes are the widespread disturbances in water and electrolyte balance. In consequence several groups of investigators have concluded that the chief function of the adrenal cortex is the control of these phases of metabolism and that any alterations in carbohydrate metabolism are of a secondary character.

On the other hand, Britton and his colleagues[95] have during the last ten years steadily upheld the view that the regulation of carbohydrate metabolism was the "prepotent" function of this endocrine gland. A final solution of this problem is not yet available but the experimental facts now clearly indicate that the alterations in carbohydrate metabolism following adrenalectomy or the injection of cortical hormone into normal animals are of such a character that they can hardly be dismissed as of minor importance. Consequently, any theory of cortical function must link both the alterations in carbohydrate and electrolyte metabolism. Such an all inclusive theory is not yet available but it would appear that the cortical hormone is related to some metabolic process which has a relationship to both these aspects of metabolism. Furthermore, consideration must be given to the observations of Long, Katzin and Fry,[96] that the cortical hormone also affects protein metabolism, particularly in fasting animals in which a marked increase in the rate of tissue protein catabolism is brought about following its injection.

The main observations indicating that the adrenal cortex participates directly in the regulation of carbohydrate and protein metabolism are as follows:

(*a*) Adrenalectomized animals suffer depletion of their carbohydrate levels in liver, muscle and body fluids.[95]

(*b*) Fasting adrenalectomized animals excrete less nitrogen than normal fasting animals.[32, 97]

(*c*) Phloridzinized-adrenalectomized rats excrete less glucose and nitrogen than intact animals.[32, 98]

(*d*) On exposure to low oxygen pressures, fasted normal rats increase their liver glycogen and urine nitrogen while adrenalectomized rats do not.[32]

(*e*) Adrenalectomy alleviates a total or partial pancreatic diabetes[91, 96] (cf. table 8).

(*f*) The injection of cortical extract or of crystalline steroids isolated from the adrenal cortex into fasting adrenalectomized or normal animals is followed by striking increases in liver glycogen and by mild hyperglycemia. Since the muscle glycogen is unchanged a new formation of carbohydrate must have taken place from noncarbohydrate sources and this source is apparently protein, for there is also found an increased nitrogen excretion of sufficient magnitude to account for the increased carbohydrate levels[95, 96] in the liver and blood.

(*g*) The mild diabetes of hypophysectomized-depancreatized or adrenalectomized-depancreatized animals can be exacerbated by injection of cortical extract. Furthermore, the diabetes of partially depancreatized rats may also be exacerbated to the point where fatal diabetic coma is precipitated.[95, 99]

(*h*) Injection of the cortical hormone or the adrenotropic hormone of the anterior pituitary will inhibit insulin convulsions in mice apparently by increasing the quantity of carbohydrate in the body.[100]

(*i*) The rapid depletion of the carbohydrate levels of fasting hypophysectomized rats may be prevented by injection of cortical extract or if these stores are already depleted they may be restored to normal. This is also accompanied by an increased nitrogen excretion.

Protein Catabolism.—The common denominator of all these varied observations would seem to be the effects on protein catabolism. Where this is proceeding at an enhanced rate as in fasting, phloridzin experiments and pancreatic diabetes, removal of the adrenal glands reduces the rate of tissue protein breakdown, thus reducing not only the nitrogen excretion but consequently the quantity of glucose made available to the organism. This is reflected by lowered carbohydrate levels in the liver and body fluids. Conversely, the injection of an excess of the hormone drives up the rate of protein breakdown, making available glucose from the catabolism of the resulting amino acids. In depancreatized animals this results in an increased glycosuria and nitrogen excretion so that it is fair to regard the cortical hormones as possessing "diabetogenic" activity.

Adrenal Cortex and Anterior Pituitary.—The relationship between the anterior pituitary and adrenal cortex in their effects on metabolism is a complicated one inasmuch as the level of activity of the cortex is controlled by the adrenotropic hormone of the pituitary. Consequently, the injection of crude extracts of the latter may not only act directly on the tissues, apparently inhibiting glucose utilization but may also by their stimulation of the adrenal cortex increase the rate of glucose formation. These two effects are, of course, found after removal of the pancreas and raise the important point that the diabetic syndrome may not only be produced by insulin deficiency but also by anterior pituitary and adrenal cortical hyperactivity.

It may be definitely concluded, however, that the adrenal cortex is an important member of the system of endocrine glands that regulate metabolism and while many questions remain unanswered it would appear to be concerned with those processes by which glucose is made available to the organism at times when either the supply from other sources is deficient or when unusual demands are made for this material.

The Thyroid and Carbohydrate Metabolism.—The thyroid hormone exerts a powerful effect on some at present unknown phase of metabolism resulting in a marked increase in the metabolic rate. Conversely, the removal of the thyroid is followed by a decreased rate of heat production and oxygen consumption.

Associated with these alterations in the metabolic rate are certain abnormalities in the metabolism of all the major foodstuffs. Thus the administration of thyroid extract or thyroxin is followed by an increased tissue protein catabolism, an accelerated utilization of fats and a reduction in the liver glycogen. In addition, glucosuria may occur, particularly after glucose feeding, and the glucose tolerance curve may show an exaggerated hyperglycemia which at times resembles that found in diabetes mellitus. It has also been found by Althausen[12] that the rate of the intestinal absorption of glucose is increased by the administration of thyroxin.

Thyroidectomy is said to be followed by an increased carbohydrate tolerance, but since Althausen has also shown that this procedure reduces the intestinal absorption of glucose it is probable that the "flat" type of tolerance curves on which this statement is based is to be attributed to this cause.

Goldblatt[101] has reported that thyroidectomized rabbits are more sensitive to insulin and in the earlier literature there will be found reports that the fasting blood glucose level is subnormal.

The work of Houssay and his colleagues and that of Lukens and Dohan[86, 102] indicates that thyroidectomy does not alleviate a total pancreatic diabetes.

While the present indications are that the thyroid hormone does not directly influence carbohydrate metabolism it should be stated that no recent systemic studies of such a possible relationship are available. Nevertheless, it would appear that such alterations as have been observed are to be attributed to the general stimulation or decline of the metabolism that follows an excess or deficiency of this hormone.

The Posterior Pituitary and Carbohydrate Metabolism.—The earlier literature contains many reports that carbohydrate metabolism is influenced by the hormones of the posterior lobe. While it cannot be denied that the injection of pharmacological amounts of this extract is followed by mild hyperglycemia and depletion of liver glycogen it has become increasingly evident that the physiological activity of this endocrine gland is not extended to the control of carbohydrate metabolism. The recent studies of Ranson and his colleagues,[103] who have shown the direct dependence of posterior lobe function on hypothalamic centers and the relation of this activity to the control of water metabolism, have been complemented by the observations of Gilman and Goodman,[105] that the probable function of this hormone is the regulation of water reabsorption by the kidney tubules. The quantity of hormone involved in this function is far below that required to influence the blood glucose level. The oxytocic activity of posterior pituitary extracts is also well known but here again the quantities which are required to produce maximal physiological effects are very much less than the quantities which are necessary to disturb the normal carbohydrate levels.

It may be concluded that the available evidence does not suggest that the posterior pituitary is a normal regulator of the metabolism of protein, fat, or carbohydrate.

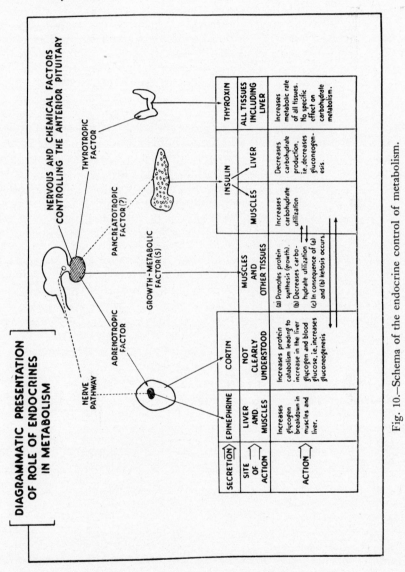

Fig. 10.—Schema of the endocrine control of metabolism.

Scheme of the Endocrine Control of Metabolism.—Figure 10 is a condensed diagram illustrating what is known concerning the main effects of certain endocrine glands upon carbohydrate metabolism.

It would appear that this control is of a balanced character. Thus the pancreatic hormone, which may or may not be regulated by a pituitary trophic factor, is opposed in its action by the secretions of the anterior pituitary and adrenal cortex. Thus, insulin accelerates the disposition of ingested carbohydrate by both oxidation and storage as glycogen and may also be concerned in the transformation of carbohydrate into fat. On the other hand, the anterior pituitary and adrenal cortical hormones inhibit carbohydrate utilization and accelerate those processes by which carbohydrate is formed from noncarbohydrate sources.

The net effect of these opposing influences is to preserve the carbohydrate levels of the body within certain limits and to maintain what is termed a normal carbohydrate metabolism. It should be emphasized that a normal metabolism is not an equilibrium but rather a steady state in which carbohydrate formation and utilization are continually proceeding. The mechanism of the action of these hormones on the cells, by which the composition of the metabolic mixture may be diverted from one consisting largely of carbohydrate oxidation to one in which fat catabolism predominates, is unknown. Although attempts have been made in the case of insulin to suggest that this hormone acts as a catalyst in the citric acid cycle,[106] this, however, is denied by others.[81]

The removal of any of these endocrine glands results in a disturbance of metabolism (a) by the removal of the influence of the hormone itself and (b) by leaving unopposed the action of its antagonist. This is well illustrated in the case of pancreatectomy where not only is the rate of carbohydrate utilization greatly diminished by the loss of insulin but in addition the unopposed effect of the anterior pituitary and adrenal cortex contribute to the effects produced. The removal of both the pancreas and pituitary (or adrenal cortex), while not reestablishing a normal metabolism, relieves the organism from many of the consequences of this displacement of the endocrine equilibrium. However, the loss of practically all humoral regulation leaves the carbohydrate metabolism in a most unstable condition and wide fluctuations between extreme hyper- and hypoglycemia are characteristic features of these doubly operated animals.

BIBLIOGRAPHY

1. Eberling, W. N., Am. J. Med. Sci., **183**: 876, 1932.
2. Scott, E. L. and Zweighaft, J. F. B., Arch. Int. Med., **49**: 221, 1932.
3. McDougall, E. J., Arb. d. 11. Abt. d. ung. biol. Forschgs., **VII**: 217, 1934.
4. Nagano, J., Pfluger's Archiv., **90**: 389, 1902.
5. Cori, C. F., J. Biol. Chem., **66**: 691, 1925.
6. Cori, C. F. and Goltz, H. L., Proc. Soc. Exp. Biol. Med., **23**: 22, 1935.
7. Verzár, F. and McDougall, E. J., Absorption from the Intestine, Longmans Green Co., New York, 1936.
8. Klinghoffer, K., J. Biol. Chem., **126**: 201, 1938.
9. Cori, C. F., Proc. Soc. Exp. Biol. Med., **23**: 125, 1926.
10. Deuel, H. J., Hallman, L. F., Murray, S. and Samuels, L. T., J. Biol. Chem., **119**: 607, 1937.
11. Magee, H. E. and Sen, K., J. Physiol., **75**: 433, 1932.
12. Althausen, T. L., Amer. J. Physiol., **123**: 577, 1938.
13. Russell, J. A., Amer. J. Physiol., **128**: 552, 1940.
14. Exton, W. G. and Rose, A. R., Am. J. Clin. Path., **4**: 381, 1934.
15. Himsworth, H. P., Clinical Science, **1**: 251, 1934.
16. Himsworth, H. P., Clinical Science, **2**: 67, 1935.
17. Bollman, J. L. and Mann, F. C., Am. J. Physiol., **96**: 683, 1931.
18. Somogyi, M., J. Biol. Chem., **78**: 117, 1928.
19. Silver, S. and Reiner, M., Arch. Int. Med., **54**: 412, 1934.
20. Greenwald, I., In Endocrinology and Metabolism, edited by Lewellys F. Barker, Vol. 4, p. 289, D. Appleton-Century Company, New York, 1922.

21. Cohen, S. L. and Marrian, G. F., Biochem. J., **30**: 57, 1936.
22. Venning, E. H., J. Biol. Chem., **119**: 473, 1937.
23. Quick, A. J., J. Biol. Chem., **70**: 397, 1926; **98**: 537, 1932; **99**: 119, 1932–33; **100**: 441, 1933.
24. Bodansky, M., Introduction to Physiological Chemistry. 4th Edition. John Wiley and Sons, Inc., New York, 1938.
25. Cori, C. F., J. Biol. Chem., **70**: 577, 1926.
26. Soskin, S., Essex, H. E., Herrick, J. F. and Mann, F. C., Am. J. Physiol., **124**: 558, 1938.
27. Soskin, S., Allweiss, M. D. and Cohn, D. J., Am. J. Physiol., **109**: 155, 1934.
28. Soskin, S. and Mirsky, I. A., Am. J. Physiol., **112**: 649, 1935.
29. Soskin, S., Mirsky, I. A., Zimmerman, L. M. and Heller, R. C., Am. J. Physiol., **114**: 648, 1936.
30. Mann, F. C., Medicine, **6**: 419, 1927.
31. Mirski, A., Rosenbaum, I., Stein, L. and Wertheimer, E., J. Physiol., **92**: 48, 1938.
32. Evans, G. T., Am. J. Physiol., **110**: 273, 1934; **114**: 297, 1936.
33. Cori, G. T., Cori, C. F. and Schmidt, G., J. Biol. Chem., **129**: 629, 1939.
34. Ostern, P., Herbert, D. and Holmes, E. G., Biochem. J., **33**: 1858, 1939.
35. Cori, C. F., Colowick, S. P. and Cori, G. T., J. Biol. Chem., **121**: 465, 1937.
36. Kiessling, C. E., Naturwissenschaften, **27**: 129, 1939.
37. Hanes, C. S., Proc. Roy. Soc. London, Series B, No. 855, **129**: 174, 1940.
38. Cruickshank, E. W. H., J. Physiol., **47**: 1, 1913.
39. Evans, C. L., Biochem. J., **19**: 1115, 1928.
40. Cori, C. F. and Cori, G. T., J. Biol. Chem., **70**: 557, 1926.
41. Parnas, J. and Wagner, R., Biochem. Zeitsch., **61**: 387, 1914.
42. Fletcher, W. M. and Hopkins, F. G., J. Physiol., **35**: 247, 1906–7.
43. Meyerhof, O., Pfluger's Arch., **182**: 284, 1920.
44. Hill, A. V., Muscular Activity. Williams and Wilkins, Baltimore, 1926.
45. Lundsgaard, E., Biochem. Zeitsch., **217**: 162, 1930.
46. Eggleton, P. and Eggleton, M. G., Biochem. J., **21**: 190, 1927.
47. Fiske, C. and Subbarow, Y., J. Biol. Chem., **81**: 629, 1929.
48. Embden, G. and Zimmerman, M., Zeitsch. Physiol. Chem., **167**: 114, 1927.
49. Lohmann, K., Naturwissenschaften, **17**: 624, 1929.
50. Abramson, H. A., Eggleton, P. and Eggleton, M. G., J. Biol. Chem., **75**: 745, 763, 1927.
51. Long, C. N. H. and Horsfall, F. L., J. Biol. Chem., **95**: 715, 1932.
52. Long, C. N. H. and Grant, R., J. Biol. Chem., **89**: 553, 1930.
53. Sacks, J. and Sacks, W. C., Am. J. Physiol., **112**: 565, 1935.
54. Hill, A. V., Long, C. N. H. and Lupton, H., Proc. Roy. Soc. London, Series B, **96**: 438, 1924; **97**: 84, 1924; **97**: 155, 1924.
55. Szent-Györgyi, A. Oxidation, Fermentation, Vitamins and Disease. Williams and Wilkins Company, Baltimore, 1939.
56. Lohmann, K. and Schuster, P., Biochem. Zeitsch., **294**: 188, 1937.
57. Krebs, H. A. and Johnson, W. A., Enzymologia, **4**: 148, 1937.
58. Stadie, W. C., Zapp, J. A. and Lukens, F. D. W., J. Biol. Chem., **132**: 411, 1940.
59. Krebs, H. A. and Johnson, W. A., Biochem. J., **31**: 645, 1937.
60. Green, D., Mechanism of Biological Oxidation. Cambridge University Press, 1940.
61. Sacks, J., Physiol. Rev., **21**: 217, 1941.
62. Katz, L. N. and Long, C. N. H., Proc. Roy. Soc. London, Series B, **99**: 8, 1928.
63. Evans, G. T., J. Physiol., **82**: 468, 1934.
64. Evans, C. L., Edin. Med. J., **46**: 733, 1939.
65. Barnes, R. H., Mackay, E. M., Moe, E. K. and Visscher, M. B., Am. J. Physiol., **123**: 272, 1938.
66. Clark, A. J. Metabolism of the Frog's Heart. Oliver and Boyd, Edinburgh, 1938.
67. Cruickshank, E. W. H., Physiol. Rev., **16**: 597, 1936.
68. Sherif, M. A. F. and Holmes, E. G., Biochem. J., **24**: 400, 1930.
69. Himwich, H. E. and Nahum, L. H., Am. J. Physiol., **90**: 389, 1929; **101**: 446, 1932.
70. Himwich, H. E. and Fazekas, J. F., Endocrinology, **21**: 800, 1937.
71. Himwich, H. E., Bowman, K. M., Fazekas, J. F. and Crenstein, L. L., Proc. Soc. Exp. Biol. Med., **37**: 359, 1937–38.
72. Wierzuchowski, M. and Ling, S. M., J. Biol. Chem., **64**: 697, 1925.

73. Lusk, G., Science of Nutrition, 4th Edition. W. B. Saunders Company, Philadelphia, 1928.
74. Drury, D. R., Am. J. Physiol., **131**: 536, 1940.
75. Stadie, W. C., Zapp, J. A. and Lukens, F. D. W., J. Biol. Chem., **137**: 63, 1941.
76. Weil-Malherbe, H., Biochem. J., **32**: 2276, 1938.
77. Stadie, W. C., Zapp, J. A. and Lukens, F. D. W., J. Biol. Chem., **132**: 423, 1940.
78. Russell, J. A., Physiol. Rev., **18**: 1, 1938.
79. Phillips, R. A. and Robb, P., Am. J. Physiol., **109**: 82, 1934.
80. Russell, J. A., Am. J. Physiol., **122**: 547, 1938.
81. Fisher, R. E. and Pencharz, R. I., Proc. Soc. Exper. Biol. Med., **34**: 106, 1936.
82. Fisher, R. E., Russell, J. A. and Cori, C. F., J. Biol. Chem., **115**: 627, 1936.
83. Soskin, S., Endocrinology, **26**: 297, 1940.
84. Houssay, B. A. and Magenta, M. A., Compt. rend. Soc. Biol., **92**: 822, 1925; **97**: 596, 1927.
85. Young, F. G., Endocrinology, **26**: 345, 1940.
86. Houssay, B. A., New Eng. J. Med., **214**: Nos. 19–23, 1936.
87. Young, F. G., Biochem. J., **32**: 513, 524, 1521, 1938.
88. Campbell, J. and Best, C. H., Lancet, **1**: 1446, 1938.
89. Richardson, K. C. and Young, F. G., Lancet, **1**: 1098, 1938.
90. Dohan, F. C. and Lukens, F. D. W., Am. J. Physiol., **125**: 188, 1939.
91. Long, C. N. H. and Lukens, F. D. W., J. Exp. Med., **63**: 465, 1936.
92. Stadie, W. C., J. Clin. Invest., **19**: 843, 1940.
93. Goldblatt, M. W., Biochem. J., **24**: 1199, 1930.
94. Cori, C. F. and Cori, G. T., J. Biol. Chem., **79**: 309, 321, 343, 1928.
95. Britton, S. W. and Silvette, H., Am. J. Physiol., **100**: 685, 693, 701, 1932.
96. Long, C. N. H., Katzin, B. and Fry, E. G., Endocrinology, **26**: 309, 1940.
97. Harrison, H. C. and Long, C. N. H., Endocrinology, **26**: 971, 1940.
98. Wells, B. B. and Kendall, E. C., Proc. Mayo Clinic, **15**: 561, 1940.
99. Ingle, D. W., Proc. Soc. Exp. Biol. Med., **44**: 176, 1940.
100. Jensen, H. and Gratton, J. F., Am. J. Physiol., **128**: 270, 1940; J. Biol. Chem., **135**: 511, 1940.
101. Goldblatt, M. H., J. Physiol., **86**: 46, 1936.
102. Lukens, F. D. W. and Dohan, F. C., Am. J. Physiol., **122**: 367, 1938.
103. Fisher, C., Ingram, W. R. and Ranson, S. W., Diabetes Insipidus, Edwards Bros., Ann Arbor, 1938.
104. Colowick, S. P., Kalckar, H. M. and Cori, C. F., J. Biol. Chem., **137**: 343, 1941.
105. Gilman, A. and Goodman, L., J. Physiol., **90**: 137, 1937.
106. Krebs, H. A. and Eggleston, L. V., Biochem. J., **32**: 913, 1938.
107. Chambers, W. H., Physiol. Rev., **18**: 248, 1938.

CHAPTER III

PROTEIN METABOLISM

By Abraham White

Advances in knowledge of protein metabolism have been made possible through the development of new experimental methods and approaches. Indeed, if a list is made of the methods which have been devised for attacking problems in protein metabolism, it will be observed that the introduction of each new method has, in reality, marked a milestone along the road which has led to the present-day understanding of the subject. It is well to consider first in more or less detail certain of these experimental methods, because an understanding of their advantages and limitations should be of considerable aid in accurately evaluating the data which each has yielded.

EXPERIMENTAL METHODS

Nitrogen Balance or Equilibrium

Method of Urine Analysis.—The accurate determination of the ingested nitrogen and of the excreted nitrogen permits the establishment of a balance sheet from which an approximation can be made of the extent or intensity of the nitrogen metabolism of the organism. Inasmuch as the element, nitrogen, characterizes proteins particularly, the information obtained regarding nitrogen metabolism may be interpreted in terms of the condition of the protein metabolism. Moreover, certain valid assumptions permit the total nitrogen content of the urine, during a metabolic period (usually twenty-four hours), to be accepted as the total nitrogen excretion. These assumptions may be briefly mentioned:

1. In the adult organism, nitrogen is not stored for significant periods of time; excess nitrogen is excreted in the urine.

2. None of the respiratory nitrogen is of metabolic origin (demonstrated by Krogh).

3. Fecal nitrogen is derived primarily from the micro-organism flora of the intestine, is not of metabolic origin, and is relatively constant in amount.

4. The nitrogen of the perspiration is insignificantly small (not more than 0.1 gm. per day, as Benedict has shown) when compared to the total nitrogen turnover.

Thus, accepting these principles, total nitrogen determinations of the food and of the urine, with a constant correction factor being employed for fecal nitrogen, make it possible to establish whether a human or an experimental animal during a given metabolic period is in nitrogen equilibrium or balance, *i.e.*, nitrogen of the diet equalling the nitrogen of the urine. When nitrogen balance does not prevail, then there may obtain a state of *negative nitrogen balance* (the nitrogen of the urine being greater than the quantity of ingested nitrogen) or a state of *positive nitrogen balance* (a retention of nitrogen as manifested by the nitrogen excretion being less than the nitrogen in the diet). Inasmuch as the Kjeldahl method for the determination of total nitrogen dates from 1883, it is evident that the method of nitrogen balance was among the earliest and remains one of the reliable procedures for studies in protein metabolism, and has served to establish the foundation of our knowledge of this subject. The introduction in the early part of this century by Folin and by Van Slyke and their collaborators of methods for determining the various *kinds* of nitrogen in the urine made it possible to derive a more detailed insight into protein metabolism from studies of the nitrogen balance. It was early established that the normal adult is in nitrogen balance, the nitrogen of the diet being equal to the nitrogen of the urine. Variations in this picture were observed to accompany deviations from the normal. Thus, a negative balance or excessive breakdown of the protein of the tissues was seen in fevers, in wasting diseases, and in response to an inadequate diet. Positive nitrogen balances were demonstrated under conditions characterized by a need for dietary nitrogen for the synthesis of new tissue protein, *e.g.*, in children, in pregnancy, in lactating animals, and after fevers.

As already mentioned, the method of nitrogen balance represents one of the first experimental approaches to problems in protein metabolism. It is quite obvious that this procedure allows only an analysis of the beginnning and the end of the story. For an insight into the intermediary chapters, other experimental methods have been elaborated.

Method of Perfusion

This technic was devised in the early part of the present century and was evolved by the independent work of Embden and of Knoop. The method consists in removing an organ, such as the liver or the kidney, from the organism and placing it in a closed system constructed so as to permit circulation of a suitable fluid under pressure from a pump. The circulating fluid may be defibrinated blood or whole blood to which a suitable anticoagulant has been added; physiologically isotonic fluids (Ringer's or Locke's solutions) have also been employed in place of blood. The advantage of this technic lies chiefly in the fact that various substances, whose metabolism it is desired to study, may be added to the perfusing fluid and analysis of the perfusate then permits conclusions to be drawn regarding the metabolic effects of the particular organ on the material being investigated. The conclusions which may be derived from this experimental method are, however, limited by the experimental conditions themselves. The results obtained represent, obviously, what the organ will do under rather abnormal conditions. The nerve supply has been severed; there are difficulties involved in exactly duplicating the normal oxygenation of blood; and, finally, the use of a circulating pump appears to be a neglect of the significance of the fundamental observations of Krogh. The latter physiologist has demonstrated that under normal circumstances the capillaries are never extended to their fullest capacity, to which they may be forced to expand under mechanical pressure. Krogh has also shown that nervous reflexes in the capillaries function to change blood flow at various times, the blood being supplied to an organ apparently according to the needs of that organ. Despite these criticisms, definite advances in information have been obtained from perfusion studies with isolated organs. This type of experimentation has indicated the metabolic potentialities of an organ and has suggested the way for further investigations.

ANGIOSTOMY TECHNIC

The angiostomy technic was devised by London and his pupils, working in Leningrad, and is an operative procedure which, literally, consists in preparing fistulas of various blood vessels. With the use of great surgical skill, London has prepared animals (dogs) in which the bases of metal (silver-nickel alloy) cannulas have been placed on one or more blood vessels and the other ends of the cannulas then brought to the outside through the body wall. For example, animals have been prepared in which there

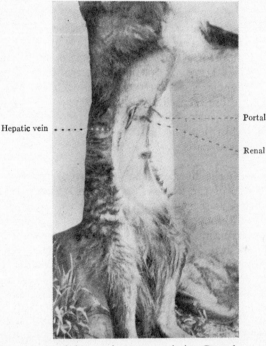

Fig. 11.–Dog prepared by angiostomy technic. Cannulas on the hepatic, portal and renal veins. (After London, E. S., Harvey Lectures, 1927–28, p. 208, Williams & Wilkins Co.)

is a cannula on each of the following blood vessels: the renal vein, the renal artery, the portal vein, and the hepatic vein. The dogs remain in good condition for several years. An illustration of an animal prepared in London's laboratory is seen in figure 11.

The advantage of the angiostomy type of preparation is very great indeed. Blood may be readily withdrawn at any time from a vessel on which there is a cannula, or injections may be made into the vessel *via* the cannula. Thus, the action of the kidney on a particular substance may be studied by injection of the compound through the cannula on the renal artery, and analysis of the blood obtained from the cannula on the renal vein. The experimental animals are normal in every respect and this is a great advantage in studies of intermediary metabolism. Although the surgical technic is very difficult, the angiostomy method has been used by several laboratories and has yielded valuable data. One of the criticisms which have been made of investigators employing the angiostomy technic is that the problem of rate of blood flow through an organ has not been adequately considered in the evaluation of the data.

PATHOLOGICAL ALTERATIONS IN PROTEIN METABOLISM, BOTH NORMALLY OCCURRING AND EXPERIMENTALLY PRODUCED

Of the organs and tissues of the body which are concerned with protein metabolism, the liver and the kidneys are among the most important. Alterations in the normal functioning of these organs, occurring as a consequence of either disease or experimental conditions, very often produce aberrations in the normal picture of protein metabolism which permit certain conclusions regarding the processes involved in the metabolism of nitrogen. Clinical pathological changes in the liver, e.g., acute yellow atrophy, cirrhosis, and fatal poisoning by chloroform, carbon tetrachloride, hydrazine, or phosphorus, produce various types of metabolic alterations which have contributed information concerning the rôle of the liver in protein metabolism. Conditions simulating those seen clinically may be produced experimentally by the use of the aforementioned poisons. Complete removal of the liver (experimental hepatectomy) in the hands of Mann and his collaborators has strikingly emphasized the nature of the normal functions of the liver in protein metabolism.

As in the case with the liver, similar approaches have been employed in determining the rôle of the kidneys in protein metabolism. Pathological changes in the kidneys, as seen clinically in the various types of nephritis, in the arteriosclerotic kidney, in mass destruction of kidney tissue, and in kidney lesions due to poisons, chiefly mercurials, result in variations in the normal protein metabolism. Studies of such clinical cases have yielded valuable data. Experimental surgery and experimental nephritis have also been used as approaches to the problem of the rôle of the kidney in protein metabolism. Uranium, mercury, or arsenic salts are effective kidney poisons. Tartrates and chromates have also been employed.

INBORN ERRORS OF METABOLISM

The group of metabolic disorders which have been labeled, by Garrod, inborn errors of metabolism, represents in some instances variations or alterations in the normal protein metabolism. The deviation from the normal is usually manifested by a failure of the organism to carry out in the usual manner some chemical metabolic process. In the case of most of these so-called errors of metabolism, no gross pathology is associated with the condition, and the individual who exhibits one or the other of these metabolic peculiarities may have a normal, and in many instances a very long, life span. The following is a list of inborn errors of metabolism which have been described:

1. Cystinuria
2. Alkaptonuria
3. Tyrosinosis
4. Phenylketonuria

5. Hematoporphyrinuria
6. Steatorrhea
7. Albinism
8. Pentosuria

Cystinuria is characterized by the excretion of the free amino acid, cystine, in the urine. As will be discussed later, cystine arising from certain sources in metabolism is not oxidized (as is normally the case) and is excreted in the urine. A cystinuric individual, therefore, becomes a valuable experimental tool for the study of the metabolic origin and reactions of cystine. *Alkaptonuria* is characterized by the voiding of a urine which, on contact with air, gradually darkens at the surface with the entire urine specimen eventually becoming a blackish color. The color is due to the oxidation of a substance, homogentisic acid, which is present in the urine of alkaptonurics and which has its metabolic origin in the aromatic amino acids, tyrosine and phenylalanine. *Tyrosinosis*, like alkaptonuria and cystinuria, is of considerable interest in protein metabolism because this inborn error is characterized by an inability to normally metabolize an amino acid, in this instance, tyrosine. In this condition, certain of the intermediates of tyrosine catabolism appear in the urine. Similarly, patients with *phenylketonuria* have yielded interesting information regarding the metabolism of the amino acids, tyrosine and phenylalanine. The data dealing with these inborn errors of metabolism will be discussed later.

The remaining inborn errors of metabolism which have been listed above are not of particular interest to the present discussion because, insofar as is known at the present time, they are not related to protein metabolism. Reference should be made to the book by Garrod for consideration of these errors.

OTHER METHODS OF STUDY

Growth Studies with the White Rat.—It is axiomatic in metabolism that no growth of new tissue normally occurs without nitrogen and inasmuch as protein, and products derived from protein, are the primary sources of nitrogen in the diet, it may be generally stated that growth is not possible without a supply of protein products. The classical studies of Osborne and Mendel served to standardize the white rat for studies of growth and nutrition. These investigators solved, in their initial investigations, the problem of the maintenance of successive generations of white rats on highly purified diets of a rather accurately known composition. On the basis of these initial experiments, it was possible to prepare diets adequate in every respect for normal growth and in which the type or nature of the protein could be varied. Experiments of this type early indicated *qualitative* differences in the nutritional value of various proteins and led to the concept of essential amino acids. The latter are amino acids which apparently cannot be synthesized by the organism in an amount adequate for normal growth and nutrition and which, therefore, must be supplied in the diet.

Study of Protein Metabolism Associated with the Biological Specificity of Protein.—The development of a condition of immunity is associated with the appearance of antibodies in the blood. This is accompanied by an increase in concentration of one of the fractions of the plasma proteins and therefore may exert a definite effect on protein metabolism. Furthermore, the biological specificity of proteins, responsible for the development of a sensitization in animals, which may be ultimately transformed into an anti-sensitization or immunity, serves as a very important method of detecting the presence of small amounts of a given, unchanged protein. Thus, immunological reactions, based upon the biological specificity of proteins, have contributed valuable information to the question of the absorption of unchanged, or native, protein from the gastrointestinal tract.

Metabolism of Tissue Slices.—Another milestone in protein metablism was reached in 1912 when Warburg introduced the manometric technique for the study of the metabolism of isolated tissue strips or slices. This procedure makes it possible to follow the metabolism of slices of a particular tissue or organ, to determine manometrically the rate of oxygen utilization and carbon dioxide production (and therefore the respiratory quotient), to study the utilization of a foodstuff or substrate which may be added to the physiological medium in which the tissue slice is placed, and to determine the nature and concentration of products of metabolism. The Warburg techniques permit the *in vitro* observation of one or more metabolic reactions which may comprise part of the total metabolic picture. A mass of valuable data has been made available as a result of the use of the Warburg methods by many investigators in problems of protein metabolism. The books by Warburg and by Dixon present a description of these methods and some of the results obtained by their application.

Studies with the Aid of Isotopes.—Within the past fifteen years a new experimental tool has been made available to investigators in metabolism, and the wealth of information which has already been obtained indicates that the introduction of this new technic will mark one of the outstanding contributions to the progress of metabolic research. Isotopes are chemical elements which differ from those commonly found in nature and in the periodic table of inorganic chemistry textbooks only in their mass or atomic weight. Their chemical behavior is quite indistinguishable from the ordinary chemical elements and, when they are employed in the usual small concentrations for physiological work, their physiological behavior also appears to be identical with that of the chemical elements which the organism is normally metabolizing. However, the variation in mass of certain of the isotopes, and the radioactivity of others, make it possible to determine accurately micro quantities of these isotopes in any particular solution, fluid, or tissue. For example, isotopic hydrogen, or deuterium, has a mass which is approximately twice that of ordinary hydrogen, and when combined with oxygen will produce water with a specific gravity considerably greater than that of ordinary water. Inasmuch as methods for determining specific gravity have been greatly refined, it is possible to determine accurately very minute concentrations of deuterium. Similarly, nitrogen of mass 15, as compared with ordinary nitrogen of mass 14, may be detected in traces by the use of a suitable physical apparatus, the mass spectrograph. Again, it is possible to detect small concentrations of compounds containing radioactive elements, *e.g.*, phosphorus, sulfur, or iron, by employing a sensitive instrument (Geiger counter) for detecting the magnitude of radiation. It is thus apparent that by incorporating one or more isotopes into a given substance the latter is labeled or tagged so that it is possible to follow and to detect the concentration of this isotope-containing substance in the organism at a particular time.

In other words, the use of isotopes in biological research, and more specifically in problems of protein metabolism, makes it possible to gain an insight into some of the intermediary chapters in the story of the metabolism of nitrogen, because these tagged elements serve to distinguish clearly the concentration of the administered material or substance from the concentration of this material already present in the organism.

PROTEIN REQUIREMENT

Before discussing in detail the experimental and clinical data which have been obtained relating to the metabolism of protein, it may be well to consider the problem of protein requirement. The demands of all living organisms for nitrogen, and of higher organisms for nitrogen in the form of protein or products derived from protein, emphasize the value of determining the minimum level of protein required in the diet. This problem is of importance from both an economical and a physiological standpoint, and assumes considerable significance in clinical conditions characterized by a wasting of body tissue and a loss of protein from the body.

The classical method of nitrogen equilibrium has been widely employed to determine the protein requirement of the adult. A great deal of heated controversy has centered around this problem. Voit first approached the subject statistically, in the middle of the last century, by a consideration of the average protein intake of the German farmer. According to Voit, 118 gm. of protein per individual per day was the desirable amount of protein in the diet.

The tradition established by Voit that a generous intake of protein was required for normal body vigor has been refuted by the careful investigations of other workers. Chittenden and his collaborators, in the early part of the present century, carried out a long series of very careful studies on a number of groups of persons engaged in various types of occupational activities, such as professional men, student athletes in training, and soldiers under military regimen. From these extensive studies Chittenden concluded that nitrogen balance could be maintained on a protein intake of 40 to 50 gm. daily with no physical impairment. Indeed, according to Chittenden, the professional group professed a greater keenness for its work, the athletic group won championships in games, and the soldiers maintained perfect health and strength, many professing a marked dislike for meat when they were given it after five months of practical abstinence.

Despite the fact that the now classical experiments of Chittenden did not include control groups of subjects maintained on the usual protein intake but otherwise existing under the same routine as the experimental groups of individuals, other data have supported the conclusion that the Voit standard appears to be rather high. On the other hand, there is no clear-cut and well-controlled evidence to indicate that high protein diets exert any deleterious effects in the normal individual. Subsequent work has strongly indicated that a protein intake somewhere between the standard established by Voit and that suggested by Chittenden furnishes an *optimum quantity of nitrogen for the maintenance of nitrogen equilibrium* and for the replenishment of nitrogen which may be lost from the body as a consequence of the continual metabolic activity of the body tissues. The careful studies of Sherman have led this investigator to suggest that in the adult the nitrogen requirement is met by the ingestion of 70 gm. of protein per day. The standard which has become quite generally accepted, assuming the average adult body weight to be 70 Kg., is 1 gm. of protein (calculated as dietary nitrogen x 6.25) per kilo body weight per day.

Although the existence of a minimum protein requirement was formerly commonly interpreted as the need of the body for protein to replace the "wear and tear" quota, modern nutritional evidence permits a rather more detailed insight into the reason for this requirement. Protein minimum has ceased to be the need of the organism for a definite quantity of protein, but rather the requirement for a definite *quality* of protein. It is the need of the body for certain specific amino acids for specialized purposes, amino acids which the organism is not capable of synthesizing at a rate commensurate with the metabolic demands. If these amino acids are not available, then the body will break down its own protein, utilizing the sought-for amino acids and catabolizing the remainder, with the usual ensuing negative nitrogen balance. It may be well at this point to consider the problem of essential amino acids and then return to conclude the discussion of protein requirement as viewed from the amino acid standpoint.

Essential Amino Acids.—The essential nature of protein in the diet has been recognized from the time of Rubner and of Voit. However, the question of whether all amino acids constituting proteins are essential was not approached until the early part of the present century. The solution of this problem was again dependent on the development of experimental techniques. The brilliant analytical work conducted on proteins in the laboratory of Osborne presented rather complete information regarding the amino acid composition of various proteins. This was made the basis for the adaptation of the white rat, by Osborne and Mendel, for growth and nutrition studies, and led to the first classical method for studying the essential nature of various amino acids. The method consisted in studying the rate of growth of the young white rat placed on a diet whose nitrogen, for the most part, was supplied by a *single protein;* the amino acid composition of the latter was known in some detail. Proteins were chosen which were incomplete in the sense that one or more amino acids were known to be absent from the molecule. If growth of the experimental rats did not take place at a normal rate, then the one or more missing amino acids were added to the ration, either singly or together. By this method it was soon demonstrated that in the absence of certain amino acids normal growth did not take place, and that the addition of the missing amino acid, or acids, to the diet caused an immediate resumption of growth. It was thus clearly established that the rat was incapable of synthesizing some amino acids and that these substances, essential to the diet, must be supplied in the food to permit normal growth and well-being. An *essential amino acid*, therefore, was defined as an amino acid which could not be synthesized but must be supplied in the diet. This technique, devised by Osborne and Mendel, has been used by a large number of investigators to study problems concerned with the rôle of proteins and amino acids in nutrition and in metabolism.

The other important experimental method of approach to the problem of essential amino acids consists in feeding the pure amino acids in various types of *synthetic mixtures*. It was early demonstrated that a protein hydrolysate, that is, a mixture of amino acids prepared by the splitting of proteins with acids, alkalis, or enzymes, could, after removal of the hydrolytic agent, substitute quite adequately for protein in nutrition and metabolism. Although success with amino acid mixtures did not, up to several years ago, approach that achieved with individual proteins, rather interesting contributions were made. One of the most striking experiments with a protein hydrolysate was that of Abderhalden[1] in 1915. This investigator fed a dog for one hundred days on a diet containing, as its sole source of nitrogen, a mixture of amino acids obtained by the complete hydrolysis of meat. During this period the dog was maintained in good health and increased almost 10 Kg. in weight. By the use of similar amino acid mixtures from which various acids had been removed, Abderhalden came to the conclusion that *tryptophane* is an essential amino acid.

The classical work with pure amino acid mixtures has been conducted by Rose and his collaborators during the past ten years. These investigations, in addition to establishing the presence in proteins of a new amino acid, have permitted a classification of amino acids into two groups. From a nutritional standpoint, one group is essential or indispensable for growth; the other includes amino acids which may be synthesized by the organism at a rate commensurate with the requirements for normal growth. This classification is shown in table 1. Rose and Rice[2] have also conducted similar experiments

TABLE 1

FINAL CLASSIFICATION OF THE AMINO ACIDS WITH RESPECT TO THEIR GROWTH EFFECTS

Indispensable	Dispensable
Lysine	Glycine
Tryptophane	Alanine
Histidine	Serine
Phenylalanine	Norleucine
Leucine	Aspartic acid
Isoleucine	Glutamic acid
Threonine	Hydroxyglutamic acid
Methionine	Proline
Valine	Hydroxyproline
*Arginine	Citrulline
	Tyrosine
	Cystine

* Arginine can be synthesized by the animal organism, but not at a sufficiently rapid rate to meet the demands of *normal* growth.

with dogs, in which nitrogen balances have been determined, and have shown that the amino acids which are dispensable for the growing rat are also dispensable for the adult dog. The significance of these findings has been clearly stated: "The fact that two widely different species require for their well-being the same components of the protein molecule, increases the probability that other mammals, including man, may manifest like responses."

The investigations of Rose and of others to be considered below would strongly suggest, therefore, that a relatively small number of amino acids is required to maintain nitrogen equilibrium in the adult animal and would reemphasize the previously made statement that a more modern view of protein requirement stresses the qualitative rather than the quantitative aspect of dietary protein. The findings of Rose and his collaborators have been confirmed independently by Corley and his colleagues[3, 4] who found that the amino acids required to maintain nitrogen equilibrium in the adult rat are the same, except for arginine, as the ones essential for growth.

Maintenance Requirements versus Growth Requirements.—Recently, Mitchell and his co-workers have carefully reinvestigated the possibility that the amino acid requirements for maintenance may in some particulars be qualitatively different from those for growth. In nitrogen equilibrium studies with adult, female rats, Burroughs, Burroughs and Mitchell[5] have presented evidence to indicate that nitrogen equilibrium may be maintained on an amino acid nitrogen supply containing only threonine, isoleucine, tryptophane, valine, methionine, tyrosine and norleucine. Phenylalanine, which is essential for growth, may be replaced for nitrogen requirements in adult animals by tyrosine. It is strongly suggested from these data that differences may exist between the physiological demands for an amino acid in growth as compared to the reconstruction of tissue constituents containing this particular amino acid and requiring its replenishment because of the continued nitrogen catabolism.

Maintenance.—The aforegoing discussion should not necessarily be interpreted as meaning that in the adult the only essential protein nitrogen components of the diet need be the few amino acids which Mitchell and his colleagues have demonstrated as being capable of maintaining nitrogen equilibrium in the adult organism. Indeed, as Rose has pointed out, such a severe limitation of the dietary intake of amino acids given without other amino acid yielding supplements may bring to light an additional requirement, under these particular circumstances, for those amino acids otherwise dispensable from the diet. It should be emphasized that nitrogen balance studies are generally short-term experiments. Mitchell and his collaborators[6] in a recent study have demonstrated that although, as stressed above, the quality of the amino acid mixture and not its quantity is of prime importance, it is possible to replace some 30 to 50 per cent of the nitrogen lost in the continual metabolism of the tissues by a variety of incomplete dietary combinations of amino acids. Further, this nitrogen loss may be prevented even by amino acid mixtures which contain none of those amino acids whose presence in the diet is essential for the attainment of nitrogen equilibrium. It would appear, therefore, that a rather substantial proportion of the nitrogen requirement for the maintenance of the integrity of the tissues is an undifferentiated one that requires for its complete satisfaction no specific amino acids. The remainder of the requirement relates to specific amino acids, and, moreover, to certain combinations of these essential amino acids. It would appear from the work of Mitchell and his group that the losses of nitrogen from the tissues in the adult animal result not from the destruction of complex amino acid aggregates of the type of proteins, but rather from the destruction of many types of nitrogenous constituents of relatively simple structure.

Growth.—Although much can be written about the nitrogen requirements of the normal, adult animal, there is relatively little known, except in the rat, regarding the nitrogen requirement of the growing individual. Rose has tentatively calculated the minimum quantity of each essential amino acid required for the normal growth of the young rat, and the total amino acid concentration arrived at comprises 5.8 per cent of the diet. It is interesting to calculate the approximate daily nitrogen intake which this represents. The average nitrogen content of the ten amino acids essential for growth is 15.58 per cent. On the basis of Rose's figure, therefore, the nitrogen required in the diet would be 0.90 per cent. If an average daily food consumption of 10 gm. be assumed for the young rat, then the nitrogen requirement, in the form of a mixture of the essential amino acids, for growth would be approximately 90 mg. per day. It is interesting to note that in Mitchell's nitrogen balance experiment, his adult animals received 80 mg. of nitrogen per day. Further, if it be assumed, for convenience of calculation, that the body weight of the young, growing test rats in Rose's experiments was in the range of 80 to 100 gm., then the amino acid nitrogen requirement per day is approximately one gram per kilo of body weight. Inasmuch as Rose's animals generally weighed less than 80 gm., this figure would be somewhat higher.

Although it is in no way intended to transfer to the human, data obtained with the rat, particularly since nitrogen requirements have been demonstrated to differ between species (the rat as compared to the chick), it may well be that the rather high protein requirement which has been empirically set for the growing child is considerably higher than necessary. Values ranging from 4 gm. of protein per kilo for children one year of age to approximately half this value for six-year-old children have been suggested by Holt and Fales[7] from a study of common dietaries. However, there is little experimental basis for this conclusion. Indeed, Mitchell has suggested that if the caloric intake of a diet be kept adequately high, then the nitrogen requirement need be only that quantity which will produce a maximum positive nitrogen balance. The tissue nitrogen metabolism of children is essentially similar to that in adult life and is of the same order of magnitude in relation to body size.

Protein Requirement in Pregnancy.—The increase in nitrogen requirement manifested by the growing organism as a consequence of the need for the synthesis of new tissue is also seen, as would be expected, in adult individuals under circumstances which demand a formation of new protein. During pregnancy the growth of the fetus representing, as it does, a synthesis of new tissue, creates an increased requirement for dietary protein and unless this is adequately met there occurs a wasting of the nitrogen of the tissues of the mother. The accelerated metabolism of the mother during pregnancy may also exert an increase in the requirements for the nitrogen metabolism of the tissues. During pregnancy there is a considerable storage of protein by the mother, provided the nitrogen intake is at a relatively high level.[8, 9]

The augmented demands of protein synthesis during pregnancy are also evident during the lactation period, when the mother must supply not only her usual metabolic requirements for protein but must also furnish enough protein for the production of an adequate supply of milk for the offspring. In meeting the requirements for protein during lactation, emphasis is again placed upon the quality of the protein inasmuch as proteins likely to be deficient in one or more of the essential amino acids will not keep the lactating mother in positive nitrogen balance. If the nitrogen requirements for lactation are not met, a curtailment of the supply of milk will generally result.

Protein Requirements in Certain Pathological Conditions.—The higher metabolism of pregnancy, with its attendant increased demand for dietary protein, is seen in a highly magnified form in *hyperthyroidism*. However, although the nitrogen requirement increases in hyperthyroid individuals, it is generally possible to meet the increased metabolic demands with increased calories. The increased total metabolism and nitrogen metabolism in fevers and acute infections also require adequate consideration of the quantity of dietary protein. The marked nitrogen excretion in these conditions is a manifestation of the increased catabolism of the tissues, and although this destruction can be minimized by an adequate supply of calories, the repair of the wasted tissue during recovery can take place only in the presence of an abundant supply of protein. The administration of twice the usual amount of protein, *i.e.*, a daily intake of 2 gm. of protein per kilo of body weight, with fat and carbohydrate in amounts sufficient to meet the calorific requirements, will keep tissue destruction at a minimum and permit adequate synthesis of new tissue proteins. As in the other instances which have been mentioned, the dietary level of protein will be largely dependent upon the severity and nature of the disease.

An increased dietary requirement for protein may also be seen in conditions in which normal absorption of dietary nitrogen from the intestine is diminished. That is evident in severe *diarrheas*, and as a consequence the protein intake should be increased to insure sufficient nitrogen for the organism.

The elevated dietary requirement for protein in conditions in which nitrogen is lost through the stool has its counterpart in the increased demand for nitrogen in clinical conditions in which protein passes through the kidney into the urine and is therefore no longer available to the body. An inadequate supply of dietary protein to *nephrosis* patients results in a depletion of the protein of the tissues inasmuch as the nitrogen lost in the urine as protein must be replaced. Similar protein losses in nephrosis and in active *chronic nephritis* may induce a plasma protein deficit of a magnitude sufficient to cause edema. In order to prevent deleterious effects attending loss of protein through the kidney, the protein intake, among other factors, must be taken into consideration and must be elevated to meet the losses and also the continuing needs of the body for dietary nitrogen. The amount of the latter will be dependent on the magnitude of the protein excretion and can be determined for each particular case.

Edema resulting from a diminished plasma protein level may result also from a restricted protein intake. In malnutrition, when, because of economical or geographical or clinical conditions, the protein of the diet is greatly restricted in quantity, the level of plasma proteins may fall to the edema level. Nutritional edema assumed epidemic proportions in famine areas and in blockaded areas during and after the last World War. Endemic nutritional edema has also been described in this country in regions in which individuals subsist on diets deficient in both protein and calories. Nutritional edema may, obviously, also arise in any chronic clinical condition in which necessary restrictions in diet may lead to hypoproteinemia.

Protein in the Regeneration of Hemoglobin.—A consideration of the rôle of protein in the diet and the requirement for this source of nitrogen is not complete without reference to the suggested function of dietary protein in the normal regeneration of hemoglobin. Although anemia itself appears to have no characteristic primary effect on nitrogen metabolism, the synthesis of new hemoglobin demands amino acids which must be derived from dietary protein or, in the absence of the latter, from the proteins of the plasma and the tissues. This occurs when stimulation of hemoglobin formation is elicited by adequate therapy. An adequate protein intake is therefore highly desirable under these circumstances in order to prevent the loss of body nitrogen. The "extrinsic" factor of Castle which is of etiologic importance in pernicious anemia is apparently dietary protein, inasmuch as the action of the "intrinsic" factor, present in the gastric juice of normal persons, on muscle protein or on beef tissue will lead to the formation of a substance or substances effective in stimulating hemoglobin formation in pernicious anemia patients. Under the stimulus of liver therapy, dietary protein must be simultaneously furnished in order to supply the nitrogen required for hemoglobin synthesis. Dietary protein must also be furnished when an adequate stimulus, *e.g.*, iron in hypochromic anemia, is used to bring about hemoglobin formation. It is also possible that the lack or absence of dietary protein, which would furnish the extrinsic factor, may be a contributing factor to the etiology of the macrocytic anemia of sprue.

Parenteral Intake of Protein.—Before concluding this discussion of the protein requirement, mention should be made of efforts to supply adequate nitrogen to the body by parenteral administration. The above considerations of the needs for dietary protein make it obvious that serious pathological changes may ensue if oral protein intake is limited or prevented because of experimental or clinical circumstances. The problem of parenteral administration of protein is, therefore, a real one and several approaches have been made toward its solution. Elman[10] has demonstrated that it is possible to maintain dogs in nitrogen equilibrium over three-day periods by the intravenous injection of an amino acid hydrolysate of casein supplemented with cystine and tryptophane. Sucrose given orally in physiological saline furnished 50 to 60 Calories per kilo of body weight per day, and a solution containing 10 per cent each of the amino acid mixture and glucose was injected hourly during six to ten hours. Elman and Weiner[11] have reported similar results in patients with good utilization of intravenously administered amino acids. The latter report is the first detailed clinical study of the utilization of parenterally administered nitrogen. Similar utilization of intravenously injected nitrogen has been recently demonstrated by Daft, Robscheit-Robbins and Whipple,[12] who were able to establish a positive nitrogen balance in dogs given a diet supplying only a very limited amount of nitrogen, and injected once or twice daily with plasma secured from healthy donors of the same species. Further confirmation of these findings has been recently reported by Shohl and his colleagues[13, 14] who found utilization of intravenously injected protein digests or of a pure amino acid mixture by normal babies. Similar data have been obtained by Farr and MacFadyen[15] in studies with nephrotic children. In the latter work, no significant immediate increase in the urinary excretion of nonprotein nitrogen, urea plus ammonia nitrogen, nor amino acid nitrogen was observed in four nephrotic children, aged five to seven years, who had received intravenously 5 gm. of an amino acid mixture from enzyme-hydrolyzed casein. It was concluded from this study that the injected amino acid mixture had been used by the patients for nutritional purposes. Altshuler, Hensel and Sahyun[16] have also recently reported the establishment of nitrogen equilibrium in both normal and postoperative patients following the subcutaneous or intravenous injection of a mixture containing all of the essential amino acids in the form of a casein hydrolysate supplemented with tryptophane and cystine.

Summary of Requirements.—To sum up, it may be said that the protein requirement for the maintenance of nitrogen equilibrium in the normal adult is, essentially, a primary requirement for a relatively few amino acids which the organism is incapable of synthesizing and which, therefore, must be supplied in the diet. The efficiency of various proteins in meeting this requirement is dependent on their quality, *i.e.*, on whether they yield on digestion the amino acids which are essential in nutrition. Although a large portion of the protein molecule may be synthesized by the body from nonnitrogenous precursors and ammonia, the construction of the whole is dependent on the dietary supply of the ten amino acids which the organism appears incapable of synthesizing at a rate commensurate with the *requirements for growth.* The actual ability of the body to synthesize any of these essential amino acids, other than arginine, *to any degree* remains to be established. The investigations of Mitchell and his group strongly suggest that the actual dietary protein requirements for *maintenance* may be very small indeed.

Any physiologically normal condition which imposes an increased nitrogen requirement on the organism, *e.g.*, growth, pregnancy, or lactation, must be met by an increased protein intake if destruction of tissue and plasma protein is to be avoided. Similarly, any abnormal circumstance which decreases the quantity of protein available to the body, whether this circumstance be inadequate protein supply, abnormal protein loss, or increased catabolic destruction of protein, will cause an increase in the protein requirement. An adequate supply of protein appears to be of importance also both as an etiologic factor in pernicious anemia and as a necessary substrate under the stimulus of adequate therapy in anemias. Finally, preliminary evidence has been obtained which suggests that parenterally administered nitrogen, derived from protein, may be utilized for physiological purposes. This fact promises to be of considerable clinical importance.

DIGESTION OF PROTEIN

Digestion in the Stomach.—The primary function of digestion is to break down complex, nondiffusible molecules to simple, diffusible compounds and ions. The digestion of protein, in addition to the above process, also serves to destroy the biological specificity of protein. The fundamental changes and agents involved in the digestion of protein in the gastrointestinal tract are adequately treated in any good textbook of physiological chemistry or physiology and it is the aim here to merely summarize the present-day information.

Gastric digestion is concerned primarily with the digestion of protein. The partial disintegration of protein which occurs in the stomach is accomplished by the enzyme pepsin in the presence of hydrochloric acid. Experiments in vitro have recently clearly refuted the commonly taught idea that peptic digestion is capable of splitting proteins only to the proteose or peptone stage. Free amino acids may be liberated from proteins under the influence of relatively lengthy peptic action.[17, 18] However, it is likely that relatively little ingested protein is broken down extensively to free amino acids during gastric digestion in the body in view of the relatively short period during which protein remains in the stomach. Studies of London and his collaborators,[19] with polyfistula dogs from which it was possible to obtain samples of gastro-intestinal contents at various places in the tract, demonstrated that 45 to 70 per cent of the dietary protein was converted to proteose by the time the food leaves the stomach. The amount converted to this stage apparently varied with the type of protein fed, inasmuch as the action of pepsin appeared to be more rapid and profound with some proteins as contrasted to others.

The *function of hydrochloric acid in the stomach* is apparently twofold: 1. It produces a conversion of pepsinogen, the precursor form of the active enzyme, to pepsin. 2. It provides an optimum acidity for peptic action. In view of these functions of the gastric hydrochloric acid, it is not surprising to find that a diminished or total lack of acid secretion will interfere with normal protein digestion and may, indeed, result in an inability to utilize dietary protein. This is seen in experimental or clinical hypoacidity and anacidity. In *achylia gastrica,* the absence of enzyme (pepsin) as well as acid from the gastric contents seriously limits protein digestion in the stomach.

Diminished Gastric Secretion.—Although the digestive secretions of the pancreas and of the small intestine are capable of completely digesting protein which may leave the stomach in unchanged form, a limited or complete lack of normal gastric secretion may be associated with pathological conditions either as possible etiologic factors or as a consequence of the subnormal gastric secretion. Anacidity is a constant phenomenon in pernicious anemia and pepsin is also usually absent in this disease. Table 2 is compiled from the data of Helmer, Fouts and Zerfas[20] and illustrates the variations in gastric juice composition seen in a patient with pernicious anemia. In view of the rôle of the intrinsic factor of gastric juice in the normal regeneration of hemoglobin, the lack of normal gastric secretion, with its attendant lack of normal protein digestion, may well be considered a prime contributing factor in certain anemias. Diminished gastric secretion under other clinical conditions, such as carcinoma of the stomach, chronic gastritis, is a consequence of the disease and not of etiologic importance.

In addition to the enzyme, pepsin, there is present in gastric juice a second proteolytic enzyme, rennin. Chemical evidence is now available establishing the nonidentity of pepsin and rennin, thus terminating a long controversy in the literature. The milk-curdling function of rennin and the suggested mechanism for this phenomenon will be found in the elementary textbooks which give a detailed account of digestion. Rennin is especially abundant in the gastric mucosa of young animals and probably plays a significant rôle in enabling these organisms to utilize ingested milk. Its function in the adult remains obscure, and the necessity of this enzyme

TABLE 2

Some Analyses of the Gastric Juice of One Normal Adult and of One Patient with Pernicious Anemia (Samples Taken at Twenty-minute Intervals Following the Injection of 0.5 Mgm. of Histamine Hydrochloride Subcutaneously)*

Subject	Specimen	pH	Volume	Total Acid per cc.	Total Acid per Specimen	Free Acid per cc.	Free Acid per Specimen	Pepsin	Total Pepsin	Rennin	Total Rennin	Chlorides	Total Chlorides	Phosphorus	Total Phosphorus
			Cc.	Cc. n/100 per cc.	Cc. n/100	Cc. n/100 per cc.	Cc. n/100	Mgm. per cc.	Mgm.	Mgm. per cc.	Mgm.	Mgm. per cc.	Mgm.	Mgm. per cc.	Mgm.
Normal.........	Fasting	4.0	21	1.4	29	.8	17	.6	13	8	168	2.7	59	0.127	2.7
	20-min.	1.4	76	6.7	506	5.2	395	1.4	106	14	1026	3.9	298	0.052	3.9
	40-min.	1.0	61	14.9	909	10.9	665	1.8	110	17	1037	5.4	326	0.020	1.3
	60-min.	1.2	45	11.7	525	8.7	392	1.3	59	10	450	3.6	164	0.038	1.7
	80-min.	1.4	23	6.1	140	5.1	117	.9	21	8	188	3.1	70	0.67	1.6
Pernicious anemia.	Fasting	8.2	37	0.0	0	0	0	0.04	1.4	Tr.	.....	2.7	100	0.15	5.4
	20-min.	8.4	83	0.0	0	0	0	0.01	0.8	Tr.	.....	1.8	150	0.11	9.1
	40-min.	8.6	62	0.0	0	0	0	0.00	0.0	0	.....	1.7	107	0.10	6.2
	60-min.	8.4	48	0.0	0	0	0	0.00	0.0	Tr.	.....	1.4	66	0.13	6.2
	80-min.	8.4	26	0.0	0	0	0	0.00	0.0	0	.....	1.0	26	0.14	3.5

* From Helmer, O. M., Fouts, P. J., and Zerfas, L. G., J. Clin. Investigation, 11: 1129, 1932.

for normal physiological functioning is questionable in view of the power-ful milk-curdling activity of pancreatic trypsin and trypsinogen.

Digestion in the Intestine.—The digestion of protein and of protein split products in the intestine is accomplished by the *proteolytic enzymes* of the pancreatic juice and of the intestinal juice.

Three proteolytic enzymes are present in the *pancreatic juice*: trypsin, chymotrypsin, and carboxypolypeptidase. The first two are secreted in their inactive forms as trypsinogen and chymotrypsinogen. Enterokinase, an enzyme of intestinal juice, activates trypsinogen; the trypsin thus formed in turn activates more trypsinogen, as well as chymotrypsinogen. Both enzymes act on native proteins, forming proteoses, peptones, and polypeptides, and, if enzymatic action proceeds long enough, are capable of liberating free amino acids from native protein. Both enzymes are also capable of clotting milk. Carboxypolypeptidase, of pancreatic juice, splits polypeptides to simpler peptides and amino acids.

The chief proteolytic enzymes of *intestinal juice* are aminopolypeptidase and dipeptidase. These enzymes were formerly called "erepsin" and the latter was considered a single enzyme until more recent studies demon-strated its dual nature. These two enzymes together are capable of hy-drolyzing polypeptides to amino acids.

Investigations[19] with polyfistula dogs permit the following conclusions regarding protein digestion in the intestine: 1. Trypsin works more rapidly and more completely if preceded by pepsin. 2. The final products of in-testinal digestion of protein are the amino acids; the latter are absorbed almost as rapidly as they are liberated.

Inasmuch as the pancreatic proteolytic enzymes play an important rôle in the digestion of protein, it is obvious that the exclusion of pancreatic juice from the intestine may result in a marked impairment in the digestion of this foodstuff. Extensive destruction of the pancreas or obstruction of the pancreatic ducts may prevent pancreatic juice from reaching the duo-denum, and under these circumstances a considerable portion of the protein of the diet is not digested and will appear in the stool.

ABSORPTION OF PRODUCTS OF PROTEIN DIGESTION

Under normal conditions, there is no absorption of protein digestion products from the stomach. Absorption takes place principally from the small intestine, and the chief products of protein digestion normally ab-sorbed are the amino acids. These enter the portal blood for the most part; to a lesser extent absorbed amino acids may pass into the lymph of the thoracic duct. The rate of absorption of the individual amino acids varies according to the particular amino acid. Quantitative data for some amino acid absorption rates have been obtained in the white rat and, in general, the average rate appears to be approximately 50 mg. of amino acid absorbed per 100 gm. of rat per hour.

Although the amino acids are the chief protein split products to be absorbed under normal conditions, there is adequate experimental and clinical evidence available to demonstrate the absorption, in relatively small quantities, of larger protein split products and also, under certain circum-stances, of native protein. London and Kotschneff,[21] by application of the angiostomy technique in dogs, have clearly demonstrated an increase in the polypeptide concentration of the blood during, and shortly following, a protein meal. These results have been confirmed by other investigators who have examined the absorption of amino acids and other protein digestion products from intestinal loops or segments.

Definite evidence also exists showing the absorption of native protein unchanged from the intestine. Ratner and Gruehl,[22] in a rather comprehensive study, found that both mature and young animals can be sensitized and shock produced by the oral administration of proteins. These results are taken to indicate the absorption of unsplit protein from the intestine. Data of this type may explain individual *idiosyncrasies* toward one or another food protein. The poor tolerance often observed in the infant to milk protein may be due to a similar sensitization because of the absorption of native protein. There are many examples of the absorption of native protein from the intestine under what may be termed normal conditions. Several factors, apparently, may influence the extent to which this occurs: the permeability of the intestines (generally greater in the young organism), the activity and efficiency of the digestive enzymes, the nature of the protein ingested, and the extent to which the dietary protein has been denatured or partially hydrolyzed during cooking. Although the absorption of native protein from the intestine may in many instances be of clinical importance, the amino acids remain the major product of protein digestion which is absorbed into the body, and the subsequent discussion of protein metabolism involves, to a considerable degree, a presentation of the fate of the absorbed amino acids.

FATE OF ABSORBED AMINO ACIDS

The amino acids which are absorbed from the intestine may have one or more of several metabolic fates. The latter may be listed as follows:

1. Temporary storage in the tissues which rapidly remove absorbed amino acids from the circulation.

2. Synthesis of absorbed amino acids into new body proteins, such as blood and tissue proteins, or other important nitrogenous substances, *e.g.*, enzymes, protein hormones, simpler nitrogenous extractives of tissue (glutathione, creatine, carnosine, etc.).

3. Deaminized and the nonnitrogenous rest either reaminated or oxidized to supply energy. The amino acids may thus serve as a source of ammonia.

4. Deaminized and the nonnitrogenous residue converted into glucose and stored as glycogen.

5. Deaminized and the nonnitrogenous residue converted to acetoacetic acid.

It is unlikely that each individual amino acid meets only one of the above suggested metabolic fates. Metabolism is in every sense a complex mixture of dynamic processes, and it is probable that no single metabolic reaction occurs in the total absence of the others. Although the absorbed amino acids may simultaneously follow several different metabolic pathways, there are of course *modifying influences*, under normal conditions, which will regulate the course which this metabolism follows. For example, the age of the organism, whether growing or adult, will regulate the extent to which new synthesis of body protein takes place. The amount of other foods in the diet, and the calorific supply of the diet, will influence the need of the body processes for protein for energy purposes, and will thus determine the quantity of absorbed amino acids which are oxidized. The nature and amount of the dietary protein will also influence the metabolism of the absorbed amino acids, inasmuch as the adaptability of these amino acids for the synthesis of necessary body constituents will be determined by the nature of the absorbed amino acids.

Although in the active metabolism of the organism it is impossible to completely dissect one metabolic reaction away from the others which are simultaneously occurring, for purposes of discussion it will be necessary to consider separately each of the suggested metabolic fates of the absorbed amino acids.

Temporary Storage in the Tissues.—The large body of experimental evidence available from nutrition studies and from studies of nitrogen equilibrium indicates that there is no real storage or deposit of protein in the tissues under normal conditions. This is in contrast with the well-established ability of the organism to store carbohydrate or fat. The fact that certain tissues rapidly take amino acids from the circulating blood was first demonstrated by the studies of Van Slyke and his colleagues. By the introduction and application of the Van Slyke amino nitrogen method for the quantitative determination of amino acids, it was shown that amino acids exist in blood and that their concentration is approximately doubled shortly after the ingestion of a protein meal. It was further found that intravenously injected amino acids disappear rapidly from the circulation with the level of amino acids in the blood returning to normal. For example, Van Slyke and Meyer[23] reported that 5 minutes after injecting 12 gm. of alanine intravenously into a dog, only 1.5 gm. remained in the circulation. This was confirmed with other amino acids, and King and Rapport[24] have more recently demonstrated that 5 gm. of tyrosine injected intravenously into a dog had disappeared from the circulation 5 minutes after the injection.

Van Slyke and Meyer also studied the *relative capacity of the various tissues* to take up administered amino acids by sacrificing the animal and extracting the tissues and organs with boiling water. The amino acid concentration of the extract was then determined. The storage was shown to be a temporary one. The liver appeared to be the first organ to be stocked with amino acids; muscle was next, having somewhat more than half as much amino acid nitrogen as liver after large amounts of amino acids had been injected. Moreover, it was also demonstrated that the liver was not only the first organ to take up amino acids but was also the first to lose them; this loss was accompanied by an increase in the concentration of blood urea. King, Simonds and Aisner,[25] in 1935, demonstrated that intravenously injected tyrosine was also taken up to some extent by the thyroid, the adrenals, and the pancreas.

Synthesis of Absorbed Amino Acids into New Body Protein or Other Nitrogenous Constituents.—The most obvious evidence that absorbed amino acids may be synthesized into new body protein is the phenomenon of growth. The increase in tissue mass necessitates the formation of new cellular protein. Even in the adult organism, the continual wear and tear metabolism involves some destruction of tissue nitrogen constituents, and in the presence of adequate dietary protein there is a replacement of these substances at the expense of the absorbed amino acids. The fact that all of the enzymes which have been studied in detail are proteins, and that many of the hormones, *e.g.*, insulin and the anterior pituitary hormones, are proteins places upon the endocrine glands which synthesize these substances a continual requirement for amino acids for the construction of these hormonal agents. Although it is indeed possible that the building of these compounds may occur from the amino acids derived from the breakdown of tissue proteins, and although in the continual metabolism of the organism it is difficult to distinguish between the amino acids which are absorbed from the intestine and those which are being liberated from tissue protein, the conservation or replacement of the latter can occur only when generous quantities of dietary amino acids are available. It is obvious also, as has already been discussed, that the level of dietary protein will in large measure determine the extent of tissue protein breakdown. It follows that under experimental or clinical conditions which impose a restriction of dietary protein, or which arouse an accentuated catabolism of tissue protein, there will be definite restrictions placed upon the extent to which synthesis of new body protein and other nitrogenous constituents is taking place.

The exact factors regulating synthetic processes, in which amino acids represent the building units, are little known at the present time. When the level of plasma proteins falls, it is said that there is a *stimulus* to plasma protein regeneration. After wasting of tissue during disease, or after experimental partial extirpation of an organ, *e.g.*, the liver, rapid regeneration and replacement of the tissue occur. The rate at which this synthesis of new tissue protein may take place is indeed phenomenal. Although the daily growth increment observed in young animals is some gross indication of the rate of protein formation, more striking data have been obtained from an examination of the rate of regeneration of various organs after partial extirpation. The study of Rous and McMaster[26] is one of the most striking observations of regeneration rate of a tissue. These investigators removed approximately 65 to 70 per cent of the total hepatic tissue in young rats (130 to 150 gm. in weight) and found that within nine to twelve days the remaining lobe mass reached the size of the entire original liver. In older animals (300 gm. or more), two-thirds of this degree of regeneration had occurred in twelve days. These data indicate a truly remarkable capacity of the organism to carry forward the synthesis of liver tissue and therefore liver protein. Similar rapid synthesis of liver, and also muscle, proteins has recently been reported by Ussing.[27] The latter maintained rats on a casein hydrolysate prepared so that deuterium (heavy isotope of hydrogen) was present as a "label" in many of the amino acids. The rate of appearance of the deuterium in the liver and muscle proteins of the animals indicated that in the course of three days, 10 per cent of the liver protein and 2.5 per cent of the muscle protein is newly formed.

There is some information available regarding the nature or type of at least one factor contributing toward the stimulation of protein synthesis, but other than this it is not possible to list other specific agents involved, except those which *a priori* seem logically concerned, nor is it possible to begin to discuss *how* these stimulating substances exert their effects. The *growth-promoting hormone of the anterior pituitary* appears logically to be either directly or indirectly concerned with the growth processes, inasmuch as in the absence of this endocrine product somatic growth ceases. The synthesis of new nitrogenous components of body tissue is, therefore, under the influence of this hormone. Replacement therapy with purified growth hormone preparations of the anterior pituitary is successful. Moreover, acceleration of the normal growth rate can be produced in intact animals by the injection of such preparations. *Gigantism* and *acromegaly*, on the one hand, and dwarfism on the other, are clinical manifestations of the overproduction and underproduction, respectively, of the growth hormone of the anterior pituitary gland. The exact mechanism by which this hormone exerts its influence on protein synthesis remains obscure. Whether this agent acts directly on suitable mixtures of amino acids in various places in the body and causes a spontaneous formation of new protein units, whether the growth hormone acts through an agent mediating synthesis and destruction of cellular protein, *e.g.*, the intracellular proteolytic enzymes, or whether the growth hormone acts indirectly by stimulating an organ or tissue to liberate some unknown catalyst which regulates protein synthesis, remain unsolved problems in protein metabolism. It is significant that the major portion of the information available regarding protein metabolism is concerned with the catabolism of protein, whereas protein anabolism remains, for the most part, the more difficult to explore and hence the least understood. A review dealing with the synthesis of protein in vivo has been recently prepared by Alcock (see list of review articles at end of chapter).

Plasma Proteins—Their Synthesis.—A portion of the absorbed amino acids may be utilized for the synthesis or regeneration of plasma proteins. Although the mechanism of this process, like that concerned with protein synthesis in vivo, is little understood, recent data have been made available regarding the factors influencing this synthesis.

It is not the purpose of the present discussion to consider the controversial problem of whether the plasma proteins are individual and characteristic components of the plasma or whether total plasma protein is a loosely aggregated mass, consisting of reversibly dissociable components which under the influence of certain experimental conditions may be separated into the plasma protein preparations described in textbooks. The bulk of the experimental and clinical evidence indicates that the plasma contains, under normal conditions, five and probably six individual proteins. These are fibrinogen, three globulins, and at least one, and probably two, albumins. The globulins of serum are the classical serum globulin, euglobulin and pseudoglobulin, which as a group are determined together for purposes of clinical diagnosis. More recently, Tiselius[28] in his electrophoretic studies of serum has called the three *globulins of serum* alpha, beta, and gamma globulins, respectively. Antibody formation in experimental animals generally leads to an increase in the gamma globulin component of the serum.[29] The average molecular weight of the serum globulins is approximately 175,000.

Serum albumin has been reported to have a molecular weight of about 70,000. Recently, Hewitt[30] has succeeded in separating highly purified serum albumin, prepared from either horse, ox, rabbit, chicken, or human serum, into two distinct proteins. One of these proteins was named seroglycoid because of its high content (up to 10 per cent) of a trisaccharide.

The other albumin was crystallized and was found to be free of carbo-hydrate. In 1938, Mann and Keilin[31] isolated a copper-containing protein from horse serum; this protein was also obtained from erythrocytes of the ox, the sheep, the horse and the human. The protein contained 0.3 per cent copper and appeared to have no catalytic activity. These same investigators have very recently reported[32] the preparation from blood of a highly purified protein containing 0.33 per cent of zinc. Moreover, this protein is shown to be identical with carbonic anhydrase, the enzyme of great importance in the transport of carbon dioxide in the blood and also re-cently suggested to be concerned with the formation of gastric hydro-chloric acid.[33]

The physiological functions of the plasma proteins and their vari-ations in health and disease can be found elsewhere and are not included in the scope of the present discussion, inasmuch as the latter is concerned with plasma protein formation, or regeneration, as a manifestation of a process dealing with absorbed amino acids and therefore involved in the metabo-lism of these digestion products. Reference is made briefly to clinical and experimental conditions in which variations in plasma proteins are pertinent to the present discussion.

There is rather good experimental and clinical evidence that the liver is the chief site of formation of the plasma proteins. Whipple and his collaborators found that damage to hepatic tissue reduces the fibrinogen content of the blood. McMaster and Drury[34] reported experiments with hepatectomized rabbits which indicated that the liver is concerned with the synthesis of plasma fibrinogen. These investigators subjected hepatec-tomized and normal rabbits to hemorrhages and then studied the rate of fibrinogen regeneration following the reinjection of defibrinated blood. Normal controls showed a 90 per cent regeneration of the removed fibrin-ogen within six hours after injection. Hepatectomized animals manifested only a slight rise in blood fibrinogen in the first four or five hours, pre-sumably derived from a small fibrinogen reserve in the tissues. In these animals, after five hours, the fibrinogen content of the blood fell until death of the animals occurred. In the absence of the liver there appeared to be no power to regenerate fibrinogen.

Whipple and his associates[35] have presented the best experimental evi-dence that the liver is actively concerned with the *fabrication of the total serum protein*. Normal dogs and dogs prepared with Eck fistulas (anas-tomosis of the portal vein and the vena cava, thus diverting from the liver blood draining the intestine; the blood supply of the liver is then wholly arterial) were subjected to low protein diets. A gradual decline in the serum proteins occurred, with the Eck fistula animals having serum protein values rapidly falling to the edema level. The normal dogs appeared more capable of maintaining the concentration of serum proteins above the edema level. Furthermore, the Eck fistula dogs had less than one-tenth the capacity of the normal dog to form new plasma protein when various food proteins were added to the diet.

This experimental evidence is in harmony with the clinical observation that patients with liver disease exhibit a depressed ability to regenerate the plasma proteins. The hypoproteinemia of hepatic cirrhosis is apparently a reflection of the inability of the liver to utilize dietary protein in the presence of an impaired synthetic mechanism for the formation of the proteins of the plasma.

Within the last decade there has been obtained a considerable body of data regarding the influence of diet on the regeneration of plasma proteins and the extent to which this synthesis may be influenced by dietary factors. The extraordinary capacity of the organism to replace the serum albumin lost in *nephritis* and *nephrosis* is seen in patients excreting 10 to 20 gm. of protein daily over a period of several months without appreciable alteration of the serum albumin content. Experimental investigations also point to a rapid regeneration of serum proteins. Elman[36] studied plasma protein regeneration following the intravenous injection of a complete mixture of amino acids in dogs depleted of plasma protein by hemorrhage and fasting; there was evident a responsive synthesis within twenty-four hours following such treatment.

Whipple and his collaborators have standardized the technique of *plasmapheresis* as an experimental approach to problems of plasma protein synthesis. The technic consists in reducing the plasma protein to a very low level by repeated bleeding and simultaneous injection of the washed blood cells suspended in a physiological medium of the type of Locke's solution. Although the regeneration of fibrinogen is a relatively rapid process, resynthesis of the serum proteins under these circumstances appears to take place gradually. Kerr, Hurwitz and Whipple[37] found that following a 50 per cent depletion of the serum proteins, seven to fourteen days were required to restore the lost protein. Regeneration was more rapid on a meat diet than on a protein-free diet, suggesting that absorbed amino acids are readily incorporated into new serum proteins. In the work from Whipple's laboratory,[38] definite differences have been observed among various proteins with respect to their capacity to stimulate serum protein synthesis. Liver protein was particularly good and gelatin very poor. However, the addition of the amino acid, tryptophane, to gelatin diets led to a marked increase of plasma protein.

Weech and Goettsch[39] have employed a different method for testing the potency of foods for serum albumin regeneration. The serum albumin of dogs is depleted by feeding a low protein diet; later, the material to be tested is added to the ration. By this method beef serum proved to be much more effective than beef muscle or casein for serum albumin regeneration. Whipple and his colleagues[40] have very recently studied the ability of individual amino acids, and combinations of amino acids, to stimulate serum protein synthesis. Cystine, tyrosine and tryptophane, administered separately, had little effect. Tyrosine and tryptophane given together also were ineffective. However, if cystine were supplemented by tyrosine or tryptophane or both, 25 to 40 per cent of the combination was converted into plasma protein, an efficiency equalling that of any protein previously tested. Methionine was incapable of substituting for cystine, or phenylalanine for tyrosine. From these data it is concluded that cystine occupies a key position among amino acids in regulating the regeneration of plasma protein.

The experimental conditions, and certain interpretations, of the Whipple work have been questioned by Melnick, Cowgill and Burack.[41] The latter investigators have subjected dogs to plasmapheresis while maintaining the animals on highly purified diets, the nitrogen content of which was care-

4

fully known and controlled. Nitrogen equilibrium was determined through-out the entire experimental period, so that the exact nitrogen turnover of the animals was known. The only variable difficult to control was the small amount of nitrogen which the animals obtained from protein liberated by the limited hemolysis which usually occurred at some stage during the plasmapheresis procedures. It was first demonstrated that fasting animals are able to resynthesize blood proteins and that therefore the products of tissue catabolism can be utilized for the formation of new serum proteins. Moreover, it was found that serum proteins, casein, and lactalbumin, studied singly in the diet, exhibited about the same ability to produce serum pro-tein regeneration after plasmapheresis. This lack of difference among pro-teins was definite and in contrast to the data of the Whipple group. Melnick, Cowgill and Burack concluded that although proteins may vary in their ability to promote nitrogen equilibrium (lactalbumin vs. serum protein), the fact that dietary proteins did not differ widely in their ability to pro-mote serum protein regeneration indicated that ingested protein is not necessarily first transformed into serum protein. Either the end-products of digestion may be synthesized to serum protein in the liver, or the dietary products may be incorporated into tissue proteins which are then the source of the plasma proteins. Conclusive evidence is presented to indicate that tissue protein synthesis may proceed independent of any plasma pro-tein formation as an intermediate. The plasma proteins are certainly not the stock proteins of the body from which nitrogen needs are met.

In summary, it would seem that absorbed amino acids may be synthe-sized in the liver to plasma proteins, or may be transported to the tissues for temporary storage or for synthesis into tissue proteins. Intravenously administered amino acids can apparently also be utilized for both of these functions. Whether individual amino acids may exert a marked effect in influencing the rate or extent of these synthetic processes remains for further experimentation to definitely establish, although nutrition studies and the investigations of Whipple and his group would strongly suggest that this is indeed the case. The exact mechanism of these synthetic proc-esses remains obscure.

CATABOLISM OF AMINO ACIDS

It should be borne in mind that protein metabolism covers a multitude of complex transformations involving eighteen to twenty, or more, dif-ferent chemical substances, the amino acids. Furthermore, these different amino acids are, for the most part, not definitely known to be intercon-vertible in metabolism, and although there are a few metabolic reactions which can be described as common to all amino acids, the changes which they undergo in the body and their functions in fulfilling the body's meta-bolic requirements are in many cases peculiar to the individual amino acids. One is immediately impressed by the remarkable fact that these amino acids, which in the laboratory are ordinarily stable at temperatures of 100 degrees or more Centigrade, are burned to very simple products in the ani-mal organism at 37 degrees Centigrade. It becomes necessary to postulate the action of enzymes which have the capacity of accelerating reactions whereby the atomic affinities of compounds are overcome and degradation ensues.

The various suggested fates of the absorbed amino acids which remain to be discussed are all, initially, catabolic processes. The first of these processes involves the deamination, or removal of the amino groups of the amino acids to be catabolized. Before considering its mechanism and the subsequent fates of the products formed, it is pertinent to discuss first the question of the site of this deamination process.

Site of Deamination of Amino Acids.—It will be recalled from the previous discussion of the work of Van Slyke and Meyer[23] that the *liver* appeared to be the first organ to take up administered amino acids and also the first organ to lose these substances. It was further demonstrated in those studies that the loss of amino acids from the liver was accompanied by an increase in the blood urea. Inasmuch as the latter's formation was known to depend on the available ammonia in the liver, Van Slyke and Meyer concluded that deamination of amino acids occurred chiefly in this organ. This conclusion is supported by a wide variety of evidence which indicates that any impairment of liver function, experimentally or clinically, generally leads to evidence of a diminished rate and extent of amino acid deamination. Lewis and Izume[42] demonstrated that amino acids injected into rabbits with severe liver poisoning, produced by hydrazine, caused an increase in the amino acid nitrogen of the blood and that this value, instead of rapidly returning to normal, remained at a high level. In addition, there was no increase in the blood urea under these experimental conditions. The clinical counterpart of these experiments is seen in patients with severe acute liver atrophy, in whom there is a diminished capacity to convert amino acids to urea.

Perhaps the most striking and conclusive experimental evidence that the liver is the chief site of deamination of amino acids is derived from the experiments of Mann and his co-workers[43] on hepatectomized animals. After complete removal of the liver in the dog, the urea of the blood and urine decrease; injected amino acids remain at a high level with an absence of an increased blood urea. Removal of the kidneys alone in the dog will produce a marked rise in blood urea. However, Mann and his colleagues demonstrated that simultaneous removal of kidneys and liver produced no rise in blood urea. In control animals in which bilateral nephrectomy was performed, the usual marked rise in the blood urea could be checked if the liver was subsequently removed. Some of the data of these experiments are illustrated in figures 12, 13 and 14. It was concluded that in the hepatectomized animal there is a failure of deamination of amino acids and urea formation.

The restriction of the deamination process solely to the liver has been questioned by a number of investigators who have presented evidence which indicates that although the liver may be the chief organ concerned with deamination, other tissues are capable of carrying out this reaction. London and his colleagues,[44] with their angiostomy technique, have obtained evidence suggesting that under normal conditions the intestinal wall is the chief site of deamination of amino acids, and that the kidney is second in importance with respect to this function. Krebs[45] has studied the deamination of amino acids by tissue slices of liver and of kidney in the Warburg apparatus. This investigator has shown that liver and kidney slices will readily deaminate amino acids and that kidney exhibits

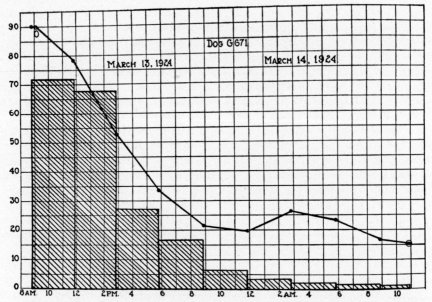

Fig. 12.—Curve showing the decrease in blood urea nitrogen and the decrease in urine urea nitrogen following removal of the liver. The line *O* represents the blood urea nitrogen in milligrams for each liter of blood. The rectangles represent the milligrams of urea nitrogen excreted during each hour of the intervals when urine was collected. (After Bollman, J. L., Mann, F. C., and Magath, T. B., Am. J. Physiol., **69:** 371 (1924).)

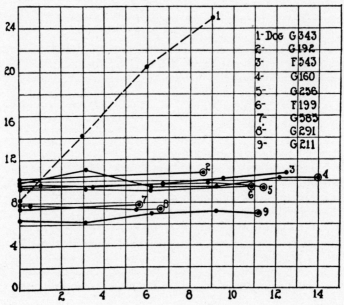

Fig. 13.—Curves showing the constant level of blood urea nitrogen following simultaneous removal of liver and kidneys. Curve *1* represents a similarly treated animal in which the kidneys only were removed. (After Bollman, J. L., Mann, F. C., and Magath, T. B., Am. J. Physiol., **69:** 371 (1924).)

a somewhat greater ability in this respect. It was found that the kidney and liver contain two distinct enzyme systems, one concerned with the deamination of the natural forms of the amino acids, the so-called *l*-isomer, and the other deaminating only the unnatural form, the *d*-isomer. As a matter of fact, kidney slices appeared to deaminate the unnatural isomers of the amino acids more readily than the naturally occurring ones. The ability of the kidney to remove the amino groups of amino acids is of considerable significance in the problem of acid-base balance in the organism, inasmuch as the ammonia formed from this source in the kidney may replace fixed base combined in salts and thus conserve this base to the body.

Recently, several investigators have studied the influence of insulin on the deamination of amino acids by liver slices. In 1937, Bach and Holmes[46] reported that deamination of amino acids by liver slices is diminished 50

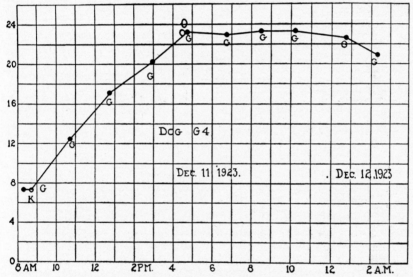

Fig. 14.—Curve showing the increase in blood urea nitrogen following removal of both kidneys at *K*, and the constant level of blood urea nitrogen maintained after removal of the liver at *O*. At points *G*, glucose was injected intravenously. (After Bollman, J. L., Mann, F. C., and Magath, T. B., Am. J. Physiol., **69:** 371 (1924).)

per cent in the presence of insulin. The amino acid studied was *dl*-alanine. This investigation was very striking because in addition to providing the first evidence of an action of insulin in vitro, it suggested one mechanism by which insulin worked in metabolism. Inasmuch as the hormone inhibited deamination of *dl*-alanine, it would therefore inhibit carbohydrate synthesis, since deamination is a prerequisite to the conversion of the glucogenic amino acids to glucose. Insulin was therefore suggested to have a regulatory effect on the processes concerned with the formation of carbohydrate from protein.

The data of Bach and Holmes were so striking that careful repetition of their work was to be expected. Experiments dealing with the problem have been reported by Stadie, Lukens and Zapp[47] in 1940. These workers found that insulin inhibits the deamination of only the *d* (unnatural) isomer of the amino acids, and has no effect whatsoever on the natural isomer. Moreover, the inhibitory effect was demonstrated with nonglycogenic as well as glycogenic amino acids, thus indicating that the hypothesis of Bach and Holmes is much too broad. Stadie, Lukens and Zapp tentatively put forward the suggestion that a possible action of insulin is to regulate protein metabolism by partially inhibiting the oxidative deamination of the d-isomers of amino acids. The exact significance of this observation remains as a matter of conjecture. Although there exists in some tissues a highly active d-deaminase, the rôle, if any, of d-amino acids in the protein metabolism of either the normal or the pathological animal is essentially unknown. The occurrence of the d-isomer in animal tissue has, as yet, not been conclusively demonstrated.

Mechanism of Deamination Reaction—Transamination.—Three simple reactions may be written to describe the mechanism of amino acid deamination. These are:

1. Reductive deamination:

$$R—\underset{\underset{NH_2}{|}}{CH}—COOH + 2H \longrightarrow R—CH_2—COOH + NH_3$$

2. Hydrolytic deamination:

$$R—\underset{\underset{NH_2}{|}}{CH}—COOH + H_2O \longrightarrow R—\underset{\underset{OH}{|}}{CH}—COOH + NH_3$$

3. Oxidative deamination:

$$R—\underset{\underset{NH_2}{|}}{CH}—COOH + O_2 \longrightarrow 2R—\underset{\overset{||}{O}}{C}—COOH + 2NH_3$$

There is little evidence to support the concept of *reductive deamination*, whereas both hydrolytic and oxidative deamination have considerable experimental basis. Of the latter two methods, the *oxidative deamination* reaction appears to be the more usual one. There is both indirect and direct evidence in support of this statement. The indirect evidence is suggested from the fact that ketonic acids are, in general, more readily oxidizable than the hydroxy acids, as revealed by the results of subcutaneous injection and by perfusion experiments with surviving livers. Moreover, keto acids resemble amino acids very strikingly with respect to their behavior in the organism, both in ease of oxidation and in their ability to meet the nutritional requirements of the body. It is true that the corresponding hydroxy acids also function to some extent in meeting nutritional requirements, particularly for growth. The direct evidence of Krebs, however, certainly points to the keto acids as the chief products of deamination, although it should be kept in mind that the relative importance of the keto and hydroxy acids in this respect may vary with different amino acids.

Krebs[45, 48] studied in detail the deamination of amino acids in vitro by kidney tissue. It was demonstrated that the presence of molecular oxygen is essential for the reaction. If the process is prevented from continuing, by poisoning the tissue with cyanide or arsenite, it is possible to show, by actual isolation experiments, the presence of the corresponding keto acid. Quantitatively, two moles of ammonia and two moles of keto acid are formed for each molecule of oxygen consumed by the tissue, thus fulfilling the theoretical requirements of the oxidative deamination equation.

It has always been more or less tacitly assumed that all amino acids in excess of those required for synthetic purposes are deaminized preliminary to the subsequent catabolism of the compounds. In 1939, Bach[49] reported that little, if any, deamination of glycine occurred when this amino acid was incubated with slices of liver, kidney, spleen, diaphragm, or brain of the rat or with tissue extracts. There was also no ammonia or urea formation in Bach's experiments. Whether these data suggest some particular rôle for glycine in metabolism remains to be demonstrated. Glycine metabolism will be considered in detail in a later section.

Intermolecular Transfer of Amino Groups.—Although it was formerly believed that the deamination of amino acids is a reaction catalyzed only by the enzyme, deaminase, recent studies have disclosed another very important mechanism by which keto acids may be formed from amino acids. Braunstein and Kritzmann,[50] in 1937, discovered a process occurring in tissues which they described as an intermolecular transfer of amino groups. The reaction could be demonstrated in muscle, heart, brain, liver, and kidney, and may be represented by the following equation:

$$l(+)\text{glutamic acid} + \text{pyruvic acid} \rightleftarrows \alpha\text{-ketoglutaric acid} + l(+)\text{alanine}$$

Other keto acids were found to act as acceptors of the amino group of glutamic acid. On the other hand, amino acids other than glutamic acid were found to readily give up their amino groups to alpha ketoglutaric acid in the presence of muscle tissue. A year later, Virtanen and Laine[51] showed that the same intermolecular transfer of amino groups occurs in plant tissues. In their early communications, Braunstein and Kritzmann claimed that the transfer of an amino group to alpha ketoglutaric acid with the formation of glutamic acid occurred in the presence of some sixteen different amino acids tested, and that this reaction was therefore a general one. Somewhat later[52] the number of amino acids was limited to fourteen. In addition, these investigators demonstrated that no amino group transfer occurs when both compounds concerned are monocarboxylic acids. Further, ketones, hydroxyketones and aldehydes cannot accept the amino group of glutamic acid. Kritzmann[53] has described a partial purification of the enzyme system concerned with catalyzing the reaction; pigeon breast muscle and pig heart are particularly good sources of the preparations. Braunstein and Kritzmann[54] suggested the term *Umaminierung* to describe the intermolecular transfer of amino groups. This has been accepted with the English equivalent of *transamination*. Braunstein has recently published a review of transamination.[55]

The discovery of the transamination reaction has attracted a considerable amount of attention, inasmuch as it affords a splendid means of explaining the mode of synthesis of many amino acids in vivo; the paucity of our information regarding amino acid and protein synthesis has already been discussed. Moreover, the intermolecular transfer of amino groups also aided in explaining some of the remarkable data which Schoenheimer and his collaborators have obtained by the use of the isotope of nitrogen with atomic mass 15. The importance of these latter investigations warrants their consideration in some detail in the present discussion of deamination and transamination, and the data also have bearing on other aspects of protein metabolism which are to be presented later.

It will be recalled that one of the methods which have been devised for the study of protein metabolism involves the use of isotopes which serve to label particular molecules or substances whose metabolic fate in the organism is to be studied. The concentration of nitrogen of mass 15 in any tissue or fluid is determined by means of a mass spectrograph and the method may be applied to one milligram of nitrogen. The method is sensitive to 0.003 per cent of heavy nitrogen.

Distribution of Heavy Nitrogen After Administration.—Schoenheimer, Ratner and Rittenberg[56] have described the results of a study in which an adult, nongrowing rat in nitrogen balance was kept for ten days on a stock diet to which had been added tyrosine containing 2.04 per cent nitrogen of mass 15. Only about half of the labeled nitrogen was recovered in the urine, while almost all of the remainder was found in the tissues. The liver contained approximately three times as much labeled nitrogen as was found in the proteins of the rest of the body. The distribution of the heavy nitrogen in the tissue proteins was determined, and for the present discussion it is interesting to note that the isotopic nitrogen was found in the alpha amino groups of a number of the amino acids which were isolated. The experiment indicates that in a healthy, nongrowing rat given an ordinary stock diet and kept in nitrogen equilibrium, the nitrogen of at least one dietary amino acid, tyrosine, is only partly excreted in the urine, while most of the remainder is deposited in tissue proteins. An equivalent amount of protein nitrogen is excreted. Only a part of the deposited nitrogen remains attached to the original carbon chain of tyrosine, and a considerable portion of the rest is used for the formation of other nitrogenous compounds, even of such amino acid molecules as were abundant in the diet.

In a later paper, the same investigators[57] have studied the metabolic activity of body proteins, using a preparation of *l*-leucine in which two isotopes, deuterium and heavy nitrogen, had been incorporated. The compound was fed over a period of three days to rats maintained in nitrogen balance. Fifty-seven per cent of the marked nitrogen was found in the body proteins. Some twenty-two different amino acids were isolated from these proteins. Among other data, it was found that the amino nitrogen of all of these amino acids, with the exception of lysine, contained a definite amount of isotopic nitrogen, suggesting the transfer of the amino group of the fed leucine and leading to a distribution of the heavy nitrogen among other amino acids. Apart from leucine, glutamic and aspartic acids had the highest isotope content. Moreover, examination of the ratio of deuterium to isotopic nitrogen in the tissue leucine fractions demonstrated that over one-third of the marked nitrogen of the dietary leucine had been replaced with ordinary nitrogen, indicating that in some process of metabolism the amino group of the leucine fed had been removed and subsequently replaced.

It is striking that in all of the experiments reported by Schoenheimer and his co-workers, relatively large amounts of the heavy nitrogen were found in the glutamic and aspartic acid fractions of the amino acids. This finding might be interpreted in support of the suggested importance of the *dicarboxylic amino acids* in protein metabolism, as indicated particularly by the in vitro work of Braunstein and Kritzmann. This concept is included in the interpretation which Schoenheimer has placed upon the findings of his group. It is believed that continuous chemical processes are occurring extensively in the tissue proteins, even under conditions of nitrogen balance. The dietary nitrogen enters the pool of these spontaneous reactions, which tend to the ultimate replacement of tissue protein nitrogen. There is therefore a continual and dynamic interchange of dietary nitrogen and tissue nitrogen.

Restriction of Transaminating Reaction.—The rather widespread ability of all amino acids to participate in the transamination reaction is not supported by the work of Cohen,[58, 59] who has made careful studies of transamination in pigeon breast muscle and also in systems in which purified extracts of pig heart and fresh pigeon breast muscle served as the sources of the transaminating enzyme. An accurate quantitative method was used for measuring the glutamic acid formed from alpha ketoglutaric acid and the individual amino acids. Cohen studied twenty-one different amino acids and confirmed the findings of Braunstein and Kritzmann with respect to $l(-)$aspartic acid and $l(+)$alanine, both of which were active in forming glutamic acid; $l(+)$valine exhibited a slight activity. None of the other amino acids tested exhibited the transaminating reaction. These data were confirmed by studying the reverse reaction, *i.e.*, the corresponding ketonic acids plus glutamic acid in the presence of the enzyme. Only oxaloacetic acid and pyruvic acid were highly active in the transaminating reaction; the other ketonic acids gave negative results. Cohen postulates three enzyme systems as being involved in the transamination mechanism:

(*a*) glutamic acid $\rightleftarrows$ alpha ketoglutaric acid
(*b*) aspartic acid $\rightleftarrows$ oxaloacetic acid
(*c*) alanine $\rightleftarrows$ pyruvic acid

Combinations of these three systems may bring about the following transaminations:

1. alpha ketoglutaric acid + alanine $\rightleftarrows$ glutamic acid + pyruvic acid
2. alpha ketoglutaric acid + aspartic acid $\rightleftarrows$ glutamic acid + oxaloacetic acid
3. oxaloacetic acid + alanine $\rightleftarrows$ aspartic acid + pyruvic acid

Evidence for reactions 1 and 2 was obtained by Cohen. Attempts to find evidence for reaction 3 were unsuccessful. Cohen has also reported[59] that cysteic acid is capable of participating in the transaminating reaction. The significance of this finding remains obscure, inasmuch as little is known regarding the metabolism of this compound. The behavior of cysteic acid may merely be a manifestation of the fact that it is a dibasic amino acid.

It would seem, therefore, on the basis of these latest data, that the intermolecular exchange of amino groups is not a generalized reaction but rather is limited to a few amino acids. Although the mechanism was attractively suited for a very prominent rôle in intermediary protein metabolism, its limitation to relatively few substrates is somewhat disappointing. It may be pointed out, however, that the substrates of reactions *a* and *b* (above) are known to play important parts in the intermediary catalytic reactions of muscle metabolism. The fact that transamination is concerned with substances involved in catalyzing metabolically important processes would indicate that the rôle of transamination is one of coupling or providing a common source or pathway for these important metabolites, or perhaps regulating the rate or direction of reversible processes with which it may be coupled. Further speculation regarding the rôle of transamination in metabolism must await future experimental work.

Fate of Ammonia Formed by Deamination of Amino Acids.—The chief end-product of protein metabolism in mammals is urea, and the major portion of this is formed in the body from the ammonia which is split off in deamination of amino acids. The evidence which has already been cited to establish the liver as the chief site of deamination may also be interpreted to support the suggestion that the liver is the principal site of urea synthesis in the body. It has already been indicated that the ammonia arising from the deamination of amino acids by kidney tissue may be used by the organism for the conservation of fixed base. The evidence is clear, however, that the ammonia arising in the liver is transformed into urea. The latter substance may perhaps be considered a detoxication product of the metabolic ammonia. Krebs[60] has demonstrated that the addition of most amino acids to rat liver tissue, in vitro, results in a measurable increase in urea formation.

Formation of Metabolic Urea.—The classical mechanism long written for the transformation of ammonia into urea postulated a combination of the ammonia with carbon dioxide to form ammonium carbonate, which, by the loss of one molecule of water, gave ammonium carbamate. The latter, by the loss of a second molecule of water, yielded urea. These reactions may be represented as follows:

$$2NH_3 + CO_2 + H_2O \rightleftarrows \underset{\substack{| \\ ONH_4}}{\overset{\substack{ONH_4 \\ |}}{C=O}} \rightleftarrows \underset{\substack{| \\ NH_2}}{\overset{\substack{ONH_4 \\ |}}{C=O}} \rightleftarrows \underset{\substack{| \\ NH_2}}{\overset{\substack{NH_2 \\ |}}{C=O}}$$

Ammonium   Ammonium   Urea
carbonate   carbamate

Although there is no concrete evidence to disprove the above mechanism as the basis for the formation of a portion of the metabolic urea, recent striking evidence has shown that another series of reactions, leading to the synthesis of urea, occurs under normal physiological conditions.

In 1932, Krebs and Henseleit[61] studied the synthesis of urea from carbon dioxide and ammonia in the presence of surviving tissue slices of rat organs. The *liver* was demonstrated to be the only tissue having a capacity to synthesize urea under these conditions. Ammonium chloride was used as the source of ammonia, a bicarbonate buffer furnished the carbon dioxide, and lactate was added as a source of energy for the reaction. The addition of *ornithine* to the system greatly augmented the urea synthesis. Ornithine apparently acted as a catalyst, since it appeared to be effective only in traces and did not disappear from the reaction mixture. No other substance tested replaced ornithine in stimulating urea synthesis. The addition of citrulline aided the urea synthesis from ammonia, but this action was not truly catalytic, since the citrulline was used up, one nitrogen atom of the latter appearing as urea. These experimental data were explained by the following three reactions:

1. The synthesis of urea follows through the combination of ornithine and carbon dioxide and ammonia to form *citrulline* and *water*:

$$NH_2-CH_2-CH_2-CH_2-CH-COOH + CO_2 + NH_3 \longrightarrow$$

$$\underset{\text{Ornithine}}{\overset{\displaystyle |}{NH_2}}$$

$$\underset{O}{\overset{H}{NH_2-\underset{\|}{C}-N-CH_2-CH_2-CH_2-\underset{\underset{NH_2}{|}}{CH}-COOH} + H_2O}$$

$$\text{Citrulline}$$

2. The second reaction of the urea synthesis postulates the combination of a molecule of citrulline with another molecule of ammonia to form *arginine:*

$$\underset{O}{\overset{H}{NH_2-\underset{\|}{C}-N-CH_2-CH_2-CH_2-\underset{\underset{NH_2}{|}}{CH}-COOH}} + NH_3 \longrightarrow$$

$$\text{Citrulline}$$

$$\underset{\underset{H}{N}}{\overset{H}{NH_2-\underset{\|}{C}-N-CH_2-CH_2-CH_2-\underset{\underset{NH_2}{|}}{CH}-COOH}}$$

$$\text{Arginine}$$

3. The last step involves the hydrolytic splitting of arginine, by the enzyme arginase, into *ornithine* and *urea.* The ornithine is thus available for another cycle:

$$\underset{\underset{NH}{\|}}{NH_2-C-NH-CH_2-CH_2-CH_2-\underset{\underset{NH_2}{|}}{CH}-COOH} \xrightarrow[\text{(Arginase)}]{H_2O}$$

$$\text{Arginine}$$

$$\underset{O}{\overset{}{NH_2-\underset{\|}{C}-NH_2}} + NH_2-CH_2-CH_2-CH_2-\underset{\underset{NH_2}{|}}{CH}-COOH$$

$$\text{Urea} \qquad\qquad\qquad \text{Ornithine}$$

There has been some criticism of the concept of Krebs and Henseleit, chiefly from the laboratory of London and his colleagues.[62, 63] Working with the *angiostomy technique* in dogs, the latter investigators were unable to confirm the findings of Krebs and Henseleit. Little urea formation was observed from arginine, and ornithine injections did not stimulate urea formation. These experiments may, however, be criticized, as may many of London's studies, because the rate of blood flow to and from the liver was not measured and therefore the rate of urea formation is not known. The failure of London and his collaborators to obtain evidence for the marked formation of urea from arginine is also surprising in view of the fact that this reaction has been demonstrated by many investigators using varied methods of experimentation.

The work of Krebs and Henseleit has been confirmed in isolated tissues by Gorter.[64] Probably the most striking confirmation, however, has been obtained by Foster, Schoenheimer and Rittenberg,[65] using isotopic nitrogen. These workers fed two rats on a low protein diet to which ammonium citrate containing labeled nitrogen was added. Arginine was isolated from the liver and was found to contain heavy nitrogen. Moreover, the exact location of the heavy nitrogen in the arginine molecule was established by hydrolysis of the amino acid with alkali into ornithine and ammonia, with a subsequent determination of the heavy nitrogen in each of the products formed. The isotopic nitrogen was found in the ammonia and was entirely absent from the ornithine portion of the arginine. Thus, the isotope had been present in the amidine portion of arginine; this portion of the molecule is liberated as urea by arginase and, according to the theory of Krebs and Henseleit, is potential urea and is involved in urea formation. As administered ammonia is generally converted to urea, this work with isotopic nitrogen is additional and rather striking proof of the Krebs-Henseleit cycle as a mechanism of urea formation from ammonia.

Fate of Deaminized Residue.—The keto acid remaining after deamination may be oxidized to supply energy, may be converted either into glucose (or glycogen) or, if ketogenic, into ketone bodies; or it may be reaminated with the formation of the amino acid. It is also possible that the keto acid may give rise to the corresponding hydroxy acid by a reductive process. The processes concerned with the transformation of the deaminized residue to glucose or to ketone bodies are discussed in the chapter on carbohydrate metabolism. The reamination of the keto acid, with the formation of the amino acid, has already been discussed under the paragraphs dealing with transamination.

The keto (or hydroxy) acids which are formed by the deamination of amino acids are essentially substituted fatty acids, and the detailed catabolism of fatty acids is considered in Chapter IV on Lipid Metabolism. For the straight chain, aliphatic fatty acids, this is apparently a straightforward process with carbon dioxide and water as the end-products of the oxidation. Certain amino acids, however, contain in their structure unusual or particular nuclei which are characteristic of the individual amino acid. The subsequent discussion of amino acid catabolism, therefore, involves a consideration of the oxidation of the aliphatic amino acids, dealt with under lipid metabolism, and a presentation of what is now known of the catabolism of the individual amino acids which, by virtue of their structural configurations, cannot be catabolized directly as fatty acids following their deamination, but which are dealt with by reactions peculiar to the particular amino acid. The first two of these amino acids to be considered are the sulfur-containing amino acids, cystine and methionine. The presence of sulfur in these compounds, and the fact that all of the sulfur of most proteins can be accounted for as cystine and methionine, makes a discussion of the metabolism of these two amino acids essentially a presentation of sulfur metabolism. Only the fundamental aspects of the latter subject will be considered. Detailed reviews are available elsewhere.[66]

SULFUR METABOLISM

THE METABOLISM OF CYSTINE AND METHIONINE

The structural configurations of the amino acids, cystine and methionine, are the following:

$$
\begin{array}{ccc}
\text{S}\!-\!-\!\text{S} & & \text{CH}_3 \\
| \quad\quad | & & | \\
\text{CH}_2 \quad \text{CH}_2 & & \text{S} \\
| \quad\quad | & & | \\
\text{NH}_2\text{CH} \quad \text{HCNH}_2 & & \text{CH}_2 \\
| \quad\quad | & & | \\
\text{COOH} \quad \text{COOH} & & \text{CH}_2 \\
& & | \\
& & \text{CHNH}_2 \\
& & | \\
& & \text{COOH} \\
\text{Cystine} & & \text{Methionine}
\end{array}
$$

In addition to these two sulfur-containing amino acids, several other substances of considerable physiological importance in the organism also contain sulfur. Vitamin B_1 (thiamine), protein hormones, *e.g.*, insulin, anterior pituitary hormones, and the tripeptide glutathione are among the more important of the sulfur-containing compounds. All of the named substances are organic and it is generally true that the metabolism of sulfur is concerned chiefly with the metabolism of organic sulfur. Relatively little is known about the physiological significance of inorganic sulfur and the factors affecting its concentration and distribution. Inorganic sulfur is of particular importance in the form of inorganic sulfate conjugated with other constituents as components of mucoitin and chondroitin sulfuric acids, two prominent constituents of connective tissue. The anticoagulant, *heparin*, has been recently demonstrated to be a mucoitin sulfuric acid compound, in which the presence of inorganic sulfate is apparently an essential factor in delaying the blood-clotting process. Inorganic sulfate also participates in certain detoxication reactions which will be discussed later.

There are other less well-defined sulfur-containing compounds occurring in the organism. Complex lipids have been described in which sulfuric acid is present in esterified form; these have been called *sulfolipids* and *sulfatides*. Thioneine, a sulfur derivative of methylated histidine, occurs in mammalian blood but its significance is unknown.

At the present time it is generally accepted that cystine and methionine account for the total sulfur of proteins. The total sulfur may be low, as in many of the plant proteins, *e.g.*, vicilin (from peas) with a sulfur content of 0.2 per cent, or may be very high in other proteins, *e.g.*, serum albumin, 1.9 per cent and insulin, 3.2 per cent sulfur, respectively. The keratins, proteins of protective tissue, are particularly high in their sulfur content; 4 to 6 per cent of this element is present in human hair.

The distribution of the sulfur of proteins between cystine and methionine varies greatly from protein to protein. The cystine and methionine contents of some proteins are shown in table 3.

TABLE 3

THE CYSTINE AND METHIONINE CONTENTS OF SOME PROTEINS

	Cystine, per cent	Methionine, per cent
Casein	0.3	3.1
Lactalbumin	3.1	2.85
Egg albumin	1.9	5.15
Edestin	1.8	2.20
Insulin	12.5	0.0
Arachin	1.3	0.5
Tobacco mosaic virus protein	0.68	0.0
Fibrin	1.64	2.59
Vitellin	1.20	2.65
Gliadin	2.74	2.03

The nutritive value of various proteins is to a degree determined by the content of the sulfur-containing amino acids. The recent work of Rose has demonstrated that methionine is an essential amino acid and that in the absence of this compound from the diet, normal growth and nutrition are not possible. Cystine, on the other hand, is not an essential amino acid and, as will be discussed later, may be synthesized in the organism from methionine. The addition of cystine to a diet containing suboptimal amounts of methionine greatly improves the nutritive value of that diet.

Distribution of Urinary Sulfur.—The total sulfur of the urine may be partitioned into three chemical types: 1. Inorganic sulfate sulfur, 2. Ethereal sulfate sulfur, and 3. Organic sulfur. The quantitative distribution of the urinary sulfur in human urine, under normal conditions, is shown in table 4.

TABLE 4

DISTRIBUTION OF URINARY SULFUR IN 24-HOUR URINE SPECIMENS OF NORMAL ADULTS*

Sex	Age	Body weight pounds	Total S mgm.	Inorganic Sulfate S		Ethereal Sulfate S		Organic S	
				Mgm.	Per cent of total	Mgm.	Per cent of total	Mgm.	Per cent of total
M......	27	165	757	622	82	55	7	135	18
M......	51	159	711	594	84	46	6	116	16
M......	25	111.5	640	505	79	33	5	135	21
F.....	28	140	621	490	79	32	5	131	21
M......	23	179	680	554	81	32	4	130	20
Average			682	553	81	39	5	129	19

* From Freyberg, R. H., Block, W. D., and Fromer, M. F., J. Clin. Invest., **19**: 423 (1940).

Approximately 80 per cent of the total sulfur excretion is in the form of inorganic sulfates, 5 per cent as ethereal sulfates and 15 to 20 per cent as organic sulfur. The inorganic sulfate sulfur arises from the oxidation of the organic sulfur (cystine and methionine) of proteins and represents, therefore, the end-product of sulfur oxidation in the body.

The ethereal sulfate sulfur fraction of urinary sulfur represents esters of inorganic sulfate and phenolic compounds. The general formula is represented by

$$RO-\underset{\underset{O}{\|}}{\overset{\overset{O}{\|}}{S}}-OH$$

in which the R group may be diversified. *Phenylsulfuric acid* was the first ethereal sulfate compound to be isolated from the urine and represents a conjugation product formed between phenol and inorganic sulfate. *Indican*, the potassium salt of indoxyl sulfuric acid,

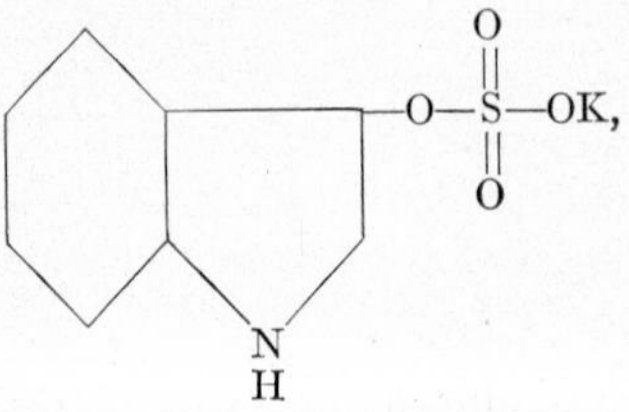

is an ethereal sulfate compound found normally in the urine. The ethereal sulfates are generally considered to be detoxication products, the body utilizing inorganic sulfate to detoxicate phenolic compounds which may be introduced into the organism either normally, from the large intestine, or under experimental or pathological conditions. It has been conclusively demonstrated that the liver is the site of *ethereal sulfate formation*. The rate of excretion of ethereal sulfates, after the administration of a given dose of thymol, has been proposed as a clinical test for liver function.

Very little is known regarding the nature of the compounds which make up the organic sulfur fraction of urinary sulfur. Small amounts of the sulfur-containing amino acids may be excreted unchanged; bile salts, containing *taurine*,

$$\overset{\displaystyle O}{\underset{\displaystyle O}{HO\overset{\|}{\underset{\|}{S}}}}-CH_2-CH_2NH_2,$$

(taurine)

may also be constituents of this fraction. The constancy of the excretion of organic sulfur is striking; the amount in the urine appears to be unaffected by diet and is therefore believed to be of endogenous origin, representing products formed by the constant wear-and-tear metabolism of the body cells.

Catabolism of Cystine.—Despite the fact that it has been recognized for years that cystine is almost completely oxidized to sulfuric acid and the sulfate rapidly eliminated by the kidneys, little is known of the intermediate reactions by which the oxidation to the final product, sulfate sulfur, is accomplished. The *first step* in the catabolism is believed to be the reduction of cystine to cysteine, a reaction which is, incidentally, reversible:

$$
\begin{array}{ccccc}
\text{S}\text{------}\text{S} & & \text{H}_2 & & \text{SH} \\
| \qquad | & & \longrightarrow & & | \\
\text{CH}_2 \quad \text{CH}_2 & & & & \text{CH}_2 \\
| \qquad | & & & & | \\
\text{NH}_2\text{CH} \quad \text{HCNH}_2 & & \text{O}_2 & & \text{HCNH}_2 \\
| \qquad | & & \longleftarrow & & | \\
\text{COOH} \quad \text{COOH} & & & & \text{COOH} \\
\end{array}
$$

Cystine   Cysteine
(disulfide sulfur)   (sulfhydryl sulfur)

The evidence for this metabolic reaction is based principally on the work of Lewis and his students,[66] who have demonstrated that administration of cystine derivatives, in which the amino group is blocked, results in the excretion in the urine of the corresponding sulfhydryl, or cysteine derivative. Inasmuch as the amino group is involved in the next step of cystine catabolism (see below), the evidence seems to warrant the conclusion that if the second step is prevented, one can obtain indication of the first, namely, the reduction of cystine to cysteine.

Data suggesting that deamination of the reduced compound, cysteine, is the *second step* in cystine catabolism are derived from the work of a number of investigators. The introduction of a substituent into the amino group of either cystine or cysteine will partially or completely interfere with the oxidation of the sulfur of the compound to inorganic sulfate. Thus, whereas as much as 80 per cent of the sulfur of cystine and cysteine appears in the urine as inorganic sulfate after administration to experimental animals, somewhat less than half of the total sulfur of cysteine appears as inorganic sulfate when the amino group is substituted by an acetyl radical as in the compound, acetylcysteine. The deamination or second reaction in cystine catabolism may then be represented as follows:

$$\text{HS}\text{—}\underset{\underset{\text{NH}_2}{|}}{\text{CH}_2}\text{—CH—COOH} \longrightarrow \text{HS}\text{—}\underset{\underset{\text{O}}{||}}{\text{CH}_2}\text{—C—COOH} + \text{NH}_3$$

Cysteine   Thiopyruvic acid

The fate of the sulfur-containing keto acid so formed remains unknown at the present time, although its ultimate conversion to inorganic sulfate has already been indicated. The possible conversion of the deaminized rest to either carbohydrate (glucose or glycogen) or acetoacetic acid is considered in the chapter dealing with carbohydrate metabolism.

Although the reactions which have been outlined probably represent the most important pathways involved in cystine catabolism, it should be pointed out that these are not necessarily the only intermediary reactions by which cystine may be converted into inorganic sulfate. Indeed, there is both direct and indirect evidence that oxidation of the sulfur portion of the molecule may occur prior to the deamination reaction. The occurrence of taurine in bile, and its suggested origin via the following reactions which have been accomplished in vitro:[67, 68]

$$\begin{array}{ccc}
\overset{\text{S}\text{——}\text{S}}{\underset{\text{CH}_2 \quad \text{CH}_2}{|\quad\quad|}} & & \\
\underset{\text{NH}_2\text{CH} \quad \text{HCNH}_2}{|\quad\quad\quad|} & \xrightarrow{\text{O}_2} & \text{HO}\text{—}\underset{\underset{\text{O}}{||}}{\overset{\overset{\text{O}}{||}}{\text{S}}}\text{—}\underset{\underset{\text{NH}_2}{|}}{\text{CH}_2}\text{—CH—COOH} & \xrightarrow{-\text{CO}_2} & \text{HOS}\text{—CH}_2\text{—CH}_2\text{—NH}_2 \\
\underset{\text{COOH} \quad \text{COOH}}{|\quad\quad\quad|} & & & & \\
\text{Cystine} & & \text{Cysteic acid} & & \text{Taurine}
\end{array}$$

necessitate the assumption that at least a portion of the cystine molecule is not deaminized. Moreover, recent evidence, which space does not permit the discussion of here, suggests that at least an open mind be held regarding other possible mechanisms for the oxidation of cystine. Enzyme systems capable of effecting an oxidation of the sulfur of cystine have been described.

Catabolism of Methionine.—Shortly after methionine was isolated for the first time from proteins by Mueller[69] in 1922, this investigator demonstrated that the compound was apparently readily oxidized in the body. This work was confirmed in dogs by White and Lewis[70] and by Pirie,[71] and recently Medes[72] has reported that 100 per cent of the sulfur of methionine appears as inorganic sulfate sixteen hours after ingestion by the human. Although methionine may be converted to cystine in the organism (see below), it is not known whether all the methionine metabolized to inorganic sulfate is transformed via cystine as an intermediate.

Deamination is apparently an early and important reaction in methionine catabolism. Virtue and Lewis[73] found that although methionine is readily oxidized in rabbits, the substitution of a benzoyl radical in the amino group of methionine completely prevents the oxidation of the sulfur of the compound. Waelsch and Borek[74] have demonstrated that methionine may be deaminated in the presence of kidney slices with the formation of the keto acid. The latter was isolated from the incubation mixture as a crystalline derivative. It would thus appear that deamination may occur as an early, and perhaps the first, step in the catabolism of methionine.

Although there is not a great amount of evidence regarding the subsequent steps in methionine degradation in the organism, there are some data which indicate that demethylation of methionine may also occur early in its catabolism. The demethylation of methionine has been carried out in vitro and results in the formation of a compound which has been named homocysteine, inasmuch as it represents the next higher homologue of cysteine, i.e., cysteine with an additional CH_2 grouping:

$$CH_3—S—CH_2—CH_2—CH—COOH \xrightarrow{\text{demethylation}} HS—CH_2—CH_2—CH—COOH$$
$$\underset{\text{Methionine}}{\overset{|}{NH_2}} \qquad\qquad\qquad \underset{\text{Homocysteine}}{\overset{|}{NH_2}}$$

The reversibility of this reaction, i.e., the conversion of homocysteine to methionine, has been demonstrated in vivo. Rose and Rice,[75] and duVigneaud and his colleagues[76] have shown that homocystine (or homocysteine) may replace methionine as an essential amino acid for growth purposes only when a source of methyl groups, e.g., the vitamin supplement,[75] or choline or betaine[76] is available in the diet. There is apparently a direct methylation of homocysteine with the formation of methionine. It is reasonable to suppose, therefore, that the reverse reaction, the demethylation of methionine with the formation of homocysteine, occurs normally in the catabolism of methionine. Rather concrete evidence that this demethylation does occur normally in vivo has very recently been presented by duVigneaud and his collaborators.[77] Synthetic methionine was prepared in which the ordinary hydrogen present in the methyl group, attached to the sulfur atom, was replaced by isotopic, or heavy, hydrogen. This compound was then fed to rats over a period of several days. The animals were sacrificed and choline was isolated from the liver tissue and creatine from the muscles. The methyl groups in both choline,

$$HOCH_2—CH_2—\overset{|}{N}—OH$$
$$(CH_3)_3$$

and creatine,

$$\overset{CH_3}{\overset{|}{NH_2—\underset{\underset{H}{\overset{||}{N}}}{C}—N—CH_2COOH,}}$$

were found to contain heavy hydrogen. Apparently, therefore, the methyl group had been removed from the administered methionine in the organism and transferred to other structures for the synthesis of choline and of creatine.

The subsequent step, or steps, between homocysteine and inorganic sulfate, via cystine or cysteine, remain obscure at the present time. On paper at least, this transformation would require the loss of a CH_2 group from either homocysteine or its keto acid. If the latter were involved, reamination would be required for the formation of cysteine, or the keto acid might be directly oxidized under circumstances in which no demand for cysteine synthesis existed. The actual synthesis of cystine from methionine in the organism has been demonstrated in two laboratories. Beach and White,[78] by determining the cystine content of whole rats reared on a diet almost devoid of cystine, showed that the animals accumulated substantially more cystine than could be accounted for by the small amount ingested. That the synthesized cystine actually originates from methionine was shown by Tarver and Schmidt[79] when they fed rats methionine containing radioactive sulfur (S^{35}) and subsequently isolated from the animals cystine containing the radioactive isotope.

SULFUR METABOLISM AND DETOXICATION REACTIONS

No discussion of sulfur metabolism would be complete without mention of the rôle of the sulfur-containing amino acids in the defense mechanisms of the organism. It has already been pointed out that many phenolic compounds are conjugated in the liver with inorganic sulfate and the ethereal sulfate compound excreted in the urine, frequently as the potassium salt. The organic sulfur of the protein serves as a source of the inorganic sulfate required for this detoxication mechanism.

In addition to the involvement of inorganic sulfate in detoxication, the amino acid cysteine is also used as a conjugating agent for certain toxic compounds. The detoxication products formed all have the general formula,

$$R-S-CH_2-CH-COOH,$$

and are termed mercapturic acids. The detoxica-

$$\mathrm{NH-COCH_3}$$

tion of bromobenzene, for example, leads to the formation of p-bromophenylmercapturic acid. Space does not permit a detailed consideration of the information which studies of mercapturic acid formation have yielded regarding sulfur metabolism.[66, 70, 80, 81]

CYSTINURIA

Cystinuria is one of the so-called inborn errors of metabolism. This condition is congenital and is characterized by the constant excretion of abnormally large amounts of the amino acid, cystine, in the urine. The excretion of this sulfur-containing amino acid in an unoxidized form results in a marked change in the distribution of urinary sulfur in a cystinuric individual. There is an increase in the organic sulfur of the urine, because of the excretion of cystine, and this increase is apparently in part at the expense of the inorganic sulfate sulfur. Protein sulfur, instead of appearing entirely in the latter fraction of urinary sulfur, augments to a considerable degree the organic sulfur of the urine. Cystinuria need not necessarily result in any pathological condition. Indeed, cystinuria has been described in individuals who have attained advanced ages, one case being recorded in a woman 87 years old. However, in rather frequent instances difficulties are encountered which are related to the abnormal cystine content of the urine. Cystine is one of the least soluble of the amino acids, and is particularly insoluble at the hydrogen ion concentration of normal urine. In some cases the crystallization of the cystine or precipitation from the urine has resulted in the deposition of *calculi* in the kidney or bladder. In fact, a number of cases of cystinuria have been encountered in patients who have come to operation for bladder and kidney calculi. Tennant, in 1923, reported the removal of fourteen cystine calculi from a young girl. The stones together weighed 73 gm.; one of the calculi had a weight of 50 gm. and on analysis was demonstrated to be practically pure cystine. Striking familial relationships exist among cystinurics.[82]

The interesting metabolic information obtained from studies with cystinuric individuals cannot be considered here because of restriction of space. Lewis[82] has reviewed the subject in detail and more recent references to the experimental investigations of cystinuria will be found in the yearly volumes of the *Annual Review of Biochemistry*. It may be here pointed out that metabolic studies of cystinuric individuals have contributed important information to our knowledge of sulfur metabolism, particularly concerning the metabolism of cystine and methionine. Certain anomalies of sulfur metabolism in cystinuria have now been explained, and the cystinuric patient remains a valuable experimental subject for further studies. It had long been known that the amount of cystine in the urine could be augmented by increasing the protein content of the diet, and it was concluded that the cystine of the protein was not metabolized normally in cystinuria and was excreted unchanged. However, the administration of the free amino acid, cystine, to a cystinuric subject was always followed by complete oxidation of the sulfur. Indeed, cystine isolated from the urine of a cystinuric person could be administered to the same individual with complete oxidation ensuing. This led to the postulation of a difference between protein cystine and the cystine from the urine of the cystinuric patient. It was also suggested that, for some reason, cystine as it existed in combined form in proteins was metabolized differently from free cystine. The discovery of another sulfur-containing amino acid, methionine, greatly aided in clarification and explanation of some experimental facts. Brand and his collaborators[83] have demonstrated that although cystine, administered to a cystinuric, is completely oxidized to inorganic sulfate, methionine given to the same individual resulted in an excretion of extra *cystine*, some 47 per cent of the administered methionine appearing in the form of cystine. Further, *cysteine* in the cystinuric subject also gave rise to extra *cystine*, and lends support to the suggestion that all cystine catabolism does not go via cysteine, since in the cystinuric person these two compounds follow different metabolic pathways. Brand and his co-workers have suggested that since *cysteine* gives rise to extra *cystine* in the cystinuric subject, whereas *administered cystine* is readily oxidized, the fundamental inborn error in cystinuria is concerned with the handling of *cysteine*.

The work of Brand and his group has been confirmed by Lewis, Brown and White.[84] The demonstration that, whereas cystine is completely oxidized in the cystinuric, methionine is excreted in part as cystine, permits ready explanation of the observation that *protein feeding* leads to augmentation of the cystinuria. It is obvious that the increase in cystine has its origin in the methionine present in the dietary protein. The work with cystinurics, therefore, offers further evidence for the metabolic conversion of methionine to cystine. The mechanism of this conversion remains for further experimentation to elucidate.

METABOLISM OF PHENYLALANINE AND TYROSINE

The amino acids, phenylalanine and tyrosine, merit special consideration in a discussion of protein metabolism. The presence in their molecules of the benzene ring, as illustrated by the formulas below,

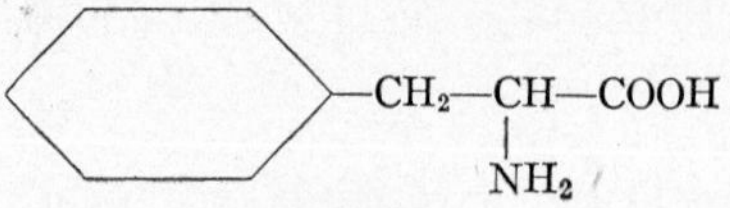

phenylalanine 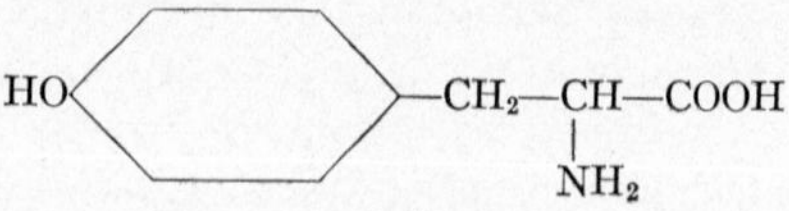   tyrosine

makes the metabolism of this ring of particular interest inasmuch as it is present only in these amino acids and, in a modified form, in tryptophane and in thyroxine.

Phenylalanine and tyrosine appear to be rather widely distributed in proteins. The chemical relationships of their structures to those of the hormone of the adrenal medulla, epinephrine, and to the thyroid hormone, thyroxine, are seen from the following chemical structures of these latter compounds:

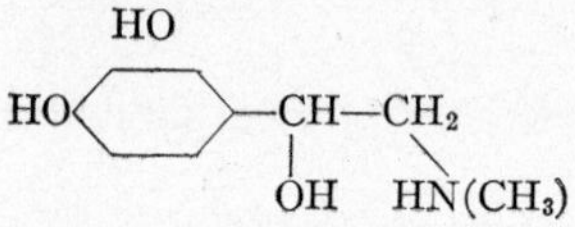

epinephrine 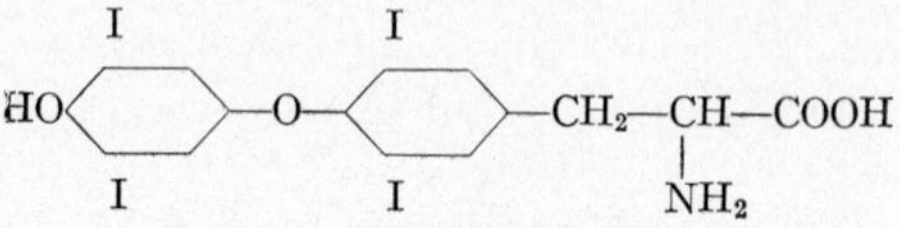   thyroxine

Another derivative of tyrosine which has assumed increased physiological significance within relatively recent times is the substance, diiodotyrosine, which has the following structure:

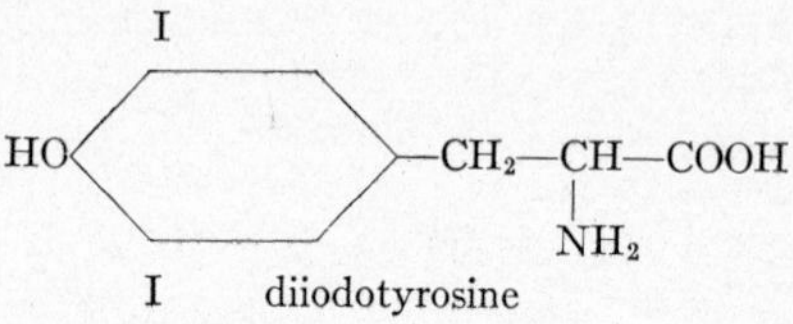

I   diiodotyrosine

A number of physiological functions have been assigned to phenylalanine and tyrosine, some of which are founded on rather suggestive experimental evidence. A derivative of phenylalanine, dihydroxy- or dioxyphenylalanine,

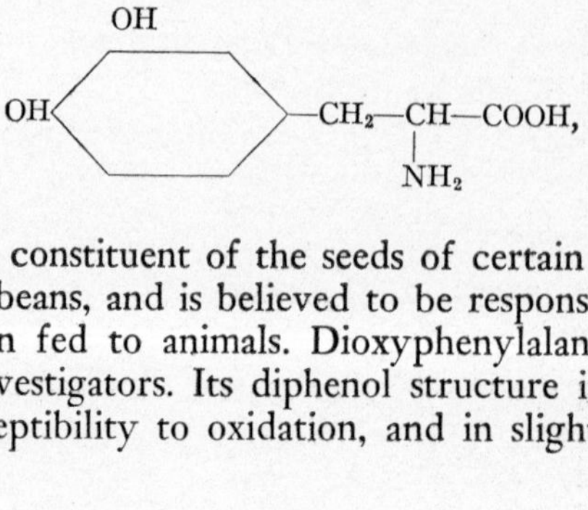

has been found as a constituent of the seeds of certain beans, e.g., Chinese and Georgia velvet beans, and is believed to be responsible for the toxicity of these beans when fed to animals. Dioxyphenylalanine has been called "Dopa" by some investigators. Its diphenol structure imparts to the compound a ready susceptibility to oxidation, and in slightly alkaline solution the substance takes up oxygen from the air and is transformed to a dark pigment. It is interesting that normal skin contains an enzyme which will catalyze the formation of a black pigment from dioxyphenylalanine. It has been claimed, notably by Bloch, that this enzyme is absent in certain diseases in which pigmentation of the skin is lacking, and this author has suggested that dioxyphenylalanine is the normal substrate for skin pigment formation. This viewpoint, however, has been questioned by other investigators.

Tyrosine has also been extensively studied as a precursor of pigment. An enzyme, termed tyrosinase and widely distributed in plant tissue, is capable of catalyzing the transformation of tyrosine into a red pigment. The latter changes spontaneously to a colorless substance which is then immediately, in the presence of air, transformed into a black, melanin-like pigment. The chemical mechanism of these reactions has been studied in detail by Raper and his co-workers[85, 86, 87] and a highly purified preparation of an enzyme catalyzing the oxidation of phenolic substances has recently been prepared by Nelson and his colleagues.[88]

The relationship of diiodotyrosine to thyroxine may be seen from a consideration of their chemical structures, and tyrosine is generally believed to be the precursor of diiodotyrosine in the organism. Recently, rather striking experimental work has supported these suggested relationships. The iodination of casein[89] and of serum proteins[90] produces materials which are capable of inducing a thyroid or thyroxine-like effect in both experimental animals and patients. These artificially iodinated proteins, on hydrolysis, yield thyroxine, which has been identified by its chemical and physiological properties. That this in vitro synthesis occurs via tyrosine and diiodotyrosine is supported by the demonstration that under suitable relatively mild laboratory conditions diiodotyrosine is converted into thyroxine.[91, 92] Diiodotyrosine has also been isolated from thyroid tissue.

Tyrosine appears to be the normal physiological precursors of epinephrine. Recent investigations[93] have shown that kidney tissue slices are capable of decarboxylating tyrosine with the formation of tyramine:

$$\text{HO}\langle\bigcirc\rangle\text{—CH}_2\text{—CH—COOH} \xrightarrow{-CO_2} \text{HO}\langle\bigcirc\rangle\text{—CH}_2\text{—CH}_2\text{—NH}_2$$
$$\qquad\qquad\qquad\underset{\text{NH}_2}{\big|}$$

tyrosine   tyramine

The subsequent reactions concerned in, and the site of formation of, the epinephrine remain unknown, although the final product arises in the adrenal glands.

Catabolism of Phenylalanine and Tyrosine.—The striking phase in the catabolism of these two amino acids appears to be the oxidation of the benzene ring. Unfortunately, little is known at the present time regarding the mechanism by which this is brought about or the nature of the products formed. The first step in the catabolism of phenylalanine appears to be its conversion to tyrosine. The early liver perfusion experiments of Embden demonstrated that the addition of phenylalanine to the perfusion fluid led to the formation of small amounts of tyrosine. Additional evidence that this transformation occurs is seen in the work of Rose, in which it has been demonstrated that phenylalanine can completely meet the requirements of the organism for growth and that tyrosine is a nonessential amino acid. This suggests that the latter amino acid is synthesized from phenylalanine.

Also, in *tyrosinosis* (see below), the administration of phenylalanine leads to an increased excretion of tyrosine. The most convincing proof for the in vivo conversion of phenylalanine to tyrosine is the very recent publication of Moss and Schoenheimer.[94] The latter investigators have prepared a synthetic phenylalanine in which the hydrogen ordinarily present in the benzene ring is replaced by heavy hydrogen, or deuterium. This phenylalanine was then fed to rats for a ten-day period and, subsequently, tyrosine was isolated from the tissue proteins. The tyrosine so obtained was found to contain a rather high proportion of heavy hydrogen, indicating the direct conversion of dietary phenylalanine to tyrosine.

On the other hand, the reverse reaction, *i.e.*, tyrosine to phenylalanine, apparently does not occur to any significant degree. The nutritional requirements for phenylalanine cannot be met by dietary tyrosine. It should also be pointed out that there is no proof that all of the phenylalanine catabolized need first be converted to tyrosine. Indeed, there is some evidence (see below) which strongly suggests that a portion of the phenylalanine and tyrosine being metabolized may follow different metabolic pathways.

The first product formed in the catabolism of phenylalanine is the keto acid, *phenylpyruvic acid*, which would arise from the oxidative deamination of the amino acid:

$$\text{phenylalanine} \quad -CH_2-\underset{\underset{NH_2}{|}}{CH}-COOH \quad \xrightarrow{O_2} \quad -CH_2-\underset{\underset{O}{\|}}{C}-COOH + NH_3 \quad \text{phenylpyruvic acid}$$

The evidence to support the occurrence of this reaction in metabolism is of several types. Krebs[48] demonstrated that the keto acid is formed from phenylalanine in the presence of kidney or liver slices. Lewis and his collaborators[95, 96] have detected the presence of phenylpyruvic acid in the urine of rabbits to which phenylalanine had been administered. Moreover, the amino acid and the keto acid appear to behave similarly in the organism. Phenylpyruvic acid, according to Rose, may replace phenylalanine for nutritive purposes in the rat and the two acids are metabolized in the same manner in the alkaptonuric individual (see below). Phenylpyruvic acid is also excreted in the urine of certain mentally deficient patients (see below), and the amount of the keto acid excreted is increased by the administration of phenylalanine.

Adequate evidence is also available to permit the conclusion that the keto acid corresponding to tyrosine is the first product arising from the catabolism of this amino acid. The excretion of the keto acid, p-hydroxyphenylpyruvic acid, in tyrosinosis (see below) is strongly suggestive of an oxidative deamination as the first step in tyrosine catabolism, particularly since tyrosine feeding in this clinical condition increased the keto acid excretion. Krebs[48] has also demonstrated keto acid formation from tyrosine by surviving tissue slices.

Following the formation of the corresponding keto acids from phenylalanine and tyrosine, there is apparently a splitting out of carbon dioxide with the formation of the corresponding substituted acetic acids:

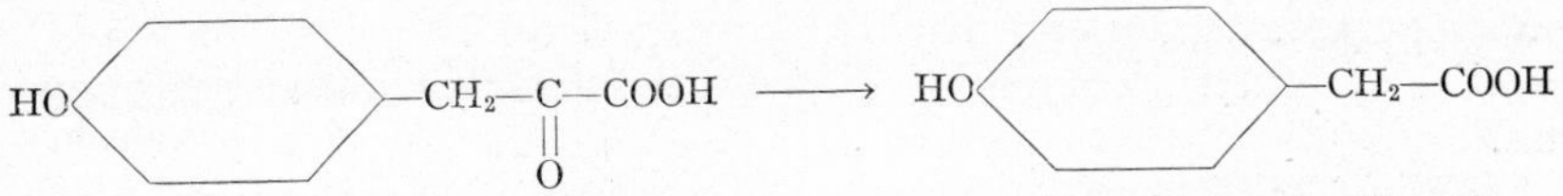

$$HO\langle\bigcirc\rangle-CH_2-\underset{\underset{O}{\|}}{C}-COOH \longrightarrow HO\langle\bigcirc\rangle-CH_2-COOH$$

p-hydroxyphenylpyruvic acid p-hydroxyphenylacetic acid

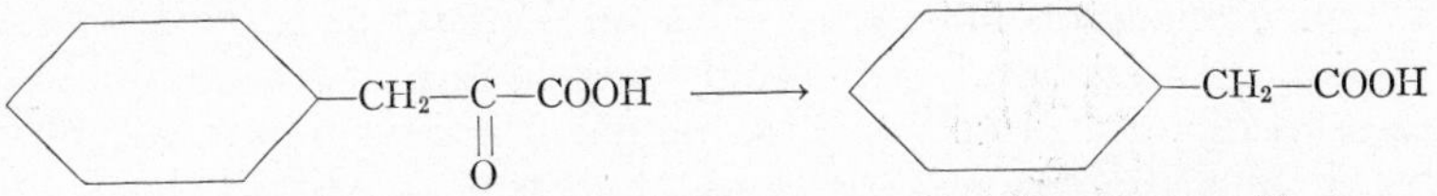

$$\langle\bigcirc\rangle-CH_2-\underset{\underset{O}{\|}}{C}-COOH \longrightarrow \langle\bigcirc\rangle-CH_2-COOH$$

phenylpyruvic acid phenylacetic acid

This metabolic reaction has been demonstrated satisfactorily for phenylalanine. Chandler and Lewis[96] found that the administration of either phenylalanine or phenylpyruvic acid to rabbits led to an excretion of phenylacetic acid in the urine. The intermediate reactions concerned with the further metabolism of the benzine ring are as yet unknown.

ALKAPTONURIA

Alkaptonuria was first described by Bödeker in 1858. The condition is characterized clinically by the excretion of a urine which becomes gradually darker in color on standing and may finally turn black. The deepening of the color will start from the surface of the urine specimen and spread through the volume of fluid, indicating that an oxidation of a constituent present in the urine is responsible for the pigmentation which results. The urine is strongly reducing and gives a violet color with dilute ferric chloride solution. The compound present in alkaptonuric urines which is responsible for these tests has been named homogentisic acid and has the following formula:

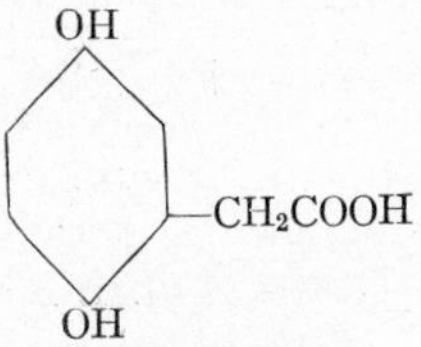

$$\underset{OH}{\overset{OH}{\langle\bigcirc\rangle}}-CH_2COOH$$

homogentisic acid

Somewhat less than 200 cases of alkaptonuria have been reported in the literature, although this number probably does not represent the total incidence. The condition has been termed an inborn error of metabolism inasmuch as it is related to an aberration in the normal picture of tyrosine and phenylalanine metabolism. The disorder shows a definite familial tendency and is inherited as a recessive Mendelian character; it is also apparently congenital.

Although in many instances of alkaptonuria there are no pathological changes present, particularly early in life, in later years abnormal pigmentation of the cartilages, fibro-cartilages, fibrous tissues and tendons may be present (ochronosis).

The metabolic abnormality in alkaptonuria involves phenylalanine and tyrosine. The administration of either of these amino acids, or their corresponding keto acids, to alkaptonuric patients results in a marked increase in homogentisic acid excretion. This is of course also true following the ingestion of proteins containing a high percentage of the aromatic amino acids.

Experimental alkaptonuria has been produced in rats by Papageorge and Lewis[97] by the continued feeding of phenylalanine. This has been confirmed by other investigators. Recently, experimental alkaptonuria has been reported[98] in two other species, the guinea pig and man. When guinea pigs or normal humans were placed on diets deficient in vitamin C and given oral doses of tyrosine, homogentisic acid could be demonstrated in the urine. The administration of vitamin C resulted in a prompt disappearance of the alkaptonuria. This would suggest that the clinical occurrence of alkaptonuria may have a vitamin C deficiency as an etiological factor. However, in one case of clinical alkaptonuria recently studied,[99] administration of vitamin C did not prevent the excretion of homogentisic acid in the urine.

It is not possible to consider here in detail the data concerning tyrosine and phenylalanine metabolism which studies of alkaptonuria have yielded. The subject has been reviewed in detail[100, 101] and more recent developments will be found referred to in the *Annual Review of Biochemistry*.

TYROSINOSIS

Although this condition has been described in only one recorded case, that by Medes[102] in 1932, its rather thorough study by the latter investigator has presented interesting further data on the intermediary metabolism of tyrosine and phenylalanine. Blatherwick[103] has examined 26,000 urines and failed to detect tyrosinosis. The case described by Medes was characterized by the excretion in the urine of the keto acid which normally arises from the oxidative deamination of tyrosine, namely, p-hydroxyphenyl-pyruvic acid. There was as much as 1.6 grams of this compound present in the patient's 24-hour urine sample even though no food was eaten during the period. The metabolic difficulty is apparently related to a failure to carry the catabolism beyond the keto acid stage. Of considerable interest is the fact that when phenylalanine was fed to this patient an increased excretion of tyrosine and of p-hydroxyphenylpyruvic acid occurred, affording further evidence that the transformation of phenylalanine to tyrosine is the first step in the metabolism of the former amino acid. The metabolic difficulty in tyrosinosis would appear to be a failure to convert the p-hydroxyphenylpyruvic acid into the 2,5 dihydroxyphenylpyruvic acid, which has been suggested, chiefly from data obtained in metabolic studies with alkaptonuric subjects, to be the next product formed in the catabolism of the aromatic amino acids.

PHENYLKETONURIA

In 1934, Fölling[104] reported the occurrence of phenylpyruvic acid in the urine of a number of mentally defective patients. This was confirmed by Penrose[105] in England and by Jervis[106] in this country. This impairment of the metabolism of phenylalanine at the stage of phenylpyruvic acid is apparently part of a clinical syndrome which has been designated by a number of names: *imbecillitas phenylpyruvica* (Fölling), *phenylketonuria* (Penrose and Quastel), and *phenylpyruvic oligophrenia* (Jervis). Excretion of phenylpyruvic acid has not been observed in normal individuals. Jervis has reported an incidence of about 0.5 per cent of phenylketonuria in a population of 8,043 inmates of an institution for mental defectives.

Jervis[107] has made a rather complete metabolic study of the condition. The excretion of phenylpyruvic acid was found to be between 1.8 and 2.1 grams daily. The administration of phenylalanine, phenylpyruvic acid, or phenyllactic acid led to an increase in the amount of phenylpyruvic acid excreted. Many other amino acids, including tyrosine, were fed but none augmented the phenylketonuria. It is interesting that here there is an apparent difference in metabolism between phenylalanine and tyrosine. The data suggest that although oxidation of phenylalanine, with the formation first of tyrosine, may be one of the principal metabolic pathways for phenylalanine, there may also occur first an oxidative deamination of phenylalanine, with the formation of phenylpyruvic acid.

In conclusion, a few remarks may be made regarding the most recent contribution to metabolism studies of phenylketonuria. Jervis and his collaborators[108] have reported a very high phenylalanine concentration in both the blood and spinal fluid of sixteen mentally deficient patients who were studied. No phenylpyruvic acid, however, was present. Significant increases in the phenylalanine content of the blood were obtained following the injection of either proteins, phenylalanine, or phenylpyruvic or phenylacetic acids, but again under these circumstances rises in phenylalanine only were demonstrable, with no determinable amounts of the other acids apparent. These observations suggest that the essential biochemical characteristic of the disease consists in a failure of the subject to dispose of phenylalanine at a normal rate rather than in a failure to break down phenylpyruvic acid, as is suggested from the earlier studies. The presence of the ketonic acid in the urine, therefore, is an incidental phenomenon which may be attributed to the active capacity of kidney tissue to deaminize a portion of the blood phenylalanine.

In concluding this discussion on tyrosine and phenylalanine metabolism, it should again be emphasized that all of the tyrosine and phenylalanine metabolized need not necessarily follow the same pathways of metabolism. In recent experiments, Butts, Dunn and Hallman[109] have reported that although tyrosine was not ketolytic in rats and did not increase the liver glycogen of normal, fasted rats, phenylalanine was definitely ketolytic and led to glycogen deposition when given orally to fasted animals. The ketolytic activity of the two amino acids was tested by determining their capacity to decrease the acetonuria produced by feeding sodium butyrate to normal, fasted rats. It would seem, therefore, that although considerable experimental evidence is available from studies of alkaptonuria, from work with phlorhizinized animals, and from investigations with perfused liver, to indicate that tyrosine and phenylalanine follow the same metabolic pathways, work with normal rats suggests that certain differences may exist in the metabolic reactions of these two amino acids. These observations are a re-emphasis of the likelihood that many of the amino acids may not be limited to a single series of metabolic reactions.

METABOLISM OF TRYPTOPHANE

Detailed information regarding the metabolism of tryptophane is lacking, particularly with regard to the fate of the indole nucleus which characterizes the tryptophane molecule. Since tryptophane is the only known naturally occurring amino acid which is an indole derivative, it has been suggested that this compound is of considerable importance in the formation of physiological substances which appear to contain the indole grouping. The rather ill-defined pigments which are grouped under the name of melanins are generally believed to be indole derivatives, and there are some instances where melanin formation may be directly attributed to tryptophane. For example, the black melanin formed during the acid hydrolysis of proteins is known to arise, to a large extent, from the tryptophane present in the protein. The melanin formed by the oxidation of tyrosine in the presence of the enzyme, tyrosinase, is a black substance whose structure has been shown by Raper to be that of an indole derivative. The exact importance of this nucleus in the formation of body pigments remains largely a matter of speculation. *Melanuria*, the term ordinarily used to describe the presence of dark pigment in the urine, may in some cases be caused by the metabolism of indole-containing substances. The extensive breakdown of hemoglobin, for example, may be the cause of a melanuria, inasmuch as the pyrrole rings in hemoglobin represent a portion of the indole nucleus. The relationship of tryptophane and the indole group to pathological formation of melanin, as in melanotic tumors, is not known. Finally, it should be pointed out that the chemical composition of melanins has been demonstrated to vary widely, and the information which is available suggests that most melanins are high molecular weight polymers. Sulfur is generally present in the molecule.

One of the well-established steps in the catabolism of tryptophane appears to be the usual oxidative deamination with the formation of the corresponding keto acid:

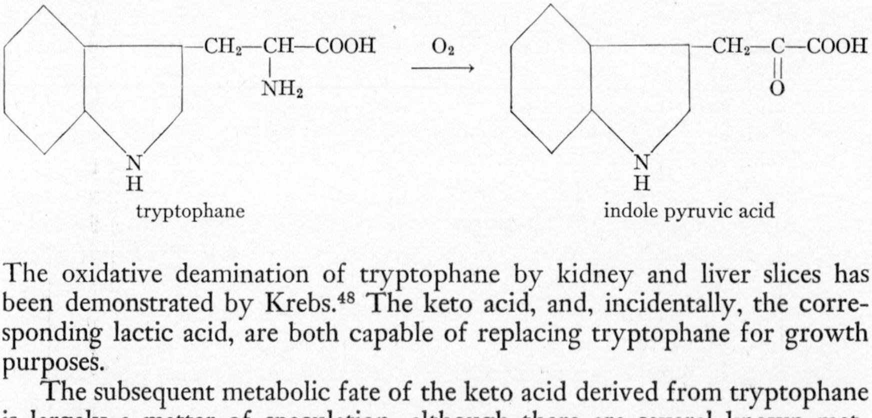

$$\text{tryptophane} \xrightarrow{\text{O}_2} \text{indole pyruvic acid}$$

The oxidative deamination of tryptophane by kidney and liver slices has been demonstrated by Krebs.[48] The keto acid, and, incidentally, the corresponding lactic acid, are both capable of replacing tryptophane for growth purposes.

The subsequent metabolic fate of the keto acid derived from tryptophane is largely a matter of speculation, although there are several known metabolic products which have been described and which are derived from tryptophane and therefore probably from the keto acid formed by the deamination of tryptophane. In 1853, Liebig isolated from the urine of a dog a compound which he named *kynurenic acid* and to which the following structure was assigned:

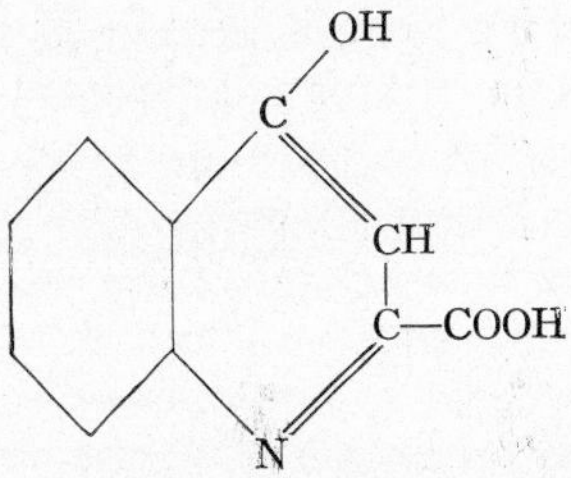

$$\text{OH} \atop \text{C}$$
$$\text{CH}$$
$$\text{C—COOH}$$
$$\text{N}$$

kynurenic acid

This compound has since been described in the urines of a number of species, either as occurring normally or as being excreted after the administration of tryptophane. Kynurenic acid has been found, generally following subcutaneous tryptophane injection, in the urine of the dog, rat, guinea pig, coyote, rabbit, fox, hyena, wolf and badger but is absent from the urine of the cat, the cheetah and several other species, including man, even after the administration of tryptophane.

Ellinger and Matsuoka[110] have suggested the following mechanism to explain the formation of kynurenic acid from tryptophane:

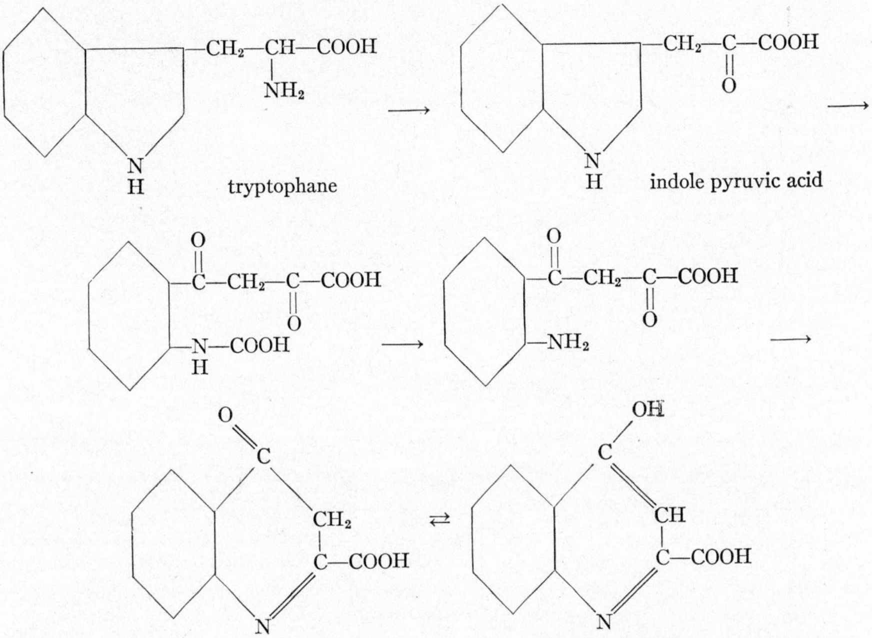

—CH$_2$—CH—COOH
      |
      NH$_2$

N
H   tryptophane   →

—CH$_2$—C—COOH
         ||
         O

N
H   indole pyruvic acid   →

—C—CH$_2$—C—COOH
 || ||
 O   O
—N—COOH
 H   →

—C—CH$_2$—C—COOH
 || ||
 O   O
—NH$_2$ →

O
||
C

CH$_2$
|
C—COOH

N   ⇌

OH
|
C

CH

C—COOH

N

kynurenic acid

Although it is true that indole pyruvic acid behaves like tryptophane in metabolism in that it augments the excretion of kynurenic acid, the remaining intermediary steps proposed by Ellinger and Matsuoka are theoretical and have no available experimental proof. Indeed, in later investigations Matsuoka[111] has suggested another mechanism for the formation of kynurenic acid, largely because he and his collaborators have succeeded in isolating from rabbit urine a compound which appears to be a likely intermediate in kynurenic acid formation from tryptophane. Following the injection of tryptophane into rabbits, there is present in the urine a substance which Matsuoka named *kynurenine*. This compound has the following structure:

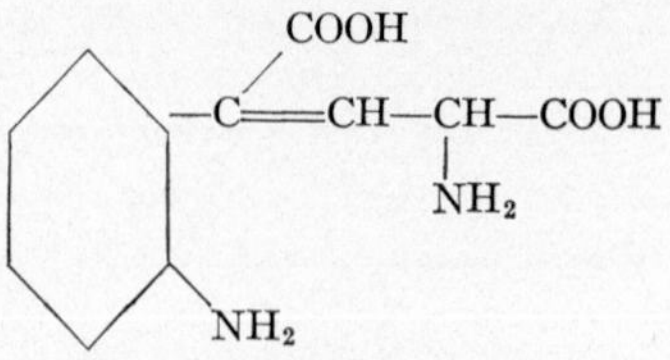

$$\text{—C}=\text{CH—CH—COOH}$$

kynurenine

Kynurenine is converted into kynurenic acid when injected into rabbits. In order to assign a metabolic rôle to kynurenine, a mechanism for tryptophane catabolism has been proposed[112] which does not include oxidative deamination as the first step. The suggested reactions are:

1.

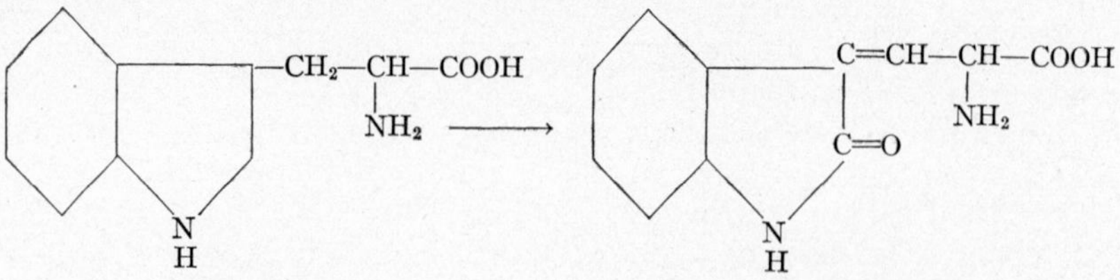

—CH$_2$—CH—COOH ⟶ C=CH—CH—COOH

tryptophane   prokynurenine

2.

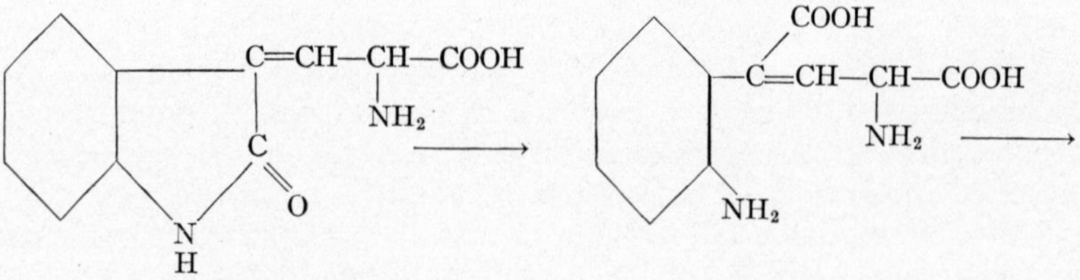

C=CH—CH—COOH ⟶ —C=CH—CH—COOH ⟶

prokynurenine   kynurenine

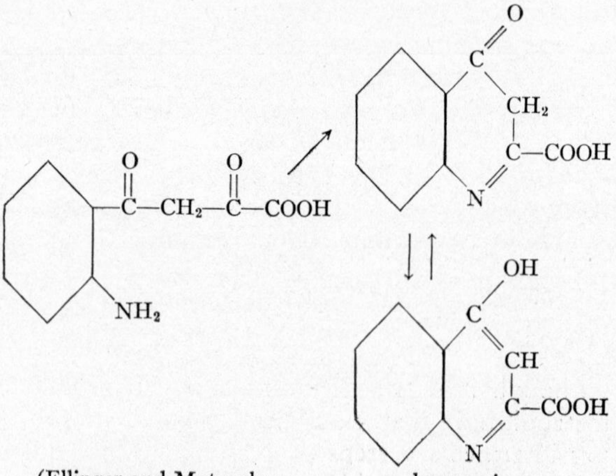

(Ellinger and Matsuoka intermediate)   kynurenic acid

It has been claimed by Kotake and his colleagues that there is present in liver an enzyme which is capable of forming kynurenine from tryptophane. When the extract is boiled, only prokynurenine is formed; therefore the second reaction is enzymatic.

It is still a matter of debate as to whether kynurenic acid is a normal product of the oxidation of tryptophane or is the end-product of a series of side reactions which take place when large amounts of tryptophane must be metabolized, *e.g.*, following injections of considerable quantities of the amino acid. That the latter view is not entirely correct appears evident from the demonstration that ingested kynurenic acid in man is disposed of readily. Either the metabolic degradation of tryptophane differs widely among several species, or there exist several metabolic pathways for the oxidation of this amino acid. The latter possibility has already been pointed out in discussing the metabolic information available for other amino acids.

METABOLISM OF ARGININE

The formula for arginine,

$$\text{NH}_2-\overset{\displaystyle \text{H}}{\underset{\displaystyle \parallel \text{NH}}{\text{C}-\text{N}}}-\text{CH}_2-\text{CH}_2-\text{CH}_2-\underset{\displaystyle \text{NH}_2}{\text{CH}}-\text{COOH},$$

indicates that this amino acid is a guanidine derivative and it is the latter group which is of particular interest in the metabolism of arginine. This amino acid is the only known constituent of proteins which contains a guanido grouping and arginine has therefore been suggested to be the precursor of several naturally-occurring compounds which contain a similar group. The best known of these compounds is creatine, and a great deal of experimental evidence is available to indicate that arginine is a precursor of creatine in the mammalian organism. Some of this evidence will be mentioned specifically in discussing the metabolism of arginine.

Oxidative deamination of arginine with the formation of the corresponding keto acid has been proposed as one of the first steps involved in the metabolism of this amino acid. This oxidative deamination has been demonstrated to occur in surviving tissue slices.[48] The keto acid behaves like arginine in increasing the glycosuria of diabetics and the urinary creatine of patients with muscular dystrophy. This similarity in metabolic behavior of arginine and the keto acid is further evidence that the latter arises early in the catabolism of the amino acid. The subsequent reactions dealing with the catabolism of the keto acid are largely hypothetical and have been described in order to account for the possible formation of creatine from arginine in metabolism. These reactions are as follows:

$$\underset{\text{arginine}}{\text{NH}_2-\overset{\text{H}}{\underset{\overset{\text{N}}{\text{H}}}{\text{C}-\text{N}}}-\text{CH}_2-\text{CH}_2-\text{CH}_2-\underset{\text{NH}_2}{\text{CH}}-\text{COOH}} \longrightarrow \underset{\alpha\text{-keto, }\delta\text{-guanido valeric acid}}{\text{NH}_2-\overset{\text{H}}{\underset{\overset{\text{N}}{\text{H}}}{\text{C}-\text{N}}}-\text{CH}_2-\text{CH}_2-\text{CH}_2-\underset{\text{O}}{\text{C}}-\text{COOH}} \longrightarrow$$

$$\underset{\gamma\text{-guanido butyric acid}}{\text{NH}_2-\overset{\text{H}}{\underset{\overset{\text{N}}{\text{H}}}{\text{C}-\text{N}}}-\text{CH}_2-\text{CH}_2-\text{CH}_2-\text{COOH}} \longrightarrow \underset{\beta\text{-keto, }\gamma\text{-guanido butyric acid}}{\text{NH}_2-\overset{\text{H}}{\underset{\overset{\text{N}}{\text{H}}}{\text{C}-\text{N}}}-\text{CH}_2-\underset{\text{O}}{\text{C}}-\text{CH}_2-\text{COOH}} \overset{\text{H}_2\text{O}}{\longrightarrow}$$

$$\underset{\text{guanidoacetic acid}}{\text{NH}_2-\overset{\text{H}}{\underset{\overset{\text{N}}{\text{H}}}{\text{C}-\text{N}}}-\text{CH}_2-\text{COOH}} + \text{acetic acid}$$

The methylation of the guanidoacetic acid would lead to the formation of creatine:

$$
\begin{array}{c}
CH_3 \\
| \\
NH_2—C—N—CH_2COOH \\
\| \\
N \\
H
\end{array}
$$

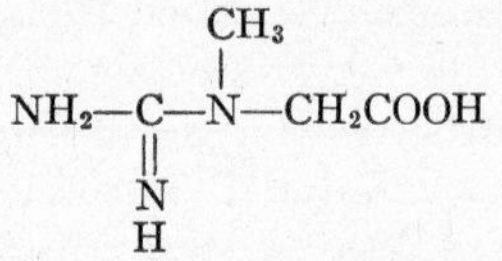

Without discussing the rather suggestive evidence indicating that arginine administration leads to creatine formation in normal metabolism, recent investigations may be cited which demonstrate that arginine does contribute to creatine synthesis in vivo but in a manner differing from that described above. The investigations of Bloch and Schoenheimer,[113] using heavy nitrogen to label administered compounds, have indicated that the carbon skeleton and one nitrogen of the guanidoacetic acid molecule arise in metabolism not from arginine but from glycine. These investigators also demonstrated that arginine furnishes the amidine group of guanidoacetic acid, a finding confirmed by the observation of Borsook and Dubnoff,[114] who have recently reported that the synthesis of guanidoacetic acid from glycine by kidney tissue takes place very rapidly in the presence of arginine. In other words, the amidine grouping of arginine is contributed to glycine, leading to the synthesis of guanidoacetic acid which is then methylated with the formation of creatine. The methyl group may arise from the demethylation of methionine,[77] as previously discussed.

On the basis of this recent work, therefore, it will be seen that the above-postulated reactions (p. 123) for the formation of guanidoacetic acid by the degradation of arginine need no longer be put forward in order to explain the synthesis of creatine from arginine. The carbon chain and one nitrogen atom of creatine are furnished by glycine and arginine contributes only the guanido grouping. The report of Borsook and Dubnoff is of a preliminary nature; it will be of great interest to know the residual product remaining after the removal of the amidine grouping of the arginine molecule. Is the keto acid formed first, prior to the transfer of the amidine group in the transamidation reaction, as it has been termed, or does this reaction take place directly with arginine itself, with a subsequent, and as yet unknown, catabolism of the remaining residue?

Ornithine in Arginine Catabolism.—One other mode of metabolism of arginine has already been considered in the discussion of the rôle of arginine in urea formation in the liver. There is present in mammalian liver an enzyme, arginase, which is capable of hydrolyzing arginine with the formation of urea and ornithine, according to the following reaction:

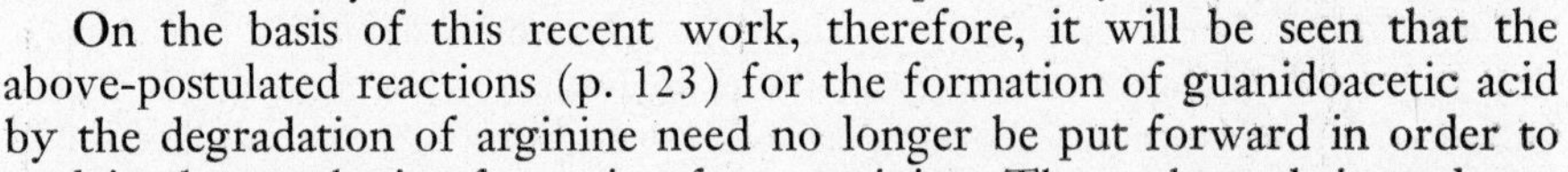

$$
\underset{\text{arginine}}{NH_2—C—N—CH_2—CH_2—CH_2—CH—COOH} \xrightarrow[\text{(arginase)}]{H_2O} \underset{\text{urea}}{NH_2—C—NH_2} + \underset{\text{ornithine}}{NH_2—CH_2—CH_2—CH_2—CH—COOH}
$$

It appears quite likely that in view of the above discussion of the transamidation reaction this hydrolysis by arginase is not the first reaction involved in the metabolism of all the arginine reaching the liver. The arginine escaping hydrolysis in the liver may serve as a creatine precursor in the tissues. Here again it appears that there may be more than one pathway for metabolizing a particular amino acid. The ornithine formed by the action of arginase on arginine is probably subsequently metabolized via an as yet incompletely known series of recently suggested reactions. The participation of a portion of the ornithine in the urea formation cycle mechanism has already been discussed in connection with the problem of the mode of urea formation in the liver. Under these circumstances, it is postulated that ornithine is ultimately reconverted into arginine. Direct evidence for this transformation has recently been furnished by Clutton, Schoenheimer and Rittenberg.[115] Ornithine was prepared in which heavy hydrogen was present as a "label" for the ornithine molecule. This ornithine was administered to normal adult mice on a stock diet. From the body proteins of these animals it was possible to isolate arginine containing heavy hydrogen. Since the deuterium of the fed ornithine was present in a stable position in the carbon chain, it is evident that the carbon skeleton of ornithine may participate in arginine formation.

Ornithine has been demonstrated to give glucose in the phlorhizinized dog but the intermediate stages are unknown. Bach[116] has recently postulated that ornithine may be oxidized in the body to glutamic acid, but has little evidence to support this view. On the other hand, the transformation of ornithine into glutamic acid does seem likely according to another mechanism proposed by Krebs.[117] The latter investigator has shown experimentally that the deaminase system in kidney tissue will act upon the non-natural (d) isomer of ornithine with the formation of α-keto, δ-amino valeric acid:

$$NH_2-CH_2-CH_2-CH_2-\underset{\underset{NH_2}{|}}{CH}-COOH \longrightarrow NH_2-CH_2-CH_2-CH_2-\underset{\underset{O}{||}}{C}-COOH$$

$$\text{ornithine} \qquad\qquad\qquad \text{α-keto, δ-amino valeric acid}$$

This keto acid was then found to be transformed into the amino acid, proline,

$$\begin{array}{ccc} CH_2 & \!\!\!\!\!\!\!\! & \!\!\!\!CH_2 \\ | & & | \\ CH_2 & & CH-COOH \\ & \diagdown \;\; \diagup & \\ & N & \\ & H & \end{array}$$

Very recently, Weil-Malherbe and Krebs[118] have demonstrated the conversion by kidney tissue of proline to α-ketoglutaric acid. The latter is the keto acid arising from the oxidative deamination of glutamic acid. There exists, therefore, a series of reactions by which it is theoretically possible to attain the formation of glutamic acid from ornithine, via proline. The experimental proof of these conversions has very recently been made available from the laboratory of Schoenheimer.[119] From the proteins of mice fed deuterium-containing ornithine, it was possible to isolate glutamic acid and proline, both of which contained deuterium in amounts indicating that a portion of these two amino acids arose from the fed ornithine. This study, together with those cited above,[115-118] offers strong proof for metabolic interrelationships between ornithine, arginine, proline and glutamic acid. The rôle of glutamic acid and its keto acid in the transamination reaction has already been considered in the discussion of the deamination of amino acids. These observations which have been presented are of great importance in that they illustrate pointedly the interrelationships between various amino acids and indicate mechanisms which the organism has available to promote the synthesis of various amino acids from other amino acid precursors.

METABOLISM OF HISTIDINE

The metabolism of histidine is peculiar to this amino acid because, like the other individual amino acids the metabolism of which has been discussed, there is present in the histidine molecule a grouping which is found only in this amino acid, namely, the *imidazole grouping*. Histidine has the following formula

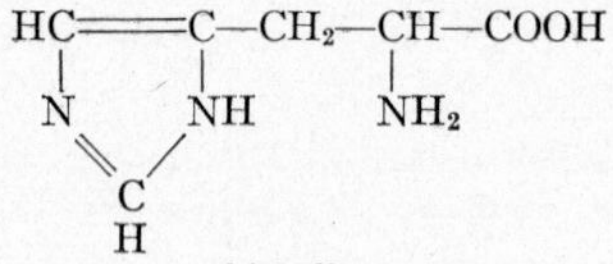

$$HC\!=\!\!=\!\!C\!-\!CH_2\!-\!CH\!-\!COOH$$

$$N \qquad NH \qquad NH_2$$

$$C$$
$$H$$

histidine

and is an amino acid which cannot be synthesized by the organism but must be supplied in the diet for normal growth and well-being.

As in the case of other amino acids, oxidative deamination with the formation of the corresponding keto acid appears to be the first step in the metabolic degradation of histidine. Keto acid formation from histidine occurs in surviving tissue slices.[48] The keto acid and the corresponding hydroxy acid are both capable of replacing histidine for growth purposes, indicating that deamination does normally occur in histidine catabolism and that this process is probably a reversible one. The subsequent steps in histidine catabolism are not well known, although suggestive evidence is available.

The organism apparently has a considerable capacity for metabolizing the imidazole ring of histidine. Leiter[120] has reported experiments in which only traces of unchanged histidine were excreted in the urine of dogs injected intravenously with as much as 5 gm. of the amino acid. The only possible intermediate in histidine metabolism which has been isolated as an excretory product following the injection of large amounts of histidine is the compound, *urocanic acid*, which has the following configuration:

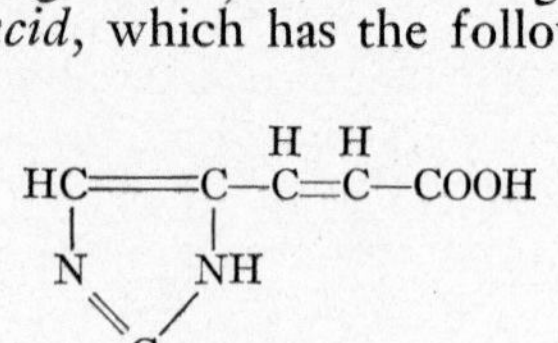

$$\overset{\text{H H}}{HC\!=\!\!=\!\!C\!-\!C\!=\!C\!-\!COOH}$$

$$N \qquad NH$$

$$C$$
$$H$$

urocanic acid

This compound was first isolated by Jaffe in 1874 from the urine of dogs fed dinitrophenol. It was later demonstrated by Raistrick to be formed by the action of *B. coli* on histidine under suitable conditions. This would appear to suggest that urocanic acid is not a normal metabolic product but may originate from bacterial action in the large intestine. More recently,

however, urocanic acid has been isolated from the urine of rabbits following intravenous administration of histidine.[121] The metabolic significance of
urocanic acid remains to be established.

Histidine is generally accepted as being the normal source of purines
in the organism. The structure of the imidazole ring and that of the nucleus
which is the basis of the purines indicate the possible relationship of histidine to *purine formation:*

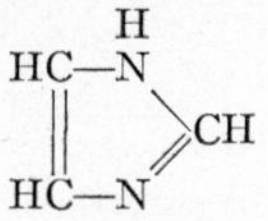

imidazole 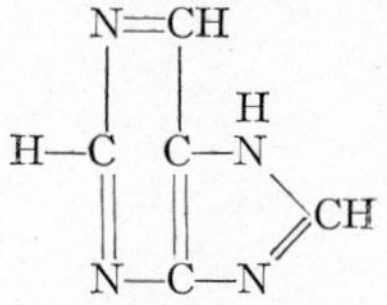   purine ring

In addition to this mere structural similarity, there is experimental evidence
to support this conclusion. The end-product of purine metabolism in rats
and mice is, for the most part, the substance allantoin:

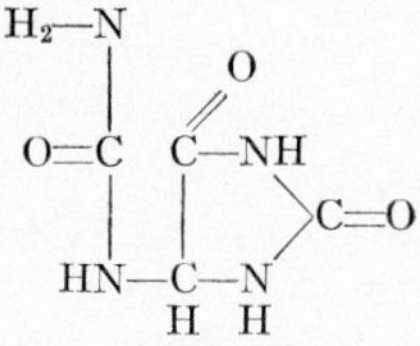

allantoin

Both Hopkins in England, working with mice, and Rose and Cook[122] in
this country, working with rats, have reported that the allantoin excretion
of animals on a histidine free diet is definitely less than that of animals
maintained on a complete diet. Moreover, the addition of histidine to the
histidine deficient diet produced an increased excretion of allantoin. Calvery[123] has studied the histidine content of chick embryos during various
periods of incubation and has reported that the histidine gradually decreases with increasing time of incubation, indicating the use of histidine to synthesize nuclear material of which purines are important components.

In 1930 Edlbacher and his co-workers[124] reported the presence in liver
of an enzyme capable of splitting the imidazole ring of histidine. The
enzyme was named *histidase* and a study of the reaction indicated that
each molecule of histidine was degraded by the enzyme with the formation
of two molecules of ammonia, one molecule of glutamic acid and one
molecule of formic acid. According to this scheme, therefore, histidine becomes concerned in the interrelationships involving glutamic acid which
have already been discussed. The only difficulty with the metabolic fate of
histidine proposed by Edlbacher is the fact that whereas glutamic acid
forms glucose in the phlorhizinized dog, histidine is neither a sugar former
nor ketone body precursor. This evidence is difficult to explain if histidine is normally converted to glutamic acid in metabolism. Again, one is
forced to conclude, assuming the validity of all data which have been as-

5

sembled, that there may be more than one metabolic pathway for histidine.

Histidinuria in Pregnancy.—A rather interesting reported occurrence of histidine in the urine of pregnancy has led to the suggestion of the use of a color test for this amino acid as a diagnosis of pregnancy. In 1930, Voge[125] reported that histidine appeared in the urine in approximately the 5th week of pregnancy, coincident with the appearance of urinary prolan. This observation was confirmed by several investigators and extended greatly by Kapeller-Adler,[126] who has had a great deal of experience with the quantitative colorimetric methods for the determination of histidine. This investigator confirmed the early appearance of histidine in the urine of pregnancy and its immediate disappearance following parturition. The injection of histidine into a pregnant woman resulted in the excretion in the urine of large quantities of the amino acid in an unchanged form. Following delivery of the offspring, the mother was again injected with the same quantity of histidine and complete metabolism of the amino acid occurred, with none appearing in the urine. It was claimed, in later studies by the same investigator,[127] that during pregnancy the histidase of the liver is inhibited by the gonadotropic hormone of the anterior pituitary and this accounts for the excretion of unchanged histidine in the urine. Several other laboratories have reported a good correlation between the urinary histidine test for pregnancy and the well-established Zondek-Aschheim test.

Criticism of the work of Kapeller-Adler has come from the study of Tschopp and Tschopp,[128] who have examined 699 specimens of urine from 300 patients. Histidinuria was found in both males and females, in health and disease. Very recently, Langley[129] has reported a careful evaluation of the urinary histidine excretion, and concludes that while the estimation of histidine in the urine cannot be recommended as a reliable test for pregnancy, it may be a valuable aid in the rapid diagnosis of, or routine testing for, pregnancy. It would appear that while histidine is usually present in the urine of pregnancy, this finding cannot be solely relied upon as diagnostic of this condition. Niendorf[130] from quantitative studies, suggests a normal daily excretion of 300 milligrams of histidine in the urine of the adult.

Origin of Histamine.—The physiologically important substance, histamine, is known to arise normally from histidine in the large intestine when this amino acid is exposed to the action of the bacteria present there. Bacteria capable of splitting carbon dioxide from amino acids are present in the large intestine. The question of whether the histamine normally present in the various organs of the body (lung, liver, muscle, gastric mucosa, etc.) has its origin in the alimentary tract, from which it is absorbed, or is actually formed in the various tissues, is a debatable one. Werle and Krautzun[131] have reported that various animal tissues, notably kidney, have the ability to decarboxylate histidine.

An enzyme capable of destroying histamine, and called *histaminase*, is rather widely distributed in the body, with the notable exception of lung tissue. This may account for the rather striking accumulation of histamine in this tissue.

Before concluding this discussion of histidine metabolism, mention should be made of several normally occurring compounds which appear to be closely related to histidine but whose metabolic significance remains obscure. The compound, *thioneine*, a sulfur imidazole derivative of histidine and having the following structure:

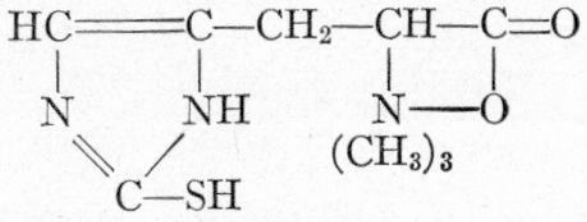

$$HC\!\!=\!\!\!=\!\!C\!-\!CH_2\!-\!CH\!-\!C\!=\!O$$

thioneine

was first isolated from ergot by Tanret in 1909. In 1927 this compound was shown to be a constituent of mammalian blood and its concentration in human blood has been reported as 5 to 10 milligrams per cent. The significance of this compound remains to be established.

Another compound of unknown metabolic significance related to histidine is a dipeptide of beta alanine and histidine. This compound, *carnosine*, is present in mammalian muscle in rather significant concentrations and has the following formula:

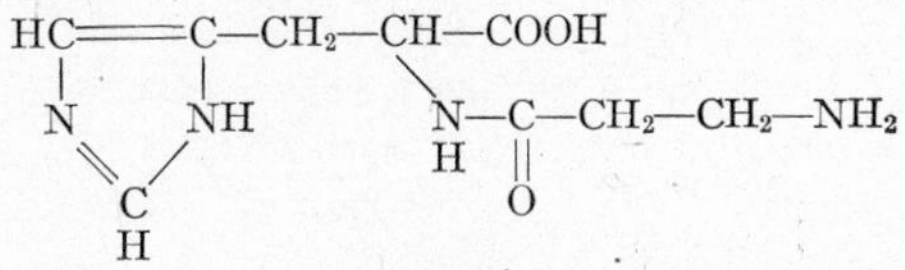

$$HC\!\!=\!\!\!=\!\!C\!-\!CH_2\!-\!CH\!-\!COOH$$

carnosine

The compound has been shown to be pharmacologically active, having a marked depressant action on the blood pressure.

METABOLISM OF LYSINE

There is a singular paucity of information regarding the metabolism of the essential amino acid, lysine. Although the formula of this amino acid, $NH_2\!-\!CH_2\!-\!CH_2\!-\!CH_2\!-\!CH_2\!-\!CH\!-\!COOH$, does not indicate the presence of any particular ring structure whose metabolism might be peculiar, lysine contains a terminal amino group in addition to the usual alpha amino group. In this respect lysine is unlike all the other amino acids which are known to occur in proteins. It is true that ornithine also contains a terminal amino group, but this compound has not been described as a product of the hydrolysis of proteins and may be considered an intermediate in the metabolism of arginine.

Lysine forms neither glucose nor ketone bodies in the phlorhizinized animal. Lysine is not deaminated in vitro by kidney and liver slices.[131a] This observation is in good agreement with animal studies described in the remainder of this section. The data which are available regarding lysine metabolism in vivo point to the extraordinary stability of this amino acid in the body in the sense that it apparently does not participate in the interreactions of the various amino acids, and does not readily lose its theoretically active groups. In the many experiments which have now been reported by Schoenheimer and his co-workers in which isotopic hydrogen and isotopic nitrogen have been administered to experimental animals with a subsequent isolation of the amino acids of the tissues, lysine has been the one amino acid which has not taken up either of the isotopes. It therefore appears that if lysine is deaminated normally in metabolism, the deamination product cannot readily undergo reamination in vivo. In this respect lysine is unique among the amino acids which have been studied. It would almost seem that the lysine synthesized by the plant is used directly for the elaboration of animal protein. Whether absorbed lysine undergoes any metabolic changes whatsoever remains a problem for future investigation. The a-N-methyl derivative of lysine,

$$NH_2—CH_2—CH_2—CH_2—CH_2—CH—COOH,$$
$$|$$
$$NH$$
$$|$$
$$CH_3$$

does not support the growth of animals on lysine deficient diets.[132] This is in contrast to the ability of the N-methyl derivatives of tryptophane,[133] histidine,[134] homocystine,[135] methionine,[135] glycine,[136, 137] cystine,[138] and phenylalanine[139] to replace their respective amino acids for growth or metabolic purposes. In this respect, then, the uniqueness of lysine metabolism finds further emphasis.

SOME ASPECTS OF GLYCINE METABOLISM

Although the comparative simplicity of its structure ($NH_2—CH_2—COOH$) would certainly not suggest any metabolic processes for glycine other than the usual ones described previously for the aliphatic amino acids in general, recent investigations have placed the metabolic pathways of glycine rather in a class by themselves. The chemical nature of glycine does not make it possible to attribute any unusual metabolic behavior of this amino acid to a peculiar type of group in the molecule and must find explanation in some as yet unknown facts.

When glycine is administered to the intact living animal, deamination with the subsequent increased production of urea occurs readily. On the other hand, glycine in vitro appears to be remarkably resistant to deamination. Although in early experiments Krebs[48] observed a slight deamination of glycine when the amino acid was incubated with kidney and liver slices, at a later time Krebs,[45] Bernheim and Bernheim,[140] and Kisch[141] all confirmed the resistance of glycine to deamination and oxidation. Neber[142] has studied the deamination of amino acids by intestinal mucosa and of all the amino acids tested, only glycine alone was not deaminized. In recent experiments, Bach[49] has reported little, if any, deamination of glycine when incubated with slices of kidney, liver, spleen, diaphragm, or brain of the rat or with tissue extracts. There was no ammonia or urea formation under the experimental conditions used. Bach has also perfused cat liver and kidney with glycine and at the end of the experiment all of the glycine was recovered, with no ammonia or urea formation having occurred. Finally, Bach made the interesting observation that glycine apparently had the capacity to combine with oxidizable substances, thus protecting them from oxidation. Pyruvic acid, for example, was found to cause the disappearance of amino nitrogen when incubated with glycine in the presence of kidney slices. Since no ammonia was formed under these conditions, it is strongly indicated that a condensation product of glycine and pyruvate was formed.

The apparent resistance of the amino group of glycine to removal has been indicated in the in vitro studies discussed in the previous paragraph. This evidence does not at first sight appear to be in good agreement with the in vivo study of glycine very recently reported from the laboratory of Schoenheimer.[143] Glycine containing isotopic nitrogen (N^{15}) was added to the food of four adult nongrowing rats ingesting an ordinary stock diet. The retained isotopic nitrogen, amounting to 60 per cent of the quantity fed, was found for the most part in the body proteins. Isolated pure samples of several amino acids (glycine, glutamic acid, aspartic acid, tyrosine, arginine) contained isotopic nitrogen. This indicated, for glycine, a replacement of glycine in protein linkage by the fed glycine. The presence of heavy nitrogen in other amino acids suggests a transfer of the glycine nitrogen to the carbon chain of other amino acids. According to this view, therefore, removal of the amino group of glycine does continually occur during the normal metabolism of this amino acid in the body. Further studies are required to elucidate the reasons for the differences observed in the in vitro and the in vivo studies of glycine metabolism, particularly with respect to the nitrogen of this amino acid. That the data are not entirely incompatible will be seen when it is recalled that Bach[49] in his experiments did observe amino acid nitrogen disappearance although there was no ammonia formation. It may well be that condensation reactions involving glycine first occur, and the subsequent removal of the amino group would not necessarily result in ammonia formation but might, ultimately, cause a metabolic turnover in glycine nitrogen. This would explain the findings of the two types of investigations. It should be kept in mind that the in vitro tissue work involves relatively short-time experiments (several hours) as contrasted to the longer periods (several days) elapsing between the feeding of glycine containing isotopic nitrogen and tissue analysis. Under the latter circumstances many metabolic reactions might take place in vivo which would not be evidenced in the in vitro studies. Certainly active removal of glycine nitrogen must at some time occur in view of the fact that this amino acid is glycogenic.

Other information regarding the metabolic behavior of glycine has been supplied recently in studies from two laboratories. This work has already been referred to in the discussion of arginine metabolism. The investigations of Bloch and Schoenheimer,[118] using heavy nitrogen to label administered compounds, have demonstrated that glycine is the precursor of guanidoacetic acid in metabolism; the latter compound is then methylated with the formation of creatine. It will be recalled that guanidoacetic acid synthesis is accomplished, according to Borsook and Dubnoff,[114] through the transfer of the amidine group of arginine to glycine. It has therefore been clearly established that in metabolism the two-carbon chain and the nitrogen atom of glycine form the basis for the creatine molecule.

Although a portion of the glycine absorbed from the intestine may be transformed into creatine, there is evidence that some of the glycine entering the organism is used for another type of reaction, namely, *detoxication*. Benzoic acid, administered experimentally, entering normally in the food, or perhaps arising metabolically, is to a large extent detoxified by conjugation with glycine and excretion as hippuric acid. This reaction may be illustrated as follows:

$$\text{NH}_2\text{CH}_2\text{COOH} + \langle\text{benzene ring}\rangle\text{—COOH} \rightarrow \langle\text{benzene ring}\rangle\text{—C—N—CH}_2\text{—COOH} + \text{H}_2\text{O}$$

hippuric acid

Glycine may also be used for conjugation with other aromatic acids. This detoxication mechanism may, therefore, be considered as a phase of the metabolism of glycine. Borsook and Dubnoff,[144] in recent in vitro studies, have demonstrated the synthesis of hippuric acid from glycine and benzoate in the presence of slices of liver or kidney. Of the many amino acids and amides tested, twenty-three in all, only glycine led to the formation of hippuric acid under these experimental conditions.

In concluding this discussion of the metabolism of glycine, the last of the individual amino acids whose catabolism is to be considered, it is well to reemphasize two points. In the first place, it is apparent that in many instances an amino acid is metabolized via more than one pathway. In the second place, many interrelationships and, indeed, interconversions exist among the various metabolic pathways of the individual amino acids, and it is these correlations which aid in the visualization of the dynamic conversions and reactions included under the term, metabolism. Moreover, evidence is now available to demonstrate not only metabolic relationships among amino acids, but also the existence of intermediates of amino acid metabolism which are likewise catabolites in intermediary carbohydrate and lipid metabolism. On this basis, therefore, it is possible to integrate the normal metabolism of the three major materials of significance in the living organism, namely, the proteins, the carbohydrates, and the lipids. Indeed, the fact that the products of digestion pass to the liver via the portal circulation serves to eliminate the distinctions which exist between carbohydrate, protein and lipid classifications, inasmuch as many of the intermediary metabolites arising in the liver are common to all three classes of foodstuff. Compounds like pyruvic acid, succinic acid, alpha ketoglutaric acid, and oxaloacetic acid, for example, may be formed from any of the three types of foodstuffs and enter the common metabolic stream.

BIBLIOGRAPHY

Books

Mitchell and Hamilton: Biochemistry of the Amino Acids. 1929. Chemical Catalog Company, Inc., New York.

Cathcart: Physiology of Protein Metabolism. 1921. Longmans-Green & Co., London.

Dakin: Oxidations and Reductions in the Animal Body. 1922. Longmans-Green & Co., London.

Annual Review of Biochemistry (Published yearly). Annual Reviews, Inc., Stanford University, California.

Chittenden: Nutrition of Man. 1907. F. A. Stokes & Co., New York.

Chittenden: Physiological Economy in Nutrition. 1904. F. A. Stokes & Co., New York.

Garrod: Inborn Errors of Metabolism. 2nd Ed., 1923. H. Frowde and Hodder and Stoughton, London.

Warburg: The Metabolism of Tumors. 1930. Constable & Co., Ltd., London.

Hindhede: Protein and Nutrition. 1913. Ewart, Seymour & Co., London.

Peters and Van Slyke: Quantitative Clinical Chemistry, Vol. II: Interpretations. 1931. Williams & Wilkins Co., Baltimore.

Dixon, M.: Manometric Methods. 1934. Cambridge Univ. Press, Cambridge.

REVIEW ARTICLES

Cuthbertson, D. P., Nutrition Abs. & Rev., **10:** 1 (1940). Quality and Quantity of Protein in Relation to Human Health and Disease.

Young, L., Physiol. Rev., **19:** 323 (1939). Detoxication of Carbocyclic Compounds.

Schoenheimer, R., and Rittenberg, D., Physiol. Rev., **20:** 218 (1940). The Study of Intermediary Metabolism of Animals with the Aid of Isotopes.

Van Slyke, D. D., Harvey Lectures, 1915–16, p. 174. The Present Significance of the Amino Acids in Physiology and Pathology. Williams & Wilkins Co., Baltimore.

Mitchell, H. H., Physiol. Rev., **4:** 424 (1924). Nutritive Value of Proteins.

Mitchell, H. H., J. Nutrition, **1:** 275 (1928). Physiological Effects of Proteins.

Thomas, K., J. Nutrition, **2:** 419 (1929). Biological Value and Behavior of Food and Tissue Protein.

London, E. S., Harvey Lectures, 1927–28, p. 208. Experimental Fistulae of Blood Vessels. Williams & Wilkins Co., Baltimore.

Rapport, D., Physiol. Rev., **10:** 349 (1930). The Interconversion of the Major Food-stuffs.

Rose, W. C., Physiol. Rev., **18:** 109 (1938). Nutritive Significance of the Amino Acids.

Alcock, R. S., Physiol. Rev., **16:** 1 (1936). The Synthesis of Proteins *in Vivo*.

Lewis, H. B., Physiol. Rev., **4:** 394 (1924). Sulfur Metabolism.

Lewis, H. B., J. Nutrition, **10:** 99 (1935). The Chief Compounds of Sulfur in Nutrition.

Madden, S. C., and Whipple, G. H., Physiol. Rev., **20:** 194 (1940). Plasma Proteins: Their Source, Production and Utilization.

ORIGINAL ARTICLES

1. Abderhalden, E., Z. physiol. Chem., **96:** 1 (1915).
2. Rose, W. C., and Rice, E. E., Science, **90:** 186 (1939).
3. Nielsen, E. K., and Corley, R. C., Am. J. Physiol., **126:** 223 (1939).
4. Wolf, P. A., and Corley, R. C., Am. J. Physiol., **127:** 589 (1939).
5. Burroughs, E. W., Burroughs, H. S., and Mitchell, H. H., J. Nutrition, **19:** 363 (1940).
6. Burroughs, E. W., Burroughs, H. S., and Mitchell, H. H., J. Nutrition, **19:** 385 (1940).
7. Holt, L. E., and Fales, H. L., Am. J. Dis. Child., **22:** 371 (1921).
8. Harding, V. J., Physiol. Rev., **5:** 279 (1925).
9. Coons, C. M., and Blunt, K., J. Biol. Chem., **86:** 1 (1930).
10. Elman, R., Proc. Soc. Exptl. Biol. Med., **37:** 610 (1937–38).
11. Elman, R., and Weiner, D. O., J. A. M. A., **112:** 796 (1939).
12. Daft, F. S., Robscheit-Robbins, F. S., and Whipple, G. H., J. Biol. Chem., **123:** 87 (1938).
13. Shohl, A. T., Butler, A M., Blackfan, K. D., and MacLachan, E., J. Pediat., **15:** 469 (1939).
14. Shohl, A. T., and Blackfan, K. D., J. Nutrition, **20:** 305 (1940).
15. Farr, L. E., and MacFadyen, D. A., Proc. Soc. Exptl. Biol. Med., **42:** 444 (1939).
16. Altshuler, S. S., Hensel, H. M., and Sahyun, M., Am. J. Med. Sci., **200:** 239 (1940).
17. Calvery, H. O., and Schock, E. D., J. Biol. Chem., **113:** 15 (1936).
18. Damodaran, M., and Krishnan, P. S., Biochem. J., **32:** 1919 (1938).
19. Abderhalden, E., Kantzsch, K., and London, E. S., Z. physiol. Chem., **48:** 549 (1906); Abderhalden, E., Baumann, L., and London, E. S., ibid., **51:** 384 (1907).
20. Helmer, O. M., Fouts, P. J., and Zerfas, L. G., J. Clin. Investigation, **11:** 1129 (1932).
21. London, E. S., and Kotschneff, N., Z. physiol. Chem., **228:** 235 (1934).
22. Ratner, B., and Gruehl, H. L., J. Clin. Investigation, **13:** 517 (1934).
23. Van Slyke, D. D., and Meyer, G. M., J. Biol. Chem., **16:** 197, 213 (1913–14).
24. King, F. B., and Rapport, D., Am. J. Physiol., **103:** 288 (1933).
25. King, F. B., Simonds, R., and Aisner, M., Am. J. Physiol., **110:** 573 (1935).
26. Rous, P., and McMaster, P. D., J. Exp. Med., **39:** 425 (1924).
27. Ussing, H. H., Nature, **142:** 399 (1938).
28. Tiselius, A., Biochem. J., **31:** 1464 (1937).
29. Tiselius, A., and Kabat, E. A., Science, **87:** 416 (1938).
30. Hewitt, L. F., Biochem. J., **31:** 1534 (1937).
31. Mann, T., and Keilin, D., Proc. Roy. Soc. London, Series B, **126:** 303 (1938).

32. Keilin, D., and Mann, T., Biochem. J., **34:** 1163 (1940).
33. Davenport, H. D., and Fisher, R. B., Am. J. Physiol., **131:** 165 (1940).
34. McMaster, P. D., and Drury, D. R., Proc. Soc. Exptl. Biol. Med., **26:** 490 (1928–29).
35. Knutti, R. E., Erickson, C. C., Madden, S. C., Rekers, P. E., and Whipple, G. H., J. Exp. Med., **65:** 455 (1937).
36. Elman, R., Proc. Soc. Exptl. Biol. Med., **36:** 867 (1937).
37. Kerr, W. J., Hurwitz, S. H., and Whipple, G. H., Am. J. Physiol., **47:** 356, 370 (1918–19).
38. Madden, S. C., George, W. E., Waraich, G. S., and Whipple, G. H., J. Exp. Med., **67:** 675 (1938).
39. Weech, A. A., and Goettsch, E., Bull. Johns Hopkins Hosp., **63:** 154, 181 (1938).
40. Madden, S. C., Noehren, W. A., Waraich, G. S., and Whipple, G. H., J. Exp. Med., **69:** 721 (1939).
41. Melnick, D., Cowgill, G. R., and Burack, E., J. Exp. Med., **64:** 897 (1936).
42. Lewis, H. B., and Izume, S., J. Biol. Chem., **71:** 33 (1926–27).
43. Bollman, J. L., Mann, F. C., and Magath, T. B., Am. J. Physiol., **69:** 371 (1924).
44. London, E. S., Dubrusky, A. M., Wassilewskaja, N. L., and Prochorowa, M. J., Z. physiol. Chem., **227:** 223 (1934).
45. Krebs, H. A., Biochem. J., **29:** 1620 (1935).
46. Bach, S. J., and Holmes, E. G., Biochem. J., **31:** 89 (1937).
47. Stadie, W. C., Lukens, F. D. W., and Zapp, J. A., Jr., J. Biol. Chem., **132:** 393 (1940).
48. Krebs, H. A., Klin. Wochschr., **11:** 1744 (1932); Z. physiol. Chem., **217:** 191 (1933).
49. Bach, S. J., Biochem. J., **33:** 90 (1939).
50. Braunstein, A. E., and Kritzmann, M. G., Enzymologia, **2:** 129 (1937–38).
51. Virtanen, A. I., and Laine, T., Nature, **141:** 748 (1938).
52. Braunstein, A. E., and Kritzmann, M. G., Biochimia, Moscow, **3:** 590 (1938).
53. Kritzmann, M. G., Biochimia, Moscow, **3:** 603 (1938).
54. Braunstein, A. E., and Kritzmann, M. G., Nature, **140:** 503 (1937).
55. Braunstein, A. E., Enzymologia, **7:** 25 (1939).
56. Schoenheimer, R., Ratner, S., and Rittenberg, D., J. Biol. Chem., **127:** 333 (1939).
57. Schoenheimer, R., Ratner, S., and Rittenberg, D., J. Biol. Chem., **130:** 703 (1939).
58. Cohen, P. P., Biochem. J., **33:** 1478 (1939).
59. Cohen, P. P., J. Biol. Chem., **136:** 565, 585 (1940).
60. Krebs, H. A., Z. physiol. Chem., **217:** 191 (1933).
61. Krebs, H. A., and Henseleit, K., Z. physiol. Chem., **210:** 33 (1932).
62. London, E. S., Alexandry, A. K., and Nedswedski, S. W., Z. physiol. Chem., **227:** 233 (1934).
63. London, E. S., and Alexandry, A. K., Z. physiol. Chem., **246:** 106 (1937).
64. Gorter, A., Acta Brevia Neerland. Physiol. Pharmacol. Microbiol., **7:** 2/3 (1937).
65. Foster, G. L., Schoenheimer, R., and Rittenberg, D., J. Biol. Chem., **127:** 319 (1939).
66. Lewis, H. B., Physiol. Rev., **4:** 394 (1924); J. Nutrition, **10:** 99 (1935).
67. Friedmann, E., Beitr. Chem. Physiol. Path., **3:** 1 (1903).
68. White, A., and Fishman, J. B., J. Biol. Chem., **116:** 457 (1936).
69. Mueller, J. H., Proc. Soc. Exptl. Biol. Med., **19:** 161 (1921–22); J. Biol. Chem., **56:** 157 (1923); **58:** 373 (1923–24).
70. White, A., and Lewis, H. B., J. Biol. Chem., **98:** 607 (1932).
71. Pirie, N., Biochem. J., **26:** 2041 (1932).
72. Medes, G., Biochem. J., **31:** 1330 (1937).
73. Virtue, R. W., and Lewis, H. B., J. Biol. Chem., **104:** 59 (1934).
74. Waelsch, H., and Borek, E., J. Am. Chem. Soc., **61:** 2252 (1939).
75. Rose, W. C., and Rice, E. E., J. Biol. Chem., **130:** 305 (1939).
76. duVigneaud, V., Chandler, J. P., Moyer, A. W., and Keppel, D. M., J. Biol. Chem., **131:** 57 (1939).
77. duVigneaud, V., Chandler, J. P., Cohen, M., and Brown, G. B., J. Biol. Chem., **134:** 787 (1940).
78. Beach, E. F., and White, A., J. Biol. Chem., **127:** 87 (1939).
79. Tarver, H., and Schmidt, C. L. A., J. Biol. Chem., **130:** 67 (1939).
80. White, J., and White, A., J. Biol. Chem., **131:** 149 (1939).
81. Stevenson, E. S., and White, A., J. Biol. Chem., **134:** 709 (1940).
82. Lewis, H. B., Yale J. Biol. Med., **4:** 437 (1932); Ann. Int. Med., **6:** 183 (1932).

83. Brand, E., Cahill, G. F., and Harris, M. M., Proc. Soc. Exptl. Biol. Med., **31**: 348 (1933–34); J. Biol. Chem., **109**: 69 (1935).
84. Lewis, H. B., Brown, B. H., and White, F. R., J. Biol. Chem., **114**: 171 (1936).
85. Raper, H. S., Biochem. J., **21**: 89 (1927).
86. Dulière, W. L., and Raper, H. S., Biochem. J., **24**: 239 (1930).
87. Evans, W. C., and Raper, H. S., Biochem. J., **31**: 2162 (1937).
88. Dalton, H. R., and Nelson, J. M., J. Am. Chem. Soc., **60**: 3085 (1938).
89. Ludwig, W., and von Mutzenbecher, P., Z. physiol. Chem., **258**: 195 (1939).
90. Lerman, J., and Salter, W. T., Endocrinology, **25**: 712 (1939).
91. Harington, C. R., and Rivers, R. V. P., Nature, **144**: 205 (1939).
92. Block, P., Jr., J. Biol. Chem., **135**: 51 (1940).
93. Schuler, W., Bernhardt, H., and Reindel, W., Z. physiol. Chem., **243**: 90 (1936).
94. Moss, A. R., and Schoenheimer, R., J. Biol. Chem., **135**: 415 (1940).
95. Shambaugh, N. F., Lewis, H. B., and Tourtellotte, D., J. Biol. Chem., **92**: 499 (1931).
96. Chandler, J. P., and Lewis, H. B., J. Biol. Chem., **96**: 619 (1932).
97. Papageorge, E., and Lewis, H. B., J. Biol. Chem., **123**: 211 (1938).
98. Sealock, R. R., and Silberstein, H. E., Science, **90**: 517 (1939); J. Biol. Chem., **135**: 251 (1940).
99. Sealock, R. R., Gladston, M., and Steele, J. M., Proc. Soc. Exptl. Biol. Med., **44**: 580 (1940).
100. Neubauer, O., "Intermediärer Eiweissstoffwechsel" in "Handbuch der normalen und pathologischen Physiologie," Berlin, p. 862.
101. Garrod, A. E., "Inborn Errors of Metabolism," 2nd Ed., 1923. H. Frowde and Hodder and Stoughton, London.
102. Medes, G., Biochem. J., **26**: 917 (1932).
103. Blatherwick, N. R., J. A. M. A., **103**: 1933 (1934).
104. Fölling, A., Z. physiol. Chem., **227**: 169 (1934).
105. Penrose, L. S., Lancet, **1**: 23 (1935).
106. Jervis, G. A., Arch. Neurol. Psychiat., **38**: 944 (1937).
107. Jervis, G. A., J. Biol. Chem., **126**: 305 (1938).
108. Jervis, G. A., Block, R. J., Bolling, D., and Kanze, E., J. Biol. Chem., **134**: 105 (1934).
109. Butts, J. S., Dunn, M. S., and Hallman, L. F., J. Biol. Chem., **123**: 711 (1938).
110. Ellinger, A., and Matsuoka, Z., Z. physiol. Chem., **109**: 259 (1920).
111. Matsuoka, Z., and Yoshimatsu, Y., Z. physiol. Chem., **143**: 206 (1925).
112. Kotake, Y., and Masayama, I., Z. physiol. Chem., **243**: 237 (1936).
113. Bloch, K., and Schoenheimer, R., J. Biol. Chem., **133**: 633 (1940); **134**: 785 (1940).
114. Borsook, H., and Dubnoff, J. W., Science, **91**: 551 (1940).
115. Clutton, R. F., Schoenheimer, R., and Rittenberg, D., J. Biol. Chem., **132**: 227 (1940).
116. Bach, S. J., Biochem. J., **33**: 1833 (1939).
117. Krebs, H. A., Enzymologia, **7**: 53 (1939).
118. Weil-Malherbe, H., and Krebs, H. A., Biochem. J., **29**: 2077 (1939).
119. Roloff, M., Ratner, S., and Schoenheimer, R., J. Biol. Chem., **136**: 561 (1940).
120. Leiter, L., J. Biol. Chem., **64**: 125 (1925).
121. Kiyokawa, M., Z. physiol. Chem., **214**: 38 (1933).
122. Rose, W. C., and Cook, K. G., J. Biol. Chem., **64**: 325 (1925).
123. Calvery, H. O., J. Biol. Chem., **83**: 649 (1929).
124. Edlbacher, S., and Kraus, J., Z. physiol. Chem., **191**: 225 (1930); **195**: 267 (1931).
125. Voge, C. I. B., Brit. Med. J., **2**: 829 (1929).
126. Kapeller-Adler, R., Biochem. Z., **264**: 131 (1933); Kapeller-Adler, R., and Haas, F., **280**: 232 (1935).
127. Kapeller-Adler, R., and Boxer, G., Biochem. Z., **293**: 207 (1937).
128. Tschopp, W., and Tschopp, H., Biochem. Z., **298**: 206 (1938).
129. Langley, W. D., J. Biol. Chem., **137**: 255 (1941).
130. Niendorf, F., Z. physiol. Chem., **259**: 194 (1939).
131. Werle, E., and Krautzun, K., Biochem. Z., **296**: 315 (1938).
131a. Felix, K., and Naka, S., Z. physiol. Chem., **264**: 123 (1940).
132. Gordon, W. G., J. Biol. Chem., **127**: 487 (1939).
133. Gordon, W. G., and Jackson, R. W., J. Biol. Chem., **110**: 151 (1935).
134. Fishman, J. B., and White, A., J. Biol. Chem., **113**: 175 (1936).

135. Patterson, W. I., Dyer, H. M., and duVigneaud, V., J. Biol. Chem., **116:** 277 (1936).
136. Abbott, L. D., Jr., and Lewis, H. B., J. Biol., **131:** 479 (1939).
137. White, A., Yale J. Biol. Med., **13:** 759 (1941).
138. Kies, M. W., Dyer, H. M., Wood, J. L., and duVigneaud, V., J. Biol. Chem., **128:** 207 (1939).
139. Carter, H. E., and Handler, P., Proc. Soc. Exptl. Biol. Med., **41:** 347 (1939).
140. Bernheim, F., and Bernheim, M. L. C., J. Biol. Chem., **109:** 131 (1935).
141. Kisch, B., Enzymologia, **1:** 97 (1936–37).
142. Neber, N., Z. physiol. Chem., **240:** 59 (1936).
143. Ratner, S., Rittenberg, D., Keston, A. S., and Schoenheimer, R., J. Biol. Chem., **134:** 665 (1940).
144. Borsook, H., and Dubnoff, J. W., J. Biol. Chem., **132:** 307 (1940).

CHAPTER IV

LIPID METABOLISM

By Abraham White

INTRODUCTION

The term "lipid" includes not only the true fats, or triglycerides, but other substances which are related to the fats by virtue of common physical or chemical properties. Although a classification of the lipids may be found in any elementary textbook of physiological chemistry, it may be well to list the substances which are generally considered to be lipids. These are:

1. Fats or Triglycerides: esters of glycerol and fatty acids, e.g., butter fat.
2. Waxes: esters of fatty acids and certain alcohols, not glycerol, and usually of a relatively high molecular weight, e.g., beeswax.
3. Phospholipids: fats which contain in addition to glycerol and fatty acids, phosphoric acid and a nitrogen-containing base (choline, amino ethyl alcohol, or sphingosine), e.g., lecithin, cephalin and sphingomyelin.
4. Cerebrosides: compounds of fatty acids, sugar and a nitrogenous base, e.g., phrenosin.
5. Sterols: high molecular weight alcohols which are cyclopentanoperhydrophenanthrene derivatives, e.g., cholesterol.

The lipids which are ingested in the diet may be represented by one or more of the above substances in varying proportions. The metabolism of lipids, therefore, is concerned with the bodily mechanisms which are involved in the handling of lipids of the type listed above. The various aspects of this metabolism will be considered in the following pages, after a preliminary discussion of the rôle of lipids in the diet and a brief review of lipid digestion and absorption from the intestine. The metabolic aspects of fats, phospholipids and sterols will be presented; little definite information is available regarding the metabolism of the waxes and the cerebrosides.

Lipids of the Diet.—Man ingests approximately 60 to 80 grams of lipid each day, and the major portion of this is in the form of fat or triglycerides. The fatty acids which occur in the food and which may enter the body if this food is eaten are grouped in table 1. The table also includes some information regarding the chemical nature and distribution of these fatty acids.

A few general remarks of some interest and importance may be made regarding the food fatty acids. It will be seen that all of the fatty acids listed in the table have an even number of carbon atoms; this is generally true of the fatty acids which occur in nature and which the organism is to metabolize. All members of the series of saturated acids, from four to twenty-four carbon atoms, are found distributed in various foods. The unsaturated acids include those of fourteen to twenty-two carbon atoms and of one to six double bonds.

Although there may be more than twenty-two fatty acids occurring in the food ingested, the common animal body fats are composed chiefly of the glycerides of palmitic, stearic, and oleic acids, and generally, in addition, small amounts of myristic acid and linoleic acid. Less frequently there are traces of arachidonic acid present. The animal phospholipids usually contain relatively large amounts of the more unsaturated acids. The special function of these phospholipids may in some manner be connected with the high degree of unsaturation of their fatty acid constituents. This point will be discussed in a later section.

TABLE 1

FOOD FATTY ACIDS

Acid	Formula	No. of double bonds	Iodine No.	Mol. Wt.	Typical occurrence in foods
Butyric	$C_4H_8O_2$	0	0	88	Butter
Caproic	$C_6H_{12}O_2$	0	0	116	Butter
Caprylic	$C_8H_{16}O_2$	0	0	144	Butter, cocoanut oil
Capric	$C_{10}H_{20}O_2$	0	0	172	Butter, cocoanut oil
Lauric	$C_{12}H_{24}O_2$	0	0	200	Butter, cocoanut oil
Myristic	$C_{14}H_{28}O_2$	0	0	228	Butter, nutmeg fat
Tetradecenoic	$C_{14}H_{26}O_2$	1	112	226	Fish oils
Palmitic	$C_{16}H_{32}O_2$	0	0	256	All fats and oils
Hexadecenoic (palmitoleic)	$C_{16}H_{30}O_2$	1	100	254	Peanut oil, fish oils
Hexadecatrienoic	$C_{16}H_{26}O_2$	3	305	250	Fish oils
Stearic	$C_{18}H_{36}O_2$	0	0	284	Tallow, lard
Oleic	$C_{18}H_{34}O_2$	1	90	282	All fats and oils
Linoleic	$C_{18}H_{32}O_2$	2	181	280	Animal lipids, semidrying oils
Linolenic	$C_{18}H_{30}O_2$	3	274	278	Rarely in foods
Octadecatetrenoic	$C_{18}H_{28}O_2$	4	368	276	Fish oils
Arachidic	$C_{20}H_{40}O_2$	0	0	312	Peanut oil
Gadoleic	$C_{20}H_{38}O_2$	1	82	310	Fish oils
Arachidonic	$C_{20}H_{32}O_2$	4	334	304	Animal lipids, fish oils
Eicosapentenoic	$C_{20}H_{30}O_2$	5	420	302	Fish oils
Docosatetrenoic	$C_{22}H_{36}O_2$	4	306	332	Brain lipids, fish oils
Docosahexenoic	$C_{22}H_{32}O_2$	6	464	328	Fish oils
Tetracosanoic (lignoceric)	$C_{24}H_{48}O_2$	0	0	368	Brain lipids

It will be noted from table 1 that two fats are exceptionally complex. Butter fat contains at least eleven fatty acids, mostly saturated, and the fish oils contain a still larger number of acids, most of the latter having three or more double bonds. Many speculations have been made in attempts to explain the complexity of these fats. The vegetable fats and oils which are ordinarily used as foods are composed chiefly of palmitic, stearic, oleic, and linoleic acids. Vegetable foods are relatively low in phospholipids.

The acids containing less than ten carbon atoms are volatile. Butyric acid is the only one soluble in water to an appreciable extent, being infinitely soluble. Caproic acid is soluble to the extent of 0.89 parts per 100 cc. of water; caprylic and capric acids are soluble to the extent of 0.079 and 0.0034 parts, respectively, per 100 cc. of water.

In summary, therefore, it will be seen that the lipids of the diet which are ultimately to be metabolized in the body consist for the most part of glycerides of fatty acids. The latter may vary in their number of carbon atoms from four to twenty-four and may be saturated or unsaturated in structure.

Rôle of Fat in the Diet.—One of the chief functions of dietary fat is to provide a large available reserve of food to the organism. This is important in view of the fact that the animal's capacity to store protein and carbohydrate is relatively limited and the fat depots therefore meet the requirement for energy reserve. Also of importance is the fact that the calorific value of fat per gram (9.3 Calories) is more than twice that for either carbohydrate (4.1 Calories per gram) or protein (4.1 Calories per gram).

In addition to providing a source of readily available energy, dietary fat serves as a vehicle for introducing the fat-soluble vitamins into the body. The potency of various fats and oils with respect to vitamins A and D has been clearly established, and the other fat-soluble vitamin, E, is present in high concentrations in wheat germ oil. The presence of these dietary essentials in fats forms a sound basis for the physiological value of fatty products like butter fat, egg yolk, and cod liver oil, which have long enjoyed a reputation for unique nutritive potency. Indeed, the normal absorption of the antihemorrhagic vitamin K from the intestine is dependent on a normal flow of bile which is stimulated by food fat.

Normal Fat Requirement.—The question of the exact amount of fat which is optimal for a normal dietary remains largely a matter of controversy. The major portion of the information available has been obtained from statistical studies of the problem and it is only within relatively recent years that it has been clearly established that *some* quantity of fat, or lipid material, is necessary in the diet. Although fat and carbohydrate can replace each other in isodynamic proportions within wide limits, other considerations make necessary some qualification of this property of *mutual replacement*. The feeling of satiety following a high fat meal is a common experience. Due to the slower absorption of fat from the intestine, this foodstuff appears to be available to the organism over a protracted period of time and to increase the so-called "staying power." The extensive replacement of fat in the diet by carbohydrate is limited by the stuffing process which is necessary and the consequent discomfort to the individual, which is often accentuated by carbohydrate fermentation in the intestine. McClendon, from observations made during a period as a visiting professor in Japan, states that he was impressed by the low fat content of the Japanese diet and the great amount of fermentative dyspepsia among the Japanese. It was also observed that Japanese men might be incapacitated for long periods of time and McClendon suggested that this might be related to the low fat content of the Japanese diet. Similar gross deleterious effects of low fat intake were observed in both England and Germany during the last World War.

Atwater proposed that in a standard dietary suitable for the average adult, fat should represent 33 per cent of the total of 3520 calories. Murlin has reported that in the diet of the United States Army soldier in the training camp during the first World War, fat represented 31 per cent of the total energy (about 3700 calories) consumed. In general, it would seem that the percentage of fat in the diets of different people varies greatly and that the influence of climate, locality, habits, work and other variables is so great as to make it impossible to suggest any one standard for fat intake on the basis of the few scattered investigations on this problem. The question of the fat intake in pathological conditions, notably diabetes mellitus, is discussed elsewhere in this book.

Essential Fatty Acids.—Although the exact and optimum requirement for fat in the diet has not been clearly established, relatively recent investigations have demonstrated that in the complete absence of dietary fat normal growth and well-being are not possible. In 1929, Burr and Burr[1] reported that rats on fat free diets did not thrive and developed a scaliness of the skin and tail. Kidney lesions were also present; in the female ovulation was irregular and male rats on a fat free diet could not be induced to mate. The syndrome which developed could be completely alleviated and the animals restored to normal health by the administration of linoleic acid ($C_{17}H_{31}COOH$). No other fatty acid tested was curative for the fat deficiency, and high-grade butter fat was also ineffective, thus supporting the view that the fat soluble vitamins were not concerned with the development of the deficiency condition. A few years later the same laboratory reported[2] that linolenic acid ($C_{17}H_{29}COOH$) is also effective in alleviating the fat deficiency manifestations. It was suggested that the capacity of the animal organism to synthesize certain unsaturated fatty acids is limited and that these fatty acids, *e.g.*, linoleic and linolenic acids, therefore, may be considered to be essential fatty acids in that they must be supplied in the diet.

The results of Burr and Burr have been confirmed in several laboratories and the concept of essential fatty acids has been extended to include the C_{20}, four double bond fatty acid, arachidonic acid ($C_{19}H_{31}COOH$). The latter was tested by Burr and Burr and reported to be entirely without effect as a curative agent for rats maintained on a fat free diet. However, both Turpeinen[3] and Hume and collaborators[4] have clearly demonstrated that arachidonic acid is also effective in curing the fat deficiency disease and, indeed, that this fatty acid is superior to the other essential fatty acids in curative power. More specifically, arachidonic acid, administered as the methyl ester, has been found to be more active than methyl linoleate when judged by weight increase of the experimental animals. The two esters are of approximately equal potency with respect to ability to cure skin lesions. The problem of the inability of mammals to synthesize certain unsaturated fatty acids will be referred to later in a discussion of the rôle of the liver in the metabolism of fatty acids.

In concluding this section, it should be pointed out that vitamins B_1 (thiamine) and B_6 (pyridoxine) have been demonstrated to be related to the essential fatty acid deficiency syndrome. Vitamin B_1 apparently influences the rate of conversion of carbohydrate to fat in animals deficient in unsaturated fatty acids. This conversion occurs at an abnormally high rate in these animals.[5] Birch[6] has suggested from his experiments that vitamin B_6 is essential for the proper utilization of the essential unsaturated fatty acids.

DIGESTION OF LIPIDS

A large body of data has been accumulated regarding the digestibility of various fats in man. These data depend upon an analysis of the feces for their lipid content during a period on a fat free diet as compared to a period during which a given amount, generally 100 gm., of fat was ingested. The results of such studies need not be discussed in detail, particularly since their experimental basis has now been demonstrated to be questionable. The work of Bloor and his pupils, notably Sperry, has clearly shown that lipids may be excreted on a fat free diet; therefore, lipid analysis of the feces must be employed with considerable reservation. These investigators demonstrated that there is a constant secretion of lipids by the intestinal mucosa, amounting to some 220 mg. of lipids per kilo of weight per week in dogs. Even under conditions of a fat free diet, the human stool may contain two grams of fat over a 24-hour period. Sperry and Angevine[7] found a large secretion of lipid into the small intestine of the dog and a relatively smaller secretion into the colon. The high sterol content of the lipids indicated that they were not of bacterial origin. Also, the amounts of lipids secreted were much greater than had been found in the feces, indicating some degree of reabsorption by the large intestine.

Although the quantity of fecal fat cannot be employed as an index of the digestibility of an ingested fat, the normal character of the stool and its lipid content indicate that a rather high proportion of ingested fat is digested and utilized by the organism. The presence in the digestive juices of enzymes which are capable of hydrolyzing fats into glycerol and fatty acids has been established, and the nature of these processes and the factors influencing them will be reviewed briefly. The following two sections will be devoted in general terms to this topic. The detailed information dealing with the digestion of lipids will be found in any introductory text of physiological chemistry.

Digestion in the Stomach.—The rôle of the gastric juice in the digestion of fats is probably insignificant. In fact, for many years it was believed that there was no gastric enzyme concerned with the digestion of fats, and that the small amounts of hydrolysis which had been reported to occur in the stomach could be explained on the basis of the digestive activity of regurgitated intestinal juice. However, in 1917 Hull and Keeton[8] clearly demonstrated the presence of a gastric lipase. These investigators prepared gastric pouches in dogs so that intestinal regurgitation was not a factor. The pure gastric juice obtained from the pouch appeared to contain a gastric lipase which, however, was readily destroyed by a 15-minute exposure to 0.2 per cent hydrochloric acid and could therefore not be detected unless the gastric juice was immediately neutralized.

It would seem, therefore, that in the adult, gastric lipase plays a negligible rôle. It is interesting that the concentration of this enzyme appears to be somewhat higher in the gastric juice of infants and children and may play some rôle in the digestion of milk fat. In cases of *anacidity* also there may be considerable activity of gastric lipase. Finally, it should be pointed out that although the strong acidity and other conditions in the stomach are not favorable to the action of lipase, there does occur a certain degree of hydrolysis in the stomach, quite apart from enzymatic action. This is particularly true if the fat reaches the stomach in a highly emulsified condition.

Digestion in the Intestine.—The presence of an enzyme in the small intestine capable of splitting fat was first described by Eberle in 1834. The demonstration of a pancreatic lipase is due to the work of Claude Bernard in 1850. This investigator was engaged in a comparison of the digestive mechanisms of herbivora and carnivora. Both types were fed fat, and Bernard observed that in the dog the lymphatics which are close to the pylorus soon became filled with a white chyme. In the rabbit, these changes took place farther removed from the pylorus. Bernard realized that the pancreatic duct of the rabbit entered the small intestine at a point farther down the gut than it did in the dog. He therefore concluded that something concerned with the digestion of fat was entering the intestine by way of the pancreatic duct. Bernard then obtained pure pancreatic juice from a pancreatic fistula and demonstrated its power to split fats. Boldyreff in 1907 reported a lipase in intestinal juice, following the observation of von Mering and Minkowski that depancreatized dogs could digest fat.

Even a brief consideration of the digestion of fats is not complete without mentioning the rôle of bile in this process. The emulsifying effect which the bile salts exert on fat entering the intestine is an extremely important factor in facilitating the digestion of this foodstuff. In addition, the bile serves the function of activating pancreatic lipase which is secreted in an inactive form, and also promotes the absorption of vitamin K.

It should be pointed out that although emphasis in this section has been placed upon the hydrolysis of fats by the digestive juices, similar changes occur with respect to other classes of the lipids, notably the phospholipids which, in addition to glycerol and fatty acids, yield phosphoric acid and either choline or amino ethyl alcohol under the influence of the digestive agents of the gastrointestinal tract. It is also probably evident that the extent of digestion of fats is determined by (1) the normal presence of the digestive fluids in the intestine, and (2) an adequate period of time for this digestive process to proceed. Thus, a marked increase in the fecal fat, or steatorrhea, is seen in conditions limiting the period of time which the fat remains in the intestine, e.g., in increased motility of the intestinal tract, in instances of exclusion of pancreatic juice from the intestine (extensive destruction of the pancreas or obstruction of the pancreatic duct), and when bile is excluded from the intestine. The latter circumstance interferes chiefly with the absorption fat; this process will be considered in the following section.

ABSORPTION OF LIPID DIGESTION PRODUCTS

Mechanism.—Inasmuch as the digestion of fats results in an hydrolysis of the molecule to glycerol and fatty acids, and since neither of these components of the fat molecule is present free in the circulating blood, it follows that during absorption a resynthesis of lipids occurs. This was early suggested by the classical experiments of Munk who had available in the clinic a young girl with a permanent lymph fistula. Munk fed this patient cetyl palmitate and then examined the lymph. Neither the cetyl palmitate nor cetyl alcohol ($C_{16}H_{33}OH$), which would arise from the hydrolysis of cetyl palmitate in the intestine, could be detected in the lymph. On the other hand, most of the palmitate found was present as the triglyceride, tripalmitin. It may be pointed out, incidentally, that Munk demonstrated that 60 per cent of the ingested fat traveled by way of the lymph stream when leaving the intestine.

Similar experiments on dogs were reported by Bloor in 1912. The administration of ethyl palmitate and ethyl stearate to dogs with a cannula in the thoracic duct led to the appearance of tripalmitin and tristearin in the lymph; the fed esters could not be demonstrated. Similar splitting and resynthesis have been established for the phospholipids by comparing the organic phosphorus of the lymph before and after the lecithin feeding. Under these circumstances there is no apparent increase in the organic phosphorus and the lecithins are therefore split before absorption and the resynthesized product does not contain the phosphorus in the form in which it was originally fed.

Rather concrete evidence of the resynthesis of lipids during the absorption of lipid hydrolysis products from the intestine has been presented by the investigations of Sinclair. In 1929 this investigator reported[9] the first of a series of studies designed to examine the problem of lipid synthesis during fat absorption from the intestine. Sinclair worked with two groups of cats; one group served as the control and was given a fat free diet. The other animals were fed a fat of known composition and animals in each group were killed at intervals after feeding. The intestinal mucosa of each cat was separated from the intestinal lumen and each tissue extracted with fat solvents. The phospholipid content of the extracts was then determined. Sinclair was able to show that regardless of the fat fed, the lecithin content in the lumen remained constant and was independent of the total amount of fat formed. After the feeding of cod liver oil, the isolated lecithin had a higher iodine number. Since the phospholipid content remained constant, Sinclair believed that this indicated a splitting of the cod liver oil followed by incorporation of its unsaturated fatty acids into lecithins. In muscle there was no iodine number change; the above transformation was limited to the intestine. Sinclair postulated the following equilibrium as existing in the intestinal wall:

$$\text{fatty acids} \leftrightarrows \text{phospholipids} \leftrightarrows \text{fat}$$

According to Sinclair there is a specific phospholipid within the intestinal mucosa which occupies an intermediary position between fatty acids and neutral fat. This general hypothesis has been supported by later work of Sinclair and Smith,[10] who "labeled" dietary fat by administering the non-natural fatty acid, elaidic acid, which is relatively resistant to metabolism and which can be quantitatively estimated. Elaidic acid in large amounts was found in the mucosa phospholipids during the absorption of this unnatural fatty acid.

The mechanism of fatty acid absorption suggested by Sinclair has been supported by evidence from other laboratories. Süllmann and Wilbrandt,[11] working in the laboratory of Verzár in Switzerland, have shown that the phospholipid content of intestinal lymph is increased during fat absorption in rabbits, and attributed this to a synthesis of phospholipid in the intestinal wall. Perlman, Ruben and Chaikoff[12] have followed the rate and extent of phospholipid synthesis in the intestinal wall by the use of radioactive phosphorus. A definite synthesis was established both in animals fed fat and in animals on fat free diets, although the extent of phospholipid synthesis was markedly less in the latter instance. The important rôle of the intestine in lipid metabolism is also stressed in the work of Sperry and his colleagues,[13, 14] who determined the extent of deposition of heavy hydrogen in the fatty acids of the tissues of rats given water containing deuterium. In all instances the intestinal fatty acids were found to have a relatively large amount of the heavy isotope of hydrogen.

It should be pointed out that cholesterol, when present in intestinal contents, is partly esterified during absorption. The sterol is not absorbed in appreciable amounts unless fat is being absorbed at the same time.

Hypothesis of Verzár.—The formation of phospholipid during the absorption of fatty acids from the intestine is a process which involves, among other reactions, an introduction of phosphoric acid by an esterification or phosphorylation process into the molecule to be formed. The importance of phosphorylation in the absorption of fatty acids has been stressed by the results of investigations from the laboratory of Verzár. In early experiments in 1934, Verzár and Laszt[15] reported that glycerol phosphate markedly increased the amount of oleic acid absorbed from intestinal segments of the rat. This absorption was hindered by mono-iodoacetic acid even if glycerol phosphate was present. The action of the halogen acid was attributed to a prevention of phosphorylation as an analogy to the effect of iodoacetic acid on muscle. The conclusion was drawn that the rate of absorption of fatty acids is dependent on the rate of phosphorylation and, therefore, phospholipid synthesis in the intestinal mucosa. Further confirmation of this interesting hypothesis was obtained by showing that the absorption rates found in isolated segments of rat intestine could also be obtained in the intact animal. The absorption of neutral fat, administered by mouth to rats, was inhibited by iodoacetic acid injection and also by the injection of phlorhidzin, a drug which has been demonstrated to inhibit the phosphorylation of glucose in the renal tubule. Even more striking has been the later work of Verzár and his colleagues[16] which has sought a relationship between the adrenal cortex and phosphorylation. Adrenalectomy in rats was found to diminish fat absorption; the administration of cortical extracts restored to normal the fat absorption of adrenalectomized animals. The conclusion is drawn that in the absence of the adrenal cortex, the synthesis of fat from fatty acids, *via* phospholipid, does not occur and that, therefore, the active phosphorylation process of the intestinal wall is under humoral control of the adrenal cortex.

This rather attractive hypothesis of Verzár awaits confirmation by other investigators. Certain criticisms of the Verzár studies have appeared. Klinghoffer[17] found severe intestinal pathology and a decreased absorption of sodium chloride and xylose in the rat following the administration of iodoacetic acid in the amounts used by Verzár. Inasmuch as the two substances whose absorption was studied do not depend on a phosphorylation process for effective absorption, Klinghoffer's data would appear to cast doubt on the validity of Verzár's interpretation of his experimental results. Lambrechts[18] has extensively investigated the effects of phlorhidzin on absorption and concluded that this drug exercises its effects not through a specific inhibition of phosphorylation but through a toxic action on cells. Finally, Deuel and his collaborators[19] showed that the absorption of glucose by adrenalectomized rats is normal if the animals are maintained in good condition by sodium chloride administration. Verzár had stated that glucose absorption, also dependent on a phosphorylation reaction, was inhibited by the experimental methods which he had employed to demonstrate diminished fat absorption.*

Rôle of Bile Salts.—There is ample experimental and clinical evidence indicating the importance of the bile salts in fat absorption. It has long been surmised that these salts increase the solubility of the fatty acids in the

---

* Further criticism and rejection of the Verzár hypothesis has recently appeared: Bruce, H. M., and Wien, R., J. Gen. Physiol., **98:** 375 (1940); Ferrebee, J. W., J. Biol. Chem., **136:** 719 (1940); Marrazzi, R., Am. J. Physiol., **131:** 36 (1940).

aqueous medium of the intestine and thereby favor diffusion through the cells and finally into the lymph vessels draining the intestine. The bile salts were considered to pass eventually to the liver, which restores them to the bile, thus participating in a continuous cycle of activity. If this cycle is interrupted by obstruction of the bile duct, by artificial drainage of bile from the organism, or by factors interfering with bile production by the liver, normal fat absorption fails.

Experiments in vitro have clearly established the importance of bile in increasing the solubility of fat digestion products. Whereas the higher fatty acids are relatively insoluble in water, they readily dissolve in an aqueous solution of bile acids or salts. The property of bile constituents in bringing an otherwise insoluble fatty acid into solution in water has been termed by Neuberg[20] an example of *hydrotropism*. This phenomenon has been studied in some detail by Verzár and his colleagues.[21, 22] The bile salts were found to be good solvents for oleic, palmitic and stearic acids. Verzár has suggested that the bile salts take up positions along the intestinal wall and facilitate the transport of fatty acids through the intestinal mucosa by exerting a hydrotropic action. This hypothesis was supported by absorption studies with intestinal segments of the rat, in which it was demonstrated that bile salts markedly increase the amount of oleic acid absorbed from isolated intestinal loops.

In summary, the following general facts appear to be available regarding the absorption of lipid digestion products from the intestine:

1. At least 60 to 70 per cent of the lipids absorbed from the intestine passes into the lymph. The remainder probably passes into the portal blood.

2. There is a general splitting and resynthesis of lipids in the intestinal wall. Bile salts and phosphorylation reactions appear to be concerned with this aspect of absorption.

3. The fatty acids appear as phospholipid and neutral fat and, to a very limited extent, as cholesterol esters in the lymph.

4. Even though fatty acids or ethyl esters of fatty acids are fed, these acids appear as neutral fat in the lymph. Glycerol is therefore supplied in the absorption process, either by direct synthesis, or from intestinal contents or from the blood.

5. The character of the fat appearing in the lymph appears to represent an average between the food fat and endogenous fat. In this connection it should be mentioned that since endogenous fatty acids may appear in the lymph, the 60 to 70 per cent fat which can be recovered from this fluid is composed of fatty acids from the two sources. Therefore, actually less than 60 per cent of the food fat can be accounted for in the lymph. It should be pointed out that the proportion of fat absorbed by way of the lymphatics has generally been deduced from a determination of the fat content of lymph obtained from the thoracic duct. Lee[23] has shown that after ligation of the thoracic duct there are established connections between the lymphatic duct and the azygos vein or its branches, and also with the right thoracic duct. Thus it would appear that the lymph, and therefore the absorbed fat, may not necessarily all enter the venous system at the base of the neck.

THE NATURE AND TRANSPORT OF BLOOD LIPIDS

Following absorption of lipids they may pass to the liver or to the tissues, depending on whether they have entered the portal or systemic blood.

Before discussing the transformations which absorbed lipids undergo, the composition of the blood lipids and the mechanism of their transport in the blood will be considered.

The application of more recently developed methods for the quantitative determination of the various types of lipids has made it possible to obtain a rather clear picture of values for plasma lipids in both health and disease. Boyd[24] has given the average values in table 2 for the lipids in the plasma of eight normal young women under controlled conditions of exercise, rest and diet.

TABLE 2

AVERAGE VALUES FOR PLASMA LIPIDS

	Milligrams per 100 cc. plasma
Total lipid	589
Neutral fat	154
Total fatty acids	353
Phospholipid fatty acids	130
Cholesterol ester fatty acids	77
Neutral fat fatty acids	146
Total cholesterol	162
Combined cholesterol	115
Free cholesterol	47
Phospholipid	196

The values given in table 2 are averages and do not indicate the rather wide variations which may occur under normal conditions. For example, the ingestion of dietary lipids will result in an increase in the total lipid content of the blood. About two hours after the administration of a lipid-containing meal, the blood lipids begin to rise and may remain at an elevated level for as long as seven hours. Under normal circumstances, factors which influence the mobilization of the lipid stores of the body will increase the concentration of lipids in the blood. Thus, starvation or exercise will elevate the level of blood lipids. During pregnancy and lactation there is also a marked rise in the concentration of the lipids of the blood. Chaikoff and his colleagues[25] have demonstrated remarkably high concentrations of lipids in the blood of laying hens. Administration of gonadotropic hormone (pregnant mare serum) or of estrin to immature females produced the same marked rise in serum lipids as was found during laying. The effect following estrin injection was seen within twelve hours. Particularly striking was the finding of a similar increase in blood lipids in male birds after treatment with estrin. These same investigators[26] have recently claimed that pancreatic juice contains a factor which causes a marked rise above normal in the blood lipid values of the depancreatized dog maintained with insulin.

Broadly speaking, alterations in values for the total lipids of the blood are generally the rule and reflect changes in the values for each of the various types of lipids, rather than striking deviations from the normal value for any particular kind of lipid. The sweeping nature of the above statement should be somewhat modified with respect to cholesterol. The concentration of the latter substance in the blood may in a few instances be markedly altered without attendant gross aberrations in the normal picture of the other blood lipids. It is not within the scope of the present discussion to discuss the influence of pathological conditions on blood lipid values. These are considered elsewhere in this book.

Transport of Blood Lipids.—Bloor and his co-workers have presented evidence which supports their suggestion that *lecithin* is the form in which fat is transported from blood to tissues and in the opposite direction. Bloor[27] fed olive oil to a dog and made microanalyses of the blood lipids. It was observed that the total fatty acids gradually rose; the increase in lecithin content appeared slightly later and the increase persisted longer than did the elevated total fatty acid value. In fasted dogs, the increased lipemia was accompanied by an increase in lecithin and in total fatty acids. Again in these experiments it appeared that lecithin was the vehicle for the transport of fatty acids.

Supporting evidence for the importance of phospholipids in the transport of fatty acids in the blood is found in the classic experiments of Meigs, Blatherwick and Carey.[28] These investigators obtained samples of mammary arterial and venous blood during lactation in the cow. Comparing the constituents of these bloods, it was found that the following two striking changes occurred in the blood during its passage through the mammary gland: (*a*) A loss in organic phosphorus, and (*b*) a gain in inorganic phosphorus. These authors calculated the amount of fat which could be produced by this transformation and the value obtained was in good agreement with the amount of butter fat produced daily by the cow. In view of their data and of the elevated phospholipid content of the blood of the lactating cow, Meigs and his collaborators concluded that almost all of the milk fat originates from blood lecithin.

While it is true that the fatty acids in the blood may in part be transported as phospholipids, an important rôle in this process is also played by the esters of cholesterol and of glycerol (neutral fat). This has already been pointed out in the discussion of the mechanism of intestinal absorption of lipids. It has also been emphasized that alterations in total blood lipids are reflected in changes in the concentration of the individual constituents which comprise the total lipid fraction of the blood.

In addition to the problem of the chemical nature of the combinations in which fatty acids are transported in the blood, the question of the physical state in which these water insoluble substances exist is an intriguing one. Gage and Fish[29] have pointed out that the absorbed fat reaches the blood in the form of tiny globules which they termed "chylomicrons." Ludlum, Taft and Nugent[30] made a careful study of the nature of these chylomicrons. They were found to be fat droplets of about one micron, or less, in diameter, and could be seen only with the aid of the microscope.

The properties of the chylomicrons strongly suggested that they are surrounded by a protective protein layer. The following properties of the droplets supported this view: (*a*) They exhibited a maximum tendency to flocculate at pH 4.8–5.2, the isoelectric point range for the blood plasma proteins; (*b*) at the above-mentioned pH values a reversal of charge on the chylomicrons appeared to occur; (*c*) coalescence to a larger drop occurred in acid or alkali at a point where the protein would be salted out. Frazer and his colleagues[31] have very recently confirmed this view and suggested that the particles seen in blood under darkfield illumination in the microscope are essentially glycerides with probably an adsorbed globulin layer. The hydrophilic protein layer around the fat particle aids in explaining the high degree of dispersion and solubility of the latter in an essentially aqueous medium like blood. Frazer has also contributed to the problem of the physiology of chylomicrons and presented detailed studies suggesting the possible absorption of unhydrolyzed neutral fat (as chylomicrons) from the intestine. The high chylomicron count of the blood, following a meal containing fat, is well established.

FATE OF ABSORBED LIPIDS

A discussion of the fate of absorbed lipids is essentially a consideration of the metabolic pathways of fatty acids, inasmuch as these are the components of lipids which characterize the latter as a group. The metabolism of the glycerol, carbohydrate, phosphoric acid, and nitrogenous constituents of the various types of lipids does not belong, strictly speaking, to lipid metabolism. The metabolism of the other important class of absorbed lipids, the sterols, will be discussed separately in a later section.

The fatty acids, following their absorption in combinations of several types from the intestine, may pass to the liver or to the tissues, depending on whether they have entered the portal or systemic blood. In consequence of this fact, three well-recognized types of transformations involving fatty acids may occur. These are:

1. Changes in the liver.
2. Oxidation.
3. Deposition as body fat.

Action of Liver Cells on Fat.—The normal liver contains about 5 per cent of lipids, the latter being approximately evenly distributed between phospholipids and neutral fat. It has been evident for some time that the liver exhibits a very active fat metabolism. During starvation there is a rapid mobilization of fat into the liver as the organism calls upon the fat depots to provide adequate energy. With a normal food intake, it is possible to demonstrate variations in the character of the food fat by alterations which take place in the type of fat present in the liver. Also, in pathological conditions of the liver (*acute yellow atrophy*) there is a marked increase in liver fat until the content of the latter may be as high as 50 per cent of the weight of the organ. These increases are accentuated normally by diets with a high lipid content. Finally, the importance of the liver in lipid metabolism is evident from recent work with fatty acids labelled with isotopic hydrogen, or deuterium. Animals given deuterium-containing fatty acids rapidly deposit them in the fat tissues and in the fat of the internal organs; the highest concentration is always found in the internal organs, particularly the liver.

Although the forces which attract fat to the liver in such large amounts are more or less obscure, relatively recent investigations have aided in the clarification of a number of variables which may influence the extent of lipid deposition in this organ. This work will be considered following a discussion of the changes which fatty acids undergo in the liver.

The early experimental evidence of Leathes and his collaborators[32] strongly suggested that the liver functions, in fatty acid metabolism, by extensively desaturating fatty acids and thus rendering them more susceptible to subsequent oxidation, inasmuch as the introduction of double bonds into a long-chain fatty acid will increase its reactivity and chemical instability.

In general, the experiments of Leathes and his co-workers consisted in administering certain fats to experimental animals and then, following a suitable time to permit digestion and absorption, the iodine number of the liver fatty acids was determined. The iodine number was invariably found to be higher than that of the food fatty acids and this was believed to indicate desaturation of the fatty acid molecules by the liver cells. This hypothesis has found some support in the work of other investigators. Hartley,[33] and Klenk and von Schoenebeck[34] have independently reported the presence in liver fat of fatty acids of a higher degree of unsaturation than those generally present in the diet. Both a C_{20} fatty acid with four double bonds, and a C_{22} fatty acid with five double bonds have been isolated. That the organism does have a definite capacity to desaturate fatty acids was conclusively demonstrated by Schoenheimer and Rittenberg[35] in 1936. These investigators fed mice synthetic saturated fatty acids containing heavy hydrogen, or deuterium. The fatty acids isolated from the entire animal were separated into saturated and unsaturated fatty acids. The high deuterium content of the latter proved conclusively that fatty acids can be desaturated readily in the organism. No separate analysis of liver fatty acids was carried out. It may be mentioned, at this time, that the reverse metabolic reaction, namely, the saturation of unsaturated fatty acids, has also been demonstrated to occur in the body. Rittenberg and Schoenheimer[36] fed mice unsaturated deuterium-containing fatty acids and isolated, from the total body lipids, deuterium-containing saturated fatty acids. There is, therefore, strong evidence that saturation and desaturation of fatty acids in the mammalian organism is a physiologically reversible process.

Notwithstanding this highly suggestive evidence in favor of the view that desaturation of fatty acids occurs in the liver, mention should be made of work which modifies the interpretation of some of this evidence. In 1934 Channon and his colleagues[37] made a careful study of liver lipids and were unable to find any evidence for the presence of the C_{20}, four double-bond-containing, fatty acid (arachidonic acid) which had been reported by Hartley. Further, the isolation from liver of a C_{22} fatty acid containing five double bonds by Klenk and von Schoenebeck may rather be indicative of a synthetic process in the liver than of a desaturation reaction. The content of C_{20} and C_{22} acids in ordinary food fats is quite insignificant, and it is therefore possible that the unsaturated fatty acid isolated was built up in the liver from smaller fatty acid residues. Also, with regard to the results obtained by Leathes and his colleagues, it may be argued that the increased unsaturation of the fat of the liver following the feeding of a fat (oils usually used) may merely be a selective deposition of certain highly unsaturated fatty acids which were present in the oils fed. Finally, although studies of metabolism repeatedly indicate the extraordinary biological specificity of reactions, it is a little difficult to understand why, if the liver readily desaturates fatty acids, certain unsaturated fatty acids (linoleic, linolenic, and arachidonic) are not synthesized by the organism but are so-called essential fatty acids and must be supplied in the diet. The latter objection should, it is realized, be modified by the possibility that the *rate of synthesis* of these essential fatty acids may not be adequate to meet the requirements of the growing organism, as has been demonstrated for the amino acid, arginine.

It is not desired to confuse the picture of the rôle of the liver in fatty acid metabolism by presentation of the above controversial evidence. Rather, the latter illustrates clearly the difficulties in unequivocally interpreting any metabolic data. The uncontrolled variables and the inability to follow substances completely through their transformations in the organism do not, however, mitigate the general conclusion that the liver participates actively in the metabolism of fatty acids. The nature of this participation may be further considered, and perhaps partially elucidated, from an inquiry into the factors known to influence the deposition of lipids in the liver.

The experimental production of livers with a high lipid content is readily achieved in a variety of ways. A diet high in lipid content is a good experimental tool in this problem. The oral administration of high levels of cholesterol is also effective in producing fatty livers. Accumulation of lipids in the liver is usually seen in the depancreatized dog and it was this phenomenon which formed the basis for modern work on factors influencing the deposition of lipids in the liver. The liver lipid increase in depancreatized animals had generally been attributed to the fact that in the absence of the external secretion of the pancreas there existed a subnormal capacity for the utilization of dietary lipids and this was reflected by the increased deposition of lipid in the liver. The general improvement in the condition and life span of depancreatized dogs following the regular feeding of raw pancreas was attributed to the supplying of the external pancreatic secretions. Depancreatized animals which had received raw pancreas in their diet generally showed less fatty livers than did operated animals which were not fed raw pancreas.

CHOLINE IN PREVENTION OF FATTY LIVERS.—About fifteen years ago, Best and his colleagues began a study of the ability of raw pancreas to prevent fatty infiltration of the livers of experimental animals. Feeding of high fat diets to rats readily produced an animal in which the effect of various dietary factors on the accumulation of liver lipids could be studied. It was early shown that the phospholipid fraction of pancreatic tissue was responsible for the prevention of fatty livers and, in 1934, MacLean and Best[38] demonstrated that choline $\left(HO-CH_2-CH_2-N \Big\langle {}^{OH}_{(CH_3)_3} \right)$ the nitrogenous basic constituent of one of the phospholipids, lecithin, would prevent fatty livers if administered to rats ingesting a high-fat diet. Choline was also found to be capable of preventing fatty livers caused by cholesterol feeding; the action of the nitrogen-containing base was shown to be effected primarily through a reduction in the triglyceride, or neutral fat fraction of the liver lipids. The effect of choline was termed a lipotropic action.

These striking observations of MacLean and Best have been confirmed by a number of investigators. Channon and his collaborators[39] also found that choline had the ability to prevent the production of fatty livers in experimental animals. Homocholine $\left({}^{HO-CH_2-CH_2-CH_2-N(CH_3)_3}_{OH} \right)$ was found to be even more effective than choline. These investigators have shown, as have Best and his colleagues[40] practically simultaneously, that the level of dietary protein administered appeared to influence the extent of liver lipid deposition. In both laboratories casein was the protein employed, although Best and his group also demonstrated that while casein has a very definite choline-like effect, gelatin exerts little, if any, rôle in preventing fatty livers. Edestin was found to act like casein. The obvious conclusion was drawn that the effect of protein was probably an amino acid effect, and this has been confirmed in several laboratories. Channon and his co-workers[41] first studied the effect of added dietary cystine on fatty liver production and found to their surprise that rather than hinder the deposition of lipids in the liver, cystine feeding greatly increased the extent to which this fatty infiltration occurred. This effect of cystine was confirmed by Tucker and Eckstein[42] who made the further very striking discovery that methionine had a marked lipotropic action, resembling that of choline. This observation has been confirmed by Channon and his group.[43]

In a later publication Tucker and Eckstein[44] pointed out that the comparative effectiveness of various proteins in preventing experimental fatty liver production was, in general, of the same order as their contents of *methionine*. Singal and Eckstein[45] report that arachin, a protein which is deficient in methionine, is without lipotropic action, although the addition of small amounts of methionine rendered arachin as active as casein. Homocystine behaved like cystine, *i.e.*, increased the already high level of liver lipids in animals ingesting a high fat diet. With respect to their lipotropic actions, therefore, cystine and methionine appear to have directly opposite actions. This is of interest in view of the generally accepted idea (see p. 112, Sulfur Metabolism) that cystine and methionine have many similarities in their metabolism and that, indeed, cystine may be formed in the organism from methionine. However, the differences in lipotropic activities of these two sulfur-containing amino acids find perhaps a more ready explanation in the recently published work by duVigneaud and his co-workers and by Rose, which were mentioned on p. 111, showing that methionine provides the methyl groups for choline synthesis. On the basis of this evidence, therefore, the lipotropic action of methionine may be understood, although the homocystine formed by the demethylation of methionine would act, according to Singal and Eckstein (see above), to promote liver lipid deposition.

Further aspects of the lipotropic rôle of choline can be more properly considered in the following section dealing with phospholipid metabolism inasmuch as the phospholipids are intimately concerned with the turnover of liver lipids. Before concluding this section dealing with the deposition of lipids in the liver, mention should be made of several other observations which indicate the complexity of the problem and serve to argue against placing all of the emphasis solely on choline, substances like choline, or compounds (*e.g.*, methionine) contributing to the synthesis of this nitrogenous base. The observations to be presented are, in some instances, isolated findings which require confirmation and further extension.

According to McHenry,[46] vitamin B_1 markedly increases the amount of fat in the livers of rats on a high fat and low choline diet. It might be mentioned, however, that a fatty liver can be the result of many unspecific factors, as is seen, for example, after experimental infection with *B. typhosus*.[47]

Fatty Infiltration of the Liver.—The effect of hormones on fatty infiltration of the liver has also been the subject of study. Best and Campbell[48] found an increase in size and fat content of livers of mice, rats, or guinea pigs following administration of the so-called ketogenic fraction of the anterior pituitary. Choline did not inhibit this pituitary effect. However, very recently, Campbell and Keenan[49] reported that the substance in anterior pituitary extracts which increases the rate of liver lipid deposition is not necessarily associated with prolactin, ketogenic or melanophore-expanding activity. Verzár and his collaborators have claimed that the action of the anterior pituitary on liver lipids is mediated through the adrenal cortex. Von Issekutz and Verzár[50] found that in rats poisoned with carbon tetrachloride or phosphorus, hypophysectomy prevented fatty infiltration. The latter did occur, however, under the same experimental conditions if cortical hormone was administered. This was in confirmation of the earlier work of Verzár and Laszt[51] who claimed that fatty livers were not produced in adrenalectomized rats by five days of phosphorus poisoning, whereas normal animals given phosphorus showed extensive accumulation of liver lipids. Also, the injection of cortical extract in adrenalectomized animals poisoned with phosphorus resulted in fatty livers. It has also been stated by LeBlond, van Thoai and Segal[52] that adrenalectomy prevents deposition of excessive quantities of fat in the liver.

LIPOCAIC.—A new hormone of the pancreas has been described by Dragstedt and his collaborators and is said to be concerned with the prevention of fatty livers. In 1936, Dragstedt, Van Prohaska and Harms[53] reported that the beneficial effect of raw pancreas feeding on fatty livers could not be attributed entirely to the lecithin or choline content of the pancreatic tissue. The tissue was fractionated and these workers obtained 1.8 to 2.5 gm. of product from 100 gm. of fresh pancreas. Oral administration of this material was effective in preventing fatty livers in depancreatized dogs. The isolated product was insoluble in ether, and soluble in alcohol, 5 per cent sodium chloride, and water. It was not present in pancreatic juice and it was suggested that the substance is a hormone. It was postulated that this hormone under normal conditions plays a rôle in the transport or further utilization of fat. The name, "lipocaic," was chosen for the substance; this name is derived from Greek roots meaning, "fat" and "I burn." Kaplan and Chaikoff[54] state that they have demonstrated in the pancreas two factors which are active in lipid metabolism. One inhibits the production of fatty livers in depancreatized dogs and is probably identical with lipocaic. It is claimed that pancreatic juice contains a factor which causes a marked rise above normal in the blood lipid levels of the depancreatized dog maintained with insulin. Channon and his colleagues[55] have also concluded that there is a lipotropic factor other than choline and protein in the pancreas. Although several investigators have questioned the existence of lipocaic, enough confirmatory evidence has accumulated which strongly suggests that pancreatic tissue does indeed contain a factor other than choline or protein, which has a preventive action on liver lipid deposition caused by feeding fat. Lipocaic apparently has no influence on the capacity of anterior pituitary extracts to produce increased liver lipid deposition in fasted rats.[56]

Before continuing with a discussion of the rôle of the liver in the metabolism, i.e., oxidation, of fatty acids, a brief consideration of phospholipid metabolism, particularly in its relations to liver fat, is essential to the completeness of the story of the deposition of lipids in the liver.

Phospholipid Metabolism.—*Relation to Liver Lipid Deposition.*—The important rôles assigned to phospholipids in the absorption of fatty acids from the intestine and in the transport of these acids in the blood have already been considered in previous sections. The relation of phospholipids to active processes involving fatty acid mobilization and turnover was evident in these aspects of lipid metabolism. Indeed, phospholipid appears to be a type of lipid intimately concerned with the metabolism of fatty acids, apparently chiefly as a representative of a readily available form of these acids. Active lipid metabolism, therefore, whether arising from normal stimuli or induced by pathological or experimental processes, is reflected in very rapid alterations in phospholipid concentration in body fluids and tissues. Bloor and his colleagues have contributed evidence emphasizing the prominence of phospholipids in supplying fatty acids as a source of energy for various types of tissues. In general, the phospholipid concentration of the tissues studied by Bloor and his group was directly related to the degree of activity of the tissue. For example, the phospholipid concentrations found[57] for the following tissues in the rabbit were in the descending order: muscles of the heart, jaw, diaphragm, and neck. In wild rabbits, the phospholipid content of the muscles of locomotion approached the values found for the respiratory-circulatory group of muscles. In contrast, the results in domestic or laboratory rabbits showed a lower content of phospholipids in muscles used in bodily movement than the figures obtained for other types of muscle. Also, the flying muscles of the breast of the pigeon showed very high values for phospholipid, compared to similar muscles in the nonflying rooster. Other similar studies by Bloor and his pupils have stressed the relation of phospholipid concentration of a tissue to the latter's metabolic activity.

In view of the above, it is not surprising that experimental work has yielded a large body of evidence regarding the phospholipid turnover in various organs and tissues. Its metabolism in the intestinal mucosa has already been discussed; its significance in the metabolism of brain and nerve tissue and in lipid deposition in the liver will now each be considered in turn.

The actual turnover of fatty acids in brain tissue appears to be relatively small (see below) when compared with this process elsewhere in the organism. McConnell and Sinclair,[58] using *dietary elaidic acid* to "label" the fat deposited in the body, found a relatively small uptake of this acid in brain phospholipids of young rats. This was interpreted to mean that the selection of fatty acids in the building of the constituent phospholipids of tissues is much more rigorous in the brain than in the liver and muscles. This problem has also been recently studied by Sperry, Waelsch and Stoyanoff[13, 14] who employed isotopic hydrogen (deuterium) to label the dietary fat administered to rats. Analysis of the brain lipids showed only traces of the isotope to be present. Inasmuch as the labeled dietary fat contained fatty acids of structures identical with those native to brain lipids, it does not seem likely that brain tissue has a more selective fatty acid requirement for the synthesis of its phospholipids, as suggested by McConnell and Sinclair. Rather, it appears that either the fatty acid turnover in the brain is relatively small, or that brain tissue has the capacity to synthesize the quantities of fatty acids required for replacement purposes. Data pertinent to the problem of the actual rate of fatty acid and phospholipid turnover in brain tissue have been obtained in several laboratories.

Sperry and his colleagues have extended their studies on brain fatty acids to include a determination of the rate of fatty acid synthesis or deposition in brain tissue. Water containing heavy hydrogen was injected into rats and the animals were subsequently given heavy water to drink in order to build up the concentrations of deuterium in the body. The deuterium content of the fatty acid fractions of various tissues, including brain, was then determined several days after the initiation of the experiment. The concentration of heavy hydrogen in the fatty acids of the brain was comparable with that found in the carcass fatty acids. It was estimated that as much as one-fifth of the brain fatty acids may be replaced in a week. This evidence definitely indicates that there is a turnover of fatty acids in brain tissue and that apparently this tissue has the capacity to synthesize fatty acids for replacement purposes inasmuch as dietary labeled fatty acids (see above) did not appear as such in the brain lipids. Confirmation of this conclusion was also obtained in studies of the deposition of lipids in the rat brain during myelination.[59] This process was again followed with the aid of deuterium as an indicator. The fatty acids deposited in the lipids of the brain during the period of most active myelination were found to be synthesized in the brain itself.

Radioactive phosphorus has been employed by Chaikoff and his group[60] to follow the phospholipid metabolism of rat brain tissue. The rate of phospholipid synthesis in the brain was found to be slower than for liver, kidney or small intestine. The synthesis of brain phospholipids was found to go forward for as long as two hundred hours after the administration of the radioactive phosphorus. Also, it was observed that the loss of labeled phosphorus from the brain is a relatively slow process.

Phospholipid metabolism in tissues actively concerned with lipid metabolism is intimately related to the problem of lipid deposition in the liver. Shifts in phospholipid concentration in liver tissue are particularly striking in the process of lipid deposition, initiated by either fat or cholesterol feeding, and following the stimulating effect of a lipotropic agent of the type of choline. Indeed, the discovery by Best and his colleagues that choline was effective in preventing fat deposition in the liver has been interpreted from the beginning as meaning that choline exerted its effect by promoting the synthesis of lecithin, of which choline is a component. This hypothesis was supported by the data, already discussed, assigning an important rôle to the phospholipids, *e.g.*, lecithin, in the metabolism of fatty acids. However, this suggestion received little confirmation in the observations from several laboratories, that the amount of phospholipid remains unchanged in the liver whether the latter be fatty or normal, or whether choline be administered or not. Indeed, this type of evidence, diametrically opposed to assigning a rôle to phospholipid in liver fatty acid metabolism, would have been impossible to refute had not a procedure been available for measuring the *turnover* of liver phospholipid. This problem can be, and has been, studied by the use of radioactive phosphorus.

Perlman and Chaikoff[61] have reported studies of the phospholipid activity of liver tissue with the aid of the radioactive isotope of phosphorus. These investigators demonstrated that the administration of choline markedly accelerates phospholipid turnover in the liver, the degree of acceleration being related to the amount of choline employed. Also of interest is the finding that the feeding of rats with cholesterol for only 30 hours decreased the phospholipid turnover in the liver, thus affording an explanation of the production of fatty livers by dietary cholesterol. The action of phospholipids and cholesterol, with respect to the problem of liver lipid deposition, is another example of the antagonistic behavior of these two types of lipids. The hemolytic action of phospholipid, as opposed to the antihemolytic effects of cholesterol, is another manifestation of this antagonism.

Chaikoff and his colleagues[62] have recently reported that each of the amino acids, cystine, cysteine and methionine, stimulates phospholipid turnover in the livers of rats. The rôle of these amino acids in the production of fatty livers has already been discussed, and it will be recalled that whereas methionine is definitely lipotropic, cystine feeding increases the extent of liver lipid deposition. In view of the latter data, it is difficult at the present time to explain adequately the similarity in the effects of these two sulfur-containing amino acids on phospholipid turnover in the liver. Further studies may indicate the significance of differences in experimental conditions employed in the two types of studies (lipid deposition vs. phospholipid turnover).

The evidence for a *continual phospholipid turnover* in the liver, made visible with radioactive phosphorus, stresses the importance of this group of lipids in fatty acid metabolism. The data are in marked contrast with the suggested constancy of the liver phospholipids. Although the total quantity of these lipids may indeed show little change, phospholipid activity is proceeding at a remarkably rapid rate. In concluding this section dealing with phospholipid metabolism, it should be pointed out that although lecithin has been the only phospholipid specifically referred to, cephalin also has been shown to participate in the processes involving phospholipid which have been discussed. The amounts of lecithin and cephalin undergoing change may vary, but considerations of total phospholipid metabolism certainly include both of these substances. The exact *mechanism* by which lipotropic agents accelerate phospholipid turnover remains to be elucidated.

Oxidation of Fatty Acids.—The action of liver cells on fatty acids has been discussed in some detail, and the importance of phospholipids in active fatty acid metabolism has been stressed. The problem of the ultimate fate of the fatty acids, and the fate of the newly-formed molecules arising in the liver turnover reactions, remains to be considered. This ultimate fate may be of a dual nature: (*a*) Oxidation with the production of carbon dioxide, water and energy, and (*b*) deposition in the tissues as body fat. The fatty acids leaving the liver are transported by the circulation to the tissues where either or both of the above types of disposal may be occurring. The nature of the predominating process is obviously markedly influenced by the balance of supply and demand of energy available and required by the tissue cells. The factors concerned in the cell for determining this balance are obscure. Further, it is uncertain whether the various types of molecules, *i.e.*, neutral fat and phospholipid, are oxidized as a whole or whether hydrolysis with liberation of free fatty acids precedes oxidation. It is quite clear that the fatty acids follow one series of degradation reactions, and the other components of the lipid molecules, *e.g.*, glycerol, choline, and phosphoric acid, follow other courses of metabolism.

Beta Carbon Atom Oxidation (Knoop hypothesis).—One of the widely-held theories of fatty acid oxidation is known to every student of physiological chemistry and is based on the classical experiments of Knoop[63] in 1904. This investigator conceived the idea of putting a non-combustible residue, or clinker, so to speak, into the fatty acid molecule and attempting to isolate the fragment which would remain following metabolism of the destructible portion of the compound. Knoop synthesized several phenyl substituted fatty acids and administered these to dogs. From the urine of these animals he succeeded in isolating two different compounds, depending on the nature of the fatty acid fed. When a phenyl substituted fatty acid with an odd number of carbon atoms in the side chain was given, hippuric acid, $C_6H_5CONHCH_2COOH$, was found in the urine. When the side chain contained an even number of carbon atoms, phenaceturic acid, $C_6H_5CH_2$-$CONHCH_2COOH$, was excreted. From these observations Knoop concluded that fatty acid degradation in the organism occurred by the loss of two carbon atoms at a time, suggesting that the initial point of oxidation attack was at the beta carbon atom, that is, the second carbon atom removed from the carboxyl group. On the basis of this mechanism, it was possible for Knoop to explain the data of his animal experiments. Knoop's suggestions are illustrated in the following two examples:

1.

$$C_6H_5CH_2CH_2CH_2COOH + O_2 \longrightarrow C_6H_5CH_2\overset{H}{\underset{OH}{C}}CH_2COOH \overset{O_2}{\longrightarrow}$$
phenylbutyric acid

$$C_6H_5CH_2\overset{}{\underset{O}{C}}CH_2COOH \overset{H_2O}{\longrightarrow} C_6H_5CH_2COOH + CH_3COOH$$
                                          phenylacetic   acetic
                                            acid   acid

$$C_6H_5CH_2COOH + NH_2CH_2COOH \longrightarrow C_6H_5CH_2CONHCH_2COOH$$
phenylacetic   glycine   phenaceturic acid
acid

2.

$$C_6H_5CH_2CH_2CH_2CH_2COOH \overset{O_2}{\longrightarrow} C_6H_5CH_2CH_2\underset{OH}{CH}CH_2COOH \overset{O_2}{\longrightarrow}$$
phenylvaleric acid

$$C_6H_5CH_2CH_2\overset{}{\underset{O}{C}}CH_2COOH \overset{H_2O}{\longrightarrow} C_6H_5CH_2CH_2COOH + CH_3COOH$$
                                            phenylpropionic   acetic
                                            acid   acid

$$C_6H_5CH_2CH_2COOH + O_2 \longrightarrow C_6H_5\underset{OH}{C}CH_2COOH \overset{O_2}{\longrightarrow} C_6H_5\overset{}{\underset{O}{C}}CH_2COOH$$
phenylpropionic
acid

$$\overset{H_2O}{\longrightarrow} C_6H_5COOH + CH_3COOH$$
               benzoic   acetic
               acid   acid

$$C_6H_5COOH + NH_2CH_2COOH \longrightarrow C_6H_5CONHCH_2COOH$$
benzoic   glycine   hippuric acid
acid

It will be seen from these examples that each fatty acid chain is shortened two carbon atoms at a time, with the production of a fatty acid of two less carbon atoms and acetic acid. The latter is then oxidized to carbon dioxide and water, and the fatty acid remaining is then again subjected to beta oxidation in the manner illustrated above.

The suggestion that fatty acids are degraded by a process of beta oxidation has been strongly supported by subsequent investigations. The production of beta hydroxybutyric acid and acetoacetic acid in diabetes mellitus is readily understood in view of the fact that the commonly ingested fatty acids all contain an even number of carbon atoms. The oxidation of these acids by the Knoop mechanism would, therefore, ultimately result in the production of the above-mentioned four carbon fatty acids which, together with acetone, are called the ketone bodies.

More direct experimental support for beta oxidation has been obtained by a number of investigators. Dakin[64] succeeded in isolating from the urine of dogs fed phenylpropionic acid the corresponding products of beta oxidation, namely, β-hydroxyphenylpropionic acid and β-ketophenylpropionic acid. Embden and Marx[65] found that if fatty acids containing an even number of carbon atoms were perfused through surviving dog liver, acetone appeared in the perfusate. The acetone was believed to arise from the degradation of acetoacetic acid. When fatty acids of an odd number of carbon atoms were perfused, no acetone was formed. "Intarvin," a commercial glyceride of margaric acid (seventeen carbon atoms), when fed to the diabetic does not increase the acetone output. Oxidation of this acid according to the Knoop mechanism should not result in ketone body production because the four carbon stage is avoided.

Further suggestive evidence in support of the Knoop hypothesis is seen in the many experiments showing that fatty acid behavior in the body generally falls into two groups, depending upon whether the acid in question has an even or odd number of carbon atoms. For example, Quick,[66] working with dogs, has determined the ratio of benzoic acid conjugated with glycuronic acid to benzoic acid conjugated with glycine. Having established this ratio for benzoic acid, longer chain phenyl substituted fatty acids were fed and the ratios determined for each of these. For benzoic acid, the ratio of glycuronic acid to glycine was 3:1. For phenylacetic acid, this ratio was 1:2. With the other acids studied, the ratio following administration of a phenyl substituted fatty acid containing an odd number of carbon atoms in the side chain was always 3 of glycuronic acid to 1 of glycine. When the side chain contained an even number of carbon atoms, this ratio was constantly 1 glycuronic acid to 2 glycine. This similarity in the two groups of acids, depending on the number of carbon atoms in the side chain, was interpreted to indicate that shortening of these side chains occurred two carbon atoms at a time. Raper and Wayne[67] obtained similar results in studying the efficiency of dogs to eliminate various phenyl substituted fatty acids. The efficiency was comparable for all the even carbon atom fatty acids, yet differing for the odd carbon atom fatty acids which resembled one another. A recent more suggestive demonstration of beta oxidation is seen in the results of Schoenheimer and Rittenberg.[68] These authors have shown that deuteropalmitic acid (palmitic acid [C_{16}] labeled with deuterium) can be isolated from the tissues of mice fed deuterostearic acid (C_{18}). The shortening of the stearic acid molecule by two carbon atoms is support for the involvement of beta oxidation in the degradation of fatty acids.

Other Modes of Oxidation.—Although the evidence supporting beta oxidation as a mechanism for fatty acid degradation is indeed strong, there is conclusive data indicating that this is not the *sole* mechanism by which fatty acids are oxidized. For example, the respiratory quotient in muscle under certain conditions is 0.71, indicating a more direct oxidation of fat. The mechanism for oxidation under these circumstances is not clear. The question of the mode of oxidation of the unsaturated fatty acids is also an unsolved one. The introduction of double bonds into the fatty acid molecule, already discussed in considering the rôle of the liver in fat metabolism, should theoretically produce points of weakness in the chain which are readily susceptible to scission by oxidation. With this in mind, Quick[69] synthesized the following two fatty acids,

$$C_6H_5CH_2CH_2CH{=}CHCH_2COOH \text{ and } C_6H_5CH_2CH_2CH_2CH{=}CHCOOH$$

and fed these to dogs. Curiously enough, the ratio of glycuronic acid to glycine, conjugated with benzoic acid in the urine, was the same with either fatty acid, indicating that the presence of the double bond had not influenced the course of the oxidation.

Modes of oxidation of fatty acids, other than the beta oxidation mechanism, have been demonstrated in several laboratories. Oxidation of the *terminal carbon atom* of the fatty acid chain, *i.e.*, the omega, or carbon atom most distantly removed from the carboxyl group, has been demonstrated[70, 71] by the isolation of dicarboxylic acids from the urine of dogs fed fatty acids, or fatty acid esters. For example, the feeding of the methyl ester of caprylic acid $(CH_3(CH_2)_6COCH_3)$ led to the excretion of suberic acid $(HOOC\text{-}(CH_2)_6COOH)$. Injection of salts of the fatty acids gave results essentially the same as those obtained in feeding experiments. The suggestion of omega oxidation has been considered as a supplementary process to beta oxidation, in which the former precedes the latter. Thus, if omega oxidation results in the formation of a dicarboxylic fatty acid, beta oxidation may then proceed simultaneously from both ends. This is illustrated below:

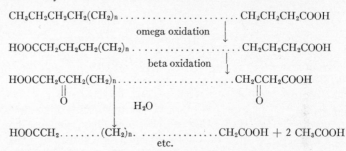

Further strong evidence is now available to prove that the Knoop hypothesis of successive beta oxidation is not the sole mechanism for explaining the ultimate formation of β-hydroxybutyric acid and acetoacetic acid. Although the problem of the *formation of ketone bodies* will be considered in detail in the following section, the *mechanism* of their formation more properly belongs to the subject of fatty acid oxidation and leads to the suggestion of yet another mode of oxidation of fatty acids. In 1916, Hurtley[72] argued that if beta oxidation were the sole means of oxidizing fatty acids, it should be possible to detect relatively large amounts of the inter-mediate fatty acids (butyric, caproic, etc.) under conditions in which ketones were being formed. However, Hurtley could find no significant amount of butyric acid in the blood or tissues of a diabetic excreting 70 grams of ketones a day. He therefore proposed the hypothesis that the fatty acid is attacked at alternate carbon atoms simultaneously along the whole length of the carbon chain, as indicated below:

$$\ldots \quad \ldots \, CH_2-CH_2-CH_2-CH_2-CH_2-CH_2 \ldots \ldots \ldots C-CH_2-C-CH_2-C-CH_2 \ldots \ldots$$
$$\xrightarrow{\quad} \quad \underset{O}{\|} \qquad \underset{O}{\|} \qquad \underset{O}{\|}$$

As a result of this process, the entire molecule breaks down into aceto-acetic acid and probably other acid products. More than a single molecule of acetoacetic acid would be expected to arise from each fatty acid mole-cule. Support for this hypothesis has been forthcoming from a number of laboratories. Jowett and Quastel[73] studied the rate and extent of formation of ketone bodies from fatty acids by liver slices in vitro. On the basis of their data, Jowett and Quastel also abandoned the successive beta oxidation hypothesis and adopted that of Hurtley which they called the *multiple alternate oxidation* mechanism. Deuel and his colleagues[74] determined the rate of excretion of ketone bodies in rats after feeding ethyl esters of fatty acids. It was found that at least 3 molecules of ketones were formed per molecule of fatty acid oxidized, thus supporting the hypothesis of multiple alternate oxidation. Finally, several investigators have compared the oxygen consumption of liver tissue with the total ketone production. Blixenkrone-Møller[75] worked with the perfused livers from diabetic cats and found a low value for the oxygen to ketone ratio. This value could be explained only by assuming that four molecules of ketones were formed per molecule of fatty acid oxidized. Similar results have been reported by Stadie and his colleagues[76] in studies with liver slices in vitro. The molecular ratio of oxy-gen consumed to ketone produced from fatty acids by the tissue was found to be close to the value 1.25 required by the multiple alternate oxidation hypothesis:

$$C_{16}H_{32}O_2 + 5\ O_2 \xrightarrow{\qquad} 4\ C_4H_8O_3$$
Palmitic acid $\qquad\qquad$ β-hydroxybutyric acid

(Molecular ratio of oxygen to ketones = 1.25 : 1)

Moreover, there was no evidence for the formation of acetic acid in similar experiments. According to the Knoop hypothesis, it would be expected that at least six molecules of acetic acid would result from the complete oxida-tion, via the beta oxidation mechanism, of each molecule of palmitic acid.

This is conclusive evidence that the higher fatty acids yield not one but probably four molecules of ketones per molecule of fatty acid oxidized. Beta oxidations occur simultaneously, therefore, at multiple alternate posi-tions along the fatty acid chain.

Before closing this discussion of the mechanism of fatty acid oxidation, mention should be made of the numerous in vitro studies of Raper and Smedley-Maclean and their co-workers. In vitro oxidation of saturated fatty acids with hydrogen peroxide has been shown to result in the formation of gamma and delta ketonic acids. It is indicated, therefore, that it is not logical to limit to one type the mode of oxidation of fatty acids in the organism.

Beta and omega oxidation have been established by animal experiments. Other types are indicated from theoretical and laboratory considerations. It is quite likely that the oxidation of fatty acids takes place through the operation of several types of reactions, in which the chain may be attacked at several places simultaneously, rather than by a single mechanism (see next section). It is evident that this mode of degradation of the fatty acid molecule makes possible the production of a wide variety of intermediate oxidation products, and is, therefore, encouraging in its support of the proposed manifold interconversions and interrelations of the various foodstuffs and metabolic processes.

Fatty acid oxidation is intimately concerned with the problem of ketone body formation, and this topic will be considered in the following section, which deals with ketogenesis and antiketogenesis. The latter term will be replaced in the following discussion by ketolysis, inasmuch as ketone body oxidation and destruction is, in reality, the process acting to balance ketone body formation. Antiketogenesis, arising from early views regarding the rôle of carbohydrate in promoting ketone body oxidation, is a misnomer since the *accumulation* of, and not the *inhibited oxidation* of, ketone bodies is the process which is occurring in ketosis.

Ketogenesis and Ketolysis.—*Formation of Ketones in Liver.*—The active rôle of the liver in lipid metabolism and the formation of four carbon fatty acids by the oxidation of naturally occurring fatty acids have already been discussed. It is not surprising, in view of these facts, to find that the liver is the chief site of formation of ketone bodies. The latter name is used to include the three substances, acetoacetic acid, beta hydroxybutyric acid, and acetone. The two acids are normal products of the degradation of longer chain fatty acids, and acetone arises secondarily, and readily, from the oxidation of acetoacetic acid. The evidence that the liver is the site of formation of these substances is conclusive. It has already been pointed out that Embden and Marx[65] demonstrated the formation of acetone in surviving liver tissue perfused with fatty acids containing an even number of carbon atoms. This work has been confirmed by other investigators. Jowett and Quastel[73] showed that the even number carbon atom fatty acids also yield acetone when incubated with liver slices in the Warburg apparatus. Stadie and his colleagues[76] have demonstrated the in vitro formation of ketone bodies in slices of liver from fasted normal and diabetic cats. Further proof for the formation of ketone bodies by the liver has been obtained from investigations with hepatectomized dogs. A high level of blood ketones, produced by either pancreatectomy in the dog[77] or by the injection of anterior pituitary extracts in the rabbit[78] is not evident in hepatectomized animals. Actual increased concentration of ketone bodies in the liver during ketosis has been demonstrated by the experiments of Harrison and Long.[79] Within six hours after the injection of phlorhidzin in rats fasted for twenty-four hours, high levels of ketones were found in the liver. In experiments in which anterior pituitary extract was injected, increased concentration of ketones in the liver cells was seen two hours after the injection. The production of ketosis by fasting, by anterior pituitary extract injection, or by phlorhidzin is therefore a stimulation of liver ketogenesis.

Crandall[80] has measured the actual proportions of β-hydroxybutyric acid and of acetone plus acetoacetic acid that are added to the blood by the liver. Working with angiostomized dogs, it was demonstrated that β-hydroxybutyric acid constitutes 25 to 93 per cent of the total hepatic acetone body output.

Formation of Ketones in Muscle Tissue.—In concluding this consideration of ketogenesis, it should be pointed out that there have been suggestions that ketones may also be formed in muscle tissue. In 1927 Krebs and Johnson[81] demonstrated ketone formation in muscle from pyruvic acid, implying that carbohydrate as well as fat may be a source of ketones. Also, Stadie, Zapp and Lukens[76] have recently reported that during experiments designed to determine the utilization of β-hydroxybutyric acid by minced muscle, an actual increase of both β-hydroxybutyric acid and total ketones was found in four of six experiments. It is not possible at this time, therefore, to exclude the muscles as a site of ketone formation.

Ketolysis.—Following the conclusion that the liver exhibits a marked capacity to produce ketone bodies from fatty acids, the problem of the disposal of these products of fat oxidation presents itself. This process, broadly termed ketolysis, evidently occurs readily and regularly under normal conditions inasmuch as there is no evidence of an accumulation of ketone bodies in the body tissues or fluids. The ketone bodies which are constantly supplied to the blood by the liver serve as sources of energy for other tissues since the latter complete the oxidation of these compounds to carbon dioxide and water. Indeed, the more recent evidence which has demonstrated the utilization of ketones by peripheral tissue has served to eliminate the necessity of an obligatory chemical coupling of the oxidation of carbohydrate and fatty acids. This latter coupling will first be discussed briefly, chiefly because of its historical interest. Following this, the present-day view of ketone body utilization and its significance in ketosis will be presented.

COUPLING OF OXIDATION OF CARBOHYDRATES AND FATTY ACIDS.—The ketonuria observed in the depancreatized dog and in the diabetic individual was early related to an altered carbohydrate metabolism. Hirschfeld[82] in 1895 showed that the factor common to all conditions of ketosis was the lack of carbohydrate in the food or, as in the diabetic, from his impaired carbohydrate metabolism. The fact that ketosis appeared to be definitely related to carbohydrate starvation led many investigators to study the quantitative relationships between dietary carbohydrate and fat, on the one hand, and the degree of ketosis, on the other. Zeller[83] in 1914 carried out studies of carbohydrate deprivation on himself and found that acetonuria appeared on a low carbohydrate diet when the food contained 80 gm. of carbohydrate and 310 gm. of fat. He therefore concluded that one part of carbohydrate is required for the combustion of four parts of fat. Lusk[84] recalculated Zeller's data and came to the conclusion that one molecule of beta hydroxybutyric acid required the presence of one molecule of a three carbon-containing compound, or triose. On the basis of this calculation, one molecule of glucose, yielding two triose molecules, had the capacity to promote the utilization of two fatty acid molecules.

From the type of investigations and calculations mentioned above, there arose the general hypothesis that the *burning of carbohydrate* in the body in some way prevents the appearance of ketosis and is therefore *antiketogenic*. The aphorism, "fats, or acetone bodies, burn in the fires of carbohydrates," became the concise description of the problem of ketogenesis and antiketogenesis. As a corollary it followed that any foodstuff which provides glucose is antiketogenic. Thus, carbohydrates, sugar-forming amino acids, and glycerol were classified as antiketogenic substances. On the other hand, fatty acids, and certain amino-acids forming ketone bodies in metabolism were classified as ketogenic substances.

Apparently rather striking in vitro confirmation of this hypothesis was provided by Shaffer[85] in 1921. This investigator demonstrated that the oxidation of acetoacetic acid by hydrogen peroxide, in alkaline solution, is catalyzed by the presence of glucose. It was established that one glucose molecule promotes the combustion of two fatty acid molecules and that glycerol would aid in the complete oxidation of one fatty acid molecule. On the basis of these data, it was concluded that one molecule of glucose is required for the complete oxidation of one molecule of fat, inasmuch as the glucose takes care of two of the fatty acids while the glycerol accounts for the third fatty acid present as a constituent of the triglyceride compound. Shaffer[86] then examined the literature and from calculations based on available clinical and experimental data found a striking correlation between the extent of ketosis in experimental animals and in patients, and the ratio of ketogenic to antiketogenic substances in the diet. From this work, theoretically practical ratios for the dietary regulation of clinical ketosis were established and used for the dietary management of diabetes mellitus in particular.

Since 1928, however, considerable evidence has accumulated in the literature necessitating a complete revision of the concept of an obligatory coupling of the oxidation of carbohydrate and fat (ketones). Snapper and Grünbaum[87] in 1928 observed a considerable disappearance of ketones from the circulation following perfusion through striated muscle of normal animals. In the same year Chaikoff and Soskin[77] studied the rate of disappearance of ketones from the blood of dogs following injection of acetoacetate. The conclusion was drawn that ketones are utilized by the muscles of the diabetic as well as the normal eviscerated dog. Similar results were reported from other laboratories. More recently, Blixenkrone-Møller[88] perfused the hind limbs of normal and diabetic cats and showed an active utilization of ketones by muscle. The extent of utilization was greatly increased in contracting muscle, and it was concluded that ketone oxidation might furnish a considerable fraction of the total energy requirements. Similar utilization and oxidation of ketones in the peripheral tissues have been shown by Harrison and Long[79] in the intact rat, following phlorhidzin or anterior pituitary extract administration, and by Stadie, Zapp and Lukens[76] in the muscle of both the normal and the diabetic cat. In the latter animals, obviously, the oxidation of ketones by muscle must be independent of the presence of insulin.

UTILIZATION OF KETONES, AND KETOSIS.—It will be seen from the foregoing evidence, therefore, that the oxidation of ketones in the peripheral tissues is a process which goes forward both in normal and in diabetic animals and is a source of energy for the organism. The utilization of ketones by the tissues of the diabetic animal, in the absence of normal oxidation of carbohydrate, clearly emphasizes the nonobligatory coupling of the oxidation of carbohydrate and ketones. Although the work of Deuel and his colleagues has demonstrated that carbohydrate, or carbohydrate formers, will abolish or diminish the ketonuria produced in normal rats by the oral administration of the sodium salts of butyric or acetoacetic acids, *it is definitely no longer tenable to postulate that ketonemia and ketonuria are a consequence of nonoxidation of ketones because of a failure of simultaneous oxidation of carbohydrate.* Rather, ketone body oxidation goes on normally under the various conditions which have been examined, including the diabetic state. However, in the latter condition the failure of carbohydrate utilization or oxidation, because of the absence of insulin, accentuates the metabolism of fat and protein in order that the organism may meet the energy requirements. Under circumstances of increased fat mobilization and oxidation there will be an increased production of ketone bodies. The latter substances will also be formed from the increased protein catabolism, since some of the amino acids are ketogenic. The rate of ketogenesis exceeds the rate of ketone oxidation in the tissues. The concentration of ketone bodies in the blood, therefore, will greatly exceed the normal levels and when the relatively low renal threshold is exceeded, ketonuria will result.

Similar circumstances adequately explain the other types of ketonemia and ketonuria which have been observed. During *starvation* the depletion of carbohydrate reserves forces the accentuation of fat and protein catabolism. The so-called ketogenic hormone of the anterior pituitary exerts its effect by mobilization of fat. It will be recalled that Best and Campbell[48] found an increase in size and fat content of livers of mice, rats, or guinea pigs following administration of ketogenic fractions of anterior pituitary extracts. Ketosis under these circumstances, therefore, is a manifestation of the increased production of ketone bodies because of the stimulated fat mobilization and catabolism.

In **summary,** ketogenesis occurs chiefly in the liver as a result of the oxidation of fatty acids. It is also possible that some ketone body formation may occur in the muscles. Carbohydrate (*e.g.,* pyruvic acid) and ketogenic amino acids may also be sources of ketones. The oxidation of the latter compounds (*ketolysis*) readily occurs in the peripheral tissues and this process thus furnishes an important source of energy to the organism. The ketolytic process is not dependent on simultaneous carbohydrate oxidation. Ketogenesis is markedly accentuated in conditions of impaired carbohydrate utilization, diminished carbohydrate supply, or accelerated fat and protein metabolism following injections of anterior pituitary extracts. Any of these circumstances augments ketone body production and is a manifestation of the increased demands which the body makes upon the metabolic processes involving fat. The ketonemia and ketonuria which may result are a consequence of ketone utilization in the peripheral tissue not being great enough to meet the increased ketone production of the liver. These views are similar to those which have recently been admirably stated by Stadie.[89] The latter investigator has reviewed and discussed the problem of fat metabolism in diabetes mellitus and its relation to ketonuria. Clinical data which had formerly been interpreted to support obligatory coupling of ketone body and carbohydrate oxidation in diabetes mellitus are reevaluated and clearly shown *not* to be supported by the quantitative data. According to Stadie, there is no significant relation between the ketone bodies utilized and the "antiketones" oxidized. This author postulates the following hypothesis as fulfilling the statistically significant facts derived from the clinical data: "Up to a certain level fat metabolism is complete and there is no ketonuria. Beyond this level fat metabolism is incomplete and part of the fat catabolized is excreted in the form of ketone bodies."

Deposition of Lipids as Body Fat.—There remains for consideration the final possible suggested fate for absorbed lipids, namely, deposition as body fat. If the energy value of the food intake exceeds that required by the body, fat is stored. Little is known regarding the mechanism of the processes or the factors influencing them. Several questions immediately present themselves:

1. What metabolic force, for example, determines whether a fatty acid molecule is burned or stored?

2. If burned, does this happen in the cells of the liver, in the blood cells, or in certain tissue cells?

3. How does an excess of total energy for the organism as a whole bring about synthesis of fat from carbohydrate?

Direct evidence for the formation of answers to these questions is not readily available, but certain experimental facts have thrown some light on the processes involved in regulating the nature and extent of fat deposition in the tissues.

Previous discussion has already pointed out that dietary lipids are rapidly and extensively deposited in the fat depots and in the fat of the internal organs. It will be recalled that this information has been conclusively established from the work of Schoenheimer and his collaborators, who have fed animals either fats or fatty acids labeled with heavy hydrogen and then determined the concentration of isotopic hydrogen in the lipids of the body. The extensive deposition of the longer chain fatty acids is observed even when the animals are held at a constant weight. The proportion of dietary fat deposited seems to be almost independent of the amount administered. Schoenheimer and his colleagues,[90, 91] have shown that even when the diet is low in fat (1 per cent) a considerable portion of the fed fat is deposited in the tissues. As much as 47 per cent of the ingested lipid was found in the fat depots, leading to the rather surprising conclusion that *even when the energy requirements of the organism are being met by diet, the dietary fat is to a considerable extent laid down in the tissues.* The fatty acids utilized for energy requirements are derived to a considerable extent from the previously stored depot fat. These experiments would suggest continual replacement of tissue fatty acids by dietary ones. Since fatty acids are not present in depot fats in the free form but in ester linkage, the presence of isotopic dietary acids in the body fats indicates changes involving continuous formation of ester linkages in normal animals. There are two reactions possible which might lead to fatty acid replacement: (*a*) A continuous breakdown into glycerol and fatty acids and resynthesis of the total fat molecule, or (*b*) continuous ester shifts. Both types of reactions are known to occur in *in vitro* experiments initiated by the enzyme, lipase. The isotopic method cannot yet determine which of these reactions (or whether both) participates in the continual fatty acid turnover of depot lipids. Evidence essentially confirming the data of Schoenheimer and Rittenberg has been reported by other investigators employing heavy hydrogen to follow the fate of the administered lipid material. Similar conclusions have been drawn also from experiments in which dietary elaidic acid was used as a "label" for following the mode of disposition of fed lipids.

It should be pointed out that the rapid deposition of dietary fatty acids occurs only when the latter are of a long chain of the type found in palmitic acid and higher fatty acids. This phenomenon is not observed when lower acids, such as butyric and caproic acids, are administered. These shorter chain fatty acids are rapidly and completely degraded. For example, Eckstein[92] fed fat-free diets and diets containing preformed fat (myristic acid, triolein, or sodium butyrate) to rats and determined the distribution of fat in the animals. The butyryl radical was apparently not deposited in the tissue, while the other two were. Eckstein confirmed his observation that fatty acids of low molecular weight are not incorporated in the body fat of rats by experiments in which tricaproin and butter fat were fed. Neither caproic acid nor butyric acid was found in the lipids of the fat depots. Confirmation of these data and evidence that the shorter chain fatty acids are oxidized, rather than stored, have been furnished by other investigators.

The marked influence of dietary fat on body fat is more readily understood in view of some of the above data. This problem has been studied rather extensively by many investigators, including workers in the laboratories of the United States Department of Agriculture. The latter division has been interested in the problem from an economic standpoint. The formation of the soft pork seen in hogs in the South receiving a high proportion of cottonseed oil was in marked contrast to the so-called hard pork of the Middle West, obtained from hogs on a corn diet. The availability of various other oils, e.g., peanut oil and soy bean oil, as by-products in industries of the South made it logical to attempt the utilization of these materials for hog feeding. In 1926, Ellis and Isbell[93] reported the results of a lengthy investigation undertaken by the Department of Agriculture. Hogs were raised on various types of diets and in addition to observing the physical nature of the body fat, iodine numbers were determined as an index to the degree of unsaturation of the depot lipids deposited. There is, of course, a definite

TABLE 3

EFFECT OF DIET ON BODY FAT

	Physical appearance of body fat	Iodine No. Diet fat	Iodine No. Lard produced
Brewer's rice + protein.....	Hard fat	53	55
Corn meal + protein.......	Hard fat	60	59
Peanut meal + corn meal..	Soft fat	90	77
Soy bean oil..............	Oily fat	90	90

relationship (inverse) between the iodine number of a fat and its melting point, and the latter in turn will determine the physical consistency of a fat. The data of Ellis and Isbell are summarized in table 3.

An extension and application of the data of Ellis and Isbell was reported by Anderson and Mendel[94] in 1928. The experiments were designed in an effort to use the southern oil products in fattening without producing a body fat which was soft and oily. These investigators used rats as experimental animals and maintained them on a basal diet in which 40 per cent of the calories were derived from dry milk powder and the other 60 per cent from one of the various kinds of fats. The rats were fed the diets until the animals' weight was 200 gm; they were then killed, the fat of the animal was rendered, and the iodine number determined. The data obtained are shown in table 4. It is evident from the table that a dietary fat with a low

TABLE 4

DIET AND BODY FAT

Type of fat supplement	Iodine No. Food fat	Iodine No. Body fat
Soy bean oil	132	123
Corn oil	124	115
Peanut oil	102	99
Crisco	79	82
Lard	63	71
Butter	36	54
Cocoanut oil	8	35
Protein	...	65
Starch	...	64

iodine number can produce a fat lower in iodine number than that produced by the animal from carbohydrate. For example, the feeding of butter produces a fat in the depots with an iodine number of only 54, as contrasted with that produced when carbohydrate is fed, leading to an iodine number of 64 for the body fat. The direct correlation between dietary fat and body fat is obvious.

In other experiments, Anderson and Mendel placed groups of rats on the same diets as above until each animal's weight was 150 gm. At this time a "hardening" diet of carbohydrate was employed until the body weight reached 250. Analyses showed that the iodine number under these conditions had dropped, for the soy bean oil diet, from 123 to 110. This experiment was repeated except that at the 150-gm. body weight mark half of the rats were fasted until 30 gm. of weight were lost and the animals were then placed on a carbohydrate diet. The values for the iodine numbers obtained are shown in table 5.

TABLE 5

INFLUENCE OF A PRELIMINARY FAST ON THE RELATIONSHIP BETWEEN DIET AND TYPE OF BODY FAT PRODUCED

	Iodine No. Body fat
Soy bean oil diet:	
Fasted animals	65
Non-fasted animals	100
Peanut oil diet:	
Fasted animals	60
Non-fasted animals	80

Therefore, by a short fast it was possible to produce in rats the same type of "hard" fat as that produced on a fat-free diet. Apparently the body stores of readily mobilizable and oxidizable unsaturated fatty acids are burned during the starvation period and the hard fat is then deposited as a consequence of the subsequent period of carbohydrate feeding. This information has been applied to the soft pork problem.

It will be seen, therefore, that dietary fatty acids may be deposited directly in the tissues as depot lipids, and that the nature of the fatty acids deposited will be related to the type of lipids ingested. Moreover, the nature of the lipids which accumulate in the tissues may be influenced by starvation, which greatly reduces the supply of depot fat, or by other dietary constituents from which fatty acids are synthesized. Dietary influences express themselves more strikingly in their effects on the type of lipids laid down in the tissues if the reserve of fatty acids is first depleted by a period of starvation. Inasmuch as the chief point under consideration in this section is the deposition of absorbed lipids in the tissues, and not factors influencing the type of depot fat deposited, the problem of possible fat formation from protein will not be considered. This is essentially another topic concerned with the interconversion of the various foodstuffs.

STEROLS: NATURE AND METABOLISM

The aspects of lipid metabolism which have been discussed have been concerned chiefly with two classes of lipids, the neutral fats (triglycerides), and the phospholipids. However, no discussion of lipid metabolism would be complete without a consideration of another group of lipids which are of great physiological importance, namely, the sterols. The literature dealing with the sterols is enormous in extent, and an effort will therefore be made to present in a cogent manner the better established facts regarding the nature and metabolism of the sterols.

Nature of the Sterols.—The term sterol was originally coined to denote a cyclic monohydroxy alcohol of high molecular weight. The organic chemists have established the chemical nature of the sterols of physiological importance, and all of these compounds are derivatives of a cyclopentanoperhydrophenanthrene nucleus. The latter structure is now known to be common to a wide number of physiologically important substances and has the following configuration:

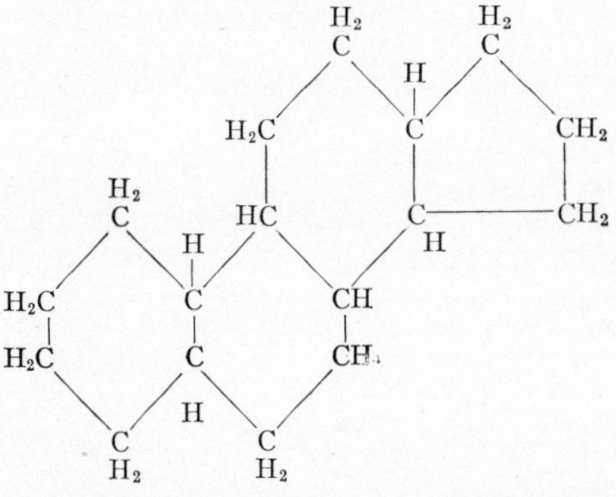

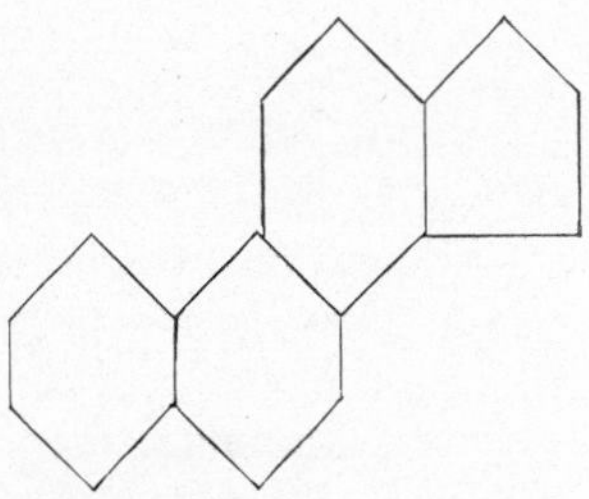

The sterols are monohydroxy alcohol derivatives of this nucleus. Inasmuch as a large number of related compounds are also derivatives of this structure, the general name of *steroid* has been suggested for the group as a whole. Some other members of this group, in addition to the sterols, are the bile acids, the sex hormones, vitamin D, the hormones of the adrenal cortex, the saponins, the digitalis glucosides, and certain toad poisons. These various steroids differ chemically from one another chiefly in the number and nature of substituents present in the above represented nucleus.

Among the most important of the naturally occurring sterols are *cholesterol*, which is the characteristic sterol of animal tissue, and the group of plant sterols which are called phytosterols. *Ergosterol*, which is recognized to be the precursor of vitamin D, is a sterol long known to be a constituent of yeast. The chemical structures for cholesterol and ergosterol are the following:

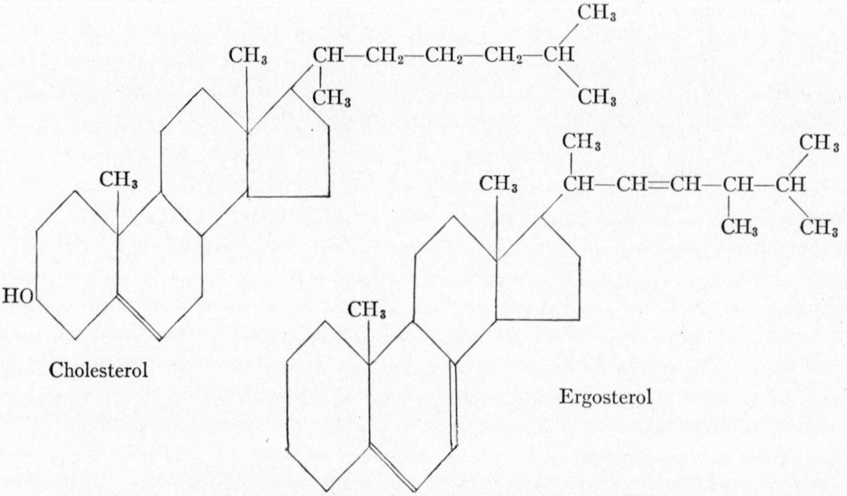

Cholesterol

Ergosterol

The presence of cholesterol in blood and its rôle in transporting fatty acids in the form of cholesterol esters has already been considered. Cholesterol is found in association with other lipids as a constituent of probably every cell; it is also present in the bile, in addition to the blood. This sterol is particularly abundant in brain and nerve tissue, and may occur free or as an ester in combination with various fatty acids.

In addition to cholesterol and ergosterol, there are several other sterols of physiological importance, each of which is closely related in structure to cholesterol. Reduction of the double bond in cholesterol yields the compound, *dihydrocholesterol*. An isomer of the latter compound is *coprosterol*, a constituent of the feces. These compounds will be referred to again in the following discussion of sterol metabolism.

Absorption of Sterols.—Schoenheimer and his collaborators[95] have studied in some detail the problem of absorption of sterols from the intestine. Although cholesterol was found to be readily absorbed from the gut of experimental animals, the plant sterols were not absorbed even when fed with bile salts to facilitate absorption. Moreover, ergosterol was also not absorbed in these experiments, although irradiated ergosterol (vitamin D) readily entered the organism from the gastro-intestinal tract. These experiments were conducted with mice, rats, rabbits and dogs, and the non-absorption of ergosterol confirmed in all species studied. In the laying hen, however, it was possible to demonstrate that small amounts of ergosterol were absorbed. *Allocholesterol*, which differs from cholesterol only in the position of the double bond in the molecule, was not absorbed by the dog or the hen. It would seem, therefore, that the number of sterols absorbed from the intestine of most species is limited to two, cholesterol and vitamin D. The specificity exhibited by the gut with respect to sterol absorption is indeed striking.

Synthesis of Sterols.—The capacity of animals to synthesize cholesterol has been clearly established in experiments with sterol-deficient diets conducted by Channon[96] and by Randles and Knudson.[97] Sterol balance studies by other investigators have also given evidence for cholesterol synthesis by the mammalian organism. The problem of the mechanism of this synthesis remains one of the important unsolved problems of sterol metabolism. The nature of the precursors is unknown. The nonabsorption of the various plant sterols eliminates one of the most obvious sources of possible cholesterol precursors. Rittenberg and Schoenheimer[98] studied the regeneration of cholesterol in mice on a cholesterol-free diet by giving the animals heavy water to drink and determining the deuterium content of the isolated sterol. The synthesis is slower than with fatty acids, requiring approximately three times as long a period of time. The amount of deuterium found in the newly synthesized cholesterol suggested that at least every second hydrogen atom in the cholesterol molecule was derived from the aqueous medium. In view of this, it is indicated that cholesterol is synthesized by condensation of small molecular units. Eckstein[99] has contributed evidence that the extent of cholesterol synthesis by rats is greater on a high fat diet than on a low fat diet. The reason for, and the source of, the excess synthesis on high fat diets remain unexplained but are in harmony with the Schoenheimer data. Further work along these lines is awaited with interest, in view of the fact that the mechanism for the synthesis of cholesterol may throw some light upon the important problem of the origin of the steroid hormones.

Metabolism of Sterols.—Despite the ubiquitous distribution of sterols in relatively high concentrations, surprisingly little is known regarding their metabolism. Cholesterol, the chief sterol of interest to the present discussion, is known to be influenced in its metabolism by the many factors which affect lipid metabolism in general. Increases or decreases in the lipid concentration of body tissues and fluids are generally a reflection of variations in the concentration of all lipids, including cholesterol. Under special circumstances, *e.g.*, cholesterol deposition in arteriosclerosis, cholesterol concentration may vary more strikingly than that of other lipids.

Although the intermediate stages of cholesterol catabolism in the organism are not known, there is adequate evidence suggesting that concomitantly with continuous cholesterol synthesis in the body, a steady destruction of this sterol also occurs. The end products of this degradation process are not known, and the balance experiments generally employed have depended on cholesterol determinations as a method of approach. In other words, evidence for the disappearance of cholesterol itself has been obtained, but proof for complete destruction is lacking. In fact, the possibility of transformation of cholesterol into a closely related compound is not excluded as an explanation for cholesterol disappearance.

Among the first reports of the *physiological destruction of cholesterol* were the experiments of Dam[100] in 1931. This investigator observed a loss of sterol in young chickens which could not be accounted for on the basis of excretion. A year later Page and Menschick[101] fed moderately large amounts of cholesterol to rabbits in the course of balance experiments. Sterol was deposited throughout the body with the exception of the brain. After all depots were accounted for, including the fur and excreta, the data indicated a destruction of cholesterol amounting to over a gram a week. Schoenheimer and Breusch,[102] in a study with mice, found that these animals which, on diets low in cholesterol, can synthesize their body content of cholesterol in a month, can also destroy five times this amount on diets rich in cholesterol. Fat in the diet had no effect on the cholesterol balance. The conclusions of these authors rather completely summarize a large portion of our present day knowledge of cholesterol metabolism: "In the tissues cholesterol is continually being formed and destroyed. Either a positive or a negative balance may be found, depending on experimental conditions, i.e., synthesis may be in excess of destruction or vice versa."

Studies of the problem of sterol excretion have produced the few data available regarding the intermediary stages of sterol metabolism. This evidence has accumulated within relatively recent times. In 1929 Beumer and Hepner[103] reported that the cholesterol concentration of the intestinal contents of a normal dog during absorption is much higher in the colon than in the ileum. These workers also studied a dog with a bile fistula after a lipid free meal and found an even more marked difference. The cholesterol concentration in the dried contents of the ileum was 0.21 per cent as contrasted to a value of 1.25 per cent for the cholesterol concentration in the contents of the colon. The results were interpreted as evidence of a secretion of cholesterol into the large bowel. In 1930, Schoenheimer and von Behring[104] examined the sterile secretion of the large intestine in dogs and found 80 per cent of the material to be sterol in nature. Dihydrocholesterol, the reduction product of cholesterol, was identified. The former sterol is evidently formed in the tissues and actually secreted through the intestinal wall. Similar endogenous excretion of sterols into the intestine has been found by Sperry and his colleagues.[7, 105] A higher excretion was found from the small intestine than from the whole intestinal tract in dogs, indicating absorption further down in the large intestine.

The other sterol excreted in addition to dihydrocholesterol is that present in the feces, namely, *coprosterol*. It is clear that the body does not eliminate cholesterol as such. Dihydrocholesterol is normally found in tissues to the extent of 2 to 3 per cent, and its formation from cholesterol with a subsequent excretion through the intestinal wall appears to be established. Inasmuch as coprosterol is not found in tissues normally but always in considerable amounts in the feces, it must be concluded, for the present, that coprosterol may be a product of bacterial action in the large intestine.

It is not within the scope of the present discussion to discuss in detail the metabolic processes and functions in which cholesterol has been implicated. The rôle of cholesterol in the absorption and transport of fatty acids in the blood has already been considered. The antihemolytic action of cholesterol and its antagonism to phospholipid both in the hemolytic phenomenon and in influencing the deposition of liver lipids are also strongly indicated. Otherwise, the suggested functions for cholesterol are largely based on circumstantial evidence and in many instances are merely theories. Among these functions and rôles for cholesterol may be mentioned the following: precursor of the bile acids, and for the steroid hormones; regulation of permeability of cells and therefore of importance in water and solute shifts in the body; insulating medium in the myelin sheath of nerves. In addition to these suggested normal functions for cholesterol, the marked variations in cholesterol concentration, particularly of blood, in various clinical conditions have been pointed to in order to emphasize further the physiological importance of cholesterol. With respect to this, it may be said that alterations in lipid concentrations are generally the cause of an altered cholesterol level which is secondary to the lipid metabolism effect. In view of the wide variation in the cholesterol concentration of the serum or plasma in health, apparent deviations from normal in the presence of disease must be interpreted with caution.

BIBLIOGRAPHY

Books

Leathes and Raper: The Fats. Longmans-Green & Co., London, 1925.
Dakin: Oxidations and Reductions in the Animal Body. Longmans-Green & Co., London, 1922.
Bull: Biochemistry of the Lipids. John Wiley & Sons, Inc., New York, 1937.
Hilditch: The Chemical Constitution of Natural Fats. John Wiley & Sons, Inc., New York, 1940.
Verzár and McDougall: Absorption from the Intestine. Longmans-Green & Co., London, 1936.
Annual Review of Biochemistry (Published yearly). Annual Reviews, Inc., Stanford University, California.

Review Articles

Frazer, A. C., Physiol. Rev., 20: 561 (1940). Fat Absorption and Its Relationship to Fat Metabolism.
Bloor, W. R., Physiol. Rev., 19: 557 (1939). Fat Transport in the Animal Body.
Bills, C. E., Physiol. Rev., 15: 1 (1935). Physiology of the Sterols, including Vitamin D.
Anderson, W. E., and Williams, H. H., Physiol. Rev., 17: 335 (1937). The Role of Fat in the Diet.
Schoenheimer, R., and Rittenberg, D., Physiol. Rev., 20: 218 (1940). The Study of Intermediary Metabolism of Animals with the Aid of Isotopes.
Schoenheimer, R., Science, 74: 579 (1931). New Contributions in Sterol Metabolism.
Verzár, F., Nutrition Abs. and Rev., 2: 441 (1932–33). The Absorption of Fats.
Smith, J. A. B., J. Soc. Chem. Ind., 58: 213 (1939). Fat Metabolism in the Animal Body.

Original Articles

1. Burr, G. O., and Burr, M. M., J. Biol. Chem., 82: 345 (1929); 86: 587 (1930).
2. Burr, G. O., Burr, M. M., and Miller, E. S., J. Biol. Chem., 97: 1 (1932).
3. Turpeinen, O., J. Nutrition, 15: 351 (1938).
4. Hume, E. M., Nunn, L. C. A., Smedley-Maclean, I., and Smith, H. H., Biochem. J., 32: 2162 (1938).
5. Wesson, L. G., J. Biol. Chem., 73: 507 (1927); 100: 365 (1933); Wesson, L. G., and Burr, G. O., J. Biol. Chem., 91: 525 (1931).
6. Birch, T. W., J. Biol. Chem., 124: 775 (1938).
7. Sperry, W. M., and Angevine, R. W., J. Biol. Chem., 96: 769 (1932).
8. Hull, M., and Keeton, R. W., J. Biol. Chem., 32: 127 (1917).
9. Sinclair, R. G., J. Biol. Chem., 82: 117 (1929).
10. Sinclair, R. G., and Smith, C., J. Biol. Chem., 121: 361 (1937).
11. Süllmann, H., and Wilbrandt, W., Biochem. Z., 270: 52 (1934).
12. Perlman, I., Ruben, S., and Chaikoff, I. L., J. Biol. Chem., 122: 169 (1937–38).
13. Sperry, W. M., Waelsch, H., and Stoyanoff, V. A., J. Biol. Chem., 135: 281 (1940).
14. Waelsch, H., Sperry, W. M., and Stoyanoff, V. A., J. Biol. Chem., 135: 291 (1940).
15. Verzár, F., and Laszt, L., Biochem. Z., 270: 24, 35 (1934).

16. Verzár, F., and Laszt, L., Biochem. Z., **278:** 396 (1935); Laszt, L., and Verzár, F., Biochem. Z., **288:** 351 (1936).
17. Klinghoffer, K. A., J. Biol. Chem., **126:** 201 (1938).
18. Lambrechts, A., Arch. intern. physiol. Suppl., **44:** 1 (1937).
19. Deuel, H. J., Jr., Hallman, L. F., Murray, S., and Samuels, L. T., J. Biol. Chem., **119:** 607 (1937).
20. Neuberg, C., Biochem. Z., **76:** 107 (1916).
21. Verzár, F., and Kúthy, A., Biochem. Z., **205:** 369; **210:** 265 (1929).
22. Verzár, F., and McDougall, E. J., Absorption from the Intestine, Longmans-Green & Co., London, 1936.
23. Lee, F. C., Johns Hopkins Hosp. Bull., **33:** 21 (1922).
24. Boyd, E. M., J. Biol. Chem., **101:** 323 (1933).
25. Entenman, C., Lorenz, F. W., and Chaikoff, I. L., J. Biol. Chem., **126:** 133 (1938); Lorenz, F. W., Chaikoff, I. L., and Entenman, C., J. Biol. Chem., **126:** 763 (1938).
26. Entenman, C., Chaikoff, I. L., and Montgomery, M. L., J. Biol. Chem., **130:** 121 (1939).
27. Bloor, W. R., J. Biol. Chem., **24:** 447 (1916).
28. Meigs, E. B., Blatherwick, N. R., and Carey, C. A., J. Biol. Chem., **37:** 1 (1919).
29. Gage, S. H., and Fish, P. A., Am. J. Anat., **34:** 1 (1924–25).
30. Ludlum, S. DeW., Taft, A. E., and Nugent, R. L., J. Phys. Chem., **35:** 269 (1931).
31. Frazer, A. C., and Stewart, H. C., J. Physiol., **90:** 18 (1937); Elkes, J. J., Frazer, A. C., and Stewart, H. C., J. Physiol., **95:** 68 (1939).
32. Leathes, J. B., and Raper, H. S., The Fats, Longmans-Green Monograph Series, London, 1925.
33. Hartley, P., J. Physiol., **36:** 17 (1907–08).
34. Klenk, E., and v. Schoenebeck, O., Z. physiol. Chem., **209:** 112 (1932).
35. Schoenheimer, R., and Rittenberg, D., J. Biol. Chem., **113:** 505 (1936).
36. Rittenberg, D., and Schoenheimer, R., J. Biol. Chem., **117:** 485 (1937).
37. Channon, H. J., Irving, E., and Smith, J. A. B., Biochem. J., **28:** 840 (1934).
38. MacLean, D. L., and Best, C. H., Brit. J. Exptl. Path., **15:** 193 (1934).
39. Channon, H. J., Platt, A. P., and Smith, J. A. B., Biochem. J., **31:** 1736 (1937).
40. Best, C. H., Grant, R., and Ridout, J. H., J. Physiol., **86:** 337 (1936).
41. Beeston, A. W., and Channon, H. J., Biochem. J., **30:** 280 (1936).
42. Tucker, H. F., and Eckstein, H. C., J. Biol. Chem., **121:** 479 (1937).
43. Channon, H. J., Manifold, M. C., and Platt, A. P., Biochem. J., **32:** 969 (1938).
44. Tucker, H. F., and Eckstein, H. C., J. Biol. Chem., **126:** 117 (1938); cf. also Tucker, H. F., Treadwell, C. R., and Eckstein, H. C., J. Biol. Chem., **135:** 85 (1940).
45. Singal, A. S., and Eckstein, H. C., Proc. Soc. Exptl. Biol. Med., **41:** 512 (1939).
46. McHenry, E. W., J. Physiol., **89:** 287 (1937).
47. Lajos, S., Z. Immunitäts-, **90:** 261, (1937).
48. Best, C. H., and Campbell, J., J. Physiol., **86:** 190 (1936); **92:** 91 (1938).
49. Campbell, J., and Keenan, H. C., Am. J. Physiol., **131:** 27 (1940).
50. v. Issekutz, B., Jr., and Verzár, F., Arch. ges. Physiol., **240:** 624 (1938).
51. Verzár, F., and Laszt, L., Biochem. Z., **288:** 356 (1936).
52. LeBlond, C. P., van Thoai, N., and Segal, G., Compt. rend. soc. biol., **130:** 1557 (1939).
53. Dragstedt, L. R., Van Prohaska, J., and Harms, H. P., Am. J. Physiol., **117:** 175 (1936).
54. Kaplan, A., and Chaikoff, I. L., J. Biol. Chem., **120:** 647 (1937).
55. Channon, H. J., Loach, J. V., and Tristam, G. R., Biochem. J., **32:** 1332 (1938).
56. MacKay, E. M., and Barnes, R. H., Proc. Soc. Exptl. Biol. Med., **38:** 803 (1938).
57. Bloor, W. R., and Snider, R. H., J. Biol. Chem., **107:** 459 (1934).
58. McConnell, K. P., and Sinclair, R. G., J. Biol. Chem., **118:** 131 (1937).
59. Waelsch, H., Sperry, W. M., and Stoyanoff, V. A., J. Biol. Chem., **135:** 297 (1940).
60. Changus, G. W., Chaikoff, I. L., and Ruben, S., J. Biol. Chem., **126:** 493 (1938).
61. Perlman, I., and Chaikoff, I. L., J. Biol. Chem., **127:** 211 (1938); **128:** 735 (1939).
62. Perlman, I., Stillman, N., and Chaikoff, I. L., J. Biol. Chem., **133:** 651 (1940); **135:** 359 (1940).
63. Knoop, F., Beitr. chem. Physiol. Path., **6:** 150 (1904).

64. Dakin, H. D., J. Biol. Chem., 6: 203, 221 (1909).
65. Embden, G., and Marx, A., Beitr. chem. Physiol. Path., 11: 318 (1908).
66. Quick, A. J., J. Biol. Chem., 80: 515 (1928).
67. Raper, H. S., and Wayne, E. J., Biochem. J., 22: 188 (1928).
68. Schoenheimer, R., and Rittenberg, D., J. Biol. Chem., 120: 155 (1937).
69. Quick, A. J., J. Biol. Chem., 77: 581 (1928).
70. Flaschenträger, B., Bernhard, K., Löwenberg, C., and Schläpfer, M., Z. physiol. Chem., 225: 157 (1934).
71. Verdake, P. E., van der Lee, J., and van Alphen, A. J. S., Z. physiol. Chem., 237: 186 (1935).
72. Hurtley, W. H., Quart. J. Med., 9: 301 (1915–16).
73. Jowett, M., and Quastel, J. H., Biochem. J., 29: 2143 (1935).
74. Deuel, H. J., Jr., Hallman, L. F., Butts, J. S., and Murray, S., J. Biol. Chem., 116: 621 (1936).
75. Blixenkrone-Møller, N., Z. physiol. Chem., 252: 117 (1938).
76. Stadie, W. C., Zapp, J. A., Jr., and Lukens, F. D. W., J. Biol. Chem., 132: 423 (1940); 137: 75 (1941).
77. Chaikoff, I. L., and Soskin, S., Am. J. Physiol., 87: 58 (1928–29).
78. Mirsky, I. A., Am. J. Physiol., 116: 322 (1936).
79. Harrison, H. C., and Long, C. N. H., J. Biol. Chem., 133: 209 (1940).
80. Crandall, L. A., Jr., J. Biol. Chem., 135: 139 (1940).
81. Krebs, H. A., and Johnson, W. A., Biochem. J., 31: 645 (1937).
82. Hirschfeld, F., Z. klin. Med., 28: 176 (1895).
83. Zeller, H., Arch. physiol., p. 213 (1914).
84. Lusk, G., Science of Nutrition, W. B. Saunders, Philadelphia, 4th Ed., 1928.
85. Shaffer, P. A., J. Biol. Chem., 47: 433 (1921); Shaffer, P. A., and Friedemann, T. E., J. Biol. Chem., 61: 585 (1924).
86. Shaffer, P. A., Harvey Lectures, The Williams & Wilkins Co., Baltimore, 1922–23, p. 105.
87. Snapper, I., and Grünbaum, A., Biochem. Z., 201: 464 (1928).
88. Blixenkrone-Møller, N., Z. physiol. Chem., 253: 261 (1938).
89. Stadie, W. C., J. Clin. Invest., 19: 843 (1940).
90. Schoenheimer, R., and Rittenberg, D., J. Biol. Chem., 111: 175 (1935); Rittenberg, D., and Schoenheimer, R., J. Biol. Chem., 121: 235 (1937).
91. Rittenberg, D., Schoenheimer, R., and Evans, E. A., Jr., J. Biol. Chem., 120: 503 (1937).
92. Eckstein, H. C., J. Biol. Chem., 81: 613 (1929); 84: 353 (1929).
93. Ellis, N. R., and Isbell, H. S., J. Biol. Chem., 69: 219, 239 (1926).
94. Anderson, W. E., and Mendel, L. B., J. Biol. Chem., 76: 729 (1928).
95. Schoenheimer, R., Science, 74: 579 (1931); Klin. Woch., 11: 1793 (1932); Schoenheimer, R., and Hrdina, L., Z. physiol. Chem., 212: 161 (1932).
96. Channon, H. J., Biochem. J., 19: 424 (1925).
97. Randles, F. S., and Knudson, A., J. Biol. Chem., 66: 459 (1925).
98. Rittenberg, D., and Schoenheimer, R., J. Biol. Chem., 121: 235 (1937).
99. Eckstein, H. C., J. Biol. Chem., 125: 99, 107 (1938).
100. Dam, H., Biochem. Z., 232: 269 (1931).
101. Page, I. H., and Menschick, W., J. Biol. Chem., 97: 359 (1932).
102. Schoenheimer, R., and Breusch, F., J. Biol. Chem., 103: 439 (1933).
103. Beumer, H., and Hepner, F., Z. ges. exptl. Med., 64: 787 (1929).
104. Schoenheimer, R., and von Behring, H., Z. physiol. Chem., 192: 102 (1930).
105. Sperry, W. M., J. Biol. Chem., 68: 357 (1926); 71: 351 (1926–27); 81: 299 (1929); 85: 455 (1929–30).

CHAPTER V

MINERAL METABOLISM

By Abraham Cantarow

CALCIUM AND PHOSPHORUS

Functions

CALCIUM

Calcium plays an important rôle in the following physiologic processes: (1) bone formation, (2) coagulation of blood, (3) maintenance of normal membrane permeability and neuromuscular excitability. It also perhaps plays a relatively minor part in the preservation of water balance and acid-base equilibrium.

Bone Formation.—Calcium constitutes about 50 per cent of the ash of bones, 85 per cent being in the form of $Ca_3(PO_4)_2$ and 12 per cent as $CaCO_3$. These are present not as a simple mixture but probably as one of the apatite series of minerals, resembling dahlite. There appears to be a nucleus of $Ca_3(PO_4)_2$, upon which is adsorbed chiefly $CaCO_3$ and also $CaHPO_4$ and $Ca(OH)_2$. These substances are deposited in the skeleton during the latter period of fetal life and increase progressively until cessation of skeletal growth. In old age the bones become richer in CO_3 and poorer in PO_4, a change which is accompanied by increase in brittleness. However, regardless of variations in total mineral content or in the form of the complex compound, the Ca/P ratio remains practically fixed at about 2.15 wherever bone is laid down or bone salts are removed.

Normal ossification involves deposition of these salts in an organic matrix in the provisional zone of calcification at the epiphyseal-diaphyseal junctions. The mechanism whereby this process is accomplished is not completely understood, but it depends fundamentally upon the presence in the surrounding tissue fluids of adequate concentrations of calcium and phosphate. These depend in turn upon their concentrations in the blood plasma and, in the case of phosphorus, probably also upon the activity of the phosphatase enzyme in liberating inorganic phosphorus from organic phosphoric esters at the site of calcification. The maintenance of normal quantities of these elements in the blood depends upon their absorption from the bowel in adequate amounts and upon the presence of adequate amounts of vitamin D and parathyroid hormone. The pH at the site of precipitation and the concentration of Mg and of vitamin C also play an important part in this process. Increased local acidity and Mg concentration tend to inhibit calcification, and vitamin C (ascorbic acid) is necessary for the normal development of osteoblasts.

The mineral constituents of the skeleton, particularly calcium and phosphorus, are readily mobilized under physiological and pathological conditions. All recent evidence indicates that the bones constitute a storehouse of available calcium and phosphorus, capable of mobilization upon demand.

Their relation to calcium and phosphorus metabolism in this respect is analogous to that of the glycogen store of the liver to carbohydrate metabolism.

Coagulation of Blood.—Calcium is necessary for normal coagulation of blood (and milk), although it may be replaced in this capacity, but less efficiently, by strontium, barium and magnesium. It appears likely that ionized calcium is essential for the formation of thrombin from its inactive precursors in the blood and tissues and that this process depends upon the formation of an intermediary colloidal complex containing prothrombin, cephalin and calcium.

Neuromuscular Irritability.—Ionic concentrations exert an important if not a controlling influence upon neuromuscular irritability, which is enhanced by an increase in Na or K ions and diminished by an increase in Ca, Mg and H ions. This relationship may be expressed as follows:

$$\text{Irritability } a \ \frac{[\text{Na}^+] + [\text{K}^+]}{[\text{Ca}^{++}] + [\text{Mg}^{++}] + [\text{H}^+]}.$$

The exact site of action of these factors in this connection is not known (nerve cell, muscle cell, or myoneural junction) but it is probably within the nervous mechanism or at the myoneural junction.

The inhibitory influence of calcium is not limited to skeletal muscle and the voluntary nervous system but extends also to unstriated muscle and autonomic nerves. Its importance in the production of normal cardiac contractions and rhythmicity has long been recognized. The *effect of calcium on the heart* resembles that of sympathetic stimulation, although recent studies suggest that it acts upon (*a*) the contractile elements, (*b*) the idioventricular centers, (*c*) the conduction system, (*d*) the cardiac nerves and (*e*) the coronary arteries.[1] The chief effects of an excess of calcium are the development of more forceful contractions, the degree of diastolic relaxation diminishing progressively until the heart stops beating in a state of tonic contraction or systolic standstill (*calcium rigor*). Withdrawal of calcium results in diastolic standstill. Studies of the relationship between the various cations and the autonomic nervous system suggest that, in general, as in the case of the heart, the effect of calcium resembles that of sympathetic stimulation, in contrast to that of K, which resembles parasympathetic stimulation.

Membrane Permeability.—There is reason to regard increase in cell membrane permeability as an intimate part of the excitatory process, inhibition, as the opposite process, being associated with decreased permeability. Since the cell membrane is impervious to cations under ordinary conditions, the action of the calcium ion is probably exerted at the surface of the cell and is probably attributable to its effect in diminishing membrane permeability and in consolidating or stabilizing colloidal systems. Sodium and potassium have an opposite effect in this connection, increasing permeability and colloidal dispersion, and normal cell function is dependent upon the presence of these and other ions in balanced proportions.[2]

PHOSPHORUS

Phosphorus is widely distributed throughout the organism, being present in all cells and body fluids in a variety of organic and inorganic combinations. It may be present in inorganic salts, phospholipids (lecithins, cephalins), nucleic acid, nucleoproteins or nucleotides, phosphoproteins (casein), or in combination as hexose phosphates, glycerophosphates, creatine phosphate and coenzymes. We are concerned here only with the metabolism of *inorganic phosphate*, which may be ingested as such or may be liberated from ester combination by the activity of phosphatase enzymes during the period of digestion or intermediary metabolism.

In addition to its obvious function in ossification of the bones (p. 174), inorganic phosphorus participates in several phases of intermediary metabolism of organic foodstuffs. For example, it has been found, by the use of radioactive isotopes of phosphorus, that administration of sodium phosphate, thus "labeled," was followed by the appearance of radiophosphorus in the casein of milk in three to four hours, and in phospholipid in the brain in one hour. This indicates that some of the P utilized in the synthesis of these and similar substances is derived from the inorganic P of the plasma. It also plays an important rôle in the intermediary metabolism of carbohydrate and of creatine in the chemical phenomena incident to muscular contraction. The formation of a hexose phosphate is a necessary step in the formation of lactic acid from glycogen in muscle (and vice versa) and the capacity for sustained contraction is dependent upon repeated breakdown (into creatine and phosphoric acid) and resynthesis of phosphocreatine.

The **phosphate buffer system,** consisting of a mixture of monosodium and disodium phosphates, is important in the regulation of the acid-base equilibrium in the tissue fluids, the addition of strong acids or alkalies to such a system causing relatively little change in the *p*H of the fluid.

REQUIREMENTS[3, 4, 5, 6]

The requirement of the organism for *calcium* varies considerably under different physiological conditions. The normal adult requires a minimum daily intake of 0.45–0.55 gm. (7–8.5 mg. per Kg.) for maintenance of equilibrium; for purposes of safety it is advisable to provide an excess of about 50 per cent above this figure (0.7–0.85 gm., Ca, 1.0–1.2 gm. CaO). The daily *phosphorus* requirement for normal adults is about 0.88–0.91 gm. (12–14 mg. per Kg.). Allowing an excess of 50 per cent, the recommended intake for maintenance of equilibrium is about 1.32–1.36 gm. daily, constituting approximately $\frac{1}{40}$–$\frac{1}{50}$ of the protein requirement.

Age.—The breastfed infant is maintained by about 45 mg. Ca per Kg. daily and the artificially fed infant by about 150 mg. per Kg. This discrepancy is due largely to the fact that 50 to 70 per cent of the calcium of human milk is retained, as compared to about 30 to 35 per cent of that of cow's milk. The requirement during childhood and adolescence is less definitely established. According to some, there is a gradual decrease from values of 70 mg. per Kg. at three years to 12 mg. at sixteen years. Others place the minimum gross requirements as follows: six months to two years, 0.8 gm. daily; two to nine years, 0.9 gm.; nine years, 1.0 gm., increasing to 2.0 gm. at fifteen to sixteen years and subsequently decreasing steadily to the adult level (0.55 gm.).

Breastfed infants require about 25 mg. P per Kg. daily (average retention 55 per cent), and artificially fed infants 95 mg. per Kg. (retention 25 per cent). These figures are based upon the assumption of an adequate vitamin D intake. As is the case with calcium, the requirement for phosphorus decreases from about 79 mg. per Kg. at three years to 35 mg. at sixteen years.

The Ca/P intake ratio is about 0.7 to 0.8 during infancy, approximately 0.77 during childhood and adolescence and about 0.53 during adult life. The high requirement of children as compared with that of adults is due largely to the necessity for providing for skeletal growth. This disproportion is actually greater than is indicated by the figures quoted above, since the percentage retention of calcium decreases with advancing years.

Food Factors.—The most important and only good natural source of calcium is represented by milk and milk products. About 0.7 gm. Ca is provided by one quart of milk or one-quarter pound of cheese. Meat is a poor source and fruits and vegetables only slightly better from a practical standpoint. Moreover, much of the calcium of vegetables is lost in the discarded water during the process of cooking. The calcium of milk is better absorbed and retained than is that of vegetables, and some variation in this regard exists among vegetables: *e.g.*, the high oxalate content of spinach and other leafy vegetables renders their calcium relatively unavailable.

Although normal nutrition depends more upon an adequate intake of both Ca and P than upon the Ca/P ratio, the latter acquires more significance as the absolute values for either element approach the minimum requirement levels. Under such circumstances, abnormally high or low intake ratios result in impaired utilization of both Ca and P. Proper assimilation is also favored by a simultaneous adequate intake of vitamins D and C. Diets unusually high in fat may tend to inhibit absorption of Ca from the intestine due to the formation of insoluble calcium soaps. Lactose appears to favor absorption of Ca, probably through the development of increased acidity by lactic acid fermentation.

Phosphorus is present in all natural foodstuffs, in largest quantity in milk and milk-products, meat, liver, egg-yolk, cereals, nuts and leguminous vegetables. Diets high in milk and protein, especially nucleoprotein, will readily provide an adequate P intake. Although there is evidence that the P of vegetables, milk and meats is capable of meeting normal requirements, probably not all forms of combination are equally well utilized. The availability depends in part upon the type of the P compound and upon other constituents of the diet. Infants retain 55 per cent of the P of human milk and 25 per cent of that of cow's milk.

Pregnancy and Lactation.—The requirement and retention of calcium are considerably increased during *pregnancy*, particularly during the late months. The quantity retained is more than can be accounted for by fetal utilization, and perhaps represents the establishment of a reserve supply which may be called upon during subsequent emergencies. The calcium content of the fetus increases from about 5 gm. at the 28th week to 30 gm. at the 40th week. It has been estimated that the Ca requirement during pregnancy is 1.5–3.0 gm. daily and that the total retention under conditions of adequate intake is about 50 gm. The excess, above that utilized by the fetus, is stored in the maternal skeleton. This storage amounts to about 200 mg. daily from the fourth to the ninth month, and 300 mg. during the last week of pregnancy. If the supply is not adequate for the needs of the fetus, its mineral requirements will be met by Ca and P mobilized from the maternal skeleton, with consequent demineralization of the latter.[2]

The onset of *lactation* is marked by a sudden change from a positive to a negative calcium balance. The loss of Ca is due not only to the large quantities present in the milk but also to excessive excretion, particularly in the feces. Negative balances may occur with daily intakes of as much as 3.0 gm. and may continue for several months after cessation of lactation. This loss of Ca may be diminished by administration of increased amounts of vitamin D.

The P requirement is also increased during pregnancy, a daily intake of 2.5–3.0 gm. being generally adequate. Under these conditions, if the supply of Ca and vitamin D is adequate, about 35–40 gm. of P are retained during the period of pregnancy. A portion of this is stored (with Ca) in the bones, the remainder participating in the intermediary metabolism of carbohydrate, fat and protein. Although a negative balance may occur with the onset of lactation, this is not so pronounced nor so persistent as in the case of Ca.

Absorption

Calcium is absorbed from the upper portion of the small intestine, especially the duodenum, and is readily assimilable whether supplied in organic or inorganic combination. As indicated elsewhere (p. 177), there is considerable variation in the facility with which the Ca of different foodstuffs is absorbed and retained. Infants absorb and retain 50–70 per cent of the Ca of human milk and 30–35 per cent of that of cow's milk. In general, the Ca of milk is better utilized than that of vegetables and, in the case of certain of the latter, the contained Ca is unavailable because of their high oxalate content.

Absorption of Ca is governed chiefly by three factors: 1. Vitamin D, 2. Other substances in the diet, and 3. Hydrogen-ion concentration within the intestine. The exact mode of action of vitamin D is not known. However, although its chief effect may be exerted in the intermediary metabolism of P and Ca and in their deposition in the bones, there is little doubt that this factor, in physiologic dosage, plays an important rôle in favoring absorption of Ca from the intestine. Excessive quantities cause abnormal mobilization of both Ca and P from the bones, with consequent demineralization, particularly if the intake is inadequate.[2, 7]

Under conditions of normal gastric acidity, compounds of Ca with weak organic acids are converted into the chloride and, if retained in the stomach for a sufficient period, even the less soluble basic phosphate may go into solution. However, solution of Ca salts by the gastric juice is not indispensable, as adequate absorption may occur in the presence of achlorhydria, or following gastrectomy or administration of alkalinizing agents. The acidity in the duodenum is of considerable importance; this ranges normally from pH 2.3 to 7.0. This factor largely determines whether the most of the Ca is in the form of the acid or the basic phosphate and, since the former is the more soluble, a higher acidity tends to facilitate absorption of Ca. Calcium chloride and acid phosphate are probably absorbed from the duodenum before the gastric acidity is neutralized and, subsequently, continued absorption may be favored by the formation of organic acids (carbonic and lactic).[3, 6]

Reference has been made to the influence of certain food factors and of the Ca/P ratio upon absorption of Ca. An excessively high P intake tends to inhibit absorption of Ca, especially if the latter is supplied in insufficient amounts. A similar inhibiting effect is apparently exerted by an excess of Mg and of K. It is important to note that calcium salts (chloride, gluconate, lactate) are absorbed most efficiently in interdigestive periods, *i.e.*, when the stomach and duodenum contain no food. When given for therapeutic purposes, therefore, these salts should be administered about one-half to three-quarters of an hour before meals and eating between meals should be avoided. Disturbance of fatty-acid absorption limits absorption of Ca, in part through formation of insoluble soaps in the intestine and also perhaps by interference with absorption of vitamin D. Inadequate absorption may also result from protracted diarrhea, due to the rapid passage of intestinal contents through the bowel.[2]

Simple phosphates (Ca, Na, K) are absorbed as such, largely in the small intestine and more readily in its upper than its lower portion. Factors which influence the absorption of calcium phosphate have been referred to previously. In the course of gastric and intestinal digestion of nucleoproteins and phosphoproteins, phosphate is split off and is absorbed as such. If ester forms are present, they must undergo hydrolysis by phosphatases prior to absorption. For example, liberation of phosphate from such substances as lecithin and the carbohydrate esters of phosphoric acid does not occur until they have been subjected to the action of pancreatic and intestinal secretions. It has been suggested that because of this fact, a considerable fraction of the ingested phosphate is absorbed later than the major part of the calcium. This permits absorption of portions of both of these elements which would not otherwise be absorbed, especially in regions of low acidity. It is also probable that a part of the phosphorus excreted into upper levels of the intestine is absorbed at lower levels.

Absorption of P is *diminished* by factors which favor the formation of poorly soluble salts of phosphoric acid. This can be demonstrated strikingly by experimental administration of beryllium which, through the formation of insoluble beryllium phosphate, prevents absorption of phosphoric acid and results in a characteristic form of rickets. Similar inhibition is produced, to a much smaller degree, by an excess of other cations, such a calcium, strontium, magnesium, barium, aluminum and thallium. It was formerly believed that absorption of P from the intestine was diminished in the presence of vitamin D deficiency, but this view is not supported by recent evidence.

EXCRETION

Calcium is excreted by the kidneys, the liver, and the epithelium of the large bowel. The fact that the fecal Ca includes that portion of the ingested Ca that has escaped absorption and has passed through the gastro-intestinal tract has rendered difficult the exact quantitative determination of intestinal excretion of Ca. With low and moderate levels of intake (0.1–0.5 gm. daily) about 30–50 per cent is eliminated in the urine, while with high levels (1.0 gm.) about 10–25 per cent is so excreted. However, considerable deviations from these values occur, dependent probably upon variable dietary, metabolic and gastro-intestinal factors. The renal threshold for excretion of Ca probably lies between 6.5 and 8.5 mg. per 100 cc. of serum, little being eliminated in the urine at serum levels below these values.[8] This threshold is raised in the presence of renal functional impairment, the urinary Ca constituting a steadily diminishing fraction of the total excretion in progressive kidney damage.

The proportion *excreted* in the feces is increased by factors which diminish absorption (p. 179); among the most important of these are steatorrhea, diarrhea and vitamin D deficiency. An increase in both urinary and fecal Ca occurs in hyperthyroidism and after administration of thyroxin. Increased urinary excretion of Ca results chiefly from the operation of factors that increase the rate of its mobilization from the bones. These include (*a*) acidosis or administration of an excess of acid-forming substances, (*b*) thyroxin, (*c*) parathyroid hormone, (*d*) excessively large doses of vitamin D (20,000 units or more). In the presence of thyroid, parathyroid and vitamin D deficiencies the urinary excretion of Ca is decreased.

Inorganic P is excreted by the kidneys and bowel, usually somewhat more in the urine than in the feces, the relative proportions varying considerably under different conditions. The source of inorganic P in the urine is the inorganic P of the plasma, although there is evidence that it may be contributed to by hydrolysis of phosphoric acid esters through phosphatase activity. The renal threshold is about 2 to 3 mg. of P per 100 cc. of plasma, excretion falling to a minimum at concentrations below this level.

On a balanced diet the urinary P constitutes about 60 per cent of the total excretion. As the Ca intake is decreased the proportion of P eliminated in the urine increases, being about 75 per cent of the total with a moderately low intake and about 85 per cent with a low Ca-moderately high P intake. The proportion excreted in the feces is increased by dietary factors which inhibit absorption, including a high intake of Ca (p. 179). In the presence of renal functional impairment, as in chronic glomerulonephritis, the urine phosphate is decreased and the fecal phosphate correspondingly increased. Urine P is increased after administration of parathyroid hormone, thyroxin, acids or acid-forming substances, dihydrotachysterol and extremely large amounts of vitamin D. Therapeutic doses of vitamin D cause a decrease in fecal P, which is increased under conditions of vitamin D deficiency.

BLOOD CALCIUM

The Ca of the blood is almost entirely in the plasma. Determinations are usually made on serum, which normally contains 9.0 to 11.5 mg. per 100 cc. During infancy and early childhood (until about twelve years) the average values approach the upper limit of this range, subsequently decreasing with advancing age. Fetal blood at term has a Ca concentration of 11 to 12 mg. per 100 cc., the maternal serum Ca being usually 9.0 to 9.5 mg. The slight fall during the last month of normal pregnancy has been attributed to the heavy drain upon the mineral reserves of the maternal organism, but it seems likely that endocrine factors participate in the production of this phenomenon.

Calcium exists in the blood, as a phosphate probably, in much higher *concentration* than would be possible in distilled water. Its solubility in plasma is dependent largely upon the following factors: 1. the *p*H, 2. the

CO_2 tension, 3. the protein concentration, 4. the total ionic strength, 5. the Mg concentration, 6. the inorganic P concentration. Their influence may be illustrated as follows: If 10 mg. of Ca and 4 mg. of P are placed in 100 cc. of distilled water (pH 7.0), only a small amount of the resulting salt will go into solution, but more will be dissolved at the pH of plasma than in a more alkaline medium. At a constant pH, its solubility is inversely proportional to the concentration of bicarbonate and phosphate ions and at constant hydrogen, bicarbonate and phosphate ion concentrations the solubility is increased by addition of other soluble ions in amounts present in normal plasma. The quantity of Ca still undissolved may be brought into solution by addition of 1–3 mg. of Mg and 4–5 gm. of albumin per 100 cc. From a practical clinical standpoint, the effects of alteration in phosphate and protein content are of greatest importance.[9]

Ca exists in the plasma in two *forms*, termed diffusible and nondiffusible accordingly as it can or cannot pass through artificial semipermeable membranes and, presumably, through living membranes. On this basis, the *diffusible fraction* normally constitutes 45 to 60 per cent of the total Ca of human serum, or 4.5 to 6.0 mg. per 100 cc., the remainder being nondiffusible. The latter is believed to be in physical or physicochemical combination with protein, chiefly albumin. This fraction is probably inert physiologically, being in an un-ionized state, and it is this portion of the serum Ca that may be diminished in the presence of a lowered plasma protein concentration. Under certain conditions (addition of large amounts of Ca or P, large doses of parathyroid hormone or vitamin D) the *nondiffusible fraction* may include a colloidal complex of calcium phosphate, but it usually consists practically entirely of calcium proteinate. Although the two fractions (diffusible and nondiffusible) may vary independently of each other under certain circumstances, there is evidence that they are in a state of rather unstable equilibrium, which is perhaps controlled to a certain extent by the parathyroid hormone.[2, 10]

The diffusible fraction contains the ionized, physiologically active portion of the serum Ca, the accurate quantitative estimation of which has encountered considerable difficulty. Despite some theoretical objection, the concept is becoming generally accepted that the diffusible Ca is practically completely ionized. On this basis the total plasma Ca is nearly all accountable as either calcium ions or protein-bound Ca, the concentration of the former at any time being the resultant of an equilibrium between the total Ca and the plasma protein. The Ca ion concentration is normally maintained within a rather narrow range (4.25 to 5.25 mg. per 100 cc.) by a process of physiological regulation in which the parathyroid hormone plays an important rôle.[11]

The parathyroid hormone and vitamin D are among the most important **physiological regulators** of the serum Ca level. The chief consequences of administration of parathyroid hormone are: (*a*) Increased serum Ca; (*b*) decreased serum P; (*c*) increased serum phosphatase activity; (*d*) increased urinary P; (*e*) increased urinary Ca. The mechanism of its action is not definitely known; there is evidence that the initial effect is the increased renal excretion of P, resulting in (*a*) a fall in serum P, (*b*) relative unsaturation of the serum with regard to calcium phosphate, (*c*) mobilization of P and Ca from the bones, (*d*) hypercalcemia, and (*e*) increased urinary excretion of Ca.[7] Others believe that the hormone acts primarily on the bones, stimulating osteoclasis and the formation of increased numbers of osteoclasts, with increased mobilization of Ca and P from the skeleton. However, regardless of the fundamental mechanism involved, the function of parathyroid hormone in maintaining the serum Ca concentration is exerted through mobilization of this element from its storehouse in the bones.

Vitamin D appears to act principally by increasing the absorption of Ca from the intestine and by facilitating the deposition of Ca and P in the bones (zones of provisional calcification). This factor exerts a greater and more immediate influence upon P than Ca in the blood serum. The mechanism of its action is not clearly understood. The view that it acts through stimulation of the parathyroid glands is contradicted by several facts. The parathyroid hormone has no antirachitic effect, causes a primary decrease in serum P and corpuscular ester P, and an increase in serum phosphatase activity and negative Ca and P balance, whereas vitamin D, in physiologic dosage, produces directly opposite effects. Moreover, the characteristic histologic picture of osteitis fibrosa cystica, which has been observed in experimental hyperparathyroidism, has not been seen in experimental hypervitaminosis D.[7]

The influence on Ca metabolism of other facts, such as the anterior hypophysis, thyroid, adrenal cortex, gonads and renal function, is evidenced chiefly under abnormal conditions, and will be considered subsequently. Ingestion of adequate amounts of soluble Ca salts in the postabsorptive state results in distinct elevation of serum Ca, which reaches a maximum in about two to three hours and returns to the previous level in about four hours. After intravenous injection, the peak is reached in a few minutes, with a subsequent fall to normal, usually within one to two hours, depending upon the quantity administered. Following intramuscular injection (Ca gluconate) the serum Ca rises to a maximum level in about one hour and falls gradually over a period of three to four hours. Intravenous or intramuscular injection of Mg salts may cause a fall in serum Ca, at times to tetanic levels.[12]

PHOSPHATASE ACTIVITY[7, 13, 14]

Definition and Distribution.—Phosphatase is an enzyme which hydrolyzes monophosphoric esters, with the liberation of inorganic phosphate. It is present in practically all tissues, body fluids and cells, including red blood cells and leukocytes. In the fetus and during the period of growth it is present in greatest concentration in the bones and teeth. It occurs in largest amount in ossifying cartilage but is absent from resting epiphyseal cartilage, from nonossifying cartilage in other situations and from bones before the appearance of ossification centers. In adults, the intestinal mucosa contains the largest amount (per unit of wet weight), followed in approximate order by the renal cortex, bone, thyroid, spleen, lungs, suprarenal glands, blood vessels and pancreas, with some variation in different species. There are two classes of phosphatases in the animal organism, *"acid"* phosphatase (liver, kidney, prostate, red blood cells) and *"alkaline"* phosphatase (bone, bile, plasma, white blood cells), varying in their optimum pH ranges of activity. The "alkaline" phosphatase is of the greatest clinical interest since it is the form present in largest amount in the blood plasma. Phosphatase is activated by a number of substances, including Mg, Fe, Mn, Co,

Ni, ascorbic acid and glycine. There is some evidence that it is inhibited by Cu, Zn and cholic acid.

The bones are apparently the chief if not the only source of the "alkaline" phosphatase of plasma, which is not appreciably reduced after removal of practically all abdominal viscera. However, some believe that other organs, especially the liver, may be additional sources of plasma phosphatase. There is also evidence that the plasma may contain "acid" phosphatase (0.5 to 2.5 units per 100 cc.) which may vary in disease states independently of alkaline phosphatase. Normal prostatic tissue appears to contain large amounts of an "acid" phosphatase. The enzyme is excreted in large amounts by the liver and also perhaps by the kidneys.

Functions of Phosphatase.—By virtue of their power to liberate inorganic phosphorus from ester combinations, phosphatases play an important part in the absorption and excretion of P and in its intermediary metabolism. It seems significant in this connection that they are usually present in large quantity in the intestinal mucosa (absorption), kidney (excretion) and bones (ossification). Phosphatases also play an essential part in fermentation reactions and in the chemical reactions in various phases of muscular activity. Their relation to the phenomenon of calcification is of particular interest.

The following hypothesis has been advanced (Robison and Soames)[15]: Osteoblasts, hypertrophic cartilage cells and certain cells of the inner portion of the periosteum in growing bones contain or can secrete phosphatase. This enzyme hydrolyzes phosphoric esters brought in the blood to the ossifying zone, with consequent local increase in the concentration of phosphate ions. The solubility product for calcium phosphate is exceeded locally and deposition of calcium phosphate occurs in or near the cells which secrete or contain the active enzyme. There are several objections to complete acceptance of this hypothesis, but there seems little doubt that this mechanism must be accorded a position of importance in any theory of calcification of bone. Other factors must be considered, such as serum Ca and P concentrations, the parathyroid hormone, vitamin D, Ca and P intake and absorption from the intestine and the state of the acid-base equilibrium.

Serum Phosphatase Activity.—According to the method of Bodansky,[16] a unit of phosphatase activity is defined as "equivalent to the actual or calculated liberation of 1 mg. of phosphorus as the phosphate ion during the first hour of incubation at 37° C. and pH 8.6, with the substrate containing sodium beta-glycerophosphate, hydrolysis not exceeding 10 per cent of the substrate." The range of normal values for plasma or serum phosphatase activity in adults by this method, is 1.5 to 4.0 units per 100 cc. and for children 5 to 14 units. Phosphatase activity is low at birth, rises to a maximum during the first month of life and remains fairly high during the second year, the values in later childhood falling gradually to adult levels. High protein diets cause a decrease and high carbohydrate diets an increase in phosphatase activity of the serum. Some observers have reported a slight increase in the last few months of pregnancy, but the statistical significance of such findings is questionable.

Increased Serum Phosphatase Activity.[17]—Serum phosphatase activity is increased chiefly in certain diseases of bone and in certain hepatic and biliary tract disorders. In the former, it appears to be related in most instances to the extent of osteoblastic activity or to the intensity of attempts at bone formation. The cause of increase in diseases of the liver and bile passages is not known, although some, probably erroneously, attribute it to retention in the blood as a result of impaired excretion.[7]

Serum phosphatase activity is consistently increased in active *rickets* (20 to 190 units). The degree of increase may be regarded as a reliable criterion of the severity of the condition, a decrease occurring within a few days after institution of antirachitic therapy and normal values being gradually restored during the period of active repair. High values (15 to 125 units) are obtained rather consistently in polyostotic forms of *osteitis deformans* (Paget's disease). Normal or slightly increased activity (to 25 units) may occur in cases with localized involvement of one or two bones. The values tend to be lower in older subjects. A moderate increase (20 to 40 units) is observed in clinical and experimental *hyperparathyroidism*. Slightly elevated values (5 to 15 units) have been reported occasionally in patients with generalized osteoporosis, marked hyperthyroidism, osteomalacia, metastatic carcinoma involving bone, osteogenic sarcoma, cases of Hodgkin's disease, lymphosarcoma and leukemia with bone involvement, polyostotic fibrous dysplasia, during the period of healing of fractures, Gaucher's disease with bone resorption and osteosclerosis fragilis generalisata (marble-bone disease), and, rarely, in renal rickets and multiple myeloma. An increase in "acid" phosphatase activity has been observed in metastasizing prostatic carcinoma, the enzyme in such cases resembling that present in normal prostatic tissue.[18]

Serum phosphatase activity is increased in a large proportion of patients with obstructive and hepatocellular types of *jaundice* (to 60 units). Values above 20 units are obtained much more often in the former than the latter form, but this factor is of limited value in differential diagnosis because of a wide overlapping of values in the two groups of cases. High figures are also observed in patients with portal cirrhosis, metastatic carcinoma involving the liver, and biliary fistula. On the other hand, normal values have been reported in infants with congenital atresia of the bile ducts. No increase occurs in hemolytic types of jaundice.

Increased serum phosphatase activity has been reported in the following conditions: during periods of calcification of hemorrhages in scurvy, in active tuberculosis and in chronic myeloid leukemia. Increased phosphatase activity has also been demonstrated in tumor cells, in heterotopic bone, in muscle and fibrous tissue in pre-ossification stages of myositis ossificans and in the liver, spleen, and kidneys in myelogenous leukemia.

HYPERCALCEMIA[2, 3, 7, 9, 17]

Hyperparathyroidism.—Increase in the serum calcium concentration is one of the most striking and constant features of hyperparathyroidism, either spontaneous or induced by administration of parathyroid hormone. Values as high as 29.5 mg. per 100 cc. have been observed. The mechanism underlying the production of this phenomenon, as well as the associated metabolic and clinical manifestations are described elsewhere (pp. 181, 189).

Hypervitaminosis D.—Hypercalcemia may result from administration of excessive amounts of vitamin D. This condition is rarely encountered clinically. However, there is a wide range of individual susceptibility to the action of this factor, and the coincident administration of large quantities of calcium increases the tendency toward the development of hypercalcemia.

Dihydrotachysterol (A.T. 10).—The administration of therapeutic doses of this substance, a photochemical derivative of ergosterol, results in an increase in serum calcium (p. 208). Its physiologic effect appears to be more closely analogous to that of parathyroid hormone than is that of vitamin D, since it causes greater urinary excretion of phosphate and rise in serum calcium than does the latter. It has no significant antirachitic properties.

Multiple Myeloma.—Hypercalcemia has been reported in about 50 per cent of cases of multiple myeloma in which mention was made of the serum Ca concentration, values as high as 20.2 mg. having been observed. Some attribute this phenomenon to the existence of a state of hyperparathyroidism, since the parathyroid glands are often enlarged. However, this hypothesis is contradicted by the frequent absence of generalized skeletal abnormality and the usually normal or elevated serum phosphorus concentration and normal serum phosphatase activity. The increase in serum Ca may be dependent upon the frequently increased serum protein concentration, but this seems unlikely as the increase in the latter is practically always confined to the globulin fraction.

Skeletal Neoplasm.—The serum Ca concentration is usually normal in the great majority of cases of primary and metastatic neoplasms of bone. However, values as high as 22 mg. per 100 cc. have been observed, particularly in cases of extensive metastatic involvement of the skeleton. In such cases, values for serum P and phosphatase activity are usually within normal limits, except in osteogenic sarcoma, in which the serum phosphatase activity may be increased.

Miscellaneous.—The serum Ca may be increased in rare instances of advanced nephritis with uremia, although any deviation from the normal in this condition is usually in the opposite direction (p. 186). This hypercalcemia is difficult to explain; some believe that chronic nephritis is accompanied by a state of hyperparathyroidism, because of the rather common observation of enlargement of the parathyroid glands (p. 187).

Hypercalcemia has been observed occasionally in leukemia and polycythemia vera, the mechanism of its production being unknown. Slight elevations may occur in conditions in which the CO_2 content of the blood is increased, thereby enhancing its capacity for maintaining Ca in solution (asphyxia, chronic emphysema, pneumonia, silicosis, congestive heart failure).

Administration of anterior hypophyseal extracts to experimental animals has resulted in hypercalcemia. This has been attributed to the action of a "parathyrotropic" principle. However, except for the possible hypophyseal origin of hyperparathyroidism due to diffuse hyperplasia or hypertrophy of the parathyroid glands, elevation of the serum Ca concentration has not been observed in uncomplicated clinical pituitary disorders. Borderline high values occur occasionally in patients with pituitary basophilism. A similar effect has followed administration of gonadotropic hormone and certain estrogens (theelin, estradiol benzoate, dihydrotheelin and theelol) to experimental animals. Marked hypercalcemia (20 to 28 mg. per 100 cc.) occurs in birds just before and during ovulation. This has been attributed to indirect stimulation of parathyroid activity through the medium of pituitary stimulation. This phenomenon has been produced by artificial distention of the oviduct.

HYPOCALCEMIA[2, 3, 9, 17]

Hypoparathyroidism.—Hypocalcemia is one of the most constant and characteristic features of diminished parathyroid function. Both diffusible and nondiffusible fractions are decreased. The clinical and metabolic features of this condition are described elsewhere (p. 202).

Vitamin D Deficiency.—Deficiency in vitamin D results in *rickets* characteristically, the serum Ca concentration being within normal limits in the great majority of instances. However, hypocalcemia occurs in some cases, with the development of infantile tetany (p. 209). The same is true of *osteomalacia*, which resembles the low calcium form of rickets in its pathologic physiology. Low Ca and normal or low P values are often obtained in rickets during recovery periods, especially if therapy has been inadequate or if vitamin D has been given in very large doses.

Steatorrhea.—This condition is encountered in celiac disease, in sprue, and occasionally in prolonged obstructive jaundice. The outstanding feature is defective absorption of fat from the intestine, as a result of which large quantities of insoluble calcium soaps are formed with consequent inadequate absorption of Ca and probably also of vitamin D. The serum Ca may be low and tetany, delayed ossification (in infants) and osteoporosis occur frequently.

Hunger Osteopathy.—This condition is due to a diet deficient in total caloric value and in Ca, P and vitamin D, and resembles a slowly progressive osteomalacia.

Hypoproteinemia.—Serum Ca values as low as 5.7 mg. per 100 cc. have been observed in association with hypoproteinemia accompanying the nephrotic syndrome, obstructive jaundice, kala-azar, malignancy, and other cachectic states. The diminution in serum Ca occurs entirely in the nondiffusible fraction and is apparently due to the decrease in serum albumin concentration and not to any disturbance of calcium metabolism. There is no significant alteration in diffusible Ca and no increase in neuromuscular excitability.

Chronic Glomerulonephritis.—Hypocalcemia is occasionally observed in non-nephrotic forms of chronic glomerulonephritis in the stage of renal functional failure. It occurs usually in the late stages of this condition and is associated with and perhaps dependent upon the increase in serum P which is present in such cases (p. 187). The concentration of Ca varies roughly inversely with that of P, values as low as 4 to 6 mg. being observed occasionally, at times with manifestations of tetany. In many cases the decrease in serum Ca is contributed to by the presence of hypoproteinemia. It is believed by some that hypocalcemia may be responsible for certain of the manifestations of uremia.

Skeletal changes may occur in chronic nephritis or in congenital urinary tract defects, their character varying from generalized osteoporosis to cyst formation and deformities, with extensive metastatic calcification. When occurring during the period of skeletal growth the condition has been termed renal rickets or renal dwarfism. A similar condition may occur in adults, with fibrocystic changes in all bones and metastatic calcification, particularly in the media of the arteries (Mönckeberg type) and in the neighborhood of joints. This has been termed *renal osteitis fibrosa cystica*, and is regarded as the adult counterpart of renal rickets. In both forms there are evidences of long-existing renal failure, usually marked acidosis, hyperphosphatemia, usually normal or slightly reduced serum Ca concentration and generally normal serum phosphatase activity. *Parathyroid hyperplasia*, involving principally the chief cells, has been found in a large proportion of such cases, being probably compensatory in nature and induced by the prolonged increase in serum P. All the parathyroid glands are increased in size when hyperplasia is present. The nature and extent of the skeletal changes are not directly proportional to the degree of hyperplasia and, indeed, may be marked in the absence of the latter, suggesting that the bone lesions are not caused by hyperparathyroidism in such cases. Some believe that there is an increase in the amount of parathyroid hormone in the blood, but this has not been demonstrated conclusively. It appears probable that the bone changes are dependent primarily upon the effects of (*a*) acidosis and (*b*) inadequate absorption of Ca resulting from the excretion into the intestine of large amounts of P which would have been eliminated in the urine under conditions of normal renal function. Differentiation of this condition from hyperparathyroidism is considered elsewhere (p. 198).

Phosphate Administration.—A fall in serum Ca, at times to tetanic levels, may follow the administration of phosphate intravenously, frank *tetany* being produced more readily by neutral and alkaline than by acid salts. A similar phenomenon may be produced by a high P, low Ca diet. These observations emphasize the usually inverse relationship between Ca and P under such conditions.

INORGANIC PHOSPHORUS IN BLOOD[3, 6, 17]

The inorganic phosphorus of the blood probably exists almost entirely in the plasma. The chief difficulty in determining its concentration in the red blood cells arises from the fact that a portion of the phosphoric esters in these cells undergoes hydrolysis in the process of analysis, with the consequent liberation of phosphate.

The *serum inorganic* P ranges from 5 to 6.5 mg. per 100 cc. in infancy and gradually diminishes until it reaches 3 to 4.5 mg. in normal adults. The concentration is usually highest in summer and lowest in winter, varying with the concentration of ultraviolet rays. A slight increase follows the ingestion of calcium and a considerable drop follows parenteral administration of Mg salts. Under normal conditions, ingestion of carbohydrate results in a progressive fall in serum P which persists during the period of increased glucose utilization, returning to normal in 4 to 5 hours. This is due to the fact that combinations of carbohydrate and phosphoric acid (hexosephosphate) play an important part in the intermediary metabolism of carbohydrate. A similar drop follows administration of insulin and epinephrin.

Hyperphosphatemia.—The serum P concentration may be increased by therapeutic and excessive doses of vitamin D. Slightly increased values are also observed in hypoparathyroidism, the degree of increase being approximately proportional to the degree of hypocalcemia. A rise also occurs at times during the period of healing of fractures. Highest values (8 to 40 mg. per 100 cc.) are observed in renal failure (chronic glomerulonephritis, pyelonephritis, nephrosclerosis, urinary obstruction, polycystic disease and destructive kidney lesions). An increase has also been reported in acute intestinal obstruction and following injection of histamine. Phosphate retention in renal failure may contribute to the development of acidosis, but the latter may exist in the absence of the former.

Hypophosphatemia.—Vitamin D deficiency is one of the most important causes of hypophosphatemia, values of 1 to 3 mg. per 100 cc. being obtained frequently in children with rickets. The exact mode of action of vitamin D is not clearly understood, but deficiency in this factor probably results in inability to utilize Ca and P properly in the process of ossification, with increased excretion of P in the feces. The fall in serum P is most marked when the P intake is inadequate. The serum Ca concentration may be normal or subnormal (p. 213). It has been pointed out that if the concentration of Ca be multiplied by that of P, each being expressed in mg. per 100 cc., a product is obtained which, in the normal child, ranges from 50 to 60. When the product is below 30, *rickets* is usually present and when it is above 40, either healing is occurring or rickets has probably not been present. These observations cannot be relied upon absolutely.

Diminished serum P concentration occurs in osteomalacia, being here, as in rickets, a manifestation of vitamin D deficiency. It occurs also in steatorrhea (sprue, celiac disease), probably as a result of defective intestinal absorption of Ca, P and vitamin D, due to the excessive amount of fat in the intestine. The characteristic fatty diarrhea in these conditions is frequently accompanied by skeletal demineralization, dwarfism, low serum Ca and P and manifestations of rickets and tetany.

Injection of *parathyroid hormone* is followed by a decrease in serum P which probably results from its increased elimination in the urine. A similar change occurs characteristically in uncomplicated clinical hyperparathyroidism (p. 195). This decrease is roughly proportional to the degree of hypercalcemia. With the supervention of renal failure in this condition, the urinary excretion of P diminishes and the serum P rises to normal or supernormal levels (p. 187).

CALCIUM AND PHOSPHORUS IN OTHER BODY FLUIDS[3, 7, 17]

The electrolyte composition of the interstitial fluid of the body is the result of a Donnan distribution between the fluid and the blood plasma. The Ca and P in this fluid are therefore in a state of equilibrium with their diffusible fractions in the plasma, plus an additional variable amount roughly proportional to the protein content of the fluid. Thus the Ca content ranges from 4.5 to 5.5 mg. per 100 cc. in the case of protein-free fluids and transudates and from 5 to 11 mg. in transudates and exudates with high protein contents and in synovial fluid, which has a protein content of 4.2 to 7.3 gm. per 100 cc. The Ca content of ocular fluid is about 6 to 7 mg. per 100 cc. and that of cerebrospinal fluid 4.5 to 6 mg. Although the latter is quantitatively identical with the diffusible fraction of serum Ca under normal conditions, this is not the case in abnormal states. For example, very little change occurs in cerebrospinal fluid Ca following parathyroidectomy, although the serum Ca concentration may be markedly diminished. In some instances the values for Ca in the serum and cerebrospinal fluid may be practically identical. This is not true of other body fluids.

The inorganic P of the blood plasma is practically entirely diffusible and, consequently, its concentration in the water of the interstitial fluids of the body is practically the same as in the water of the plasma. The actual concentration is slightly higher than in equivalent volumes of plasma because of the relatively high protein content of the latter. The P content of aqueous humor and of cerebrospinal fluid averages about 50 per cent of that of the plasma, suggesting that these fluids are not in diffusion equilibrium with the blood.

CLINICAL MANIFESTATIONS OF ABNORMAL CALCIUM AND PHOSPHORUS METABOLISM

The most important clinical conditions characterized by disturbance of Ca and P metabolism are those dependent upon or associated with abnormalities of *parathyroid function* and of *vitamin D supply* or utilization. In these conditions, characteristic changes in the metabolism of these elements can usually be demonstrated. There are many other clinical disorders, not primarily dependent upon disturbance in Ca or P metabolism, in which significant changes may occur in the Ca content of and distribution in various tissues. In certain of these, as in renal disease and hyperthyroidism, the pathogenesis of these changes is fairly well understood. In others, however, as in certain skeletal disorders (osteitis deformans, polyostotic fibrous dysplasia, marble-bone disease, fragilitas ossium, *etc.*) and in calcinosis universalis, little or no disturbance of Ca and P metabolism can be demonstrated. The former will be discussed in detail and the latter mentioned only briefly in their relation to problems of differential diagnosis.

HYPERPARATHYROIDISM[2, 3, 9, 17, 19]

Excessive secretion of parathyroid hormone has been demonstrated in association with (*a*) adenoma of one or more parathyroid glands and (*b*) diffuse hyperplasia or hypertrophy of all parathyroid glands. These may be regarded as primary forms of hyperparathyroidism, although it has been suggested that diffuse hyperplasia may be the result of hypophyseal hyperfunction, with excessive stimulation of the parathyroids, presumably by the parathyrotropic principle of the pituitary gland.

The existence of a state of hyperparathyroidism has been implied or affirmed in a number of other conditions in which parathyroid hyperplasia is present occasionally or consistently. These include:

1. Chronic glomerulonephritis and other forms of renal disease associated with "renal rickets."

2. True rickets and osteomalacia.

3. Certain cases of senile osteoporosis, multiple myeloma, pituitary basophilism, metastatic malignancy involving the skeleton, osteogenesis imperfecta, chronic hypertrophic arthritis, acromegaly, and "marble-bone disease."

In some of these conditions, *e.g.*, renal rickets, renal disease, rickets, and osteomalacia, the existence of hyperparathyroidism has been predicated on the basis of the apparent determination of an increase in parathyroid hormone in the blood by means of the rabbit hypercalcemia test of Hamilton and Schwartz.[22] However, the validity of interpretations based upon results obtained by this procedure is open to question. Moreover, it is obvious that enlargement of the parathyroid glands occurring as a secondary phenomenon in response to either elevation of the serum P concentration or active skeletal demineralization may not necessarily be accompanied by an actual increase in parathyroid hormone secretion. This enlargement should probably be regarded as a condition of *compensatory hyperplasia* rather than hyperfunction. Hyperparathyroidism has also been implicated as an etiologic factor in *scleroderma*. This association has been predicated on the basis of the occasional occurrence of calcinosis in scleroderma and the experimental production of scleroderma-like lesions by administration of parathyroid hormone. However, there is no substantial evidence that this condition is accompanied by a state of hyperparathyroidism.

A state of hyperparathyroidism (*primary hyperparathyroidism*) is the functional basis for the development of the condition variously designated as generalized osteitis fibrosa cystica, von Recklinghausen's disease of bone, parathyroid osteosis, osteodystrophia cystica and osteodystrophia fibrosa. The term "hyperparathyroidism" is to be preferred inasmuch as it indicates the essential nature of the disorder and not only do the other designations emphasize only a single aspect of the pathologic changes, but they may give an erroneous impression of the character of the skeletal lesions. Moreover, all of these lesions may occur in other conditions in which the factor of hyperparathyroidism is not implicated.

Etiology.—The condition has been produced in experimental animals by administration of parathyroid hormone. Excessive secretion of this hormone is the cause of the subjective and objective manifestations of clinical forms of the disease. It is due to either (1) focal hyperplasia (adenoma) of one or more parathyroid glands or (2) hyperplasia or hypertrophy of all parathyroid glands. The latter may possibly be due to primary pituitary hyperfunction (parathyrotropic principle).[19]

Pathology.[20]—One or more parathyroid glands are practically invariably involved in a neoplastic, hyperplastic or hypertrophic process. Adenomas have been found in about 86 per cent of cases and diffuse hyperplasia in about 14 per cent. In the neoplastic group, a single gland is involved in over 90 per cent of instances, the lower parathyroids being affected about five times as frequently as the upper. Tumors of aberrant parathyroid tissue have been found within the thyroid and the thymus glands and in the mediastinum (retrosternal). A few cases have been reported of *metastatic carcinoma* of the parathyroid glands accompanied by metabolic features of hyperparathyroidism. Whether or not these may be regarded as true examples of the condition is questionable. Occasionally the syndrome may occur in the absence of demonstrable morphologic abnormality of the parathyroids, but in such cases the possibility of aberrant parathyroid tissue must be considered. It should also be emphasized that enlargement of these glands (hyperplasia) frequently occurs as a secondary phenomenon, without clinical or metabolic manifestations of hyperparathyroidism, in such conditions as rickets, osteomalacia, renal disease, skeletal carcinomatosis, multiple myeloma, and pregnancy.

In cases of diffuse hypertrophy or hyperplasia the total *weight* of the parathyroid glands may be as great as 19 gm., more than 100 times normal. Adenomatous glands weighing as much as 300 gm. have been reported, but characteristic manifestations have been observed with tumors only twice the size of a normal gland. In contrast to the neoplastic cases, in those with diffuse hyperplasia or hypertrophy there appears to be a distant correlation between weight of parathyroid tissue and degree of hyperparathyroidism. Histologically, these glands are characterized by the uniformity of their structure, the enormous size of the cells, the extreme clearness of the cytoplasm (wasserhelle Zelle) and the tendency to glandular formation. Rarely the dominant cell type is the so-called "chief cell." In the localized tumors, involving a portion of one gland, a whole gland or, occasionally, portions of two glands, the histologic picture is much less uniform. The tumors may be composed almost entirely of chief cells, wasserhelle cells or oxyphil cells or any combination of these elements, with gland formation in one area, broad anastomosing cords in another and solid cell masses elsewhere.

The *skeletal lesions*[21] vary considerably and include generalized demineralization, multiple foci of osteitis fibrosa with or without benign giant cell tumors and single or multilocular cysts, hemorrhages, cortical thinning, and localized expansion of the bones leading to fracture and deformity, which may be of extreme grade. Every conceivable variation may occur, from mild osteoporosis, with slight fibrosis, to extensive cystic change with giant cell tumor. The periosteum may be thinned and the medullary cavity filled with grayish-white fibrous tissue interspersed with fine reticulated bone. Decalcification may be of so extreme a grade that the affected bones can be readily cut with a knife. The long tubular bones are usually the seat of earliest and most extensive involvement. Next in order of involvement are the vertebrae, sacrum, pelvis, skull, jaw-bones, flat bones of the thorax and the short tubular bones of the hands and feet.

On histologic examination there is an increase in the number of osteoclasts, connective tissue proliferation, and fibrosis of the marrow. These areas of fibrosis may contain giant cells, fresh or old extravasated blood, single or multiple cystic spaces, giant cell tumors and finely reticulated bone. In the long bones, the greatest amount of regeneration and repair usually occurs in the diaphyses, the epiphyses showing no change or only osteoporosis.

Changes may occur in other tissues. The majority result from the direct action of excessive amounts of parathyroid hormone or from precipitation of calcium phosphate, or are the consequences of these phenomena. In acute forms of hyperparathyroidism, which are rare clinically, degenerative changes may be found in the renal tubular epithelium, heart muscle and gastric mucosa. Calcific deposits, probably erroneously termed "metastatic" calcification, may occur in these situations and also in the lungs and walls of the arteries. Serious pathologic changes in the kidneys are perhaps the most common of the extraskeletal lesions, occurring in about 50 per cent of cases. These consist of nephrolithiasis (calcium phosphate calculi), pyelonephritis, and calcific deposits in the lumen of the tubules and in the peritubular and interstitial tissue, with interstitial fibrosis and contraction.[19]

Compression of the spinal cord has been observed as a result of collapse or fracture of thoracic or lumbar vertebrae. Decubitus ulcers, pneumonia and urinary tract infection may develop in the terminal stages.

Clinical Features.—Sex and Age. About 70 per cent of the reported cases have been in women, the predominance of females over males being slightly greater in the adenoma than in the hyperplastic group. The condition occurs most commonly between the ages of 20 and 60 years, but has been

7

TABLE 1*

SEX INCIDENCE OF HYPERPARATHYROIDISM

	Per Cent	
	Females	Males
Total cases..............................	70	30
Adenoma (88 per cent).......................	70.6	29.4
Hyperplasia (12 per cent)....................	66.7	33.3

* After Castleman and Mallory.[20]

TABLE 2

AGE INCIDENCE OF HYPERPARATHYROIDISM

Age in Years								
	0–9	10–19	20–29	30–39	40–49	50–59	60–69	70–79	80–89
Total cases.......	0	12	29	29	46	45	12	8	1
Adenoma.........	2	11	26	27	39	40	11	5	1
Hyperplasia......	0	1	3	2	7	5	1	3	0

TABLE 3

SYMPTOMS OF HYPERPARATHYROIDISM

	Per Cent	
	Early	Late
Skeletal....................................		
Pain in back or extremities.................	47	40
Deformities.............................	27	35
Fractures...............................	18	24
Difficult gait...........................	15	14
Muscle weakness.........................	14	15
Bedfast.................................	2	18
Enlarged skull...........................	0	1
Renal		
Polyuria, polydipsia......................	6	8
Colic...................................	6	2
Gastro-intestinal		
Nausea, vomiting, anorexia................	8	14
Epigastric pain..........................	2	4
Miscellaneous		
Marked weight loss.......................	8	12
Deafness................................	0	1
Paresthesias.............................	0	2

observed at 2 years of age, probably beginning in the first year. Such cases are rare.

The frequency of most important early and late symptoms and signs is outlined in table 3.

SKELETAL CHANGES.—There may be no symptoms referable to the skeleton. In the majority of instances, however, one or more of the following are present: bone pain and tenderness, bone tumor, kyphosis or other deformity, spontaneous fractures, clubbing of the fingers (due to loss of supporting substance), waddling gait and limp. At times, the earliest clinical indication of the presence of this condition is the discovery of a giant cell tumor of the jaw (*epulis*). Pain may be severe and, being frequently referred to the joints of the lower extremities and to the spine, is often erroneously regarded as arthritic. Demonstrable changes may be minimal or absent in early stages or in the rarely encountered instances of rapidly progressive acute hyperparathyroidism. There is reason to believe that the extent of bone involvement is an index of the duration rather than of the severity of the disease.

The x-ray is of great value in diagnosis, but it must be emphasized that the findings are not pathognomonic, except perhaps in advanced and classical forms of the disease.[9] The important *radiographic manifestations* include generalized osteoporosis, cysts, fractures, tumors, deformities and a granular, mottled appearance of the calvarium. There may be no demonstrable skeletal abnormality, or only a slight degree of demineralization. In advanced cases the most marked changes are usually observed in the long bones. The order of involvement of the remainder of the skeleton is as follows: vertebrae, pelvis, calvarium, jaw bones, thorax and bones of the hands and feet. Obviously, the effect of the hyperparathyroid state in promoting mobilization of Ca and P must be exerted upon the entire skeleton and, therefore, more or less generalized decalcification is an absolutely essential feature of the x-ray picture, regardless of the presence or extent of other changes.

The *long bones* show cortical thinning, the trabeculae becoming indistinct and the shadow light and homogeneous, or the medullary cavity may appear to be expanded. If new trabeculae are formed, the bone may present a finely-mottled, granular appearance. There may be single or multilocular cysts, often accompanied by marked localized expansion and surrounded by only a thin shell of bone. Fractures are common and tend to unite readily. Giant-cell tumors are not uncommon in both long and short tubular bones. Cysts, too, are seen in the small bones of the hands and feet. These changes may be associated with a variable degree of deformity. Similar manifestations may be observed in the spine; biconcavity of the vertebrae may result from extreme softening.

The calvarium may be thinned and porotic, it may present a finely mottled, granular appearance, or it may be irregularly or generally thickened, resembling the changes in Paget's disease. The remainder of the skull usually shows evidence of osteoporosis, occasionally with cysts and giant cell tumors in the mandible and maxillae. The pelvis and scapulae often show decalcification and cyst formation, with deformities and fractures in the former, due probably to the excessive strain to which it is subjected.

Calcific deposits may be observed in soft tissues, especially in the kidneys and lower urinary passages (calculi) or, occasionally, in the arteries.

GASTRO-INTESTINAL SYMPTOMS.—Anorexia and constipation are often troublesome features, due probably to the existing hypercalcemia, with consequent gastro-intestinal atony. There may be periodic, recurring bouts of nausea and vomiting, at times with severe abdominal pain, these attacks usually lasting for a few days to two weeks. These manifestations are generally attributed to acute parathyroid intoxication.

URINARY TRACT SYMPTOMS.—These include polyuria, polydipsia, frequency of urination, enuresis, nocturia, dysuria, renal colic, hematuria, pyuria, ureteral obstruction and other manifestations of stone in the urinary passages or renal failure. These symptoms are due primarily to the increased excretion of Ca and P by the kidneys and, perhaps, to deposition of calcium salts in the kidneys as a result of hypercalcemia and degenerative changes in the tubular epithelium. Renal complications have been reported in 30 to 70 per cent of cases of hyperparathyroidism. These may be classified under three headings:

1. Precipitation of calcium phosphate in the renal pelvis with calculus formation and resulting pyelonephritis.

2. Precipitation in the uriniferous tubules (nephrocalcinosis), with resulting nephrosclerosis, contraction and renal functional impairment, with or without hypertension. In some cases the calcium deposits in the kidneys are demonstrable by x-rays.

3. Precipitation in the kidneys as a part of the process of precipitation in various soft tissues, with acute renal failure and death in a few hours or days. This seldom occurs clinically, and only in very acute forms of hyperparathyroidism. Death in such cases is associated with circulatory collapse; this feature and the rapidly progressive renal failure have been attributed to dehydration and marked plasma sodium and chloride deficit resulting from the excessive loss of these elements in the urine.

It is important to note that these renal lesions can occur in the absence of demonstrable skeletal changes, the former being an index of the severity and the latter of the duration of the disease. It has been estimated that hyperparathyroidism is the etiologic factor in about 0.3 per cent of cases of urinary lithiasis. The latter may be the first clinical evidence of this condition.

MISCELLANEOUS SYMPTOMS.—Lassitude and muscular weakness are common early symptoms, and there may be difficulty in muscular coordination. These are probably dependent upon muscular hypotonia due to hypercalcemia. This is evidenced objectively by diminished electrical excitability of muscles and nerves (p. 175). Another interesting manifestation is shortening of the R-T interval in the electrocardiogram, which may be reduced to about 0.22 second (normally 0.26–0.28 second; in hypocalcemic tetany, 0.30–0.34 second).

Loss of appetite and loss of weight are nearly always present and may lead to profound emaciation. There may be extreme dehydration and base deficit as a result of prolonged polyuria and loss of sodium and other electrolytes in the urine. Respiratory difficulty and reduction in height may result from deformities in the thorax (kyphosis and scoliosis) and extremities (bowing, knock-knee, etc.), due to softening and fractures. Stunting of growth has been observed in cases in which the skeletal changes had progressed before full physiologic growth had been attained. Occasionally, a parathyroid tumor may be palpable in the neck, but owing to their position behind the thyroid or in the mediastinum, even extremely large parathyroid glands may not be visible or palpable from the surface. The trachea or esophagus may be displaced by enlarged glands. Metastatic calcification and visceral hemorrhages may occur in very acute phases of the disease.

Metabolic Manifestations.—The characteristic, indeed almost pathognomonic metabolic manifestations are: (*a*) hypercalcemia, (*b*) hypophosphatemia, (*c*) increased urinary excretion of Ca and (*d*) increased serum phosphatase activity. It is the combination of all of these rather than the presence of any one that is of diagnostic significance.

In typical cases the serum Ca has ranged from 12.5 to 29.4 mg. per 100 cc. Values above 20 mg. are rare. Occasionally, the serum Ca may be within normal limits, but repeated determinations usually reveal hypercalcemia at some time during the course of the disease. Hypercalcemia is probably invariably present during periods of progression of the skeletal lesions and in the presence of active symptoms. It is possible that there may be periods of temporary latency of the condition, as in the case of hyperthyroidism; under such circumstances the characteristic metabolic features will be lacking and accurate diagnosis may be impossible. There is also experimental basis for the possibility that the serum Ca concentration may return to normal or even subnormal levels following a period of hypercalcemia with exhaustion of the mobilizable Ca reserves in the bones, particularly if the Ca intake is inadequate. Occasionally, relatively low or normal values may be obtained in cases complicated by renal failure, with high serum P levels. Similar difficulty in producing hypercalcemia by parathyroid hormone has been reported in nephrectomized animals. Accurate diagnosis is difficult under such circumstances (p. 196).

The *serum inorganic P concentration* is subnormal in typical uncomplicated cases, ranging from 1.0 to 2.5 mg. per 100 cc. in adults and to 3.5 mg. in young children. This finding is not as constant as is hypercalcemia, due chiefly perhaps to the frequent coexistence of a variable degree of renal functional impairment, which tends to produce an increase in serum P. In advanced renal failure, increased concentrations may be observed, accompanied by nitrogen retention and a tendency toward lowering of the previously elevated serum Ca values, at times to subnormal levels. Under such circumstances the condition may be confused with "renal rickets" (p. 198).

The *serum phosphatase activity* is characteristically increased, usually ranging from 6.5 to 25 Bodansky units, and occasionally as high as 60 units. The relatively slight increase in the majority of instances (as compared, for example, to the findings in Paget's disease) contrasts strikingly with the extent of the skeletal changes. This is due to the fact that the phosphatase activity is probably a reflection of the degree of osteoblastic activity, which is usually rather low in hyperparathyroidism.

Abnormally large amounts of Ca are eliminated in the urine, especially under conditions of low Ca and comparatively low P intake. Under such circumstances the urinary Ca may exceed the quantity ingested and may constitute 70–90 per cent of the total output. The organism is in a state of negative Ca and usually also negative P balance, this being most readily demonstrated when the intake of these elements is maintained at a low level for test periods of at least three days (calcium 0.11 gm. and phosphorus

0.4 gm. daily). In contrast to other conditions accompanied by negative Ca and P balance (rickets, osteomalacia), the loss occurs chiefly by way of the kidneys rather than the bowel.

Other Laboratory Findings.—Extensive fibrosis and cystic changes in the bone-marrow may result in an aplastic type of anemia, with leukopenia and, occasionally, thrombopenia. During periods of severe acute hyperparathyroidism there may be manifestations of hemoconcentration (increased plasma protein concentration and increasing hematocrit values), hypochloremia, and evidences of renal failure (hyperphosphatemia, nitrogen retention, acidosis). Prolonged vomiting may be accompanied by oliguria. Bence-Jones proteinuria occurs occasionally. In the presence of urinary tract complications the urine may contain albumin, casts, leukocytes, red blood cells and bacteria. Small calcium phosphate calculi may be passed.

Prognosis.—Hyperparathyroidism is an insidious disease, usually of long duration. Except in rare instances of the very acute form, death results usually from complications such as renal failure, respiratory and urinary tract and other infections, cardiac failure, inanition, etc. Temporary spontaneous remissions may occur, but the condition tends to become progressively worse unless proper treatment is instituted. In many reported instances of apparently spontaneous remission there is considerable question as to the accuracy of the diagnosis. Permanent and complete cure, with healing of the bone lesions, has followed surgical removal of affected glands.

Diagnosis.—Cases of hyperparathyroidism may be roughly classified under four headings on the basis of the predominant clinical manifestations[19]:

1. Classical Hyperparathyroidism (von Recklinghausen). In this form there are pain, spontaneous fractures, skeletal deformities, bone cysts and tumors and generalized decalcification.

2. Osteoporotic Form. The bone changes in this type are practically identical with those of hyperthyroidism, osteomalacia, inactivity or senile osteoporosis. Significant symptoms may be absent.

3. Renal Form. The presenting symptoms may be those of urinary lithiasis, pyelonephritis, or renal functional insufficiency. Skeletal changes may be absent, minimal, or extreme. Diffuse nephrocalcinosis may be demonstrable by the x-ray.

4. Acute Hyperparathyroidism. This form is rarely encountered clinically. The manifestations are those of acute experimental parathyroid intoxication, and include nausea, vomiting, prostration, hematemesis, melena, diarrhea, visceral hemorrhages, the shock syndrome and renal failure.

Because of the variability of the clinical manifestations and skeletal changes, the diagnosis of hyperparathyroidism must rest finally upon demonstration of the characteristic group of metabolic features, namely, (*a*) hypercalcemia, (*b*) hypophosphatemia, (*c*) excessive calcinuria on a low Ca, relatively low P intake, (*d*) increased serum phosphatase activity and, although unsatisfactory in our experience, an excessive quantity of parathyroid hormone in the blood (Hamilton and Schwartz).[22] In the absence of one or more of these findings, particularly the first three, accurate diagnosis is difficult. This difficulty arises most commonly in those cases accompanied by advanced renal insufficiency, in which the serum Ca may be normal or subnormal, the serum P increased and urinary Ca excretion relatively low.

The condition must be differentiated from a number of skeletal disorders with which it may be confused if careful metabolic studies are not made, and also from other conditions accompanied by hypercalcemia.

POLYOSTOTIC FIBROUS DYSPLASIA.[23, 24]—This condition has been described in the literature under a variety of designations, including osteodystrophia fibrosa unilateralis, osteitis fibrosa localisata, osteodystrophia fibrosa cystica generalisata, fibrous osteodystrophy, and osteitis fibrosa disseminata. It is probably much more common than hyperparathyroidism and the majority of cases have undoubtedly in the past been erroneously regarded as the latter, to which it is entirely unrelated etiologically. The following features differentiate it from hyperparathyroidism:

1. It occurs most often in children and young adults, more frequently in females.

2. Symptoms commonly date back to early childhood, the condition evolving very slowly over a period of years or decades.

3. The characteristic pathologic feature is apparently a disturbed development or function of the bone-forming mesenchyme, resulting in filling of the medullary cavity of the affected bones by fibrous tissue, with areas of collagenous differentiation, hyaline cartilage or spicules of primitive fiber bone. These bones may present an x-ray picture indistinguishable from that of true osteitis fibrosa cystica (hyperparathyroidism). Epiphyses as well as diaphyses may be affected.

4. The progress of the condition tends to become less active with advancing years and a condition of equilibrium may be established, with restoration of function, although the normal bone structure is not restored.

5. The involvement is predominantly unilateral, but lesions may occur on the opposite side.

6. Unaffected portions of the skeleton show no evidence of demineralization, except that resulting from disuse.

7. In girls, there may be precocious puberty and some cases have shown areas of cutaneous pigmentation having a distribution related to the osseous changes.

8. Except for the very occasional occurrence of slight hypercalcemia and slightly increased serum phosphatase activity, there is no evidence of abnormality of Ca or P metabolism.

MULTIPLE MYELOMA.—Multiple myeloma may simulate hyperparathyroidism clinically, roentgenographically, and chemically. However, the distribution of the skeletal lesions is usually somewhat different and demineralization is rarely if ever generalized. Hypercalcemia may be present, often to a marked degree, but it is frequently accompanied by increase in serum protein, especially the globulin fraction. The serum P concentration is rarely subnormal and is frequently increased (renal failure). The serum phosphatase activity is rarely increased. Excessive calcinuria may occur in the presence of hypercalcemia. Bence-Jones proteinuria is present to a marked degree in the majority of cases, while it is observed only occasionally and in small amount in hyperparathyroidism. Secondary enlargement of the parathyroid glands has been described. In doubtful cases, marrow puncture or bone biopsy is the only certain way to establish the correct diagnosis.

GENERALIZED SKELETAL XANTHOMATOSIS.—Typical forms of the Hand-Schüller-Christian syndrome present no difficulty in diagnosis. Cases of xanthomatosis involving only the long bones, pelvis or calvarium may, however, be confused with hyperparathyroidism on the basis of the x-ray appearance of the bones and the occurrence of spontaneous fractures. However, diffuse demineralization is absent, as are the usual metabolic manifestations of hyperparathyroidism, there is often an increase in plasma cholesterol esters, cutaneous lesions are common and histologic examination of the affected bones (biopsy) reveals the characteristic vacuolated "foam" cells containing cholesterol.

The bone changes in *Gaucher's* and in *Niemann-Pick's* disease may present an x-ray picture resembling that of hyperparathyroidism. These conditions, however, usually present other characteristic features, including splenomegaly, hepatomegaly and pulmonary involvement, there is rarely evidence of abnormality of Ca and P metabolism, the serum phosphatase activity is normal, and examination of material obtained by marrow or splenic puncture or bone biopsy usually reveals the lipid-containing cells typical of those conditions.

RENAL RICKETS.—Renal rickets may present all of the cardinal clinical and laboratory features of the osteoporotic type of hyperparathyroidism complicated by renal functional impairment. It usually differs from the latter, however, in the following respects:

1. The renal impairment antedates the bone changes and, frequently, there is a long history of renal disease, often with hypertension and its attendant cardiovascular manifestations. If the onset occurs in early childhood, growth may be stunted (dwarfism).

2. The underlying cause is usually chronic glomerulonephritis, chronic pyelonephritis or renal hypogenesis. Consequently, urinary lithiasis or nephrocalcinosis are rare in this condition, whereas they constitute a common basis for the development of advanced renal functional impairment in hyperparathyroidism.

Parathyroid hyperplasia, at times of marked degree, may occur in advanced renal insufficiency. It has been regarded as a response to hyperphosphatemia and the skeletal demineralization has been attributed to chronic acidosis, the excretion of abnormally large amounts of Ca and P by the bowel and, perhaps, to the development of a state of secondary hyperparathyroidism, especially in cases of congenital urinary tract defect, when the exact time of onset of renal functional impairment cannot be established. Metastatic calcification, especially in the arteries, has been observed in renal rickets and, occasionally, there may be changes in the bones resembling the cysts and giant cell tumors of osteitis fibrosa cystica. The serum Ca concentration is usually normal or subnormal, and the serum P concentration is increased. However, the significance of these findings in differential diagnosis is diminished by the fact that the supervention of renal failure in true primary hyperparathyroidism tends to produce an increase in the previously low serum P and a fall in the previously elevated serum Ca concentration. Frequently the only possible means of differentiating the two conditions is to decipher the course of events leading to the combination of skeletal lesions and renal impairment.

OSTEOMALACIA.—The term osteomalacia, which was formerly applied to a variety of dissimilar bone disorders, should now be applied only to that condition dependent upon and associated with deficiency in Ca, P and vitamin D. It is the adult counterpart of childhood rickets (p. 213). The parathyroid glands may be somewhat enlarged. It differs from hyperparathyroidism in the following respects:

1. The serum Ca is normal or subnormal, the urinary Ca excretion is not increased, and excessive amounts of Ca and P are lost in the feces.

2. Although the appearance of the bones may resemble superficially that in the osteoporotic form of hyperparathyroidism, fibrosis is minimal, the trabeculae have wide osteoid borders and there are few osteoclasts.

3. Osteomalacia responds promptly to administration of adequate amounts of Ca, P and vitamin D, which have no beneficial effect on the course of hyperparathyroidism.

The skeletal lesions of late rickets in adolescent children may resemble osteitis fibrosa cystica, particularly in bowing of the lower extremities and widening of the metaphyses. The criteria useful in differential diagnosis are identical with those outlined for osteomalacia.

PAGET'S DISEASE (OSTEITIS DEFORMANS).—Until recently, osteitis deformans and osteitis fibrosa cystica were regarded by many as variants of the same fundamental process. This opinion was based largely upon occasional superficial similarities in the x-ray appearance of the bones; among these are thickening and mottling of the calvarium, and diffuse sclerosis, cortical thickening, and coarsely striated trabeculation at times observed in the bones of the extremities in hyperparathyroidism. In some instances confusion has undoubtedly resulted from the coexistence of the two conditions. However, there is no valid evidence that the parathyroids are implicated in the pathogenesis or etiology of Paget's disease. Hypercalcemia and hypophosphatemia do not occur, Ca and P balances are normal, serum phosphatase activity is usually greatly increased (in the polyostotic form), the skeletal lesions are localized, the periosteum is almost always involved, giant cell tumors are usually absent, and the cortex of the long tubular bones is usually lamellated. Enlargement of the parathyroid glands is rare and fractures seldom occur.

METASTATIC MALIGNANCY.—Metastatic malignancy of the bones may be mistaken for hyperparathyroidism. This, as in other skeletal lesions, is due chiefly to the x-ray appearance of the bones, but also in some cases to the occurrence of hypercalcemia, increased serum phosphatase activity and parathyroid enlargement. However, the differentiation should be made readily on the bases of (a) age, (b) demonstration of a primary site of the malignant process, (c) distribution of the skeletal lesions, which are seldom below the knees or elbows in metastatic carcinoma, (d) the normal appearance of the rest of the skeleton and the absence of hypophosphatemia. In rare instances the parathyroid glands may be the seat of metastases.

OSTEOPOROSIS OF OTHER ORIGIN.—The osteoporotic lesions of hyperparathyroidism may be simulated roentgenographically by similar changes resulting from a variety of causes. These include senile osteoporosis and that associated with disuse or inactivity, hyperthyroidism, pituitary basophilism and hypercorticoadrenalism. In the great majority of instances these conditions present few if any diagnostic difficulties.

In *senile osteoporosis* the serum and urinary Ca and P and serum phosphatase activity are normal. The skeletal lesion is characterized by chronic atrophy of the marrow, absence of osteoid borders, and occasionally brown

areas of hemosiderin and oil cysts in the long bones resulting from liquefac-
tin of the fatty marrow. The parathyroid glands may be slightly enlarged.
In *pituitary basophilism*, adrenal cortical tumor and hyperthyroidism, the
diagnosis is usually made readily on the basis of the characteristic features of
those conditions. The urinary Ca excretion may be increased but the other
metabolic manifestations of hyperparathyroidism are lacking. Hyperplasia
of the parathyroid glands has been reported in pituitary basophilism; in this
condition and in cortical tumor, osteoporosis is usually confined chiefly to
the vertebrae.

MISCELLANEOUS CONDITIONS.—Localized skeletal lesions may simulate hyperparathyroidism roentgenographically. These include solitary giant cell
tumors, focal osteitis fibrosa cystica, solitary cysts and multiple enchondromata. In these disorders there is no evidence of abnormality of Ca or P metabolism, and serum phosphatase activity is normal, as are the bones except
for the areas involved in the local processes.

Osteoporosis and other lesions of hyperparathyroidism may be simulated roentgenographically by bone changes in certain cases of leukemia,
Hodgkin's disease, polycythemia vera, erythroblastic and hemolytic anemias,
osteomyelitis, radium poisoning and osteogenesis imperfecta. In certain experimental animals the administration of large doses of parathyroid hormone
over long periods may result in skeletal changes resembling those of "marble-
bone" disease (Albers-Schönberg), in which condition parathyroid hyperplasia has been reported.[25] This has prompted the suggestion that this rare
disorder may represent a special form of hyperparathyroidism, but there is
no metabolic evidence that such is the case. Hypercalcemia may occur occasionally in leukemia and in polycythemia vera. However, with occasional
exceptions, none of these conditions is accompanied by abnormality of Ca
or P metabolism, and their differentiation from hyperparathyroidism can
usually be made readily on the basis of the rather typical clinical and laboratory manifestations in each instance.

Treatment.—*Roentgen therapy* has been practically entirely unsatisfactory in cases due to adenoma, resulting in neither symptomatic nor metabolic improvement. There is some indication, however, that better results may
be obtained in those due to generalized hyperplasia or hypertrophy. Unfortunately, the distinction between the two forms can be made only by surgical exploration. It has been suggested that irradiation therapy may be useful
under the following conditions: (*a*) when operative procedures are contraindicated; (*b*) when a tumor has not been found at operation; (*c*) when
part of an adenoma has been left behind at operation.

Medical treatment consists essentially in administration of a diet high in
Ca and P, usually supplemented by Ca and P salts. This has resulted in
some cases in definite improvement in the skeletal lesions, which is usually
only temporary. Moreover, it is not without danger, since it aggravates
the existing tendency toward deposition of lime salts in soft tissues, the
development of renal complications, dangerous hypercalcemia and circulatory failure. The treatment of acute fulminating hyperparathyroidism
(p. 196) consists essentially in intravenous administration of solutions of
sodium chloride and dextrose for the purpose of replenishing Na and Cl
and maintaining renal function.

Surgical treatment offers the only hope of permanent benefit. Because of the great difficulty of locating and identifying a parathyroid tumor at operation, it is advisable to attempt to locate it preoperatively by means of roentgenograms designed to demonstrate (a) calcification of the capsule, (b) displacement of the trachea or (c) displacement or filling defect of the esophagus (after swallowing barium). Moreover, it must be realized that parathyroid glands may be present anywhere from the pharynx to the mediastinum, and may be buried in the thyroid gland. At operation, a frozen section from a biopsy specimen should be examined to determine (a) whether it is parathyroid tissue and (b) whether it is normal, adenomatous or hyperplastic. If adenomatous, the affected gland should be removed providing no normal glands had been removed previously. If this had been done, a piece of the gland somewhat larger than a normal gland should be left and its location marked by a silver suture to facilitate subsequent removal, if necessary. If histologic examination reveals hyperplasia, an attempt must be made to locate all parathyroid glands since all are involved in such cases. It appears advisable to remove about three-fourths of the parathyroid tissue identified.

Postoperative Course.—Improvement occurs promptly following removal of diseased parathyroid tissue. Within a few hours the urinary excretion of Ca and P diminishes sharply, as does the urine volume. There may be transitory anuria with manifestations of renal failure. The serum Ca falls rapidly, reaching normal or subnormal levels in twelve to twenty-four hours. The normal serum P and phosphatase activity are restored more gradually, usually after a period of several weeks or months. Subjective improvement is likewise prompt. The skeletal lesions gradually disappear over a period of months, bone cysts being the only permanent abnormality, apart from pre-existing deformities. Nephrocalcinosis and other renal and urinary tract changes also persist, as do other calcific deposits in soft tissues.

Tetany is the most common complication of parathyroidectomy. It may occur even in cases in which adequate amounts of parathyroid tissue were left and at serum Ca levels as high as 8 mg. per 100 cc. The development of tetany may be dependent upon (a) the extremely rapid fall in serum Ca, (b) atrophy and functional insufficiency of the remaining parathyroids after sudden removal of a hyperfunctioning gland, (c) inadequate amounts of Ca or an excess of P in the diet, and (d) removal of too much parathyroid tissue. Except when due to the latter, the condition is transitory. Treatment is essentially the same as in all forms of parathyroid tetany (p. 207) except that larger amounts of Ca should be administered because of the excessive demand incident to the necessity for skeletal recalcification. Even in the absence of tetany, calcium should be administered orally and parenterally if a large portion of the parathyroid tissue has been removed. Parathyroid hormone or dihydrotachysterol may be required (p. 208). During the period of skeletal recalcification, an optimal or high Ca intake (1 to 1.5 gm.) and an optimal P intake (0.75 to 1.0 gm.) should be provided, supplemented by 3 to 5 gm. of secondary calcium phosphate ($CaHPO_4$) or other Ca salts (gluconate or lactate) if the bone changes have been extensive. Phosphorus should be administered cautiously in the presence of tetany or hypocalcemia (p. 207). In the absence of the latter, vitamin D may be administered in conjunction with Ca salts in an attempt to facilitate recalcification of the skeleton.

HYPOPARATHYROIDISM AND TETANY[2, 9, 17]

Tetany is the outstanding clinical manifestation of hypoparathyroidism. Since this symptom complex may be produced by a variety of causes, it seems advisable to consider it here as a clinical entity and to discuss its varied etiology from the standpoint of differential diagnosis.

Tetany is a syndrome characterized by an abnormally increased reaction of the somatic and autonomic motor and sensory nerves to stimuli and by painful, tonic spasms of groups of muscles or even of the entire musculature of the body. This hyperirritability is dependent upon or associated with one or more of the following phenomena: (*a*) Hypocalcemia, with a decrease in the ionized fraction of the serum Ca and also in the non-diffusible fraction; (*b*) hyperphosphatemia, the increase in serum P perhaps operating to bind and thus inactivate a portion of the serum Ca; (*c*) alkalosis, which acts probably by depressing Ca ionization; (*d*) depression of Ca ionization by other factors, such as administration of citrate; (*e*) hypomagnesemia, which may produce hyperirritability in itself or may act through the medium of causing a portion of the Ca to be bound by phosphate ordinarily bound to Mg.

Clinically, all forms of tetany may be divided into two stages—latent and manifest. The former presents no frank symptoms, but these may be elicited by stimulation of peripheral nerves; the latter is manifested by spontaneous muscular spasms and other manifestations of nervous hyperirritability.

Latent Tetany.—The presence of this condition is demonstrated by mechanical or electrical excitation of the hyperexcitable nerves.

Erb Phenomenon.—This important sign depends upon the fact that the neuromuscular response to galvanic stimulation can be obtained with weaker currents in tetany than under normal conditions. Measurements are usually made on the peroneal or median nerves, the indifferent electrode (50 sq. cm.) being placed on the abdomen and the stimulating electrode (3 sq. cm.) over the nerve. The galvanic battery should be graduated in fifths up to 5 milliamperes. Contractions occur by making or breaking the current (closing or opening contractions) and vary according to the different poles employed (anode or cathode). There are, therefore, four different types of response, *viz.*, cathodal closing (C.C.C.), anodal closing (A.C.C.), cathodal

TABLE 4

ELECTRICAL THRESHOLDS IN MILLIAMPERES

Age	C.C.C.	A.C.C.	C.O.C.	A.O.C.
Under 6 months............	3.5	7.0	10.0	9.0
1–2 years.................	2.5	5.0	8.0	6.0
Over 5 years.............	1.8	4.0	6.5	3.5

opening (C.O.C.) and anodal opening (A.O.C.) contractions. Typical electrical thresholds in normal subjects are presented in table 4.

Clinically, the C.O.C. is the most useful reaction, a contraction elicited by less than 5 ma. being highly suggestive of tetany. The A.O.C. is more delicate but more difficult to interpret. Attainment of an A.O.C. with currents less than that required to produce an A.C.C. (anodal reversibility) is also of significance up to the fifth year. These reactions are not infallible. They may vary considerably from time to time and even in normal subjects, and bear no consistent relation to the serum Ca concentration. Nevertheless, the Erb phenomenon is of great value in the diagnosis of latent tetany.

Chronaxie.—Chronaxie is the length of time necessary to elicit a reaction when a current is employed, the strength of which is twice the rheobase. The rheobase is the minimal galvanic current which, continued indefinitely, suffices to produce a reaction. Normally, it takes about 0.00024 second (24 sigma) to elicit a reaction from the flexor pollicis. In tetany it may take only 12–14 sigma; in hyperparathyroidism it may take as long as 50 sigma.

Chvostek Sign (Facial Phenomenon).—Hyperexcitability of the facial nerve to mechanical stimulation is elicited by tapping the trunk of the facial nerve (*a*) immediately anterior to the external auditory meatus or (*b*) just below the zygomatic process. A positive reaction consists in momentary contraction of the lip, the lip and nose, or the entire side of the face. This sign is most dependable before the second year, after which time it may occur in normal subjects. It may occur also in meningitis. Dorsal flexion and abduction of the foot may be produced by tapping the peroneal nerve on the lateral surface of the fibula just below the head (peroneal sign).

Trousseau Phenomenon.—This sign is elicited by making pressure upon the blood vessels and nerves of the upper arm (tourniquet or sphygmomanometer) with sufficient force to stop the circulation. A positive reaction consists in the production of the typical "tetanic" contraction of the fingers and hand in the obstetrical position. A bilateral response may follow application of the pressure to one arm. This sign is not pathognomonic of tetany and is less reliable than the Chvostek sign.

Other Signs.—A number of other signs have been described, depending on stimulation of various nerves or muscles. Dimpling of the tongue may be produced by tapping it lightly (also in myotonia). Plantar flexion of the foot and spasm of the extensor muscles of the knee may be produced by grasping the ankle and forcibly flexing the thigh at the hip joint (tension of sciatic nerve). Carpal spasm may follow forcible abduction of the arm (tension of brachial plexus).

Hyperexcitability of sensory nerves is also present, but is not easily demonstrated. The "Hoffman phenomenon" consists in the manifestation of hyperirritability of peripheral sensory nerves to galvanic and faradic currents. Hypersensitivity of the optic, acoustic, vagus, glossopharyngeal, and other nerves has been demonstrated.

Chemical changes in the blood are among the most significant features of all forms of tetany. Inasmuch as the changes in latent tetany differ from those in manifest tetany only in degree, they will be described subsequently in the discussion of that condition.

Manifest Tetany.—*Acute Tetany.*—After a variable period of latency, neuromuscular irritability increases to the point where spontaneous manifestations appear. Among the most important of these are carpopedal spasm, laryngospasm, and convulsions. These may be preceded and accompanied by paresthesias and intense pain.

In *carpal spasm* the thumb is inserted into the palm, the fingers, extended at the distal joints, are flexed at the metacarpophalangeal joints ("obstetric hand"), and the wrist is flexed and the hand drawn to the ulnar side. In pedal spasm the feet are bent downward, often in the position of equino-varus. There may be stiffness or spasm and pain in other muscle groups of the extremities. Facial spasm may produce stiffness and rigidity, with a fixed expression ("tetany facies"), the corners of the mouth being drawn downward ("carp mouth"). There may be rigidity of the entire body, especially of the neck and back, strabismus, nystagmus, inequality of the pupils and difficulty in speech and swallowing.

Laryngospasm occurs most frequently in children and is precipitated by very slight reflex irritation (cold, emotional disturbance, sudden awakening, etc.). It is characterized by a loud inspiratory crow due to spasm of the glottis. The attacks vary in severity and frequency and, if repeated, may be accompanied by dyspnea, cyanosis, coma, and respiratory failure, which may terminate fatally. Usually the glottic spasm relaxes in a few minutes. Diaphragmatic spasm may cause inspiratory or, rarely, expiratory apnea, which may cause death. Bronchotetany may produce attacks simulating asthma; in severe cases there is dyspnea, with areas of pulmonary atelectasis and emphysema. This condition responds well to calcium but is not relieved by epinephrin.

Autonomic nerves and smooth muscles may be extensively involved. Spasm has been observed in the iris, ciliary muscle, esophagus, throughout the gastrointestinal tract (often with pain, vomiting, constipation or diarrhea), the bladder (with urinary retention or enuresis), the bronchi and the heart. *Cardiac spasm* (probably vagus stimulation) may cause sudden death, with precipitate pallor and apnea. Palpitation, tachycardia, and cardiac irregularity occur frequently. The R-T interval may be prolonged to 0.30 to 0.34 second (normal, 0.26–0.28 second). *Angiospasm* results in pallor, especially of the fingers and toes, dermographia and muscle pain. There may be localized areas of puffiness of the skin or frank edema, usually limited to the face or the dorsum of the hands and feet, but at times generalized. This occurs more frequently in young infants than in adults.

Convulsions, usually generalized, but sometimes limited to one side of the body (hemitetany) or to single muscle groups, occur most frequently in infants. They may appear suddenly and spontaneously or may be precipitated by slight stimulation. Premonitory manifestations may occur, including paresthesias, joint pains, muscular twitching, carpopedal spasm, laryngospasm, etc. Death may occur if the convulsions are prolonged and repeated frequently (status eclampticus).

There may be *mental symptoms,* such as irritability, apprehension, disorientation, hallucinations and confusion, moodiness, loss of memory, and dulness. These phenomena are usually of brief duration and, since they occur most frequently in tetany following thyroidectomy, they may be dependent in part upon a state of hypothyroidism. Loss of consciousness during convulsions occurs rarely if ever.

Chronic Tetany.—Chronic tetany develops most commonly in conditions which do not respond particularly to specific forms of therapy. Hypoparathyroidism is the most important of these, although recently introduced therapeutic measures have greatly diminished the chronicity of tetany in this condition, as in infantile tetany, sprue, celiac disease and osteomalacia. However, in cases of very mild or latent tetany, particularly in hypoparathyroidism, the progress of the metabolic abnormalities characteristic of chronic tetany may escape recognition because of the absence of acute manifestations. These consist largely in trophic changes in structures of ectodermal origin, notably the hair, skin, nails, teeth, and the crystalline lens of the eye.

The hair becomes coarse in texture and is lost in patches or almost completely. The skin is thickened and roughened and the nails become brittle, ridged and may be shed. These changes are believed to be due to spasm of the vessels of the nail-beds. Defects appear in the dentin and enamel of the teeth, which may exhibit small pits and horizontal grooves. These changes are particularly striking in infantile tetany, in which the disturbance in Ca and P metabolism occurs during the period of dental development. They are observed much less commonly at present than formerly, because of the introduction of improved methods of treatment and diagnosis. Lenticular opacities, both nuclear and cortical, have been observed in a large proportion of cases, their true incidence being appreciated more widely with the increased use of the slit lamp for their early demonstration.

Etiologic Classification of Tetany.[2, 9]—The several forms of tetany may be classified as follows (Shelling):

I. Tetany due to reduction in concentration or inactivation of a portion of the serum Ca.

(*a*) Parathyroprivic tetany, idiopathic and postoperative.

(*b*) Infantile tetany, usually associated with rickets.

(*c*) Osteomalacic tetany.

(*d*) Maternal tetany.

(*e*) Tetany due to loss or lack of absorption of calcium, as in sprue, celiac disease and other forms of steatorrhea.

II. Tetany due to inactivation or precipitation of calcium, as in citrate, oxalate and phosphate tetany.

III. Tetany due to alkalosis. Hyperventilation, bicarbonate and gastric tetany.

IV. Tetany due to magnesium deprivation.

(*a*) Experimental Mg deprivation.

(*b*) "Grass tetany" of cattle.

Parathyroprivic Tetany (Hypoparathyroidism).—Clinically, this occurs in two forms, (*a*) postoperative, following thyroidectomy or parathyroidectomy, and (*b*) idiopathic, a condition analagous to spontaneous hypothyroidism. A third variety may follow hemorrhage or inflammation in the deep cervical tissues or in the glands themselves; this form is rare.

Postoperative tetany may result from accidental removal of one or more parathyroid glands during thyroidectomy, or from excision of too much parathyroid tissue in parathyroidectomy for hyperparathyroidism. In most cases, however, following thyroidectomy, it is probably due to temporary suppression of parathyroid function, as a result of trauma, edema or hemorrhage or interference with the blood supply. In such cases the condition is usually mild and of brief duration.

Manifestations of latent or manifest tetany appear usually within a few hours or days after operation. In some instances in which an interval of several days to a few weeks elapses, disturbance of blood supply to the parathyroid glands is often due to fibrous organization of inflammatory exudate or hemorrhagic extravasations, and the tetany is frequently prolonged or even permanent. *Idiopathic hypoparathyroidism* (juvenile or adult) is a comparatively rare condition. Its cause is unknown, although it has been attributed to inflammation of or hemorrhage into the glands. It is practically always chronic in nature and presents essentially the same clinical and metabolic features as are seen in postoperative tetany. Tetany following parathyroidectomy for hyperparathyroidism is due in many instances to the fact that the remaining glands are in a state of atrophy or functional suppression as a result of the presence of a hyperfunctioning adenomatous gland. This condition is usually transitory.

The characteristic *metabolic features* of parathyroprivic tetany are: (a) hypocalcemia, (b) normal or increased serum P concentration, (c) decreased urinary excretion of Ca and P, with positive Ca and P balances, (d)

TABLE 5

METABOLIC FEATURES IN CLINICAL FORMS OF TETANY[2]

Type	Calcium	Blood Phosphorus	pH	Urine Calcium	Feces Calcium
Parathyroid....	Low	High	Normal	Low	Normal
Infantile......	Low or normal	Usually low; may be high or normal	Normal	Low	High
Osteomalacic...	Low	Usually low; may be normal	Normal	Low	High
Steatorrhea....	Low	Usually low; may be normal	Normal	Low	High
Maternal......	Low	Variable	Normal	Low	Variable
Alkalotic......	Normal	Normal	High	Normal	Normal
Nephritis......	Low	High	Low	Low	High

normal serum phosphatase activity, (e) normal acid-base equilibrium, and (f) no significant skeletal abnormality.

One of the most important manifestations is the diminished serum Ca concentration. This is usually between 7 and 8 mg. per 100 cc. in latent and between 4 and 6 mg. per 100 cc. in manifest tetany. However, this close parallelism between the severity of symptoms and the degree of hypocalcemia is not constant. Latent tetany may be present at normal or at low (6 to 7 mg. per cent) serum Ca levels and manifest tetany may occur at concentrations as high as 8 mg. per 100 cc. Such discrepancies indicate that other factors must participate in the pathogenesis of neuromuscular hyperirritability in this condition. Perhaps the most important of these is the serum P concentration. This is at times normal, but is usually increased (5 to 10 mg. per cent). Even when it is not elevated, the serum Ca/P ratio is decreased. It appears likely that this absolute or relative increase in serum P plays a significant rôle in determining the precipitation of clinical symptoms of tetany. From the standpoint of differential diagnosis, particularly from tetany due to vitamin D deficiency, the elevated or normal serum P concentration, positive Ca and P balances, normal serum phosphatase activity and absence of skeletal abnormality are of paramount importance.

Treatment.—Rational therapy consists in correction of the existing metabolic errors: (*a*) hypocalcemia, (*b*) phosphate retention and hyperphosphatemia and (*c*) parathyroid deficiency. This may be accomplished by (1) administration of Ca salts, (2) restriction of intake of P, (3) specific substitution therapy (parathyroid transplants or parathyroid hormone administration), and (4) administration of dihydrotachysterol (A.T. 10).

CALCIUM THERAPY.—Calcium salts may be administered orally (chloride, lactate, gluconate, intramuscularly (gluconate) or intravenously (chloride, gluconate). The chloride contains 36 per cent, the lactate 18 per cent and the gluconate about 9 per cent calcium. The phosphate may be administered orally, but is much less effective because of the effect of the phosphate ion. Oral Ca administration constitutes the mainstay of the therapeutic regimen in parathyroid tetany. The usual dosage for adults is: gluconate, 4 gm., chloride and lactate, 2 gm., four times daily. To ensure maximum absorption, calcium salts should be given in interdigestive periods, that is, about one-half to three-quarters of an hour before meals and at bedtime. The chloride is perhaps the most effective but is also the most irritating, and the gluconate can usually be taken over long periods with a minimum of gastrointestinal disturbance.

In the presence of acute spastic or convulsive phenomena, Ca should be given intravenously, the chloride in doses of 5 to 10 cc. of a 10 per cent solution, the gluconate in doses of 10 to 30 cc. of a 10 per cent solution and the glucogalactogluconate, 10 to 20 cc. of a 20 per cent solution. These, given at a rate of 2 to 3 cc. per minute, produce prompt relief (within a few minutes), but the hypercalcemic effect usually lasts only about one to two hours. The injection may be repeated three or four times daily, if necessary, and should be supplemented by oral or intramuscular therapy. Calcium gluconate (10 per cent) may be given intramuscularly (10 to 20 cc.), the hypercalcemic response being obtained in fifteen to thirty minutes and lasting four to eight hours. This route may be employed twice daily, if necessary to prevent acute manifestations, or if oral therapy is not feasible.

LOW PHOSPHORUS THERAPY.—Increase in P intake causes an increase in the requirement for both Ca and parathyroid hormone in hypoparathyroidism. Consequently, it is advisable to restrict the daily intake of P to 0.3 to 0.6 gm., according to the total caloric and protein intake. For this reason, milk, despite its high Ca content, often causes an exacerbation of tetanic manifestations and increased refractoriness to parathyroid hormone, since each quart contains about 0.93 gm. P. It is therefore not advisable to use milk or milk products as a source of extra Ca in such cases.

In the author's opinion, the same is true of vitamin D, although there is considerable difference of opinion in this regard. One of the chief effects of this agent is to produce increased retention of P, which is already retained in abnormal amounts in hypoparathyroidism, the serum P being increased in typical cases. Although there is little doubt that tetany subsides in many cases following administration of large doses of vitamin D, the use of this factor appears illogical. Many instances of apparent "refractoriness" to parathyroid hormone are probably due to the simultaneous use of vitamin D and a high P intake.[9, 26]

PARATHYROID THERAPY.—Transplantation of parathyroid tissue has not met with great success, although some cases have been reported in which excellent results have been obtained, particularly following growth of parathyroid tissue in the plasma of the recipient.[27] In the great majority of instances, substitution therapy consists in the subcutaneous or intramuscular administration of parathyroid hormone. One unit of the hormone is defined as "one one-hundredth of the amount which produces, on an average, 1 mg. rise in the blood serum Ca in 20-kilogram dogs, over fifteen hours." One cubic centimeter contains 100 such units. The dosage depends upon the degree of hypocalcemia and the severity of the manifestations of tetany. This agent is most effective when the intake of Ca is increased and that of P is maintained at a relatively low level (0.3 to 0.6 gm.). If the hormone is administered over long periods, simultaneous administration of Ca salts is essential to prevent demineralization of the skeleton. In very acute cases, 500 units (5 cc.) of the hormone may be given daily in divided doses of 100 units. The quantity needed for maintenance must be determined in each case by repeated determinations of the serum Ca concentration, which may increase rapidly and to dangerous levels, especially if the hormone is injected at relatively short intervals. The usual maintenance dose, except in cases of virtual aparathyroidism, is from 50 to 200 units daily. If more than 100 units are required, it is advisable to administer equal doses at 12-hour intervals.

The increase in serum Ca occurs gradually, reaching a maximum in eight to fifteen hours, and then subsides, reaching preinjection levels in about twenty-four hours. A step-ladder effect may be obtained if the hormone is injected repeatedly at intervals of four to eight hours, and dangerous hypercalcemia may result. It has been observed that symptomatic relief may occur at times within one hour after injection, although there is little or no change in serum Ca concentration at that time. This may be due to the possibility that the primary effect is to increase the diffusible, ionized fraction in the blood and tissue fluids at the expense of the nondiffusible fraction. It is generally believed that a state of "refractoriness" or "immunity" to the effects of the hormone develops in subjects to whom it has been given continuously over long periods. This may be true to a certain extent, but in many instances this apparent refractoriness may be due in large measure to the maintenance of a relatively high P intake or to the simultaneous administration of vitamin D. The chief objections to the prolonged use of the parathyroid hormone are (a) that it must be given parenterally and (b) that spontaneous activity of remaining parathyroid tissue may be suppressed or inhibited.

DIHYDROTACHYSTEROL (A.T. 10).[19, 36, 37, 38]—Dihydrotachysterol is a photochemical derivative of ergosterol which has a pronounced hypercalcemic effect but practically no antirachitic properties. It is effective when given orally in an oil solvent (5 mg. per cc.) and therefore represents a distinct advance in the therapy of tetany of parathyroid origin. It appears to increase absorption of Ca from the bowel and to increase urinary excretion of phosphorus, resembling vitamin D in the former respect and parathyroid hormone in the latter.[19] As is the case with the hormone, its hypercalcemic effect is so marked that, until the dosage necessary for maintenance has been established, the level of serum Ca must be determined frequently if danger-ous hypercalcemia is to be avoided. The necessity for this procedure may be diminished, if it is not feasible, by the daily application of a qualitative test for Ca in the urine (Sulkowitch).[19] If no precipitate (calcium oxalate) ap-pears, there is no Ca and the serum Ca is probably below 7.5 mg. per cent. If there is a fine white cloud, the serum Ca concentration is probably within normal limits, while if a dense milky precipitate appears hypercalcemia is present.

The *dosage* varies considerably, depending upon the degree of hypo-calcemia. Ca salts should be given simultaneously. Initially, 3 to 10 cc. may be required daily for two or three days, then 1 to 2 cc. daily for one or two weeks, depending upon the degree of elevation of serum Ca. In many cases, after the latter has returned to normal, it may be maintained within satisfac-tory limits by as little as 1 to 2 cc. two or three times weekly, or even by smaller amounts.

MISCELLANEOUS.—Many recommend the use of vitamin D in rather large doses (50,000 to 300,000 I.U. daily), in conjunction with a high Ca, low P intake. The most effective means of securing this high dosage is by use of crystalline preparations, which contain 20,000 to 40,000 I.U. per milligram. In many cases this has resulted in restoration of normal Ca and P concen-trations in the serum. However, as stated above, the use of this agent seems illogical and, in our experience, the serum P not infrequently rises and tetany may be aggravated, particularly if smaller doses are employed and the P intake is not rigidly restricted. Calcium salts must be given in adequate dosage if a satisfactory increase in serum Ca is to be maintained.

Administration of thyroid extract is of value in raising the serum Ca in hypoparathyroidism, probably by accelerating its mobilization from the bones. The addition of lactose to the diet is also of benefit in many cases. It acts perhaps by furthering Ca absorption by increasing intestinal acidity and by lowering the plasma phosphate (increased carbohydrate utilization).

Although seldom necessary, sedatives such as chloral hydrate, phenobar-bital or sodium amytal, may be beneficial in relieving severe convulsions or dangerous laryngospasm.

Because of its depressant action, magnesium is used at times in the treat-ment of severe parathyroid tetany (0.5 to 1.0 gm. $MgSO_4$ intravenously, in 2 to 5 per cent solution; 0.2 cc. of 8 per cent $MgSO_4$ solution per Kg. intramuscularly). A syringe containing 10 cc. of 10 per cent calcium chloride or gluconate must be available for administration promptly if cir-culatory or respiratory embarrassment develops. However, the use of magnesium is not advisable and, in the experience of the author, may ac-tually precipitate tetany by further lowering the serum Ca concentration.

Infantile Tetany.—This is due characteristically to vitamin D deficiency and inadequate intake of calcium. It is usually associated with rickets, but may occur in the absence of clinical manifestations of that condition. The serum Ca is decreased. The serum P is usually subnormal in the presence of rickets, but may be normal or elevated in its absence. The Ca and P balances are negative or subnormal, due to excessive loss of these elements in the feces. The serum phosphatase activity is usually increased in proportion to the severity of the skeletal lesions, which vary from simple demineralization to typical rachitic manifestations.

As for *treatment*, this condition usually responds well to the addition of extra amounts of Ca to the antirachitic regimen. It is given in the same manner as in hypoparathyroidism (p. 207). Vitamin D may be given in the form of cod-liver oil or other fish-liver oils, irradiated ergosterol or ultra-violet irradiation of the skin. The action of cod-liver oil is rather slow and it is usually necessary to employ more concentrated forms of the vitamin (p. 416). The quantity required naturally varies with the severity of the deficiency; 10,000 to 100,000 international units may be required daily. In the majority of cases a high P intake is advisable. It is essential that Ca be given, particularly in the first several days of vitamin D administration, since otherwise there is a primary fall in serum Ca, with aggravation of tetanic manifestations, due probably to rather sharp elevation of the serum P concentration.

Osteomalacic Tetany.—This form of tetany is due to Ca and vitamin D deprivation and, occurring in adults with osteomalacia, may be regarded as the counterpart of infantile tetany. In the past, occurring most commonly during the winter months and in the early spring, and in subjects living and working under conditions which deprived them of adequate nutrition and exposure to sunlight, this condition was variously termed idiopathic tetany, workmen's tetany, shoemaker's, tailor's, seamstresses', carpenter's, housemaid's tetany, etc. The metabolic manifestations are the same as those of infantile tetany, although the serum P concentration is more consistently subnormal and x-ray examination reveals generalized skeletal demineralization. Treatment is essentially the same as in infantile tetany.

Maternal Tetany.—The physiologic changes in Ca and P metabolism in pregnancy have been described elsewhere (p. 177). The requirement for these elements and for vitamin D is increased and the occurrence of parathyroid hyperplasia indicates increased demand upon those structures. Under normal conditions the serum Ca does not fall to subnormal nevels, but it may do so occasionally, particularly in the late months and during lactation, accompanied by manifestations of tetany, mild or latent. These consist usually of muscle cramps, insomnia, irritability, tingling or burning sensations and other paresthesias in the extremities, and the signs of latent tetany (p. 202). The etiology of this condition is not clear, but it appears to be dependent, in some instances, upon deficiency in Ca and vitamin D intake and in others upon parathyroid deficiency operating alone or in conjunction with the other factors. The interesting condition of "tetany of the newborn" appears to be related to the existence of tetany in the mother. It is perhaps due to inability of the maternal parathyroid glands to compensate fully for the fetus and to the fact that the fetal parathyroids are not fully functioning at birth in such cases. The condition appears to differ from the more common form of infantile tetany, which rarely occurs before the third or fourth month.

Maternal tetany is best *prevented* or *treated* by administration of Ca salts (orally or parenterally) and vitamin D in adequate dosage. In cases in which the serum P concentration is increased, parathyroid hormone or dihydrotachysterol may be employed, as in parathyroid tetany. Tetany of the newborn usually responds well to administration of Ca salts parenterally and, if necessary, parathyroid hormone.

Tetany in Steatorrhea.—Tetany, latent or manifest, is a rather common manifestation of celiac disease, sprue and so-called "idiopathic" steatorrhea. It is due to impaired intestinal absorption of fats, resulting in the formation of relatively insoluble calcium soaps and, therefore, inadequate assimilation of calcium. There is probably also inadequate absorption of vitamin D. Impaired absorption is also contributed to by the increased intestinal motility. These abnormalities eventuate in osteoporosis, rickets, dwarfism, osteomalacia, hypocalcemia and tetany. The serum P concentration is also frequently diminished and excessive amounts of Ca and P are lost in the feces. These conditions are usually easily differentiated from other forms of tetany by the characteristically high fat content of the feces, the presence of anemia of various types, and gastro-intestinal abnormalities.

Treatment of tetany of this variety consists primarily in treatment of the underlying steatorrhea, plus administration of vitamin D and calcium salts, parenterally if oral administration is not feasible. Dihydrotachysterol may be useful in refractory cases.

Phosphate, Citrate and Oxalate Tetany.—Parenteral administration of soluble oxalates and of citrates produces tetany, the former by the production of hypocalcemia through the formation of insoluble calcium oxalate, the latter by formation of a poorly ionizable calcium citrate compound, without hypocalcemia. Tetanic manifestations may also follow the intravenous injection of neutral, alkaline or slightly acid sodium phosphate, with a concomitant fall in serum Ca concentration. That tetany does not occur after injection of acid sodium phosphate even though the serum Ca falls, is probably due to an increase in ionization of Ca incident to the accompanying acidosis. There is evidence that increase in serum P in various forms of tetany is accompanied by increase in neuromuscular irritability and, in parathyroid tetany, by increased resistance to parathyroid hormone. This suggests a relationship between hypocalcemia and hyperphosphatemia and the severity of tetany, which is due to the possibility that phosphate, like bicarbonate and citrate, depresses Ca ionization. Tetany occurs occasionally in advanced forms of renal failure. It is associated with hypocalcemia and hyperphosphatemia, the latter probably being the cause of the former. This condition thus probably represents a true primary "phosphate" tetany. In this condition, manifestations of tetany are often absent, despite the low serum Ca concentration, because of the almost invariably accompanying acidosis.

Alkalotic Tetany.—As is indicated in the formula,

$$\text{Irritability } \alpha \ \frac{[Na^+] + [K^+]}{[Ca^{++}] + [Mg^{++}] + [H^+]},$$

decrease in the hydrogen ion concentration results in increased neuromuscular irritability with no accompanying change in serum Ca concentration. Thus, tetany may be present in alkalosis. This may occur clinically in the following conditions: (*a*) following ingestion of excessive quantities of alkali, especially bicarbonate; (*b*) after prolonged periods of pulmonary hyperventilation, with lowering of alveolar and plasma CO_2 tension (voluntary, hysteria, certain cases of encephalitis); and (*c*) after excessive gastric lavage or protracted vomiting (gastric tetany), as in pyloric or upper intestinal obstruction. The excessive loss of HCl results in lowering of the plasma Cl and increase in bicarbonate, with consequent tendency toward a more alkaline reaction in the blood and tissue fluids.

In bicarbonate and gastric tetany, in addition to the history and clinical findings, significant observations include: increase in plasma CO_2 combining power, decrease in plasma Cl concentration (gastric tetany), increase in pH of the blood, and normal serum Ca concentration.

In hyperventilation tetany, the significant chemical changes are: fall in alveolar and plasma CO_2 combining power, increase in plasma pH, increase in alkalinity and decrease in ammonia in the urine, and normal serum Ca concentration.

Treatment of these types of tetany is, of course, removal or correction of the underlying cause. Administration of sodium chloride, by restoring the normal plasma Cl, promptly relieves tetany due to excessive vomiting or gastric lavage. It is seldom necessary to resort to the use of acidifying agents such as dilute HCl or ammonium chloride. If desirable, ammonium chloride may be given in doses of 1 to 2 gm., three or four times daily, and HCl, in N/10 solution, mixed with milk or fruit juices, in divided doses up to 250 cc. daily.

Low Magnesium Tetany.—As has been indicated (irritability formula, p. 211), the magnesium ion has essentially the same effect as the calcium ion upon neuromuscular irritability. Hyperexcitability, convulsions, and low serum Mg concentration have been produced in experimental animals (rat and dog) by feeding diets practically free of magnesium.[28] A similar condition, accompanied by defective ossification, occurs spontaneously in cattle grazing on pastures poor in Mg ("grass tetany"). No comparable disorder has been reported in man. Hypocalcemia occurs occasionally but not consistently. The tetany may be due directly to the hypomagnesemia or, indirectly, to relative inactivation of Ca by an excess of P which would normally have been bound by Mg. The condition is cured by administration of adequate amounts of magnesium.

Conditions Simulating Tetany.—Manifestations of nervous hyperirritability, including convulsions, may occur, particularly in infants and young children, at the onset of acute infectious diseases. In the absence of vitamin D deficiency or of alkalosis, which may follow prolonged vomiting, these have no relation to true tetany, from which they may be differentiated by the absence of the characteristic chemical findings. The same is true of such conditions as meningitis, tetanus, uremia, and poisoning with chemical agents, including atropine, strychnine, lead and guanidine.

VITAMIN D (ANTIRACHITIC VITAMIN)[29]

The rôle of vitamin D in nutrition and the clinical manifestations of deficient and excessive supply of this factor are described elsewhere (p. 400). It is necessary here only to summarize its influence upon Ca and P metabolism.

The multiple nature of vitamin D is now well established, at least ten different sterol derivatives having been shown to possess antirachitic properties in varying degree. The two of greatest practical significance are vitamin D_2 (calciferol, irradiated ergosterol of yeast, viosterol) and vitamin D_3 (activated 7-dehydrocholesterol, present in cod-liver oil and produced by irradiation of milk or of the skin). The various forms of vitamin D have qualitatively the same effect physiologically, and can be detected only by their action in the prevention or cure of rickets. Consequently, the mode of action of this factor can be best illustrated by reviewing the consequences of its withdrawal from the diet and of its subsequent readministration.

Vitamin D Deficiency.—Under ordinary conditions, vitamin D is necessary for normal calcification of bone, although this is not the case in vitro. The absence of adequate amounts from the diet results in the development of rickets in infants and osteomalacia in adults, other factors, particularly the Ca and P intake and the rate of body growth being also of great importance.

Rickets.—In normal, growing long bones, the epiphyseal cartilage is a narrow plate, supported by transverse trabeculae or a thin fenestrated plate of bone on the epiphyseal side and uniformly penetrated by capillaries on the diaphyseal side. Growth takes place by continuous proliferation of orderly columns of cartilage cells on the epiphyseal side and by simultaneous degeneration of matured cartilage cells on the diaphyseal side. The latter are replaced by capillaries and osteoblasts, which are responsible for the deposition of the bony matrix (zone of preparatory calcification). One of the characteristic features of normal growth is the presence, on the diaphyseal side of the plate of cartilage, of a continuous layer of clear cartilage cells in an almost straight line.

The *first visible changes* in rickets are the cessation of degeneration in the diaphyseal cartilage cells, the absence of a straight layer of clear cells, and the absence of capillaries and osteoblasts in this zone. The proliferating epiphyseal cartilage becomes wider and its diaphyseal border irregular, the cells losing their columnar arrangement. Cartilage cells and osteoid tissue (poorly calcified) extend toward the shaft of the bone. These changes, *i.e.*, defective calcification at the points of growth and enlargement of the epiphyseal cartilages, result in softening of the bones and the development of the characteristic rachitic deformities (p. 410). In experimental animals these changes may be demonstrated histologically and by means of the *"line test."* The latter consists essentially in staining the split bone with silver nitrate to demonstrate the line of new calcification. Chemical analysis of rachitic bone reveals a decrease in calcium, phosphate and carbonate, and an increase in magnesium and organic matter (normal ratio of ash to organic matter, 3:2; rachitic, 1:2 or 1:3).

Clinically, the diagnosis is made on the basis of clinical findings (p. 411), x-ray examination and chemical studies. The bone shadows are less dense than normally and the ends of the bones present a moth-eaten appearance, the outline being indistinct and the ends frequently concave rather than straight or convex. The *serum Ca and P concentrations* vary considerably in different stages of the disease and under different conditions of Ca and P intake. In the majority of cases in infants on modified milk diets, the serum Ca is essentially normal and the serum P is low, frequently 1 to 3 mg. per 100 cc. The ester P of the red blood cells is low also. During the initial stage of recovery, particularly if vitamin D is given inadequately and the Ca intake is relatively low and the P intake high, the serum Ca may be low and the serum P elevated and tetany may develop (p. 209). Occasionally, especially in premature infants, the serum Ca and P are both low. In experimental animals, by varying the Ca/P ratio in the diet, rickets may be produced with high Ca, low P or low Ca, high P values in the serum.

The serum phosphatase activity is increased in rickets, being perhaps the earliest metabolic manifestation of the condition. The degree of increase is roughly indicative of the severity of the defect. Repair is accompanied by a decrease in this factor, normal values being restored usually only after all other manifestations have disappeared. Ca and P balances are subnormal and may even be negative in severe cases. The excretion of P and Ca in the feces is considerably increased and the urinary Ca and P decreased. It is of interest that the parathyroid glands frequently enlarge and the cells hypertrophy. The significance of this observation is questionable.

When vitamin D is given to rachitic subjects the metabolic abnormalities are corrected and the zones of provisional calcification reassume a more normal appearance. Histological evidence of beginning repair may be noted within twenty-four to forty-eight hours. The manner in which vitamin D produces this effect is not clearly understood. The hypothesis that it operates through stimulation of parathyroid activity has no basis in fact. Metabolic studies indicate that it increases absorption of Ca from the intestine, increases retention of P in the organism and facilitates utilization of both Ca and P in the process of calcification of bone. Recent studies suggest that it aids also in the liberation of inorganic P from organic compounds, thus rendering more available for bone formation. Vitamin D appears to be necessary for the occurrence of the proper type of cartilage degeneration preliminary to normal calcification and, in clinical rickets, for the maintenance of a Ca and P content of the blood plasma and tissue fluids favorable for the deposition of the normal calcium-phosphate-carbonate complex in the osteoid matrix (p. 174).

Late Rickets and Osteomalacia.—Rickets usually occurs before the second year, during the period of most active bone growth and development. Occasionally it may occur in older children (four to sixteen years); then it is termed late or *juvenile rickets.* The etiology, pathogenesis, metabolic features and morphologic changes are essentially the same as in infantile rickets except that the histologic changes in the bones are modified by the difference in the stage of their development.

Deficiency in vitamin D, Ca and P intakes in adults results in osteomalacia, which may be regarded as *adult rickets.* It differs from ordinary rickets in that, skeletal growth having been completed, the characteristic rachitic abnormalities occurring in the zones of provisional calcification are, of course, lacking. The entire bone is softer than in rickets, the mineral content being greatly diminished, although the Mg is usually increased, constituting a state of generalized skeletal demineralization. This is evident by x-ray examination. The serum Ca and P concentrations are lowered and fecal excretion of Ca and P is increased. Changes in Ca metabolism are usually more pronounced than those in P metabolism and tetany may develop (p. 209). Marked deformities may develop as a result of the extreme pliability of the bones. This condition has become rare in civilized countries, but still occurs in times of famine and under other conditions of inadequate vitamin D and Ca intake, especially when exposure to sunlight is simultaneously restricted. Osteomalacia, like rickets, is cured by an adequate supply of vitamin D, Ca and P.

Miscellaneous.—Rachitic and osteomalacic changes may occur in infants with celiac disease and in adults with sprue or "idiopathic" steatorrhea. The skeletal abnormalities in these conditions are dependent upon inadequate absorption of Ca and probably of vitamin D, which results from impaired absorption of fat and increased intestinal motility (fatty diarrhea). The essential features with regard to Ca and P metabolism and skeletal changes are the same as those of rickets, in children, and osteomalacia, in adults. Tetany may develop (p. 211). Successful treatment depends upon correction of the underlying condition, but administration of Ca and vitamin D is frequently beneficial.

Absorption and utilization of vitamin D are impaired in the presence of hepatocellular damage and in the absence of bile salts from the intestine (obstructive jaundice and bile fistula). In the latter case, absorption of Ca is also interfered with because of the disturbance of fat digestion and absorption, with consequent formation of insoluble calcium soaps. When these hepatic or biliary tract disturbances occur in children (congenital or juvenile cirrhosis), growth is stunted (hepatic rickets).

The condition known as renal rickets is described elsewhere (p. 198). It is dependent primarily upon retention of phosphorus, with high serum P concentration, increased P excretion into the intestine and consequent interference with Ca absorption. Acidosis also contributes to the development of skeletal demineralization. When renal functional insufficiency occurs during the period of skeletal growth, growth is stunted (renal dwarfism). Deficiency of vitamin D is not involved in the pathogenesis of this condition.

Hypervitaminosis D.—Manifestations of vitamin D excess have been rarely encountered clinically in the past because of the wide margin between ordinary therapeutic and toxic doses. However, with the increasing employment of very large amounts of this agent in various conditions, evidences of hypervitaminosis are observed occasionally. Toxic manifestations should be watched for in infants receiving more than 30,000 international units, in children receiving more than 50,000 international units, and in adults receiving more than 200,000 international units daily over protracted periods. As much as 1,000,000 international units daily has been given for several weeks with little or no evidence of toxicity.

The concentrations of Ca and P in the blood and their excretion in the urine are increased, the Ca and P balances becoming negative unless large amounts of these elements are administered. In children, there is increased deposition of lime salts in the zones of provisional calcification. If the intake is inadequate, demineralization occurs in the shafts of the bones, with continued deposition at the epiphyses. Thus, in infants, osteoporosis may progress simultaneously with the healing of rachitic lesions. In experimental animals, bone changes have been produced which superficially resemble those of hyperparathyroidism but are not histologically identical with the latter. Degenerative changes occur in renal tubular epithelium, blood vessels, heart, stomach, intestines, liver and bronchi, with metastatic or dystrophic calcification in many of these tissues (pp. 218, 219). Degeneration and abnormal calcification are most readily produced when the diet is high in P and adequate in Ca. The *symptoms* of vitamin D excess include nausea, vomiting, anorexia, loss of weight, diarrhea, headache, polyuria, increased urinary frequency, weakness, urinary abnormalities (albumin, casts, hematuria) and evidences of renal functional impairment.

Miscellaneous.—By virtue of its relationship to the state of "intercellular material," vitamin C (ascorbic acid) plays an important part in growth and repair of bones and teeth (p. 217). It appears to be necessary for the proper functioning and development of osteoblasts (also ameloblasts and odontoblasts), which in its absence are unable to form osteoid tissue and revert to their prototype (fibroblasts). The resulting bone lesions are quite characteristic and the diagnosis of scorbutic skeletal lesions may usually be made readily by x-ray or histological examination (p. 462). There is no evidence of disturbance of Ca or P metabolism in vitamin C deficiency and serum phosphatase activity is normal, except during periods of calcification of hemorrhagic extravasations. Mention is made here of this condition because it may at times complicate the picture of rickets.

Lead resembles calcium in its deposition in and mobilization from the bones and, in both of these respects, it is influenced in the same manner by factors which influence the latter. In other words, the deposition of lead in the bones is favored by factors which favor the deposition of Ca (high Ca and P intake, adequate vitamin D intake) and its liberation is facilitated by factors which accelerate mobilization of Ca (parathyroid hormone, excessive doses of vitamin D, inadequate Ca and P intake, acidosis, thyroxin). The *administration of lead* has no significant effect on Ca or P metabolism that can be demonstrated by alteration in Ca and P balance or excretion, or in serum Ca and P concentrations. During the process of deposition of lead in the skeleton, Ca is liberated from the calcium phosphate of the bones and is replaced by lead, which is retained as the relatively inert and insoluble (at resting pH) tri-lead phosphate. Flat bones (skull, pelvis, scapula) contain more lead than tubular bones, the ends of long bones containing more than the shafts and the teeth (principally in the dentin) proportionately more than the bones. During the period of active growth, lead is deposited chiefly in the zones of provisional calcification and in the subperiosteal zones. In *children* with lead poisoning this is evidenced by the x-ray as a series of transverse lines in the diaphyses and linear rings of density in ossification centers of the epiphyseal cartilages and carpal bones. These may resemble changes that occur in healing rickets. In *adults*, the distribution resembles that in children, but the characteristic changes in the zones of provisional calcification are, of course, lacking, and retention in the bones does not occur as avidly as in embryonal or growing bone. It is stored in relatively high concentration in the trabeculae, especially at the epiphyses. These facts are taken advantage of in the treatment of lead poisoning. During acute episodes, the flow of lead toward the bones, where it is stored in inert form, is stimulated by high Ca and P intake. After subsidence of acute manifestations, if gradual mobilization and excretion of lead is desired, this may be accomplished by administration of a diet low in Ca and P, acids or acid-forming substances (dilute HCl or ammonium chloride) or parathyroid hormone, among other agents.

Radium resembles lead in its storage in and mobilization from the skeleton. It is deposited most readily in newly formed trabeculae and undergoes gradual mobilization and redeposition until it is redistributed throughout the bones. It differs from lead, however, in that, because of its destructive action, prompt removal from the body is desirable. This may be facilitated by the use of agents which favor mobilization and excretion of Ca and lead, but their effect is not so striking as in the case of these elements.

MINERAL METABOLISM AND TEETH

In considering the effects of disturbances of mineral metabolism on dental structure, one must draw a distinction between the period of dental development and that of adult tooth structure. Calcification of growing teeth may be influenced by a number of factors. Hypoparathyroidism (parathyroid tetany) may be accompanied by defective calcification of the dentin and enamel hypoplasia (p. 205). In experimental animals, hypophysectomy or adrenalectomy result in rather characteristic changes in calcification of the dentin, which is denser than normal. Similar changes have not been described in man. *Vitamin A deficiency* in rats and guinea-pigs results in atrophy and metaplasia of the enamel-forming organ, atrophy and depression of function of odontoblasts, cessation of enamel formation and defective formation of dentin. Similar changes have been described in the tooth germ during infancy, and it seems probable that vitamin A is of the greatest importance in contributing to normal dental development during the formative period. Vitamin C deficiency in animals is characterized by *defects in enamel, cementum and dentin.*[30] This factor appears to be necessary for proper development and functioning of odontoblasts and ameloblasts (enamel). In C deficiency, the pulp becomes atrophied and hyperemic, odontoblasts show evidence of degeneration, with small cysts and foci of abnormal calcification and, in complete deficiency, the matrix is undifferentiated. Although evidence of similar changes in humans is meager, the consensus of opinion is that an adequate intake of vitamin C is essential for normal dental growth and structure. There seems to be no doubt that vitamin D deficiency *in infancy* may result in defective calcification, hypoplastic defects and caries in deciduous teeth. It probably has little or no influence upon the development of caries in permanent teeth although, since the latter develop during the entire period of growth, there may be enamel hypoplasia and abnormal calcification of dentin.

It is generally believed that the adult tooth is a fixed structure, unaffected by metabolic factors which influence the Ca and P deposits in the bones. This question has aroused considerable discussion, especially in its relation to the important problem of dental caries. The statement seems justified that there is no substantial evidence that adult teeth are subject to active withdrawal of calcium, even in such extreme conditions as experimental and clinical hyperparathyroidism, in which enormous quantities of Ca and P may be withdrawn from the skeleton. On the other hand, it has been found that radium, which is deposited in situations and in a manner similar to that of calcium, is deposited in adult teeth. Furthermore, when radioactive P is administered, a very small amount enters the nongrowing tooth, and it has been calculated that 1 per cent of the P content of a human tooth is replaced by P from the food in about 250 days. Therefore, it cannot be maintained that the teeth are metabolically inert. However, the available evidence suggests that the fully erupted adult tooth, unlike bone, is not significantly subject to modification in structure or calcification by changes in Ca or P metabolism.

The teeth may be affected by other minerals. *Lead* is known to be deposited in the teeth in relatively high concentration in lead poisoning. Its relation to the occurrence of dental defects has not been established. Ingestion of excessive amounts of *fluorine* (fluorosis) results in a condition known as "mottled enamel." The occurrence of this disorder is related to the amount of fluorine in drinking water and is endemic in certain districts.[31] The fluorine is retained also in the bones, and the Ca balance has been found to be diminished and the serum phosphatase activity lowered. In acute fluorine poisoning the serum Ca concentration may be diminished (formation of calcium fluoride). Although *chronic fluorosis* exerts a marked effect on skeletal development, enzyme action, body growth, respiration and reproduction, the growing tooth shows the most striking effects. These teeth, as well as adult teeth, become an opaque, chalky white and then brown, and the enamel becomes pitted. The enamel-forming cells (ameloblasts) are first affected and enamel formation is disturbed, probably by the deposition of calcium fluoride instead of the normal phosphate and carbonate, and perhaps by disturbance in the phosphatase mechanism. Deciduous teeth are affected only by much larger doses of fluorine than are required to produce characteristic changes in permanent teeth.

PATHOLOGICAL CALCIFICATION[32]

Calcification may occur in abnormal situations under a variety of circumstances. These may be classified as (1) metastatic calcification, (2) dystrophic calcification, (3) calcinosis, (4) arterial calcification, (5) lithiasis (renal, biliary, salivary, *etc.*), and (6) heteropic bone formation. Abnormalities of Ca and P metabolism are implicated in the etiology of certain forms of metastatic and dystrophic calcification and perhaps also in calcinosis.

Metastatic Calcification.—This term is applied to the deposition of lime salts in tissues which have not been the site of preceding regressive changes. The lesions occur chiefly in the kidneys (especially tubular epithelium), gastric mucosa (chiefly about acid-secreting glands), and lungs (alveolar walls and vessels); less frequently there is calcification of the pulmonary veins and wall of the left auricle and, rarely, of the peripheral arteries, trachea and liver. Occasionally, virtually all tissues are affected. In some instances, especially in cases of renal "osteitis fibrosa" (p. 198), there is an extreme degree of calcification of practically the entire arterial system, readily demonstrable by the x-ray. Occasionally the media is primarily or exclusively involved (Mönckeberg's sclerosis). These deposits have approximately the same mineral composition as bone, except perhaps for a slightly higher Ca/P ratio. In some instances actual bone formation may occur.

It is significant that the tissues most commonly affected (kidneys, stomach, lungs) are those in which acid secretion takes place, the cells themselves being relatively alkaline in reaction. This relatively high local alkalinity favors precipitation of Ca and P from the blood plasma in the form of calcium phosphate. Obviously, if the previous condition of the tissues is assumed to be normal, precipitation of Ca and P from the plasma presupposes that the capacity of the latter for maintaining them in solution has been exceeded. Phenomena that might produce this effect are (*a*) increase in the concentration of Ca or P or of both, (*b*) increased alkalinity, and, perhaps, (c) decrease in total electrolyte concentration and (d) decrease in protein content of the plasma. Impairment of renal function may also be a contributory factor, the accompanying acidosis increasing mobilization of Ca from the bones and the elevation of serum P probably increasing the quantity of colloidal calcium phosphate in the blood.

Metastatic calcification has been observed clinically in the following conditions: hyperparathyroidism, hypervitaminosis D and renal rickets and renal "osteitis fibrosa," and, less frequently, in multiple myeloma, myelogenous leukemia, extensive skeletal metastases of sarcoma and carcinoma, "marble-bone disease" and widespread osteomyelitis. Although no cases have as yet been reported, it may also follow administration of excessive amounts of dihydrotachysterol (A.T. 10). These are generally regarded as examples of true metastatic calcification. However, although conditions favorable for the occurrence of this phenomenon are often present in such conditions, *i.e.*, hypercalcemia, hyperphosphatemia, destructive bone lesions and renal functional impairment, it is probable that frequently local tissue changes precede and facilitate the precipitation of lime salts. Under such circumstances, the condition should be regarded more properly, in part at least, as one of dystrophic calcification. Thus, regressive changes in the renal tubular epithelium, heart muscle and other tissues have been found to precede the occurrence of demonstrable calcification in these situations in experimental hyperparathyroidism and hypervitaminosis D.[33]

Dystrophic Calcification.—This term is applied to deposits of lime salts in dead, degenerated, or devitalized tissue, as in infarcts, areas of necrosis and fatty degeneration, inspissated collections of pus, hyalinized scar tissue, caseating tubercles, and atheromatous patches in the intima of vessels. This constitutes the most common types of pathological calcification, may occur in any organ or tissue and, in the vast majority of cases, is not dependent upon or associated with abnormality of Ca or P metabolism. However, as stated above, precipitation of lime salts in the soft tissues in hyperparathyroidism and hypervitaminosis D may represent a process of dystrophic calcification superimposed upon one of true metastatic calcification. It is believed that deposition of calcium phosphate is facilitated in dead or devitalized tissues by virtue of the lowered CO_2 tension and increased alkalinity in such areas. Naturally, this phenomenon becomes more marked and more extensive in the presence of such aggravating factors as hypercalcemia, hyperphosphatemia, destructive bone lesions and renal functional impairment, such as occur in hyperparathyroidism, hypervitaminosis D, renal osteitis fibrosa, and after administration of dihydrotachysterol.

Calcinosis.[34, 35]—In this rather rare condition, lime salts are deposited in and beneath the skin. Two forms have been described: (1) *Calcinosis circumscripta*, the more common, in which calcification is superficial, localized to the skin, occurs at any age, almost invariably in the upper extremities, particularly in the fingers and, because of the resemblance of the deposits to tophi, has been called "calcium gout." (2) *Calcinosis universalis*, occurring most frequently in the first two decades, in which, in addition to the skin, widespread deposits occur subcutaneously and in the connective tissue of muscles, tendons, fascia and nerves, with serious impairment of health. Calcification has also been observed in the capsules of lymph nodes, but not in the usual visceral situations in which metastatic calcification is usually observed. The nodules often coalesce and may break down and ulcerate, extruding a chalk-like material. True bone formation may occur. When the muscles are extensively involved the condition is termed "myositis ossificans." The etiology is unknown. Scleroderma, or manifestations of the Raynaud syndrome occur in a large proportion of cases. Although evidence of previous tissue damage has not been demonstrated, it seems significant that this process involves portions of the body liable to trauma and most subject to muscular activity. Serum Ca and P concentrations and serum phosphatase activity are normal, but balance studies have revealed a striking tendency to retain Ca and P. This has been ascribed to an increased affinity of the affected tissues for these elements. It may be significant that increased phosphatase activity has been demonstrated in muscle and fibrous tissue in pre-ossification stages of myositis ossificans. Spontaneous disappearance of the calcific deposits has been reported, rarely, however, in the generalized form. The course is chronic, with spontaneous remissions and exacerbations. Calcinosis circumscripta causes little or no interference with function, but in calcinosis universalis contraction of tendons and muscles interfere with joint and muscle function and ulcerations of the skin may lead to local infections, septicemia, or bacteremia.

Treatment is unsatisfactory. Attempts have been made to mobilize the abnormal deposits of calcium by the production of acidosis (ketogenic diet, ammonium chloride), parathyroid hormone, low Ca intake and administration of di-sodium hydrogen phosphate. Physical therapy, heliotherapy, radiotherapy, insulin, acetylcholine and pilocarpine have been used, without consistently significant effect.

BIBLIOGRAPHY

1. Berliner, K., Am. Heart J., **8**: 548, 1933; Am. J. Med. Sci., **191**: 1, 1936.
2. Cantarow, A., Calcium Metabolism and Calcium Therapy, Lea & Febiger, Philadelphia, Ed. 2, 1933.
3. Schmidt, C. L. A. and Greenberg, D. M., Physiol. Rev., **15**: 297, 1935.
4. Leitch, I., Nutrit. Abst. and Rev., **6**: 553, 1937.
5. Jeans, P. C., Stearns, G., McKinley, J. B., Goff, E. A. and Stinger, D., J. Pediat., **8**: 403, 1936.
6. Shohl, A. T., Mineral Metabolism, Reinhold Publishing Corp., New York, 1939.
7. Cantarow, A., Internat. Clin., **1**: 230, 1936.
8. Albright, F., J.A.M.A., **112**: 2592, 1939.
9. Shelling, D. H., The parathyroids in health and disease, C. V. Mosby Co., St. Louis, 1935.
10. Cantarow, A. and Haury, V. G., Am. J. Physiol., **126**: 66, 1939.
11. McLean, F. C. and Hastings, A. B., Am. J. Med. Sci., **189**: 601, 1935.
12. Haury, V. G. and Cantarow, A., Proc. Soc. Exper. Biol. and Med., **43**: 335, 1940.
13. Kay, H. D., Physiol. Rev., **12**: 384, 1932.
14. Robison, R., Herter Lectures, New York University Press, New York, 1932.
15. Robison, R. and Soames, K. M., Biochem. J., **18**: 740, 1924.
16. Bodansky, A., J. Biol. Chem., **101**: 93, 1933; **104**: 473, 1934.
17. Cantarow, A. and Trumper, M., Clinical Biochemistry, W. B. Saunders, Philadelphia, 2nd Ed., 1939.
18. Gutman, A. B. and Gutman, E. B., J. Clin. Invest., **17**: 473, 1938.
19. (a) Albright, F., Aub, J. C. and Bauer, W., J.A.M.A., **102**: 1276, 1934.
    (b) Albright, F., Bloomberg, E., Castleman, B. and Churchill, E. D., Arch. Int. Med., **54**: 315, 1934.
    (c) Albright, F., Baird, P. C., Cope, O. and Bloomberg, E., Am. J. Med. Sci., **187**: 49, 1934.

(d) Albright, F., Sulkowitch, H. W. and Bloomberg, E., Arch. Int. Med., **62**: 199, 1938; Am. J. Med. Sci., **193**: 800, 1937.

(e) Albright, F., Drake, T. G. and Sulkowitch, H. W., Bull. Johns Hopk. Hosp., **60**: 377, 1937.

20. Castleman, B. and Mallory, T. B., Am. J. Path., **11**: 1, 1935.
21. Jaffe, H. L., Arch. Path., **16**: 63, 236, 1933.
22. (a) Hamilton, B. and Schwartz, C., J. Pharmacol. and Exper. Ther., **46**: 285, 1932.
    (b) Hamilton, B. and Highman, W. J., Jr., J. Clin. Invest., **15**: 99, 1936.
23. Lichtenstein, L., Arch. Surg., **36**: 874, 1938.
24. Horwitz, T. and Cantarow, A., Arch. Int. Med., **64**: 280, 1939.
25. Selye, H., Endocrinol., **16**: 547, 1932.
26. Cantarow, A., Stewart, H. L. and Morgan, D., Endocrinol., **24**: 556, 1939.
27. Stone, H. B., Owings, J. C. and Gey, G. O., Am. J. Surg., **24**: 387, 1934.
28. Greenberg, D. M. and Tufts, E. V., Am. J. Physiol., **121**: 311, 1938.
29. Bills, C. E., Physiol. Rev., **15**: 1, 1935.
30. Dalldorf, G., J.A.M.A., **111**: 1376, 1938.
31. Greenwood, D. A., Physiol. Rev., **20**: 582, 1940.
32. Barr, D. P., Physiol. Rev., **12**: 593, 1932.
33. Cantarow, A., Stewart, H. L. and Housel, E. L., Endocrinol., **22**: 13, 1938.
34. Rothstein, J. L. and Welt, S., Am. J. Dis. Child., **52**: 368, 1936.
35. Bauer, W., Marble, A. and Bennett, G. A., Am. J. Med. Sci., **182**: 237, 1931.
36. (a) Albright, F., Bloomberg, E., Drake, T. and Sulkowitch, H. W., J. Clin. Invest., **17**: 317, 1938.
    (b) Albright, F., J.A.M.A., **112**: 2592, 1939.
37. Snapper, I., Lancet, **1**: 728, 1934.
38. MacBryde, C. M., J.A.M.A., **111**: 304, 1938.

MAGNESIUM METABOLISM[1,2]

Experimental observations in recent years have thrown considerable light upon the rôle of magnesium in animal nutrition. However, little is known as yet of its functions in the human organism and of the relation of disturbance of Mg metabolism to clinical observable abnormalities in man. The few such disturbances that have been demonstrated and the possibility of future developments in this field justify a brief resumé of present knowledge of this subject.

FUNCTIONS

These cannot be stated definitely but must be merely inferred from the physiologic properties of Mg as demonstrated experimentally. Mg is present in all cells and body fluids, its chief deposits being in the bones and muscles. It is a probably important constituent of bone, constituting 0.5 to 0.7 per cent of the ash. An excess has been shown to inhibit calcification, in vivo and in vitro. In other respects, too, it acts as an antagonist to calcium (pharmacologically). It activates the alkaline phosphatase of plasma, bone, etc., and may thus play a part in the functioning of many enzyme systems concerned with the intermediary metabolism of phosphorus and carbohydrate and in muscular contraction. Muscle contains much more Mg than Ca, but the significance of this fact is not apparent. It plays a rôle similar to that of Ca in the control of neuromuscular irritability (see equation, p. 211) but, peculiarly, its action in this respect is counteracted by Ca. For example, the narcosis produced by parenteral injection of Mg salts may be prevented or relieved by administration of Ca. Moreover, the effects of Mg deficiency in experimental animals are enhanced by Ca administration and ameliorated by a simultaneous low Ca intake.

The *absorption* of Mg from the bowel resembles that of Ca in many respects (p. 178). It is diminished by a high intake of fat, phosphate, Ca and alkalis, due probably to their influence on the solubility of Mg salts. Vitamin D apparently exerts no influence upon absorption of Mg.

Under normal conditions, 50 to 80 per cent is *excreted* in the feces (bile and intestinal secretions) and the remainder in the urine. The quantity in the urine is increased somewhat following administration of acidifying substances (HCl, NH_4Cl), and slightly and very temporarily after parathyroid hormone. No significant alteration occurs in hyperthyroidism or hyperparathyroidism, indicating an essential difference between Ca and Mg metabolism. After parenteral administration of Mg salts, 70 to 90 per cent is eliminated in the urine.

The *requirement* for Mg is not known exactly, since equilibrium may be established, in adults at least, on relatively low or high intakes, whereas infants and children show extremely variable balances regardless of the intake. It has been estimated, however, that 0.2 to 0.6 gm. daily is adequate for adults. Due to the high Mg content of chlorophyll, green vegetables constitute an important dietary source of this element.

BLOOD MAGNESIUM

Mg is present in both red cells and plasma, about 5.4 to 7.8 mg. per 100 cc. in the former and 1.8 to 3.6 mg. in the latter. A decrease has been reported during menstruation and in the late months of pregnancy. About 75 to 90 per cent (average 85 per cent) of the serum Mg is in diffusible form, the remainder being probably bound to protein (see Calcium, p. 181). The Mg content of cerebrospinal fluid is higher than that of blood serum, averaging about 3.3 mg. per 100 cc.

Little is known regarding the factors involved in the regulation of Mg metabolism or the Mg content of the blood. The latter is relatively unaffected by phosphate, protein, vitamin D or parathyroid hormone, although the last apparently causes a slight and brief elevation of serum Mg. There is in some respects a reciprocal relationship between Mg and Ca in the serum; *e.g.*, in oxalate poisoning, the decrease in serum Ca is accompanied by an increase in Mg, while the hypermagnesemia induced by parenteral administration of Mg salts is accompanied by a fall in serum Ca concentration, even to tetanic levels.

Slight *increases* have been reported in chronic infections, atherosclerosis, hypertrophic arthritis, essential hypertension and oxalate poisoning. A slight decrease has been reported in uremia, epilepsy, rickets and hypervitaminosis B. However, many of the values regarded as abnormal by some fall within the range regarded as normal by others, and the general opinion is that significant deviations from the normal do not occur consistently enough to be of clinical importance. Increase in serum Mg occurs rather frequently in renal failure, but rarely to values more than twice normal. The danger has been emphasized of administration of Mg salts as purgatives or for other reasons in such cases because of the possibility of consequent elevation of the serum Mg to dangerous levels.[3] It seems questionable whether this occurs frequently enough to constitute a real hazard. *Hyper-*

magnesemia is accompanied first by sedation and mild hypnosis (at 5 mg. per 100 cc.) and later by profound coma (18 to 20 mg. per 100 cc.). This effect may be counteracted by parenteral administration of soluble Ca salts. The rise in Mg is usually accompanied by a fall in Ca and an increase in blood sugar, with glycosuria.

Marked *decrease* in serum Mg concentration (to 10 per cent of normal) has been produced in experimental animals by virtual withdrawal of Mg from the diet; it occurs also in the so-called "grass tetany" of cattle.[4] These conditions are accompanied by manifestations of increased neuromuscular excitability (electrical reactions, restlessness, convulsions) and later coma. In the experimental animals the chief manifestations include vasodilatation, hyperemia and hyperexcitability and, later, cachexia, kidney damage (nephrosis, periglomerular fibrosis, calcification) and myocardial degeneration and fibrosis. The Ca content of the soft tissues is increased (50 to 100 per cent in heart and muscle; fifteen times normal in kidney). Although no such condition has yet been observed in man, these observations indicate the indispensability of Mg for the animal organism. There is a relative increase in the Mg content of the ash of bones in rickets and osteomalacia. An increase in nondiffusible Mg has been reported in hyperthyroidism and a decrease in hypothyroidism.[5] The significance of these changes is not known.

BIBLIOGRAPHY

1. Schmidt, C. L. A. and Greenberg, D. M., Physiol. Rev., **15:** 297, 1935.
2. Shohl, A. T., Mineral metabolism, Reinhold Pub. Corp., New York, 1939.
3. Hirschfelder, A. D. and Haury, V. G., J.A.M.A., **102:** 1138, 1934; J. Biol. Chem., **104:** 647, 1934.
4. Greenberg, D. M. and Tufts, E. V., Am. J. Physiol., **121:** 311, 1938.
5. Soffer, L. J., Cohn, C., Grossman, E. B., Jacobs, M. and Sobotka, H.: J. Clin. Invest., **20:** 429, 1941.

IRON METABOLISM[1, 2]

Function.—Although present in the body in relatively small amounts, iron is of great importance to the life and function of all cells and of the organism as a whole. It is an essential component of hemoglobin and chromatin material and its chief functions lie in the transport of oxygen to the tissues (hemoglobin) and in cellular respiration or oxidation processes (cytochrome).

REQUIREMENT, ABSORPTION, EXCRETION

Normal adults may be maintained in approximate iron equilibrium with intakes of as little as 5 mg. daily, but it is believed that 10 to 15 mg. constitutes a more satisfactory allowance. This amount appears to be adequate to meet the demands of menstruation, pregnancy and lactation in the absence of digestive disturbances that might interfere with absorption of iron. Young children (four to eight years) require daily about 0.6 mg. per Kg. of weight and infants (up to one year) 1 to 2 mg. per Kg. Under normal conditions the requirement may be met by the iron of foodstuffs, particularly liver, meats, egg-yolk, green leafy vegetables and legumes.

Iron is *absorbed* chiefly in the first portion of the duodenum. The degree of absorption of inorganic iron salts compares favorably with that of iron in foods, but ingested hematin iron is not available for utilization by the animal organism. Ferric is probably reduced to ferrous iron in the intestine, the latter being most likely the form in which simple iron salts are absorbed. A number of factors may render absorption difficult[2]: 1. The relatively high pH in the duodenum facilitates the formation of insoluble basic iron com- pounds. 2. The alkalinity of pancreatic juice and the relative insolubility ot iron salts of bile acids probably interfere with the absorption of iron. 3. Absorption of iron appears to be hampered by the absence of free HCl and of bile and is also influenced unfavorably by administration of alkalis. 4. The presence of relatively large quantities of phosphate facilitates the formation of insoluble iron phosphate compounds. Absorption may also be decreased in the presence of increased intestinal motility. There is evidence that, in experimental animals at least, the normal organism absorbs iron only in pro- portion to its need, the quantity absorbed being determined by the magni- tude of the body reserves of this element. It would appear that the intestinal mucosa is the tissue responsible for its acceptance or rejection, being per- haps conditioned by the iron content of the circulating blood, anemic ani- mals absorbing and utilizing iron very efficiently.

Relatively little iron is *excreted* from the body, the largest portion of the iron content of the feces, which varies with the amount ingested, repre- senting that which has escaped absorption from the intestine. That which is excreted is eliminated chiefly in the bile, to a lesser extent by the bowel mucosa and to a very slight extent by the kidneys. It seems likely that the organism controls its iron stores by regulating absorption rather than excre- tion of this element.

BLOOD IRON

The normal iron content of the blood is 40 to 60 mg. per 100 cc., aver- aging about 52 mg. in males and 45 mg. in females. Practically all of this is in the red blood cells in the form of hemoglobin (15.6 gm. per cent), which contains about 0.33 per cent of iron. The inorganic iron content of whole blood averages only about 1 to 1.7 mg. per 100 cc. There is a small amount of inorganic iron in the plasma or serum, 0.08 to 0.17 mg. per 100 cc., ap- parently entirely in the ferric form. This value is rather constant in the fasting state and is probably an index of the activity of the intermediary metabolism of iron, particularly hemoglobin destruction and production. About 90 mg. of iron are liberated daily by normal breakdown of erythro- cytes.

After ingestion of *inorganic iron salts,* the plasma iron concentration rises to maximum levels of about 3 to 4 times the fasting level in about 2 to 4 hours, subsequently declining gradually over a period of 6 to 12 hours, de- pending on the dosage. Thus, the plasma appears to be the medium of trans- portation of iron from the intestinal tract to the tissues in which it is further utilized or stored. Absorbed iron is transferred to the erythrocytes with remarkable rapidity, having been demonstrated (radioactive iron) in these cells in anemic dogs within a few hours after its oral administration.[3]

The *plasma iron* is influenced by and may be regarded as a measure of (1) the quantity of iron absorbed from the intestine, (2) the adequacy of the iron reserves of the tissues, (3) the capacity of the bone-marrow to utilize iron in hemoglobin synthesis and (5) the activity of hemolytic processes.[4]

INTERMEDIARY METABOLISM AND STORAGE

Iron is absorbed probably in the form of ferrous salts and is transported in the plasma as ferric iron. As has been indicated, the endogenous supply of iron (about 90 mg. daily), representing the breakdown of about 29 gm. of hemoglobin, is much greater than the exogenous, and practically all of it is retained in the body. This is true even under conditions of excessive hemolysis. During the course of destruction of red blood cells in the cells of the reticuloendothelial system, hemoglobin is decomposed into globin and hematin, and the latter into iron-containing hemosiderin and a series of iron-free pigments terminating in bilirubin, which is eliminated in the bile. The iron thus liberated is partly stored or reconverted to hemoglobin in situ, or is transported in the blood plasma (*a*) to storage depots, (*b*) to the bone-marrow for hemoglobin synthesis, or (*c*) to the tissues for participation in processes of cellular respiration.

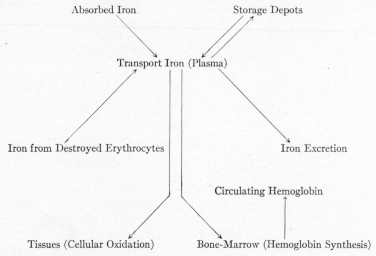

Fig. 15.—Intermediary metabolism and storage of iron. (After Moore, Doan and Arrowsmith.[4])

Following its absorption, iron is carried to the liver, where it apparently exists in two functionally different forms, (*a*) parenchyma iron and (*b*) available storage iron. The distribution of the approximately 3 gm. of iron in the body is about as follows: (1) blood hemoglobin iron, 57 per cent; (2) muscle hemoglobin iron, 7 per cent; (3) parenchyma iron (muscle and other tissues), 16 per cent; (4) available tissue storage iron (liver, spleen, bone-marrow), 15 per cent; (5) available iron of other tissues, 5 per cent. Thus, about 65 per cent of the body iron is in the form of hemoglobin, 15 per cent as functional iron of the tissues and 20 per cent stored in available form. Muscle hemoglobin and parenchyma iron as not available for blood hemoglobin production and are not drawn upon, regardless of how urgent the demand due to anemia. There is some evidence that blood hemoglobin may constitute an important source of iron necessary for growth. In the presence of an increased demand for iron (anemia, dietary restriction), it is mobilized readily from the tissue depots.

ABNORMAL IRON METABOLISM

Disturbances in the metabolism of iron are evidenced by (a) decreased hemoglobin formation, (b) decrease in circulating hemoglobin, or (c) abnormal deposition of iron-containing pigment in the tissues (hemosiderin). A consideration of the pathogenesis and treatment of the various types of anemia is beyond the scope of the present discussion (see p. 351). It must be pointed out, however, that certain forms of hypochromic and microcytic *anemia* are dependent upon inadequate supply or absorption of iron, the latter occurring particularly in the presence of gastric anacidity. Iron deficiency may also occur as a result of *hemorrhage*, with consequent exhaustion of the available tissue reserves of this element. Low values for plasma or serum iron have been reported in hemorrhagic and hypochromic types of anemia. High values are present in forms of anemia characterized by diminished hemoglobin formation not due to iron deficiency (pernicious anemia).

Because they are absorbed more readily from the intestine, ferrous salts are more effective than ferric salts (with the exception of iron and ammonium citrate) in the *treatment* of iron-deficiency anemias. The usual daily dosage of the preparations employed most commonly are: iron and ammonium citrate, 6 gm. (1000 mg. iron); reduced iron, 3 gm. (2800 mg. iron); ferrous carbonate, 4 gm. (360 mg. iron); ferrous sulfate, 1 gm. (200 mg. iron).

Deposition of excessive amounts of iron-containing pigment (hemosiderin) in the tissue occurs (a) as a result of excessive breakdown of red blood cells in hemolytic types of anemia, (b) in conditions in which hemoglobin synthesis is inadequate due to factors other than iron deficiency (pernicious anemia) and (c) in hemochromatosis, the cause of which is unknown. In the latter condition, relatively enormous amounts of iron may be deposited in the tissues, particularly in the liver, pancreas and retroperitoneal lymph nodes, over 50 gm. having been found in the body (exclusive of the blood) in some cases.[5] Studies of iron balance have revealed no significant abnormality, but it is possible that a slight degree of abnormal retention may exist over a period of many years.

BIBLIOGRAPHY

1. Schultze, M. O., Physiol. Rev., **20:** 37, 1940.
2. Hahn, P. F., Medicine, **16:** 37, 1937.
3. Hahn, P. F., Bale, W. F., Lawrence, E. O. and Whipple, G. H., J. Exper. Med., **69:** 739, 1939.
4. Moore, C. V., Doan, C. A. and Arrowsmith, W. R., J. Clin. Invest., **16:** 627, 1937.
5. Sheldon, J. H., Hemochromatosis, Oxford University Press, London, 1935.

IODINE METABOLISM[1-6]

The only known significant function of iodine lies in its relation to the formation of thyroid hormone. Consequently, the state of iodine metabolism is largely dependent upon and intimately related to that of thyroid function. Iodine occurs in the body in two types of combination, inorganic and organic. The first is probably in the form of iodide; two forms of organically bound iodine have been identified in the body: thyroxine (iodinated thyronine, a tetraiodo derivative of a compound of tyrosine and phenol) and diiodotyrosine (iodinated tyrosine). The former contains about 65 per cent, the latter about 58.6 per cent iodine. Thyroid protein, iodo-thyroglobulin, appears to be a composite molecule, containing diiodo-tyrosine and thyroxine in peptide combination. Other organic combinations probably exist naturally but have not as yet been demonstrated.

NORMAL IODINE METABOLISM

Absorption.—Iodine and iodides can be absorbed from any portion of the alimentary tract, but most readily perhaps from the small intestine. free iodine and iodates being probably first converted to iodide. Organic iodine compounds, such as diiodotyrosine and thyroxine are in part absorbed as such and in part broken down in the stomach and intestine with the formation of iodides. Absorption can also occur from other mucous membranes and from the skin after application either in aqueous solution or in the form of ointments. Iodine is taken in through the lungs, the quantity varying considerably (0.4-20 gamma* daily), depending upon the iodine content of the atmosphere, which is greatest near the sea and lowest inland and at high altitudes.

Requirement and Sources.—As would be anticipated on the basis of the extremely small amount of iodine in the body (20 to 50 mg.), the daily requirement is very low. Balance studies indicate that equilibrium may be maintained in normal subjects by as little as 25 gamma daily. It seems best, however, to place the daily requirement for normal adults at 100 to 200 gamma, for children at 50 gamma and for infants at 20 to 40 gamma. The requirement is apparently increased during pregnancy.

Iodine is ordinarily taken into the body chiefly from foods and drinking water, a relatively small and variable amount entering in the inspired air. In the absence of iodine supplementation, the quantity present in food and water is determined chiefly by geographical location. In general, the largest amounts are found in marine plants and sea foods and in plants and animals raised in coastal areas. The iodine content of plants and water is determined chiefly by that of the soil. Potable water usually contains very small amounts (0.2 to 2.0 gamma per liter), although water from deep mineral springs may contain relatively large quantities (185 gamma per liter. As a rule, garden vegetables contain more than fruits and cereals do. The iodine content of cow's milk depends upon that of the soil and water.

Excretion.—Iodine is excreted by the kidneys, liver, intestine, skin, and lungs, and also in the milk and saliva. Under ordinary conditions it is almost entirely inorganic and may be either endogenous (mobilized from stores in the body or from destruction of thyroxin or diiodotyrosine) or exogenous (intake in food, water, and air). No thyroxine is demonstrable in the excreta (except after administration) and the question of the presence of diiodotyrosine has not been settled.

The quantity excreted under normal conditions naturally varies considerably depending upon the intake. About 40 to 80 per cent of the total is ordinarily eliminated by the kidneys, chiefly by the tubular epithelium, the daily range being about 20 to 70 gamma in adults and 20 to 35 gamma in children. It is almost entirely in the form of inorganic iodide and, perhaps, at times a small amount of diiodotyrosine, being chiefly exogenous

* 1 gamma = 0.001 mg.

and partly endogenous. The proportion excreted in the urine is greatest when the intake is lowest, and diminishes as the amount ingested increases. The urinary iodine is increased by exercise and other factors that increase metabolism, except in the event of profuse perspiration, when the amount in the sweat is greatly increased. Urinary iodine is also increased during pregnancy. After administration of iodides, the excess is eliminated chiefly in the urine, the most marked increase occurring within the first six hours, the remainder being lost in diminishing amounts during the next four days.

Iodine excreted in the *feces* is almost entirely exogenous, consisting of that which passes through the alimentary tract unabsorbed and that eliminated in the bile and by intestinal secretions. It normally varies from 2 to 11 gamma daily, constituting 3 to 27 per cent of the intake. The quantity in the feces diminishes to almost nothing (0 to 0.4 gamma) after fasting for forty-eight hours and increases markedly with a high intake or under conditions of increased intestinal motility (diarrhea). The bile contains about 9 gamma per 100 cc. in the resting state and an average of 50 gamma per 100 cc. after eating. A portion of this is reabsorbed from the intestine, constituting an enterohepatic circulation of iodine. Iodine in the *bile* is chiefly of alimentary origin but is also in part endogenous, since it does not disappear during periods of fasting. After intravenous injection of a large quantity of thyroxine, some may be excreted unchanged by the intestine. The concentration in the saliva may vary from 0 to 350 gamma per 100 cc.

The part played by the *skin* in excretion of iodine varies considerably. At high altitudes, low temperatures and low humidity, the amount eliminated by this route may be negligible, but with profuse perspiration (heat, humidity, exercise), as much as 30 per cent or, according to some, 60 per cent of the total may be excreted by the skin (0 to 68 gamma daily).

The quantity in the *expired air* varies enormously, but may be as much as 10 to 30 gamma daily. The amount present in *mother's milk* is of importance because of its obvious relation to the requirement of the new-born infant. Colostrum, on the first day, contains 8 to 40 gamma per 100 cc., and on the fifth day 2 to 3 gamma. In late lactation the concentration may fall to 1 to 2 gamma per 100 cc. This, as in the case of cow's milk, depends upon the iodine intake and may be increased by administration of iodine. It is practically all in inorganic form.

Iodine in Blood and Body Fluids.—There is no complete unanimity of opinion regarding the amount, form of combination or distribution of iodine in the blood and body fluids. It is absorbed from the intestine either into the lymph or the portal blood. In the resting state the concentration in the lymph of the thoracic duct averages about 40 gamma per 100 cc., increasing after eating to about 250 to 400 gamma (after milk). The discrepancy in values reported for the blood may be due to differences in analytic method and in geographical location (intake). It may be safe to assume that the outer limits of normal (fasting) are probably 3 to 20 gamma per 100 cc. According to some, the average normal is about 6 gamma and according to others about 12 gamma per 100 cc. It increases after ingestion of iodine, is somewhat higher in the summer than the winter (denied by some), varies with geographical situation (intake), and appears to increase slightly after the age of 50 (climacteric?). A sharp rise occurs within a few minutes after vigorous exercise, with a return to normal after about two hours of rest. An increase (16 to 40 gamma per 100 cc.) may occur at times during the latter half of pregnancy and the first day of menstruation. The greater part is in the plasma (about 60 to 70 per cent), but there is some evidence that the concentration is the same in the water of the plasma and of the red blood cells.

In the *fasting state*, a portion of the blood iodine is in inorganic form (2 to 3 gamma per 100 cc.), a small fraction is perhaps bound to lipid and the remainder (about 50 to 70 per cent) is in organic combination. There are 2.9 to 4.8 gamma per 100 cc. or more of thyroxin or a thyroxin-like substance, constituting 25 to 30 per cent of the total and 40 to 60 per cent of the organic fraction. The nature of the remainder of the organic fraction is problematical; it apparently contains no thyroglobulin and may consist entirely of diiodotyrosine. It seems clear that the circulating form of the thyroid hormone differs from the storage form (iodothyroglobubin), none of which has been demonstrated in the blood, even in thyrotoxicosis.

The **blood iodine concentration** is the resultant of several factors, among which are the intake, ease of absorption, intestinal motility and the state of renal and thyroid function. After ingestion of potassium iodide, the blood iodine concentration rises, reaching a peak in thirty to ninety minutes (depending on the dose) and returns to normal only after about forty-eight hours. After intravenous injection, the added iodine disappears from the blood more rapidly. Removal from the circulation depends chiefly on normal functioning of the thyroid gland and in part on passage of iodine into the tissues and its excretion by the kidneys and, to a lesser extent, by the liver, skin, bowel, lungs. *etc.* During the rise in blood iodine the inorganic fraction increases sharply and the organic decreases; during the subsequent decline in blood iodine the inorganic fraction falls and the organic rises, the normal concentrations and proportions being restored after about forty-eight hours. The primary decrease in the organic fraction of blood iodine is probably due to depression of thyroid function.

Oral administration of thyroglobulin, thyroid substance or thyroxin is followed in about two hours by a simultaneous and practically equal increase in both organic and inorganic fractions in the blood. This is believed to be due to the disintegration of a portion of these substances in the intestine or the liver, with the consequent entrance of both organic and inorganic iodine compounds into the blood. When thyroxin is given intravenously, the increase in blood iodine occurs only in the organic fraction, which returns to the normal level in about two hours.

The iodine content of cerebrospinal fluid is lower than that of whole blood, ranging usually from 2 to 10 gamma per 100 cc. Its nature is not known, but the thyroid hormone is probably not present in this fluid.

Iodine in Tissues and Endocrine Glands.—The total iodine content of the body, under normal conditions, is 20 to 50 mg., the major portion being distributed approximately as follows: muscles 50 per cent, thyroid 20 per cent, skin 10 per cent, skeleton 6 per cent. It is present in much higher concentration in the thyroid (10 to 40 mg. per cent) than in other tissues, the next highest concentration occurring in other endocrine glands.

Muscles.—The muscles which, by virtue of their bulk, contain the largest store of iodine in the body, have a concentration of only about 0.03 mg. per cent. The amount in all tissues diminishes when the supply is lowered, but the normal thyroid retains its capacity for preferential trapping and storing iodine, even under such circumstances. The normal adult body contains about 12 to 14 mg. of *thyroxin*.

Other Tissues.—The liver usually contains 500 to 2300 gamma of iodine, marked variation occurring during periods of absorption and excretion. It exerts its influence upon both exogenous and endogenous iodine. That entering the portal vein from the intestine in part passes through the liver into the systemic circulation and in part is excreted in the bile. Organic iodine, whether exogenous or endogenous (thyroxin, diiodotyrosine), is partly or wholly broken down in this organ.

After administration of inorganic iodine, apart from the enormous increase in the thyroid, temporary storage occurs in the liver, kidneys, skin, heart and lungs (few days). The iodine of simple organic compounds tends to be retained particularly in the skin, while after thyroxin, in addition to its selective accumulation in the thyroid and, perhaps, the anterior hypophysis and tuber cinereum, the excess iodine remains in small amounts in the liver, skin and muscles. However, except for storage in the thyroid, the tissue increment usually disappears after a few days.

Thyroid.—The normal adult thyroid gland usually contains about 2 to 28 mg. of *iodine*, the concentration varying from 0.1 to 0.55 per cent of dry weight. It is present practically entirely in the colloid, and varies with the iodine intake, geographical location, season and state of endocrine function. The effect of these factors is similar to that upon the blood iodine (p. 229). The quantity increases from birth to puberty, reaching a maximum at about twenty years and usually decreasing after fifty years of age. The higher content in maritime regions is attributed to the greater iodine content of the soil, water and air.

By far the largest part of the thyroid iodine is in organic form, the question of the presence of inorganic iodine being still unsettled. Although there is some difference of opinion in this connection, it seems probable that thyroid protein (*thyroid hormone*), iodothyroglobulin, is a composite molecule containing thyroxin and diiodotyrosine in peptide combination. About 25 to 35 per cent is in the form of thyroxin (or thyroxin-like substances) and 60 to 65 per cent as diiodotyrosine. According to some observers, there may be as much as 7 per cent inorganic iodine and perhaps a small amount in lipid combination. The thyroid may contain 0.2 to 9 mg. of thyroxin and 2 to 11 mg. of diiodotyrosine. Some believe that diiodotyrosine is a precursor of thyroxin, being converted to the latter in accordance with the requirements of the organism. Certainly, iodothyroglobulin is not a chemical entity, since its iodine content may range from practically zero to 1 per cent and the relative proportions of thyroxin and diiodotyrosine in its molecule may also vary considerably, the ratio (T:D) being lowered when the total iodine content is low. Thyroxin is probably liberated from this peptide linkage by the action of proteolytic enzymes. Whether it is the natural active thyroid principle or an intermediate stage in the formation of the latter is not known. The process of *synthesis of thyroxin* is not clearly understood. There is some evidence that it is formed from tyrosine through the intermediate stage of diiodotyrosine, the latter being itself synthesized in the organism since it does not occur in ordinary foodstuffs. Synthesis of these substances probably takes place chiefly if not entirely in the thyroid.

The remarkable affinity of the thyroid colloid for iodine is evidenced by the fact that the normal gland is surfeited with new iodine within fifteen minutes after administration of radioactive iodine.[7] The added amount is quickly incorporated in the thyroid protein molecule, being perhaps transformed progressively into diiodotyrosine and thyroxin. A portion, depending upon the storage capacity of the gland at the time, diffuses back into the blood so that little or no inorganic iodine remains in the thyroid after twenty-four to forty-eight hours. However, an "iodine-starved" gland may retain 10 to 20 per cent of a single therapeutic dose and, after repeated doses, the iodine content may increase to over 1 per cent of the dry weight.

It has been estimated that about 0.33 mg. of thyroxin is liberated into the *blood* in twenty-four hours. This secretion probably varies in response to nervous (sympathetic) and hormonal (thyrotropic) stimulation. Thus, the thyroid gland regulates iodine metabolism in two ways: (1) it fixes iodine by incorporating it within the organic molecule of iodothyroglobulin and (2) it releases portions of this molecule into the circulation in accordance with physiologic needs of the organism. By virtue of these properties it also maintains the blood iodine within normal limits (see iodine tolerance, p. 242). The regulatory action of the thyroid is also indicated by the fact that after thyroidectomy other tissues, particularly the endocrine glands, lose their capacity for storing iodine.

Other Endocrine Glands.—The relatively high concentration of iodine in the anterior lobe of the *hypophysis* is of interest because of the relation of the thyrotropic principle elaborated by this gland to the activity of thyroid function. Administration of this hormone causes hyperplasia of the thyroid gland, with increased mitosis and a decrease in colloid. These changes are accompanied by manifestations of thyrotoxicosis, an increase in blood iodine concentration and urinary iodine elimination and a decrease in the iodine content of the thyroid gland. These phenomena subside after a few days, due probably to depression of anterior pituitary thyrotropic secretion by the excessive amount of thyroid hormone in the circulation. After hypophysectomy, the blood iodine increases for about two weeks (to 50 gamma per 100 cc.) and then falls gradually to normal, with similar changes in urinary iodine, the thyroid atrophies and the iodine concentration in the colloid increases.

The concentration of iodine is considerably higher in the tuber cinereum than in the remainder of the brain, but the significance of this fact is not apparent. The iodine content of the ovary, 30 to 250 gamma per cent in adults, is lower before puberty and after the menopause. The changes in blood iodine that occur during menstruation and pregnancy (p. 229) may be dependent upon ovarian or anterior hypophyseal influences or upon both.

ABNORMAL IODINE METABOLISM[1, 2, 4, 5]

Because of the dominant rôle of the thyroid in the maintenance of normal iodine metabolism, it is natural that abnormalities in the latter should be dependent upon or associated with disturbances of thyroid function.

These may be due to processes arising primarily in the thyroid gland or resulting from extrinsic influences, the most important of which, perhaps, are abnormalities of anterior pituitary function (thyrotropic hormone) and nervous stimulation.

SIMPLE GOITER

This type of goiter, also known as colloid, endemic, sporadic colloid, nontoxic, and "iodine-want" goiter, occurs sporadically and endemically. In certain regions practically the entire population, including lower animals, is goitrous. Most of the important endemic goiter belts lie in mountain districts (Alps, Himalayas) but others do not, as in the Lombardy plains and the Great Lakes district. The lowest incidence in this country is along the Atlantic coast and the Gulf of Mexico. It is now well established that the essential cause of the condition, and the factor common to districts in which it is endemic, is a low concentration of iodine in the environment (soil, water, air).

Etiology.—Simple goiter is due to an inadequate supply of iodine to the organism. The deficiency may be absolute or relative. In the latter case, an otherwise normal intake is inadequate to meet added demands incident to such factors as pregnancy and puberty. Some believe that infection may be important in some instances, but the evidence in favor of this hypothesis is not convincing. Evidence is accumulating in support of the view that, in addition to the well-recognized "negative" factor of iodine lack in etiology of simple goiter, certain "positive" factors may be of importance. Perhaps the best studied is cyanide, which, as such or as a constituent of cabbage and related vegetables (cauliflower, Brussels sprouts), has definite goitrogenic properties. This substance acts probably by retarding tissue oxidation and thus increasing the demand for thyroid hormone. This form of goiter can be prevented by administration of iodine just as in the case of those due to absolute iodine deficiency.

Pathology and Pathogenesis.—According to Marine, the thyroid undergoes a definite cycle of morphologic changes as a result of iodine deficiency (thyroid cycle of Marine).[8] According to this hypothesis, the primary effect of iodine deficiency is hypertrophy of the gland. This is characterized chiefly by increase in the blood supply, increase in height of the lining epithelium (cuboidal to columnar) and decrease in iodine and stainable colloid. If the stimulus continues there may be infolding and plication of the lining epithelium and active mitosis (*hyperplasia*). This series of events constitutes a response to a demand for increased activity as a result of inadequate iodine supply and consequent difficulty in hormone production. One of two things may happen subsequently. If the difficulty persists, atrophy may occur (*exhaustion atrophy*). On the other hand, at any time, a decrease in iodine demand or an increase in supply results in involution. This consists in reversal of the processes of hypertrophy and hyperplasia and is characterized by enlargement of the gland, diminution in its blood supply, distention of the follicles with colloid, decrease in height of the epithelium to cuboidal or flat cuboidal form, and an increase in total iodine content, although the concentration is low. This is the stage of colloid goiter, which may again undergo hypertrophy and hyperplasia or exhaustion atrophy. In later years (early middle life), there is a distinct tendency toward nodule formation, the nodules being local areas of colloid swelling, "fetal adenomata" or cysts. Malignancy of these nodules is a rare occurrence.

Clinical Manifestations.—In endemic goiter regions the incidence increases to the age of puberty, after which it decreases in males but persists or increases in females. In such districts, there is little difference in sex incidence, but sporadic goiter is more common in females.

The thyroid enlargement is symmetrical and the gland is of uniform, rather soft consistency. Particularly in girls, the enlargement increases to the age of fourteen to eighteen years, with temporary further increase during periods of emotional stress, menstruation and pregnancy. Occasionally, exhaustion atrophy may occur during pregnancy, with manifestations of mild hypothyroidism. The enlarged gland tends to become nodular in middle life, and these nodular goiters may later become toxic (p. 247). Malignancy occurs in a very small proportion of cases. Uncomplicated simple goiter is accompanied by no symptoms other than a sense of fullness in the neck and those due to pressure if the enlargement is marked. There may be dysphagia, cough, hoarseness and aphonia (recurrent laryngeal nerve paralysis). In endemic goiter districts, after several generations of simple goiter, cretinism appears and the incidence of hypothyroidism increases in children and adults.

Iodine Metabolism.—Despite the probability that simple goiter represents a response to an absolute or relative deficiency in iodine intake, demonstrable abnormalities of iodine metabolism do not occur consistently. This is probably due to the fact that in this condition the potential metabolic defect is successfully compensated by the changes in the gland. As a rule the total *iodine content of the gland* is within normal limits, but its concentration (per cent dry weight) is usually diminished. It has been reported that the iodine content of the thyroglobulin is considerably lower than that of normal thyroglobulin, as is the relative amount present in the form of thyroxin. The *blood iodine concentration* remains within normal limits but the urinary and fecal iodine excretion may be low (in presence of absolute deficiency).

Treatment.—There is little doubt that simple goiter can be eradicated by adequate *prophylactic iodine therapy*. Several methods of administration have been proposed, including iodinization of the water supply 1:100,000,000) and, much more satisfactory, iodinization of table salt (1 part potassium iodide to 100,000 of salt). It may be preferable to give iodine in endemic goiter regions only during childhood (until puberty) and during periods of unusual stress (pregnancy), in doses of 2 to 4 mg. of potassium iodide or 1 to 2 drops of Lugol's solution weekly. This procedure has been advocated because of the occasional ill effects following the use of relatively large amounts of iodine, particularly in subjects with nodular (adenomatous) goiter.

Iodine therapy is usually of little value after simple goiter has developed and has reached the colloid stage. However, it may be administered in the dosage mentioned above, particularly to children, but not in the presence of nodular goiter. *Surgical removal* is indicated if the enlargement is disfiguring or causes pressure symptoms. Thyroid extract should be given only when manifestations of hypothyroidism develop.

HYPOTHYROIDISM (CRETINISM—MYXEDEMA)

The manifestations of hypothyroidism vary according to the age at which the condition occurs, being more severe during the period of most rapid development (infancy) than during adult life. Consequently, from a clinical standpoint, four varieties of the hypothyroid stage may be distinguished: (1) Infantile myxedema or cretinism, (2) juvenile myxedema, (3) adult myxedema (Gull's disease) and (4) hypothyroidism accompanying certain hypopituitary states (Simmonds' disease).

Adult Myxedema.—*Etiology.*—The immediate cause is athyreosis, *i.e.*, usually complete or practically complete absence of thyroid function. This may result from (*a*) primary atrophy of the thyroid, (*b*) destructive or inflammatory lesions (chronic thyroiditis) of the thyroid, or (*c*) total thyroidectomy (artificial myxedema; cachexia strumipriva).

Operative myxedema is rare in this country but has been encountered more frequently in recent years because of the performance of total thyroidectomy as a therapeutic procedure in congestive heart failure and angina pectoris and, occasionally, in diabetes mellitus and leukemia. Chronic thyroiditis or other thyroid lesions constitute unusual causes of myxedema. It also occurs occasionally as a result of, or at least at the end of the clinical course of toxic goiter. The etiology of primary atrophy of the thyroid, the most common form of spontaneous myxedema, is not known. The occurrence of a similar process in some cases of marked pituitary hypofunction, as in Simmonds' disease, suggests the possibility of a pituitary basis for this condition. However, there is no evidence to support this hypothesis. In fact, there is some evidence that the opposite is the case, that the pituitary is overactive and produces an excess of thyrotropic hormone in myxedema.

Pathology.—The morphologic changes in the *thyroid* consist essentially in disappearance of the parenchyma, removal of disintegrating and dying cells and colloid by phagocytes and replacement fibrosis. In rare instances (postinflammatory) there may be residual evidence of antecedent inflammatory processes. In uncomplicated cases the other endocrine glands show no consistent abnormalities. Prolonged thyroid therapy may cause a varying degree of atrophy of the anterior hypophysis and the latter may result in atrophy of the adrenal cortex. Occasionally there may be hyperplasia of the parathyroids and pancreatic islet cells.

The *heart* is often enlarged, due primarily to interstitial edema and fibrosis and probably also to swelling of the muscle fibers. True hypertrophy may result from complicating hypertension in older subjects. Arteriosclerosis is frequently present but the relation of myxedema to this condition is uncertain.

The *skin* is edematous and contains an excess of mucin, with associated degenerative and atrophic changes in the epidermis and hyperkeratosis of the hair follicles and ducts of the sweat glands. The skeletal muscle fibers are edematous as are many of the viscera, including the brain.

Pathological Physiology.—(*a*) METABOLIC RATE. Decrease in the metabolic rate is the most significant and consistent functional consequence of diminished production of thyroid hormone. The extreme range of variation in basal metabolic rate in patients with hypothyroidism is −5 per cent to −45 per cent, but values above −35 per cent are unusual in the presence of the classical picture of myxedema. It should be emphasized that low basal

metabolic rates due to causes other than thyroid deficiency are not accom-
pained by this clinical picture. The rate of fall in basal metabolism following removal of the thyroid is more rapid than is the rate of development of characteristic symptoms (myxedema), which appear only after
the former has dropped to from −35 to −45 (about eighty days).

(*b*) CARBOHYDRATE AND LIPID METABOLISM.—The fasting blood sugar
concentration tends to be slightly lower than normal and glucose tolerance
is somewhat increased. It is interesting that, despite the relatively insignificant effect of thyroidectomy upon the carbohydrate metabolism of
previously normal subjects, it has been found to exert a distinctly beneficial
effect upon that of certain patients with severe diabetes.

The concentration of cholesterol and other lipids in the blood is characteristically increased in hypothyroidism, the degree of hyperlipemia being
roughly proportional to the decrease in basal metabolic rate.[9] Cholesterol
values of over 400 mg. per 100 cc. have been obtained in some cases. Hypercholesterolemia is not present in all cases, but when it is, it usually disappears rapidly after thyroid administration, simultaneously with improvement
in the clinical condition.

(*c*) PROTEIN METABOLISM.—There is characteristically a decrease in
endogenous protein metabolism, with retention of protein in intercellular
fluid and to a certain extent also in the blood plasma and other body fluids,
including the cerebrospinal fluid. The low urinary excretion of nitrogen is
a reflection of the low rate of protein catabolism. Excretion of creatine is
diminished. This is apparent during childhood but not in adults, since
creatinuria is insignificant in the latter except during pregnancy. However,
the increased retention of creatine may be demonstrated by observing the
urinary excretion of this substance after ingestion of a fixed quantity (1.32 to
2.64 gm. creatine hydrate), a smaller proportion (5 to 15 per cent) being
excreted by hypothyroid than by normal subjects (20–30 per cent) (see
p. 241).[10, 15]

(*d*) IODINE METABOLISM.—The iodine content of the thyroid gland is
decreased and the blood iodine concentration tends to be low, being generally subnormal in cases of severe deficiency. As in hyperthyroidism, there is
no consistent parallelism between changes in the basal metabolic rate and
in blood iodine concentration. There is not sufficient information available
regarding the state of the organic fraction in hypothyroidism to permit
any conclusion as to the presence or absence of any close correlation between this factor and the basal metabolic rate. It is significant, however,
that *a marked fall in blood organic iodine,* to practically zero, has been
observed after thyroidectomy. Under ordinary conditions of normal iodine
intake little if any deviation from the normal can be observed in the amount
excreted, since the latter depends largely upon the supply. However, in
the fasting state there is a much more marked decrease in urinary iodine
than occurs in normal subjects. It has also been stated that after oral administration of iodine the increase in blood iodine concentration and also
in urinary excretion is greater and more prolonged than normal. These
observations suggest that the atrophic thyroid gland is unable to take up
iodine as completely as the normal gland. This is in sharp contrast to the
markedly increased affinity of the gland for added iodine in the hyperthyroid state.

(e) MISCELLANEOUS.—The osmotic pressure and viscosity of the blood plasma are increased, due probably to the increase in plasma protein concentration. There is a fall in pulse rate, pulse pressure and minute volume output of the heart, roughly in proportion to the decrease in basal metabolic rate. Urinary excretion of calcium and phosphorus is subnormal. Gastric anacidity is present in the majority of cases and may be related in some instances to the development of anemia.

Clinical Manifestations.—Women are affected more frequently than men, in the ratio of about 4 to 1, with the highest incidence between the ages of forty and fifty years. The onset is usually gradual and insidious and seldom can be related to any possible cause, except in those cases that follow thyroidectomy, toxic goiter, or thyroiditis. Occasionally the onset is apparently related to pregnancy, the menopause or an acute infection, but such relationships may be purely coincidental. As the metabolic rate falls to about —20 per cent, symptoms appear which are dependent upon the low metabolic rate per se; these consist chiefly of slight increase in weight, decreased perspiration and increased susceptibility to cold, dryness and coldness of the skin, with a sensation of chilliness even at moderate external temperatures. The specific manifestations of thyroid deficiency, especially nonpitting edema, begin to develop when the basal metabolic rate falls to below —30 per cent. This may occur after a period of years of the above phenomena. The presenting symptoms vary considerably. Among the most common are mental dulness, fatigue, slowing of speech and muscular movements, loss of memory, constipation, puffiness of the skin, especially of the face, falling hair, weight gain, pallor or menstrual disturbance.

SKIN.—There is a firm, inelastic swelling of the skin, which is dry, roughened and cold. The subcutaneous tissues are thickened but do not pit on pressure, except in some cases in the lower extremities. There is an increase in subcutaneous fat, especially above the clavicles. The nails are brittle and thick. The hair is coarse, dry, brittle, and tends to fall, especially that of the scalp, eyebrows, and face. The rate of growth of hair and nails is slowed, as is healing of the skin following injury (retarded growth). Perspiration is generally much decreased. The thickening of the skin and subcutaneous tissues of the face, thickening of the lips, broadening of the nose, often with a yellowish pallor and reddish patch over the cheeks, constitute the characteristic rather expressionless and heavy physiognomy of patients with myxedema.

ALIMENTARY TRACT.—The tongue is broad and thick and frequently smooth. The enlargement of the lips and tongue may cause difficulty in articulation. Anorexia, constipation and tympanites are common. Achlorhydria is present in the majority of cases.

CARDIOVASCULAR SYSTEM.—There is a tendency toward bradycardia and, to a lesser extent, hypotension and lowered pulse pressure. The heart is usually enlarged, due probably to edema and dilatation, the sounds are feeble and the electrocardiogram shows small P waves and QRS complexes, with low or inverted T waves. Myocardial insufficiency of mild grade may develop and, occasionally, precordial pain which, however, occurs more frequently during thyroid therapy than in untreated cases.

NEUROMUSCULAR.—Muscular weakness, and stiffness, with pain on motion or pressure, are present almost invariably. The gait is characteristically slow and heavy and may have an ataxic quality. All muscular movements are slow and tendon reflexes are sluggish.

There may be a variety of sensory disturbances, including pain, paresthesia (numbness and tingling in the extremities) and diminution in sensory perception. Deafness is a common complaint; this may be due to changes in the nervous mechanism or to myxedematous changes in the middle or internal ear. The latter may cause vertigo, which may also be of cerebellar origin.

Mental symptoms, which occur frequently, include loss of memory, inability to concentrate, drowsiness, decreased irritability and general lowering of the emotional level. Delusions and hallucinations and even true psychoses occur occasionally.

MISCELLANEOUS.—A very characteristic feature is a husky, low voice and slow, often slurred speech. The urine volume is often low, albuminuria is frequently present, but renal function is normal in uncomplicated cases. Libido is decreased and menorrhagia occurs often and amenorrhea seldom. Bleeding from other sources is not unusual (hemoptysis, epistaxis, purpura). *Anemia* of varying degree is present in the majority of cases; it is usually of the hypochromic variety, but occasionally has all of the characteristics of true pernicious anemia. The thyroid gland is small and fibrous. The characteristic laboratory findings have been reviewed in the consideration of the pathological physiology of hypothyroidism (p. 234).

Course and Prognosis.—If untreated, the condition becomes progressively more severe over a period of ten to fifteen years. Death is usually due to intercurrent infection (pneumonia, tuberculosis, *etc.*) or to cardiovascular or other complications. In uncomplicated cases there eventually develops a picture of cachexia, with extensive edema, mental and physical lethargy and finally coma. Cases of apparent spontaneous recovery have been reported but, if authentic, must be extremely rare and must be dependent upon hyperplasia of vestiges of still functioning thyroid tissue.

Diagnosis.—Diagnosis offers little difficulty in typical cases. The appearance of the patient may suggest nephritis or pernicious anemia. Low basal metabolic rates may be present in pituitary cachexia (Simmonds' disease), Addison's disease, and starvation. However, the combination of the characteristic clinical features and the very low metabolic rate are pathognomonic of myxedema. *Hypercholesterolemia* is a feature of particular diagnostic significance in infants and children, in whom it may be difficult to obtain accurate basal metabolic readings.

Juvenile Myxedema.—This is a condition of athyreosis acquired by a previously normal child prior to attainment of full growth (Means). The clinical picture is, therefore, intermediate between that of cretinism and adult myxedema, resembling the former or the latter in accordance with the age at which the thyroid insufficiency appears. It may be differentiated from cretinism by the criteria enumerated below.

Infantile Myxedema (Cretinism).—*Etiology.*—Cretinism, or infantile myxedema, is a condition of athyreosis which probably exists in utero but becomes manifest first usually in the early months of extrauterine life. There are two forms, endemic and sporadic, which some believe to be identical although they differ clinically in certain respects. The incidence of endemic cretinism is highest in endemic goiter districts and increases in proportion to the number of generations in which endemic goiter has existed. It is therefore most prevalent in old goiter regions, as in Switzerland, and represents the most advanced stage of goitrousness in an endemic goiter district (Means). The etiology of sporadic cretinism is unknown, but it is apparently not dependent upon simple goiter or hypothyroidism in the mother. It is interesting in this connection that cretinism has occurred in one of twin children, the other being normal.

Pathology and Pathological Physiology.—The pathologic features are the same as those of adult myxedema plus evidences of retarded development. The thyroid gland may or may not be enlarged in the endemic form but is not atrophic and fibrosed in the sporadic variety. Whether enlarged or not, it is functionally inadequate. The chief developmental abnormalities are hypoplasia of the brain, delayed dentition, delayed epiphyseal union and ossification, and dwarfism. Hypertrophy of the anterior hypophysis occurs frequently.

Clinical Manifestations.—The cretinous child is usually overweight at birth. Characteristic symptoms usually begin to appear at three to six months. Growth and mental development are retarded. At one to two years the manifestations are marked, the characteristic features being as follows: *dwarfism*, with a large head, open fontanelles, relatively short arms and legs; protuberant abdomen; umbilical hernia, and imbecility. The *face* is large and puffy, with a dull expression, harsh, thick, dry, pasty yellow skin, broad nose, thick lips, open mouth, and protruding tongue. The *voice* is harsh, the neck short and thick, and dentition is delayed. The *skeletal development* is arrested in the infantile stage and muscular weakness and sexual infantilism occur commonly. Other features are essentially the same as in adult myxedema except that the thyroid may be enlarged in the endemic form.

Diagnosis.—The condition should be suspected in infants overweight at birth who do not develop normally during the first year of who manifest peculiarities of appearance or behavior. A low basal metabolic rate is of great diagnostic value but is determined only with difficulty during infancy. Hypercholesterolemia may be of distinct aid in diagnosis, as is x-ray evidence of retarded skeletal development. After the characteristic clinical picture has developed there is little difficulty in diagnosis. The condition must be differentiated from mongolism and other forms of dwarfism and imbecility. It differs from all of these in that manifestations of hypothyroidism (myxedema) are lacking in all other conditions, and in that striking improvement follows thyroid therapy particularly if begun within the first few years. Cretinism may be differentiated from juvenile myxedema on the basis of the history and the stage at which mental and physical development has been arrested. In this connection the x-ray is of particular value in determining the bone age.

Treatment.—Treatment of uncomplicated myxedema consists essentially in administration of desiccated thyroid or thyroxin in proper dosage. According to the U.S.P. XI, desiccated thyroid should contain 0.17 to 0.23 per cent iodine in thyroid combination. It has been found that 1½ grains (0.1 gm.) of U.S.P. thyroid is equivalent to approximately 0.35 mg. crystalline thyroxin. The *potency of commercial thyroid preparations* varies considerably, a fact which must be kept in mind in prescribing this substance (*e.g.*, 1½ grains [0.1 gm.] U.S.P. thyroid is equivalent to 1 grain [0.65 gm.] Parke Davis thyroid and to 5 grains Burroughs and Wellcome thyroid). The following scheme has proven of value in determining the required dosage (Means): (*a*) ½ grain (0.03 gm.) U.S.P. thyroid daily should keep the basal metabolic rate of a myxedematous subject at about —20; (*b*) 1 grain (0.065 gm.) daily should keep the rate at about —10; (*c*) 1½ grains (0.1 gm.) daily should keep the rate at about —5 per cent; (*d*) 3 grains (0.2 gm.) daily should keep the rate at about standard normal.

For oral therapy, desiccated thyroid is superior to pure thyroxin because the contained hormone is assimilated more readily, thyroxin being relatively poorly soluble. In those rare cases in which intravenous therapy is required, thyroxin may be employed. One milligram causes an average increase of 2.8 per cent in the basal metabolic rate, the peak being reached in three to ten days, with a subsequent decline. It has been estimated that thyroxin is destroyed or lost at the rate of 0.2 to 0.4 mg. daily, so that the therapeutic and maintenance doses can be calculated readily on this basis. Because of untoward reactions (nausea, vomiting, palpitation, restlessness, insomnia, delirium and precordial and muscle pain) and the necessity for intravenous injection, thyroxin has no place in the routine treatment of patients with myxedema.

The success of thyroid therapy in cretinism depends largely upon how early it is instituted. Adequate treatment begun in the first few months may be followed by absolutely normal development in every respect. The extent of restoration of normal development decreases with increasing age at the institution of treatment and little or no benefit may be expected in cases untreated until seven to ten or more years of age. The dose of U.S.P. thyroid at two to four months is about $\frac{1}{10}$ grain (0.01 gm.) daily, increasing in proportion to age until about four to twelve years, at which time the requirement is approximately the same as that of adults (1 to 3 grains daily). The criteria of adequate dosage are maintenance of normal metabolic rate and normal growth.

Thyroid medication may be accompanied by certain rather characteristic *symptoms;* these include cardiac symptoms, especially palpitation and precordial pain, at times actually anginal, muscular pains, and cramps in the extremities. These untoward symptoms appear most frequently when excessive amounts are given at the beginning of treatment. If these occur, thyroid administration should be discontinued and resumed after several days in about one-half the previous dosage.

HYPERTHYROIDISM[1, 4, 5]

There are two main clinical forms of the hyperthyroid state, (*a*) *exophthalmic goiter* (Graves', Parry's or Basedow's disease; toxic goiter) and (*b*) *toxic nodular goiter* (toxic adenoma), the former being referred to at times as primary and the latter as secondary hyperthyroidism. There are two main schools of thought with respect to the pathogenesis of these conditions. According to one, there is excessive secretion of thyroid hormone in both forms of thyrotoxicosis, whether dependent fundamentally upon factors residing without or within the thyroid gland. According to the other, toxic nodular goiter (toxic adenomatous goiter) is accompanied by a state of true hyperthyroidism (excessive secretion of normal thyroid hormone); in exophthalmic goiter, however, the gland not only secretes an excess of normal hormone but also forms an abnormal substance which is presumably incompletely saturated with iodine. Although no definite statement can be made in this connection at present, the bulk of evidence is against the latter hypothesis.

EXOPHTHALMIC GOITER (TOXIC GOITER; GRAVES' DISEASE)

Etiology.—The cause of toxic goiter is not known. Its incidence and distribution do not coincide with those of simple goiter. In many cases the onset appears to be related directly to severe psychic trauma (worry, fright, mental shock, *etc.*), acute infections, puberty, menopause and pregnancy. It may occasionally follow the taking of thyroid extract for reduction purposes. The general belief is that probably these factors act merely as "trigger mechanisms" or as activating episodes rather than as fundamental causes. Experimental production of a state of hyperthyroidism resembling clinical toxic goiter has been produced by administration of anterior pituitary extract (thyrotropic hormone). However, there appears to be little conclusive evidence of hypophyseal abnormality in clinical hyperthyroidism, although some believe that this mechanism may be implicated in some instances. Others feel that adrenal and gonadal disturbances may be involved. There appears to be a family predisposition in some instances and a thymicolymphatic constitution is often present in subjects with toxic goiter.

Toxic goiter occurs at all *ages*, the highest incidence being between the ages of twenty and forty years. *Females* are affected much more frequently than males, in the proportion of approximately 4 to 1, although lower ratios have been reported in endemic goiter regions.

Pathology.—The essential morphologic feature consists in parenchymatous hypertrophy and hyperplasia of the thyroid, involving either the entire gland or limited portions. In the latter case the remainder of the thyroid usually presents the picture of either simple or adenomatous goiter (p. 247). The features characteristic of hyperplasia include a change from a cuboidal to a columnar type of epithelium, redundancy and infolding of the follicular walls, increased vacuolization, and diminution in amount of colloid, increased vascularity, and cytologic evidence of increased cellular activity. The thyroid gland is usually but not necessarily enlarged. Persistent thymus and increase in other lymphoid tissue occur in about 50 per cent of cases and hyperplasia of the adrenal cortex has been reported in some instances. In the absence of complicating factors, enlargement of the heart and spleen is seen only occasionally. Many believe that degenerative and fibrotic changes (focal and central necrosis, subacute atrophy, cirrhosis, fatty change) occur in the liver in a large proportion of cases. This is denied by others.

Pathological Physiology.—(*a*) METABOLIC LEVEL.—The metabolic rate is invariably increased in the presence of thyrotoxicosis (increased oxygen consumption). It must be realized, however, that with normal limits for basal metabolism of +15 to —15 per cent, certain individuals who fall within the lower range may have an increase of 20 to 30 per cent in their basal metabolic rate and still be within the range regarded as normal. In moderately severe hyperthyroidism the basal metabolic rate may be +30 to +60 per cent and in extreme cases more than +100. In addition to an increased basal metabolism, the thyrotoxic patient responds to muscular work and emotional excitement by an abnormally high expenditure of energy. In other words, the energy cost of work and emotion is increased.

(*b*) CARBOHYDRATE METABOLISM.—The tolerance for glucose is diminished. This is evidenced by an abnormally high and prolonged blood sugar curve following administration of glucose and by glycosuria. The fasting blood sugar level is sometimes slightly or moderately increased. Hepatic glycogen appears to be diminished in amount, due perhaps to acceleration of its mobilization from the liver. There is also evidence that galactose is absorbed from the intestine more rapidly than normally in the presence of hyperthyroidism.

(*c*) LIPID METABOLISM.—Changes in blood cholesterol are not so striking nor so constant in hyper- as in hypothyroidism (p. 235). However, there is a tendency toward a decrease in plasma cholesterol concentration in thyrotoxicosis, particularly in severe cases. The cause is unknown, but there is some evidence that it is perhaps dependent more upon abnormality of anterior pituitary than of thyroid function.

(*d*) PROTEIN METABOLISM.—As would be expected in the presence of an increased metabolic rate, protein catabolism is increased. The urinary excretion of nitrogen is abnormally high, as is that of sulfate and phosphate.

Particular interest is attached to a rather constant abnormality of creatine metabolism in thyrotoxicosis. *Spontaneous creatinuria* occurs in a large proportion of cases, and is regarded as an evidence of disturbance in the chemistry of muscular contraction that is probably related to the prominent symptom of muscular weakness. Several observers have demonstrated a rather striking decrease in creatine tolerance, *i.e.*, abnormally low retention of ingested creatine, which returns to normal after administration of iodine and after subtotal thyroidectomy.[10, 11, 12, 14]

(*e*) CALCIUM AND PHOSPHORUS METABOLISM.—In hyperthyroidism there is characteristically an increased excretion of Ca and P in the urine. This is dependent upon increased mobilization of these elements from the bones, and may result in osteoporosis.

(*f*) IODINE METABOLISM.—The iodine content of the thyroid gland is diminished, approximately in proportion to the decrease in colloid and the degree of hyperplasia. The iodine concentration falls below 0.1 per cent of the dry weight and may be as low as 0.02 per cent. The organic fraction, especially its thyroxin component, is particularly affected. This phenomenon is due to inability of the thyroid gland to store iodine under existing conditions, and not to decreased formation of thyroid hormone.

As a result of the impaired storage capacity of the gland, increased quantities of iodine enter the circulation. In the majority of cases (about 70 per cent) the *blood iodine concentration* is increased, the average values in large series of cases (12–27 gamma per 100 cc.) being about twice the normal values (6–12 gamma). Values as high as 100 gamma have been reported, but concentrations above 50 gamma are unusual. Both organic and inorganic fractions participate in this increase. According to some observers, the organic (particularly thyroxin) increases proportionately more than the inorganic, but results obtained by different methods are not in agreement on this point. In some cases of severe hyperthyroidism the blood iodine is normal or even subnormal. In some instances this may be due to previous administration of iodine. It has been suggested that in others it may be due to the fact that existence of the hyperthyroid state for long periods of time may, as a result of excessive excretion of iodine (p. 227), so deplete the reserve stores of this element that its concentration in the blood and urine falls to normal or subnormal levels. The consensus of opinion is that there is no consistent direct relationship between the blood iodine concentration and either the basal metabolic rate or the severity of the clinical manifestations of thyrotoxicosis. This relationship may be closer if the organic fraction alone is considered, but technical difficulties have prevented the accumulation of sufficient data in this connection.

The increased blood iodine is accompanied by a corresponding increase in its *excretion* by the kidneys, liver, intestine and, according to some, the skin. The daily urinary excretion may reach 40 to 950 gamma, depending upon the level in the blood and the intake. In some cases a negative balance of as much as 200 gamma daily has been demonstrated. Under such circumstances the body reserve of 20 to 50 mg. would be exhausted in a relatively short time. However, it is probable that the urinary excretion and probably also the blood iodine concentration decrease before this occurs.

The state of iodine metabolism in exophthalmic goiter may be summarized as follows: (1) increased mobilization of iodine from the thyroid gland, resulting in (2) depletion of thyroid iodine, (3) increased concentration of iodine in the blood, (4) increased excretion of iodine in the urine, feces and perspiration, and (5) negative iodine balance.[13, 16]

Iodine Tolerance Test. That the thyroid gland has not lost its ability to take up iodine, however, is indicated by the phenomena that follow administration of a comparatively large amount of iodine. The following procedure (iodine tolerance test) may be employed to illustrate these changes (Perkin, Lahey and Cattell).[13] After withdrawing a control blood sample, 6 minims of Lugol's solution (37 mg. iodine) are taken in a little milk. Blood samples are obtained for iodine determination at one-half, one and one-half, and two and one-half hours. In nonthyrotoxic subjects the blood iodine concentration rises to over 80 gamma per 100 cc. (usually over 100 gamma) at one-half hour and remains at this level or, at least, considerably above normal during the test period. In hyperthyroidism the rise in blood iodine is relatively slight, the maximum being less than 80 gamma per 100 cc.

It has also been found that intravenously injected iodine (250 gamma per Kg.) disappears from the blood more rapidly than in normal subjects (Watson). Since it has been shown that the failure of the normal blood iodine to rise to levels attained in normal subjects is not due to increased excretion, it seems logical to assume that it may be due to increased affinity of the thyroid for the added iodine.

This is also indicated by chemical and histologic changes that occur during the therapeutic administration of iodine to patients with exophthalmic goiter. The colloid-poor acini, lined by columnar epithelium thrown into folds, quickly assume a more normal appearance, with accumulation of a large amount of colloid in acini lined by flattened, inactive epithelial cells (involution changes). Simultaneously, there is a sharp increase in the concentration of iodine in the thyroid, which may reach 1 per cent of the dry weight. In the blood, the total and inorganic iodine concentrations rise but the organic iodine fraction falls. In about 90 per cent of cases this period of involution is accompanied by clinical evidences of amelioration of the thyrotoxic state.

(g) VELOCITY OF CIRCULATION.—Both the velocity of the circulation and the minute volume output of the heart are increased in thyrotoxicosis, to a degree approximately proportional to the increase in basal metabolic rate. Moreover, the degree of increase in these factors incident to the performance of muscular work is abnormally great.

Clinical Manifestations.—The onset is usually gradual (weeks or months), but it may be abrupt, occasionally within a few days after a sudden emotional shock. In some cases there are few or no significant subjective manifestations. One or more of the following are among the first prominent symptoms: thyroid enlargement, exophthalmos, tremor, palpitation, loss of weight and nervousness. Weight loss, which is a common manifestation, may be absent in some cases due to increased appetite. There may be slight fever.

GOITER.—Thyroid enlargement is usually but not invariably present. It is generally diffuse and symmetrical, but occasionally one lobe may be larger than the other. A considerable portion of the enlarged gland may be behind the sternum and not detectable by palpation (substernal goiter). This possibility must always be investigated by x-ray examination. The gland is firm in consistency and, in typical cases, a systolic thrill is palpable and a systolic murmur audible, particularly over the upper poles. Pressure symptoms may be present, but are less common than in nodular goiter; they include dysphagia, cough, stridor, hoarseness, aphonia and venous engorgement (face, neck and anterior chest wall).

EYE SIGNS.—Prominence of the eyes (exophthalmos), one of the most characteristic features of the disease, may impart a wild, staring expression of terror or apprehension. Exophthalmos may occasionally be unilateral or more marked on one side. Other eye signs include (a) lag of the eyelids behind the eyeballs on downward or upward rotation, (b) imperfect or unequal convergence, (c) failure of the forehead to wrinkle when looking upward, and (d) infrequent winking. In cases of marked exophthalmos there may be conjunctival irritation, blepharitis or corneal ulceration with pain, burning and photophobia. Horner's syndrome may occur in cases in which pressure is exerted upon the sympathetic trunk (enophthalmos, ptosis, pupillary contraction). Any one or all of these eye signs may be absent.

CIRCULATORY SYMPTOMS.—Tachycardia and palpitation are almost constantly present, the pulse having a bounding quality. The pulse pressure is characteristically increased, due to a disproportionate rise in systolic pressure. The diastolic pressure may be actually decreased. There may be precordial pain or anginal attacks. The heart frequently appears to be enlarged by physical examination, but this is usually not confirmed by x-ray examination. The heart sounds are loud and ringing, systolic murmurs being commonly and diastolic murmurs occasionally heard. Paroxysmal or persistent auricular fibrillation occurs in about 10 per cent of cases. Some believe that thyrotoxicosis may of itself cause myocardial damage and cardiac decompensation. Others maintain that the latter, occurring not infrequently in such patients, is dependent primarily upon preexisting cardiac disease (rheumatic, luetic, arteriosclerotic, *etc.*), being precipitated or exaggerated by the increased burden thrown upon the circulation during the hyperthyroid state. In some instances myocardial damage may be due to thiamine (vitamin B_1) deficiency.

NEUROMUSCULAR SYMPTOMS.—Nervousness, irritability, restlessness and exaggerated reaction to all stimuli are present in typical cases. Emotional disturbances are common and psychoses develop occasionally. The extreme hyperactivity may be accompanied or followed by asthenia and fatigability. Muscular weakness may be profound and there is often muscle atrophy of varying degree. In typical cases there is a fine tremor of the fingers, most apparent when they are separated and extended. Tremor may also be noted in the protruded tongue.

GASTRO-INTESTINAL SYMPTOMS.—The tongue is often red and smooth. This has been ascribed to vitamin B deficiency by some observers, and is frequently associated with achlorhydria. The pharyngeal lymphoid tissue, including the tonsils, is often hyperplastic. The appetite is usually increased but anorexia occurs occasionally. Achlorhydria or hypochlorhydria is common. Diarrhea occurs frequently and nausea and vomiting may occur in severe thyrotoxicosis. According to some, hepatic complications (with hyperbilirubinemia or frank jaundice) are present in a large proportion of cases.

MISCELLANEOUS SYMPTOMS.—Among the most common complaints are increased susceptibility to heat and preference for a cold environment. The skin temperature is raised and active sweating occurs with relatively slight exertion and at relatively low temperatures. The palms are often hot and moist. There is marked vasomotor lability and often distinct flushing of the face and neck. Brownish pigmentation occurs occasionally, at times approaching that seen in Addison's disease. There may be increased libido and disturbances of menstrual function, the most common being amenorrhea or oligomenorrhea.

Laboratory Findings (see also pp. 240–243).—The most important is the increase in basal metabolic rate, which is proportional to the degree of hyperthyroidism. Establishment of a consistently high or a rising rate is of much greater diagnostic value than isolated determinations. This is particularly true in borderline cases.

Increase in blood iodine, in urinary iodine and in iodine tolerance occurs in the majority of cases. The characteristic findings have been discussed elsewhere (p. 241). The general opinion at the present time is that, although of immense importance in improving our understanding of the pathological physiology of thyroid disease, they have little clinical value in diagnosis or prognosis. It has been shown repeatedly that the blood iodine concentration bears no consistent relation to the basal metabolic rate, although it has been suggested that a closer correlation is obtained when the organic iodine fraction alone is considered and logarithmic rather than actual values are employed. More extensive application of the iodine tolerance test may show it to be of greater clinical value than the blood iodine concentration.

Particular mention should be made of the *creatine tolerance test*. As has been stated (p. 241), spontaneous creatinuria and decreased creatine tolerance occur rather consistently in hyperthyroidism. The latter is evidenced by abnormally high creatine excretion after oral administration of a standard test dose (1.32 or 2.64 gm. creatine hydrate). About 70–80 per cent of this is retained (during the succeeding twenty-four hours) by normal adult subjects, whereas those with hyperthyroidism excrete 40 to 50 per cent or more in the urine.[11, 12, 14]

Fasting hyperglycemia, glycosuria and decreased glucose tolerance occur frequently. A galactose tolerance test has been proposed as an aid in differential diagnosis, based upon the premise that this sugar is absorbed from the intestine more rapidly than normally in the presence of hyperthyroidism. After the ingestion of 40 gm. of galactose, its concentration in the blood normally reaches a maximum of 20 to 30 mg. per 100 cc. after thirty to sixty minutes in the great majority of normal subjects (occasionally to 50 mg.); much higher values (40 to 100 mg. or more) are obtained in hyperthyroidism.[17]

Other laboratory findings include increased urinary excretion of calcium (p. 241) and a tendency toward a decrease in plasma cholesterol concentration. These are of little diagnostic significance. *Hyperbilirubinemia* or other manifestations of impaired liver function (bromsulfalein excretion, hippuric acid synthesis, urobilinuria) may occur in a fairly large proportion of cases. In the absence of complicating factors anemia is rare. The white blood cells are usually within normal limits, characteristically with an increase in the percentage of lymphocytes and monocytes.

Course.—The clinical course is extremely variable, with spontaneous remissions and exacerbations and a definite tendency toward self-limitation. In untreated cases spontaneous recovery has occurred after periods of several months or years. However, liability of relapse is always present in such cases. The term "burning-out" is frequently applied to spontaneous recovery from thyrotoxicosis, which is probably dependent upon either subsidence of the causative stimulus or inability of the thyroid to respond due to functional exhaustion. The latter may result in or be accompanied by a state of myxedema, which follows hyperthyroidism in occasional instances. The course of the condition may be punctuated by sudden fulminating episodes (*thyroid crises*) which occur at times following operation and constitute the chief cause of death. The cause is not known, but these episodes appear to be most effectively prevented by administration of adequate amounts of glucose and iodine. *Congestive heart failure* and *auricular fibrillation* occur rather frequently; some believe that the former practically invariably depends upon the existence of antecedent cardiac damage, aggravated by increased circulatory demands and perhaps also by relative vitamin B_1 deficiency. The requirement for thiamine is increased in hyperthyroidism in proportion to the increase in basal rate and to the increased consumption of carbohydrate.

Diagnosis.—Typical cases are recognized easily. Exophthalmos of mild degree may occur in bronchial asthma and unilateral exophthalmos in local orbital lesions (aneurysm, tumor, *etc.*). Cases of autonomic imbalance may present many features of borderline hyperthyroidism, but the basal metabolic rate is normal and the skin temperature is usually subnormal or normal. Accurate diagnosis usually depends upon careful observation and study of patients with unexplained tachycardia, diarrhea, nervousness or loss of weight. The combination of one or more of the typical symptoms, increased basal metabolic rate, low creatine tolerance, and other laboratory findings, and the rather prompt response to iodine therapy usually establish the diagnosis of toxic goiter. A low plasma cholesterol concentration may be of some diagnostic value in children, in whom metabolic rates may be difficult to obtain.

Treatment.—The patient should be placed at complete physical and mental *rest*, insofar as this is possible. Removal from all sources of irritation or worry is essential and sedatives (phenobarbital, bromides, chloral hydrate) are useful if required to secure adequate rest. The *diet* should be adequate to meet the increased demand incident to the increased metabolic rate. The increase should be largely in the form of carbohydrate, both because of its protein-sparing action and because of the desirability of maintaining an adequate store of hepatic glycogen. Glucose should be administered intravenously if necessary (thyroid crisis; postoperatively, *etc.*). The protein intake should be kept at 0.75 to 1.0 gm. per Kg. since large amounts increase metabolism unduly by virtue of its specific dynamic action. The *vitamin B intake* (particularly B_1, thiamine) should be increased. The advisability of doing so is based largely upon three premises: 1. It is well known that the requirement for thiamine is increased in the presence of heightened metabolism (Thiamine requirement (I.U.)= Calories $\times$ 0.00142 weight in kilograms). 2. The administration of a high carbohydrate diet also increases the requirement for this factor. 3. There is some evidence that there is an antagonism between thiamine and thyroxine.

Belladonna, ergot and quinine hydrobromide have been used extensively, but the necessity for medication of any sort seems questionable since the introduction of iodine therapy. With the possible exception of bed rest, this constitutes the most important aspect of the medical management of thyrotoxicosis. Iodine is usually given in the form of saturated solution of potassium iodide, 5 minims (230 mg. iodine) once daily or Lugol's solution (compound solution of iodine), 3 to 5 minims, one to three times daily. The basal metabolism usually reaches a low level after ten to fourteen days of this therapy, at which time subtotal thyroidectomy offers the best hope of permanent cure. About 4 per cent of cases fail to respond to the administration of iodine.

Occasionally iodine therapy alone may suffice to maintain the patient in a satisfactory condition through the natural course of the disease. However, although by no means entirely satisfactory, *subtotal thyroidectomy* in a completely iodinized patient constitutes the best therapeutic procedure at present. Permanent cure may thus be anticipated in about 80 per cent of cases. Some believe that iodine should be given only in preparing for operation because of the frequency of severe relapse during its continued administration. There is a difference of opinion on this point. It is generally agreed, however, that its prolonged use should be restricted to relatively mild cases.

Digitalis should be employed only in the presence of congestive heart failure. Quinidine may be useful if auricular fibrillation persists after operation. The incidence of postoperative thyroid crises or storms is relatively low in patients receiving iodine before and during operation and during convalescence. Glucose should be given intravenously before and after operation. In the event of a "thyroid crisis," the patient should be placed in an oxygen tent, the body surrounded with cold packs or ice-bags, and glucose solution and iodine given intravenously. The iodine may be added directly to the glucose solution, in the form of sodium iodide (15 grains to one liter of solution) or Lugol's solution (1 cc. to one liter of solution).

Roentgen therapy as a substitute for subtotal thyroidectomy may be employed in cases in which operation is refused or is otherwise contraindicated. Since the introduction of iodine therapy as a method of preoperative preparation, with the attendant decrease in operative risk and mortality, the employment of the x-ray as an elective therapeutic procedure has steadily declined.

TOXIC NODULAR GOITER (TOXIC ADENOMA)

This condition is essentially one of hyperthyroidism developing in patients with previously nontoxic nodular goiter. The nodules may be of two types: fetal and colloid. Their designation as adenomas may be erroneous since their neoplastic nature has not been established. The histology of colloid nodules resembles that of colloid goiter, *i.e.*, large follicles, lined by low epithelium and distended with colloid. This form develops on the basis of simple colloid goiter. In the fetal type follicles are small, the epithelium taller and the colloid scant in amount. There is considerable controversy regarding the pathogenesis of both varieties. Apparent nodules may also be cysts or areas of inflammation, calcification, or malignancy. Nodules may be single or multiple, the former showing more apparent evidence of being neoplastic and the latter being colloid in nature. Hyperthyroidism develops in 10 to 25 per cent of cases of nodular goiter, the incidence increasing in increasing age groups. Opinion is divided as to whether this form of thyrotoxicosis is essentially the same as that of exophthalmic goiter. Some believe that in this condition there is an increased production of normal thyroid hormone, whereas in exophthalmic goiter the gland liberates a toxic intermediary product not normally present in the circulation.

Clinical Features.—As a rule thyrotoxicosis develops after the age of forty years and after many years of thyroid enlargement. Sudden onset of symptoms is far less common than in exophthalmic goiter; eye signs, including exophthalmos, occur rarely, vasomotor, psychic and emotional disturbances and tachycardia are less marked, but hypertension and cardiac abnormalities are more common, due to the later age incidence. In general, the increase in basal metabolism is not so great as in the "primary" form of hyperthyroidism. The metabolic features are essentially the same, qualitatively, but are usually less pronounced. Symptoms due to pressure on adjacent structures occur more frequently, including displacement of the trachea. The thyroid is irregularly enlarged, the surface being nodular (single or multiple nodules), and pulsation, thrill and murmur are not often elicited over the gland.

Treatment.—The most important form of treatment is prophylactic, *i.e.*, the prevention and treatment of simple colloid goiter, which constitutes the basis for perhaps the majority of cases of nodular goiter. Surgical removal is the only effective form of treatment of toxic nodular goiter. In fact, many surgeons believe this is indicated in all nontoxic cases. Despite some contrary opinion, it is generally believed advisable to administer iodine preoperatively as in exophthalmic goiter. However, continued iodine therapy is not advisable if operation is not to be performed, since it is almost invariably unsuccessful. Some believe that hyperthyroidism may be induced in nontoxic nodular goiter (iod-Basedow) by administration of iodine. This is questionable.

IODINE METABOLISM IN OTHER DISEASES

Significant abnormalities of iodine metabolism occur in very few conditions other than those associated with disturbances of thyroid function. A decrease in the iodine content of the thyroid gland and increased urinary and cutaneous (perspiration) excretion have been reported in certain acute infections, the concentration in the blood being usually within normal limits. An increase in blood iodine has been found in about 40 per cent of cases of *lymphatic leukemia* and occasionally, according to some observers, also in *myeloid leukemia*. This increase is not related to the basal metabolic rate. Conflicting findings have been reported in other conditions accompanied by elevated basal metabolic rates, *viz.*, essential hypertension and congestive heart failure. Elevated blood iodine values have been observed in occasional cases of lymphosarcoma, carcinoma of the breast, stomach and kidney, and during periods of remission in pernicious anemia. It has been suggested that the increased urinary iodine in acute febrile and infectious diseases may be dependent upon increased thyroid activity. Marked increase in urinary iodine excretion has been noted during periods of excitement and after a variety of surgical procedures. In the latter, the blood iodine concentration also rises, these phenomena appearing within a few minutes and often persisting for several days, depending upon the extent of the trauma. No evidence is available as to the source of this iodine, *i.e.*, whether it has its origin in the thyroid or in the traumatized tissues. An increase in blood iodine has been reported in cases of biliary stasis and hepatic functional insufficiency.

BIBLIOGRAPHY

1. Salter, W. T., The Endocrine Function of Iodine, Harvard University Press, Cambridge, 1940.
2. Salter, W. T., Physiol. Rev., **20**: 345, 1940.
3. Cantarow, A. and Trumper, M., Clinical Biochemistry, W. B. Saunders Co., Philadelphia, Ed. 2, 1939.
4. Means, J. H., The Thyroid and Its Diseases, J. B. Lippincott Co., Philadelphia, 1937.
5. Elmer, A. W., Iodine Metabolism and Thyroid Function, Oxford University Press, London, 1938.
6. McClendon, J. F., Iodine and the Incidence of Goiter. University of Minnesota Press, Minneapolis, 1939.
7. Hertz, S., Roberts, A., Means, J. H. and Evans, R. D., Am. J. Physiol., **128**: 565, 1940.
8. Marine, D. and Williams, W. W., Arch. Int. Med., **1**: 349, 1908.
9. Hurxthal, L. M., Arch. Int. Med., **51**: 22, 1933; **52**: 86, 1933; **53**: 762, 825, 1934.
10. Thorn, G. W., Endocrinol., **20**: 628, 1936.
11. Shorr, E., Richardson, H. B. and Wolff, H. G., J. Clin. Invest., **12**: 966, 1933.
12. Sohval, A. R., King, F. H. and Reiner, M., Am. J. Med. Sci., **195**: 608, 1938.
13. Perkin, H. J., Lahey, F. H. and Cattell, R. B., N. Eng. J. Med, **214**: 45, 1936.
14. Richardson, H. B. and Shorr, E., Trans. Assoc. Amer. Phys., **50**: 156, 1935.
15. Poncher, H. G., Visscher, M. B. and Woodward, H., J.A.M.A., **102**: 1132, 1934.
16. Perkin, H. J. and Lahey, F. H., N. Eng. J. Med., **216**: 501, 1937.
17. Althausen, T. L., Am. J. Med. Sci., **199**: 342, 1940; J.A.M.A., **115**: 101, 1940.

SODIUM, CHLORIDE AND POTASSIUM METABOLISM

The metabolism of these substances is intimately related to the water balance and acid-base equilibrium of the body, which are considered in detail elsewhere (p. 270). These aspects of the subject of Na, Cl, and K metabolism (dehydration, edema, acidosis, alkalosis) will, therefore, be mentioned here only briefly, and the present discussion will be restricted chiefly to other specific and fundamental disturbances in the metabolism of these elements.

Functions in the Organism.—Na, Cl and K are concerned in at least four important fundamental physiologic processes: (1) the maintenance of normal water balance and distribution; (2) the maintenance of normal osmotic equilibrium; (3) the maintenance of normal acid-base balance (physiological neutrality); (4) the maintenance of normal muscle irritability.

The maintenance of normal hydration and osmotic pressure depends primarily upon the total base content of the body fluids. Since Na constitutes the largest fraction (142/155) of the total base of the extracellular fluids, it plays a dominant rôle in this connection (p. 278). At any given H_2CO_3 concentration, the hydrogen ion concentration of the plasma and other extracellular fluids depends upon the bicarbonate concentration $\left(H^+ = K \frac{H_2CO_3}{BHCO_3}\right)$. Since the bicarbonate content depends upon the amount of total base present in excess of anions other than H_2CO_3, and since Cl constitutes by far the largest fraction (103/155) of the total acid of the plasma, it is obvious that the maintenance of the normal pH depends largely upon the presence of normal concentrations of Cl and Na (p. 278). The importance of a proper balance between Na, K, Ca, and Mg in the maintenance of normal neuromuscular irritability and excitability is well known and has been referred to elsewhere (p. 175). It may be expressed as follows:

$$\text{Irritability } a \ \frac{[Na^+] + [K^+]}{[Ca^{++}] + [Mg^{++}] + [H^+]}$$

Potassium is the chief cation of the muscles and of most other cells (intracellular fluid), whereas Na is the chief cation of extracellular fluids of the body. Although some movement of K and water occurs from cells to plasma, particularly when excessive amounts of NaCl and water are lost from the body and in disturbances of acid-base balance, the K is usually excreted promptly in the urine. Any considerable replacement of Na by K in the extracellular fluids is accompanied by serious disturbances and is eventually fatal. Moreover, no other cation can entirely replace K in the intracellular fluid without interfering to a certain extent with the functional activity of the cell. In low concentrations K is excitatory and in higher concentrations it is inhibitory,[1] these effects being particularly important in relation to nerve synapses or myoneural junctions.[1] Under normal conditions, its effects resemble those of parasympathetic stimulation, and are usually inhibited by Ca (*e.g.*, neuromuscular excitability). The K/Na ratio is also important in this connection. K and Ca modify the most fundamental properties of protoplasm and cells, including the permeability of cell membranes, and thus they play a significant rôle in almost all "vital" processes.

Requirement, Absorption, Excretion.—As a rule, diets adequate in other respects are liberally adequate in regard to Na, Cl and K. The average American diet contains about 4 to 6 gm. Na, 6 to 9 gm. Cl and 2 to 4 gm. K daily, but normal function can be maintained by a normal organism with much smaller intakes. The requirement for K is greatest during periods of rapid growth because of its predominance in intracellular fluids. In adults, the K requirement is minimal, while a relatively high intake of Na and Cl is desirable throughout life.

These elements are readily and rapidly absorbed from the intestine after ingestion, and from subcutaneous tissues and serous cavities following parenteral administration. There is some evidence that absorption of Na and Cl from the intestine is diminished in the absence of adequate amounts of the adrenal cortical hormone.[2]

From a quantitative standpoint, Na and Cl are the most important mineral constituents of the normal extracellular fluids of the body. The electrolyte composition of these fluids is illustrated in figure 16.[3] Under conditions of normal renal and gastro-intestinal function and in the absence of excessive perspiration, about 95 per cent of the excreted Na and Cl and 90 per cent of the excreted K are eliminated in the urine, the actual quantity

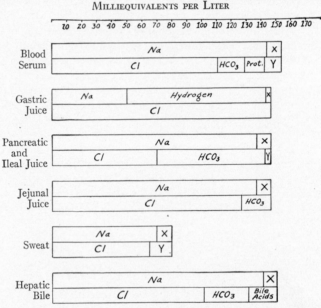

Fig. 16.—Electrolyte composition of body fluids. **X** = unnamed basic radicles. **Y** = unnamed acid radicles. (After McCance.)

depending upon the amount ingested during the preceding few days. Cl is one of the so-called "threshold substances," which, after passing through the glomeruli, are reabsorbed into the circulation in order to maintain their normal concentration in the body fluids. As the plasma NaCl concentration falls to 560 mg. per cent, the excretion of Cl in the urine diminishes, and finally ceases, except under unusual circumstances (e.g., Addison's disease, lobar pneumonia, chronic glomerulonephritis). If a normal subject is kept on an adequate NaCl intake, the sudden addition of a large quantity is usually followed by the complete elimination of the excess in forty-eight hours. However, if the previous intake has been low, the body retains the added salt with greater tenacity, and its excretion may be delayed for several days.

The Na and Cl contents of the various digestive fluids vary within wide limits (Fig. 16), while their concentration in the perspiration is probably approximately the same as in blood plasma (550 to 650 mg. per cent, as NaCl). Under normal conditions, almost all of the NaCl of the digestive fluids is reabsorbed in the intestine, but large amounts may be lost by excessive vomiting or in diarrhea (p. 264). Similarly, excessive sweating may result in the loss of considerable quantities of NaCl, the amount eliminated in the urine being usually correspondingly decreased, except under conditions of forced diuresis (p. 264). Inasmuch as Na is the chief base of extracellular fluid, deviations from the normal ratio of Na to K in the excreta are utilized as indices of variations in extra- and intracellular fluids (p. 275). Administered K salts are much less readily retained in the body than are Na salts, being eliminated in the urine much more rapidly and provoking more copious diuresis.

Intermediary Metabolism.—Potassium is the predominant base in the cells and Na predominates in the blood plasma and other extracellular fluids of the body (lymph, edema fluid, cerebrospinal fluid). The exact significance of this inequality of distribution and the mechanism whereby it is preserved are not clearly understood. It is clear, however, as stated by Peters and Van Slyke,[4] that K is prevented from diffusing out of the cells by a membrane or some other restraining factors present in the cellular and extracellular media. It also appears that the same or similar factors tend to prevent the undue passage of Na into the cells under normal physiological conditions.[4] There is evidence, however, that this "impermeability" of cells, at least to K, and perhaps also to Na, is by no means complete,[1] and it is certainly not so in a variety of abnormal conditions. Present knowledge regarding this subject may be summarized as follows[1]:

1. K is not fixed in its predominantly intracellular position, but can move about in the body rather freely, according to the demands of shifting membrane equilibria.

2. It probably moves in or out of cells when the usual state of static equilibrium is disturbed by acid-base imbalances.

3. It moves into cells when protoplasm grows and out when protoplasm disintegrates.

4. It passes from cells to extracellular fluids, including the plasma, when excessive quantities of Na and water are lost from the body, as in hemorrhage, shock, adrenocortical insufficiency, intestinal obstruction and intestinal, biliary or pancreatic fistulas.

5. It moves into the blood plasma during periods of increased muscular activity and increased metabolism, and in the opposite direction during rest or anesthesia.

6. It appears to follow the carbohydrate cycle from muscle to liver, and back again, i.e., it moves from muscle to liver with lactic acid and from liver to muscle with glucose.

7. It often rises and falls, in the plasma, with the lactic acid content, as in muscular exercise, hemorrhage and asphyxia, and also frequently with the sugar content, falling after insulin and rising, temporarily, after epinephrine.

Distribution.—Chloride is present in all cells and body fluids, and it is generally assumed that it is readily diffusible through cell membranes. However, there is some evidence that this is not true of muscle cells.[5, 6] Its concentration is slightly higher in the lymph and serous fluids than in the plasma, its concentration in these fluids varying roughly inversely as their protein content. It is present in considerably lower concentrations in the erythrocytes and muscle cells (about 50 per cent and 30 per cent of the plasma Cl content, respectively). The low Cl content of the red-blood cells and probably other cells, is attributed to (1) their relatively low water content and (2) the fact that a considerable portion of the base (chiefly K) is combined with hemoglobin and other proteins, leaving only a comparatively small balance to combine with Cl and HCO_3.[7, 8]

The distribution of K, Na, Cl and water between intracellular and extracellular fluids of the body is profoundly influenced by the adrenal cortical hormone (cortin) (p. 261). The effect of this agent in this connection can be best indicated by enumerating the changes that occur in adrenocortical insufficiency: (a) increased urinary excretion of Na, Cl and water, (b) decreased urinary excretion of K, (c) increased serum K concentration, and (d) decreased serum Na and Cl concentrations, with consequent (e) hemoconcentration and (f) renal and circulatory failure and their attendant manifestations (p. 253). These phenomena are corrected by administration of the hormone. Administration of the latter to normal subjects causes (a) retention of Na, Cl, and water, and (b) potassium diuresis.[9, 10] The mechanism of action of cortin in this connection is not known, but it is probably exerted upon cell membranes in general and not upon the kidneys alone,[11] maintaining their normal "permeability" or "impermeability" to K and Na and thus preserving the normal distribution of these electrolytes and water between the extracellular and intracellular phases.

The concentration of electrolytes in the blood serum is expressed in either milligrams per 100 cc. or milliequivalents per liter (milliequivalents per liter = milligrams per liter times the valence, divided by the atomic weight). In terms of milliequivalents per liter, the distribution of acid and base elements in the blood serum is approximately as follows:

$$\text{Total Base} = \underset{155}{\text{Na}} + \underset{142}{\text{K}} + \underset{5}{\text{Ca}} + \underset{5}{\text{Mg}} \text{ equals} \atop 3$$

$$\text{Total Acid} = \underset{155}{\text{Cl}} + \underset{103}{\text{HCO}} + \underset{28}{\text{PO}_4} + \underset{2}{\text{Protein}} + \underset{16}{\text{SO}_4 \text{ and Organic Acids}} \atop 6$$

The concentration of Na in normal blood serum ranges from 315 to 340 mg. per cent (average 330 mg.). The K concentration is 16 to 22 mg. per cent (average 19 mg.). There is little or no Na in the red corpuscles, whereas the average concentration of K in these cells is about 420 mg. per cent. The Cl content of the whole blood normally ranges from 270 to 300 mg. per cent (450 to 500 mg. per cent NaCl). The distribution of Cl between plasma and cells is similar and intimately related to that of HCO_3, in accordance with Donnan's law governing the distribution of diffusible monovalent ions. This physicochemical equilibrium plays an important part in the maintenance of the normal acid-base balance.

ADDISON'S DISEASE

Addison's disease is a condition characterized clinically by pigmentation, languor, asthenia, hypotension, gastro-intestinal and nervous system disturbances and certain characteristic disturbances of electrolyte and water metabolism.

Etiology and Pathology.—A lesion of the adrenal glands is present in the great majority of cases. Guttman,[12] in a review of 566 cases, found the following lesions, in order of frequency: (1) tuberculosis (69.72 per cent), (2) atrophy, (3) amyloid disease, (4) neoplasms, (5) vascular lesions, (6) fatty degeneration and (7) pyogenic infections. Syphilis, metastatic lesions, pressure atrophy, hypoplasia and trauma are mentioned as rare possibilities. Until recently it was generally conceded that tuberculosis accounted for 80 to 90 per cent of cases of Addison's disease and atrophy for the vast majority of the remainder. In recent years this ratio appears to be changing, atrophy accounting for 50 to 60 per cent of reported cases. The reason for this is not readily apparent and the cause of the atrophy is not known.[13] Wells[14, 15] has emphasized the increasing importance of selective cortical necrosis of the adrenals as a cause of this conditions, suggesting that it may be due to the action of chemical agents (*germanin*).

Rarely, Addison's disease is due to neoplasms (carcinoma, sarcoma, melanotic tumors), infarction, echinococcus disease and congenital malformations. Both glands are usually involved. In tuberculosis, the process appears to begin in the medulla or midcortex and to progress toward the periphery, while atrophy begins in the cortex and compresses the medulla. Experimental and clinical evidence indicates that practically all of the clinical and metabolic features depend on decreased function of the cortex alone.[16] Pigmentation may be due to medullary disturbance.

Changes have been described in other organs, none of which is consistently present. In about 30 per cent of cases due to tuberculosis, the only active tuberculous lesion is in the adrenal glands.[17] In the remainder, there is tuberculosis of the lungs, genito-urinary tract, bones, peritoneum, *etc.* The adrenals may be extensively calcified, a point of importance in diagnosis. Changes in the sympathetic ganglia and nerves have been reported (inflammation, pressure or pigmentation atrophy, fibrosis, tuberculosis). The heart is often small (brown atrophy). The intestines may be the seat of tuberculosis and congestion, and ecchymoses and lymphoid hyperplasia are seen frequently. Pigmentation of the skin and mucous membranes occurs commonly, consisting in deposition of excessive amounts of melanin in the cells of the rete Malpighii or in the corium of the skin and in similar portions of the mucous membranes.

Pathological Physiology.—The essential features of the clinical picture of Addison's disease can be produced experimentally by adrenalectomy and adrenalectomized animals can be maintained in a normal state by administration of extracts of the adrenal cortex. These extracts contain one or more hormones, collectively termed "cortin," one of the most potent of which has been identified as corticosterone.[18] Perhaps the most dramatic effects of this hormone are exerted upon Na, K and water metabolism and upon the metabolism of carbohydrate.

The following changes in salt and water metabolism occurring during periods of crisis in patients with Addison's disease and animals with acute adrenal insufficiency are due to insufficiency of adrenal cortical function (cortin)[19, 20]:

1. Increased concentration and total elimination of Na and Cl in the urine.

2. Decreased concentration of Na and Cl in the blood serum.

3. Decreased elimination of K in the urine.

4. Increased serum potassium concentration.

These changes in electrolyte balance and distribution are accompanied by evidences of loss of fluid from the plasma:

5. Decreased plasma volume (30 to 45 per cent decrease in terminal stages).

6. Increased hematocrit values and red blood cell count (30 to 40 per cent increase in terminal stages).

7. Increased plasma protein concentration (increase of 15 to 20 per cent in terminal stages).

8. Increased oxygen capacity of the blood (increase of 2 to 5 volumes per cent in terminal stages).

This decrease of circulating plasma volume results in:

9. Progressive decrease in the circulatory minute volume (blood flow), which is perhaps responsible for (10) the progressive impairment of renal function, as evidenced by the steadily rising NPN concentration of the blood (100 to 500 per cent increase in terminal stages) and (11) the final circulatory collapse, with marked fall in blood pressure.

There is also (12) a gradual diminution in oxygen consumption and (13) a lowering of body temperature in the terminal stages.

The *mechanism* of the production of these changes is not definitely known. Some believe that they are due primarily to increased urinary excretion of Na, Cl and water and retention of K. Others believe that the decreased plasma volume and hemoconcentration are due to three factors: (1) passage of extracellular fluid into the tissue cells, (2) drainage of plasma water into the extracellular fluids outside of the vascular compartment, and (3) increased excretion of urine.[21] Others believe that the most important fundamental action of the adrenal cortical hormone is in the regulation of K metabolism.[22]

Inadequate adrenal cortical function results also in significant disturbances of carbohydrate metabolism. These appear to be due largely perhaps to diminished gluconeogenesis from protein and are characterized by (*a*) a tendency toward fasting hypoglycemia, (*b*) increased sensitivity to insulin, (*c*) increased tolerance to glucose and (*d*) diminished glycogen storage in the liver.[23] These changes are considered in detail elsewhere (Chapter II).

Clinical Manifestations.—Addison's disease is not common (16 in 100,000 patients at the Mayo Clinic).[24] It occurs about twice as frequently in males as in females in cases due to tuberculosis, this ratio being reversed in cases of primary atrophy. The highest *age incidence* is between thirty and fifty years.

The onset is usually insidious, with increasing weakness and loss of weight for several weeks or months, often beginning, according to the patient, with some respiratory tract infection. Other prominent presenting symptoms include gastro-intestinal symptoms (nausea, vomiting, anorexia, constipation, diarrhea), pain (epigastric, abdominal, back), circulatory manifestations (syncope, dyspnea), and pallor and pigmentation of the skin.

Gastro-intestinal Manifestations.—These occur in about 90 per cent of cases. Anorexia is common, but at times the appetite is good. Constipation is the rule early in the disease, but may be followed later by periodic attacks of diarrhea. Nausea and vomiting occur late, usually preceded by a sensation of fulness after meals, hiccough and gaseous eructations. Epigastric or generalized abdominal pain sometimes occur. Hypochlorhydria or achlorhydria are common and the vomitus or stools may contain blood during acute attacks of vomiting and diarrhea.

Cardiovascular Manifestations.—Weakness of the heart and circulation are characteristic features of the disease. Syncope, vertigo, numbness and tingling of the hands and feet, dyspnea and palpitation on slight exertion are common. There may be anginal pain. The heart sounds are distant and of poor quality and the pulse is small, soft, and usually rapid. The systolic and diastolic blood pressures are characteristically low, with the average reading about 95/65. These are lower in the erect than in the recumbent posture. The pulse pressure is often as low as 20 mm. Hg. Normal or even slightly elevated blood pressures have been observed occasionally. During acute exacerbations (crises) the systolic blood pressure almost invariably falls to very low levels (60 to 70 mm. Hg or less), with accompanying manifestations of shock.

Pigmentation.—This is one of the most striking of the objective manifestations of Addison's disease, and is present to some degree in an overwhelming majority of cases. It may occur before any other symptoms have been noted and is often observed first by friends of the patient. The color varies, having been described as light to dark brown or even negroid, amber, tan, yellow, olive, gray or bluish, bronze, sooty, *etc.* The intensity of pigmentation varies considerably in different cases and in different areas in the same patient. The order of frequency of involvement of different areas of the skin surface is as follows: exposed surfaces (face, neck, hands, arms), flexor surfaces of joints, normally pigmented areas (nipples, axillae, genitalia), median line between pubes and umbilicus, points of pressure by clothing (belt, garters, *etc.*), areas of friction (gluteal folds), and prominences over spinous processes and knuckles, knees and elbows. The palms and soles are seldom affected, with the exception of the creases and folds. Scars may be unusually deeply pigmented. There may be small areas of intense pigmentation, resembling large freckles or moles, especially on the back of the neck, ears, hands, and feet. Areas of leukoderma or vitiligo are frequently distributed throughout pigmented regions. Discoloration of the nails has been described, and the hair may become darker. Pigmentation of mucous membranes occurs almost invariably, particularly on the lips, gums, tongue, buccal mucosa, palate, conjunctivae, and labia. The pigmentation is usually not diffuse, but occurs in streaks and spots.

The intensity of pigmentation may diminish during periods of remission, but it usually tends to increase as the disease progresses.

Mental and Nervous Manifestations.—Progressive asthenia and fatigability are among the most prominent symptoms. There is often apathy, loss of power of concentration, loss of memory, drowsiness and depression. On the other hand, there may be insomnia, restlessness, apprehension, and irritability. In advanced stages the patient may become disoriented, confused and delirious and develop hallucinations and delusions. Headache occurs commonly and dizziness, tinnitus, areas of paresthesia and anesthesia occasionally. Vision may be blurred temporarily, speech may be slurred and slow, and hearing and taste impaired. There is often pain in the abdomen, back, and extremities, which may be continuous or paroxysmal, and the abdomen

9

may become rigid. Such attacks have been mistaken for peritonitis, biliary or lead colic, perforated peptic ulcer, and tabetic crises.

Crises.—Acute relapses may occur without recognizable cause or following dietary indiscretion, intercurrent infection, or trauma of any nature, including surgical operation. Their incidence is highest with the onset of hot weather. The earliest symptoms are usually anorexia, vomiting, epigastric discomfort, increasing asthenia and lethargy or insomnia and irritability.[25] There may be severe pains in the abdomen, back or legs. The extremities are cold and the temperature is subnormal. The blood pressure falls to very low levels, urinary volume diminishes, and coma may develop within a few hours. In other cases, coma may be preceded by restlessness, muscular twitching, irregular breathing and dyspnea, mental disorientation, and irritability or depression.

Laboratory studies reveal evidence of hemoconcentration (hyperproteinemia, polycythemia, low plasma volume), renal functional impairment (increasing blood urea concentration), subnormal serum Na and Cl and elevated K concentrations. Death occurs unless adequate treatment is instituted promptly (p. 259).

Miscellaneous.—The temperature is usually subnormal, although hyperthermia has been reported, especially in terminal stages. There is usually a progressive and often a considerable loss of weight during periods of progression of the disease, although as a rule the patient does not appear emaciated. This may be due to the fact that elasticity of the skin is not lost. There are few or no urinary symptoms except during crises, when renal failure occurs, with all of its attendant manifestations. Dysmenorrhea is common, and occasionally there may be menorrhagia or amenorrhea. Atrophy of the testes has been observed, with occasional loss of libido and potentia.

Laboratory Findings.—The *urine* often contains small amounts of albumin and a few hyaline casts and the specific gravity tends to be low. If renal tuberculosis is present the urine may contain red and white blood cells in excessive numbers and also tubercle bacilli. In advanced stages of the disease and during exacerbations there is oliguria or anuria, the urine being of low specific gravity, and renal failure occurs, as evidenced by decreased phenolsulfonephthalein excretion, low urea clearance and increased concentration of nonprotein nitrogenous elements in the blood. Creatinuria has been observed.

The *fasting blood sugar concentration* tends to be low, glucose tolerance is increased and there is increased sensitivity to insulin. These findings are exaggerated during exacerbations of the disease.

There are characteristic alterations in Na, Cl and K metabolism. The urinary excretion of Na and Cl is increased and that of K diminished. This is demonstrated most readily under conditions of low NaCl and high K intakes[26] (see p. 257). Particularly during critical phases, the serum K is elevated and the concentrations of Na and Cl lowered; these latter changes are often not striking.

The *basal metabolic rate* tends to be low, values as low as — 34 per cent having been reported. This, however, is not a constant finding. Gastric hypochlorhydria or achlorhydria is present in the majority of instances. Blood and plasma volume are normal except during crises and in terminal stages, when both, particularly the plasma volume, are lowered. Under such circumstances there is an associated state of hemoconcentration, with high hematocrit, hemoglobin and red blood cell values, increased blood viscosity, increased plasma protein concentration and increased blood oxygen capacity. Anemia of more than moderate degree is not common. Leukocytosis (11,000 to 17,000) occurs occasionally and there may be a moderate lymphocytosis or mild eosinophilia. Calcific deposits in the adrenal glands may be demonstrated by the x-ray in a rather large proportion of cases due to tuberculosis, approximately 30 per cent of one large series.[27]

Diagnosis.—The diagnosis may be apparent in typical cases presenting the cardinal features, namely, asthenia, pigmentation, gastro-intestinal disturbances and hypotension. If these are not present in characteristic form, the diagnosis can rarely be established definitely without the aid of metabolic studies, except possibly in cases in which calcification of the adrenal glands can be demonstrated by x-ray. Pigmentation of the skin and mucous membranes is almost indispensable for certain diagnosis since, in its absence, the possibility of Addison's disease is rarely considered sufficiently to warrant detailed metabolic study. **Differential diagnosis** of this condition therefore resolves itself essentially into its differentiation from other causes of similar pigmentation. These include pregnancy, malaria, carcinoma, tuberculosis, hemochromatosis, arsenic poisoning, jaundice, argyria, hyperthyroidism, chronic glomerulonephritis, vagabond's disease, pernicious anemia, melanoma, scleroderma, acanthosis nigricans, ochronosis and generalized neurofibromatosis (von Recklinghausen). In the great majority of instances, differentiation from these conditions presents little or no difficulty. *Asthenia,* often profound, is of the utmost diagnostic importance, as is the rather characteristic type and distribution of the pigmentation. However, difficulty may be encountered in early cases or in normally dark-skinned subjects. Under such circumstances, one or more of the following tests may be of assistance, particularly the chloride excretion test[26] and the symptomatic response to a period of administration of a diet low in Na and Cl and high in K.

During exacerbations (crises), the sudden occurrence of such symptoms as severe abdominal pain, nausea and vomiting, may suggest some acute intra-abdominal disease, such as acute cholecystitis or appendicitis, and perforating peptic ulcer.

Skin biopsy may aid in excluding arsenic and silver poisoning, hemochromatosis, acanthosis nigricans, and scleroderma.

Salt-Free Diet.—Restriction of Na and Cl intake in patients with Addison's disease, especially if the K intake is increased simultaneously, results in exacerbation of symptoms and metabolic abnormalities (decrease in serum Na and Cl, increase in serum K, hemoconcentration, renal failure, *etc.*) which might previously have been latent. Typical manifestations of adrenal crisis may be produced in this manner. This procedure, which must obviously be employed only with great caution and with provision for prompt treatment (p. 262), may be useful as a means of diagnosis in doubtful cases.[28]

Urinary Excretion of Electrolytes.—It has been found that under standard conditions the concentration of Cl or Na in the urine is of great diagnostic significance. The test procedure is as follows[26]: A diet is administered containing 0.95 gm. of Cl ion, 0.59 gm. of Na and 4.1 gm. of K daily. Free drinking of water is encouraged during the first day, on the afternoon of which the patient is given potassium citrate in a dosage of 42 mg. per pound (33 mg. K per Kg.). On the second day the fluid intake is 40 cc. per Kg. and the dose of potassium citrate is repeated in the morning. On the third day, 20 cc. of fluid per Kg. are given before 11 A.M., the test period ending at noon of that day. Urine is collected from 8 A.M. to 12 noon of the third day for chemical examination.

It has been found that in normal subjects the *concentration of Na* in this four-hour specimen ranges from 6 to 85 mg. per cent, with a mean of about 22 mg., and the concentration of Cl from 15 to 150 mg. per cent, with a mean of about 55 mg. The corresponding values in patients with Addison's disease were 160 to 285 mg. per cent (Na) and 225 to 360 mg. per cent (Cl). Because of the ease of its determination, estimation of the chloride concentration suffices for practical purposes. Under the conditions of the test, a urinary *concentration of Cl* in excess of 225 mg. per cent may be regarded as indicative of inadequate adrenocortical function and values below 125 mg. per cent as evidence of normal function, in the absence of impaired renal function.

The significance of results obtained with this procedure is questionable in the presence of complicating conditions such as glomerulonephritis and uncontrolled diabetes. The patient must be watched carefully during the test period for evidences of acute adrenocortical insufficiency, in which case NaCl, dextrose and cortical hormone therapy must be instituted promptly (p. 262). This test procedure has proven of great value in the detection of early or latent states of adrenocortical hypofunction.

Glucose Tolerance.—Although by no means specific for adrenocortical insufficiency, increase in glucose tolerance, in conjunction with other features, may aid in diagnosis. The fasting blood sugar level may or may not be subnormal, but the increase following administration of glucose tends to be less pronounced than normal and the subsequent fall usually continues over a period of three to six hours (after ingestion of glucose), at times to levels low enough to be accompanied by manifestations of hypoglycemia. This phenomenon may be demonstrated best by the intravenous injection of 0.5 gm. of dextrose per kilogram of body weight in 20 per cent solution over a period of thirty minutes.[29]

Other Blood Studies.—Except during periods of crisis, or in terminal stages, significant abnormalities in the blood may be lacking. Serum Na, Cl and K are usually within normal limits. A potassium tolerance test has been proposed[30] as a means of diagnosis during early stages of adrenocortical insufficiency, but it has not proven satisfactory clinically.[31] In crisis, a series of changes is initiated by the development of acute severe adrenocortical insufficiency, which consists essentially of hemoconcentration and its consequences, serum Na and Cl deficit, increased serum K and manifestations of impaired renal function. These have been described in discussing the pathological physiology of Addison's disease (p. 253).

Course and Prognosis.—The natural course of the disease, until the recent introduction of specific therapy, was usually progressively downward, with acute exacerbations at irregular intervals. There may be spontaneous remissions, lasting weeks, months or years, and spontaneous recovery has apparently occurred occasionally.[32]

In a study of 566 reported cases,[12] it was found that the average duration of life in patients with Addison's disease due to tuberculosis was about thirteen months, as compared with about thirty-four months in cases due to atrophy. A large proportion of patients with tuberculosis of the adrenals have tuberculosis elsewhere (kidneys, lungs, bones, peritoneum, *etc.*), which naturally affects the course of the condition unfavorably. Untreated patients with Addison's disease are unable to withstand unusual stress and strain as well as otherwise normal subjects (infection, trauma, pregnancy, operation, *etc.*). Before the introduction of specific therapy, successful gestation in these patients was practically unheard of. It has often been observed that the duration of life is longer and severe crises are less frequent in patients in whom pigmentation is the predominating feature and gastrointestinal symptoms and asthenia are less marked.[28] Apart from those cases in which death is due to tuberculosis elsewhere than in the adrenals, intercurrent infection or some other coincidental malady, the majority of patients who succumb to this condition do so during an acute crisis of adrenocortical insufficiency. Until recently, the outlook in such cases was practically hopeless. At present, if adequate treatment can be instituted promptly the majority of patients can be carried through periods of crisis safely.

With the introduction of improved methods of treatment, the prognosis of Addison's disease has altered considerably, and in many cases not alone is life saved, but also the patient is enabled to resume his normal occupation and activities, and he can withstand surgical operations and intercurrent infections. However, these therapeutic measures have not been in use for a sufficient period of time to allow a definite statement concerning their ultimate effect upon the duration of life, which is extremely variable in untreated cases. There seems little doubt that it is greatly prolonged. Early enthusiasm regarding these measures has not been entirely justified, but this is due in large measure to inadequate treatment. There can be no doubt of the efficacy of specific treatment during periods of crisis, and it seems probable that the success of present methods of treatment should depend upon their adequacy in any given case, accuracy of diagnosis, cooperation on the part of the patient and the nature of the lesion in the adrenals. However, some patients with Addison's disease die despite energetic treatment, for reasons that are not apparent at present.

Treatment.—Treatment of Addison's disease is based upon three principles: (1) correction of the physiologic disturbances that result from adrenocortical insufficiency, the rôle of medullary insufficiency being apparently of little importance; (2) specific replacement of adrenal cortical hormones; (3) avoidance of conditions known to aggravate Addison's disease.[33]

Some patients may be maintained in satisfactory condition under ordinary circumstances by dietary regulation alone, with added NaCl and, perhaps, restriction of K. This should be attempted in all cases except when the patient is seen first in acute crisis or during a period of unusual stress (infection, trauma, pregnancy, operation, *etc.*), at which time prompt and energetic treatment is indicated (p. 262). If these measures prove inadequate, natural or synthetic hormone therapy must be resorted to, as outlined below. If *desoxycorticosterone* acetate is administered, the addition of NaCl and restriction of K are not essential, but the former materially reduces the daily hormone requirement but also increases the incidence of untoward complications (p. 262), which must be watched for carefully. It is probably best not to restrict the K intake unduly if desoxycorticosterone acetate is given, for the same reason (p. 262).

Diet.—The important principles of dietotherapy consist in providing a *high intake of Na, carbohydrate, and total calories, and a low intake of K.* Many patients with Addison's disease can be maintained in fairly good condition with no other medication than 10 to 20 gm. of NaCl daily in addition to that in their food.[33] This may be taken most readily in the form of 1 gm. tablets (preferably enteric coated), or by drinking large amounts of salt solution. Some believe that sodium citrate or bicarbonate (5 gm.) should be given in addition to sodium chloride (10 gm.), because of the frequent deficiency in bicarbonate as well as chloride in adrenocortical insufficiency. However, this is seldom necessary except, perhaps, in cases with persisting renal functional impairment. A high carbohydrate intake may be ensured by taking sugar, candy or sweetened orange juice between meals and at bedtime. These supplementary feedings tend to prevent the development of hypoglycemia, which occurs not infrequently in patients with Addison's disease three to six hours after a high carbohydrate meal.

Adrenal cortical insufficiency is accompanied by a state of not only Na deficiency but also K retention (p. 253). For this reason, and because an increase in K intake increases the requirement for Na and adrenal cortical hormone,[34] a low K intake (less than 2 gm.) is desirable, if it can be accomplished without the sacrifice of an adequate caloric intake. Such a diet may be arranged as follows[35]:

1. Limit the selection of bread, cereal and sugar to highly refined products.

2. Avoid those soups, broths, and gravies which contain meat stock or meat extracts, catsup, chili sauce, mustard, and other meat sauces and seasonings, dried fruits and vegetables, bran, molasses, Postum, and chocolate.

3. Restrict moderately the use of milk, meat, fruit, vegetables, and condiments.

4. Meat and vegetables should be cooked by a special method whereby their K content is lowered. The latter and meat should be cut into small pieces and cooked in six to eight times their bulk of water in Patapar (parchment paper) bags. By this method the K content of vegetables may be reduced 60 to 70 per cent and that of meats about 75 per cent.

Adrenal Cortical Hormones.[36, 37, 38, 39]—Commercial extracts of adrenal cortex in aqueous or saline solution are available for parenteral administration. The effectiveness of these extracts is unquestionable, but the average patient with Addison's disease requires so much extract (20 to 50 cc. daily) for maintenance that the cost of such therapy is practically prohibitive. Most of the discouraging reports regarding the efficacy of these preparations have been due largely to inadequacy of treatment. Several crystalline compounds have been isolated from these extracts, including corticosterone, dehydrocorticosterone and desoxycorticosterone. The latter has been synthesized and is available commercially (desoxycorticosterone acetate in sesame oil) at a cost far below that of natural extract.[40] It has been estimated that 1 mg. of this substance, in oil, injected intramuscularly once daily, is equivalent to approximately 3 cc. of a potent extract of adrenal cortex injected subcutaneously in divided doses.[41] It is as effective as the natural extracts in correcting the defect in Na, K and water metabolism, in maintaining life and in the treatment of crisis, but has a much less marked effect, if any, upon the abnormality in carbohydrate metabolism. Pellets of crystalline desoxycorticosterone acetate may also be implanted subcutaneously under local anesthesia.[42]

Oral Therapy.—Cortical extract in aqueous solution is destroyed in the gastro-intestinal tract. Preparations effective by oral administration have been made by adsorption upon charcoal[43] and by preservation with glycerol.[44] They have been used successfully in the treatment of patients with Addison's disease,[45] but the requirement is at least three times that of extracts administered subcutaneously. Moreover, it cannot be given orally in doses large enough for the adequate treatment of adrenal crisis. This form of therapy too is impractical at present because of the cost. Adequate absorption of desoxycorticosterone has been reported following its administration in propylene glycol sublingually,[79] the requirement being essentially the same as with subcutaneous injection. The preparation contains 10 mg. per cubic centimeter and is given in divided doses of 0.1 cc. each. This constitutes a great advance in hormone therapy.

Subcutaneous, Intramuscular and Intravenous Therapy.—Extracts of adrenal cortex are usually given subcutaneously or intramuscularly. They may be given intravenously in the treatment of crisis (p. 262), but their effect after intravenous injection is transitory. The daily requirement varies in different patients, but in the majority of cases in which hormone therapy is essential it ranges from 20 to 50 cc., given usually in two to three equally divided doses. As has been stated, the cost of such therapy is almost prohibitive.

Satisfactory results have been obtained by intramuscular injection of synthetic preparations of desoxycorticosterone acetate in oil (5 mg. per cc.).[41, 46] The daily requirement for the majority of patients is 2 to 5 mg., except during periods of unusual stress or crisis, when 10 to 25 mg. may be required. The simultaneous addition of NaCl (6 to 8 gm.) to the diet and moderate restriction of K reduces the hormone requirement but increases the incidence of manifestations of overdosage (p. 262). There should be an immediate gain in weight and clinical improvement, with retention of Na, Cl, and water, and restoration of the normal plasma volume. Failure to gain weight within forty-eight to seventy-two hours indicates insufficient dosage of the hormone, while excessive gain in weight (more than 0.5 Kg. daily during the first week or more than 0.3 Kg. daily subsequently) indicates overdosage.[46]

Implantation of Pellets of Desoxycorticosterone Acetate.—This procedure has been found to constitute an effective and economic substitute for intramuscular hormone therapy, but the pellets of crystalline desoxycorticosterone acetate are not yet available commercially.[42, 46] It is recommended that subcutaneous implantation of pellets (infrascapular region) may be considered after the patient has been maintained in good condition by intramuscular injection over a period of four to eight weeks, during which time the daily requirement is determined with a constant NaCl intake (4 to 8 gm. daily, in addition to that in the food). One pellet of about 125 mg. is implanted for each 0.4 to 0.5 mg. of material required for maintenance daily. As many as fifteen pellets have been inserted through one incision, and pellets of this size should provide effective therapy for nine to twelve months. The mean daily absorption from a pellet weighing about 100 mg. is about 0.3 mg.[42]

Complications of Desoxycorticosterone Therapy.—Manifestations of local irritation, due to the sesame oil, may occur at the site of injection. Edema and hypertension have been observed, and are almost invariably due to the simultaneous administration of excessive quantities of NaCl. Both usually respond readily to (*a*) withdrawal of added NaCl, (*b*) reduction in the dose of hormone or (*c*) the administration of K salts (10 to 20 cc. of 10 per cent solution of potassium citrate added to fruit juice two or three times daily). Evidence of circulatory embarrassment (dyspnea, pulmonary edema) may develop after prolonged therapy as a result of increase in plasma volume, blood pressure and activity, usually in patients with antecedent cardio-vascular disease. Hypoglycemia may occur during periods of prolonged fasting or three to six hours after a meal high in carbohydrate. There have been a few reports of abnormal lowering of the serum K concentration, with symptoms resembling those of familial periodic paralysis (p. 265), *viz.*, mus-cular weakness and transient paralysis of the extensor muscles of the hands, feet and neck. This may occur in patients in whom the K intake has been unduly restricted and NaCl has been given in large amounts. It responds readily to administration of potassium citrate, withdrawal of added Na and reduction in hormone dosage. Adrenal cortical atrophy has been reported following administration of both synthetic and natural hormones of adrenal cortex.

Desoxycorticosterone Therapy of Adrenal Crisis.[46]—FIRST 24 HOURS.—(1) Place the patient immediately in a warm bed and give 0.5 cc. of 1:1000 epinephrine solution subcutaneously if the systolic blood-pressure is less than 70 mm. Hg.

(2) Inject intramuscularly 25 to 35 mg. of desoxycorticosterone acetate in oil, the total quantity being divided and injected in four different sit-uations.

(3) Inject subcutaneously, in three divided doses, 25 cc. of adrenal cortical extract in aqueous or saline solution.

(4) Administer by slow venoclysis 1000 cc. of 1.5 per cent NaCl solu-tion and 1000 cc. of 5 to 10 per cent dextrose solution, to which has been added 25 cc. of aqueous cortical extract.

SECOND 12 HOURS.—(1) Slow venoclysis of 500 to 1000 cc. of physiologic NaCl solution and 500 to 1000 cc. of 5 to 10 per cent dextrose solution.

(2) If they can be tolerated, give fruit juices and ginger ale by mouth.

SECOND DAY.—(1) Inject intramuscularly 10 to 20 mg. of desoxycortic-osterone acetate in oil.

(2) Inject by slow venoclysis 1000 cc. of physiologic NaCl solution and 1000 cc. of 5 to 10 per cent dextrose solution.

(3) Frequent small feedings of sweetened fruit juice, dextrose tablets or candy should be given. If this is not feasible, maintain the blood sugar level by continuous parenteral administration of dextrose solution.

THIRD DAY.—(1) Inject intramuscularly 5 to 15 mg. of desoxycortic-osterone acetate.

(2) If possible, administer 3 to 6 gm. of NaCl (as 1 gm. enteric coated tablets) by mouth. If this is not tolerated, an equivalent amount of NaCl

should be given parenterally. If edema appears, the quantity of both NaCl and desoxycorticosterone should be reduced promptly.

Results of Treatment.[46]—Adequate treatment, as outlined above, usually results in striking clinical and metabolic improvement, with increase in weight and plasma volume and restoration of (a) normal renal functional activity, (b) normal Na and Cl balances, (c) normal plasma Na, Cl, K and NPN concentrations, and (d) elevation of the blood pressure and improved strength and sense of well-being. Intercurrent infections and surgical operations are better tolerated. The intensity of pigmentation may diminish in some cases; in others it is unchanged. Decrease in pigmentation has been observed by some following administration of ascorbic acid.[47, 48] In the majority of cases, the characteristic abnormality of carbohydrate metabolism (pp. 254, 258) is not influenced significantly by desoxycorticosterone acetate therapy, but is corrected by extracts of adrenal cortex, dehydrocorticosterone and corticosterone, in adequate dosage. However, some improvement in the oral glucose tolerance curve may occur after the use of desoxycorticosterone acetate.[49]

ACUTE ADRENOCORTICAL INSUFFICIENCY

Acute adrenal insufficiency, with manifestations similar to those of acute crisis in Addison's disease (p. 256), may occur occasionally in the absence of the latter condition. It has been observed following removal of adrenal tumors or after adrenalectomy for hypertension. This condition is probably responsible for death in newborn infants with bilateral adrenal hemorrhage, which is probably traumatic in origin in the majority of instances. The *Waterhouse-Friderichsen syndrome* is the term applied to acute adrenal insufficiency resulting from extensive adrenal hemorrhage during the course of acute infections, such as meningococcemia, diphtheria, scarlet fever, pneumonia, pemphigus and poliomyelitis.[50] The *treatment* of these types of acute adrenal insufficiency is identical with that of adrenal crisis (p. 262).

ADRENOCORTICAL HYPERFUNCTION

Inasmuch as the adrenal cortex produces a substance or substances exerting a marked effect upon electrolyte and water metabolism, it would be anticipated that clinical states of adrenocortical hyperfunction would be accompanied by changes similar to those produced by administration of these agents (p. 252). Evidence is accumulating that this is the case. Hypercorticoadrenalism[51] is evidenced clinically by one or both of two groups of manifestations included under the designations (a) adrenogenital syndrome and (b) Cushing's syndrome. The former is characterized by a tendency toward sex-reversal or precocious maturity and the latter by adiposity limited to the face, neck and trunk ("buffalo type"), hypertrichosis (females and adolescent males), arterial hypertension, kyphosis, vertebral osteoporosis, sexual dystrophy, reddish linea atrophica, erythremia, plethora, edema of the lower extremities, acrocyanosis, purpuric manifestations, hyperglycemia, and glycosuria, susceptibility to infection, and polyphagia, polydipsia, and polyuria.[52] *Cushing's syndrome* has been observed in association with basophil tumors of the pituitary, hyperplasia and adenoma of the adrenal cortex, tumor of the thymus and arrhenoblastoma of the ovary. In the case of pituitary basophilism, at least, it is probable that the syndrome is mediated by the adrenal cortex.

Detailed consideration of this subject is beyond the scope of the present discussion, which deals only with the associated abnormalities of electrolyte metabolism. From a theoretical standpoint, an excess of adrenal cortical hormone (salt and water hormone) should result in (*a*) diminished urinary excretion of Na, Cl and water, (*b*) increased urinary excretion of K, (*c*) increase in serum Na and Cl and (*d*) decrease in serum K concentration (p. 252). In a few cases of Cushing's syndrome studied from this standpoint the following findings have been obtained: decreased serum K and Cl concentrations, inconstantly increased serum Na concentration, with increase in total base, and, in advanced cases, increased plasma bicarbonate.[51, 53, 54, 55] It has also been found that subjects with this disorder have a subnormal capacity for concentrating Cl in the urine when maintained on a standard high intake of NaCl.[56] Lowering of serum K and retention of Na are in accord with present knowledge regarding the effects of cortical hormone on the distribution of these elements, but the decrease in plasma Cl and increase in bicarbonate, constituting a state of alkalosis, are difficult to explain. The latter are corrected by administration of potassium chloride or citrate but not by ammonium chloride, suggesting that disturbance in K regulation may be a factor in the mechanism underlying this abnormality. Certain of the clinical features of hypercorticoadrenalism may be dependent upon these electrolyte changes. They may contribute to the development of plethora, edema and hypertension.

In the *treatment* of this disorder, in addition to measures directed toward eradication or suppression of activity, if possible, of the underlying lesion, an attempt should be made to counteract the existing disturbance in electrolyte metabolism. This may be best accomplished by limitation of intake of Na and administration of potassium chloride (10 gm. daily) or potassium citrate (15 gm.). In some instances this has resulted in clinical improvement, with a significant fall in blood pressure.

DEHYDRATION

Among the most important clinical conditions that may be accompanied by hypochloremia and/or hyponatremia are those associated with excessive loss of various body fluids which contain large amounts of these elements. These include excessive vomiting (pyloric obstruction, intestinal obstruction, gastric irritation, uremia, "toxemia of pregnancy"), protracted diarrhea, intestinal, pancreatic or biliary fistula, excessive and prolonged diuresis (diabetes mellitus, chronic glomerulonephritis, acute hyperparathyroidism) and profuse perspiration (especially if salt-free water is ingested simultaneously). The relative degrees of Na and Cl depletion depend upon the relative amounts of these substances in the fluids lost (Fig. 16, p. 250). For example, in pyloric obstruction, if the gastric juice contains a large amount of free HCl, there may be a marked plasma Cl deficit, with comparatively little loss of Na. The excessive loss of electrolytes is accompanied by a simultaneous loss of water, with consequent dehydration (p. 289). The resulting hemoconcentration may mask the extent of plasma deficiency in these elements and their concentrations in the plasma or serum may be altered only slightly.

This subject, including the alterations in acid-base balance which accompany the loss of electrolytes from the body fluids, is considered in detail elsewhere (p. 285). However, certain therapeutic considerations may be mentioned here for the sake of emphasis. Dehydration due to the excessive loss of body fluids is almost invariably accompanied by either acidosis or alkalosis, depending up the extent to which the fixed base (chiefly Na) exceeds the sum of the concentration of acid radicles (Cl, HPO_4, SO_4, organic acids) other than bicarbonate, *i.e.*, upon the ratio of carbonic acid to bicarbonate. Clinical changes in this ratio in conditions of dehydration are in the great majority of instances secondary to alterations in Cl, and whether the ratio increases (acidosis) or decreases (alkalosis) depends largely upon whether the decrease in Cl is relatively smaller or greater than that in Na. In view of these facts, it is apparent that dehydration and excessive loss of Na and Cl should be treated by administration of NaCl solution, irrespective of the direction of the associated abnormality of acid-base balance.[57] Unless renal function is seriously impaired, the excess of Na or Cl will be eliminated in the urine and the normal electrolyte pattern restored. In the presence of impaired renal function or ketosis, glucose solution should be administered in addition to salt solution. Dehydration and NaCl depletion may be increased by administration of dextrose solutions alone and can be repaired only by salt solution (p. 346).

FAMILIAL PERIODIC PARALYSIS

This rare condition is characterized by recurrent temporary attacks of flaccid paralysis affecting chiefly the muscles of the trunk and extremities, during which the deep reflexes disappear and the muscles become inexcitable to electrical stimulation.

Etiology, Pathology, Pathological Physiology.—The cause is not known. Heredity is an important factor, since the majority of cases reported have been in family groups.[58, 59] It may be transmitted through either males or females, who may themselves be free from the disease. Some believe that many members of the family who do not have the disease may have migraine, but this is denied by others. Factors mentioned as possibly capable of precipitating an attack include exposure to cold, muscular exertion, fatigue, worry and excitement, menstruation, dietary indiscretion and lack of exercise. It has also been suggested that this condition may bear some relation to the sudden attacks of muscular weakness that occur in thyrotoxicosis (*Basedow's paraplegia*).[59]

In some cases no significant morphological lesion could be demonstrated. In others there has been reported waxy degeneration and hypertrophy and vacuolization of muscle fibers, the significance of which is doubtful. Some regard the condition as a muscular dystrophy.

Recent studies have revealed interesting metabolic abnormalities that throw some light upon the *pathogenesis* of this disorder. The most important observations have been that the serum K concentration falls during the attack and that the latter are relieved by administration of K salts.[60-64] During the paralytic phase the serum K concentration varies considerably in different cases, being usually below 14 mg. per cent and at times as low as 7.6 mg. per cent, although values as high as 17.4 mg. per cent have been observed. Weakness has been observed to begin, in one case, whenever the serum K fell below 16 mg. per cent,[46] but lower levels have been well tolerated by other subjects. Attacks may be induced by agents that cause a lowering of the serum K concentration, including dextrose, insulin, thyroid extract, epinephrine and ephedrine. The urinary K excretion may decrease markedly during an attack,[63] suggesting that the K is not lost from the body but perhaps undergoes redistribution between the plasma, tissue fluids and cells. The exact part played by this abnormality of K distribution in the production of the paralysis is not clear since, after administration of K, a considerable degree of recovery may occur before the serum K concentration is demonstrably altered. Moreover, serum K values as low as 7.6 mg. per cent have been produced in normal subjects[64] without evidence of paralysis, suggesting that some abnormality of the neuromuscular mechanism is present in familial periodic paralysis in addition to the abnormal lability of serum K. It appears that the underlying chemical defect is in the central nervous system and not in the muscles[63] and that the condition is an inborn error of metabolism.

Excessive *creatinuria* is another apparently significant metabolic abnormality observed during attacks.[63, 65] It has also been found that the serum inorganic P falls during the period of recovery after administration of K salts, suggesting the implication of some mechanism involving hexosephosphate.[64] Inconsistent elevation of the serum Ca concentration and lowering of the CO_2 combining power have been reported. Metabolic studies in intervals between attacks reveal no significant abnormality.

Clinical Manifestations.—The disease occurs about twice as frequently in males as in females. Attacks usually begin during early childhood or adolescence and tend to become less frequent in later life. However, first attacks have been reported after thirty years of age. The attacks usually come on during sleep without premonitory warning, but there may at times be prodromal symptoms such as numbness and fatigue. The paralysis is flaccid and may involve all of the voluntary muscles in extreme cases. The muscles of the face, eyes, tongue, and organs of speech and deglutition are seldom affected. Bladder and bowel functions are maintained. The deep and superficial reflexes in the affected areas are lost. Although there are no objective sensory disturbances, sensations of numbness, formication and heaviness may precede and continue throughout an attack. In severe attacks there is complete absence of reaction to faradic and galvanic stimulation, with a return to normal during intervals between attacks in the great majority of cases. There are wide variations in the distribution and severity of the paralysis. The attacks may last only one-half to one hour, but usually persist for a few hours to a few days. Motor power and reflexes usually return gradually and the patient feels perfectly well. Occasionally the paralysis develops slowly, over a period of a few hours.

Course.—As stated previously, the frequency and severity of the attacks tend to diminish after middle life. Sudden death may occur during an attack. In some instances muscular degeneration and atrophy have been observed to develop over long periods of time, with disabling muscular weakness. The introduction of potassium salts into the therapeutic management of this disorder has been too recent to allow an evaluation of its effect upon the clinical course of the disease.

Treatment.—Oral administration of potassium chloride or citrate usually results in return of ability to move in one-half to one hour and to walk in about two hours. After intravenous injection, movement may begin to return in five to ten minutes and recovery may be complete in one-half to one hour. Potassium chloride may be given orally in doses of 5 to 10 gm. in water, and intravenously in doses of 50 cc. of a 2 per cent solution (1 gm.) injected over a period of ten minutes. Potassium citrate may be given in the same or slightly larger dosage. Prompt recovery from attacks has also been observed after injection of 25 mg. of acetyl-beta-methyl-choline chloride (mecholyl) and, less consistently, after 0.5 to 1.5 mg. of prostigmine methylsulfate.[63]

MISCELLANEOUS

Decrease in serum Cl, with or without diminution in serum Na concentration, may occur in certain *acute infections*, including lobar pneumonia, rheumatic fever and meningitis. The cause is not known. Similar but less marked changes may occur in other febrile disorders, such as erysipelas, typhoid fever and pulmonary tuberculosis, and they have also been reported in pulmonary carcinoma and congestive heart failure. In *lobar pneumonia* there is a simultaneous fall in the urinary elimination of Cl and Na which, as well as the serum Cl and Na, increase abruptly at the time of crisis.[66] In the other conditions the chloride depletion appears to result from, in part at least, an ability on the part of the patient to excrete Cl readily in the urine at levels of serum Cl at which the urinary excretion of this ion normally virtually ceases.[67] In this respect these disorders resemble Addison's disease and chronic glomerulonephritis. Patients with lobar pneumonia and severe toxemia have been apparently benefited by administration of salt solution.

Severe, acute *mercury poisoning* is almost invariably accompanied by a marked fall in the serum Cl and Na concentrations. This may be due in part to vomiting, but probably cannot be explained on this basis alone in all instances. Slight and inconstant decrease in Na and Cl has been reported in acute hepatic necrosis, shock due to various causes, ether anesthesia, congestive heart failure, and following repeated withdrawal of ascitic fluid in patients with *cirrhosis of the liver* receiving a low NaCl and relatively high K intake. The practical significance of such changes in these disorders is questionable. In the case of cirrhosis, however, the occasionally marked serum Na and Cl deficit and an associated increase in serum K may contribute to a more rapid fatal termination, which may be delayed by less rigid restriction of NaCl and decreased intake of K.

An increase in serum Na and Cl is seldom observed clinically, but one or both may occur at times in the following conditions: (*a*) excessive administration of NaCl in cases of *urinary suppression, obstruction or oliguria;* (*b*) nephrotic stages of *glomerulonephritis*, especially during periods of rapidly disappearing edema; (*c*) *hypercorticoadrenalism* (basophilic adenoma of pituitary; Cushing's syndrome, or adrenal cortical tumor or hyperplasia) (p. 263); (*d*) *congestive heart failure;* (*e*) *excessive sweating*, with simultaneous restriction of fluid intake.

In addition to severe adrenal insufficiency (p. 256), elevated serum K values have been reported in some cases of *uremia, intestinal obstruction and fistula, shock* due to a variety of causes, *asphyxia* and *hemorrhage*.[68-71] Attention has been directed toward the possible rôle of adrenal insufficiency in these conditions and to the apparently beneficial effects of administration of adrenal cortical hormone and NaCl and restriction of K intake. Other observers have obtained contradictory findings.[72]

Decrease in plasma Cl has been observed in individuals *exposed to high external temperatures,* who perspire freely and drink large quantities of salt-free water.[73] The symptoms in severe cases resemble those of mild adrenal cortical insufficiency. This phenomenon appears to be the basis for the production of so-called "miners' " or "stokers' " cramp, a severe, localized muscle spasm, brought on particularly by exertion, and often preceded by weakness of the affected muscles.[74, 75, 76] This condition may be prevented or cured by administration of NaCl. Na and Cl deficit has been reported in heat stroke, but negative findings have been obtained by recent observers.[77]

It has been found that normal women gain weight and exhibit retention of Na, Cl and water during the *intermenstrual* and *premenstrual* periods. These phenomena, often accompanied by latent or mild, frank edema, may be dependent upon increased secretion of estrogenic hormone during these phases of the menstrual cycle. The onset of menstruation is associated with increased renal excretion of Na, Cl and water.[78]

Decrease in the Cl content of the body fluids occurs in *bromide intoxication,* the latter ion replacing Cl. Administration of chloride hastens the elimination of the bromide.

BIBLIOGRAPHY

1. Fenn, W. O., Physiol. Rev., **20:** 377, 1940.
2. Clark, W. G., Proc. Soc. Exper. Biol. and Med., **40:** 468, 1939.
3. Cantarow, A. and Trumper, M., Clinical Biochemistry, W. B. Saunders Co., Philadelphia, Ed. 2, 1939, p. 259.
4. Peters, J. P. and Van Slyke, D. D., Quantitative Clinical Chemistry, Williams and Wilkins Co., Baltimore, Vol. 1, 1931.
5. Cameron, A. T. and Walton, C. H. A., Trans. Roy. Soc. Canada, **22:** 1, 1928.
6. Banus, M. G. and Katz, L. N., Am. J. Physiol., **81:** 628, 644, 1927.
7. Van Slyke, D. D., Wu, H. and McLean, F. C., J. Biol. Chem., **56:** 765, 1923.
8. Warburg, E. J., Biochem. J., **16:** 153, 1922.
9. Thorn, G. W. and Harrop, G. A., Science, **86:** 40, 1937.
10. Thorn, G. W., Engel, L. L. and Eisenberg, H., J. Exper. Med., **68:** 161, 1938.
11. Cantarow, A. and Rakoff, A. E., Endocrinol., **27:** 652, 1940.
12. Guttman, P. H., Arch. Path. and Lab. Med., **10:** 742, 895, 1930.
13. Snell, A. M., Proc. Staff Meet. Mayo Clinic, **9:** 57, 1934.
14. Wells, H. G., Arch. Path., **10:** 499, 1930.
15. Wells, H. G., Humphreys, E. M. and Work, E. G., J.A.M.A., **109:** 490, 1937.
16. Brenner, O., Quart. J. Med., **22:** 121, 1928.
17. Gsell, O. and Uehlinger, E., Beitr. z. Klin. d. Tuberk., **83:** 121, 1933.
18. Mason, H. L., Endocrinol., **25:** 405, 1939.
19. Cantarow, A. and Trumper, M., ibid., p. 262.
20. Harrop, G. A., J. Exper. Med., **58:** 17, 1933.
21. Swingle, W. W., Am. J. Physiol., **119:** 557, 1937.
22. Zwemer, R. L., Endocrinol., **21:** 40, 1937.
23. Long, C. N. H., Medicine, **16:** 215, 1937.
24. Rowntree, L. G. and Snell, A. M., A Clinical Study of Addison's Disease, W. B. Saunders Co., Philadelphia, 1931.
25. Hartman, F. A., Thorn, G. W., Lockie, L. M., Greene, C. W. and Bowen, B. D., J.A.M.A., **98:** 788, 1932.
26. Cutler, H. H., Power, M. H. and Wilder, R. M., J.A.M.A., **111:** 117, 1938.
27. Ball, R. G., Greene, C. H., Camp, J. D. and Rowntree, L. G., J.A.M.A., **98:** 954, 1932.

28. Harrop, G. A., Weinstein, A., Soffer, L. J. and Trescher, J. H., J.A.M.A., **100:** 1850, 1933.
29. Thorn, G. W., J. Clin. Invest., **19:** 813, 1940.
30. Zwemer, R. L. and Truszkowski, R., Endocrinol., **21:** 40, 1937.
31. Greene, J. A., Levine, H. and Johnston, G. W., Endocrinol., **27:** 375, 1940.
32. Rowntree, L. G., Greene, C. H., Swingle, W. W. and Pfiffner, J. J., J.A.M.A., **96:** 231, 1931.
33. Loeb, R. F., J.A.M.A., **112:** 2511, 1939.
34. Wilder, R. M., Kendall, E. C., Snell, A. M., Kepler, E. J., Rynearson, E. H. and Adams, M., Arch. Int. Med., **59:** 367, 1937.
35. Rynearson, E. H., J.A.M.A., **111:** 897, 1938.
36. Greene, C. H., Arch. Int. Med., **59:** 759, 1937.
37. Grollman, A., The Adrenals, Williams and Wilkins Co., Baltimore, 1935.
38. Loeb, R. F., J.A.M.A., **104:** 299, 1935.
39. Thorn, G. W., Am. J. Med. Sci., **197:** 718, 1939.
40. Miescher, K., Fischer, W. H. and Tschopp, E., Nature, **142:** 435, 1938.
41. Thorn, G. W., Howard, R. P. and Emerson, K., Jr., J. Clin. Invest., **18:** 449, 1939.
42. Thorn, G. W., Howard, R. P., Emerson, K., Jr., and Firor, W. M., Bull. Johns Hopk. Hosp., **64:** 339, 1939.
43. Grollman, A., Firor, W. M. and Grollman, E., J. Biol. Chem., **109:** 189, 1935.
44. Hartman, F. A. and Pohle, W. D., Endocrinol., **20:** 795, 1936.
45. Thorn, G. W., Emerson, K. and Eisenberg, H., Endocrinol., **23:** 403, 1938.
46. Thorn, G. W. and Firor, W. M., J.A.M.A., **114:** 2517, 1940.
47. Szent-Gyorgyi, A. V., Am. J. Physiol., **90:** 536, 1929.
48. Szule, D., Deutsch. med. Wchnschr., **59:** 561, 1933.
49. Thorn, G. W., Koepf, G. F., Lewis, R. A. and Olsen, E. F., J. Clin. Invest., **19:** 813, 1940.
50. Aegerter, E. E., J.A.M.A., **106:** 1715, 1936.
51. McQuarrie, I., Johnson, R. M. and Ziegler, M. R., Endocrinol., **21:** 762, 1937.
52. Cushing, H., Bull. Johns Hopk. Hosp., **50:** 137, 1932.
53. Willson, D. M., Power, M. H. and Kepler, E. J., J. Clin. Invest., **19:** 701, 1940.
54. Anderson, E., Haymaker, W. and Joseph, M., Endocrinol., **23:** 398, 1938.
55. Anderson, E. and Haymaker, W., Proc. Soc. Exper. Biol. and Med., **38:** 610, 1938.
56. Cantarow, A., Science, **90:** 375, 1939.
57. Gamble, J. L., N. Eng. J. Med., **201:** 909, 1929; Bull. Johns Hopk. Hosp., **61:** 151, 1937.
58. Holtzapple, G. E., J.A.M.A., **45:** 1224, 1905.
59. Shinosaki, T., Ztschr. f. d. ges. Neur. u. Psychiat., **100:** 564, 1926.
60. Herrington, M. S., J.A.M.A., **108:** 1339, 1937.
61. Aitken, R. S., Allott, E. N., Castleden, L. I. M. and Walker, M., Clin. Sci., **3:** 47, 1937.
62. Gammon, G. D., Proc. Soc. Exper. Biol. and Med., **38:** 922, 1938.
63. Pudenz, R. H., McIntosh, J. F. and McEachern, D., J. Clin. Invest., **17:** 530, 1938; idem: J.A.M.A., **111:** 2253, 1938.
64. Allott, E. N. and McArdle, B., Clin. Sci., **3:** 229, 1938.
65. Ferrebee, J. W., Atchley, D. W. and Loeb, R. F., J. Clin. Invest., **17:** 504, 1938.
66. Sunderman, F. W., J. Clin. Invest., **7:** 313, 1929.
67. Winkler, A. W. and Crankshaw, O. F., J. Clin. Invest., **17:** 1, 1938.
68. Scudder, J. and Zwemer, R. L., Surgery, **2:** 519, 1937.
69. Scudder, J., Zwemer, R. L. and Truszkowski, R., Surgery, **1:** 74, 1937.
70. Zwemer, R. L. and Scudder, J., Surgery, **4:** 510, 1938.
71. Scudder, J., Zwemer, R. L. and Whipple, A. O., Ann. Surg., **107:** 161, 1938.
72. Bisgard, J. D., McIntyre, A. R. and Osheroff, W., Surgery, **4:** 528, 1938.
73. McCance, R. A., Lancet, **1:** 704, 1936.
74. Moss, N. K., Proc. Roy. Soc. B., **95:** 181, 1923–1924.
75. Derrick, E. H., Med. J. Australia, **2:** 612, 1934.
76. Talbott, J. H. and Michelsen, J., J. Clin. Invest., **12:** 533, 1933.
77. Ferris, E. B., Jr., Blankenhorn, M. A., Robinson, H. W. and Cullen, G. E., J. Clin. Invest., **17:** 249, 1938.
78. Thorn, G. W., Nelson, K. R. and Thorn, D. W., Endocrinol., **22:** 155, 1938.
79. Anderson, E., Haymaker, W. and Henderson, E., J.A.M.A., **115:** 2167, 1940.

CHAPTER VI

WATER BALANCE IN HEALTH AND IN DISEASE

By John P. Peters

PHYSIOLOGIC CONSIDERATIONS

In spite of our feeling of solidarity our bodies must be regarded as aggregations of solutions, divided into compartments by boundaries which, in their native state, are far less substantial than artificial preparations lead us to believe. Even our backbones shift continuously in the tides of fluid that course through and about them. Seventy per cent of the weight of the average human being is water. So dependent are all chemical reactions which occur in the body upon the presence of this universal solvent that it may be considered the greatest common divisor of life. Although it has, as the order of subjects in this book indicates, become linked with electrolyte and acid-base equilibrium, it is quite as essential for the processes of intermediary metabolism which have been discussed in earlier chapters.

The Elements of Water Metabolism.—Water metabolism is naturally divided into: (1) the exchanges of water between the organism and its environment; (2) movements of water within the organism.* Exchange with the environment in turn involves the processes of (a) absorption and (b) excretion. The water made available to the body by absorption from the gut is derived from two *sources:* preformed water and water of oxidation. The former includes not only obvious liquids which are imbibed, but also the water which is contained in apparently solid foods, which may equal or even exceed the amounts taken as beverages. Water of oxidation is the water formed in the oxidation of foods to CO_2 and H_2O. It must be recognized that water continues to be formed by this means from endogenous sources even when neither food nor fluids of any kind are taken. Water is *excreted* by four channels: the skin, the lungs, the kidneys and the bowels. The excretory function of the lungs and skin is exercised chiefly in behalf of regulation of the body temperature. Water lost in the feces may be regarded as waste incurred because of the necessity that unabsorbable residua of ingesta and intestinal secretions be diluted sufficiently to permit their convenient ejection. To the kidneys, in mammals, is entrusted the task of excreting excessive quantities of particular solutes which may accumulate in the body to excess, while retaining those which require conservation, in order to maintain in the internal environment a constant and optimal volume and chemical composition.

The Objectives of Water Metabolism.—If the purpose or effect of the exchange of water is to maintain within the body an approximately constant state that is favorable to the operation of vital activities, the subject may best be approached by an examination of the properties of the internal

* The participation of water in chemical reactions, such as hydrolysis, has an insignificant effect on its overall metabolism and is not germane to the purposes of this chapter.

environment in relation to water and its movements in this environment. The statement that the osmotic pressure of the fluids in the body varies only within narrow limits is unimpeachable; but its constant reiteration, by centering attention too much upon this single colligative property, has fostered the conception that movements of water to and from and within the body are actuated entirely by anxiety to prevent divagations of osmotic pressure. The osmotic pressure of a solution is a measure of the concentration of active chemical components in this solution; it is, therefore, an expression of the proportion of water to solutes or the degree of dilution. Consequently, the preservation of a fixed osmotic pressure is, in the broadest sense, the maintenance of a constant internal environment. However, stated in terms of osmotic pressure, it implies that the aggregate concentration of solutes in this environment is given precedence over the concentrations of all its individual components. This is not the case except in so far as the interests of a group are likely to prevail over the interests of any single member of the group. Exchanges of water within the body and between the body and its environment are determined by a great variety of equilibrium reactions, so interrelated that their combined effect is to minimize distortions of the temperature, volume, composition, and distribution of the body fluids. To avoid extreme dislocation of the system in one direction it is necessary, if one of these linked equilibria be disturbed that all the associated equilibria undergo readjustments of a compensatory nature.

FUNCTIONAL DIVISIONS OF THE BODY FLUIDS

Their Common and Individual Properties.[110]—Within the body all media, extracellular and intracellular alike, in equilibrium states, have the same osmotic pressure. This is merely an inevitable consequence of the fact that all membranes separating these fluids appear to permit water to traverse them without restraint. Local activities of one kind or another may set up temporary osmotic gradients, but these are minimized by various mechanisms and disappear rapidly when the activities which produced them cease.[111]

The body may be divided roughly into two great *compartments,* the intracellular and the extracellular. The latter in turn is subdivided into the intravascular portion, consisting of the circulating blood and lymph, and the extravascular portion, or interstitial fluid proper. The intravascular fluids, as they are propelled about the body, transport materials from one organ or tissue to another; the interstitial fluids distribute them or collect them within each organ for the ultimate consumers, the cells.* All the membranes within the body seem to permit the unobstructed passage, not only of water, but also of a certain number of organic compounds of small molecular size, of which urea and monosaccharides are outstanding examples.† At the opposite end of the scale lie proteins, lipids and other compounds of great molecular size, which are not free to cross any membranes by simple processes of diffusion. Between these two extremes fall a variety

* Such special cases as the cerebrospinal fluid and the fluids of the eye play a negligible part in gross water exchanges and will, therefore, receive no consideration.

† It cannot be inferred that molecular size is the only property which determines the ability to penetrate cellular membranes. The contrast between the universal distribution of urea and the segregation of the chloride ion defies any such simple explanation.

of materials, among which electrolytes are the most important, that can pass freely across the walls of the blood and lymph capillaries, but are obstructed by cellular membranes.[111]

General Consideration of Osmotic Equilibria.—If into two compartments, separated by a semipermeable membrane and so perfectly elastic that their contents are free from external pressure, are placed two solutions of different composition, equilibrium will be reached when the concentration of active chemical components—*i.e.*, the osmolar concentration* or osmotic pressure—in the two compartments is identical. The distribution of water between them will depend upon the relative quantities in each of the two media of those solutes which can not traverse the membrane. If the fluids in the system contain a solute to which the membrane is freely permeable, this will distribute itself uniformly throughout the water of both compartments under all circumstances, contributing always the same amount to

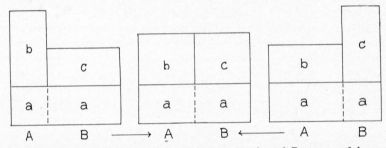

Fig. 17.—In each drawing are two compartments, A and B, separated by a membrane. In all osmolar concentrations (or osmotic pressures) are represented by vertical dimensions, volume by horizontal dimensions. *a* represents a solute to which the membrane is permeable, as indicated by the broken line; *b* and *c* are solutes which can not traverse the membrane. The central drawing represents an equilibrium state that will be attained from either of the initial conditions depicted by the drawings which flank it. Fluid is drawn in each instance to the compartment which contains in highest concentration one of the immobilized solutes, *b* and *c*, from the compartment that contains the lowest concentration, until the concentrations of *b* and *c* are the same in both compartments. The concentration of the freely diffusible solute, *a*, remains always uniform throughout both compartments and is without influence upon their volumes. Nevertheless, it does contribute to the total osmotic pressure, in every instance.

the osmotic pressure of each, but it will have no influence upon the partition of water between them. This will be determined not by the total osmotic pressure, but by the partial osmotic pressures of those solutes to which the membrane is impermeable. This relation is graphically illustrated in figure 17. It was long contended, but has been quite definitely disproved, that accumulations of urea and glucose in the blood lead to compensatory reduction of the concentrations of sodium and chloride. If they were reciprocally related, urea and sodium chloride could have no mutually compensatory effect on the distribution of water within the body, since urea enters freely cells from which sodium and chloride are excluded.

* *Osmolar concentration* connotes the concentration of osmotically active components in a solution in terms of chemical equivalents. For example 1 millimol of glucose is equal to 1 milliosmol because glucose is not dissociated; but 1 millimol of NaCl is equal to 2 milliosmols, and 1 millimol of Na_2SO_4 to 3 milliosmols, because these salts dissociate into 2 and 3 ions, respectively.

Exchanges Between Blood and Interstitial Fluid.[84, 110]—Blood plasma differs from interstitial fluids chiefly in containing more protein and lipids, substances of great molecular size that ordinarily do not traverse the capillary walls. The lipids appear to exert a negligible osmotic pressure, probably because of their slight solubility in water and because they are adsorbed upon the proteins. The proteins, however, have a definite osmotic effect. Since the capillary walls permit the passage of all other chemical components, the serum proteins would tend to draw the interstitial fluid into the vessels continuously were their force not opposed by the hydrostatic force of the blood pressure in the capillaries (see Fig. 18). In the following table

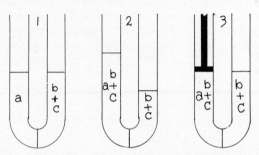

Fig. 18.—At the bottom of each U-tube, separating the two arms, is a membrane which is permeable to solutes *b* and *c*, but not to *a*. Starting from 1, with *a* entirely in the left arm, *b* and *c* in the right, water will flow from right to left until the height of the column on the left exceeds that on the right by an amount equal to the osmotic pressure exerted by *a*. At the same time *b* and *c* will distribute themselves uniformly through the water in both arms. If a piston is inserted in the left arm the fluid in the 2 arms can be brought to the same level again if the pressure on the piston equals the osmotic pressure exerted by *a*. Again *b* and *c* will distribute themselves uniformly throughout the fluid in both arms.

are listed the forces which tend to control the motions of fluid between the blood stream and the interstitial fluids about them:

Driving fluid from capillaries	*Driving fluid into capillaries*
Capillary blood pressure	Tissue tension
Interstitial fluid proteins	Blood serum proteins

Fluid moves out of the capillaries under the force of the intracapillary blood pressure (it must be clearly recognized that this is not necessarily directly related to the arterial blood pressure), assisted by the osmotic pressure of the proteins in the interstitial fluid. The latter is usually negligible in subcutaneous tissues, but may become quite appreciable if the permeability of the capillaries is increased as it may be by anoxemia, surgical shock, and certain poisons. There is, however, reason to believe that in certain parts of the circulation, the liver, and possibly the intestinal tract, the interstitial fluids regularly contain considerable concentrations of protein, either because the capillaries in these regions are unusually permeable or because the interstitial fluids in them contain preformed protein. Tending to drive fluid back into the capillaries are the osmotic pressure of the proteins of the plasma and the tension or elasticity of the tissues which offers resistance to expansion of the interstitial spaces.

The **osmotic pressure** of proteins in normal human plasma amounts to about 30 cm. of water or 22 mm. of mercury.* Because of its smaller molecular size, albumin, per unit of weight, contributes more than globulin does to the osmotic pressure. The osmotic pressure of 1 gm. of serum albumin per 100 gm. of water in human serum is estimated at about 5.2 cm. of water (3.9 mm. Hg), while that of globulin in the same concentration is about 1.9 cm. H_2O (1.4 mm. Hg).†

Both **capillary blood pressure** and tissue pressure probably vary greatly from tissue to tissue and from organ to organ. Moreover, the former is gradually dissipated as the blood passes from the arterioles to the venules, while the osmotic pressure of the proteins increases by reason of the loss of water to the tissue. At the arteriolar end of the capillaries, under average conditions, the capillary blood pressure must exceed the osmotic pressure of the plasma proteins or the very existence of the interstitial fluids would be threatened. At the venous end of the capillaries the blood pressure is probably usually so low that some fluid is drawn back into the capillaries. This creates a continuous circulation between the blood stream and the interstitial fluids which serves to stir the latter.

The impermeability of the capillaries to proteins and lipids cannot be absolute. There is probably a more or less continuous leakage, varying from place to place and from time to time. In addition there must be some provision by which these substances can be moved, upon demand, in quantities, to and from the blood stream. The nature of this provision is not known, but without its existence the movements of fats to and from their repositories and the rapid removal from the blood stream of injected homologous proteins could not be explained. It may be presumed that these movements involve cellular activities and possibly chemical transformations.

It must not be supposed that movements of solutes which can diffuse across the capillary walls are limited by the movements of water that have been described. Diffusion is determined by the concentration gradients of the individual diffusible solutes. For example, if potassium is being discharged from the cells of a given area into the interstitial fluid, it can diffuse into the arterial end of the capillary against the current of emerging fluid, to enter the blood stream where its concentration is lower. Besides maintaining the volume of fluid in the interstitial spaces by the opposing forces of capillary blood pressure and the osmotic pressure of the proteins, therefore, the blood in the capillaries distributes to and removes from the interstitial fluid by diffusion, diffusible solutes of all kinds, which follow the direction of their individual concentration gradients. By this means

* This value, like those given below for the individual protein fractions, represents the observed osmotic pressure exerted by the proteins of human serum in the osmometer. This includes, in addition to the true osmotic pressure of the proteins, a small increment contributed by the Gibbs-Donnan effect.

† About the specific osmotic pressure of the protein fractions there is much dispute which probably arises from several sources, the chief of which are: differences in methods of measurement, the heterogeneous nature of the globulin fraction, effects of albumin on the osmotic pressure of globulin, and the influence of dilution on the osmotic pressure of proteins. The figures here given are from Wies and Peters,[162] in which a brief general discussion of the subject may be found. It should be noted that they are stated in terms of gm. protein per 100 gm. of water, rather than per 100 cc. of serum. The water of serum may be estimated by the equation: Water = 98.40 − 0.718 Protein, water and protein being represented in terms of gm. per 100 cc.

waste materials find their way to the blood, while nutritive substances pass in the opposite direction.

Exchanges Between Interstitial Fluid and Lymph.[31, 84, 110]—The lymphatics offer an alternative route for the removal of fluids and solutes from the interstitial spaces. But in addition they appear to possess the specialized function of ridding the interstitial fluids of substances which, because of their magnitude or configuration, are excluded from the capillaries: proteins, dyes, lipids and particulate matter of all kinds. Having found their way into the lymph capillaries by those mysterious processes known as cellular activities, these materials are apparently unable to escape. The fluid which accumulates with them, presumably because of their osmotic pressure, is propelled along the lymph vessels by tissue tension, especially muscular activity, aided by valves, to find its way back, ultimately, to the blood stream.*

Exchanges Between Cells and Interstitial Fluid.[110, 111, 112]—*General Patterns of Intracellular and Extracellular Fluids.*—Some of the most characteristic distinctions between cellular and extracellular fluids are listed below.

Interstitial Fluid		*Intracellular Fluid*
Protein	$<$	Protein (more highly differentiated)
Na	$>$	$(Na)^1$
K	$<$	K
Ca	$>$	$(Ca)^2$
Mg	$<$	Mg
Cl	$>$	$(Cl)^3$
HCO₃	$<$	HCO₃
P (inorganic)	$(=)^4$	P (inorganic)
P (organic)	$<$	P (organic)
Creatine	$<$	Creatine
Creatinine	$(=)^5$	Creatinine
Urea	$=$	Urea
Glucose	$(=)^6$	Glucose
Amino acids	$(=)^6$	Amino acids
O		Glycogen
		Nucleotides, etc.
Enzymes, coenzymes, etc.	$<$	Enzymes, coenzymes, etc.

[1] Under ordinary circumstances most of the highly differentiated tissue cells seem to contain negligible quantities of sodium.

[2] There is some controversy about the concentrations of calcium in highly differentiated tissue cells, but the preponderance of evidence indicates that they are extremely low in the tissues that have been most intensively studied.

[3] Chloride seems to be more completely excluded than any other inorganic element from muscle and liver, but is probably a normal component of connective tissue cells and perhaps brain. It is also found of necessity in the cells of the gastric mucosa which secrete hydrochloric acid, the cells of the intestinal mucosa which form secretions containing chloride, and in the tubular cells of the kidney which reabsorb chloride. In most of these cells it may be associated with a certain amount of sodium.

[4] There appears to be considerable variability in the distribution of inorganic phosphorus, probably because it varies so greatly with cellular activities.

[5] The concentration of creatinine in cells cannot be measured with extreme accuracy because of the nonspecificity of analytical methods.

[6] Glucose and amino acids in the cells are subject to great variation by the metabolic activities of the cells. The equality sign indicates merely that there is reason to believe that they can diffuse without restraint through cellular envelopes.

Extracellular fluid, when compared with intracellular fluid, appears to have a relatively simple chemical structure. This lack of differentiation

* This is the theory of lymph formation which seems to the author[110] most compatible with known facts. Drinker has proposed a different theory for which the reader is referred to his monograph.[31]

enables it to minister to every cell in the body. Nevertheless, it could not achieve this object unless it contained all the chemical substances essential for the elaboration of cellular contents. The cells contain far more protein, potassium, magnesium, and phosphate, but much less sodium, calcium, chloride, and bicarbonate, than do extracellular fluids. They also contain glycogen and a variety or organic compounds, some of which are listed at the bottom of the table, which are entirely or almost entirely absent from serum. These are synthesized by the cells from the simpler structural materials in the fluids about them. This differentiation of composition, a property which is indispensable if there is to be functional specialization, implies highly selective permeability of the cell membranes. It is, however, equally essential that the impermeability of the cell walls be facultative, not absolute or permanent. Some means must be provided by which chemical substances, to which it usually opposes a barrier, may enter or leave the cell to meet the demands of its changing activities. An understanding of the nature of the forces by which both segregation and exchange of solutes are effected is prerequisite to the comprehension of the movements of water with which they are associated.

Osmotic Pressure of Interstitial Fluids and its Influence on Cellular Water.[110, 111]—The presence of a distinct, homogeneous body of extracellular fluid, normally comprising from one-fifth to one-fourth of the total body mass and containing most of the sodium and chloride in the body, has been established by a variety of methods. The most convincing are the total analyses of animals made by Darrow and his associates,[63] analyses of muscle tissue by Fenn, the Eggletons, and Eichelberger and Hastings,[33, 70] * and the demonstration that a variety of substances, when injected into the body, distribute themselves through approximately the same proportion of the body water. Among these substances are sucrose, sulfate, thiocyanate,[87] magnesium,[144] and bromide.[17, 142, 168] Recently more direct evidence concerning sodium has been secured by injections of the radioactive isotope of this element.[79] The exclusion of sodium and chloride from cells is not complete. Both elements are found in red blood cells; chloride, possibly with some sodium, is a constituent of connective tissue cells[94] and maybe of brain cells. In addition chloride appears in relatively high concentration in the cells of the gastric mucosa, and the concentrations of both chloride and sodium are higher in intestinal mucosa and the kidney than they are in other tissues.[95] It could hardly be otherwise, since these elements are found in variable proportions in the secretions of the gastro-intestinal tract and are reabsorbed by the cells of the renal tubules. Muscle and liver cells appear to be particularly devoid of sodium and chloride; but the former seems to be able to enter even muscle cells when these become depleted of their normal base, potassium.[75] Although the exceptions to the generalization that sodium is confined to the extracellular fluids may seem formidable, their practical effect on the exchange of water and salt in the body is relatively small.

If all cell membranes permit the free passage of water, but not of sodium and chloride, changes of the concentration of the latter in interstitial fluid must result in transfers of water to and from cells. If the concentration of

* For a further discussion of this evidence and bibliographical references the reader is referred to the previous reviews by the author.[111, 113]

sodium falls, the cells must swell; if it rises they must shrink.[111] Such changes in the water of cells entail alterations in the dilution of all cellular constituents; it need cause no surprise, then, that they are attended by disorganization of physiologic processes. The demonstration that cells swell or contract in a predictable manner in response to variations of the concentration of sodium in the serum and interstitial fluids justifies the inference that the sodium salts in these fluids may be regarded as completely dissociated into osmotically active ions.*

The State of Solutes in Cells.—Because of their large molecular size, proteins, glycogen and certain other organic compounds occupy a space which is enormous in proportion to their osmolar concentration. It is, therefore, essential, in comparing osmolar concentrations in biological media, to estimate them, not with relation to total volume of solution, as osmols per liter, but with relation to the quantity of water in this volume of solution, as osmols per kilogram of water. If the concentrations of known solutes in cells and in interstitial fluid are compared on this basis, it is impossible to strike any reasonable balance, although the existence of identical osmotic pressures requires that the total concentrations of active chemical components in the two media be identical. The difficulty is enhanced when it is recognized that none of these calculations include a complete list of the cellular constituents.† Moreover, although changes in the concentration of sodium in the interstitial fluid provoke movements of water to and from the cells, the concentrations of potassium and organic phosphate in cells can vary considerably without comparable disturbances in the distribution of water.[111, 112] This can mean only that the whole or some fractions of these substances within the cells are not osmotically active, presumably because they form undissociable compounds with proteins or other organic compounds within the cells.[145] That this should be true of the phosphate esters might have been suspected, since the intervention of certain proteins is essential to the orderly transfers of phosphate that occur in the chemical reactions of cellular intermediary metabolism. It has also been demonstrated that potassium and magnesium may be more subject than sodium to restraint or inactivation by proteins.

The Transfer of Solutes Across Cellular Membranes.—If two entirely dissimilar solutions were separated by a semipermeable membrane that allowed the free passage of water, but of none of the solutes in either solution, osmotic equilibrium, once established, could be maintained without expenditure of energy. But such extreme differentiation could not be produced *de novo* without initial expenditure of energy; nor could it be maintained without continuous expenditure of energy unless the impermeability of the membrane to the solutes in the two solutions was complete.

The problem of *cellular differentiation*, therefore, resolves itself into the pertinent question whether potassium, phosphate, etc., in interstitial fluids are in equilibrium with the same substances in cells at any or all times. That in the two media of blood potassium cannot be in equilibrium at all times

---

* This statement applies strictly only to protein free ultrafiltrates of serum.

† Rapoport and Guest[127] have recently made a new attempt to calculate the osmotic equilibrium between blood cells and serum. With the aid of certain assumptions they have succeeded in achieving a plausible balance; but some of their assumptions are distinctly open to criticism.

has long been evident, since large increments of potassium *in vitro* remain confined to the plasma so long as metabolic processes in the cells are kept in abeyance by reduction of the temperature. The same is true of the other inorganic bases, of phosphate and of sulfate.[111, 112] Furthermore, the radioactive isotope of potassium, if added to blood under the same conditions remains entirely in the plasma.[35] On the other hand, in the incubator, where cellular metabolism is accelerated, potassium and phosphate enter and leave the cells, the direction and magnitude of their movements depending upon the nature of the metabolic activities of the cells.[112] By indirect methods evidence has been adduced that in their general behavior tissue cells resemble blood cells. Although magnesium is found predominantly in cells, if its salts are injected intravenously in animals, serum magnesium increases to an extent that suggests that the exogenous magnesium remains chiefly in the extracellular fluid.[144] Phosphate and potassium, or their radioactive isotopes, if administered in the same manner, do not distribute themselves as they would if these substances were free to diffuse through all the fluids of the body, nor do they follow the pattern of distribution of the endogenous phosphate and potassium.[163, 168]

The implications of all this evidence are clear. The membrane of the resting cell appears to oppose an insuperable barrier to the passage by simple diffusion of inorganic bases and most inorganic acids, as well as a variety of other chemical substances that give the cell contents their distinctive characteristics. The inorganic substances are, however, enabled to enter and leave the cells in conjunction with certain metabolic activities of the cells. The energy evolved in the chemical reactions which constitute these activities could provide the force needed to produce and to maintain the unequal distribution of solutes between cells and extracellular fluids. Water distributes itself by simple diffusion in proportion to the amounts of osmotically active chemical components in these two media. The cells, however, can vary their load of essential materials without disturbance of their osmotic pressure, because variable proportions of potassium, phosphate, and probably other chemical units can apparently exist within the cells in an osmotically inactive state. It is possible, then, to conceive of conditions in which potassium, phosphate, or other components of cells may increase or diminish with or without proportionate deviations of the osmotic pressure of the contents of the cells and, therefore, with or without proportional variations of the cellular load of water; whereas comparable changes in the concentrations of sodium, chloride, and other constituents of the interstitial fluid to which cell membranes are impermeable, will inevitably provoke osmotic disturbances with consequent transfers of water.

In general, dislocations of the sodium balance betoken or give rise to disturbances of the water exchange; dislocations of the potassium balance are likely to originate from or to denote disorders of cellular metabolism.

THE ACID-BASE PATTERNS OF THE BODY FLUIDS

All the fluids within the body are slightly alkaline; but the divergence from neutrality is so slight that the sum of basic cations in these fluids is practically equal to the sum of acid anions. In figure 19, which represents the pattern of normal *serum*, it will be noted that sodium makes up the major part of the base, with potassium, calcium and magnesium playing relatively insignificant rôles. On the acid or anion side of the balance chloride predominates, with bicarbonate an important second. As far as *interstitial fluids* are concerned the concentrations of these three ions so far outweigh those of the other electrolytic components that they determine the osmotic exchanges between cells and interstitial fluid.*

Because the *p*H of serum is on the alkaline side of the isoelectric point of the plasma proteins, the latter act chiefly as anions. Phosphate, sulfate and organic acids together fill out the small remainder of the anion column. The acid-base balance within the cells can be set up with no such accuracy. From the nature of cellular contents it may be deduced that potassium is the most important basic cation, that organic phosphates must make up a large part of the anion column to which, because of their higher concen-

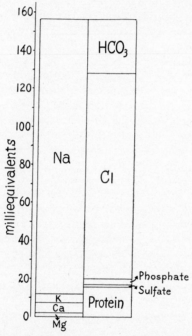

Fig. 19.–Electrolyte pattern of normal human serum.

tration in cells, proteins must also contribute far more than they do in serum. The *p*H of intracellular fluids appears to be slightly lower than that of the extracellular, but the reactions of the two fluids are related. Variations of intracellular *p*H will, therefore, be reflected in changes of the *p*H of interstitial fluid.†

Internal Mechanisms for the Maintenance of Acid-Base Equilibrium and *p*H.–(For a more adequate discussion the reader is referred to Peters

* This is the more true since a large proportion of the calcium, and fractions of magnesium and potassium appear to be undissociably united with protein.

† *p*H is the negative logarithm of the hydrogen-ion concentration–*i.e.*, $pH = \log \frac{1}{[H^+]}$. It follows that the two terms are inversely related. When acidity increases, the hydrogen-ion concentration [H^+], rises, but *p*H falls.

and Van Slyke,[124] pp. 868–1002.)—*Buffers.*—The devices by which the balance of cations and anions and the *p*H of the blood can be simultaneously preserved are inseparably connected with the mechanism for osmotic regulation which has just been described, and with the water balance. Like the latter they can be roughly divided into those which are inherent in the internal environment and those which depend upon exchanges with the exterior. The first of the internal devices is *dilution.* It is quite possible for the acid-base pattern or *p*H of the fluids in one part of the body to deviate considerably from normal without producing a detectable change in the blood of the systemic circulation, because the mixing effects of diffusion, aided by the blood stream, rapidly dissipate the disturbance by distributing it throughout the whole volume of fluid in the body. The second of the internal devices resides in the *buffers*, salts of weak acids, which mitigate changes of reaction. The chief buffers in the body are proteins, ably seconded by bicarbonates, and supported by phosphates. The mode of action of these buffers is illustrated in the following equations:

$$
\begin{array}{llll}
\textit{Strong acid} + & \textit{Buffer salt} & \rightleftarrows \textit{Neutral salt} + & \textit{Weak acid} \\
\text{HCl} & + \text{Na}_n \text{ Protein} & \rightleftarrows \quad \text{NaCl} & + \text{Na}_{(n-1)}\text{Protein} \\
\text{HCl} & + \text{NaHCO}_3 & \rightleftarrows \quad \text{NaCl} & + \text{H}_2\text{CO}_3 \\
\text{HCl} & + \text{Na}_2\text{HPO}_4 & \rightleftarrows \quad \text{NaCl} & + \text{NaH}_2\text{PO}_4
\end{array}
$$

The combination of a highly dissociated strong acid with a salt of a weak acid (the buffer) forms a neutral salt and a slightly dissociated weak acid. Since proteins occur in higher concentration in cells than in serum, the buffer defense is more intracellular than extracellular.

Carbonic acid has peculiar advantages as a buffer. It is formed by solution in water of carbon dioxide

$$\text{CO}_2 + \text{H}_2\text{O} \rightleftarrows \text{H}_2\text{CO}_3$$

which is continually produced in the normal metabolism of the tissues. At the same time it is volatile and therefore can be eliminated through the lungs. The concentration, or pressure of CO_2, which determines the concentration of H_2CO_3 in solution, depends upon the rate at which CO_2 is produced in the tissues compared with the rate at which it is discharged by the lungs. Carbonic acid reacts with salts of weaker buffer acids to form bicarbonates by reactions similar to the following:

$$
\begin{array}{l}
\text{H}_2\text{CO}_3 + \text{Na}_n \text{ Protein} \rightleftarrows \text{NaHCO}_3 + \text{Na}_{(n-1)}\text{Protein} \\
\text{H}_2\text{CO}_3 + \text{Na}_2\text{HPO}_4 \quad \rightleftarrows \text{NaHCO}_3 + \text{NaH}_2\text{PO}_4
\end{array}
$$

It is, therefore, continually competing with these other buffers for the possession of base. From the mass law for the dissociation of acids, Lawrence Henderson[74] proved that the hydrogen ion concentration of a solution containing a mixture of a buffer acid and its salt varies directly with the ratio of acid to salt in the mixture.* For carbonic acid this relation is expressed by the equation:

---

* The mass law equation for the dissociation of an acid is

$$\frac{[\text{H}^+] \times [\text{A}^-]}{[\text{HA}]} = \text{K, or } [\text{H}^+] = \text{K} \frac{[\text{HA}]}{[\text{A}^-]},$$

in which the brackets indicate molar concentrations, H^+ and A^- the dissociated cations and anions respectively, HA the undissociated fraction of the acid, and K the dissocia-

$$H^+ = K \frac{[H_2CO_3]}{[NaHCO_3]}$$

in which K is the dissociation constant of carbonic acid. Since H_2CO_3 is directly related to the pressure or concentration of CO_2 in the solution, it follows from this equation that, with a given amount of bicarbonate, the hydrogen ion concentration will vary directly (the pH inversely) as the pressure of carbon dioxide in the blood. If the production of CO_2 increases or its elimination diminishes, the blood will become more acid; if the production of CO_2 diminishes or its elimination increases, the blood will become more alkaline. The reactions of the respiratory system are so attuned that they tend automatically to prevent deviations of the blood pH. When the pH falls, pulmonary ventilation increases and CO_2 is driven off; when it rises, ventilation diminishes and CO_2 is retained.

The quantity of bicarbonate in the body fluids depends upon the base available for formation of bicarbonate, that is, the base not combined with acids stronger than carbonic. This corresponds, in figure 19, to the base already combined with bicarbonate and a large part of that combined with proteins and phosphates. It can evidently be altered by a change of either the total base of the serum or the acids stronger than carbonic. Since it constitutes the denominator of the Henderson equation, the *concentration of bicarbonate* is inversely related to the hydrogen ion concentration. If bicarbonate increases, therefore, the hydrogen ion concentration will fall (pH will rise) unless the carbonic acid concentration (the pressure of CO_2) rises accordingly. If the total base rises because of ingestion of sodium bicarbonate or other alkaline salts,* or if extra base is made available for combination with bicarbonate by loss of chloride in acid vomitus, bicarbonate in the serum will increase and alkalosis will result. The change of pH can be prevented by reduction of the respiratory output of CO_2. If the total base of the body fluids becomes depleted by diarrhea or other means, or if acids stronger than carbonic, such as mineral acids, lactic acid or β-hydroxybutyric acid, accumulate in the serum, bicarbonate will diminish and acidosis will result. The change of pH can be prevented by increased respiratory output of CO_2. The respirations, therefore, by regulating the carbonic acid concentration of the body fluids (the numerator of the Henderson equation) compensate, as far as pH is concerned, changes in the concentration of bicarbonate (the denominator of the Henderson equation).

Such compensation is seldom quite complete: reduction of bicarbonate usually entails some reduction of pH; increase of bicarbonate is usually asso-

---

tion constant. Weak acids are so slightly dissociated and their salts so completely dissociated, that in a mixture of an acid with its salt it may be assumed that all the acid present is undissociated, while all the dissociated anion is derived from the salt. Therefore, in a solution containing the acid HA and its salt BA, [BA] may be substituted for the term $[A^-]$ in the equation above, which then becomes $[H^+] = K \frac{[HA]}{[BA]}$. For mathematical convenience this equation is commonly used in the negative logarithmic form proposed by Hasselbalch,[60] who elaborated Henderson's theory.

$$pH = pK + \log [BA] - \log [HA]$$

* As far as the acid-base equilibrium is concerned, the administration of salts, such as sodium lactate, in which an inorganic cation is combined with an organic anion that can be oxidized, has the same effect as the administration of an equivalent amount of the same inorganic base as bicarbonate.

ciated with some increase of pH. Below are listed in tabular form the various general measures by which the pH of the blood may be shifted in the direction of either acidity or alkalinity:

Tending toward acidosis, *reduction of pH,* *and requiring overventilation*		*Tending toward alkalosis,* *augmentation of pH,* *and requiring underventilation*
1. { Increased CO_2 production { Diminished CO_2 output	2.	{ Diminished CO_2 production { Increased CO_2 output
3. Increase of acids stronger than carbonic		4. Loss of acids stronger than carbonic
5. Reduction of base		6. Increase of base

Numbers 1 and 2 concern primarily the respiratory mechanism and affect the numerator of the Henderson equation. They are best termed *primary CO_2 excess* and *primary CO_2 deficit*, respectively. Numbers 3, 4, 5 and 6 affect the denominator of the Henderson equation and only secondarily influence the respiratory mechanism. Numbers 3 and 4 may be spoken of as *acid excess* and *acid deficit* respectively; while 5 and 6 may be correspondingly named *base deficit* and *base excess*. Numbers 3 and 5 will lead to compensatory secondary CO_2 deficit, 4 and 6 to secondary CO_2 excess.

Internal Transfers of Water in Response to Changes of pH.—Measures which increase the hydrogen ion concentration of the body fluids (reduce its pH), will cause the passage of a certain amount of water from the interstitial fluids into the cells; reduction of the hydrogen ion concentration will have an opposite effect. The reason for these transfers is found in the greater concentration of proteins in the cells. In the equation

$$H_2CO_3 + Na_nProtein \rightleftarrows NaHCO_3 + Na_{(n-1)}Protein$$

the two terms on the left of the equation are both only slightly ionized, one being a weak acid, the other being a protein salt; the bicarbonate salt on the right is, however, highly dissociated. Therefore, as the reaction proceeds to the right the osmolar concentration must increase because instead of the two osmotically active components, H_2CO_3 and $Na_nProtein$, there are three, the ions Na^+ and HCO_3^- and the protein salt. Therefore acidification of a solution containing protein salt increases its osmotic pressure. Since there is more protein in cells than in interstitial fluid the former will be more affected than the latter by these reactions; the osmotic pressure of their contents, therefore, will increase more than that of the surrounding fluids and, consequently, will withdraw water from the latter.

Losses of Fluids and Solutes by the Skin and Lungs.[110]—The air in the alveolar depths of the lungs has approximately the same temperature as the circulating blood and, because of its intimate exposure to the large area of moist alveolar epithelium, is almost completely saturated with water vapor at this temperature. This means that in atmospheric conditions prevailing in temperate climates it contains far more moisture than is in the environmental air which is ordinarily inspired. Respiration, therefore, involves continuous loss of water from the body, the amount lost varying directly with the difference in temperature between the subject and his environmental air and inversely as the vapor pressure of the latter. It will also vary with the volume of the respiratory exchange and the nature of the respirations. For a given minute volume of respiration the loss of water will tend to vary inversely with the number of respirations per minute, because rapid, small respirations contain a larger proportion of air from the respiratory dead spaces which has not reached complete temperature equilibrium with the body. The expired air carries with it, besides CO_2, negligible quantities of solutes, consisting almost entirely of volatile substances, such as anesthetics, alcohol and acetone.

A certain amount of water is continuously dissipated by evaporation at the surface of the body. This, together with the water discharged through the lungs, constitutes the insensible perspiration. Vaporization of insensible perspiration is one of the means by which the body gives off heat. Under normal resting conditions about 24 per cent of the total heat produced in the body is lost through this process, approximately half through the lungs and half from the skin. The water of insensible perspiration is not produced by activity of the sweat glands and appears to contain no appreciable amounts of solutes. If the temperature of either the environment or the body becomes unduly elevated, the sweat glands burst into activity to provide more water for evaporation. True sweat contains considerable quantities of sodium and chloride, which must emanate from the interstitial fluids. Excessive sweating, therefore, will deplete the body of water, sodium and chloride.

Exchanges of Fluids and Solutes in the Alimentary Canal.[44, 110]—Normally the main channel for the admission of water is the alimentary canal. The sense of thirst is apparently most delicately regulated to satisfy automatically the bodily requirements.[2] The chief stimuli to drinking appear to be a deficiency of water or a relative excess of salt in the body fluids.*

In the middle of the last century Bidder and Schmidt,[9] by extensive collections and analyses of gastro-intestinal secretions, demonstrated that enormous quantities of fluid were poured into the stomach and intestines daily, only to be reabsorbed, and pointed out the general resemblances between these fluids and serum. Schmidt[132] also disclosed the depletion of water and salts that occurs in cholera and other diarrheal states and the beneficial effects of salt in these conditions. It is to Gamble,[44] however, that we are chiefly indebted for what organized knowledge we possess concerning the relations of gastro-intestinal function to water and salt metabolism. Diverse as are their chemical patterns, all the secretions of the gastro-intestinal tract from the stomach to the colon inclusive, as well as bile and pancreatic juice, appear to have the same osmotic pressure—i.e., the same osmolar concentration—as the fluids within the body proper. This is illustrated in figure 20, in which the chemical patterns of these fluids are compared with that of serum. Sodium is the chief cation in all these fluids except the acid secretion of the fundus of the stomach, in which it is largely replaced by the hydrogen ion; the chief anions are chloride and bicarbonate. Chloride predominates in the acid contents of the stomach, but progressively gives way to bicarbonate as the secretions become more alkaline in the descent of the intestine. From the preponderance of sodium, chloride, and bicarbonate, it is evident that these secretions must be derived from the interstitial fluids.

Not only are all the native gastro-intestinal and digestive secretions in osmotic equilibrium with the body fluids; but all materials introduced into

* Or, possibly, more particularly in the blood.

the alimentary canal, before or during the process of absorption, become
isotonic with the blood serum. Moreover, they tend to assume an electrolyte
pattern similar to that of the secretions of that part of the gastro-intestinal
tract in which they happen to be. This adjustment is effected by additions of
salt and water. It matters not whether the substance introduced is plain
water or a solution of organic or inorganic compounds, nor whether the
solutes in it can be absorbed or not. For example, if a solution of glucose
is introduced into the gut, its volume first increases and, as the glucose disappears, the concentrations of sodium and chloride in the solution increase.
Although osmotic equilibrium is established and maintained between the
gastro-intestinal contents and the interstitial fluids, secretion and absorption

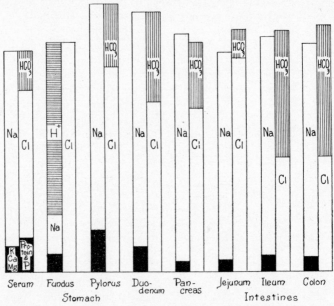

Fig. 20.—Electrolyte patterns of gastro-intestinal secretions, compiled from the literature.[113] The pattern of normal serum is represented for comparison on the left. The
figure indicates the differences in composition of the normal secretions, and especially
in the relative proportions of Na, Cl and HCO3. The uniformity of osmolar concentrations is not so evident because of the miscellaneous sources from which the data were
derived. See Gamble.[44]

must be accomplished by some more complicated processes than simple
diffusion. Diffusion alone could not remove glucose from the intestine completely when the concentration of glucose in the interstitial fluid is 100 mg.
per cent or more, especially when its removal appears to be unaffected by
the concentration of glucose in the blood.[99]

In the course of the day liters of fluid containing salt are poured into
the alimentary canal from the interstitial fluids only to be withdrawn to
their source again. Since the gut lacks the power to concentrate its contents
above the osmolar concentration of the body fluids, unabsorbable solutes
that gain access to the intestines will retain and ultimately remove from the
body with them as much water as is required to dilute them to isotonicity
with the body fluids. This is the *modus operandi* of saline cathartics. If, by

vomiting or diarrhea, or through fistulae, alimentary contents are discharged before they are absorbed, they will take with them sodium, chloride, bicarbonate, and water derived from the interstitial fluid. This will tend to reduce the volume of the interstitial fluid and to deplete it of its chief basic cation and an equivalent quantity of anions. Its osmotic pressure will, therefore, fall. The relative deficits of chloride and bicarbonate will depend on the locality from which the alimentary contents are withdrawn: loss of acid gastric contents will result in chloride depletion and will lead to bicarbonate excess with alkalosis; losses of pancreatic juice or fluid from the lower bowel will deplete both chloride and bicarbonate, but especially the latter, inducing a relative chloride excess and a bicarbonate deficit with acidosis.

REGULATION OF WATER BALANCE, ELECTROLYTE AND ACID-BASE EQUILIBRIUM BY THE KIDNEY[44, 45, 110]

The contributions of lungs, skin and gastro-intestinal tract to the conservation of the volume and chemical composition of the body fluid seem to be almost adventitious. These organs appear to be quite ruthless in their disregard for these essential properties, so intent are they upon their own highly specialized functions. There is, to be sure, evidence that the process of acclimatization to extremely hot temperatures consists of teaching the skin not to put so much salt into its sweat,[30] but the chief preoccupation of the skin is the maintenance of body temperature. The lungs do not, if they can, make any attempt to economize water. They do pump off any excess of CO_2, but this procedure is largely subsidiary to the elimination of the CO_2 produced in metabolism and to the oxygenation of hemoglobin. The gastro-intestinal tract does kindly serve as a channel for the reception and absorption of food and fluids; but, if the current in the channel is reversed or greatly accelerated, neither stomach nor intestines make any effort to stem the abnormal excretory tide of water and salt in behalf of their impoverished host. The stomach continues unconcernedly to secrete hydrochloric acid long after the chloride of serum has fallen below the lowest normal limits.[91]

Upon the kidneys falls the great brunt of responsibility, not only for the excretion of abnormal substances that find access to the blood or normal products that accumulate in the body to excess, but also for the preservation of the volume and composition of the body fluids. These conservative functions are at least as important as the excretory functions. For example, urea, which is continually being formed in the body by the degradation of protein, must be eliminated with great efficiency; its concentration in the urine greatly exceeds that in the blood. On the other hand, sodium and chloride, which must be secured from the environment, need be expended with great economy; they usually appear in lower concentration in the urine than in the blood serum. Consideration of the renal control of water balance and acid-base equilibrium has been deferred to this point because these belong among the properties which the kidneys protect. To understand how these organs succeed in adjusting so many different equilibria while simultaneously performing their purely eliminative functions it is necessary to examine briefly some of the details of renal physiology. For a more extensive treatment of the subject the reader is referred to reviews by the author,[110, 112] by Richards,[128] and by Smith.[140, 141]

It has now been established almost beyond dispute that, by the force of the blood pressure in the capillaries of the glomerular tuft, a protein-free ultrafiltrate of plasma is driven into the glomerular capsule and down the tubules. In the latter most of the water, all the glucose, some of the urea, and a large proportion of the salts in this ultrafiltrate are reabsorbed, while a number of other solutes are added. These secretory increments in some instances—*e.g.*, creatinine—merely augment the concentrations of materials already present in the ultrafiltrate; in others they may represent original contributions.

The kidney is distinguished from all other secretory or excretory organs in the mammal by its ability to elaborate a solution with an osmotic pressure greater than that of the internal environment. By virtue of this power, which seems to reside in the loop of Henle, it is peculiarly adapted to the *conservation of water*. The magnitude of this conservative activity can be best appreciated if it is realized that under normal conditions 99 per cent or more of water and sodium salts filtered through the glomeruli is absorbed by the tubules. Because the kidney can perform osmotic work and because this particular function appears to be the first to suffer when renal substance is reduced, it does not follow that the osmolar concentration of the urine is the ultimate determinant of the amount of water that can be reabsorbed from the tubules. Such an inference would imply that solutes of all kinds would compete with one another for water in the urine and that if the concentration of one was greatly increased the concentrations of the others would be proportionately reduced. There may be competition on these grounds among certain solutes, but there is probably no such competition among all solutes. It has been shown by Gamble and associates[46, 47] and by Gilman[55] that the osmolar concentration of urea in the urine can be driven far higher than that of sodium chloride. Furthermore, when both substances are given together, each can be concentrated quite as much as it can when it is given alone. The osmolar concentration of urea + sodium chloride combined may, therefore, become more than twice as great as the osmolar concentration that can be attained with sodium chloride alone. Gamble *et al.*[46] found that a variety of inorganic ions (sodium, chloride, potassium, and bicarbonate) did impose upon one another mutual restraints. There appears to be, then, an irreducible minimum to the amount of water required for the excretion of each solute, but this minimum varies from solute to solute, depending somewhat upon the mechanisms by which the various solutes are excreted.

The kidney also possesses the power to eliminate a urine more dilute than an ultrafiltrate of serum. Dilution necessitates work just as concentration does. From the standpoint of the glomerular filtrate in the tubules it is a process of concentration in the direction of the blood. Indeed, much confusion might be avoided if it were recognized that secretion and absorption need not differ in character, but only in direction. The urine volume may be increased by change of either glomerular filtration or reabsorption; dilution *per se*, however, is achieved by reduced absorption of water. Although, upon demand, the kidneys can excrete enormous volumes of water, their protective powers are not absolute; there appears to be some limit to dilution as there is to concentration.

The Meaning of "Clearances."—Since elimination of water is conditioned by elimination of solutes, it cannot be comprehended until the mode of excretion of the latter is analyzed. To those who are somewhat mathematically-minded this analysis may be facilitated by the use of "clearance equations." The clearance of any substance represents *the amount of blood (or better, plasma) which would be entirely freed of this substance in a given time by the activities of the kidney.* Differently stated it tells *the amount of plasma that would be required in this period to provide the quantity of the substance which appears in the urine.* This is expressed by the term $\dfrac{UV}{P}$, in which U and P represent the concentrations of the substance in urine and blood plasma respectively, V the volume of urine excreted in a given unit of time, conventionally cc. per minute.

The Excretion of Organic Compounds.—The glomerular filtrate seems to contain all the solutes of the serum except the proteins and lipids and substances which are adsorbed upon them. Of these solutes some escape reabsorption entirely and are not secreted by the tubules. The importance of such solutes to physiology is that their clearances are equal to the rate of glomerular filtration, that is $\dfrac{UV}{P} =$ rate of *glomerular filtration.* The excretion of such a substance is dependent entirely upon the rate of filtration. Creatinine belongs to this class of solutes in most species, but not in man. In humans, in fact, no one of the substances normally excreted in the urine is known to behave in this simple manner. If it is desired to measure glomerular filtration in man it is necessary to resort to the foreign compound inulin, which must be injected intravenously.

Another group of substances, of which urea and foreign sugars are the best known members, are partly reabsorbed in the tubules in quantities proportional to the amounts which are filtered. Their clearances are lower than, but ordinarily bear a constant relation to, those of purely filtered substances. That is, $\dfrac{UV}{P} \times K =$ the rate of glomerular filtration, when K is a constant characteristic for the substance in question. For example, K for urea is usually about 0.5, K for xylose is about 0.9. This means that about 50 per cent of filtered urea and about 10 per cent of filtered xylose are reabsorbed in the tubules. K is truly constant only at average urinary volumes, falling off slightly when the rate of urine excretion becomes extremely small, rising slightly when it becomes extremely large. There is reason to believe that solutes of this group find their way back to the blood from the tubular fluid by a simple process of diffusion. In this case they must diffuse back with less facility than water, since the concentration of urea may be as much as one hundred times as great in urine as it is in an ultrafiltrate of serum.

There is another class of substances, to which *creatinine* in man and certain dyes in all species belong, which is excreted both by secretion and filtration. In this case $\dfrac{UV}{P}$ is greater than the rate of glomerular filtration, although in humans the creatinine clearance closely parallels the inulin clearance under ordinary circumstances. Comparison of the excretion of certain of these substances (creatinine and phenol red, especially) with that of

10

inulin and urea permits a differential evaluation of glomerular and tubular functions. *Diodrast,* which is commonly used to visualize the urinary tract for intravenous pyelography, is excreted so rapidly that Smith[141] has concluded that the renal tubules probably withdraw it from the blood plasma completely. In this case the diodrast clearance becomes a method for the measurement of renal blood flow. $\frac{UV}{P}$ for diodrast = rate of flow of blood plasma through the kidney.

Glucose is excreted by a different principle. It finds free access to the glomerular fluid, but is ordinarily almost completely reabsorbed in the tubules. It was long held that glucose appeared in the urine only when its concentration in the blood reached a certain limit. Shannon and Fisher[135] have shown that it is not the concentration of glucose in the plasma that determines the occurrence of glycosuria, but the amount of glucose that is proffered to the tubules. These are apparently unable to absorb more than about 200 mg. of glucose per minute; quantities in excess of this pass into the urine. This is a peculiarly happy expedient to prevent wastage of an essential material while insuring against its excessive accumulation in the body. *Phlorhizin* produces glycosuria by inhibiting the reabsorptive activities of the tubule cells, presumably by interfering with the metabolic processes by which reabsorption is effected. Renal glycosuria probably arises from impairment of the same processes. Ascorbic acid seems to belong among the substances which are treated like glucose;[72, 126] creatine may also belong in this class.

The substances thus far discussed are all organic compounds. All except those of the class of glucose normally appear in higher concentration in the urine than in the blood. They are, therefore, excreted with great efficiency, their elimination being determined largely by the rate of glomerular filtration and being but little affected by reabsorption. They ordinarily exert little influence upon the excretion of water because they are not offered to the kidneys in quantities that surpass the concentrating powers of these organs. When they accumulate in the blood in high concentrations, however, and are therefore offered to the tubules in unusually large quantities, a greater amount of water is required for their excretion because the kidneys can not concentrate them beyond a certain limit. In this case, unless extra water is taken, they will draw upon the water stores of the body, causing dehydration. The only native solutes that are produced in sufficient quantities to have such an effect are urea in conditions associated with extreme destruction of protein, and glucose in diabetes or severe renal glycosuria. However, sucrose, sorbitol and other sugars which can not be utilized, when injected intravenously in large quantities in high concentration, cause diuresis by similar means, as does urea when given in large doses by mouth.

Because the excretion of urea depends predominantly upon filtration, increases of its concentration in the blood denote either increased destruction of protein, diminished filtration, or both. Since the rate of filtration is determined chiefly by the blood pressure in the glomerular capillaries, retention of urea is observed in conditions of circulatory collapse, such as surgical shock.

The mode of excretion of the organic compounds thus far discussed is epitomized as follows:

EXCRETION OF ORGANIC COMPOUNDS

By filtration alone
  Creatinine in most species, inulin in man

$$\text{Clearance}, \frac{UV}{P} = \text{rate of glomerular filtration}$$

By filtration and reabsorption by back-diffusion
  Urea and foreign sugars
    Clearance a linear function of filtration

$$\frac{UV}{P} K = \text{rate of glomerular filtration. } K < 1$$

For urea K is about 0.50

By filtration and tubular secretion
  Creatinine, phenol red
    Clearance usually a linear function of filtration

$$\frac{UV}{P} K = \text{rate of glomerular filtration. } K > 1.$$

Diodrast, completely cleared from plasma

$$\text{Clearance } \frac{UV}{P} = \text{rate of plasma flow through kidney}$$

By filtration and limited reabsorption
  Glucose, ascorbic acid (creatine)
    All glucose offered to tubules above a certain quantity
    rejected and passed into urine

$$\frac{UV + A}{P} = \text{glomerular filtrate, where A is the}$$

maximum amount of the substance which can be absorbed per minute, in the case of glucose about 200 mg.

The Excretion of Water and Electrolytes.—It devolves upon the kidneys to maintain in a reasonably constant state, at one and the same time, not only the total quantity of fluid in the body, but also the osmolar concentration and the detailed acid-base pattern of the interstitial fluids. This requires that these organs be so equipped that they may, within wide limits, excrete water and salts independently, and further that they may be able, in the process of elimination, to draw distinctions between cations and anions. The inorganic elements of the serum, with the exception of a fraction of the base, chiefly calcium, which forms undissociated combinations with protein, are freely diffusible and therefore enter the glomerular filtrate. This is true also of most organic acids of importance which gain access to the blood. Since the volume of glomerular filtrate is ordinarily one hundred times as great as the volume of urine, all demands for variation in the excretion of water and salts can be met merely by changing the quantities of these materials reabsorbed in the tubules. The outputs of water and salt can, apparently, vary independently over a wide range. The excretory responses of the kidney are automatically regulated to correct the disturbances of the internal environment by which they are elicited and are quantitatively proportioned to the stimulus. This quantitative relationship may not be obvious unless the degree of the disturbance is measured in all its dimensions. For example, a simple change of volume will not be so potent as a simultaneous change of volume and osmotic pressure or acid-base equilibrium. If a large quantity of water is ingested, the volume of urine increases with great rapidity. The urine during this diuresis is quite dilute, containing less than the usual concentration of solutes of all kinds. Unless the diuresis is extreme the extra water is selectively discharged. Evidently glomerular filtration is not appreciably affected; reabsorption of water by the tubules has been checked, while reabsorption of salt has continued as before. If hypertonic salt solution is given there is also prompt and speedy diuresis of urine containing salt in high concentration; reabsorption of salt is retarded, while water continues to be withdrawn from the tubules. When an equal volume of isotonic sodium chloride solution is taken it is also eliminated, but at a slower rate. Both the pure water and the hypertonic saline have disturbed the internal environment in two dimensions, volume and concentration, thereby evoking a more vehement response than the isotonic saline, which has altered only volume.

The Excretion of Water.—The preferential excretion of water as such—or rather, the reabsorption of water by the tubules—is controlled in large part by the activity of the hormone of the posterior lobe of the pituitary gland. If this gland or the hypothalamic centers or tracts through which it is controlled are destroyed, a condition of diabetes insipidus ensues in which enormous volumes of extremely dilute urine are eliminated and thirst increases proportionately. In spite of the quantities of water that are lost, a comparatively small amount of electrolytes or other solutes is sacrificed. Reabsorption of water seems to be almost specifically inhibited.* That the diuresis is aggravated by administration of extra salt and somewhat relieved by salt restriction, proves that it is not entirely uninfluenced by factors that normally affect urine volume. It can be checked promptly by the administration of pitressin.† If pituitrin is given to a normal subject after the administration of a large volume of water, diuresis is greatly delayed, but the excretion of other solutes continues unchecked. On the other hand, pituitrin has little effect upon the rate of urine flow when no extra water is given or when salt solution is substituted for plain water. Gilman[54] found that the urine of dehydrated rats with oliguria had antidiuretic activity and gave reactions like those of pitressin. This observation has been confirmed in rats, but not in other species.[159] All the evidence combined, however, seems to point to the fact that the antidiuretic principle of the posterior pituitary controls water reabsorption. It apparently acts directly upon the tubular cells since it works upon the denervated or even upon the isolated kidney. The slight and irregular alterations of glomerular filtration that follow its use are probably adventitious effects of the vasopressor principle.

Urine volume is determined not only by the amount, but also by the availability, of water in the body. Ordinarily, with free access to water, an animal will drink enough to replace water lost by extrarenal channels and to permit the excretion of those solutes that require elimination. With kidneys, circulatory system, and the composition of the body fluids intact, extra fluid and solutes are rapidly dispersed through the body and excesses quickly find their way to the kidneys and thence to the urine. Circumstances may arise, however, in which water becomes unavailable to the kid-

---

* Pituitrin exerts no antidiuretic effect upon those orders of the animal kingdom that do not possess the loop of Henle, suggesting that the posterior pituitary hormone acts specifically upon this segment of the renal tubules.

† Or an active principle of pitressin. Heller[73] has adduced evidence that vasopressor and antidiuretic principles of pitressin are not identical.

neys because it has been segregated in certain tissues or structures. The commonest example of such segregation is *subcutaneous edema* resulting from a loss of balance between the blood pressure and the osmotic pressure of proteins in the serum. Whether the capillary blood pressure is increased, as it is in heart failure, or the plasma proteins are reduced, as they are in the nephrotic syndrome or malnutrition, the effect is the same. Fluid escapes from the blood stream into the interstitial spaces and the total fluid in the body increases because it is diverted from the kidneys. That the kidneys are not altogether directly to blame is proved by the fact that restoration of the proper balance (in heart failure by digitalis, in nephrosis or malnutrition by infusion of acacia or suitable protein solutions) results in diuresis with delivery of the edema. Fluid may become segregated in a similar manner in more restricted areas because of venous or lymphatic obstruction. In all such instances the kidneys appear to be quite indifferent to the disturbance. The impression is given that they are concerned rather with the blood volume than with the volume of the body fluids as a whole.

In these conditions the kidneys themselves are not seriously affected by the disturbances; their inherent ability to eliminate water when it is offered to them is not impaired. The situation is different when the kidneys participate in the circulatory disorder, as they may in severe heart failure and in circulatory collapse or surgical shock. In the latter condition the capillary blood pressure in the glomeruli falls, hence filtration diminishes. Oliguria or even anuria ensues; urea and other nonprotein nitrogenous constituents are imperfectly excreted and, therefore, accumulate in the blood. Extreme passive congestion of the kidneys has a somewhat similar effect.*

If the intake of water is restricted, not only do losses by extrarenal channels continue unchecked, but also the kidneys are forced to excrete a certain amount of water to enable them to eliminate waste products. This will obviously lead to depletion of the water in the body. Were there no associated reactions, the concentration of electrolytes in the internal environment would rise. To avoid this, the kidneys respond by excreting an amount of salt roughly equivalent to the water lost, thereby preserving the osmolar concentration of electrolytes in the interstitial fluids at the expense of the volume of fluid.

A similar sequence of events is initiated if the kidneys are put under compulsion to excrete water by any other means. If, for example, an animal is given large amounts of urea without adequate quantities of water, or large intravenous injections of highly concentrated sugar solutions, it is forced to draw upon its own fluid reserves for the water required to excrete these substances in concentrations that are within the capacity of the kidneys. Again these organs, in behalf of the electrolyte osmotic pressure, excrete with the water which is sacrificed the salts which were dissolved in this water. If the process of dehydration is pushed to extremes by these means, compensation becomes less and less complete because the animal gives up water with progressively increasing reluctance. Urea and even salt are incompletely excreted and accumulate in the body. At this point the circulation is imperfect and filtration is impaired. Urea is usually retained

* The mechanism in this case is not entirely clear. Glomerular congestion should, and within limits will, increase filtration pressure. However, when venous congestion becomes extreme it apparently engenders back-pressure in the tubules and glomeruli.

more than salt because its excretion is more dependent upon filtration and it must be concentrated far more than salt in the process of excretion. The retention of urea in states of water depletion bespeaks a degree of dehydration profound enough to compromise the circulation.

If salt is withdrawn from the diet, but free access to water is given, excretion of sodium and chloride does not cease at once; consequently a certain amount of the normal salt of the body is lost. In response to this, and again to prevent reduction of the concentration of electrolytes in the internal environment, an equivalent volume of water from the interstitial fluids is sacrificed. Restriction of salt, therefore, results in depletion of water. This, however, never becomes great because the conservative activities of the kidneys rapidly come into play. After a surprisingly short interval the excretion of sodium and chloride diminishes, equilibrium is established and salt wastage ceases. If salt depletion is pushed to greater extremes by the combined effects of restricted intake and excessive elimination by extrarenal channels, while water intake remains undiminished, osmotic pressure is not completely preserved at the expense of fluid volume. A compromise is reached in which the sodium concentration and the volume of the interstitial fluids both yield. In this state the blood urea is likely to rise. McCance[96, 97, 98] has shown that when salt depletion becomes extreme glomerular filtration falls strikingly. Paradoxically enough, at the same time the diuretic response to ingested water also becomes retarded.*

The Excretion of Electrolytes.—Under normal conditions the inorganic elements are continuously excreted in the urine as they enter the body, so that both the quantity and the concentration of each in the interstitial fluid remain relatively constant. The rate of excretion is not, however, so closely related to the serum concentration as it is in the case of urea and other organic solutes discussed above. Moreover, the kidneys are not regularly called upon to concentrate inorganic elements as much as they do these organic substances. In fact some, like sodium and chloride, usually appear in lower concentration in urine than in serum; they are reabsorbed more completely than water.

The electrolytes are subject to certain restraints from which neutral organic solutes are free.† Although the kidneys exercise the greatest discrimination in the selective excretion of ions, they cannot violate the principles of electroneutrality by excreting individual ions separately. The anions, chloride and bicarbonate, can be excreted in varying proportions; but neither can be excreted without taking with it an anion. The excretion of any ion is, therefore, to some extent conditioned by its mate. To maintain in the interstitial fluids a constant concentration of ions that are supplied at an irregular rate, there must be provisions by which superfluous accessions may be promptly eliminated, while the normal stores are conserved.

The operation of these various restrictions can be best shown by a series of examples. Inorganic sulfate is continually supplied, not only in the pre-

* The reasons for these reactions are not entirely clear. They are not necessarily associated with demonstrable evidence of circulatory failure.

† For the following description the author has drawn upon his monograph *Body Water*,[110] articles by Adolph[1] and studies made in his own laboratory by Winkler and associates,[166, 169] and unpublished experiments.

formed state, but also from the products of protein metabolism; nevertheless its concentration in the serum is extremely low, about 1 mg. per cent of S. Normal clearances of inorganic sulfate are high; it is excreted with great efficiency, as if it were a foreign material of which the body wished to rid itself entirely. For this reason it was placed by Cushny[24] among the "non-threshold" substances. If extra inorganic sulfate is given to an animal, the rate of excretion rises rapidly and out of proportion to the concentration of sulfate in the serum. This is illustrated in figure 21 A. With moderate in-

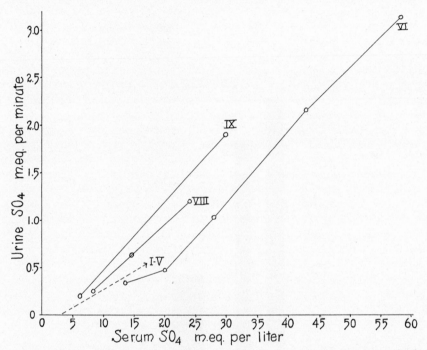

Fig. 21 A.—The effect of the injection of sulfate salts upon the composition of urine. A. The relation between the excretion of sulfate in the urine and its concentration in the serum of dogs after intravenous injections of sulfate salts. The line I–V represents the average curve of excretion of moderate quantities of the sulfates of magnesium, potassium, and sodium. The lines VI, VIII and IX illustrate the effects of injections of large quantities of sodium sulfate. No. VI depicts the course of excretion of about 1000 cc. of twice physiologically normal sodium sulfate. No. VIII shows the excretion of sulfate after injection of 1000 cc. of physiologically normal sodium sulfate, containing an equivalent amount of sodium chloride. For no. IX the same quantity of sodium sulfate was injected with twice as much sodium chloride.

crements of sulfate, the concentration in the serum appears to bear a linear relation to the rate of excretion. If this line is extrapolated (see Fig. 21 A, I–V), it is found to intersect the serum concentration at a positive value, approximately the normal concentration of inorganic sulfate in serum. Obviously the exogenous increment of sulfate is excreted quite differently from the endogenous fraction, as if it were a true threshold substance. If enormous quantities of sulfate are given the rate of excretion becomes still greater in proportion to the serum concentration, as if the threshold had risen further, (Fig. 21 A, VI, VIII, IX). As far as the subject can be investigated, the rate of elimination of sulfate is but little influenced by the cation with which it is combined.

There is no great difference in the curves describing the excretion of sodium, potassium or magnesium sulfate. If the excretion of these companion ions is studied, it is found that their exogenous increments are excreted almost at the same rate as the sulfate with which they were combined, although their endogenous rates of excretion differ greatly. The additions appear to have been excreted, not by the laws that govern the excretion of

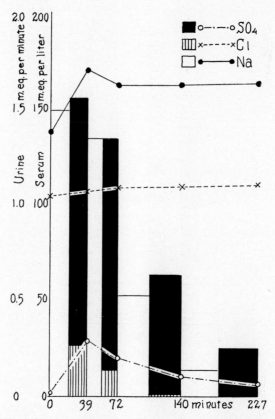

Fig. 21 B.—The rate of excretion of sodium, sulfate and chloride by the dog after intravenous injection of about 1000 cc. of a solution containing equimolecular concentrations of sodium sulfate and sodium chloride, the combined concentrations yielding a twice physiologically normal solution. This is the experiment depicted in A, VIII. The columns represent urinary excretion, the lines, concentrations in the serum.

their component ions, but as so much foreign matter. There are detectable differences between the cations, but they are relatively small in the case of the ions which have been mentioned. When calcium sulfate is given, the calcium is excreted far more slowly, proving that the cations do not entirely surrender their individuality to sulfate. With the exception of calcium, the inorganic ions which exist in low concentration in the serum, Mg, K, and inorganic phosphate, resemble sulfate in their excretory behavior.

The *elimination of sodium* follows somewhat different principles. Its

normal concentration in the serum is extremely high in proportion to its
rate of excretion. If the exogenous supply is cut off or if elimination by

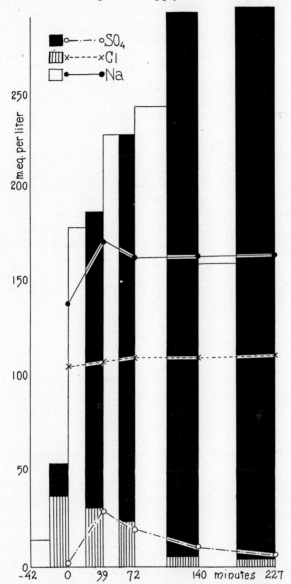

Fig. 21 C.—The concentrations of sodium, sulfate and chloride in the urine, compared with the concentrations of the same substances in the serum in the course of the
experiment illustrated by B. A illustrates the acceleration of the excretion of sulfate as
its concentration rises in the serum and the further accelerating effect of the simultaneous
administration of chloride. B and C demonstrate the selective excretion of sulfate and
the extent to which it suppresses urinary chloride even when the concentration of the
latter in the serum rises to extreme heights.

extrarenal channels is increased, urinary excretion of the ion becomes
negligibly small before its concentration in the serum has fallen significantly.

If large quantities of sodium chloride are given the excretion of sodium rises promptly, but the increment is not eliminated nearly as rapidly as an equivalent amount of sodium sulfate or sodium phosphate. If equivalent amounts of the chlorides of potassium and sodium are given, potassium is excreted more rapidly than sodium. The kidneys appear to be less sensitive to increases of sodium in the serum than they are to increases of ions which usually occur in lower concentration. Sodium appears from the excretory point of view to occupy a mendicant position towards these other ions. Actually this means that it is preferentially reabsorbed, that the kidneys are more reluctant to let it escape. More careful analysis reveals that after administration of sodium sulfate, the increment of sodium is excreted perceptibly slower than the sulfate increment. Finally if sodium chloride and sodium sulfate are given simultaneously, excretion of sulfate is greatly accelerated, while that of chloride is retarded or even suppressed. The sodium which was combined with chloride and part of that which was combined with sulfate is also held back. The concentrations of sodium and chloride in the serum may rise to extremely high levels. (See Fig. 21 *A, B* and *C*.)

If anions are compared it is found that chloride follows the pattern of behavior of sodium. Chloride is excreted more rapidly when it is given as the potassium salt than when it is combined with sodium. At the same time, after administration of potassium chloride, the potassium increment finds its way into the urine more promptly than the chloride increment. The kidneys also appear to distinguish imperfectly the two halides, chloride and bromide, retaining and excreting them quite indifferently in proportion to their relative concentrations in the serum and their relative rates of diffusion.[71, 143] *

Knowledge of the intimacies of the procedures by which the kidneys make adjustments among electrolytes is altogether inadequate; but from the relations described the tubules appear to reject with especial vigor those ions which are foreign to the serum or which occur in the serum in low concentration and to reabsorb selectively those which make up the bulk of the salt in the interstitial fluids. If confronted with the necessity of making a choice they will allow the latter to accumulate to excess in the serum for the sake of eliminating the less favored ions. The kidneys must resort to discriminative selection when there is insufficient water available to permit the excretion at the same time of all the ions which demand elimination. It has already been pointed out that urea and salts do not compete with one another for the possession of water in the urine; the kidneys can concentrate either one without consideration of the other. The four ions, sodium, potassium, chloride and bicarbonate, on the other hand, impose mutual restraints upon one another. The extent to which any one of them can be concentrated depends upon the simultaneous concentrations of the others; the ultimate limit of concentration is determined by the aggregate osmolar concentration of the four.[1, 46, 47] Other ions, such as sulfate and phosphate, also exert a restraining influence, but the nature and extent of this influence has not yet been precisely defined.

* This lack of discrimination is not confined to the kidneys. Davenport and Fisher[20] have shown that the stomach also substitutes the bromide ion for chloride when the former gains access to the blood.

Preservation of the Acid-Base Equilibrium by the Kidney.[44, 110, 112]—
The mechanism for the maintenance of the acid-base equilibrium of the
body fluids, which were described earlier, the buffers, and the respiratory
system, can make only minor or temporary adjustments. The kidneys are
responsible for the ultimate rectification of major disturbances of the acid-
base balance. This they accomplish by three principal devices: 1. variation
of the reaction of the urine; 2. substitution of ammonia for inorganic base in
the urine; 3. excretion of inorganic base as bicarbonate.

Blood serum is slightly alkaline and its reaction is quite constant. Even
in the most profound disorders its pH seldom departs from the narrow
limits 7.0 to 7.6. The pH of urine, however, may vary from about 4.0 to
8.0. This enables the kidneys to excrete buffer acids with variable amounts
of base. In normal serum, with a pH of 7.3, for example, 80 per cent of
inorganic phosphate exists in the form of the alkaline salt, Na_2HPO_4, only
20 per cent as the acid salt, NaH_2PO_4. In an acid urine, with a pH of 5.0
practically all is in the acid form, NaH_2PO_4; while at a pH of 8.0 it is
almost all in the alkaline form, Na_2HPO_4. In a serum, at a pH of 7.4, 90 per
cent of β-hydroxybutyric acid is neutralized by base, in a highly acid urine
as much as 50 per cent exists as the free acid. The following calculations
will give an idea of the economy of base which may be achieved in the
excretion of acids in this manner:

		Serum $pH = 7.3$	Urine $pH = 5.0$	Base saved
Phosphate	$\begin{cases} Na_2HPO_4 \\ NaH_2PO_4 \end{cases}$	0.80 / 0.20	0.00 / 1.00	44 per cent
β-hydroxybutyrate	$\begin{cases} Na\text{—}OOC \cdot CH_2 \cdot CH(OH) \cdot CH_3 \\ H\text{—}OOC \cdot CH_3 \cdot CH(OH) \cdot CH_3 \end{cases}$	0.90 / 0.10	0.50 / 0.50	40 per cent

The kidneys regulate the reaction of the urine, apparently, by reabsorbing
carbonic acid and bicarbonate in varying proportions. The tubules possess
the power to reabsorb bicarbonate, while opposing the passage of CO_2.
The pressure of CO_2 in the urine may be as great as 200 mm. Hg, compared with 40 to 60 mm. Hg in the blood.[93, 134] The reactions involved in
the acidification of urine may be depicted thus:

$$CO_2 + H_2O = H_2CO_3 \begin{cases} H_2CO_3 + Na_2HPO_4 & \overset{\text{absorbed}}{=} NaHCO_3 + \overset{\text{excreted}}{NaH_2PO_4} \\ H_2CO_3 + Na \cdot OOC \cdot CH_2 \cdot CH(OH) \cdot CH_3 = NaHCO_3 + HOOC \cdot - \\ (\beta\text{-hydroxybutyric}) & CH_3 \cdot CH(OH) \cdot CH_3 \end{cases}$$

The second defense against acidosis lies in the substitution of ammonia
for inorganic base in the urine. Ammonia is produced by the kidney and
secreted by the tubular cells into the urine. The reactions involved may be
represented by the following equations:

$(\beta\text{-hydroxybutyric})$ reabsorbed excreted

$$H_2CO_3 + (NH_4)_2CO_3 + 2NaOOC \cdot CH_2 \cdot CH(OH) \cdot CH_3 = 2NaHCO_3 + 2NH_4 \cdot OOC \cdot - \\ CH_2 \cdot CH(OH) \cdot CH_3$$

$$H_2CO_3 + (NH_4)_2CO_3 + 2NaCl = 2NaHCO_3 + 2NH_4Cl*$$

Ammonia production does not usually come into active play until acidosis

* Obviously this reaction could not take place in the tubules just as it has been
depicted. Some intermediary reaction, probably in or at the surface of the tubular
cells, would have to be hypothecated, by which Na and Cl could be separated, similar
to that by which hydrochloric acid is manufactured by the cells of the gastric mucosa.

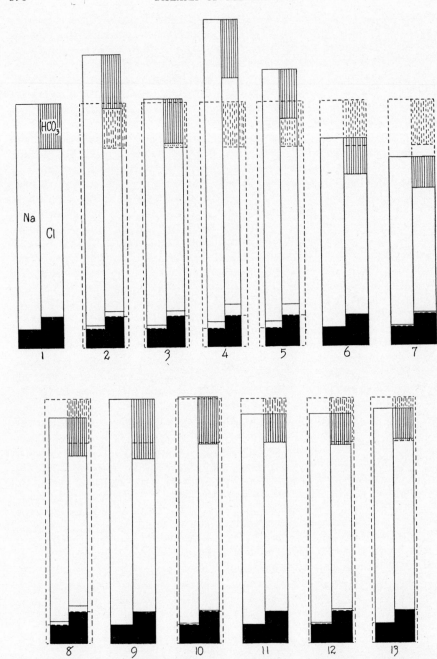

Fig. 22.—Disturbances of electrolyte equilibria and compensatory adjustments. In each pair of columns the vertical dimension represents osmolar concentration, the horizontal dimension, volume. The broken lines in each pair represent the pattern of normal serum for comparison. 1. The pattern of normal serum. 2. The result of removing one-sixth of the water without salt. 3. Compensation by sacrifice of one-sixth of the sodium chloride and sodium bicarbonate. 4. The result of removing one-fourth of the water without salt. 5. Partial compensation by sacrifice of one-sixth of the sodium chloride and the sodium bicarbonate. 6. The result of removing one-sixth of the sodium chloride

has persisted for an appreciable length of time. By means of these two reactions, acidification of the urine and substitution of ammonia, the body is effectively protected against base depletion. The defense is not, however, complete. In severe acidosis some inorganic base is sacrificed.

If the concentration of either total base or base combined with bicarbonate becomes excessive, the kidneys excrete the surplus as bicarbonate in an alkaline urine. In other words they reabsorb less bicarbonate than usual and excrete more base combined with buffer acids.

In figure 22 some of the relations between electrolytes and water have been diagrammatically illustrated. The pairs of columns in each case represent the volume and composition of interstitial fluid or serum. The horizontal dimension indicates volume of interstitial fluid; the vertical dimension, concentration of electrolytes in the serum in terms of chemical combining equivalents per kilogram of water. As far as the important ions— sodium, chloride and bicarbonate—are concerned, combining equivalents have the significance of osmolar equivalents. No. 1 represents the normal pattern. In No. 2 the concentration of electrolytes has been greatly increased by the loss of one-sixth of the water in the interstitial fluids. In No. 3 the osmolar concentration has been restored by the sacrifice in the urine of an equal proportion of sodium chloride and sodium bicarbonate, but the volume of fluid remains low. It is evident that chemical analysis of the serum in this case would give no evidence of the depletion of electrolytes. In No. 6 one-sixth of the sodium chloride and one-sixth of the sodium bicarbonate have been lost. If osmotic compensation were established by the sacrifice in the urine of the same proportion of water the result would be identical with No. 3 in which the same amounts of the same components were lost in the reverse order.

In No. 4 the concentration of electrolytes has been enormously increased by the loss of one-fourth of the water from the interstitial fluids. In No. 5 compensation has been only partial; a compromise has been reached between volume and osmotic pressure by the sacrifice of one-sixth of the sodium bicarbonate and one-sixth of the chloride. The volume of the interstitial fluid is greatly reduced, the concentrations of sodium, bicarbonate and chloride are moderately increased. The degree of hemoconcentration is denoted by the high concentrations of the proteins. This picture is relatively rare because few conditions cause loss of fluid in excess of salt and because there is seldom difficulty in excreting excessive amounts of salt which may accumulate in the body fluids.

In No. 7 one-fourth of the sodium, chloride, and bicarbonate have been lost, without change of the volume of the interstitial fluid. In No. 8 compensation has been incompletely established by the sacrifice of one-sixth

and the sodium bicarbonate without water. (Compensation would be established by sacrifice of one-sixth of the water, giving the same pattern as 3.) 7. The result of removing one-fourth of the sodium chloride and the sodium bicarbonate. 8. Partial compensation by sacrifice of one-sixth of the water. 9. The effect of losing 10 millimols of Cl in acid vomitus and replacement of the Cl by HCO_3. 10. Partial compensation by excretion in the urine of 10 millimols of $NaHCO_3$ and 5.4 per cent of the water. 11. The effect of losing 10 millimols of $NaHCO_3$ in diarrheal stools. 12. Imperfect compensation by excretion in the urine of 10 millimols of NaCl and 5.4 per cent of the water. 13. Better, but still incomplete compensation by excretion in the urine of 5 millimols of NaCl and 5 millimols of Cl as NH_4Cl with 5.4 per cent of the water.

of the water. This has partly restored the osmolar concentration. This is the kind of compromise between volume and concentration that is most commonly observed in states of dehydration. Chemical analysis of the serum gives an imperfect impression of the true degree of salt depletion.

In No. 9, owing to vomiting of acid gastric juice, enough chloride has been lost to reduce its concentration in the serum by 10 milliequivalents and the sodium formerly combined with the chloride has been converted to bicarbonate. In No. 10 the concentration of electrolytes has been restored almost to normal by the simultaneous sacrifice in alkaline urine of enough sodium bicarbonate to reduce the original concentration by 10 milliequivalents and of 5.4 per cent of the water from the interstitial fluids.

In No. 11, enough sodium bicarbonate has been lost in diarrheal stools to reduce the concentrations of both sodium and bicarbonate 10 milliequivalents. It is evident from No. 12 that compensation cannot be established as it was in the last case by the sacrifice of equivalent amounts of sodium chloride and water, because this only exaggerates the deficiency of base. The substitution of ammonia for half the sodium combined with the chloride which is excreted, by permitting the retention of the remaining sodium, partially preserves the total osmolar concentration (see No. 13), but does little to reestablish the proper proportions of chloride and bicarbonate. The explanation for this anomaly lies in the relative quantities of these two ions in the body fluids. Since there is three to four times as much chloride as there is bicarbonate in serum, loss of a given quantity of chloride causes less distortion of the composition of the serum than does the loss of an equal quantity of bicarbonate.

Further examples of disturbances and compensatory reactions could be given; however, these should suffice to establish the principles which govern interchanges of water and electrolytes and to permit the reader to comprehend the more complex phenomena encountered in disease.

Methods for the Measurement of Water and Electrolyte Exchange.— The accurate measurement of total exchanges of water and salts in health and disease requires extremely complicated procedures. For descriptions and discussions of the methods by which they can be effected the reader must be referred to monographs and reviews dealing specifically with the subject.[86, 88, 104, 110] Only certain practical simplifications will be considered in this chapter.

Measurement of the Salt Exchange.—Potassium and phosphate are relatively unimportant in connection with water exchanges and acid-base equilibrium. Being ubiquitous in foods and being supplied during starvation by destruction of tissues, they are always available. It is sufficient, therefore, to know the exchanges of sodium and chloride. For the most part these are ingested in the form of table salt which is added in the preparation of food. The average adult ingests from 7 to 15 gm. of sodium chloride per day. If no salt is added in the preparation of food or at the table this can be reduced to 1.5 to 3 gm. per day, depending upon the total amount and variety of food eaten.* Fairly accurate estimates of the amounts of sodium and chloride in raw food-stuffs can be made with the aid of standard dietary tables[136]; amounts added in the preparation of food may be measured.

* Canned and ready prepared foods must be used with caution, because salt is frequently introduced in the process of manufacture.

In the absence of gastro-intestinal disorders or sweating, sodium and chloride are excreted almost entirely in the urine. Moreover, because they are taken chiefly in the form of sodium chloride, the quantities of the two elements in the urine ordinarily parallel one another so closely that the excretion of sodium may be deduced from the excretion of chloride, which is more easily measured. Unless there is diarrhea, feces contain only minute amounts of sodium and chloride. Both feces and vomitus can, however, be analyzed without great difficulty if exact information is desired. Insensible perspiration contains negligible quantities of salt; but sweat presents a serious problem. It lends itself neither to collection nor to analysis, but may contain large amounts of sodium and chloride. If there is profuse sweating, loss of these elements by the skin must be calculated indirectly.

(Salt intake + salt originally in the body) — (Salt output in urine, feces and vomitus + salt finally in the body) = Salt lost in the sweat.

The quantities of sodium and chloride in the body can be estimated only if both the concentrations of these elements in the body fluids and the volume of fluid in which they are dissolved are known.*

Measurement of the Fluid Compartments of the Body.—Methods for measurement of the *volume of the circulating blood* depend upon two principles: (1) the dilution of substances added to blood plasma which escape with difficulty from the blood vessels; (2) the distribution and dilution of red blood cells which have been labelled by some means that permits their identification. The first methods presumably measure directly the volume of the plasma; those of the second class, the volume of the red blood cells, in circulation. In either case the volume of the second phase and the total volume of the blood can be calculated, if the relative volumes of plasma and cells are determined by means of the hematocrit. For direct measurements of plasma various dyes have been used. These are injected intravenously and, after a sufficient interval has elapsed to permit complete admixture with the blood, a sample of blood is withdrawn and the plasma is analyzed for the material. The quantity injected ÷ the concentration found = the volume of the circulating blood plasma. Relatively simple techniques and analytical procedures adapted to photoelectric colorimetry and utilizing Evans blue (T 1824) have been developed by Gregerson[59] and Gibson.[50] For direct measurements of red blood cell volume carbon monoxide has been most frequently and successfully employed.[21] Because of their greater simplicity the dye methods have been more extensively employed, although there are theoretical reasons for preferring the carbon monoxide method. The latter gives consistently lower values than the dye methods, probably because the dyes employed are not confined strictly to the blood stream, but diffuse rapidly into the lymph of the thoracic duct system.[139] Results by the dye methods may, therefore, be influenced by

* Analyses of biological fluids for sodium are so time consuming and technically difficult that they are more suited to investigative than clinical purposes. Since, however, sodium makes up most of the base, while chloride and bicarbonate make up the major part of the acids of serum, the concentration of sodium can be inferred with a sufficient degree of accuracy for most purposes from the combined concentrations of bicarbonate + chloride. The only conditions in which false inferences may be drawn are those in which a large fraction of bicarbonate has been replaced by foreign acid—*e.g.*, severe diabetic acidosis.

variations in the volume of this system, about which little is known. Although measurements of plasma or blood volume have proved useful, they must be interpreted with some consideration of the weaknesses of the methods.

The *volume of the extracellular fluids* can be measured by studying the dilution of various substances introduced into the body which diffuse through the extracellular fluid without entering the cells. Time must be given for dissemination of the test substance and a correction must be applied for the amounts excreted in the urine. Suitable substances for this purpose are sucrose, sulfate, bromide and thiocyanate.[17, 87, 142, 144, 168] The last is most to be recommended because it is excreted extremely slowly. It is, however, known to enter red blood cells and fluids in the gastro-intestinal tract. Moreover it diffuses slowly into large aggregations of fluid such as pleural transudates.[52] The method gives information of importance and might be employed to advantage more frequently; but, like the blood volume method, it must be interpreted with a certain amount of reserve and with due consideration of all other available evidence.

For measurement of the *total volume of fluid in the body* there is, as yet, no convenient procedure. However, fluctuations of body water involve chiefly the extracellular fluids; the intracellular ones are affected principally by variations of osmotic pressure in their environment. The general state of hydration of the body can, therefore, be evaluated by knowledge of the volume and concentration of sodium in the extracellular fluids. Such clinical aids as the elasticity of the skin and subcutaneous tissues, the blood pressure and other criteria of the state of the circulation should not be neglected. Distinctions should be drawn between hemoconcentration and depletion of the volume of the interstitial fluid. When hydration is changing rapidly information of great value can be secured from comparisons of body weight with blood counts or the concentrations of protein in the serum, the latter serving as measures of the variation of water in the blood.

Measurement of the Water Balance.—The intake of water consists of the preformed water in foods or fluids which are ingested and the water formed by the oxidation of foods; the output consists of the losses in urine, feces, vomitus, sweat and insensible perspiration. The difference between intake and output represents the change of water in the body. Direct measurement of all these terms is an extremely difficult matter, quite inapplicable to the general problems of the clinic. Some idea of the relative magnitude of all the variables is, nevertheless, essential for the intelligent evaluation of the water requirements of patients, even if calculation of the water exchange is not contemplated.

The preformed water of the diet is not confined to obvious fluids; apparently solid foods contain large quantities of water. This can be measured by drying aliquots or duplicates of the diet, or can be estimated roughly from the weight and general character of the diet. It is important to remember that reduction or withdrawal of food entails reduction of intake of water. The water produced by the oxidation of foods depends on the nature and quantity of food stuffs burned in the body, which is not always equal to the diet given. The water produced in the combustion of one gram of each of the food stuffs is: for protein, 0.41 gm.; carbohydrate, 0.60 gm.; fat, 1.07 gm. In an adult the total produced in a day, with extreme variations of metabolism, will seldom vary beyond the limits of 200 to 600 gm. per day.

The water lost in urine, feces and vomitus can be measured without great difficulty. Insensible perspiration, on the average, amounts to about 0.45 times the calories produced (not the diet eaten) in the metabolic processes. 0.45 Cals. = IP. If there is sensible perspiration no such estimation can be made. The best approximation can be reached, when facilities are available and the condition of the subject permits, by weighing subject, ingesta, and excreta at intervals. By this means the insensible loss,* IL, may be determined:

$$IL = (W_1 - W_2) + (w_f - w_e)$$

where W_1, W_2, w_f and w_e stand respectively for initial and final body weights and weights of ingesta and excreta. IL includes not only sweat and insensible perspiration, but also the net exchange of gases $(O_2 - CO_2)$ through the respiratory system. For general practical purposes of estimating gross water exchanges, this last item may be neglected.

Water and Salt Requirements.—Under ordinary circumstances, if an animal is given free access to water, its instincts will direct it to take what it requires. However, conditions arise not infrequently in disease in which either instincts have not free play or some disorder prevents the normal assimilation of water. In this case it becomes necessary for the physician to provide water in optimum quantities. If the subject is in complete possession of his senses and has no gastro-intestinal disorder to interfere with the ingestion and absorption of water, he need be given only the opportunity to follow the dictates of his own thirst. This is especially true if he is receiving a full diet and if he is not sweating. When the diet is greatly reduced and especially when he is receiving only fluids, the situation is altered. Thirst in most animals is somewhat conditioned to the ingestion of food. In addition, reduction of the diet usually entails a variable reduction of the salt intake and, if carried to the extreme, involves also elimination of carbohydrate. The latter may lead to ketosis, the former to a certain degree of salt depletion. Both ketosis and salt depletion promote dehydration and salt deficiency also abates thirst. Care should be taken, therefore, to provide always enough carbohydrate and salt to prevent these disorders. In most instances 100 gm. of sugar and 5 gm. of sodium chloride will meet these demands. Sweating enhances the need for salt. Moss,[102] Haldane,[61] Dill,[30, 150] and others have clearly demonstrated that the cramps which afflict persons laboring at high temperatures are induced by drinking water after extreme sweating. Large quantities of salt as well as water are lost in the sweat. When water alone is taken to replace these deficits, the salt of the body fluids becomes diluted to hypotonic concentrations. This is the condition known as *water intoxication*. If salt is given as well as water, to slake the thirst after sweating, no cramps or other symptoms appear. Water intoxication of varying degrees is not uncommon in the clinic. Its incidence may be diminished if care is taken to provide extra salt to patients who sweat excessively.

---

* The term insensible loss cannot be applied with strict propriety to sensible sweat, but the distinction between sensible and insensible perspiration is of minor importance in the measurement of gross water exchanges.

In the subject who has no impairment of the ability to burn carbohydrate and no inherent defect of renal function, administration of 100 gm. of carbohydrate daily and enough salt and water to provide 1500 cc. of urine containing chloride in moderate concentration (from 0.05 to 0.5 per cent of chloride, estimated as NaCl) will meet all ordinary requirements.

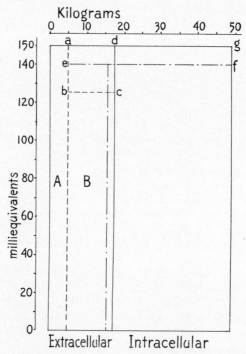

Fig. 23.—The transfer of water from the extracellular to the intracellular compartment after the loss of sodium salts. In the diagram the vertical dimension represents osmolar concentration while the horizontal dimension represents the volume of the body fluids of a 70 Kg. man, divided into extracellular and intracellular compartments by the solid vertical line. Both salt and water of area *A* are removed together and in addition enough sodium salt to reduce the osmolar concentration of the remaining extracellular fluid 50 milliosmols, the area *abcd*. The remaining extracellular fluid is defined by the rectangle *B*. Because the osmotic pressure of *B* is lowered, water is transferred to the intracellular compartment until the osmotic pressures in extracellular and intracellular fluids are again identical. This involves expansion of the intracellular compartment at the expense of the extracellular, to the extent indicated by the dot-dash vertical line. The ultimate osmolar concentration in both compartments is given by the line *ef*. It will be found that the area *aefg* equals *abcd*. In other words, although no salt has traversed the membrane, the removal of salt from the extracellular compartment has the same apparent effect on osmolar concentrations in both compartments as would the removal of an equivalent amount of salt from both compartments.

The special needs of patients with renal disease or diabetes will be considered later.

At times it becomes necessary to repair the effects of *antecedent dehydration*. In this case the same criteria may be employed. The deficiencies must be made up by the administration of sodium chloride and water in proportions to restore the electrolyte concentration as well as the volume of body fluids. Usually this can be effected by the use of normal salt solution. When salt has been more greatly depleted than water, reparation may be accelerated by the introduction of an appropriate quantity of hypertonic (2 per cent) solution of sodium chloride. Election of the proper amounts of salt and water may be facilitated by analyses of the serum for chloride and bicarbonate. From figure 19 (p. 279) it will be seen that the sum of the concentrations of these two amount to about 136 milliequivalents per kilogram of water, while sodium exceeds this by about 8 milliequivalents. To make up a reduction of the concentration of sodium it is necessary to add the quantity of sodium salt which would be required to increase the concentration of sodium in the entire mass of fluid in the body by the required amount. Water in the normal individual makes up about 70 per cent of the weight of the body.

On first thought it may seem strange that, if sodium is confined to extracellular fluids it is necessary in the face of a deficit of sodium to give enough sodium to provide for a deficit in the cells as well; but consideration of a concrete problem will explain the apparent anomaly. The solid lines in figure 23 represent the fluids of a normal 70-Kg. individual, the horizontal dimension indicating volume and the vertical dimension the osmolar concentration of electrolytes. The total fluid volume is 70 per cent of the weight or 49 liters, of which 17.5 liters or 25 per cent of the body weight consists of extracellular fluid. The fluids in both compartments contain electrolytes in a concentration of 300 milliosmols.* Let it be supposed, now, that the subject loses in sweat or vomitus or by any other means 5 liters of fluid and the electrolytes within it, pictured in A, and enough sodium salts besides to reduce the osmolar concentration of electrolytes in the remaining 12.5 liters of extracellular fluid from 300 to 250 milliosmols. The extracellular fluid would then be defined by the rectangle B. Whereas it originally had a volume of 17.5 liters with an electrolyte concentration of 300 milliosmols, and therefore contained $17.5 \times 330 = 5250$ milliosmols, it now has a volume of 12.5 liters with an electrolyte concentration of 250 milliosmols, or a total of $12.5 \times 250 = 3125$ milliosmols. Since its osmolar concentration is now less than that of the cells, the latter will withdraw water from the extracellular fluid until the electrolyte concentration in the two compartments is equal. This means that the intracellular fluid will grow at the expense of the extracellular. The original volume of the intracellular fluid was 31.5 liters, with an osmolar concentration of 300 milliosmols, or a total content of $31.5 \times 300 = 9450$ milliosmols. The final volume of the system is 44 liters and its osmolar content $3125 + 9450 = 12,575$ milliosmols. In order that the osmolar concentration may be the same throughout both compartments it must be $12,575 \div 44 = 285.8$ milliosmols. This requires that its volume increase from 31.5 liters to $9450 \div 285.8 = 33.1$ liters, while the extracellular fluid contracts to the same extent, 1.6 liters. The end result is illustrated by the dot and dash lines. If the figure be examined it will be seen that (1) by the transfer of water the deficit of osmotic pressure in the extracellular fluid has been reduced from 50 to 14 milliosmols, and (2) the quadrangle $abcd$, which represents the loss of elec-

* This is equivalent to a normal salt solution with a sodium chloride concentration of 150 millimols. The osmolar concentration is twice as great as the molar concentration because NaCl in solution is dissociated to the ions Na^+ and Cl^-.

trolyte without its associated water, has the same area as the rectangle *aefg*, 625 milliosmols. To restore the electrolyte concentration of the extracellular fluid, therefore, it is necessary to introduce enough sodium to fill the rectangle *aefg*, that is, enough to bring the concentration of the whole volume of fluid in the body to normal. To restore *A* it is only necessary to administer 5 liters of normal saline.

Diuretic Measures and Their Modes of Operation.—Diuretic measures may be divided into three classes:

1. Those which merely increase the volume of urine without altering the fluid content of the internal environment.

2. Those which cause the volume of urine to increase under any circumstances, provoking thirst and tending to deplete body fluids.

3. Those which cause the volume of urine to increase only when the fluids of the body are unusually large or abnormally distributed.

Class 1.—The only important member of the first class is water. Under normal conditions the volume of urine excreted varies with the quantity of water taken. Although the administration of enormous amounts of water may lead to temporary excessive hydration or, by exaggerating urine volume tremendously, may sweep some salt and solutes out of the body, no such disturbances follow the ingestion of water under natural impulses, because thirst and water needs are so closely associated. Attention has already been called, however, to the advisability of giving extra salt if the fluid intake is pushed to extremes for the sake of insuring an unusually large urinary output, in infections of the urinary tract, for instance. The salt not only protects the subject against remote possibilities of water intoxication; by increasing thirst it enables the subject to drink the desired quantities of water with less discomfort.

Class 2.—*Measures which cause the volume of urine to increase under any circumstances, and which provoke thirst* and tend to deplete body fluids can be called obligatory diuretics. They can be divided into several categories. In the first belongs ablation of the function of the posterior lobe of the pituitary, which has been described above. Destruction of the adrenal cortex has a somewhat similar result, which will be discussed (p. 313) in connection with the problems of Addison's disease.

In the second category may be placed those chemical substances which gain their effect by distorting the pattern of the internal environment. Among these are organic substances such as urea and foreign saccharides, which are filtered freely through the glomeruli and only partly reabsorbed by back-diffusion. The tubules are unable to concentrate these substances beyond certain limits and are, therefore, forced to relinquish a certain amount of water if the quantities demanding excretion are excessive. Neutral salts may act in the same manner. As might be inferred from what is known of their mode of excretion the most effective salts for this purpose are those which contain ions foreign to the body or ions which normally occur in low concentration in the interstitial fluids. Sodium sulfate and potassium chloride are more effective than sodium chloride. If it is desired to deplete the fluids of the body, not merely to insure a large urine flow, it is necessary to give all diuretics of this class with *a minimum of water.*

More active diuresis is provoked by salts which alter acid-base equilibrium as well as electrolyte balance. The commonest of these are the acidifying diuretics, calcium and ammonium salts of mineral salts. Those most commonly used are calcium chloride and ammonium chloride. When calcium chloride is given the calcium ion is excreted by the gut, while the chloride ion is absorbed and must be eliminated in the urine. In the case of ammonium chloride, the ammonia is converted to urea, leaving the chloride ion to combine with base. In both cases the net effect is equivalent to the administration of a certain amount of hydrochloric acid. The reactions with NH_4Cl can be pictured in the following manner:

$$2NH_4Cl + H_2CO_3 = 2HCl + \overset{\text{urea}}{(NH_2)_2CO} + 2H_2O$$

$$HCl + NaHCO_3 = NaCl + H_2CO_3$$

Bicarbonate is displaced from combination with sodium by chloride, producing an acidosis. To rectify this disturbance the excretion of chloride by the kidneys is increased. Since chloride is a strong mineral acid it takes with it a certain amount of sodium. This, in turn, reduces the concentration of sodium in the interstitial fluids. To restore the electrolyte osmotic pressure, therefore, it is necessary to sacrifice an equivalent amount of water. Ammonium nitrate, which was first proposed by Keith[80] appears to be even more effective than the chloride, presumably because it not only causes acidosis, but also introduces a foreign ion. These salts are seldom used by themselves as diuretics because large doses, 20 gm. or more daily, are required. Such doses are likely to produce unpleasant gastric symptoms. In addition, if, instead of provoking diuresis, the chloride is retained, severe acidosis may result. The acidifying diuretics can be used to advantage, however, in moderate doses (6 to 10 gm. of NH_4Cl daily) to supplement the action of mercurial or purine diuretics. In normal persons alkalinizing salts also act as diuretics, but are far less effective than the acidifying salts. The reason for their relative failure may be that they do not distort the electrolyte pattern to the same extent. The salts used are sodium bicarbonate and sodium salts of organic acids that can be oxidized by the tissues and, therefore, from bicarbonate. The commonest of these is the citrate. Potassium salts might have a stronger effect, but cannot be given in large enough quantities to disturb the electrolyte pattern of the interstitial fluids.

Certain diuretic drugs, of which the most important are mercurials and members of the purine group, appear to act principally by inhibiting the reabsorption of water and sodium chloride, especially the latter, by the cells of the renal tubules.[8, 56, 89, 108, 133] By this reaction the tubules are protected from injurious concentrations of these drugs. If they do not produce diuresis, symptoms and signs of intoxication are prone to occur. It is, therefore, advisable, before administering either purine or mercurial diuretics, to see that the therapy is in all other respects disposed to favor diuresis.

Class 3.—*Measures that cause the volume of urine to increase only when there is abnormal retention or distribution of fluids in the body.* When salt is withdrawn from the diet of a normal individual, only small amounts of salt and water are lost before the conservative powers of the kidney are brought into play and the elimination of sodium and chloride is curtailed. If, however, there is an excessive accumulation of fluid in the body, withdrawal of salt, by putting a compulsion upon the kidney may lead to the discharge of part or all of the excessive fluid. There is no single measure which is so generally useful in the treatment of edema of all kinds as restriction of salt. Even if it does not of itself initiate diuresis it predisposes to diuresis and, therefore, should be part of the stage setting for all other diuretic measures. It removes one of the essential components of edema fluid, sodium. Furthermore, it makes restriction of the other chief essential, water, unnecessary, since it reduces thirst.

Drugs of the *digitalis* group have a diuretic action only when they relieve or abolish heart failure. Besides improving the circulation in the kidney, they promote absorption of edema fluid into the blood stream by reducing venous congestion and capillary blood pressure.

When serum albumin becomes reduced by reason of malnutrition or the profuse albuminuria of the nephrotic syndrome, edema ensues because the osmotic pressure of the proteins in the blood stream is low in proportion to the capillary blood stream. The only ultimate remedy for this condition is restitution of the serum proteins by dietary measures or disappearance of the albuminuria. However, temporary relief may be secured by introducing into the blood stream as a substitute for the depleted serum albumin, some colloid that will not escape from the capillaries. The foreign colloid which has been used most extensively for this purpose is *gum acacia*, which can be secured in sterile ampoules.* There can be no doubt that acacia may be effective in many cases. It may be employed to advantage in the treatment of shock when blood or other blood substitutes are not available; it may also be used in rare acute states when edema *per se* has become a menacing factor. After considerable experience, however, the author has abandoned it in the treatment of the edemas of nephritis, because of its tendency to produce untoward reactions of the urticarial or angioneurotic type. Sometimes these occur upon the first injection. More often they appear later. Acacia seems to have definite antigenic properties; a small test dose should, therefore, be given before a full therapeutic dose is injected.†

Injections of ascitic fluid,[27] and blood plasma or serum in native or concentrated form[3, 4] serve a similar purpose, are more effective and are attended by less danger. If the protein depletion is associated with anemia, blood transfusion is to be preferred.

The last diuretic measures that have been mentioned are directed to the reparation of some existing disorder; those which were discussed in the earlier categories aimed to disturb one equilibrium or another in such a direction that the kidneys would be put under compulsion to excrete more than the usual quantities of salt and water. All these measures are synergistic. Intelligent therapy consists in selecting that combination of diuretic procedures which is best adapted to the problem of the particular subject under treatment.

---

* This was originally put up as a 30 per cent solution in concentrated sodium chloride, to be diluted with sterile distilled water to an 8 per cent solution in normal saline. Since this necessitated the introduction of an undesirable quantity of salt, ampoules were prepared which contained acacia in distilled water. Such solutions, when mixed with blood, cause distinct hemolysis and, in the author's experience, are productive of untoward reactions. If salt free acacia is used, therefore, it should be diluted with glucose solution instead of water to give a final concentration of 8 per cent acacia in 5 per cent glucose.

† Intracutaneous tests are of no value. Because of its colloidal nature acacia attracts fluids and produces a nonspecific local reaction in persons who are not allergic to it.

CLINICAL DISORDERS OF WATER METABOLISM AND ACID-BASE EQUILIBRIUM

To consider clinical disorders of water metabolism and acid-base equilibrium entirely in relation to diseases would lead to confusion and endless repetition, because these disorders are not related to diseases themselves, but to certain phenomena that may attend these diseases. With the exception of certain conspicuous diseases in which these disorders dominate the clinical pictures, therefore, they will be considered in relation to the general functional disturbances with which they may be associated in diseases in general.

EDEMA

Local Edemas of Vascular or Lymphatic Origin.—*Lymphedema.*—Obstruction to the lymphatics of a part, most commonly the lower extremities, may result from chronic inflammation or trauma which is sufficiently extensive to destroy or obstruct the lymphatic trunks leading from the part. Occasionally the obstruction is caused by neoplasms, especially malignant neoplasms. There is an accumulation, distal to the obstruction, of fluid having a characteristic composition. Unlike the fluid usually found in hypostatic edema, it contains large quantities of protein. According to analyses by Drinker[32] and by the author[116] the concentration of protein in lymphedema, usually approaches 4 per cent. This is approximately the maximum to which Iversen and Johansen[77] have estimated that protein can be concentrated in the interstitial spaces by the interplay of capillary blood pressure and the osmotic pressure of the proteins, if these two opposing forces have their normal magnitude and the permeability of the capillaries is not altered. This is the point at which the effective osmotic pressure of the proteins (osmotic pressure of serum proteins — osmotic pressure of interstitial fluid proteins) equals the venous capillary blood pressure. With the lymphatics obstructed, proteins which gain access to the interstitial spaces are unable to escape, while the water and salts with which they were associated can be reabsorbed into the capillaries. The protein, consequently, becomes concentrated to a maximum extent. As it continues to accumulate it draws more and more fluid from the vessels. A state of equilibrium is reached when the tissue tension becomes sufficiently high to lift the fluid in the interstitial spaces to regions where the lymphatics are intact. If the affected part is elevated the edema can be made to disappear. In lymphedema of the lower extremities, for example, if the legs and hips are elevated the edema will first be transferred to the back, whereupon copious diuresis will follow. This proves conclusively that the fluid can move in the subcutaneous tissues freely under the force of gravity and that it is reabsorbed when it enters an area with uninjured lymphatics. Diuretic measures have little effect on lymphedema.

Obstruction of the thoracic duct at any point has a similar effect, but the transudation will, in this case, affect the peritoneal or pleural cavities or both, causing chylous ascites or pleuritic effusions. The fluid in these transudates will contain not only protein, but also lipids, in high concentration, because lymph coming from the intestines contains lipids. Although local accumulations of fluid of this nature are not usually regarded as problems of water metabolism, these edemas have the general composition of extracellular fluids and changes in their volume cause perceptible variations of water and salt balances.

Obstruction of the Venous Trunks.—This condition causes transudation in the tissues drained by these veins, but the edema does not attain the proportions of lymphedema because, so long as the lymphatics are intact, protein in the fluid does not reach such high concentrations.[85] If edema does become massive it may be suspected that there has been some obstruction of lymphatics as well. Motions of the legs, by increasing the flow of lymph, favor reabsorption of fluid, while they have a negligible influence upon lymphedema. The application of bandages to increase tissue tension may be of some benefit in both conditions, but offers less in lymphatic than in venous obstruction. General dehydrating or diuretic measures are not justified in such local disorders because they do so little good in proportion to the distress which they cause. For lymphedema only *surgical procedures* offer any permanent relief. The edema of venous thrombosis may be helped by bandaging and by the adoption of proper habits. Those afflicted with the condition should be taught to keep the limb warm and to hold it in the elevated position whenever it is motionless. If the lower extremity is affected they may walk, but never stand still nor sit with the leg dependent.

Edema of Portal Obstruction.—In advanced cirrhosis and other conditions which cause widespread destruction of the liver and replacement by scar tissue, ascites is prone to develop, and later, edema of the lower extremities. These have been generally attributed to obstruction of the portal venous system. Although portal obstruction undoubtedly plays a part, it is not the sole agent responsible for the edema. It has long been recognized that the appearance of ascites in cirrhosis is not directly related to the severity or the duration of the condition. In some instances it appears early as a transitory incident, to recur only in the terminal stages of the disease; in others it is not evident until the end approaches. Recent studies have disclosed that the serum proteins are characteristically altered in cirrhosis, the albumin fraction being reduced, while globulin is irregularly increased. Ascites and edema make their appearance when serum albumin falls.[19, 121] The albumin deficiency need be relatively slight to permit the development of ascites because it serves only as a contributory factor. In animals with experimental cirrhosis Bollman[15] has shown that both the reduction of serum albumin and ascites may be prevented by a diet consisting chiefly of easily assimilable carbohydrate and milk proteins. Icterus and other signs and symptoms of impairment of hepatic function are prevented or allayed by the same means. In humans, too, diets high in protein and carbohydrate, but low in fat, appear to have a favorable influence on the course of cirrhosis. Administration of large quantities of vitamin B has also been recommended.

These measures are aimed to retard the progress of the disease and eliminate or prevent ascites and edema by the restoration of serum albumin. In the presence of *ascites*, however, it may be necessary to resort to more active treatment. In fact, ascites may so far interfere with appetite and digestion as to defeat all dietary therapy. In this case paracentesis cannot be avoided. Nevertheless, efforts should be made continuously to prevent or delay reaccumulation of fluid. In addition to the dietary measures already mentioned, salt should be restricted. Urea, in doses of 20 to 60 gm. per day, may be given to promote diuresis. Ammonium chloride, in the author's experience, too often destroys appetite and provokes indigestion. The mercurial diuretics have been recommended, but should be used with caution (see discussion under heart failure, below, p. 328) and only when ascites and edema cannot be abolished or minimized by combination of the other procedures which have been mentioned.

Angioneurotic Edema.—Angioneurotic edema would require no particular mention were it not that it not infrequently occurs in diseases which affect water metabolism. The term "angioneurotic edema" is used to denote swellings of an urticarial character or local edemas of vascular origin whether or not they are allergic in origin. It is not sufficiently appreciated that such swellings are attended by perceptible retention of salt and water. Govaerts[57] has shown that the fluid in angioneurotic transudates contains protein in relatively high concentration, from which he concludes that the capillaries of the affected part lose their normal impermeability to protein.

Malnutrition Edema.—The incidence of edema in famine areas has long been recognized, but commanded particular attention in the World War of 1914–1918. Since then it has been established conclusively that this condition arises from deficiency of protein in the diet which leads to depletion of serum albumin.[110, 160] It can be reproduced in animals by diets which contain insufficient amounts of protein or by plasmapheresis. The latter procedure consists of withdrawing blood, separating the cells from the serum, and reinjecting them suspended in saline. By this means the plasma proteins are reduced without loss of blood cells. In plasmapheresis as well as in protein starvation the globulins of serum do not diminish appreciably; only albumin suffers. Apparently the capacity of the body to regenerate globulins is almost unlimited.

The mechanism of malnutrition edema should require little comment after the physiological discussion above. When the concentration of albumin falls, the protein osmotic pressure diminishes, reducing the usual resistance to the transudative force of the capillary blood pressure. A deficiency of albumin is particularly conducive to transudation because albumin is the most osmotically active fraction of the plasma proteins. Edemas referable solely to plasma albumin deficiency are seen in the clinic, but it is far commoner to find slight plasma albumin deficits acting as contributory causes of edema in conjunction with other disorders. Such a combination has just been mentioned in connection with cirrhosis of the liver. The appropriate treatment of malnutrition edema is obviously the administration of adequate amounts of protein in the diet. If this is not feasible recourse may be had to intravenous injection of plasma. The edema is responsive to salt restriction which may well be employed until diet has had an opportunity to do its work. Diuretics are seldom indicated and are too apt to have a deleterious influence on appetite and digestion.

Weech[160] has demonstrated that reduction of the concentration of serum albumin is not the most serious, but only the most obvious result of prolonged deprivation of protein. This might have been surmised, since protein is the most indispensable constituent of all tissues. Hemoglobin and red blood cells are greatly reduced, but their fall is somewhat masked by a coincidental diminution of blood volume. For the same reason the reduction of the concentration of protein in the serum is an inadequate measure of the actual albumin deficit. As the albumin diminishes the plasma volume shrinks, presumably because the protein osmotic pressure drops. As the process continues a compromise is, as usual, reached between plasma volume and protein concentration by the interaction of compensatory mechanisms. Analysis of the bodies of animals reveals the fact that the tissues are the greatest sufferers of all. Before serum albumin becomes sufficiently depleted, therefore, to cause edema, the tissues and organs throughout the body have been drained of protein.

With the discovery that malnutrition edema was referable to protein deficiency, it was for a time rather generally believed that the edema of beri-beri (avitaminosis B_1) had the same origin. Undoubtedly a large proportion of the patients seen in American clinics with vitamin B deficiency are also suffering from varying degrees of protein starvation. Frequently the edema in these cases responds rapidly to the administration of adequate amounts of protein. There are, however, reports of authentic cases of *beri-beri edema* in which the serum proteins have been normal or so nearly normal that they could not be held responsible for the edema. In these cases the edema can be attributed to heart failure arising specifically from deficiency of vitamin B_1, thiamine.[161] It is important that the two conditions be differentiated. Heart failure of beri-beri is an urgent indication for intensive thiamine therapy; it marks an advanced and critical stage of the disorder. The characteristic neuritis is the most important differential criterion. Nevertheless, the existence of a concomitant serum albumin deficiency should not be overlooked. In this, as in every other disease, edema may be produced by the summation of a number of disturbances, each one so small that individually it would be quite innocent.

Anemia.—Strauss and Fox[148] have recently shown that even moderate anemia is attended by a demonstrable retention of fluid. The explanation for this phenomenon is not entirely clear, although it may be surmised that it resides in a disturbance of the balance between capillary blood pressure and the osmotic pressure of the proteins. It is of relatively little importance *per se* because the retention of fluid seldom attains the proportions of clinical edema; however it throws some light on earlier observations that in the presence of anemia reductions of serum albumin so slight that they would ordinarily have no significance, are regularly accompanied by edema.[121] Anemia, therefore, acts as one of the numerous contributory causes of edema.

If anemia becomes sufficiently profound, the tendency to transudation of fluid from the capillaries becomes great enough to produce gross edema by itself. This is probably referable to lack of oxygen and to circulatory changes. In addition it has been demonstrated that colloids, whether acacia or protein, when added to perfusion solutions will not prevent continuous escape of fluid from the capillaries unless they are accompanied by a certain proportion of red blood cells.[131] The latter seem to be necessary to preserve the integrity of the capillaries.

The problems of acute hemorrhage will be discussed in connection with surgical shock, below (p. 319).

THE INFLUENCE OF THE ENDOCRINE GLANDS ON WATER METABOLISM AND
ACID-BASE BALANCE

From time to time attempts have been made to implicate every one of the glands of internal secretion in the control of water metabolism and acid-base balance, but there is definite evidence to involve only the pituitary, adrenal cortex and thyroid.

Pituitary Gland.—The rôle of the posterior lobe of the pituitary has been discussed above and needs only passing mention here. The most satisfactory treatment of diabetes insipidus, in our experience, is the insufflation of powdered pituitary gland.[157] This is far more economical and convenient than injections of pituitrin. The powder is sniffed up the nose, the size and frequency of the doses being regulated in accordance with the symptoms.

Edema of pituitary origin is frequently mentioned in the literature, but there is little evidence in most of the reports to indicate that the posterior lobe of the pituitary is at fault. There is no theoretical reason why this gland should not become hyperactive as other endocrine organs do. Hyperactivity of the pituitary should, however, cause not only retention of fluid, but a particular kind of retention of fluid, one which involves water, but not salt. Most of the cases described and those which have been referred to the author do not conform to this pattern; they are peculiarly susceptible to the influence of sodium chloride. The only case which bears the stamp of authenticity is one reported by Grassheim[58] with a cystic tumor of the midbrain.

Both diuretic and antidiuretic properties have been imputed to the anterior lobe of the pituitary, but no convincing evidence has been adduced that this portion of the hypophysis has any direct action upon the kidneys. It does appear to have been reasonably well established that removal of the posterior lobe will not cause diabetes insipidus unless the anterior lobe is intact. In other words the diuretic action of ablation of the posterior lobe is conditioned by the presence of the anterior lobe.

The Suprarenal Glands.—Epinephrine, through its action on the circulation, may vary the volume of urine; but this is of no great clinical significance. Because it acts upon the arterioles, it affects chiefly glomerular filtration. In urticaria or angioneurotic edema of allergic origin, epinephrine, by alleviating the edema, may exert a transient diuretic effect.

It has long been recognized that in the shock which marks the crises of **Addison's disease** the blood becomes inspissated and that in the agonal stages of the disease urine excretion ceases. It was assumed quite naturally that these disturbances of the distribution and elimination of water were merely sequelae of hypotension and comparable to the disturbances encountered in traumatic shock. It was discovered by Loeb[90] in 1932 and rapidly confirmed by numerous other investigators that removal of the adrenals is followed by characteristic changes of water and salt equilibria. Reabsorption of sodium salts by the renal tubules is strikingly diminished, consequently the concentration of sodium in the interstitial fluids falls. There is a coincident reduction of the concentration of chloride + bicarbonate of serum, in which the two ions participate to a varying degree. In some cases bicarbonate bears the brunt of the deficiency; in the majority chloride suffers most. By the administration of large quantities of sodium chloride and bicarbonate (or its equivalent, citrate) it may be possible to mitigate or prevent the serum sodium deficit. If chloride is withdrawn from the diet, on the other hand, excretion of sodium and chloride does not cease promptly as it does in normals, but continues unabated after the concentration of these ions in the serum has fallen far below normal. In consequence serum sodium falls precipitately and a crisis is likely to ensue. Crises may also be induced by vomiting, diarrhea, or other conditions in which sodium salts are wasted through extrarenal channels.

With the initial diuresis of sodium salts a certain amount of water is also sacrificed, but the depletion of sodium regularly exceeds that of water.[64] As the condition proceeds and signs and symptoms of circulatory collapse appear, the urine volume diminishes and finally ceases. Sodium deficiency is not alone responsible for this collapse. It may be impossible to revive a patient from collapse by the most vigorous administration of salt solution. Patients may die suddenly in the course of the disease when serum sodium is quite normal.

In the premortal state the concentration of potassium in the serum may rise, though seldom to the levels at which potassium poisoning is likely to occur. Nevertheless, the metabolism of potassium is disturbed. During the early sodium diuresis the urinary excretion of potassium diminishes, although its concentration in the serum does not rise until far later.[64] The retained potassium must remain in the tissue cells. During recovery from a crisis, urinary potassium rises, while sodium diminishes.

The symptoms of collapse cannot be due to dehydration since, during recovery, water is swept out with potassium. Nilson[105] and Kendall[5] have shown that dogs can be maintained indefinitely with both adrenals removed if they are given diets containing excessive quantities of sodium and restricted amounts of potassium. Wilder and associates[164] advocate similar diets for the treatment of Addison's disease and have demonstrated that reduction of potassium in the diet of patients suffering from this disease diminishes the wastage of sodium.

Reduction of the concentration of sodium and thereby of the osmotic pressure of the interstitial fluids should cause the cells in the body to swell. Accumulation of potassium in the cells should exaggerate this tendency. Harrison and Darrow,[62] however, found that the increase of cellular potassium in animals is not attended by a proportional accession of water, suggesting that the extra potassium is not osmotically active. The metabolic abnormalities of Addison's disease or adrenalectomy are not confined solely to water and the electrolytes; they involve also carbohydrate and protein. It seems quite probable that the derangement of potassium is connected with dislocations of the vital chemical processes within the cells.

In the *crises* of Addison's disease the fluid exchange between capillaries and interstitial fluid is also disturbed. As the pressure falls the blood becomes more and more inspissated, plasma proteins, hemoglobin and blood count rising progressively. In this respect adrenal cortical shock resembles traumatic shock. However, there seems to be less tendency for proteins to escape with plasma filtrate from the capillaries. The administration of saline at this stage may fail entirely to reinstitute urine flow, to restore the blood pressure, or to produce a sustained increase of blood volume; it may only escape rapidly into the interstitial fluids to form edema. Transfusions are of little value. In other respects the circulatory collapse of Addison's disease is distinctive: it is usually attended by elevation of temperature and often by signs of peripheral vasodilatation in contrast to the peripheral constriction and subnormal temperature of traumatic shock.

Although the metabolic disorders of Addison's disease may aid in the diagnosis of the condition, none have the pathognomonic significance that has been attributed to them. Reduction of the concentration of sodium and failure to retain administered sodium salts are common in advanced renal insufficiency and in certain diseases of the lungs which are discussed below. Withdrawal of sodium from the diet does not, in these conditions, provoke such serious symptoms as it does in Addison's disease; but it is extremely hazardous to precipitate a crisis merely to establish a diagnosis. Sodium restriction in doubtful cases should be practiced with the greatest caution and with assiduous attention to the concentration of chloride + bicarbonate in the serum. A rising blood nonprotein nitrogen may give a clue; but the appearance of azotemia is a danger signal, denoting the onset of renal failure and impending circulatory collapse. The occurrence of hypoglycemia in the postabsorptive period or after test doses of glucose is valuable corroborative evidence.[155] Ultimately in this, as in most other diseases, diagnosis must depend on analysis of all the clinical evidence available; it cannot be established by the laboratory alone.

Treatment.—This involves administration of enough sodium chloride and bicarbonate to balance the sodium lost in the urine and to maintain a normal concentration of sodium (or chloride + bicarbonate) in the serum. In the presence of vomiting, diarrhea, or any symptoms that prevent ingestion of salt, sodium chloride must be given subcutaneously, or intravenously in hypertonic solution, if the sodium deficit is great. The dosage must be adjusted to the needs of the individual patient and may vary from 5 to 10 gm. in addition to that in the diet to 30 or 40 gm. Part may be added to the food, the rest given in tablets, capsules, tomato juice, soups, and other fluids, or even as normal saline. Carbohydrate should also be given in generous quantities at frequent intervals to prevent hypoglycemia.

A number of steroids have been isolated from the adrenal cortex which are more or less effective in preventing or relieving the symptoms and signs of Addison's disease or experimental adrenalectomy. Of these, corticosterone appears to replace most completely the endogenous hormone. Several potent extracts are available on the market. These should be employed without delay, when a crisis is present or imminent, in frequent and massive doses (25 to 50 cc. of a potent extract every four to six hours). It is probably advisable, when possible, to use smaller doses, 5 to 20 cc. daily, for maintenance treatment as well. With this aid less salt is required. Furthermore, it may prevent the sudden collapse which has carried off many patients unexpectedly when salt, water, and blood sugar seem perfectly regulated. A synthetic product, desoxycorticosterone, has been prepared which closely resembles in chemical structure and physiological action, the extracted product, corticosterone.[146] Unlike the latter it has little or no influence on carbohydrate metabolism, although it relieves the electrolyte disorder completely. Nevertheless, it has been used successfully over long periods for the treatment of Addison's disease.[153] Apparently, if the balance of water and electrolytes is preserved, hypoglycemia is not prone to occur. Thorn and his associates[153, 155] have shown that patients with Addison's disease may be kept in good health for long periods by the implantation beneath the skin of solid pellets of this material.

Thorn[154] has shown that the administration of large doses of *adrenal cortical extracts* or corticosterone in normal men is followed by a temporary reduction of the excretion of sodium salts and water. Ragan, Ferrebee, Phyte, Atchley and Loeb[125] have reported that excessive doses of desoxycorticosterone give rise to a condition resembling diabetes insipidus. It might be expected that a condition the reverse of Addison's disease would result from tumors or hyperplasia of the adrenal cortex with functional hyperactivity. McQuarrie[100] has reported a case in which serum sodium was abnormally high, but such cases must be rare. In these conditions, as in pituitary basophilism, the author has been unable to detect any anomalies of salt and water metabolism that could not be imputed to the heart failure and renal insufficiency which patients with these conditions usually develop.

Sexual Hormones.—Thorn[152] claims that a variety of sexual hormones chemically resembling corticosterone have a similar, but lesser, effect on salt and water excretion. He has also presented certain data, not entirely consistent or convincing, suggesting the existence of fluctuations of salt and water balances bearing a rough relation to the menstrual rhythm.[156] Beyond this there is no evidence that the gonads have any influence upon the metabolism of salt or water. Zuckerman's[106] demonstration of retention of water and salt by some female apes during heat is not relevant to human physiology, because these animals are endowed with "sexual skin" which swells greatly during the period of sexual activity. There are, nevertheless, authentic reports of women who regularly develop edema of varying degree during or about the menstrual period.[7] By some these edemas have been attributed to disorders of the pituitary; others would relate them directly to abnormal activity of the ovaries.

Thyroid.—Ord,[107] in 1878, called attention to the accumulation of a gelatinous type of fluid in the interstitial tissues of a patient who died of myxedema. It is from this characteristic that the disease acquired its name. This edema is rapidly discharged when active thyroid preparations are given. During this diuresis Boothby and associates[16] found that nitrogen was lost in the urine in such proportions to weight as to indicate that the edema fluid contained about 2 per cent of protein. With the diuresis sodium is swept out, with a minimum of potassium[20]; the fluid, therefore, is presumably lodged in the extracellular compartment. In keeping with the idea that there is an accumulation of fluid containing protein in the interstitial spaces, are (a) the observation by Deusch[29] that the serum proteins are elevated and (b) the discovery by Thompson[151] that the blood volume is low and rises after thyroid therapy.

Although there is a definite retention of salt and water in myxedema, there is no clear evidence of an opposite condition in hyperthyroidism. Abnormally large blood volumes reported by Blumgart, Gargill and Gilligan[14] may be only effects of vasodilatation and accelerated circulation. Claims that thyroid has a specific diuretic action, advanced by Eppinger[37] are not substantiated by his own experimental protocols. There is some evidence that the thyroid may have an influence upon experimental diabetes insipidus of dogs.[92]

Hyperthyroid subjects eliminate more than the usual proportion of heat produced in metabolism by vaporization of water through insensible perspiration.[78] In addition they are particularly prone to sweat. Conversely myxedematous patients lose less than the normal proportion of heat by insensible perspiration.[53] Measurement of insensible perspiration as a means of estimating basal metabolism in these conditions, as has been recommended, is, therefore, subject to variable and not inconsiderable error.

EXCESSIVE SWEATING

The effects of excessive sweating in depleting the body of salt and water have been discussed above. The evils of sweating lie not only in the immediate dehydration which it causes; but in the reduction of the concentration of sodium and electrolyte osmotic pressure that follows subsequent attempts to restore the water without salt under the compulsion of thirst. Toxic symptoms and collapse may be induced in fever therapy if care is not taken to provide patients with sufficient salt and water.[51] In all febrile or other pathological states attended by excessive sweating not only water, but also salt, should be given in sufficient quantities to replace losses by the skin.

PULMONARY DISEASES ACCOMPANIED BY SALT DEPLETION

Lobar Pneumonia

It was early recognized that in lobar pneumonia urinary excretion of chloride may diminish almost to the vanishing point. With this reduction of chloride excretion the concentrations of chloride and sodium in the serum are found to be depressed. From studies of Sunderman[149] and Wilder and Drake[165] it appears that for some reason, the subject with lobar pneumonia tends to maintain the concentration of sodium and chloride in the interstitial fluids at an abnormally low level. If salt is withheld, chloride, sodium and water are wasted through the kidneys. If the patient receives salt poor fluids, according to the customary therapeutic regimens, the usual compromise is made between fluid volume and osmotic pressure. There is some dehydration with greater salt depletion. If excessive amounts of salt are given, the concentrations of sodium and chloride cannot be forced quite to the normal level. Instead water is retained and edema may result. Sputum and sweat serve as additional vehicles for the elimination of salt. Bicarbonate is little affected by these disturbances. Clinical experience indicates that administration of enough salt during the acute stages of the disease to replace and prevent losses influences the course of the disease favorably. For adults 10 to 15 gm. of sodium chloride daily is usually sufficient; for infants and children Wilder and Drake[165] recommended about 0.2 gm. per Kg. of body weight per day. After the crisis salt and water balances rapidly become normal. Similar phenomena have been noted in a variety of other acute febrile diseases, such as typhus fever and acute rheumatic fever, but in these diseases they do not occur so consistently. Partly because of the salt wastage, administration of adrenal cortical extracts has been advocated for the treatment of lobar pneumonia. Newburger,[103] however, was unable to alter the chloride balances of patients with pneumonia by means of cortical extract.

Pulmonary Emphysema

In pulmonary emphysema and other conditions associated with severe impairment of the respiratory gas exchange, especially when there is obstruction of the upper respiratory passages, the tension of CO_2 in the blood increases. Under these circumstances compensation of the pH disturbance is established by increase of serum bicarbonate, which, in turn, displaces chloride.[119] This is a true condition of primary CO_2 excess (*vide supra*). Water balance, the volume of fluids in the body and the concentration of sodium in these fluids are not appreciably altered. A certain amount of chloride in the interstitial fluid is replaced by bicarbonate, the sum of the two remaining normal.

Tuberculosis and Other Chronic Conditions of the Lungs

In certain patients with advanced *pulmonary tuberculosis* or other chronic diseases of the lungs, Winkler and Crankshaw[167] noted reduction of the concentration of chloride in the serum without a concomitant increase of bicarbonate. Hypochloremia had been reported previously in such conditions. There were no associated symptoms that could be directly related to the salt deficiencies, but most of the patients who exhibited the phenomenon were extremely ill. If no salt or only the usual quantity was given the concentrations of sodium and chloride fell to extremely low levels; but in none of the patients did signs of collapse appear. Large amounts (10 to 20 gm.) of sodium chloride, given by mouth, subcutaneously or intravenously, were excreted with great rapidity. Only by administration of as much as 20 gm. of sodium chloride daily was it possible to maintain normal concentrations of chloride and sodium in the serum with a balanced intake and output. The bicarbonate of serum was not consistently disturbed, nor was any disorder of water metabolism demonstrated.* Special interest attaches to these cases because their reactions in so many respects resemble those of patients with Addison's disease. The combination of tuberculosis, sodium wastage, and frequently low blood pressure, certainly suggests adrenal cortical deficiency. Nevertheless, autopsies in some of these patients revealed intact suprarenal glands. The absence of any striking clinical change when the intake of salt is varied aids in the exclusion of Addison's disease. In a few instances administration of large doses of cortical extract has had no effect on the salt exchange or the serum chlorides.[116] If this should prove to be regularly true, the reaction to such extracts would be a valuable diagnostic aid.

Hyperventilation.—Breathing in excess of the physiological requirements tends to pump carbon dioxide out of the blood, thereby producing alkalosis by increasing the ratio $\dfrac{H_2CO_3}{NaHCO_3}$ in the serum and in the interstitial fluids. If the pH is driven far in the alkaline direction *tetany* results. The first symptoms of tetany are usually tingling of the fingers or toes, followed by typical carpopedal spasm, and ultimately by general spasms or convulsions. Acute hyperventilation is not uncommon, occurring especially in unstable persons under sudden emotional stress. It seldom reaches serious proportions.

* The condition of the patients made studies of water balance difficult, however; and no definite conclusions can properly be drawn in this respect until the subject has been more carefully investigated.

In patients who have a preexisting alkalosis from other causes, such as vomiting or excessive alkaline therapy, only moderate hyperventilation is required to precipitate severe tetany. It is for this reason that the vomiting patient is likely to burst into overt gastric tetany only when excited. Primary overventilation tetany ceases as soon as the respirations are quieted or the breath is held. Rebreathing into a paper bag is an effective way to check it. The treatment of gastric tetany or the tetany of primary alkali excess should be directed toward rectification of the abnormal serum electrolyte pattern by removal of its cause.

Chronic hyperventilation is occasionally encountered in patients with lesions of the basal ganglia in the region of the midbrain, especially individuals suffering from the postencephalitic syndrome. The overventilation of these patients may be so extreme and continuous that the carbon dioxide tension is persistently lowered. This leads to a compensatory excretion of bicarbonate in the urine and replacement of serum bicarbonate by chloride: primary CO_2 deficit with secondary bicarbonate deficiency.[120] Tetany may be absent or intermittent, depending on the degree of compensation.

The Nature of "Shock" and Its Effect on Water Distribution

Although it embodies a fallacy, the best working definition of shock is *any condition in which the volume of circulating blood is too small in proportion to the size of the vascular bed.* The fallacy or paradox lies in the fact that in an elastic system filled with fluid, the volume of fluid must always equal the volume of the system in which it moves. The definition, however, implies relative vasodilatation with stagnation in the peripheral parts of the circulation. Shock can be produced by hemorrhage, by extreme loss of fluid, or by any condition that leads to the accumulation and stagnation of a large amount of blood in a particular part of the circulation. In the last class may be placed the shocks occasioned by distention of the pericardium or by occlusion of a coronary artery. A general discussion of the circulatory phenomena of shock is not relevant to the purpose of this chapter; but certain features of the condition can not be neglected because they involve profound changes in both the internal and external exchanges of water and salt. Most of these can be best illustrated by a general discussion of the effects of hemorrhage.

The loss of a moderate amount of blood is followed by a transient drop of blood pressure. Peripheral vasoconstriction promptly takes up the slack in the vascular bed and subsequently fluid is withdrawn from the interstitial spaces to restore the blood volume. A falling blood count after hemorrhage is a favorable sign if there is certainty that bleeding has ceased. If the hemorrhage is larger compensation is neither so prompt nor so complete; the blood pressure remains low longer, the blood volume is more slowly restored and does not reach the normal magnitude. Finally, if the hemorrhage is very large, the blood pressure, after the initial drop, rises only slightly and temporarily, thereafter gradually falling again progressively to reach levels incompatible with life. Anuria and loss of consciousness are parts of the terminal picture.

The temporary collapse that follows moderate hemorrhage may be spoken of as primary collapse. Recovery in this stage may be accelerated by replacing the fluid lost with saline solution. The progressive fall of blood

11

pressure that follows more severe hemorrhage may be termed secondary shock. In primary shock, if blood loss is not too great, blood volume can be spontaneously restored by withdrawal of water and salt from the interstitial fluids. In secondary shock fluid tends to escape from the blood stream, further reducing the blood volume. Rising of hemoglobin and red blood cells after hemorrhage constitutes a danger signal. At first the concentration of proteins in the plasma also rises, further evidence of inspissation of the blood; but as the condition progresses the concentration of proteins may fall. The capillaries have now become more pervious and protein is leaking through their walls.

Blalock and his associates,[10,11] have shown that if solutions containing salt or other diffusible materials are injected intravenously when the blood pressure is falling in shock, they are not retained in the blood stream, but rapidly escape into the tissues and, furthermore, carry proteins with them. Although, while the solution is flowing into the vein the blood volume may be kept up and the blood pressure sustained, the end result of such infusions in this state is deleterious, not beneficial. Only a solution containing colloids can reverse the flow of fluid and permanently reconstitute the volume of the circulating blood. For this purpose acacia may be used in emergency with the precautions prescribed above, but it is distinctly inferior to blood plasma. If shock from any cause, but especially from hemorrhage, is profound, nothing is so efficacious as *transfusion of whole blood*. In case of internal hemorrhage transfusions are frequently withheld lest, by increasing blood pressure, they cause renewed bleeding. It is doubtful whether fears on this score are entirely justified. In shock there is a peripheral vasoconstriction, but probably congestion and even paralysis of the visceral circulation.[42, 43] Transfusion restores not only the volume, but also the proper distribution of the circulating blood. In the last analysis, however, these philosophical questions are of relatively little importance; there is no reason to prefer death from shock to death from hemorrhage. If the former is to be avoided, transfusion of blood or plasma is imperative before the vicious cycle of transudation of fluid and protein becomes irreversible. If the integrity of the circulatory system can be maintained, hemorrhage can be attacked by direct surgical procedures.

Saline should be given to replace fluid lost; but while the blood pressure is low or falling, subcutaneous injection is to be preferred to intravenous. If or when competence of the circulation is established, the fluid will be absorbed into the blood stream and redistributed. Until the circulation is competent no danger of depleting blood proteins is incurred. Glucose, on the other hand, should be given intravenously, because when it is given subcutaneously it is not absorbed rapidly and tends at first to draw water and solutes into itself from the rest of the body.* In order to minimize transudation, the glucose should be given as a concentrated solution in a small volume of water, not more than 500 cc. of 10 per cent glucose at one time (50 to 100 cc. of 50 per cent glucose may be used). Never should hypertonic solu-

---

* Glucose diffuses more slowly than sodium chloride. When, therefore, glucose solution is injected into the subcutaneous tissues, salt diffuses into the pool of solution more rapidly than glucose diffuses out. The osmotic pressure in the pool is thereby raised, attracting water, which temporarily increases the volume of the pool at the expense of the other fluids in the body.

tions be given subcutaneously, because they tend to draw into them fluid from other parts of the body.

What has been said of the shock of hemorrhage holds equally for other types of shock. Transfusions of blood plasma or whole blood should be used if the blood pressure falls, even if there has been no actual loss of blood. Nor should these measures be delayed until the blood pressure has reached the critical point. The time to act is before or during the drop of pressure, while the process is reversible. One of the principal reactions to shock is constriction of the peripheral vessels, evidenced in the cold, pale skin. This is an emergency measure to shunt as much blood as possible into the more important parts of the circulation. For the moment it also sustains the blood pressure. Freeman[42, 43] has shown that this reaction is not altogether beneficial because it sacrifices certain tissues or organs for the sake of others. To be successful, therapy must restore the circulation before the emergency reaction fails or leads to irreversible injury.

THE EFFECTS OF DISEASES AND DISORDERS OF THE GASTRO-INTESTINAL TRACT ON WATER METABOLISM AND ACID-BASE BALANCE

The disturbances of water and salt metabolism and acid-base balances associated with disorders of the alimentary canal are all implicit in gastro-intestinal physiology. Nevertheless, it is the unfortunate truth that they are often exaggerated or even induced by well-intentioned but misdirected efforts of physicians. Most deplorable is the tendency to follow routine regimens in the treatment of certain diseases without consideration of the distinctive features which different individuals exhibit. Meulengracht,[101] with his liberal diets for the treatment of peptic ulcer, represents a healthy revolt against the recurrent evil of multiple meals of an unbalanced and inadequate type with unlimited doses of alkali. It is only this last feature which need engage our immediate attention. Since there have been simple clinical methods for the measurement of serum bicarbonate it has been repeatedly demonstrated that these regimens give rise to serious alkalosis in a proportion of patients, more often those in the older age group who have a certain amount of arteriosclerosis and renal disease.[34, 36] To escape this difficulty many clinicians have abandoned sodium bicarbonate, adopting in its stead alkaline salts of the bivalent metals. These are, however, given in such large doses, that they may be quite as harmful.[22] There is no particular virtue in treating all patients with peptic ulcers by milk mixtures every hour or two. Redistribution of more normal feedings to conform to the incidence of pain in each individual case, with interpolation of extra feedings at night and to break the longest interval between meals during the day, will allay symptoms in most cases and at the same time avoid the production of deficiency states. Belladonna, if given in the same individualized manner, is extremely useful. If recourse must be had to alkalis for relief of pain or symptoms, it is usually a sign that other therapeutic measures have been ineptly prescribed.

Vomiting.—A moderate degree of vomiting may interfere with nutrition, but has little effect on water and electrolyte exchange so long as the subject continues to ingest food and fluids. If there is doubt about the severity of vomiting, useful information may be secured by analyzing the urine for acetone and chloride and the serum for chloride and bicarbonate. If, after vomiting has persisted twenty-four hours or more, the urine contains no acetone and normal amounts of chloride, especially if serum chloride and bicarbonate are also normal, it may be inferred that, in spite of emesis, the patient must have retained and absorbed enough carbohydrate to preserve hepatic glycogen stores and enough salt and water to prevent sodium depletion and serious dehydration.

Vomiting may disturb electrolyte and acid-base equilibrium in two ways. By interfering with the assimilation of carbohydrate, it may give rise to starvation ketosis. The β-hydroxybutyric acid thus produced will displace bicarbonate from combination with sodium, giving rise to acidosis. On the other hand, the vomitus will remove from the body chloride and sodium in varying proportions, depending upon the concentration of hydrochloric acid in the gastric secretions. If the vomitus is strongly acid, chloride will become depleted, and will be replaced by bicarbonate to produce alkalosis. In adults with normal gastric secretory function chloride depletion and bicarbonate excess with alkalosis are most frequently encountered. In infants and pregnant women *starvation acidosis* dominates the picture because both infants and pregnant women apparently use available carbohydrate more lavishly and wastefully than do nonpregnant adults, and therefore develop earlier and more intense *starvation ketosis*. In addition the gastric secretions in pregnancy contain less than normal quantities of free hydrochloric acid. Patients with achlorhydria also tend to develop acidosis rather than alkalosis.

Whether bicarbonate or chloride suffers most, sodium is always sacrificed by the vomiting subject, in the vomitus and in the urine. Gastric secretions are seldom so acid that they contain no sodium and in achlorhydria may contain as much sodium as chloride. But if only chloride is lost in the vomitus, sodium is excreted in the urine to aid in elimination of ketone acids and to mitigate bicarbonate excess and consequent alkalosis. With this sodium water is also sacrificed in behalf of the electrolyte osmotic pressure. The loss of sodium, however, almost invariably exceeds the loss of water; the concentration of sodium in serum and interstitial fluids, therefore, falls. The explanation for this discrepancy lies in the fact that if water is taken by mouth, chloride and sodium are added to it in the stomach in the usual manner to bring its osmotic pressure to that of the serum. These elements are then lost in the vomitus.

Pyloric Obstruction.—The classical example of vomiting is found in pyloric obstruction, which has been exquisitely analyzed by Gamble.[44, 48] Its effects on the serum and interstitial fluids and the manner in which they are brought about are represented in the diagrams of figure 24. For the sake of clarity the various reactions have been pictured as occurring serially in a stepwise fashion, whereas in point of fact they merge into a continuous progression. For purposes of simplification only sodium, chloride, and bicarbonate are shown and the concentration of sodium is arbitrarily represented as equal to the concentration of chloride + bicarbonate, whereas it is actually greater. As usual the vertical dimension indicates concentration, the horizontal dimension, volume of interstitial fluid. Below the various pairs of columns are set down the quantities of materials lost in vomitus and urine, expressed in per cent of the quantities originally in the subject. *A* represents the original normal state. In *B*, 10 per cent of the chloride has been vomited and the sodium with which it was united has combined with carbonic acid to form bicarbonate. There is, therefore, a bicarbonate excess or alkalosis. Actually there would be a simultaneous loss of some water and sodium and development of ketosis. The last would involve only the substitution of a small amount of β-hydroxybutyric and aceto-acetic acids for part of the bicarbonate. In *C*, by the excretion in an alkaline urine of 5 per cent of the sodium, in the form of bicarbonate, about two-thirds of the bicarbonate excess has been eliminated, but at the same time a deficit of sodium, and hence of electrolyte osmotic pressure has been produced. In *D*, by excretion in the urine of 5 per cent of the water from the interstitial fluids, the concentration of sodium and electrolyte osmotic pressure have been restored; bicarbonate is slightly elevated and chloride slightly depressed, but the acid-base balance is not grossly distorted. This may be called the stage of osmotic

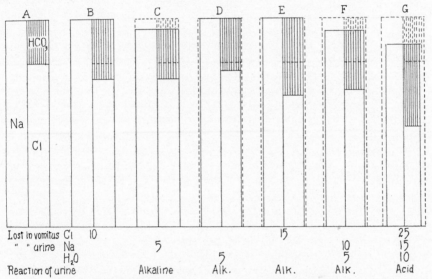

Fig. 24.—A schematic representation of the effect of vomiting in pyloric obstruction on the electrolyte pattern and volume of the extracellular fluids. In each pair of columns the vertical dimension represents osmolar concentration, the horizontal dimension, volume of fluid. For purposes of simplification only Na, Cl and HCO₃ are depicted. The broken lines in each case indicate the pattern of normal interstitial fluid for comparison. Below the diagram are given in per cent the proportions of Cl, Na and water that have been lost at each interval.

compensation. In *E*, vomiting has made new inroads upon Cl, to the extent of 15 per cent, bicarbonate increasing to an equivalent degree. In *F*, further sodium as bicarbonate and water has been excreted, but compensation this time has been less complete; volume has not been altogether sacrificed for osmotic pressure or acid-base balance; a compromise has been reached in which sodium (electrolyte osmotic pressure), fluid volume, and the balance between chloride and bicarbonate have all had to yield somewhat. In *G*, loss of Cl has advanced another 25 per cent and compensation has been still more incomplete. The body is clinging tenaciously to base and fluid to the neglect of acid-base equilibrium. In this stage, when dehydration and depletion of sodium and chloride are extreme, a peculiar anomaly is observed:

As early as *C* chloride practically disappeared from the urine, which had become alkaline and loaded with bicarbonate. This state continued through F and into G. In spite of this valiant attempt to restore acid-base balance, serum bicarbonate excess steadily increased. Nevertheless, when the extreme condition of G is reached, the urine becomes acid and free from bicarbonate.[48, 67] The kidneys refuse to sacrifice any more sodium to preserve the concentration of bicarbonate and the pH at the expense of electrolyte osmotic pressure. Parenteral administration of sodium chloride at this juncture, while it reduces bicarbonate and tends to lower the pH of the serum, causes the reappearance of alkaline urine containing bicarbonate. When sodium is made available in combination with chloride to restore electrolyte osmotic pressure, the body can afford to release some sodium with bicarbonate into the urine to mitigate alkalosis.

It should be unnecessary to point out the variants in this sequence of events and in the ultimate patterns of the interstitial fluids that attend vomiting of neutral gastric contents, or losses of alkaline secretions through fistulae of the pancreas or intestines. The differences between them lie chiefly in the relative proportions of bicarbonate and chloride which are lost. In the vomiting of achlorhydria sodium chloride is withdrawn as such, consequently bicarbonate excess and alkalosis are not so prominent. With fistulae of the pancreas or intestines more bicarbonate than chloride is lost, therefore a bicarbonate deficit with acidosis ensues, while chloride is relatively increased. In all disorders that lead to discharge of gastro-intestinal contents, ultimately sodium and water become greatly depleted. Sodium invariably suffers more than water, principally because ingestion of water tends to wash out extra salt. As dehydration and salt depletion progress, circulation and renal function deteriorate. The final stages are marked by shock and anuria. But before this point has been reached the blood nonprotein nitrogen may rise as the result of the interplay of a variety of factors. Protein catabolism is increased, the circulation of the kidneys may be impaired, and little water is available for the formation of urine. Finally McCance[96, 97, 98] has discovered that in states of salt depletion glomerular filtration diminishes and water is excreted less promptly than usual.

The Treatment of Obstruction of the Gastro-intestinal Tract.[113]—Obstruction of the gastro-intestinal tract not only prevents progress of food and fluids through the lumen of the canal; it also seems to inhibit absorption. Secretions and other materials therefore tend to accumulate and to cause distention. This impairs the circulation to the gut, thus further embarrassing function. In addition the distention leads to vomiting with all the resultant disorders that have been described above. Treatment is logically directed to removal of the obstruction, relief of distention, and restoration of the salt and water supplies of the body. Immediate operative interference may be inadvisable either because the general condition of the patient does not warrant operation or because there is reasonable hope that the obstruction may be overcome without operation. In any case preliminary treatment to relieve the distention is desirable. Current procedures for this purpose consist of introducing tubes through the nose and mouth which permit removal of accumulated fluids and gas and, if desired, lavage of the obstructed viscus. The introduction of foreign matter, however, provokes motor and secretory activity and the removal of products of secretion promotes the dehydration and salt depletion which it is desired to check.

Foster[41] demonstrated that after ligation of the pylorus dogs vomit but a short while. If no foods nor fluids were given by mouth, after this preliminary period all activity of the stomach ceased. If only enough saline was given to replace the electrolyte and water lost in the initial vomitus such dogs lived quite as long as dogs without pyloric obstruction who were deprived of food and water. That the same procedure may be practised successfully in humans with pyloric obstruction has been demonstrated by the author.[113] *Withdrawal of fluid must be absolute;* not even cracked ice or sips of water should be allowed. Vomiting subsides rapidly, to cease entirely within forty-eight hours. Thus far, in a small series of cases failure has been recorded only once, and then in an elderly patient with a large ulcerating carcinoma that bled continuously. The blood in this case may have served as a stimulus to maintain gastric secretory activity. It may be advisable to introduce a tube to empty the stomach, if it is greatly distended, at the very outset of treatment; but after this the use of a tube is quite unnecessary. It is not improbable that the same principle could be employed for obstructions lower down in the gastro-intestinal tract; but this has not yet been studied in a series of cases sufficiently large and varied to justify any conclusions. There is reason to believe that secretory activity of the whole digestive tract is evoked only by the presence of food or fluid in the stomach or gut.

If it is elected or proves necessary to use lavage or to introduce fluid of any kind, care should be taken that this fluid is made isotonic with serum by means of salt. Crider and Thomas[23] have shown that isotonic solutions of glucose or saline when placed in the gut elicit no secretory response from the pancreas or intestine, whereas water does. It was pointed out in the discussion of gastro-intestinal physiology above that before water can be absorbed it must be brought into osmotic equilibrium with serum by the addition of salt from the blood, and that extra water is secreted with this salt. It has been demonstrated that lavage with isotonic salt solution withdraws minimal quantities of salt and fluid from the body, while lavage with water withdraws enormous amounts.[113] It is especially important to avoid the use of water if the tube lies in the ileum, because it has been found by Dennis[28] that water has an injurious effect upon the ileal mucosa. In postoperative treatment the same principles obtain. In patients with fistulae or enterostomies the administration with foods and fluids of enough salt to make these materials isotonic with blood serum may also allay motor activity of the intestines, reduce the volume of discharge from the stoma and thus promote absorption. In general these measures serve to reduce not only discharges from the gastro-intestinal tract but also drainage of salt and water from the interstitial fluids.

The restoration and maintenance of the salt and water of the interstitial fluids require little special attention in this particular connection. The principles which determine the quantities of salt, water, and glucose which are required in states of dehydration and salt depletion are the same quite irrespective of the channels through which salt and water have been lost. They have been adequately discussed under water and salt requirements above. The treatment of shock has also been described. For replacement of electrolytes only sodium chloride is required. No special attention need be given to the readjustment of the details of the acid-base pattern. If enough sodium chloride and water are given to replace the deficits of sodium and water and to permit the kidneys to work efficiently, these organs will soon make the necessary rearrangements of details by excreting chloride or bicarbonate selectively. If bicarbonate deficit or excess persists it may be inferred that the gross deficiency of salt has not been fully repaired. It would, of course, be possible to give a semblance of normality to the electrolyte pattern in F of figure 24 by administration of relatively small amounts of ammonium chloride. This would overcome the bicarbonate excess and restore chloride, but dehydration and sodium depletion would remain untouched. Gratification of chemical esthetics is a poor substitute for the satisfaction of physiological needs.

Diarrhea.—Because feces normally are alkaline, it is usually held that diarrhea produces bicarbonate deficit and acidosis. This, indeed, appears to be its commonest effect in infants[65]; bicarbonate is usually reduced, chloride excessively high. In adults, however, there seems to be less consistency in the acid-base disorder[116]; even frank bicarbonate excess with alkalosis is not uncommon. The difference in reaction may be related to the greater tendency of infants to develop acidosis under any circumstances, even after vomiting, which was referred to above. It may also be connected with differences in the functional disorders behind various diarrheas. The subject requires more careful analysis. The *treatment*, besides measures to check the diarrhea itself, consists of replenishing and maintaining the salt and water supplies of the body. For this purpose Hartmann[66] recommended, in infants, the use of alkali as well as sodium chloride, to combat the acidosis. The alkali which he advocates is sodium lactate. The sodium of this salt becomes available for the formation of bicarbonate when the lactate is oxidized; the lactate serves as a substitute for carbohydrate. If a suitable lactate solution is convenient, the combination of saline and lactate lends elegance to the therapy. However, Hoag and Marples[76] have demonstrated that satisfactory results can be secured with sodium chloride alone, or better with sodium chloride and glucose, if enough fluid is given to overcome dehydration and salt depletion and to establish an adequate flow of urine. Again it should be emphasized that it is more important to correct the gross defects of water and salt balance than to attempt the adjustment of minor derangements of the ionic pattern of the serum.

Gastro-intestinal Hemorrhage.—A word of caution was given in the discussion of shock (p. 320) against the tendency to delay transfusion after massive gastro-intestinal hemorrhage for fear of precipitating fresh bleeding. Shock is an imperative indication for appropriate therapy and the medical treatment of gastro-intestinal hemorrhage is essentially that of shock. It has been repeatedly noted that after massive hemorrhage into the stomach or intestines the blood nonprotein nitrogen rises. The most fanciful explanations have been advanced for this *azotemia*, some of them involving hypothetical toxic products generated in the intestines. There is no obvious reason for dragging in such hypotheses. Massive hemorrhage gives rise to increased destruction of protein and is followed by circulatory disturbances that diminish glomerular filtration. This may occur long before the blood pressure falls to irreversible shock levels.[147] Too often the dilatory tactics of the physician influenced by fear exaggerate the circulatory collapse. Digestion of blood and reabsorption of its nitrogenous products probably play, at most, a minor contributory rôle. Raw blood appears to be quite irritative to the human gastro-intestinal tract and is usually rapidly expelled by vomiting or diarrhea or both. Moreover, the quantities of protein in even a massive hemorrhage should be disposed of without difficulty by normal persons. A liter of normal blood contains only about 200 gm. of protein.

DISTURBANCES OF ACID-BASE EQUILIBRIUM, AND OF WATER AND SALT METABOLISM IN HEART FAILURE

Acid-base Equilibrium in Heart Failure.—In compensated heart disease water and salt metabolism and acid-base balance are essentially normal. In heart failure a great variety of disturbances of the electrolyte pattern of the blood plasma is encountered, depending upon the nature and intensity of the functional disturbances in any given case. For a detailed discussion of the subject and references to original studies the reader is referred to Peters and Van Slyke[124] (p. 990 ff.); only the salient points will be presented here. The causes of disturbances of acid-base equilibrium in heart failure are: (1) circulatory stasis and venous congestion in the tissues, (2) impairment of the exchange of gases in the lungs, and (3) reduction of the efficiency of the kidneys. Circulatory stasis and venous congestion have two effects. *First*, by damming back blood they increase the capillary blood pressure and thus promote transudation with the formation of edema. *Second*, because they retard the flow of blood, the venous blood leaves the tissues with less than the usual amount of oxygen and more than the usual amounts of carbon dioxide and lactic acid. The most consistent abnormality in heart failure is exaggerated oxygen unsaturation, carbon dioxide pressure, and lactic acid concentration in the venous blood. This means that there must be a similar oxygen deficiency and heaping up of CO_2 and lactic acid in the tissues. The respiratory system responds to the accumulation of CO_2 and lactic acid by overventilation. If the facilities for the exchange of gases in the lungs are reasonably sound the carbon dioxide tension may be brought not only to, but below the normal point. Under these circumstances there may be primary carbon dioxide excess and acid excess with acidosis in the venous blood, primary carbon dioxide deficit with alkalosis in the arterial blood. Bicarbonate sometimes diminishes, while chloride rises proportionately. If, by reason of congestion of the lungs, pleuritic effusions, *etc.*, the exchange of gases in the lungs is greatly impaired, on the other hand, oxygenation of the arterial blood suffers and carbon dioxide heaps up in the arterial as well as the venous blood, giving a primary carbon dioxide excess. In this case bicarbonate increases and chloride falls, just as they do in pulmonary emphysema and other diseases of the respiratory system which impede the aeration of blood in the lungs. Since adjustments between chloride and bicarbonate are made by the kidneys, these organs also play their part in determining the ultimate acid-base pattern of the blood plasma. With such a large number of factors operating, many of which work in opposite directions, it is not surprising that the proportions of bicarbonate and chloride and the pH of serum in heart failure vary in the most capricious manner. Greater attention to these variations might aid in the evaluation of symptoms and the direction of therapy.

Water-balance in Heart Failure.[137]—Edema in heart failure owes its existence primarily to venous congestion causing a backing up of pressure in the capillaries. The mean capillary blood pressure comes to exceed the osmotic pressure of the proteins. Fluid is diverted from the kidneys into the interstitial spaces. As far as the kidneys themselves are concerned, venous congestion, *per se*, should increase the capillary pressure, and consequently filtration, in the glomeruli. In keeping with this, with moderate degrees of heart failure, clearances of urea and other organic filtrable substances, though they do not rise above normal, are not significantly below normal. In the most advanced or profound failure, however, these clearances do fall and blood nonprotein nitrogen rises. Through experimentation it has been demonstrated most definitely by Winton[170] that extreme increases of pressure in the veins of the kidney cause so much congestive swelling that the tubules become compressed, the flow of urine is impeded, and the pressure in the glomerular capsule rises. In addition the glomerular tuft may become so distended that it obliterates the capsule. Therefore, although slight or moderate venous congestion may facilitate filtration, severe congestion impedes it.

The principal feature of *cardiac edema* is displacement of fluid from the circulation. The abnormalities of the composition of the fluid and serum which were described above are of minor importance. *Diuresis,* with delivery of the edema, can best be accomplished by abolishing venous congestion. Bed rest reduces the demands upon the circulation and diminishes venous pressure in the lower extremities by removing part of the influences of gravity. *Digitalis* is the most beneficial drug. Although edema originates from a dislocation of the normal balance between capillary blood pressure and the osmotic pressure of the proteins of the plasma, like all other transudative processes it can be influenced by disturbances of other equilibria. *Restriction of salt*, for example, is most effective and may be used to advantage in all cases to accelerate the action of rest and digitalis. Acidifying diuretics, such as ammonium chloride or ammonium nitrate are useful aids, but should not be given in large enough doses to upset the digestion. Moreover their administration should not be continued if they fail to induce diuresis or after edema has disappeared, because they are likely to produce severe, sometimes fatal, acidosis.[81] The introduction of highly effective and relatively innocuous mercurial preparations has fostered an unfortunate tendency among physicians to rely too largely upon diuretic drugs. It is possible with some of the newer preparations to induce diuresis before cardiac compensation is established. The consequence is that rest, restriction of salt, and even digitalis are neglected. By the intermittent injection of one of these drugs it is possible to effect a "week-end" diuresis, but since the underlying causes of the edema are not removed, it continues to recur. Both purine and mercurial diuretics should be reserved until rest, diet, and digitalis have been given an opportunity. This minimizes dangers of poisoning and gives more assurance of permanent relief from the edema.

Just as diuresis in heart failure may be facilitated by a variety of procedures that do not impinge directly upon its cause, so edema may be favored by any associated disorder that promotes transudation. In cirrhosis of the liver a slight measure of cardiac decompensation may determine the appearance of ascites. Anemia heightens the tendency to edema. Of greatest clinical importance is the coexistence of a serum albumin deficiency. Loss of appetite and digestive disorders, common symptoms of heart failure, lead to limitation of food and this, in turn, to malnutrition with depletion of serum albumin. Too often the physician abets the process by dietary restrictions. Hypoalbuminemia is frequent among patients with chronic heart disease; frequently it is accompanied by anemia.[109] These patients are likely to have intractable edema, unresponsive to digitalis and salt restriction. They make up many of the "week-end" diuresis victims. If, by proper attention to diet, they can be induced to eat enough, especially protein, not only will the edema often disappear, but the general condition will improve as well. Even restriction of salt should not be pushed to the destruction of appetite. However, palatability need not be sacrificed altogether if attention is given in the selection of foods to variety and the tastes of the patient. Frequent small meals, an extra feeding at night, and other expedients may be employed to enable them to take enough protein and calories without uncomfortable distention.

DISTURBANCES OF WATER AND SALT METABOLISM AND ACID-BASE BALANCE IN NEPHRITIS AND OTHER DISEASES OF THE KIDNEYS AND URINARY TRACT

(FOR GENERAL REVIEWS SEE REFERENCES 110, 114, 124)

The Effects of Reduction of the Functioning Mass of the Kidneys.—Removal of a single kidney has no lasting demonstrable effect upon renal function. The remaining kidney, after it has undergone hypertrophy, can carry on the necessary activities without difficulty. Only after a considerable portion of the second kidney has been removed are there any noticeable symptoms. The first of these is *polyuria:* the kidneys tend to excrete large volumes of dilute urine and cannot be made to concentrate the urine to the normal extent by either restriction of fluid or administration of pitressin. The polyuria is associated with increased thirst and if water is restricted, leads to a certain degree of dehydration. This polyuria and inability to concentrate may be regarded as the first signs of renal insufficiency.

Theoretically, *concentration tests* should be the most delicate criteria of renal functional impairment; practically they may be extremely deceptive because they are so susceptible to extraneous influences. The simplest concentration tests consist of limiting the fluid intake for twenty-four hours, allowing no fluids at all in the last twelve to sixteen hours of this period. The last urine voided in this period and the first urine voided after the period, but before the subject has drunk any fluid, are collected. The specific gravity of these specimens is used as a measure of concentrating powers; it should be 1.026 or higher, after correction for albumin.* If the subject has been overhydrated before fluids were limited, more than twenty-four hours may be required to eliminate the excess fluid and bring him to pass a concentrated urine. Concentration tests are almost valueless in the presence of edema, because limitation of fluids may only initiate diuresis. If the protein metabolism is low or if the salt intake is restricted there may not be enough solutes requiring excretion to necessitate concentration. In diabetes insipidus, severe anemia, and cirrhosis of the liver concentrating powers are impaired even when the kidneys are sound. For these reasons, a high specific gravity

---

* Protein has an effect on specific gravity out of all proportion to its molecular concentration and osmotic pressure. If there are considerable amounts of protein in the urine, therefore, specific gravity should be corrected for its presence by subtracting 0.0029 for each gram per cent of protein at 20° C.

may be interpreted as an indication that renal function is comparatively well preserved; but low specific gravity in the concentration test cannot be interpreted as evidence of impaired function, unless all symptoms and signs and circumstances attending the test are taken into consideration.

Loss of concentrating powers is not necessarily accompanied by retention of urea and other nitrogenous products or significant reduction of the excretion of phenol red. The polyuria may be regarded in a certain sense as a compensatory reaction. The nonprotein nitrogen of the blood may even be low at this stage. Urea or creatinine clearances, especially if extra urea is given, may be lowered as renal destruction advances. Nonprotein nitrogen begins to rise only when the excretory powers are so reduced that the kidney is no longer able to excrete the required amount of urea unless its concentration in the blood is elevated. This may be looked upon as the sign of *renal decompensation*, the point at which the kidneys are no longer able to excrete nitrogenous waste products rapidly enough to prevent some accumulation of these substances in the blood and tissues. The distinction between insufficiency and decompensation is important from another point of view: just as it is possible to have insufficiency without decompensation, so may there be decompensation without insufficiency. Numerous examples of this latter state have already been cited above; conditions in which, despite inherently sound kidneys, blood nonprotein nitrogen rises because of circulatory failure, fall of blood pressure, or lack of available fluid, with or without augmented protein metabolism. The nonprotein nitrogen of the blood is the resultant of the rate of protein catabolism compared with the rate at which its products, especially urea, are excreted by the kidneys. It cannot, therefore, be used as a specific measure of the extent of renal damage. Even urea clearances will not serve this purpose, because they, too, are affected by circulatory disturbances. However, they give more accurate and rapid information about the immediate functional state of the kidney than can be obtained from mere knowledge of blood urea or nonprotein nitrogen because they are not influenced by the rate of nitrogen catabolism. Moreover, they give an instantaneous cross-section of the state of function, whereas blood nonprotein nitrogen gives a record of the immediately antecedent events. It takes a measurable time for nitrogen retention to raise the concentration of nonprotein nitrogen in the blood.

The conservative functions of the kidneys suffer quite as much as the excretory functions. Among the components of the body fluids that the kidneys treat with especial economy are sodium salts. These usually appear in lower concentration in the urine than in the serum; that is, they are reabsorbed in the tubules even more than water is. As renal function fails, reabsorption of sodium becomes less efficient. At just what stage of kidney destruction this begins has not yet been ascertained. Certain it is, however, that in the terminal stages of renal failure sodium is wasted in the urine, and, unless it is given in generous quantities to meet this wastage, its concentration in the body fluids falls. As usual this leads to loss of water, but, if water intake is not limited, sodium is lost in excess of water. The net result is a state of dehydration with a greater sodium deficit. With the sodium, chloride is also sacrificed. In the face of these facts the too common practice of limiting salt in the diets of all patients with renal disease or hypertension is greatly to be deplored. With dehydration and salt depletion physiologic functions become disorganized, the circulation suffers, and azotemia itself increases. The administration of salt may work rapid improvement. Care must be taken, however, not to push salt therapy too far and not to limit fluids. The greatly damaged kidney is not only unable to reabsorb sodium and chloride to the normal extent; it is also unable to concentrate it adequately. In fact, in the last stages of insufficiency, the concentrations of sodium and chloride in the urine appear to approach those in the serum. For this reason excessive amounts of salt, especially with insufficient water, may drive the concentrations of sodium and chloride in the serum above normal and provoke edema.

Not only do the abilities to reabsorb or to concentrate chloride and sodium suffer in advanced renal failure; with them goes the discriminatory power by which finer adjustments of the acid-base balance are normally effected. Chloride and bicarbonate cannot be selectively excreted, nor can the reaction of the urine be varied over so wide a range. Finally, ammonia production fails. In consequence, bicarbonate deficit with acidosis develops. The total sum of water and electrolyte disorders, then, in untreated renal failure, includes dehydration, and sodium, chloride, and bicarbonate deficits.* In other conditions administration of sodium chloride and water in adequate quantities would suffice to rectify such a state, because the kidneys could be trusted to excrete the extra chloride, leaving the sodium to form the necessary bicarbonate. In renal failure, however, the kidneys are unable to make this adjustment; therefore, both sodium chloride and sodium bicarbonate must be given in appropriate proportions to restore the electrolyte pattern.

Total removal of the kidneys is not attended by edema or other striking indications of disturbed water or salt exchange. If renal function is entirely ablated and free access to fluids and food is permitted, enough water is apparently taken to prevent gross changes of the water content of the body; there is no desire to drink more and efforts to force further drinking are thwarted by nausea and vomiting. By parenteral injection of saline the volume of water in the body may be abnormally expanded, and it is even possible to produce edema. Within limits this appears to prolong life.

Between the polyuria of renal insufficiency and the anuria of renal ablation a stage of subtotal renal destruction might be expected in which oliguria and edema resulted simply from the incapacity of the kidneys to excrete fluid which was ingested. The author is unaware that any such condition has ever been experimentally produced. It is highly probable that the spontaneous drinking of animals in this state, as in the normal state, is regulated to keep the volume of fluid in the body constant, and that, in consequence, fluid ingestion falls with fluid excretion. The edema frequently seen in the terminal stages of diseases of the kidney is not relevant to the subject, because patients in this state invariably present disorders of function and anatomical derangements that cannot be referred to destruction of the kidneys alone.

Acute Glomerulonephritis (Acute Hemorrhagic Nephritis).—Acute glomerulonephritis, following scarlet fever or other streptococcus infections, may run its course without any appreciable disturbance of water or salt

---

* Changes of calcium, phosphorus, potassium, etc., are neglected, because they have no important relation to water metabolism and acid-base balance.

metabolism. Signs of the disease may be confined to hematuria, albuminuria, and hypertension. In the majority of patients, however, sometime in the course of the disease oliguria and retention of water and salt can be demonstrated even if there is not frank edema. At this time serum proteins, both total and fractions, may be quite normal; the edema cannot, therefore, be attributed to low serum albumin. Blood nonprotein nitrogen is usually variably elevated, urea clearance reduced.

From the preceding discussion of the effects of destruction of kidney substance it is clear that the edema cannot be connected with these signs of renal decompensation. The *edema* differs in distribution from most generalized edemas in certain respects. It is less subject to the influence of gravity. The face or a hand may suddenly swell while the patient is sitting upright, without any increase of the edema of the feet or back. Careful analysis of the *vascular reactions* of these patients reveals a peculiar vasomotor instability. They respond in an abnormal manner to all kinds of intravenous injections and are particularly prone to develop reactions resembling urticaria. These may be provoked by substances with known antigenic properties, but cannot be definitely stigmatized as allergic because they are sometimes precipitated by indifferent solutions. They have been observed after injections of sucrose, occasionally after transfusions of compatible blood. The author was led to abandon the use of *acacia* in acute nephritis, because even the first injections provoked severe angioneurotic edema and exacerbation of symptoms in a number of cases. The edema fluid in acute nephritis also seems to contain more protein than does the edema fluid in nephrosis and other noninflammatory transudative processes.[118] All these phenomena suggest the existence of a diffuse vascular disorder which involves derangement of vasomotor control. Other evidences of general vascular involvement are found in the hypertension, the variability of blood pressure, and retinal hemorrhages.

It is being increasingly recognized that the *heart* also is frequently affected by the disease. Rapid changes in the size of the heart may be detected, with sudden acute dilatations; electrocardiographic abnormalities are common; venous pressure is often abnormally high. The edema of acute nephritis, then, seems to be produced by a combination of heart failure and peripheral vascular disorders, the latter resembling those seen in angioneurotic edema. Increased permeability of the blood vessels may contribute, but need not be regarded as a primary factor; it may be only a secondary result of abnormal vasomotor activity.

There is no characteristic disturbance of the electrolyte pattern of the *serum*. The commonest abnormality is, perhaps, elevation of serum Cl with slight reduction of bicarbonate. The kidneys, therefore, cannot be completely exonerated. Vomiting, which is common, may sometimes be sufficiently severe to cause sodium and chloride depletion. Bicarbonate excess and alkalosis seldom result because the vomitus usually contains little or no free acid.

Treatment.—At the very onset of the disease, before edema has appeared, administration of liberal amounts of fluid seems to be indicated. If nausea and vomiting prohibit drinking and eating, parenteral glucose solution should be given; dehydration may be the determining factor in precipitating suppression of urine. The fluid intake must be regulated to the needs of the patient according to the principles outlined above, with due appreciation that the volume of urine is no longer a reliable criterion. There is no reason to promote edema. Salt may well be restricted from the outset; but it may be a wise precaution to analyze the serum at intervals for chloride + bicarbonate, especially if the patient is vomiting. There are no contraindications to feeding whatever the patient is willing to take without salt. There is little danger that the acute nephritic will take too much protein, if this is deleterious (which is highly doubtful), because anorexia is usually a striking symptom of the early stages of the disease. Nausea and vomiting should be avoided. If the latter becomes serious all food and fluids by mouth may have to be withdrawn for an interval and parenteral fluids substituted. If serum sodium and chloride fall as a result of vomiting it may even be necessary to inject normal saline or small amounts of 2 per cent sodium chloride, but this must be done with great circumspection. Symptoms and signs of heart failure should be treated by appropriate measures. Digitalis may be given and occasionally seems to have a beneficial effect.

The appearance of edema is no indication for radical revision of the therapeutic regimen. There is too much tendency to treat edema to the neglect of the patient. Salt restriction is more imperative and may be made more rigid. Water need not be limited. Without salt thirst diminishes. Diuretics are seldom efficacious and are likely to produce untoward symptoms. Stimulation of elimination by extrarenal channels is frequently advocated and practised. Sweating has happily fallen into disrepute, but vigorous catharsis is still commonly employed. The bowel is physiologically ill adapted to assume the functions of the kidney. Profuse catharsis may only divert from the kidneys water that might be used to better purpose for the formation of urine.

Magnesium sulfate has enjoyed a special reputation which has been enhanced by the discovery of its utility in the treatment of hypertensive crises and convulsions. Given intravenously in adequate dosage, it has a sedative and anticonvulsive action and a transitory hypotensive effect.[12, 13*] In addition it may be mildly diuretic. Its action depends directly upon the concentration of magnesium in the serum; it is quite independent of diuresis or any transfer of water within the body. It is an invaluable weapon in the prevention or treatment of convulsions or sudden hypertensive crises, but beyond this has no demonstrable effect upon the course of the disease. Magnesium sulfate given by mouth has an entirely different effect. Only a small part of the magnesium is absorbed. In fact, its cathartic action depends on the fact that it is not absorbed and therefore carries out in the feces with it water withdrawn from the interstitial fluids of the body. It does not take with it an equivalent amount of sodium salt. In the author's experience it often produces hemoconcentration associated with exacerbation of toxic symptoms, but has little or no effect on the edema. It has been necessary to resort to injections of glucose solution to relieve the symptoms produced

---

* A detailed study of the effects of magnesium on animals and patients has been conducted in the author's laboratory, chiefly by Alexander Winkler, Jr., which, it is hoped, may be published shortly. The statements below are derived largely from this investigation.

by the catharsis. To distress a patient to remove water that must be restored is not an altogether logical procedure.

After diuresis has occurred and edema has disappeared, there is no reason to prolong salt restriction. It makes no essential difference in this respect whether the diuresis marks regression or advance of the disease, as it may. It is usually advisable to restore salt to the diet gradually in order to avoid recurrence of edema. A convenient procedure is to permit the patient to add increasing amounts of salt to his food, while weight and urine volume are carefully observed. Two extra grams may be allowed at first for two or three days. If this has no ill effect 5 grams may be given. If this proves equally innocent, salt may be used in the preparation of the food. At any point if urine volume falls sharply or weight increases, salt should again be withdrawn.

The Nephrotic Syndrome.—This is not the place to discuss the pathological significance of the nephrotic syndrome. The term is here used to denote a clinical symptom complex characterized by profuse albuminuria, hypoalbuminemia, and edema, without serious renal insufficiency or hypertension. It is regularly encountered in amyloid degeneration of the kidneys. It is also one of the stages through which glomerulonephritis may progress, toward either recovery or disaster. Whether it may occur as an independent disease entity is still a controversial question. In any case its effects on water and salt metabolism are essentially the same regardless of its origin. For this reason it will be considered only as it appears in the evolution of glomerulonephritis.

If acute nephritis does not resolve rapidly with complete recovery, it may after a time take on a nephrotic complexion. Hypertension gradually subsides, hematuria disappears or becomes insignificant, blood nonprotein nitrogen and renal functional tests become normal; only profuse proteinuria persists. Under the stress of albuminuria the serum albumin becomes greatly depleted. Consequently, edema persists or may even increase. The disease may pass into this stage quite imperceptibly from the acute stage, and during the transition all the phenomena of acute nephritis may persist to a variable degree. In general it may be said that, if acute nephritis with profuse albuminuria persists as long as five weeks, by the end of this time a serious serum albumin deficiency may be expected.[118] Although vasomotor disturbances and heart failure may continue to play a part in the production of edema, reduction of the protein osmotic pressure now becomes the most important factor. In the most characteristic form of the syndrome the correlation between edema and the concentration of albumin in the serum is extremely consistent. It may be predicted with a high degree of certainty that it will be difficult or impossible to eliminate edema completely if serum albumin falls below 2 per cent, while if albumin is higher than this it should be possible by rest and salt restriction to keep it in abeyance.[40, 117]

The edema owes its presence, then, chiefly to accelerated transfer of fluid from capillaries to interstitial spaces due to an abnormally low protein osmotic pressure of the serum in proportion to the capillary blood pressure. This effectively removes the fluid from the province of renal control. Robinson and Farr[129] have reported that nephrotic urine has antidiuretic activity. If this could be taken as an indication that there are excessive quantities of antidiuretic agents in the circulating blood, the kidneys would have to share the onus for the edema.* The concentration and partition of electrolytes in the serum are not characteristically affected. Sodium is commonly normal or slightly reduced; chloride is usually normal or slightly elevated, with bicarbonate comparably depressed. There are, however, distinct exceptions to this rule, cases in which serum bicarbonate tends to remain persistently high, with chloride correspondingly low. No explanations for these differences have been discovered.

Treatment.—As far as the disorder of water and salt metabolism is concerned, treatment consists of (1) general measures aimed to promote diuresis, and (2) attempts to remedy the underlying hypoalbuminemia. Among the general measures restriction of salt is, as usual, preeminent. Urea is the diuretic of choice because it is bland towards both the gastro-intestinal tract and the kidneys. It may be given in doses of 20 to 80 gm. daily in 20 per cent solution. The acidifying diuretics enjoyed a vogue, but have declined in popularity, because of their tendency to destroy appetite, upset digestion, and sometimes produce acidosis without diuresis. Purine diuretics are seldom effective. Mercurials have been recommended and are rather generally employed, but are not without danger. As usual, they should be given only after other measures which may be conducive to diuresis have been taken, in order to favor their action as much as possible. They should not be given if renal function, as measured by phenolsulfonephthalein excretion, is seriously impaired. It is a wise precaution to give a small test dose first (0.5 cc. of salyrgan or mercupurin). If this causes no untoward symptoms and increases the urine volume, a more adequate dose may be given after an interval of two or three days. The principal objection to these drugs is that their effects are so transient. The edema rapidly recurs and it is necessary to repeat the dose at frequent intervals. Ordinarily, in the nephrotic syndrome, the total quantity of protein excreted is more constant than the concentration of protein in the urine. Protein enters urine with the glomerular filtrate. The actual quantity is, therefore, proportional to the volume of filtrate, which is relatively constant. Since the ultimate urine volume is determined chiefly by the proportion of filtrate which is reabsorbed, it should have a negligible influence upon the amount of protein excreted. Mercurial diuretics should have a particularly indifferent effect if, as is supposed, they act entirely upon tubular reabsorption. Nevertheless, in certain patients proteinuria is correlated to a variable extent with urine volume. In these cases mercurial diuretics increase proteinuria and therefore abet protein wastage. Although they may, for the moment, give relief from the edema, they aggravate the condition which is fundamentally responsible for the edema. Efforts should be directed mainly to the elimination of this defect, towards restoration of serum albumin, and anything which diverts or detracts from this object must be avoided.

The primary measure is the provision of enough protein in the *diet* to replace both the protein which is catabolized and that which is excreted as

* It does not follow, however, that these organs are primarily responsible for the edema. The specific nature of the normal antidiuretic stimulus has not yet been unequivocally established. If it should be the volume of circulating fluid or any function of this volume, a condition in which the volume of circulating fluid was being continually drained by excessive transudation might elicit antidiuretic activity quite as effectively as would the withdrawal of circulating fluid through any other channel.

protein in the urine, and in addition to supply some for reconstruction of wasted tissues. It is possible in most instances, in this way, to establish a positive nitrogen balance. As dietary protein is increased, successive increments are utilized with progressively diminishing efficiency, until a point is reached at which further increments are entirely wasted. No advantage is gained by feeding more protein than can be effectively utilized. In fact, Farr[38] has found that if more than optimum quantities are given nitrogen storage may actually decrease. Children could take as much as, but not more than, 3 gm. per Kg. to advantage. In the author's experience adults will seldom tolerate such large quantities. It is the exceptional patient who will take more than 150 gm. daily. To insure the most efficient utilization of the protein it should be accompanied by ample calories in the form of carbohydrate and fat. Despite the most assiduous efforts, even after prolonged positive nitrogen balances, serum albumin may fail to rise. If the urine contains more than 10 gm. of protein a day it is rarely possible, if more than 15 gm. it is almost invariably impossible, to increase the concentration of serum albumin by diet. This has tended to discredit the use of *high protein* diets without due reason. It has already been pointed out that the presence of a serum albumin deficit betokens a more serious deficiency of protein in the tissues. It would seem to be advantageous to replace these losses even if the serum albumin deficiency is not immediately reparable. Further than this, reconstitution of serum albumin may for a time escape notice because as the albumin increases it draws from the tissues a proportional amount of fluid to expand the volume of the circulating blood. Finally, even if diet is powerless to replace serum albumin it may sustain it against the ravages of proteinuria. If albuminuria abates or ceases, serum albumin rises and edema disappears with surprising rapidity. Since the nephrotic syndrome represents a pathologic process that is essentially reversible, everything should be done to conserve the general health and the nutritive state of the patient in the hope that nature may eventually come to the rescue.*

Intravenous injections of *colloids* to restore the colloid osmotic pressure and thus remove the cause of the edema should be reserved for those especial occasions when edema itself becomes intolerably distressing or menacing. This is especially true of unnatural substitutes like acacia. Foreign colloids of this kind can be used only in limited quantities for short periods because of their antigenic properties and other deleterious effects. In addition they should not be given if the serum albumin is extremely low, *i.e.,* less than 1 per cent. The expansion of the circulation that follows injection of acacia dilutes serum albumin so that its concentration falls. There is some recent evidence that the total amount of circulating protein may also decrease after acacia. In any case, a minimal concentration of serum albumin appears to be essential. If the concentration of serum albumin is driven below this by acacia, edema is not diminished and the general condition suffers.

Transfusions of fresh serum or solutions of properly dried or concentrated serum are a highly effective means of inducing immediate diuresis. With a severe nephrotic syndrome, however, with profuse albuminuria, the

---

* Intravenous injections of protein hydrolysates have been used in the treatment of nephrosis. It is not a practical method of administering a substitute for protein over long periods, but may, according to Farr,[39] have a more specific effect on some of the adventitious disorders associated with the disease.

injected protein is excreted with great rapidity. Such injections are so expensive that they are prohibitive except as emergency procedures for the average person. Transfusion of whole blood is the procedure of choice if there is anemia.

Chronic Progressive Glomerulonephritis.—The edema of acute nephritis or the nephrotic stage of glomerulonephritis may gradually disappear, not because the disease regresses, but because it advances. As destruction of the kidneys progresses, proteinuria usually diminishes, partly because glomerular filtration decreases, perhaps also because there is a change in the character of the injury to the glomeruli which makes them less pervious to protein. The concentration of albumin in the serum consequently rises. At the same time the polyuria of renal insufficiency appears as an added diuretic force. As this transformation proceeds therapy must be modified accordingly. Salt restriction first must be abandoned; later, when the tendency to waste salt sets in, salt must be added to the diet; finally, bicarbonate may also be required to combat the acidosis of the terminal stages of the disease.

Treatment.—The appearance or persistence of a serum albumin deficit at these stages of the disease usually betokens malnutrition. Edema can be attributed to malnutrition, anemia, and heart failure in various degrees, and should be treated appropriately. It is not uncommon to find the concentration of sodium, chloride, and bicarbonate in the serum low in the presence of massive edema in the terminal stages of the disease. Administration of salt in this state may increase edema without appreciably changing the electrolyte pattern of the serum. If salt is withdrawn, on the other hand, serum sodium may fall further without any considerable diuresis. At the same time the subjective state of the patient may change for the worse. Sometimes small intravenous injections (250 to 500 cc.) of 2 per cent sodium chloride work improvement. Success, however, depends on the elimination of the causes of edema which were enumerated above. Diuretic drugs are not only useless, but harmful. Urea is supererogatory, as the kidneys are already working under the stimulus of a high endogenous blood urea. Acidifying diuretics only aggravate the existing acidosis. Purines and mercurials are not only ineffective; they are likely to poison the few remaining vestiges of functional renal tissue.

Nothing is more intractable and disastrous than the *vomiting* which attends extreme renal insufficiency. It prevents feeding and contributes to wastage of salt and water. It does not lead to bicarbonate excess because the vomitus contains no free hydrochloric acid. When it first makes its appearance it is prone to occur in the morning, before or after the first meal. In this case it is usually associated with a rather characteristic sequence of symptoms. The patient awakens early to void, conscious of acute thirst and hunger. In the interval between waking and breakfast, this hunger gives way to nausea, often accompanied by headache. The ingestion of food or fluid immediately upon awakening, when hunger and thirst are acute, frequently relieves the syndrome completely, eliminating nausea, headache and vomiting. A glass of hot water occasionally suffices; a carbohydrate drink is more effective; sometimes the addition of a small amount of food containing salt gives more certain relief. It is not unlikely that the symptoms are referable to dehydration and salt wastage from the nocturnal polyuria. Nausea at other times of day in rare instances may be allayed by drinking small quantities of cold hypertonic salt solution (50 cc. of 2 per cent sodium chloride).

As renal failure progresses the vomiting becomes more and more intractable, resisting all therapeutic efforts. The nausea and vomiting of advanced nephritis are almost unique in their failure to respond to complete withdrawal of food and fluids. Ultimately the sole support is parenteral fluids. By carefully proportioning sodium chloride, bicarbonate, glucose and water it may be possible to establish and maintain some semblance of normality in the volume and composition of the body fluids.

Nocturnal polyuria may give rise to other symptoms, the commonest being muscular cramps. These usually come in the early morning and can be relieved by the addition of salt to the diet. They may be akin to miners' or stokers' cramps, evidences of sodium depletion. Patients sufferings from such cramps should be directed to take some salt with water when they arise to urinate during the night.

Mixed Syndromes.—In the gradual progress of nephritis various combinations of the nephrotic syndrome and signs of renal destruction are encountered. Albuminuria and hypoproteinemia may be prolonged into the stage of renal insufficiency. Acute nephritis may pass rapidly to chronic progressive renal insufficiency without the intervention of a nephrotic stage. In this case there is no intermission of hypertension; urea clearances deteriorate and blood nonprotein nitrogen rises continuously. Recessions and exacerbations are common and may take on various complexions. The problems presented by such mixed types of cases, however, are only variants or combinations of those that have been discussed above under the headings of acute nephritis, the nephrotic syndrome and chronic progressive nephritis. Treatment, as far as water, salt and acid-base balances are concerned, depends upon the meticulous analysis of the functional capacity and metabolic defects in each case and the choice of appropriate measures to remedy these defects.

Too much emphasis has been placed upon the mere measurement of the excretory competence of the kidneys by conventional methods such as the blood nonprotein nitrogen or blood urea nitrogen, phenolsulfonephthalein excretion and urea clearance. Importance attaches not only to what a kidney can do, but what it is doing at a given time. Excretory powers are no more important than conservative powers. It is the preservation of a normal internal environment that is desired and the principal constituents of this environment are salt and water. The clinical conduct of nephritis would be measurably advanced if estimations of fluid volume, serum proteins, chloride and bicarbonate were more frequently utilized as guides for the direction of therapy.

Nephrosclerosis.—This term is employed in a broad sense to include diseases of the arteries associated with hypertension. These diseases affect water and salt metabolism and acid-base balance only when they destroy kidney tissue or give rise to heart failure. There is nothing distinctive about the disturbances which they engender, nor the therapy which they require. Restriction of salt has been recommended as a general measure for the treatment of all hypertensive states, on not entirely convincing grounds. Whether it has or has not a place in the treatment of uncomplicated hypertension, it should not be practised when destruction of the kidneys has progressed to the point of renal insufficiency and salt wastage. It is incumbent upon the physician to analyze renal and cardiac function with the greatest care in all cases of hypertension. If both kidneys and heart are functionally sound, no especial attention need be given to the regulation of the intake of salt and water. At the first signs of incompetence of kidneys or heart, treatment should be instituted along the lines prescribed in the sections on heart failure (p. 328), renal insufficiency (p. 332), and chronic progressive nephritis (p. 337).

Surgical Conditions of the Kidneys and Urinary Tract.—Under this heading come infections of the kidneys, ureters, or bladder, and obstructive lesions. Any general discussion of these conditions is irrelevant to the purposes of this chapter; but certain disorders arising from them and some therapeutic procedures that are commonly employed deserve mention. Treatment should be directed toward the elimination of infection or obstruction when this is feasible. If it is not, palliative treatment is indicated. For infections a regimen of "forced fluids"—*i.e.*, ingestion of large quantities of water—is often ordered. If this is done care should be taken that the patient receives a suitable amount of salt. Without this precaution excessive drinking is not only disagreeable, but may even be harmful, especially if there is renal insufficiency with a tendency to waste salt.

Incomplete or intermittent obstruction of the urinary tract causes dilatation of the pelvis and progressive destruction of the kidney. If the obstruction is bilateral and sufficiently great, evidences of renal insufficiency may precede serious or irreversible anatomical lesions.

Mercury Poisoning.[122]—Although mercury is a general protoplasmic poison, the obvious lesions which it produces, irrespective of the route of administration, are usually restricted to the gastro-intestinal tract and the kidneys, in which it causes epithelial necrosis. Local lesions at the site of administration, where mercury may have an opportunity to act in high concentration for a considerable time, must, of course, be excepted from this general rule. When mercury gains access to the blood stream it is, apparently, rapidly diluted to innocuous concentrations. It speedily finds its way to the kidneys, where it passes into the glomerular filtrate. As water is withdrawn from the filtrate in the tubules the concentration of mercury increases enough to coagulate the epithelial protein. The alimentary lesions probably owe their origin to a similar process. The most significant feature of the lesions is their superficial character. Since they are confined almost, if not quite, to the epithelial layers and do not extend to the basement membranes, they are reparable. Even the most complete degeneration of the tubular epithelial cells, with calcification, appears to be reversible.

Treatment should be directed, therefore, to prevent absorption of the metal, to provide initially a large enough volume of urine to insure its dilution to innocuous concentration in the tubules, and finally, if efforts in these directions fail, to sustain the victim until the gastro-intestinal and renal lesions have had an opportunity to heal. The drug itself, if taken by mouth, usually acts as a prompt and efficient emetic. If the stomach happens at the time to be full of fluid and food, the major part of the mercury may waste its coagulating powers on the protein of the stomach contents and be ejected before it has caused serious injury. Egg white, milk or other proteins may be introduced to promote this process and immediate lavage may be practised. Sodium formaldehyde sulfoxylate, proposed by Rosenthal,[130] may be added to the lavage fluid if it is at hand. Like all other antidotes which have been offered, however, it is of no value after the mercury has been absorbed. Lavage itself is useless unless it is practised promptly; it may even be vicious because it tends to remove from the body fluid that is needed for the formation of urine and because it diverts attention from more imperative needs.

The vomiting induced by mercury removes fluid and salt from the body. Far more is probably poured into the stomach and gut in response to the intensely irritant action of the drug. These factors, the trauma of the gut, and possibly the systemic effects of the drug combine to produce early circulatory collapse. Nothing could be less conducive to the excretion of a large volume of urine than the combination of dehydration, hemoconcentration, and shock. It was demonstrated by Haskell[68] that the tolerance of animals to mercury could be greatly enhanced by previous intravenous injection of sodium chloride. This is the most exigent therapeutic indication. Even lavage should not be allowed to delay the institution of *intravenous infusion of saline*. If, when the patient is first seen, symptoms and signs of shock are already evident, blood transfusion should be given as promptly as possible. In any case preparations should be made for transfusion. If the blood pressure is well sustained as much as 2000 to 3000 cc. of saline may be injected into the vein. If the blood pressure is falling it is advisable to give only a small amount of the saline intravenously until it is possible to inject blood, giving the remainder of the saline subcutaneously. If these measures are instituted sufficiently early urine excretion may never fail and serious effects of the poison may be entirely averted.

After the initial lavage no food nor fluids of any kind should be given by mouth. The common practice of frequent lavage merely maintains irritation of the stomach and bowels and withdraws further water and salt from the already depleted victim. Lavage of the bowel is equally pernicious. Vomiting and diarrhea cease almost immediately if nothing is introduced into the stomach. The major part of the mercury in any case appears to be eliminated by the kidneys quite early. The small traces which may be excreted into the gut subsequently are of little moment. The mouth must be kept scrupulously clean to prevent stomatitis, but the patient should not be permitted to swallow any of the solutions used for cleansing purposes.

Treatment after this consists of restoring and maintaining the normal volume and composition of the body fluids by the parenteral administration of proper quantities of water, salt, and glucose, and by sustaining the circulation with transfusions of blood. Under this treatment patients have remained practically symptomless and have recovered completely in spite of periods of complete anuria and total obstipation as long as five to seven days. In the first twenty-four hours as much as 5000 to 7000 cc. of saline, depending on the volume and duration of vomiting, may be given to advantage. If the urine volume never falls, vigorous administration of fluid may be prolonged for forty-eight to seventy-two hours, always with provision of adequate amounts of salt. At the appearance of oliguria or anuria the fluid intake should be reduced to the amounts required to provide for the urine excreted and replacement of losses by extrarenal channels. No evil comes from keeping the volume of fluid in the body slightly above normal, but nothing is gained by giving gross excesses of water or salt. If the blood pressure is not sustained or if the blood count falls, as it usually does, further transfusions are indicated. Enough glucose (100 gm. daily) should be given to prevent excessive protein catabolism or ketosis. It is best administered in two doses daily.

The concentrations of chloride and bicarbonate in the serum should receive the most assiduous attention. With the kidneys no longer active serum bicarbonate tends to fall. It is, therefore, necessary to give bicarbonate—or some substitute such as sodium lactate—as well as chloride to preserve the acid-base equilibrium.

After vomiting and diarrhea have ceased for twenty-four, or probably forty-eight hours, peroral administration of fluids, and later carbohydrate foods, may be cautiously attempted, but must be stopped again at the first sign of nausea or vomiting.

Mercury poisoning deserves this long and detailed consideration, not because of its intrinsic importance, but because it is representative of a variety of toxic conditions which are characterized by gastro-intestinal irritation, shock, and oliguria. Among them belong the effects of a great many poisons, blackwater fever[158] and transfusion reactions. The treatment of all these conditions, so far as the regulation of fluids and salts is concerned follows the general principles outlined for the treatment of acute mercury poisoning.

It is claimed that mercury, taken in small doses over a long period, may also induce a true *nephrotic syndrome*. The treatment of this condition, besides removal of the etiological factor, does not differ from the treatment of the nephrotic syndrome from any other cause.

Toxemias of Pregnancy.—(This section is largely based upon published and unpublished observations of the author[115, 116, 171].) In consideration of water and salt metabolism the classification of the toxemias, a highly controversial subject, may be neglected. The disturbances of water and salt metabolism and acid-base equilibrium in these conditions are not specifically related to etiological factors or to any particular category of toxemia with the exception of the pernicious vomiting of early pregnancy. The *treatment* of this condition is, as far as fluid exchange and acid-base equilibrium are concerned, that of vomiting and starvation acidosis. Because the pregnant woman has an unusual tendency to exhaust liver glycogen and to develop ketosis, emphasis should be laid on the liberal administration of glucose in frequent doses. This is especially indicated if, as is suspected, there may be behind the vomiting a disorder of hepatic function. The vomiting usually responds to withdrawal of all food and fluids, which is the best treatment if palliative measures fail. Parenteral administration of those vitamins which can be procured in suitable form should not be neglected. It may be necessary to terminate pregnancy if the vomiting cannot be checked.

Whatever may be the cause of the other toxemias, they resemble in symptomatology and functional disturbances the nephritides. Pregnancy seems to bestow a peculiar predisposition to reactions of this nature in the kidneys and vascular system. The woman who is already suffering from renal or vascular disease or who develops acute nephritis early in pregnancy is almost certain to have an exacerbation during pregnancy and this is likely to assume a particularly explosive character. This can be differentiated from the true toxemias, if the two conditions are distinctive, only by the fact that it may manifest itself earlier in the course of pregnancy. The cause of this predilection in the pregnant woman is not clear. It may be, as some believe, referable to an imbalance of the hormones which control the natural evolution of pregnancy; it may lie in certain anatomical and chemical transformations that are associated with pregnancy. The first of these is a hypertrophy of the lower segment of the ureters which results in partial obstruction and hydronephrosis. During the course of pregnancy serum sodium and bicarbonate diminish slightly[83]; serum albumin also falls.* Whether these disorders contribute to the incidence of renal and vascular disorders of pregnancy or not, their occurrence must be recognized.

In the last analysis termination of pregnancy is still the only universally trustworthy method of resolving toxemias. There are circumstances, however, in which it may not be immediately practicable for personal or social reasons. Sometimes the condition of the patient does not warrant immediate interference. It is in these situations that regulation of salt and water metabolism assumes major importance. Hypertension and albuminuria alone require no particular attention except as they forebode more serious complications. The addition of dependent edema should increase anxiety. Rest, restriction of salt, and a high protein diet are indicated, with digitalis if there are any symptoms or signs of heart failure.

The major problem is found in the toxemias usually termed preeclamptic or *eclamptic,* in which edema and hypertension appear or become exaggerated rather rapidly. The edema, like that of acute nephritis, is usually not confined to the dependent parts, but affects hands, face, and trunk as well. Headache, visual disturbances, and vomiting too often are preludes to convulsions which may prove fatal.

Careful questioning in these cases discloses the fact that the swelling was ushered in with dyspnea. On examination the heart is usually found enlarged, râles at the bases of the lungs are common. Dyspnea and orthopnea are not uncommon. Venous pressure is abnormally high. All these symptoms and signs bespeak heart failure. Those patients who succumb, either after convulsions, in labor, or after delivery, present a terminal picture of circulatory collapse or "shock" together with cardiac dilatation, cyanosis and pulmonary edema. The whole suggests a combination of heart failure and shock, a pooling of the blood in the visceral veins with peripheral vasoconstriction and venous congestion. If the blood is examined at intervals serum proteins and hemoglobin are seen to rise during the crisis—evidence that fluid is escaping from the circulation as it does in other types of shock. In nephritis convulsive seizures are associated with a similar sequence of phenomena. Both in toxemias and in nephritis vomiting is likely to precipitate explosions. They may be precipitated also by any trauma, including delivery.

Treatment.—This should be directed as early as possible to restoring the competence of the circulation in order that pregnancy may be safely terminated. At the very outset salt should be sharply restricted. If the condition is very mild a high protein diet may be helpful. The subject should be put to bed and given adequate digitalis. Hypertonic glucose solution intravenously will provide necessary carbohydrate if there is vomiting.

---

* It has been claimed that this hypoalbuminemia and the anemia that accompanies it are not obligatory features of pregnancy, but only the result of insufficient protein and iron respectively in the diet.

These measures may succeed in reestablishing circulatory competence and evoking diuresis. If they do not, transfusion of blood is indicated. Transfusion is a wise precaution at or before delivery in any case and an urgent necessity if the blood pressure falls or other signs of circulatory collapse appear. For the convulsions themselves intravenous injections of magnesium sulfate are most effective.

Beyond this treatment follows the principles prescribed for the management of nephritis.

Water and Salt Metabolism and Acid-Base Balance in Diabetes.—The disturbances of water and salt balances in diabetes are of three kinds: (1) the diuresis of profuse glycosuria, (2) the edema of malnutrition, (3) the phenomena of diabetic acidosis. The first and second require brief attention, chief interest centers in the last.

The *polyuria which accompanies profuse glycosuria* in diabetes is the classical example of a diuresis which depends upon the limited concentrating powers of the kidney. Glucose is filtered freely through the glomeruli, but not more than about 200 mg. per minute can be reabsorbed by the tubules. If the concentration of glucose in the blood is abnormally high and the volume of filtrate large, as it is in diabetes, glucose is offered to the tubules at a rate far exceeding this. A large proportion of the glucose, therefore, escapes reabsorption. The extent to which glucose can be concentrated by reabsorption of water is also limited. Consequently, as the blood glucose rises, not only glycosuria, but also the volume of the urine increases. This results in a certain degree of dehydration and provokes thirst. The severity of both polyuria and polydipsia varies with the quantity of glucose that must be excreted and the concentrating powers of the kidneys. Whether the diuresis of glycosuria of clinical proportions of itself necessarily takes with it salts and other solutes is uncertain. If the ingestion of water and the excretion of urine were exactly synchronized it might be possible to prevent such losses. Actually, however, while urine formation is a continuous process, drinking is intermittent. At night, when the interval between drinks is especially long, dehydration becomes significant and salt is probably lost with the water. This explains *nocturnal cramps* in the legs which may be relieved by taking salt and water before retiring or on arising to urinate. In the most profuse glycosuria there is probably some constant dehydration, since elimination of the glycosuria almost invariably results in an immediate slight, persistent increase of body weight. The proper treatment of the polyuria, of course, consists in the elimination or reduction of the glycosuria by proper regulation of diet and, when necessary, administration of insulin. Whether glycosuria *per se* is deleterious is open to argument; when it reaches symptomatic proportions argument ceases.

If diabetes becomes sufficiently grave to interfere with nutrition, serum albumin falls and edema appears.[18] While glycosuria persists its diuretic effect may be great enough to keep the edema in abeyance. The edema is most likely to make its appearance when diabetes is first brought under control. Like other nutritional edemas it is aggravated by salt and responds to salt restriction and diuretics. In most instances it requires no special treatment, because it disappears spontaneously as malnutrition is overcome. Occasionally, when it assumes embarrassing proportions, salt restriction and, possibly, administration of urea are justified. Patients with malnutrition sometimes manifest an inexplicable craving for salt, which provokes or aggravates edema. Restraint of this craving may be enough in these cases to prevent or eliminate the edema. After recovery from acidosis edema may appear without demonstrable hypoproteinemia. The cause of this edema is not entirely clear. It has been suggested that it owes its origin to a slight bicarbonate excess and alkalosis with which it is usually associated. This heightens, rather than solves, the mystery, because the alkalosis itself requires explanation.

Diabetic Acidosis.—The patient with advanced diabetic acidosis presents extreme dehydration, hemoconcentration, depletion of sodium, chloride, and bicarbonate of the serum and interstitial fluids, and replacement of further bicarbonate by ketone acids, with resultant acidosis. The blood pres-

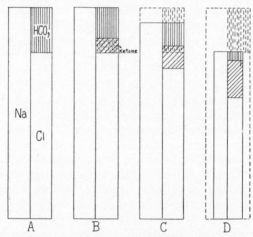

Fig. 25.—A schematic representation of the effect of diabetic acidosis on the volume and composition of the extracellular fluids. In each pair of columns the vertical dimension represents osmolar concentration, the horizontal dimension, volume of fluid. For purposes of simplification only Na, Cl and HCO_3 are depicted. The broken lines in each case indicate the pattern of normal interstitial fluid for comparison. For detailed description see text.

sure may be low and the temperature subnormal—signs of circulatory collapse or "shock." [82, 123]

The sequence of events which leads to this profound disorganization has been traced by Atchley, Loeb, et al.[6] It follows the general course described by Gamble, Ross, and Tisdall[49] for starvation, but proceeds further. It is outlined diagrammatically in figure 25. When no exogenous carbohydrate is available the organism is forced to subsist entirely on fat and protein, chiefly the former. When the glycogen stores of the liver are exhausted the only carbohydrate available is that which is derived from protein. It is now recognized that fat is first converted to β-hydroxybutyric acid and aceto-acetic acid in the liver. These acids are then conveyed by the blood stream to the tissues, where they are burned. When the metabolism is turned over chiefly to fat, therefore, the concentration of these acids in the blood must increase. Since they are acids they displace bicarbonate from combination with sodium, as is depicted in *A*. This results in the excretion of some sodium with the ketones in the urine and of some displaced CO_2 by the lungs (see *B*). In starvation these reactions are always moderate. When, however, the ability to oxidize carbohydrate is destroyed, as it is in diabetes, even the glucose formed from protein escapes combustion. In this case the liver seems to pour out ketone acids in great excess. Atchley, Loeb et al.[6] found that at the very onset of ketosis sodium chloride was, for some inexplicable reason, also swept into the urine. With the sodium sacrificed with ketone acids and with chloride water too is lost; dehydration begins at the very onset of the condition. In fact, sodium chloride and water may be lost in the preacidotic stage. Ammonia production does not become accelerated until acidosis is measurably advanced and never reaches proportions that protect the subject entirely from loss of sodium. Furthermore, chloride continues to pour into the urine after its concentration in the serum is greatly reduced (see *C*). The patient with diabetic acidosis is consumed with thirst, but is seldom able to retain food or fluids because of nausea and vomiting. Drinking and vomiting add to the salt depletion and dehydration. Overventilation in the attempt to eliminate CO_2 and thus restore pH of the blood to normal further aggravates the dehydration and, in addition, promotes heat loss. There is no condition in which dehydration, hemoconcentration and salt depletion can reach such extremes. The ultimate state of the body fluids is suggested by *D*.

Two features of this last diagram are particularly worthy of attention. First, although bicarbonate suffers the greatest absolute reduction, sometimes approaching extinction, the base with which it was combined is to a great extent preserved. It has only transferred its allegiance to the ketone acids; if these could be removed, a large part of bicarbonate would be at once reconstituted. Since restoration of carbohydrate combustion by means of insulin retards ketone production to its normal rate and permits oxidation of the accumulated ketone acids, the ketone fraction of the anions in the body fluids may be considered as potentially bicarbonate. The deficit of chloride and the sodium which has gone with it, on the other hand, must be considered as total losses which can be replaced only from extraneous sources. Furthermore, the chloride deficit, although relatively smaller than the bicarbonate deficit is actually much larger. The major deficiency derives from contraction of the interstitial fluids as a whole. Since the concentration of chloride in these fluids is four times as great as that of bicarbonate, contraction of the fluid volume will involve the loss of 4 parts of chloride to one of bicarbonate, if the general chemical pattern of the fluids is retained.[82, 123]

Treatment.—This treatment of diabetic acidosis should be directed to the reversal of the processes which have been described. Before turning to specific therapy, however, a word about general therapy is in order. No food nor fluids should be given by mouth until the patient is well on the way to recovery and free from nausea. Earlier they can only provoke vomiting, thereby furthering dehydration and salt depletion. Initial lavage is frequently recommended, but in the author's experience is unnecessary. If nothing is given by mouth, nausea rapidly subsides and the contents of the stomach and gut are reabsorbed, where they are more useful than in the emesis basin. *Circulatory collapse* is the gravest feature of diabetic acidosis, the source of the coma and other most serious symptoms, and the cause of most fatalities. Every patient with diabetic acidosis must be treated as an actual or potential victim of shock. Warmth is imperative. The blood pressure should be watched as closely as the blood sugar. Transfusion of blood is indicated if the blood pressure does not rapidly return to and remain at safe levels. Large volumes of fluid should not be given intravenously. Especial care should be taken that during recovery the blood sugar does not fall too precipitately to superimpose the shock of hypoglycemia upon the shock of dehydration.

The first consideration is to restore the glycogen stores of the liver and the ability to burn sugar by administering glucose and insulin. An initial dose of 50 units of insulin with a slow intravenous injection of 500 cc. of 10 per cent glucose meets these indications.* Thereafter glucose should be given at intervals, to provide about 10 gm. per hour, with frequent doses of insulin. About 20 units per hour at this stage is usually satisfactory; but the blood sugar should be examined at frequent intervals and the dose of insulin modified according to the course of the glycemia. Urine examinations are of little value because the patient may be unable to void at sufficiently frequent intervals. The use of an inlying catheter is hardly justifiable when analysis of the blood for glucose is such a simple procedure and gives so much more precise information. The blood sugar usually does not fall for an appreciable interval, sometimes 2 to 4 hours. When it does head downwards it may drop precipitately. It is at this time that hypoglycemic shock is likely to occur if the physician is not alert, with disastrous results. As soon, therefore, as the blood sugar takes a decided turn downwards, the dosage of insulin should be reduced, while that of glucose is increased. About 10 units of insulin and 20 gm. of glucose per hour is a safe average formula. It matters little at this juncture whether hyperglycemia and glycosuria persist, so long as ketonemia is abolished. For further regulation of the diabetes the reader is referred to the chapters that deal directly with this subject.

The dehydration and salt depletion are quite as serious as ketosis itself and must be vigorously combated from the outset by subcutaneous injections of normal saline. This should be instituted immediately. The quantities to be given depend upon the degree of dehydration. They should be sufficient to provide a free flow of urine in order that the kidneys may be enabled to readjust the acid-base pattern of the serum and interstitial fluids.

Bicarbonate and lactate have been recommended to facilitate this adjustment. Although there can be no reasonable objection to their use, they are not essential and should be given in moderate quantities. It has already been pointed out that the actual deficit of bicarbonate is far less than the apparent deficit, because the sodium combined with ketones is potentially bicarbonate. Attention has been called further to the fact that the deficiency of chloride exceeds the deficiency of bicarbonate in all cases. This is true even in those rare instances in which the concentration of chloride in the

* The use of glucose at this time has been challenged on the ground that there is enough glucose in the body fluids to meet the needs of the body. This argument was open to physiological objections even when the ketolytic action of glucose still prevailed. Since it is now proven beyond peradventure that, to check ketosis, glucose is required for the formation of liver glycogen as well as oxidation in the tissues, apologies need no longer be offered for the use of glucose.

serum is not reduced. Therefore, administration of bicarbonate is of secondary importance—chloride is the prime requisite.

If sufficient saline is given, the kidneys will rapidly adjust the acid-base pattern of the serum as soon as the gross deficiencies of water and salt have been replaced. In the course of treatment with saline alone serum chloride may for a time become unduly elevated. This seems to have no evil effect. The hyperchloremia disappears as soon as dehydration has been overcome. On the other hand, the mere restoration of a normal acid-base pattern by the administration of balanced amounts of sodium chloride and bicarbonate too small to restore the losses of fluid which have been sustained, will benefit the patient little. If the circulation and kidneys are competent, the appearance or persistence of a disproportionate partition of sodium between chloride and bicarbonate, in diabetic acidosis, as in the other diseases and disorders which have been discussed above, betokens that dehydration and gross salt depletion have not yet been entirely abolished.

BIBLIOGRAPHY

1. Adolph, E. F., Am. J. Physiol., **74:** 93 (1925).
2. Adolph, E. F., Am. J. Physiol., **125:** 75 (1939).
3. Aldrich, C. A., and Boyle, H. H., J. Am. Med. Assoc., **114:** 1062 (1940).
4. Aldrich, C. A., Stokes, J., Jr., Killingsworth, W. P., and McGuinness, A. C., J. Am. Med. Assoc., **111:** 129 (1938).
5. Allers, W. D., and Kendall, E. C., Am. J. Physiol., **118:** 87 (1937).
6. Atchley, D. W., Loeb, R. F., Richards, D. W., Jr., Benedict, E. M., and Driscoll, M. E., J. Clin. Invest., **12:** 297 (1933).
7. Atkinson, A. J., and Ivy, A. C., J. Am. Med. Assoc., **106:** 515 (1936).
8. Bartram, E. A., J. Clin. Invest., **11:** 1197 (1932).
9. Bidder, F., and Schmidt, C., Die Verdauungssäfte und der Stoffwechsel. G. A. Reyher, Mitau und Leipzig (1852).
10. Blalock, A., and Beard, J. W., J. Clin. Invest., **11:** 311 (1932).
11. Blalock, A., Beard, J. W., and Thuss, C., ibid., 267.
12. Blackfan, K. D., and Hamilton, B., Boston Med. Surg. J., **193:** 617 (1925).
13. Blackfan, K. D., and McKhann, C. F., J. Am. Med. Assoc., **97:** 1052 (1931).
14. Blumgart, H. L., Gargill, S. L., and Gilligan, D. R., J. Clin. Invest., **9:** 69 (1930).
15. Bollman, J. L., and Mann, F. C., Ann. Int. Med., **5:** 699 (1931-32).
16. Boothby, W. M., Sandiford, I., Sandiford, K., and Slosse, J., Ergebn. Physiol., **24:** 728 (1925).
17. Brodie, B. B., Brand, E., and Seymour, L., J. Biol. Chem., **130:** 555 (1939).
18. Bruckman, F. S., D'Esopo, L. M., and Peters, J. P., J. Clin. Invest., **8:** 577 (1930).
19. Butt, H. R., Snell, A. M., and Keys, A., Arch. Int. Med., **63:** 143 (1939).
20. Byrom, F. B., Clin. Sci., **1:** 273 (1934).
21. Chang, H. C., and Harrop, G. A., Jr., J. Clin. Invest., **5:** 393 (1928).
22. Cope, C. L., Clin. Sci., **2:** 287 (1936).
23. Crider, J. O., and Thomas, J. E., Proc. Soc. Exp. Biol. Med., **44:** 299 (1940).
24. Cushny, A. R., The secretion of urine. Longmans Green and Co., New York (1917).
25. Darrow, D. C., Harrison, H. E., and Taffel, M., J. Biol. Chem., **130:** 487 (1939).
26. Davenport, H. W., and Fisher, R. B., Am. J. Physiol., **131:** 165 (1940).
27. Davis, H. A., and Blalock, J. F., Jr., J. Clin. Invest., **18:** 219 (1939).
28. Dennis, C., Am. J. Physiol., **129:** 171 (1940).
29. Deusch, G., D. Arch. klin. Med., **134:** 342 (1920).
30. Dill, D. B., Hall, F. G., and Edwards, H. T., Am. J. Physiol., **123:** 412 (1938). Dill, D. B., Jones, B. F., Edwards, H. T., and Oberg, S. A., J. Biol. Chem., **100:** 755 (1933).
31. Drinker, C. K., and Field, Madeline E., Lymphatics, lymph and tissue fluid. Williams and Wilkins Co., Baltimore (1933).
32. Drinker, C. K., Field, Madeline E., and Homans, J., Am. J. Physiol., **108:** 509 (1934).
33. Eichelberger, Lillian, and Hastings, A. B., J. Biol. Chem., **118:** 197, 205 (1937).

34. Eisele, C. W., Arch. Int. Med., **63:** 1048 (1939).
35. Eisenman, Anna J., Ott, L., Smith, P. K., and Winkler, A. W., J. Biol. Chem., **135:** 165 (1940).
36. Ellis, A. W. M., Quart. J. Med., **17:** 405 (1924).
37. Eppinger, H., Zur Pathologie und Therapie des menschlichen Ödems zugleich ein Beitrag zur Lehre von der Schilddrüsenfunktion. Eine klinischexperimentelle Studie. J. Springer, Berlin (1917).
38. Farr, L. E., Am. J. Med. Sci., **195:** 70 (1938); Am. J. Dis. Child., **58:** 935 (1939).
39. Farr, L. E., J. Pediatrics, **16:** 679 (1940).
40. Farr, L. E., and Van Slyke, D. D., Am. J. Dis. Child., **57:** 306 (1939).
41. Foster, W. C., J. Am. Med. Assoc., **91:** 1523 (1928).
42. Freeman, N. E., Shaffer, S. A., Schecter, A. E., and Holling, H. E., J. Clin. Invest., **17:** 359 (1938).
43. Freeman, N. E., Shaw, J. L., and Snyder, J. C., J. Clin. Invest., **15:** 651 (1936).
44. Gamble, J. L., Chemical anatomy, physiology and pathology of extracellular fluid, a lecture syllabus. Spaulding-Moss Co., Boston, Mass. (1939). Also Johns Hopkins Hosp. Bull., **61:** 151 (1937).
45. Gamble, J. L., Johns Hopkins Hosp. Bull., **61:** 174 (1937).
46. Gamble, J. L., McKhann, C. F., Butler, A. M., and Tuthill, E., Am. J. Physiol., **109:** 139 (1934).
47. Gamble, J. L., Putnam, M. C., and McKhann, C. F., ibid., **88:** 571 (1929).
48. Gamble, J. L., and Ross, S. G., J. Clin. Invest., **1:** 403 (1925).
49. Gamble, J. L., Ross, S. G., and Tisdall, F. F., J. Biol. Chem., **57:** 633 (1923).
50. Gibson, J. G., 2d, and Evans, W. A., Jr., J. Clin. Invest., **16:** 301 (1937).
51. Gibson, J. G., 2d, and Kopp, I., J. Clin. Invest., **7:** 219 (1938).
52. Gilligan, D. R., and Altschule, M. D., J. Clin. Invest., **18:** 501 (1939).
53. Gilligan, D. R., and Edsall, G., J. Clin. Invest., **14:** 659 (1935).
54. Gilman, A., and Goodman, L., J. Physiol., **90:** 113 (1937).
55. Gilman, A., and Kidd, N. E., Am. J. Physiol., **123:** 77 Soc. Proc. (1938).
56. Govaerts, P., Compt. rend. Soc. biol., **99:** 647 (1928).
57. Govaerts, P., ibid., 339.
58. Grassheim, K., Klin. Woch., **11:** 1257 (1932).
59. Gregerson, M. I., and Gibson, J. G., 2nd, Am. J. Physiol., **120:** 494 (1937).
60. Hahn, L. A., Hevesy, G. C., and Rebbe, O. H., Biochem. J., **33:** 1549 (1939).
61. Hancock, W., Whitehouse, A. G. R., and Haldane, J. S., Proc. Roy. Soc. Lond., **105B:** 43 (1929).
62. Harrison, H. E., and Darrow, D. C., J. Clin. Invest., **17:** 77 (1938).
63. Harrison, H. E., Darrow, D. C., and Yannet, H., J. Biol. Chem., **113:** 515 (1936).
64. Harrop, G. A., Nicholson, W. M., and Strauss, M., J. Exp. Med., **64:** 233 (1936).
65. Hartmann, A. F., Am. J. Dis. Child., **35:** 557 (1928).
66. Hartmann, A. F., and Senn, M. J. E., J. Clin. Invest., **11:** 337 (1932).
67. Hartmann, A. F., and Smyth, F. S., Am. J. Dis. Child., **32:** 1 (1926).
68. Haskell, C. C., Carder, J. R., and Coffindaffer, R. S., J. Am. Med. Assoc., **81:** 448 (1923).
69. Hasselbalch, K. A., Biochem. Z., **78:** 112 (1917).
70. Hastings, A. B., and Eichelberger, Lillian, J. Biol. Chem., **117:** 73 (1937).
71. Hastings, A. B., Harkins, H. N., and Liu, S. K., ibid., **94:** 681 (1932).
72. Heinemann, M., J. Clin. Invest., **17:** 751 (1938).
73. Heller, H., J. Physiol., **89:** 81 (1937).
74. Henderson, L. J., Am. J. Physiol., **21:** 427 (1908).
75. Heppel, L. A., Am. J. Physiol., **127:** 385 (1939).
76. Hoag, L. A., and Marples, E., Am. J. Dis. Child., **42:** 291 (1931).
77. Iversen, P., and Johansen, E. H., Klin. Woch., **8:** 1311 (1929); ibid., 309.
78. Jores, A., Z. ges. exp. Med., **77:** 734 (1931).
79. Kaltreider, N. L., Meneely, G. R., Allen, J. R., Van Voorhis, S. N., and Downing, V. F., J. Clin. Invest., **19:** 769 Soc. Proc. (1940).
80. Keith, N. M., Whelan, M., and Bannick, E. G., Arch. Int. Med., **46:** 797 (1930).
81. Klinghoffer, K. A., International Clinics, **1:** series 4, J. B. Lippincott (1941).
82. Kydd, D. M., J. Clin. Invest., **12:** 1169 (1933).
83. Kydd, D. M., Oard, H. C., and Peters, J. P., J. Biol. Chem., **98:** 241 (1932).
84. Landis, E. M., Harvey Lectures, **32:** 70 (1936–37).

85. Landis, E. M., Jonas, L., Angevine, M., and Erb, W., J. Clin. Invest., **11**: 717 (1932).
86. Lavietes, P. H., ibid., **14**: 57 (1935).
87. Lavietes, P. H., Bourdillon, J., and Klinghoffer, K. A., ibid., **15**: 261 (1936).
88. Lavietes, P. H., D'Esopo, L. M., and Harrison, H. E., ibid., **14**: 251 (1935).
89. Lindeboom, G. A., D. Arch. klin. Med., **175**: 74 (1933).
90. Loeb, R. F., Proc. Soc. Exp. Biol. Med., **30**: 808 (1933); Science, **76**: 420 (1932).
91. Lyall, A., and Nicol, B. M., J. Physiol., **96**: 21 (1939).
92. Mahoney, W., and Sheehan, D., Am. J. Physiol., **112**: 250 (1935).
93. Mainzer, F., Z. klin. Med., **111**: 1 (1929).
94. Manery, Jeanne F., Danielson, I. S., and Hastings, A. B., J. Biol. Chem., **124**: 359 (1938).
95. Manery, Jeanne F., and Hastings, A. B., ibid., **127**: 657 (1939).
96. McCance, R. A., Proc. Roy. Soc. Lond., **119B**: 245 (1936).
97. McCance, R. A., Lancet, **1**: 643, 704, 765, 823 (1936).
98. McCance, R. A., and Widdowson, E. M., J. Physiol., **91**: 222 (1937).
99. McDougall, E. J., Magyar Biol. Kutató Intezet Munkái, **7**: 217 (1934); Chem. Abstr., **29**: 3011 (1935).
100. McQuarrie, I., Johnson, R. M., and Ziegler, M. R., Endocrinology, **21**: 762 (1937).
101. Meulengracht, E., Brit. Med. J., **2**: 321 (1939).
102. Moss, K. N., Proc. Roy. Soc. Lond., **95B**: 181 (1923–24).
103. Newburger, R., Personal communication.
104. Newburgh, L. H., and Johnston, Margaret W., The exchange of energy between man and the environment. Charles C. Thomas, Springfield, Ill. (1930).
105. Nilson, H. W., Am. J. Physiol., **118**: 620 (1937).
106. Ogston, A. G., Philpot, J. St. L., and Zuckerman, S., J. Endocrinol., **1**: 231 (1939).
107. Ord, W. M., Med.-Chirurg. Trans. London, **61**: 57 (1878).
108. Page, I. H., J. Clin. Invest., **12**: 737 (1933).
109. Payne, S. A., and Peters, J. P., ibid., **11**: 103 (1932).
110. Peters, J. P., Body Water. Charles C. Thomas, Springfield, Ill. (1935).
111. Peters, J. P., Bull. N. Y. Acad. Med., **14**: 299 (1938); Harvey Lectures, **33**: 112 (1937–38).
112. Peters, J. P., Chemistry and Medicine, Univ. Minn. Press, Minneapolis, Part I, p. 30 (1940).
113. Peters, J. P., Ann. Surg., **112**: 490 (1940); Symposia on Med. Sciences, Univ. Penn. Bicentennial Conference (1940).
114. Peters, J. P., Medicine, **11**: 435 (1932).
115. Peters, J. P., Yale J. Biol. Med., **9**: 233, 311 (1937).
116. Peters, J. P., and associates. Unpublished data.
117. Peters, J. P., Bruckman, F. S., Eisenman, A. J., Hald, P. M., and Wakeman, A. M., J. Clin. Invest., **10**: 941 (1931).
118. Peters, J. P., Bruckman, F. S., Eisenman, A. J., Hald, P. M., and Wakeman, A. M., ibid., **11**: 97 (1932).
119. Peters, J. P., Bulger, H. A., and Eisenman, A. J., ibid., **3**: 497, 511 (1927).
120. Peters, J. P., Bulger, H. A., Eisenman, A. J., and Lee, C., J. Biol. Chem., **67**: 175 (1926).
121. Peters, J. P., and Eisenman, A. J., Am. J. Med. Sci., **186**: 808 (1933).
122. Peters, J. P., Eisenman, A. J., and Kydd, D. M., ibid., **185**: 149 (1933).
123. Peters, J. P., Kydd, D. M., and Eisenman, A. J., J. Clin. Invest., **12**: 355 (1933). Peters, J. P., Kydd, D. M., Eisenman, A. J., and Hald, P. M., ibid., 377.
124. Peters, J. P., and Van Slyke, D. D., Quantitative Clinical Chemistry, Interpretations. Williams and Wilkins Co., Baltimore (1931).
125. Ragan, C., Ferrebee, J. W., Phyte, P., Atchley, D. W., and Loeb, R. F., Am. J. Physiol., **131**: 73 (1940).
126. Ralli, E. P., Friedman, G. J., and Rubin, S. H., J. Clin. Invest., **17**: 765 (1938).
127. Rapoport, S., and Guest, G. M., J. Biol. Chem., **131**: 675 (1939).
128. Richards, A. N., Methods and results of direct investigations of the function of the kidney. Williams and Wilkins Co., Baltimore (1929); Harvey Lectures, **30**: 93 (1934–35); Croonian Lectures, Proc. Roy. Soc. Lond., **126B**: 398 (1938).
129. Robinson, F. H., Jr., and Farr, L. E., Ann. Int. Med., **14**: 42 (1940).
130. Rosenthal, S. M., J. Pharm. Exp. Therap., **54**: 34 (1935).
131. Schade, H., Claussen, F., and Birner, M., Z. klin. Med., **108**: 581 (1928).

132. Schmidt, C., Characteristik der epidemischen Cholera gegenüber verwandten Trans-sudationsanomalieen. Eine physiologisch-chemische Untersuchung. G. A. Reyher, Leipzig und Mitau (1850).
133. Schmitz, H. L., J. Clin. Invest., 11: 1075 (1932).
134. Sendroy, J., Jr., Seelig, S., and Van Slyke, D. D., J. Biol. Chem., 106: 479 (1934).
135. Shannon, J. A., and Fisher, S., Am. J. Physiol., 122: 765 (138).
136. Sherman, H. C., Chemistry of Food and Nutrition, Macmillan Company, New York (1937).
137. Smirk, F. H., Clin. Sci., 2: 317 (1936).
138. Smith, F. J., J. Am. Med. Assoc., 102: 660 (1934).
139. Smith, H. P., Johns Hopkins Hosp. Bull., 36: 325 (1925).
140. Smith, H. W., The Physiology of the Kidney. Oxford Univ. Press, New York (1937).
141. Smith, H. W., Harvey Lectures, 35: 166 (1939–40).
142. Smith, P. K., and Walker, D. W., J. Pharm. Exp. Therap., 63: 35 (1938).
143. Smith, P. K., and Winkler, A. W., ibid., 69: 303 Soc. Proc. (1940).
144. Smith, P. K., Winkler, A. W., and Schwartz, B. M., J. Biol. Chem., 129: 51 (1939).
145. Solomon, R. Z., Hald, P. M., and Peters, J. P., ibid., 132: 723 (1940).
146. Steiger, M., and Reichstein, T., Helv. Chim. Acta, 20: 1164 (1937).
147. Stevens, R. J., Schiff, L., Lublin, A., and Garber, E. S., J. Clin. Invest., 19: 233 (1940).
148. Strauss, M. B., and Fox, H. J., Am. J. Med. Sci., 200: 454 (1940).
149. Sunderman, F. W., J. Clin. Invest., 7: 313 (1929).
150. Talbott, J. H., and Michelsen, J., ibid., 12: 533 (1933).
151. Thompson, W. O., ibid., 2: 477 (1926).
152. Thorn, G. W., and Engel, L. L., J. Exp. Med., 68: 299 (1938).
153. Thorn, G. W., and Firor, W. M., J. Am. Med. Assoc., 114: 2517 (1940).
154. Thorn, G. W., Garbutt, H. R., Hitchcock, F. A., and Hartman, F. A., Endocrinology, 21: 213 (1937).
155. Thorn, G. W., Koepf, G. F., Lewis, R. A., and Olsen, E. F., J. Clin. Invest., 19: 813 (1940).
156. Thorn, G. W., Nelson, K. R., and Thorn, D. W., Endocrinology, 22: 155 (1938).
157. Vigdoff, B., ibid., 16: 289 (1932).
158. Wakeman, A. M., Morrell, C. A., Eisenman, A. J., Sprunt, D. L., and Peters, J. P., Am. J. Tropical Med., 12: 407 (1932).
159. Walker, A. M., Am. J. Physiol., 127: 519 (1939).
160. Weech, A. A., Bull. N. Y. Acad. Med., 15: 63 (1939); Harvey Lectures, 34: 57 (1938–39).
161. Weiss, S., and Wilkins, R. W., Ann. Int. Med., 11: 104 (1937).
162. Wies, C. H., and Peters, J. P., J. Clin. Invest., 16: 93 (1937).
163. Wilde, W. S., J. Biol. Chem., 128: 309 (1939).
164. Wilder, R. M., Kendall, E. C., Snell, A. M., Kepler, E. J., Rynearson, E. H., and Adams, M., Arch. Int. Med., 59: 367 (1937).
165. Wilder, T. S., and Drake, T. G. H., J. Clin. Invest., 7: 353 (1929).
166. Winkler, A. W. et al., Unpublished studies.
167. Winkler, A. W., and Crankshaw, O. F., J. Clin. Invest., 17: 1 (1938).
168. Winkler, A. W., and Smith, P. K., J. Biol. Chem., 124: 589 (1938).
169. Winkler, A. W., Smith, P. K., and Schwartz, B. M., Am. J. Physiol., 129: 498 Soc. Proc. (1940).
170. Winton, F. R., J. Physiol., 72: 49 (1931).
171. Zimmerman, H. M., and Peters, J. P., J. Clin. Invest., 16: 397 (1937).

CHAPTER VII

NUTRITIONAL AND METABOLIC ASPECTS OF DISORDERS OF THE BLOOD

By LEANDRO M. TOCANTINS

The term disorders of the blood, as it is generally understood, covers those disturbances that may be detected by standard hematological methods. Reasons of convenience and similarity in methods of study and treatment have led to grouping together so many diseases of entirely diverse etiology and pathogenesis.

The discussion in this chapter will be restricted to those disorders which may be influenced or complicated by or which find their origin in defects or deficiencies in body metabolism.

ANEMIAS

General Considerations.—The number of red blood cells in the peripheral blood is kept at the normal level by a balance between the organs for production of these cells (hematopoietic tissues) and the forces and organs of destruction (spleen, lymph nodes). External loss of blood as in hemorrhage is perhaps the most common upsetting factor in this balance; the introduction of blood as by transfusion is the quickest and, perhaps, the most commonly used method for the reestablishment of this balance.

Investigations of the past ten years have demonstrated the great importance of nutritional factors in blood formation. Both the number and quality of the regenerated red blood cells depend to a large extent on the food ingested and the functional integrity of many organs, chiefly the liver and gastro-intestinal tract. Mineral elements such as iron and perhaps copper, organic materials such as certain proteins and amino acids are, among other substances, required for the formation of erythrocytes. Deficient intake of these substances or their incomplete digestion and absorption by the stomach and intestines or their improper mobilization and utilization by organs such as the liver and bone marrow end sooner or later by affecting red cell production.

Since this treatise deals with diseases of metabolism, only those anemias in which a clear nutritional or metabolic disorder is involved will be discussed. Even though the metabolic defect may not be the principal etiological factor, the various anemias will be arranged and discussed chiefly from that viewpoint.

The red blood cell is a biconcave disc composed of water (about one-half of its volume), protein (of which hemoglobin accounts for about one-third of the cell volume), lipids, and salts. Red cells are formed in the bone marrow at the rate of about a trillion per day while a corresponding number is normally destroyed or lost. Many substances are necessary for the formation of red cells but, of only two is sufficient known to allow

12 351

rational conclusions to be drawn concerning them. For the formation of the stroma a substance known as the *erythrocyte maturation factor*, found chiefly in the liver but present also in other organs, is required; for the production of hemoglobin, *iron* is necessary. In addition to these, copper, vitamin C and thyroxin are also essential for the maturation of the red blood cell. The degree of activity of the blood making cells is regulated by the oxygen tension of the blood in the bone marrow, when all necessary materials are available.

Laboratory Examinations.—Though the results of laboratory examinations are often more descriptive than explanatory, they supply accurate evidence which, with other facts, contributes to the proper classification and understanding of the pathogenesis of the anemias. It is, therefore, highly desirable that in the study of the anemic patient the descriptive constants for the erythrocyte be carefully determined. Standard methods for these and other hematological determinations are described in textbooks on hematology and will not be described here.

Determination of the *number* of reticulocytes (young red blood cells) in the blood is a useful means of measuring the degree of activity of the bone marrow in regenerating erythrocytes. It is employed not only to test the efficacy of a therapeutic agent but also as an important diagnostic and prognostic point. Absence or decreased number of reticulocytes in a patient with severe anemia is a bad omen. Conversely an increase in the number of reticulocytes, especially if accompanied by increases in the number of leukocytes and of platelets, is a sign of heightened activity in the bone marrow. This activity may not always result from a normal orderly stimulus, but from pathological stimuli, as for example, in instances of metastatic tumor invasion of the marrow.

In modern evaluation of hematological problems some dependence must be placed upon the cytological examination of the *bone marrow*. In most instances a sample of the marrow can be obtained from the manubrium or the body of the sternum by simple puncture with an appropriate needle; a small amount of the blood-marrow mixture is withdrawn, spread on a slide, and examined after staining. The information to be obtained is necessarily limited by the fact that the histological structure of the marrow is not preserved. It is possible, however, to ascertain certain facts by this method, namely, leukemic infiltration, hyperplasia or hypoplasia of erythroid or granulocytic elements, relative increase in the number of megakaryocytes, and megaloblastic or myeloblastic proliferation. Those changes, though not in themselves specific, may be valuable in supporting or excluding a clinical diagnosis.

The metabolic studies of disorders of the blood should properly include an estimation of the blood *iron* and determination of the blood, urinary and fecal pigments. Of the latter, bilirubin and urobilin are the most commonly studied. Their level may supply, along with the number of reticulocytes, some indication of the activity of the blood destroying and blood regenerating forces of the body. Measurement of the excretion of the porphyrins has yielded information of value in pernicious anemia, lead poisoning and hemolytic jaundice. It seems, from analysis of excretion of coproporphyrin I, that this porphyrin bears some relationship to the erythropoietic activity of the marrow. So far, however, knowledge of porphyrin metabolism is too limited to permit its use in drawing definite conclusions regarding the pathogenesis of hematological disorders.

Analysis of Case.—Once in possession of the information supplied by the laboratory studies, the clinician can then proceed to a rational analysis of the causes of the type of anemia found. Besides all the modern hematological methods now available for the study of the blood and hematopoietic tissues (marrow, spleen, lymph nodes) a careful investigation into the diet and medicinal drugs ingested by the patient is often of great help in arriving at a correct etiological diagnosis. For this purpose it is essential to go in detail into the number and composition of the meals taken by the patient, habits of eating, and foods disliked or avoided. Since the problem consists in accounting for the anemia, special attention should be paid to the detection of any existing channels for loss of blood from the body as for example through the gastro-intestinal tract. Fractional analysis of the gastric juice, examination of the stools and measurement of the basal metabolic rate are also helpful in elucidating possible mechanisms for the production or perpetuation of anemia. In a few instances measurement of the fragility of the red cells and of the blood ascorbic acid level may offer a clue to the disorder.

CLASSIFICATION OF ANEMIAS

A classification of the anemias according to the size and hemoglobin content of the erythrocyte is useful principally because it often indicates the direction wherein lies the cause for the anemia. Measurements of size and hemoglobin content of the red cell as calculated from determinations of number of red cells, hemoglobin content and packed cell volume of the blood allow a subdivision of the anemias into several "types," as follows: (1) Macrocytic: the volume of the red cell may be almost twice the normal. (2) Normocytic: the individual volume and hemoglobin concentration of the red cell are normal; the number of cells alone is diminished. (3) Microcytic: the volume of the red cell is reduced to about three-fourths of normal, though its individual hemoglobin concentration is normal. (4) Hypochromic: the hemoglobin concentration of each erythrocyte is reduced to as much as one-half the normal.

With few exceptions, due usually to the presence of complicating factors, a given set of etiological agents produces a certain "type" of anemia with great regularity. It is, therefore, of great clinical help to determine these various types and thereby have a clue to their probable etiology.

Though etiological considerations should naturally occupy the most important place in the classification of anemia, restrictions imposed by the scope of this treatise make it necessary to group the various disorders chiefly according to their clinical manifestations which make them more readily recognized by the physician.

Anemias Due to Nutritional Deficiencies.—In this group are found anemias of the *hypochromic* and those of the *macrocytic* types. Generally speaking these hypochromic anemias are caused by *deficiencies in the intake or absorption of iron and other hemoglobin producing substances*. There may be either a lack or a diminution in the ingestion and absorption of substances required for the normal needs of the body or their intake in insufficient amounts to cope with increased demands on the hematopoietic organs, as after a hemorrhage, hemolytic crisis, or infection. In estimating the degree of a deficiency with a view to correction, it should always be kept in mind that at any time intrinsic changes may take place in the body which alter its requirements for certain substances, thereby accentuating or making obsolete any existing deficiencies.

Hypochromic Anemia.—About 25 gm. of hemoglobin are formed daily by the marrow in adults. In order to maintain this rate of hemoglobin production about 100 mg. of iron are required (available chiefly from destroyed hemoglobin) and of this amount about 15 mg. are lost each day. The amount of iron contained in most foods is so small that it barely replaces this daily loss. When extraordinary demands are placed on the mechanism of hemoglobin production the usual daily iron intake proves insufficient and a hypochromic anemia supervenes. Such conditions are observed in a variety of clinical states. It is this type of anemia that may appear during periods of active growth, during pregnancy or lactation. The hypochromic anemia of infancy and childhood belongs in this group. This anemia is rarely observed before the tenth week of life; it is made more severe if in addition to a deficient intake of iron the infant is troubled with gastro-intestinal disorders and consequent poor digestion and absorption of food. Its therapy is essentially like that of hypochromic anemia of adults. Care should be taken to distinguish it from erythroblastic anemia or leukemia. The hypochromic anemia of *pregnancy* results partially from a deficiency of iron. In many patients however, an associated hypochlorhydria or achlorhydria aggravates the deficiency and often renders iron therapy ineffective.

HCl AND IRON ABSORPTION.—Absorption of ingested iron is thought to take place chiefly in the duodenum. Such absorption is much influenced by the amount of hydrochloric acid present in the stomach. A diminution or absence of HCl interferes with absorption of iron, particularly when in an insoluble form, thereby producing a deficiency. Such, in part, is the pathogenesis of the "idiopathic hypochromic anemia" of middle aged women almost always associated with other nutritional deficiencies. Such patients often display the signs of vitamin B deficiency: sore tongue, fissured lips, paresthesias, brittle, concave finger nails. In a certain group designated as the Plummer-Vinson syndrome[1] there is, in addition, difficulty and pain in swallowing.

Structural defects in the esophagus, stomach, or intestine (stricture, resection, anastomosis, fistula) by affecting the intake, digestion and absorption of food, may contribute to the production of an iron deficiency. In diseases accompanied by diarrhea, as in dysentery and ulcerative colitis, the reduced intestinal absorption leads to the same results. In all these instances the anemia as well as the deficiency is often made worse by blood loss, an inadequate diet, or the presence of infection or parasites such as hookworm. In the disorder of fat digestion designated as *idiopathic steatorrhea*, a hypochromic anemia is often found.

The hypochromic anemia sometimes seen *in young women* yields readily to iron therapy and must be considered to belong in this group of anemias. Its occurrence may be traced to a combination of factors among which are an inadequate diet, decreased gastric secretions and excessive blood loss at menstruation. Under these circumstances, the great demands for iron by the body are not satisfied and a deficiency follows. Substantially the same syndrome in a more exaggerated form was designated chlorosis by the old writers.

Macrocytic Anemias.—Nutritional deficiencies may also account for anemias of the macrocytic type. These deficiencies lead to a *diminished function of the bone marrow* due to a lack of certain elements necessary for normal blood formation. In the case of the macrocytic anemias these

TABLE 1

ANEMIAS DUE PRIMARILY TO NUTRITIONAL OR METABOLIC DEFECTS

Etiology	Type of Anemia	Treatment (Specific and/or Supportive)
Deficiency of the erythrocyte maturation factor: Pernicious anemia Defects or disorders of the gastro-intestinal tract (stricture, resections, anastomosis, obstruction, diarrhea, steatorrhea, fish tapeworm infestation) Pellagra Sprue Tropical anemia of pregnancy	Macrocytic Usually macrocytic Usually macrocytic Usually macrocytic Macrocytic	Liver extract orally or parenterally. Correction of defects. Nutritious diet high in protein and including Brewer's yeast
Deficiency of iron: Anemias of infancy and childhood Chlorosis Idiopathic hypochromic anemia of adolescent and of middle aged women Anemia of pregnancy Disorders of the gastro-intestinal tract (strictures, resections, anastomosis, obstructions, diarrhea, steatorrhea, and parasites, *e.g.*, hookworm)	Hypochromic, sometimes microcytic Hypochromic, sometimes microcytic Hypochromic, sometimes microcytic Hypochromic, sometimes microcytic Hypochromic, sometimes microcytic	Iron as ferrous sulfate, ferrous chloride or ferrous carbonate. Blood transfusion* (small, frequent). Dilute hydrochloric acid if achlorhydria exists Correction of defects
Deficiency of thyroid secretion	Usually normochromic	Thyroid substance
Deficiency of vitamin C	Usually hypochromic	Ascorbic acid
Metabolic disorders: Chronic nitrogen retention Primary xanthomatosis Osteosclerosis Disease of the liver	Normocytic or macrocytic Normochromic or hypochromic Normochromic or macrocytic Macrocytic	Transfusion* (great care!) Transfusion* Transfusion* Liver extract sometimes effective. Transfusion.

* Transfusions of whole blood.

elements are the ones found in certain extracts of liver. In *Addisonian pernicious* anemia there is an achlorhydria of the gastric contents and along with that an absence of a thermolabile constituent designated by Castle[2] as the intrinsic factor. This factor when combined with an extrinsic factor to be found in meat, eggs, yeast and other substances forms a substance which is required for the normal maturation of cells in the marrow. Neither the extrinsic or intrinsic factors nor the anti-anemic factor resulting from their interaction has been identified or isolated in pure form. It has been known for many years that the gastric mucous membrane in patients with pernicious anemia is atrophied and this fact along with the resulting imperfect secretion of gastric juice is the fundamental defect responsible for the development of Addisonian pernicious anemia. Alterations have been found in the constituents of the blood other than the cell elements, in this disease; a few of these are probably a result of the anemia and, as such, bear no relation to the cause of the disease. It is well to bear in mind that many disorders (chronic nephritis, myxedema, chronic cholelithiasis) have been confused with pernicious anemia, with which they have many clinical points of similarity.

A macrocytic anemia indistinguishable from that of pernicious anemia is observed in *sprue* and in a *tropical anemia of pregnancy*. In both of these disorders a diet rich in sources of the extrinsic factor (meat, autolyzed yeast, eggs) leads to the rapid disappearance of the anemia.

Dietetic and possibly gastric defects are probably also the underlying reasons for the macrocytic anemia observed occasionally in association with infestation with the *fish tapeworm*.

Defective absorption of the end product of the interaction of the gastric and food factors may be responsible for the appearance of a macrocytic anemia in patients with chronic intestinal obstruction, intestinal anastomosis, prolonged attacks of diarrhea and idiopathic steatorrhea.

Combined Deficiencies.—Many of the circumstances surrounding the development of an iron deficiency may also entail a deficiency in the extrinsic hematopoietic factor. In treated pernicious anemia the accelerated output of red cells may after a time, disclose a lag in hemoglobin production from insufficiency of available iron. It is possible, therefore, to have in the same patient, within short periods of time, manifestations of two deficiencies ordinarily observed as distinct entities. The complex nutritional disorder that leads to pellagra is sometimes accompanied by a macrocytic anemia. Though substances effective in treating pernicious anemia are likewise curative of pellagra there does not seem to exist sufficient evidence that the pellagra preventive factor and the extrinsic anti-pernicious-anemia factor are one and the same.

A *lack of vitamin C* in the diet may, according to some authors lead to an anemia, normochromic in type, but with a wide variation in size of the red cells, sometimes suggesting pernicious anemia. Prompt reticulocyte responses follow administration of ascorbic acid. The anemia of scurvy, when not complicated by excessive hemorrhage, appears to result from diminished production of erythrocytes by the marrow.

In *deficiencies of the secretion of the thyroid gland*, particularly if they are accompanied by myxedema, it is not uncommon to find an anemia, usually of the normochromic type. Occasionally the anemia is hypochromic or even macrocytic; in these patients there is usually in addition to the myxedema a deficiency of iron or of the liver active principle. The anemia of myxedema is probably due to a depression of hematopoiesis as a result of the low oxygen consumption of the tissues in general, including the bone marrow. In uncomplicated myxedema the anemia is usually corrected by the proper administration of thyroid substance alone. In those patients in whom the anemia is of the hypochromic type, iron should be given in addition to thyroid therapy. In patients with myxedema and a macrocytic type of anemia, liver extract should be added to the glandular medication. Examination of the cytological composition of the marrow as obtained by sternal puncture may yield information in this respect. While in uncomplicated myxedema the bone marrow is either normal or slightly hypoplastic in so far as any evidence of red cell regeneration is concerned, in the macrocytic and hypochromic anemias there is usually a megaloblastic or a normoblastic hyperplasia, respectively.

In *chronic nitrogen retention* resulting from many types of renal impairment a normocytic, normochromic anemia, refractory to liver or iron therapy, is often observed. The anemia appears to result from a toxic depression of the bone marrow produced by substances so far unknown but probably associated with nitrogen retention.

A group of anemias remains to be discussed which displays many signs of an advanced metabolic disorder but about which little is known. These anemias result from reduced hematopoietic activity of the marrow due to *osteodystrophies* of one kind or another (myelosclerosis, osteofibrosis, multiple myeloma, carcinomatosis). The metabolic findings in anemia complicating these diseases are not sufficiently constant to be of any help in elucidating the mechanism of the disorder.

Primary disorders of lipid metabolism (the xanthomatoses) often lead to anemia by interfering with hematopoiesis. The presence in the marrow of large cells loaded with lipid material, that may later be replaced by fibrosis interferes with the functional activity of the marrow.

The widespread osteoporosis and other changes in the bones commonly found in association with sickle cell anemia, and the erythroblastic anemias of childhood suggest that there may exist in these diseases a deficiency or defect in a factor required both for hematopoiesis and ossification. There are no indications, however, where this deficiency may lie.

TREATMENT OF THE ANEMIAS

The following measures are most generally used in correcting the anemic state:

1. If the cause is known and can be removed it should, of course, be removed.

2. Part of the deficit in blood formation may be temporarily corrected by giving the patient a transfusion of blood.

3. If the diet is deficient, care should be taken to make it nutritious and well balanced.

4. In the anemias of the *macrocytic* type liver extract should be tried though not all may respond to it. Eating of partly cooked liver should be encouraged. If the anemia proves refractory to powdered liver extract taken by mouth, the extract should then be given parenterally in doses proportional to the degree of the anemia. If the anemia is moderate, 15 units of liver extract three times a week for two weeks should constitute a fair trial. In marked anemia this dose should, of course, be given oftener and for a longer period.

5. In the *microcytic* and *hypochromic* anemias iron is indicated. The ferrous salts are now inexpensive and readily available. Iron may be given as ferrous sulfate, dose 0.65–1.0 gm. (10–15 grains) daily, or as ferrous

chloride 0.325–0.65 gm. (5–10 grains daily) or as ferrous carbonate (Blaud's pill) dose 2.6–4.0 gm. (40–60 grains) daily. Sometimes iron is either not absorbed when taken by mouth or produces much irritation of the gastrointestinal tract. Patients with achlorhydria are said to require, in addition to iron, the administration of dilute hydrochloric acid, 15 to 30 minims t.i.d. to aid in the absorption of the metal. Other times, though rarely, iron ammonium citrate in doses of 30 mg. daily, intramuscularly, will produce the desired results.

Correction of existing deficiencies such as hypothyroidism will often influence the anemia favorably. The administration of vitamin B complex and of vitamin C is of value in some instances.

POLYCYTHEMIA

The etiology of true polycythemia is still in dispute. There are indications that in this disease, as in pernicious anemia, one is dealing with a metabolic disturbance. The disorder may consist of a poorly or improperly compensated excess of substances required for erythropoiesis. It has been shown that the high red cell mass found in this disease is favorably influenced by repeated bleedings and the administration of an iron deficient diet.[3] By these means the factors that are known to operate in the production of hypochromic anemia are brought to bear in polycythemia. The bleedings are carried out twice a week until the hemoglobin is reduced to about 80 per cent, the red cell count to about 5 millions and the hematocrit to about 42 per cent. This may require 6 to 8 venesections. The patient is then given a diet containing only about 6 mg. of iron per day. Red meats, meat soups, liver, eggs, rye bread and brown cereals are not permitted. Fowl once a week, fish twice a week, cheese, milk and legumes supply sufficient proteins. Alkaline powders may be prescribed to counteract the acidity of the gastric juice. Acetylphenylhydrazine, a drug which destroys erythrocytes, is also effective in reducing the red cell count. It should be given cautiously, under close supervision, in doses at the start of 0.1 gm. (1½ grains) daily until 1 gm. (15 grains) has been taken. The doses to follow will depend on the reaction of the patient to this first course. As little as 0.1 gm. (1½ grains) once a week may be sufficient to maintain the red cell count at a normal level.

DISORDERS OF LEUKOCYTES

These disorders may be grouped for the purposes of this discussion under two main headings:
(1) Leukopenias.
(2) Leukemias.

So far as present knowledge goes there are few clinical entities involving disorders of leukocytes which can be traced to a nutritional or metabolic origin.

At present very little is known concerning the substances necessary for the formation of leukocytes. As with the erythrocytes it is likely that specific substances are required for their formation. The granulocytes of the blood are formed in the bone marrow and are thought to last from a few hours to as long as four or five days after entering the circulation. The leukocyte count in the blood is an expression of the balance between the utilization of the granulocytes by the tissues and the regular formation of these cells by the marrow.

LEUKOPENIAS

Knowledge of the leukopenias is today at an undifferentiated stage, analogous to that of knowledge of the anemias two or three decades ago. The fruitful results of the past ten years in the study of anemias from the pathophysiological viewpoint indicate the desirability of directing studies of disorders of leukocytes along similar lines. Decrease in number of leukocytes probably results as in the anemias, from either an increase in the loss or destruction of leukocytes or from an insufficient production of these cells in the marrow. Most of the leukocytes may be considered as cells in transit in the blood. This is in contrast with the erythrocytes and platelets, which perform all their functions in the circulating blood itself where they remain normally.

In the presence of ulcerative or necrotizing lesions a lasting leukopenia should be taken as evidence of failure of *myelopoiesis*.

In studies with normal animals it has been found that nucleic acid and its derivatives produce a myeloid hyperplasia of the marrow and leukocytosis in the peripheral blood. The demonstration of the presence of pentose nucleotides in normal human blood and of their apparent stimulative effect on normal marrow led to the use of that nucleotide in malignant leukopenias. The available evidence does not allow the conclusion that these substances have been proven effective in leukopenias. In the monkey and the dog neutropenias have been induced by giving the animals a diet deficient in some substance that is present in liver extract, meat, yeast. No such relationship, however, has been clearly demonstrated in man. Considering, however, how common it is to obtain a history of nutritional deficiency in patients with malignant leukopenia, it seems that a *diet* rich in meat with additions of yeast and liver extract may be administered to such patients with profit.

A few of the persistent leukopenias seem to be the result of, or at least influenced by a prolonged period of a diet inadequate in many essential substances, added to the ingestion of sedatives, especially those containing amidopyrine. One patient who came under our observation had been taking a compound containing amidopyrine daily for several months while at the same time his diet had been restricted because of "colitis." It was only after about one month following discontinuance of the drug and the administration of a protein rich diet supplemented by yeast and liver extract that the white cell count remained above 3,000 and all ulcerations disappeared.

LEUKEMIAS

There is abundant evidence available pointing to widespread changes in metabolism in the leukemias. The *basal metabolic rate* is uniformly elevated above normal, sometimes quite markedly. This change may be helpful in distinguishing between the leukemias and transitory leukemoid states. A high basal metabolic rate is observed in both lymphogenous and myelogenous leukemias and parallels generally the severity of the disease and the number of immature leukocytes in the blood. Though in this respect leukemia and hyperthyroidism are similar, there are marked differences in the type of metabolism of the two diseases. In leukemia there seems to be economy of *muscular movement* (tremors and other evidences of deranged muscular action are absent in leukemia) while in hyperthyroidism there is excessive muscular activity. Irritability, nervousness and insomnia are not common in leukemia. The *specific dynamic action of proteins* is diminished in the leukemias, the more severe the disease the less the action. It has been suggested that protein catabolism is the main factor responsible for the increased oxygen consumption and consequently the increased metabolic rate in leukemia. The immediate effect of *roentgen ray therapy* in leukemia is an increase in the metabolic rate, a result perhaps of an increased destruction of leukocytes. Furthermore, measures effective in controlling hyperthyroidism have not succeeded in leukemia. In leukemia there is also retention of nitrogen by the body. A high uric acid content in the blood is a regular occurrence in leukemia, often helpful in differential diagnosis between this disease and leukemoid states. When roentgen ray therapy is followed by diminution in the size of the spleen and number of leukocytes, there is an increase in the excretion of total nitrogen, uric acid, ammonia and phosphorus. The diminution in nitrogen excretion is thought to be an indication that in leukemia there is a decrease in the normal breakdown of cells, or as others propose, nitrogen is retained because of excessive demands for it in the formation of new cells.

Marked elevation of the total blood phosphorus is common in leukemia, due almost entirely to an increase in total phosphorus content of the corpuscles, particularly in the immature forms. The total phosphorus content of the plasma is usually normal, and the inorganic phosphorus of plasma or corpuscles is not altered. Other changes commonly found are an increase in blood glutathione, occasional appearance of Bence-Jones protein in the plasma or urine, and moderate decreases in the plasma albumin.

Leukemic cells display an increased consumption of oxygen and a type of metabolic activity similar to that of malignant tissue cells. This type of activity may be observed even in the tissue cells, sometimes preceding the manifestations of the disease in the blood.

Though much information is available concerning the metabolic changes in leukemia it has served little in clarifying the fundamental nature of the disorder or in offering an efficacious method of treatment. Dependence is still placed today on arsenic and roentgen ray therapy as palliative measures.

DISORDERS OF BLEEDING

For a proper understanding and treatment of disorders of bleeding it is necessary to have a clear conception of the forces involved in the production and arrest of bleeding. Wherever it happens to take place, bleeding is a result of an upset of the balance between the hemostatic forces of the body that keep the blood within the vessels and the stresses, internal or external, that tend to drive it out of them. A rational handling of the problem of excessive bleeding must always take into consideration the existence of these stresses which are chiefly mechanical in nature. By external stresses are meant traumata of any type (blows, incisions, etc.), or even the traumata to which the tissues are exposed in every-day life and which they are ordinarily able to overcome. Internal stresses are those placed on the vessels by certain forces—the blood pressure, tissue contraction and stretching (heart and intestines), changes in posture, and alterations in the pressure surrounding organs such as the lungs. The hemostatic forces are intended to overcome the effect of the operation of such stresses so far as they may give rise to loss of blood from the vessels.

While not enough information is available to work out satisfactorily a grouping of hemorrhagic disorders based on changes in the various factors responsible for normal hemostasis, enough is known to warrant making an attempt at forming such a group. Abnormal bleeding may result from:

1. Failure of a defective hemostatic mechanism to overcome ordinary stresses placed on the vessels.
2. Failure of a normal hemostatic mechanism in overcoming abnormal stresses.

Mention of the second group is made to emphasize the fact that not all abnormal bleeding results from a defect in hemostasis. In the second group are perhaps the most commonly met instances of excessive bleeding, regardless of its location. There is good reason to believe, however, that even abnormal bleeding due purely to excessive or widespread trauma may, if sufficiently prolonged, be complicated by impairment in hemostasis which will further prolong the bleeding.

Methods of Investigation.—The methods in common use for the investigation of disorders of bleeding are: measurement of the coagulation time of venous blood, retraction of the blood clot, number of platelets, amount of prothrombin and fibrinogen and less frequently the amount of antithrombin. These methods have as their main object an analysis of the main factors concerned in hemostasis. The bleeding time, and the test for the petechial reaction of the skin after prolonged venous congestion of an extremity, are actual tests of the ability of the body to react to increased external or internal stresses; when properly performed and interpreted they supply valuable information.

Failure of the mechanism responsible for the arrest of bleeding may come about in a variety of ways. This failure is usually a result of a temporary or permanent alteration in one or more of the factors that play a part in normal hemostasis. These factors may be of three different types: 1. extravascular factors, 2. vascular factors, and 3. intravascular factors.

Extravascular Factors.—Abnormalities in hemostasis due to alterations in extravascular factors (content of thromboplastin of surrounding tissues, tissue rigidity, tissue tension, tissue elasticity), are not clearly understood. Their importance in conditioning and influencing bleeding is not to be minimized however. The loss of tone and elasticity of the skin in certain debilitating diseases is probably related to the ease by which hemorrhages are produced in patients with such diseases.

Vascular Factors.—Alterations in the vessels themselves may give rise to manifestations of excessive bleeding. The chief example of this is scurvy. An adequate intake of vitamin C (ascorbic acid) is evidently required for the proper formation and maintenance of blood vessels. The vitamin probably regulates the deposition of collagen between the cells, though the morphological changes in support of that fact that have been detected in the capillaries are not conclusive. The effect of the deficiency is probably on the sheath or the cement substance surrounding the endothelial cells of the capillary. The hemorrhagic manifestations of scurvy are like all hemorrhagic manifestations determined to a large extent by the type or degree of stress applied to the part. The hemorrhages usually take on the form of fine petechial eruptions, particularly in the lower extremities; there is also associated bleeding from the gums and occasionally from the gastro-intestinal tract. The deficiency may be purely dietetic or the result of increased demands for the vitamin because of an infection, high metabolic rate, rapid growth, etc. There is predilection of the hemorrhages for infected areas, such as, infection at the roots of the teeth. In the skin the hemorrhage is usually around the hair follicles. Blood stained effusions may appear in the serous cavities. The production of an increased venous pressure in the arm by application of pressure up to the diastolic level will, after three or four minutes, give rise to a petechial rash below the point of constriction.

Vitamin C is also known to affect blood formation. Patients with a vitamin C deficiency often have anemia which is a result not only of blood loss, but of deficient blood production. A vitamin C deficiency may occasionally appear in the course of other hemorrhagic disorders. Administration of the vitamin is often followed by such a marked diminution in the bleeding as to make it seem that a specific effect has been produced. If the patient is taking an adequate diet and still displays signs of a deficiency in vitamin C, the vitamin should be given intravenously (100 mg. of ascorbic acid daily).

In some hemorrhagic disorders resembling scurvy it has been pointed out that the use of a flavin obtained from lemon rinds is effective in correcting the disorders. This substance has been called vitamin P (hesperidin and eriodictyol glucoside). Two patients with Schoenlein-Henoch's purpura that have come under our observation were free of recurrences while taking the vitamin. The rebelliousness of this disorder to any form of treatment makes it desirable to try the effect of this vitamin.

Intravascular Factors.—Disorders of bleeding may also result from a delayed coagulability of the blood or from defects in the physical properties of the clot. In many hemorrhagic disorders the rate of coagulation of the blood is but slightly altered; the poor quality of the formed clot accounts for its inefficacy in checking the blood flow. Two factors play leading parts in endowing the clots with the properties of rigidity, adhesiveness and rapid contractility: the amount of prothrombin in the plasma and the number and agglutinability of blood platelets.

Diminished Plasma Prothrombin.—An increasingly large number of instances of abnormal bleeding is being found in which the main defect is an alteration in the coagulability of the blood due to a diminished plasma prothrombin. Metabolism of prothrombin is closely related to vitamin K (see Chap. VIII). An insufficient amount of prothrombin in the blood results in a deficiency in thrombin and an impaired coagulability of the blood. In such instances, not only is there a prolongation of the clotting time but the clot itself is soft and inadequate from the standpoint of checking blood flow. A low plasma prothrombin may result from:

1. *Diminution in the ingestion of vitamin K in the diet.* The vitamin is

fat soluble and is found principally in green vegetables (spinach), hog liver fat, yeast, and in some cereals. Instances of pure vitamin K deficiency of dietetic origin are not common, the deficiency being usually found in association with other deficiencies.

2. *Interference with the digestion of food.* This is found in many disorders of the gastro-intestinal tract. The little food that is taken in is not properly digested and is allowed to pass through the rest of the bowel almost unchanged. In resections of the stomach, anastomosis of bowel, strictures, obstructions, etc., such may be the case. In diseases of the liver accompanied by diminution in the amount of bile flowing into the intestines, or in patients with insufficient pancreatic secretion, digestion of fat is so impaired that no vitamin is freed in the intestine for absorption.

In obstructive jaundice the absence of bile from the intestine interferes with the digestion of fat and the proper absorption of vitamin K. The low plasma prothrombin in these cases is partially due to inadequate intake; diets of patients with gallbladder disease are often made deliberately low in fat. If the obstructive jaundice is not of long duration and the function of the liver is not markedly impaired, there is a prompt response to the administration of vitamin K.

3. *Defective absorption by the gastro-intestinal tract.* In these patients though the vitamin is present in adequate amounts the essential elements fail to be absorbed because of some defect of the gastro-intestinal tract—(prolonged diarrhea, vomiting, obstruction, intestinal fistula, sprue, etc.).

4. *Imperfect synthesis of the vitamin by the liver.* Prothrombin is formed almost entirely in the liver. Though prothrombin requires vitamin K for its formation, vitamin K itself has no prothrombin activity. In diseases of the liver accompanied by marked functional impairment of this organ, there is a diminution in the plasma prothrombin, sometimes quite marked. Administration of the various forms of vitamin K to these patients fails to produce any significant increase in the plasma prothrombin. Should these patients bleed excessively the only recourse as far as hemostasis is concerned is a blood transfusion which will supply a limited amount of prothrombin. A transfusion of approximately 400 cc. of blood will lead, however, to only approximately 10 per cent increase in prothrombin in the blood. The effect is, therefore, one of simple addition of an already made substance, from the outside.

Substitutes for Vitamin K.—There are now available two effective synthetic substitutes for the natural vitamin K. One of them 2-methyl-1,4-naphthoquinone is the ideal source of vitamin K when administered by mouth, 1–2 mg. daily.[4] Its low solubility in water makes it less desirable for parenteral use. The other substitute, 4-amino-2-methyl-1-naphthol hydrochloride, though apparently not as potent, is more soluble in water, more stable in solution and therefore better adapted for intramuscular and intravenous use. The dose is 2 mg. by intramuscular or intravenous injection.

Diminished Plasma Prothrombin in the Newborn.—The newborn infant has a low plasma prothrombin during the first three to five days of life.[5] This circumstance is responsible in a large measure for the hemorrhagic disorders of early infancy and perhaps for many of the hemorrhagic accidents at birth. The mother usually has an increased amount of prothrombin in her blood and this explains the efficacy of the still reliable method of treating the hemorrhagic disorders of infants by giving the baby *injections of maternal blood*. A simpler method of correcting this deficiency, however, is to give the baby the vitamin K synthetic substitute in oil 2-methyl-1,4-naphthoquinone, 1 mg. daily, by mouth immediately after birth. Giving the substitute to the mother for two or three weeks before delivery is also helpful to the baby.

In case there is reason to believe that the vitamin is not being absorbed, intramuscular administration is indicated. In these instances the vitamin K substitute 4-amino-2-methyl-1-naphthol hydrochloride, 1 mg. in aqueous solution, is indicated. The bleeding stops promptly, sometimes within three hours after administration of the drug.

HEMOPHILIA

This condition, which is an inherited disposition of males to bleed, though a relatively uncommon disorder of bleeding, is one of the most difficult to treat. Many of its manifestations suggest a disturbance of metabolism, as the underlying cause for the deficiency in thromboplastin and the resultant impaired coagulability of the blood. The hemophilic, like the diabetic patient, lacks an essential principle at all times, but in varying degrees. The present treatment of hemophilia consists in supplying this deficient principle in the form of blood transfusions. In the future, the hemophilic may have this deficiency corrected by frequent administration of that essential principle in a concentrated form.

THROMBOPENIA

The tendency toward excessive bleeding from the skin and mucous membranes is often a result of a diminution in the number or absence of platelets in the blood. There are certain indications that nutritional factors play important rôles in certain types of thrombopenia. After liver therapy, the moderate thrombopenia observed in pernicious anemia gives place to a rapid thrombocytosis, the initiation of which often precedes the rise in reticulocytes. Transient phases of thrombopenia appear sometimes during nutritional disorders complicating derangements of the gastro-intestinal tract. Administration of thiamin chloride and nicotinic acid to one patient who, besides a B avitaminosis developed thrombopenic purpura during recovery from an operation for intestinal obstruction (the plasma prothrombin was not altered), led to a prompt cessation in the bleeding and an increase in the number of platelets. Though a relationship appears to exist between certain thrombopenias and nutritional defects, the attempts of a few authors to establish a connection between specific vitamins (A, D and the hypothetical T) and the production of platelets remain unconvincing.

BIBLIOGRAPHY

1. Graham, G. and Johnson, R. S., Anemia with dysphagia, Quart. J. Med., **25**: 41, 1932.
2. Castle, W. B. and Minot, G. R., Pathological physiology and clinical description of the anemias (Reprinted from Oxford Loose-Leaf Medicine), N. Y., Oxford, 1936.
3. Dameshek, W. and Henstell, H. H., Diagnosis of Polycythemia, Ann. Int. Med., **13**: 1360, 1940.

4. Tocantins, L. M. and Jones, H. W., Hypoprothrombinemia: Effect of peroral and parenteral administration of a synthetic vitamin K substitute (2-methyl-1, 4-naphthoquinone), Ann. of Surg., **113**: 276, 1941.
5. Tocantins, L. M., The probable mechanism of the "physiologic" hypoprothrombinemia of the newborn, Amer. J. Dis. Child., **59**: 1054, 1940.

USEFUL TEXTS FOR CONSULTATION

Vaughan, J. M., The Anemias, 2nd ed., N. Y., Oxford, 1936.
Haden, R. L., Principles of Hematology, 2nd ed., Philadelphia, Lea & Febiger, 1940.
Forkner, C. E., Leukemia and Allied Disorders, The Macmillan Co., New York, 1938.
A Symposium on the Blood and Blood Forming Organs, University of Wisconsin Press, Madison, Wis., 1939.

CHAPTER VIII

VITAMINS AND AVITAMINOSES

By Tom D. Spies and Hugh R. Butt

INTRODUCTION

The achievements in the young and vigorous science of nutrition promise to be the most significant of all that have been made in modern medical science. We could not hope to list, let alone adequately describe, the various ramifications of the newer knowledge concerning vitamins. Vitamins are organic food substances which, in however small quantities, are necessary for maintaining proper growth and continued health of the body. The quantities required are indeed so ridiculously small as to make it probable that they act as catalysts or that they help to form such in the body. In fact, a number have been shown to be involved in the systems governing oxidation of carbohydrates, proteins, and fats. They are frequently called accessory food factors, and often differ widely in chemical structure from one another. Though the body cannot make them, it must have them. The word "vitamin" has reference to the fact that they are essential to life, and it would seem to the authors that every living cell of the human body probably requires these substances.

In the specific treatment of vitamin deficiency diseases the changes effected by the administration of indicated vitamins are miraculous, and the judicious use of them in the clinic is revolutionizing medicine. Much less dramatic, but probably more beneficial, would be the application of the principles of nutrition toward the prevention of deficiency diseases. Certain it is that the vitamins are necessary for the health and vigor of the higher forms of life. In other sections of this book, minerals and other important elements of the dietary are described. These materials have functional interrelationship to the vitamins.

It is known to nutritionists that a superior breed of rats has come into existence through improvement of diet over many generations. These rodents are longer lived, heavier, more fertile, and more energetic than the rat of twenty-five years ago. The growth, health and well-being of children and young adults have been greatly benefited by improvement in their diets. It appears that this physical superiority is attributable mainly to better nutrition. The modern science of vitamins, though it seems to promise miracles, offers no elixir of life and no panaceas. It is a fruitful science that already constitutes one of the most fascinating chapters in the history of the practice of medicine, and it promises even more far-reaching results in the near future. It is making the practitioner more receptive to the lessons coming from other sciences. Many patients near death have been restored to health by synthetic vitamins.

The story of the vitamins is that of the growth of a great science. One can recognize the many aspects which have a closely underlying unity of purpose. As much as we intellectually abhor "polypharmacy," there is a logical basis for including sufficient amounts of a variety of vitamins in a single therapeutic preparation. The vitamins occur together in nature, and the progress of medicine will be greatly enriched by full realization that deficiency diseases tend to occur as complexities rather than as single entities. The clinical, laboratory and dietary studies indicate that the specific deficiency syndromes occurring from inadequacy of water soluble vitamins are so interrelated as to suggest that the same general biochemical systems are disturbed. The authors find in the day-to-day practice of medicine that convalescence of the patient is greatly shortened by administering the water soluble vitamins together and the fat soluble vitamins together, rather than by treating the patient with a single chemical substance (see Fig. 26).

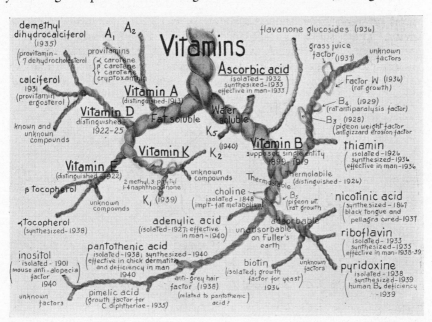

Fig. 26.—This diagram portrays many of the known vitamins and undifferentiated compounds with vitamin-like activity in foods. They are separated on the basis of physiologic, physical, and chemical properties. Heavy lettering indicates that the structural formula of the compound is known and that the substance is important in human nutrition. The formulas of these compounds are shown in the text. Factors of unidentified structure are indicated by small lettering.

So far as feasible, every section within this chapter has been written as a separate unit. Theories have been discussed with as little prejudice as a personal opinion allows. The authors were restricted in giving references to the literature and selections have of necessity been most arbitrary. Many papers have been omitted and the writers are greatly indebted to unspecified monographs and reviews too numerous to mention. Colleagues and friends have given invaluable assistance.

VITAMIN E

When compared to the other vitamins, vitamin E assumes a rather unimportant position since it has never been demonstrated that a deficiency of this substance occurs in man. As early as 1922 the necessity of this factor (then called "factor X") was recognized in animals, and in spite of a host of brilliant chemical and physiologic discoveries, attempts at clinical application of this knowledge have resulted only in controversy.

CHEMISTRY

The formula for *alpha tocopherol* was proposed by Fernholz on the basis of oxidative degradation with chromic acid. Synthesis was later accomplished independently in three laboratories. At the present time three antisterility factors have been isolated from natural material, namely, alpha, beta, and gamma tocopherols (Fig. 27).

Beta tocopherol and gamma tocopherol, which are homologues of the natural substance, have almost identical properties but slightly less biologic activity. These substances are readily soluble in lipid solvents but only slightly soluble in water. Although stable at high temperature (200° C.) they rapidly lose their activity in the presence of ultraviolet light or mild oxidizing agents. The long recognized resistance to rancidity of vegetable

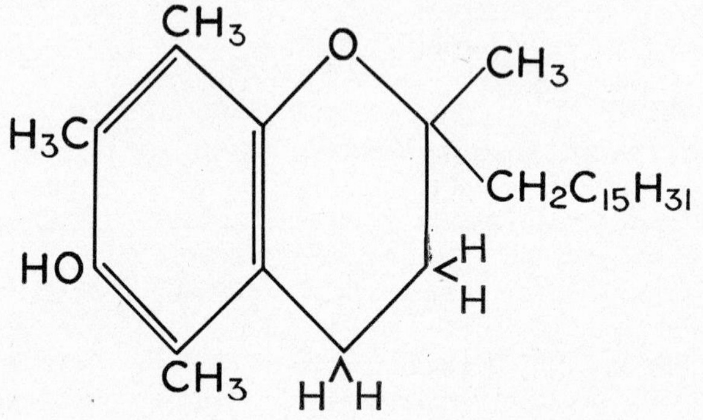

Fig. 27.—Structural formula of alpha tocopherol.

oil that contains vitamin E might be cited as an everyday example of its oxidation inhibiting quality. It is likewise this antioxidation activity which has led investigators to postulate the possible rôle of vitamin E as a *respiratory enzyme* in the living organism.

Whereas most vitamins require a rather specific structure for their activity, of the 130 compounds tested, more than forty exhibit vitamin E activity but they do so in limited fashion when compared to tocopherol. The tocopherols themselves have a certain structural specificity and the removal of a methyl group from the aromatic nucleus or the aliphatic side chain greatly diminishes the E activity of these substances. The acetate of tocopherol is equal in biologic activity and possesses the added advantage of increased stability over tocopherol. Several methods exist for the chemical and biologic estimation of vitamin E but these are of little importance to the clinician.

PHYSIOLOGY AND PATHOLOGY

In animals a lack of vitamin E manifests itself chiefly by changes in the reproductive mechanism; it was from this observation that the terms "antisterility vitamin" and "reproductive vitamin" were derived. This would appear to be a rather unfortunate choice since vitamin E has never been shown to bring about reproductive ability in cases of primary sterility. In the presence of vitamin E deficiency, conception occurs in the female rat but it is followed by "resorptive sterility." In the male rat degeneration of the germinal epithelium and spermatozoa develops to the point of complete loss of reproductive power.

In the absence of vitamin E in the diet of animals, muscular dystrophy and a characteristic paralysis of the hind quarters have been shown to develop. The relation of these disorders to human muscular dystrophy is by no means clear although some investigators claim that the microscopic changes in the muscles are indistinguishable in the two conditions. This remains an intriguing subject for further investigation. Vitamin E appears to be intimately related to growth, but to advance a theory for a vitamin as a growth factor has become almost trite. The possible relation of vitamin E to the glands of internal secretion has stimulated a great amount of experimental work but results are completely controversial. This is likewise the state of our knowledge regarding vitamin E in the occurrence and growth of tumors.

CLINICAL USE

Habitual Abortion.—A cursory appraisal of the current literature may lead the credulous physician to believe that in vitamin E he has an invincible weapon for his attack on habitual abortion. A critical analysis of the numerous reports, however, tends to stem one's enthusiasm in rather large measure. In fact, the prevalent view was well stated by Taussig: "In this country where all the needed constituents of a well balanced diet are obtainable dietary deficiencies probably do not play a very great part in abortions except in domestic animals." In attempting to arrive at a logical evaluation of any statistical report, two very important factors must be considered before reaching any conclusion. The first of these is in the correctness of diagnosis, and in the consideration of habitual abortion one is immediately confronted with the obstacle of distinct lack of a standard criterion. The diagnosis of habitual abortion is not justified until a woman has had at least two consecutive abortions in which the possibility of artificial induction or organic disease has been excluded. It is true that some reports show rather striking evidence of curative action of vitamin E in cases in which women have had even three or more consecutive abortions but in only about half of these cases was it possible to ascertain that these abortions were spontaneous and previous abortions actually have been observed in only a very small percentage of the reported cases. The other difficulty in obtaining evidence of the effect of vitamin E in preventing habitual abortion arises when one realizes that knowledge of the outcome in the absence of treatment is completely lacking. There is a marked tendency to spontaneous cure of repeated abortion; for example, it can be predicted from certain statistical studies that if a woman has had two consecutive abortions the chances are about one to three that she will not have another.

Considering these factors, one is impressed with the almost complete futility of attempting to arrive at any justifiable conclusion as to the effect of vitamin E on habitual abortions. The reported "75 per cent cures" must be greatly modified. On the other hand, in seeking to temper their enthusiasm physicians must not become iconoclastic but must keep an open mind on this subject and await results from further study, remembering that the current reports are sufficiently encouraging to warrant further clinical study. The physician confronted with a case in which the diagnosis of habitual abortion is established should not be discouraged from the use of wheat-germ oil but he must not be led into the error of promising dramatic cures.

Abruptio Placentae.—A unique theory has been presented by Shute for the rôle of vitamin E in cases of abruptio placentae. This is based on the excessive antitryptic activity of the blood serum, which he said prevents the normal penetration of the fetal villi into the maternal decidua. He has described a method for the chemical estimation of this antitryptic activity and said that this affords an index of vitamin E nutrition. This work has not been substantiated and there is no convincing clinical datum to support his statement that the administration of vitamin E relieves the symptoms of abruptio placentae within twenty hours.

Other Diseases of the Reproductive System.—Vitamin E has been used in the treatment of various other disorders of the reproductive system, including male and female sterility, menstrual disorders, toxemias of pregnancy, faulty lactation, and vaginal pruritus. The reported results are at variance and cannot be accepted until further evidence has been accumulated.

Myoneurogenic Disorders.—If the literature on the relation of vitamin E to reproductive disorders seems confusing, it reverts to utter chaos when one comes to a consideration of its use in cases of muscular dystrophy and related conditions (amyotrophic lateral sclerosis, muscular dystrophy and muscular atrophy). Without digressing too far into the field of this controversy one may observe that the number of "induced remissions" does not outnumber the complete failures.

Since this field has been only recently explored there doubtlessly will be more light thrown on this problem in the next few years. Until that time physicians must completely reserve their answer to the question "what can we expect of vitamin E in the treatment of human myoneurogenic disorders?"

REQUIREMENTS AND SOURCES

As might be construed from what has already been observed in regard to vitamin E, the human requirements are completely unknown. Apparently vitamin E occurs in most foods and it is noteworthy that one of the greatest obstacles which investigators encountered was in obtaining a diet deficient in this vitamin. Wheat-germ oil is the richest source of vitamin E but this substance also is found in considerable amounts in cotton seed oil, lettuce oil, rice-germ oil and other seed-germ oils.

Various authors have used wheat-germ oil in doses varying from 0.25 to 6 cc. daily, and it may be of significance that any apparent success was the same in spite of any variation in dose. No toxic reactions have been reported in cases in which small doses were administered, and large doses of wheat-germ oil have given rise to only minor symptoms. The danger of production of neoplasms appears to be nonexistent.

REFERENCES

Butt, H. R. and Leary, W. V., Diseases of Nutrition: Review of Certain Recent Contributions, Arch. Int. Med., **67**: 411–465 (Feb.) 1941.

American Medical Association Council on Pharmacy and Chemistry: The Treatment of Habitual Abortion with Vitamin E., J.A.M.A., **114**: 2214–2218, 1940.

Smith, L. I.: The Chemistry of Vitamin E, Chem. Rev., **27**: 287–329, 1940.

Evans, H. M.: The William Henry Welch lectures, I. New Light on the Biological Rôle of Vitamin E, J. Mt. Sinai Hosp., **6**: 233–244, 1940.

VITAMIN K

HEMORRHAGIC DIATHESIS OCCURRING IN PATIENTS WHO HAVE JAUNDICE AND CERTAIN INTESTINAL DISORDERS, AND IN THE NEWBORN INFANT

To observe certain patients bleed to death in spite of all known forms of treatment has been the unhappy experience of physicians and surgeons for many generations. This experience in the past was most common among patients who had jaundice and who underwent some surgical operation. It was fairly common, however, among patients who had surgical treatment for various intestinal disorders, and fatal hemorrhage in the newborn infant has been a sad experience of many physicians from time immemorial. All these instances of death were unusually shocking because the physician had no satisfactory form of treatment—the cause was unknown. It is a pleasant and gratifying thought to know that during the past few years most of these perplexing problems have been solved. These advances have been brought about during the past five years by the isolation, synthesis, and clinical application of vitamin K.

The introduction of vitamin K in clinical medicine came as a result of the observation of Dam and his associates of Copenhagen, Denmark. They showed that a deficiency disease could be produced in chicks by a diet washed in ether and could be cured by the administration of an antihemorrhagic material present in hog liver fat, hemp seed, and certain cereals and vegetables. Later it was shown by these investigators that deficiency in this dietary factor resulted in diminution in the amount of prothrombin in the circulating blood which led to a fatal hemorrhagic diathesis. The term vitamin K was proposed by Dam as an abbreviation of the name "Koagulations vitamin" to apply to the substance that was necessary for the prevention of a nutritional deficiency disease in chicks. Soon it was suggested by Quick of this country that deficiency in vitamin K might be present in patients who had obstructive jaundice and it was demonstrated by this author and his associates that a deficiency of prothrombin did exist in the blood of patients who had obstructive jaundice. These suggestions have now been amply confirmed and extended and within a relatively short time various workers in this country and abroad have demonstrated that vitamin K under most circumstances is a specific remedy for deficiency of prothrombin.

CHEMISTRY

In early attempts at isolation of vitamin K, concentrates of alfalfa, rich in the vitamin, were employed. Several attempts were made to crystallize the vitamin from these potent but impure concentrates but it was not until the spring of 1939 that it became apparent that more than one compound possesses vitamin K activity. From alfalfa was isolated a compound called vitamin K_1 and from putrefied fish meal a compound called vitamin K_2.

It was suggested by MacCorquodale and McKee that vitamin K_1 has a quinoid structure. For the final isolation and synthesis of vitamin K_1, Doisy and his associates, Almquist and Klose, and Fieser and his associates are responsible. Experiments from their laboratories demonstrated conclusively that the structure of vitamin K_1 is represented correctly by the formula 2-methyl-3-phytyl-1,4-naphthoquinone (Fig. 28). This vitamin is identical with 2-methyl-1,4-naphthoquinone with the exception that vitamin K_1 has a phytyl side chain in the three position; the synthetic product also is identical with natural vitamin K_1 which is obtained from alfalfa. Exposure to sunlight destroys the vitamin activity of alfalfa within several hours, although if artificial light is used little destruction is observed within twenty-four hours. The pure preparations, however, are destroyed by both sunlight and artificial light. A large part of the activity of concentrates of vitamin K is destroyed by alkali, by strong acids and by aluminum chloride. The vitamin is fat soluble and at low temperatures forms yellow crystals.

Vitamin K_2 was first isolated from putrefied fish meal. The empiric formula, $C_{41}H_{60}O_2$, has been proposed to represent its structure. Available data indicate that the structure may be 2,3-difarnesyl-1,4-naphthoquinone.

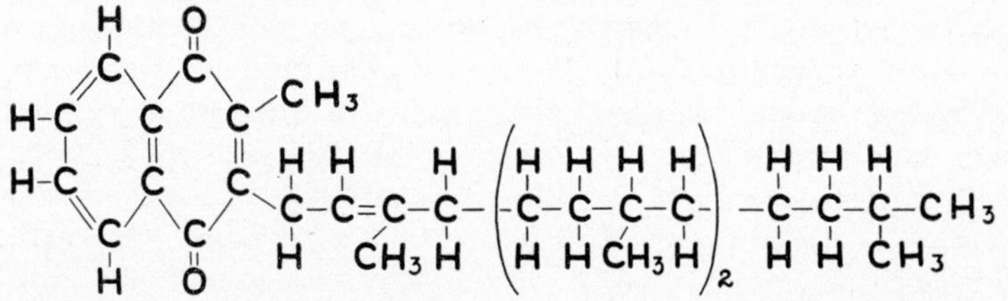

Fig. 28.—The structural formula of vitamin K_1 (2-methyl-3-phytyl-1,4-naphthoquinone).

This compound is also fat soluble and has been obtained as light yellow, crystalline flakes. Its potency is found to be about 60 per cent of that of vitamin K_1.

After it was demonstrated that vitamin K is of a quinoid structure a large number of investigators began to study the known substances which possess a quinoid nucleus. It was first reported by Almquist and Klose that *phthiocol* (2-methyl-3-hydroxy-1,4-naphthoquinone) possesses physical and chemical properties similar to those of pure vitamin K and also possesses marked antihemorrhagic activity. Phthiocol is the yellow pigment found in the human tubercle bacillus. Many other derivatives of naphthoquinone have since been investigated and of all of these studied *2-methyl-1,4-naphthoquinone* has proved to possess the most marked antihemorrhagic activity. It is thought that this synthetic compound is even more active than vitamin K_1 itself. This material is very slightly soluble in water. In solution its activity is impaired by sterilization with steam; therefore, it is rather unstable unless special precautions are taken. This compound is so active that several investigators have suggested that it be adopted as a basic standard for assay of vitamin K.

Many other compounds have been tested for vitamin K activity. Most of those which have such activity are basically 1,4-naphthoquinone or the corresponding hydroquinone; a few, however, are not. The compounds, 4-amino-2-methyl-1-naphthol hydrochloride and 2-methyl-1,4-naphthohydroquinone-3-sodium sulfonate, are both water soluble and, therefore, have proved of considerable use clinically. These compounds are not as active as 2-methyl-1,4-naphthoquinone but they are active enough to produce desired clinical results. Both of these compounds are now available commercially.

PHYSIOLOGY

Pure vitamin K has not been available long enough to allow complete knowledge of its physiologic action to be collected. Unlike some of the water soluble vitamins, little is known of the relation of vitamin K to the enzyme systems or to cell respiration but it is known that it is associated intimately in some way with the integrity of the hepatic parenchyma and with the metabolism of prothrombin.

Absorption.—Many investigators have shown that the presence of bile in the intestinal tract is essential for proper absorption of the fat soluble vitamin K, and there is furthermore some evidence to suggest that these fat soluble compounds are absorbed better if other fats are present in the intestinal tract. Clinically it is well established that the presence of bile, or more correctly the presence of adequate amounts of bile salts, is required for the proper absorption of vitamin K. The exact point of absorption in the intestinal tract is not known but our own experience indicates that concentrates of vitamin K are not absorbed through the colon or upper part of the ileum but that they are absorbed readily through the upper part of the small intestine.

Storage.—The vitamin is not stored readily in the body but it has been found in the livers of lower animals in relatively small amounts. Greaves has shown that in the liver of the rat vitamin K is not stored in appreciable quantities. Clinical work would indicate that the same observations are applicable in the human being.

Excretion.—Insofar as is known vitamin K is not present in the urine. It can be demonstrated in the feces but whether it is there because the feces hold the organisms which are known to contain vitamin K or whether the presence of the vitamin in feces is referable to real excretion of vitamin K remains to be established. The vitamin is not present in human bile collected under sterile conditions. In chicks on a normal diet the spleen, red muscle, gizzard, bone marrow, and pancreas were found to contain relatively large amounts of vitamin K while the liver and lungs were found to contain somewhat less. It would be most interesting to determine whether or not vitamin K is present in human breast milk.

Metabolism.—Little is really known of the metabolism of vitamin K but it might be assumed that it is absorbed as a bile acid compound. What happens when it enters the blood stream is not yet known. Some have suggested that the compound is carried as a prosthetic group with the prothrombin molecule and others have suggested that vitamin K acts in some capacity in the formation of prothrombin, but all of this is certainly hypothetical. That proper response to vitamin K depends upon the integrity of the hepatic parenchyma is now a well established fact.

Insofar as is known at the present time, vitamin K has no relation to immunity, infection, pregnancy and lactation, the nervous system, gastro-intestinal tract, or cardiovascular system, but it is intimately associated with normal physiologic function of the liver and with proper coagulation of the blood. Its exact rôle in blood coagulation is not known. It is known to be necessary for proper formation of prothrombin, but in what manner this is accomplished remains to be determined. A deficiency of vitamin K from any cause produces a deficiency of prothrombin in the circulating blood and in all instances except those in which there is severe hepatic damage this deficiency of prothrombin can be corrected by the proper administration of vitamin K.

EFFECT OF DEFICIENCY OF VITAMIN K

In Animals.—In chicks fed on a diet deficient in vitamin K there develop subcutaneous, intramuscular, and internal hemorrhages, profuse bleeding from minor abrasions, and a delayed clotting time associated with a low level of plasma prothrombin. Injuries in a wide sense may determine the occurrence and severity of these hemorrhages. Studies of the plasma prothrombin level in hemorrhagic chick disease by many investigators show that hemorrhages do not occur until the level of prothrombin has declined to about 10 to 15 per cent of normal. It has been indicated that the clotting time is delayed only if the prothrombin level has declined to less than 30 or 40 per cent of normal. Thus, early in the course of the disease when deficiency of the vitamin is less severe, the level of plasma prothrombin may be reduced considerably and yet the clotting time will remain normal. This is extremely important as a clinical factor. As has been mentioned repeatedly in the literature, determinations of the plasma prothrombin are essential if any but the more severe grades of deficiency are to be detected. Deficiency of prothrombin has also been produced in rats, mice, ducklings, young geese, pigeons, canaries, and rabbits that were fed diets deficient in vitamin K.

It has been long known that in dogs which have biliary fistulas, in addition to many pathologic complications an abnormal tendency to bleed also develops. Furthermore, it has been pointed out that continuous subsequent feeding of bile to such animals will correct this abnormality. This tendency of dogs which have biliary fistulas toward bleeding was shown later to be caused by deficiency of prothrombin which could be corrected by the administration of vitamin K. In rats which have renal biliary fistulas there is likewise a diminution in the circulating prothrombin which can be corrected by the administration of vitamin K.

In Man.—*Inadequate Diet.*—The production of a diminished level of prothrombin in the circulating blood of man resulting from inadequate intake of vitamin K has never been accomplished. However, several cases of scurvy, chronic alcoholism, pellagra or a combination of the three have been reported in which there was a significant decrease in the level of plasma prothrombin. It is assumed that this resulted from the simple nutritional deficiency of vitamin K. These decreased levels of prothrombin were increased following the administration of vitamin K. This work remains to be adequately confirmed.

Biliary Fistula.—Clinically it is well known that among patients who have chronic biliary fistulas an abnormal tendency to bleed sometimes develops. It has been demonstrated that in these instances there is an associated deficiency of prothrombin in the circulating blood which can be corrected by the administration of vitamin K.

Obstructive Jaundice.—It is now well established that the absence of bile from the intestinal tract of man from any cause is capable of producing a deficiency of prothrombin in the circulating blood which is corrected by the administration of vitamin K, providing there is an intact hepatic parenchyma. This work also has been confirmed adequately by experiments on animals.

Intestinal Lesions.—It is obvious that normal absorption of a fat soluble material from the intestine cannot take place unless an adequate and physiologically intact intestinal surface is available. It is also obvious that an adequate dietary intake of vitamin K and the presence of bile in the intestinal tract are prerequisites to the proper metabolism of vitamin K, and that both factors may be altered seriously by various intestinal disorders. Many persons, because of the disease from which they suffer, have been compelled to

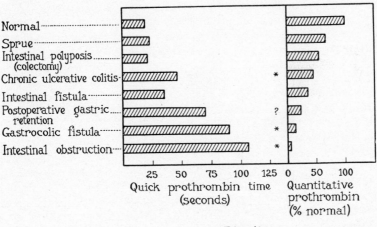

* Bleeding

Fig. 29.—The various intestinal disorders with which may be associated a deficiency of prothrombin which is readily corrected by the proper administration of compounds with vitamin K activity. (Butt and Snell, *Vitamin K*, W. B. Saunders Company.)

remain on limited diets. For others it is necessary to withhold food and to establish intestinal intubation in order to control symptoms of obstruction. Profuse discharge from ileac stomas further complicates the situation in many other cases. All patients, however, may be affected by both morphologic and functional disturbances involving the small intestine. However, a number of patients who have had anorexia and nervous vomiting have been studied and the plasma was not strikingly deficient in prothrombin. A previously deficient diet, continued vomiting or diarrhea, however, may lay the groundwork for a deficiency state in respect to vitamin K but some other factor such as an abdominal operation may be required for its precipitation. Under such circumstances adequate amounts of vitamin K may not be absorbed and in various intestinal disorders, such as sprue, chronic diarrhea, short-circuiting operation of the small and large intestine, and intestinal obstruction, deficiency of vitamin K and subsequent development of deficiency of prothrombin may ensue (Fig. 29).

Newborn Infants.—During the first few days of an infant's life some deficiency of prothrombin in the circulating blood apparently exists. The cause of this deficiency is debated. It has been suggested by many that lack of a reserve of prothrombin in the blood of the newborn infant is the result of a deficiency of vitamin K, since a normal level of prothrombin can be restored by the parenteral administration to the infant of a concentrate of the vitamin or by the oral administration of this accessory food substance. Others believe that in the blood of the normal infant a moderate deficiency of vitamin K develops during the first few days of life and that it arises from an insufficient supply of vitamin K from the intestine (Fig. 30). To explain the return of the value of prothrombin to normal by the end of

A COMPARISON OF THE PLASMA PROTHROMBIN CONCENTRATION AND THE BLEEDING AND COAGULATION TIMES IN THE INFANT DURING THE FIRST SIX DAYS OF LIFE

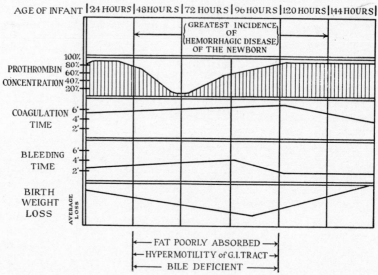

Fig. 30.—A composite chart taken from the work of Grossman which shows the level of prothrombin in the circulating blood at birth and during the subsequent six days of life.

the third day it must be assumed that the infant after birth receives a supply of vitamin K which was not present at birth.

It has been suggested that as soon as the presence of bacterial flora of the intestinal tract is established the infant is capable of synthesizing vitamin K, a fact which is well proved experimentally. This explanation, however, does not explain the delay of four days in the return to normal of the value for prothrombin, a delay which occurs in many infants. A normal value is reached usually by the fifth day. To explain this phenomenon it must be recalled that the liver of the newborn infant is unable to secrete sufficient bile, that absorption of fat is very limited and that gastro-intestinal hypermotility is the rule. Thus, even though vitamin K is present proper absorption of the vitamin is unlikely until the digestive function approaches normal. This occurs on about the third or fourth day of life. To support the suggestion that the presence of bacterial flora in the intestinal tract is intimately connected with the return of the value for prothrombin to normal at the end of the third day, some investigators have shown that extra feeding, started within two hours after delivery of the infant, can prevent the subsequent development of hypoprothrombinemia.

Hepatic Injury.—By injury to the hepatic parenchyma, deficiency of prothrombin can be produced in both man and animal in the presence of adequate amounts of vitamin K. This result must be considered not as a deficiency of vitamin K but rather as a disruption of the organ which is responsible for proper metabolism of the substance known as prothrombin. Intoxication with chloroform produces in animals a marked deficiency of prothrombin and results in hemorrhagic diathesis. It has also been shown that injury of the liver by carbon tetrachloride produces a tendency to bleed and that this tendency is not corrected by the administration of vitamin K if hepatic damage has been too great. All these experimental facts have been well established clinically.

To recapitulate, it appears now well established that a deficiency of prothrombin can occur if certain animals are sustained on diets which are lacking in certain fat soluble substances, and that such a deficiency can occur in experimental animals which have external or renal biliary fistulas and in dogs of which the livers have been injured by chloroform. All these conditions are associated with a well-marked hemorrhagic tendency and it is interesting that in each, one or a combination of these conditions may exist: bile is excluded from the bowel, the liver is injured by toxic substances, or a state of nutritional deficiency exists. The probable relationship of a deficiency of vitamin K to a deficiency of prothrombin in the plasma of dogs which have biliary fistulas or obstructive jaundice, or the plasma of human beings who have these conditions is reasonably clear, since bile acids are required for the normal absorption of fat soluble substances from the bowel and since, in the conditions mentioned, bile usually is excluded completely from the bowel. Two factors, therefore, the presence of bile in the bowel, and vitamin K, are known to be of importance in the maintenance of a normal concentration of prothrombin. A third and equally important factor is the liver; its importance in the synthesis of prothrombin already has been mentioned.

TOXICITY

No serious untoward reactions have been observed in the human being receiving reasonable therapeutic doses of either natural concentrates of vitamin K, synthetic vitamin K_1 or quinone derivatives exhibiting antihemorrhagic activity. No effect has been noted on the blood pressure, respiration, capillary permeability or urinary excretion following the administration of any of these compounds.

Concentrates of alfalfa have been administered to human beings both orally and intramuscularly in single doses as large as 2 gm. without the occurrence of untoward reaction. Doses of the various synthetic compounds exhibiting antihemorrhagic activity have been administered orally in doses of 25 to 50 mg. and intravenously in doses of 5 to 10 mg. without any untoward reaction.

It has been observed that large doses of 2-methyl-1,4-naphthoquinone (180 mg.) administered orally to human beings result in vomiting and porphyrinuria. A dose of 30 mg. of the substance per Kg. of body weight injected intramuscularly into a dog caused vomiting, porphyrinuria, and albuminuria. Others have noted that large doses of this compound administered to rats produced a decrease in the number of erythrocytes and in the quantity of hemoglobin. These doses, however, are obviously greater than those employed for therapeutic use in man and to date no one has noted any untoward reaction in man after administration of reasonable therapeutic doses of any of these compounds.

HUMAN REQUIREMENTS

Distribution.—Vitamin K is distributed widely in nature; among its richest sources are *green leaves* of different kinds. Alfalfa and spinach are very rich in it and cabbage, cauliflower, kale, carrot tops, chestnut leaves, soy bean oil, and seaweed are all good sources of this vitamin. Less potent are tomatoes, orange peel, and hemp seed. Seeds, fruits, and roots contain in general considerably less vitamin K than do green leaves of different kinds. The parts of the plant which contain chlorophyl usually have the largest amounts of vitamin K and because of this it was postulated early that vitamin K_1, like chlorophyl, probably would contain a phytyl group.

Vitamin K is found also in a number of *bacteria*. Apparently during the growth of the bacteria the vitamin K is synthesized and is retained within the bacteria since the filtrate of the culture medium which is free of the bacteria contains none of the vitamin. Dried human feces, both normal and acholic stools, are also rich in the vitamin but the vitamin K activity of feces undoubtedly results from the bacterial content within them.

Nothing is known of the minimal requirements of vitamin K for infant, child, mother, or normal adult. This lack of knowledge undoubtedly will be corrected as soon as methods are developed by which vitamin K can be measured in biologic fluids.

Although minimal requirements for the normal individual in respect to vitamin K are still unknown, it is known that pure vitamin K_1 or synthetic compounds exhibiting vitamin K activity in doses of 1 to 2 mg. are capable of correcting deficiency of vitamin K in most instances. However, apparently depending on the degree of hepatic damage, this dose may have to be increased considerably in order to produce the desired result. It is known that diarrhea and inadequate intestinal absorptive surface will increase the need for vitamin K. Similar increased requirements are found in such diseases as sprue and celiac disease.

ASSAY METHODS AND UNITAGE

Like every new vitamin, vitamin K possesses numerous methods of assay and standards of unitage. There are primarily two methods of assay which have been employed to measure the antihemorrhagic activity of a given material. One method is known as the *preventive method*. In this, foodstuffs are assayed by rearing chicks for a month on a diet deficient in vitamin K and rearing other chicks for a like period on a diet in which test material has been incorporated. A protective action which these materials afforded is determined by measurement of the coagulation time of the blood of the chick. If the coagulation time of the blood of chicks fed the diet containing the test material is found to be shorter than that of the controls which had received unsupplemented rations the material assayed is said to contain vitamin K.

One of the other most favored methods, known as the *curative method*, is based on the observation that animals which suffer from deficiency of vitamin K become normal with reference to the clotting time of their blood within three days of their beginning to ingest sufficient food containing vitamin K. Other reliable assays have since been developed and with each new assay there has developed a standard of unitage. The subject of the correct unit to use is still controversial and the matter is so involved that it here warrants no discussion. Obviously there is considerable disagreement among the various investigators working in the same field as to the exact definition of a unit and the best method of assay. It has been suggested that 2-methyl-1,4-naphthoquinone be adopted as a standard of reference for vitamin K. Obviously this would greatly simplify the various and diversified systems now employed. One of the most commonly used unit systems at the present time is that developed by Thayer and his associates, in which 1 mg. of pure vitamin K_1 contains 1000 Thayer-Doisy units.

METHODS OF MEASURING DEFICIENCY OF PROTHROMBIN

To have a proper evaluation of hemorrhagic diatheses the reader must be conversant with at least the fundamental properties of blood and also with the current hypothesis by means of which attempts are made to explain the normal coagulation of blood. Suffice it to say here that present evidence indicates that the phenomenon of coagulation of blood involves two consecutive reactions: (1) the interaction of calcium, prothrombin and platelets (or tissue extract) to form thrombin and (2) the reaction of fibrinogen with thrombin to form fibrin.

Methods designed in the past for the measurement of the tendency of a jaundiced patient to bleed have been almost as uncertain as have been the conclusions derived from some of the older studies on the mechanism of bleeding. Most determinations of coagulation time and of bleeding time are of little or no value for determination of the potential danger of hemorrhages afflicting a patient who has jaundice. The usual methods employed for measurement of the ability of the blood to coagulate give little evidence of deviation from the normal until the patient is on the verge of experiencing hemorrhage. Several excellent methods for measuring deficiency of prothrombin in the blood of man have been described but in our experience the method developed by Quick and his associates has been found well adapted for general use in the clinical laboratory. This method as modified by Magath has proved in our hands to be very satisfactory. When the expressions "prothrombin time" or "prothrombin clotting time" are used subsequently they will refer to the clotting time of recalcified plasma to which optimal amounts of thromboplastin have been added as determined by the *method of Quick*.* This method requires as much as 4.5 cc. of venous blood of the patient. The necessity of obtaining this much blood, particularly among premature infants, often is a real obstacle, especially if the tests are to be repeated at frequent intervals upon the same individual. For this reason several micromethods for the determination of prothrombin have been suggested. Details of these methods can be found in the literature mentioned in the references.

* See Addendum, p. 502, first item.

The so-called *bedside method* has received considerable use and although my experience with this method is very limited, it has been reported that it is of great value particularly for the general practitioner. The *principle* of the "bedside" test for determination of the content of prothrombin of plasma of man is that blood freshly drawn and placed in a small tube containing a measured amount of thromboplastin will clot, under these conditions, within twenty-five to forty seconds. If the content of prothrombin is unduly low the clotting time will be prolonged. The degree of prolongation is used as a measure of the reduction in the content of prothrombin. Smith has suggested that a physician's small kit can be arranged so that it will contain all the equipment necessary for performance of the test except the needle and syringe, which are used to withdraw the blood. The equipment consists of a tube of dried thromboplastin (extract of lung tissue prepared in dried form by means of the lyophile technic, now available commercially), a pipet with a capacity of 0.1 cc. and several small test tubes which are calibrated in the 1 cc. scale.

The tube containing dried thromboplastin is opened and water is added to a mark which indicates the level of 2 cc. The tube is inverted back and forth over the finger until the thromboplastin dissolves; two or three minutes may be required for this procedure. The solution should be kept in the refrigerator prior to use and should be used the same day on which it is prepared. With the aid of the pipet, 0.1 cc. of thromboplastin is then placed in one of the small test tubes. Blood is drawn from a vein of the patient into a clean syringe; as much care as possible should be exercised to avoid the forming of bubbles. If bubbles form, if delay is encountered, or if the sample becomes unduly soiled with tissue juice, the sample so affected should be discarded. The needle is removed rapidly from the syringe and the blood is expressed gently into the test tube until its level reaches the 9 cc. mark etched on the side of the tube. The tube is then inverted over the finger to effect immediate mixing of the blood and thromboplastin. The tube is next gently tilted every second or two until clotting occurs. The time which has elapsed after contact of the blood with the solution of thromboplastin is noted. It is best to conduct a control test in which the blood of a normal person is used. This test should be performed with each new tube of thromboplastin, for the potency of the different preparations varies somewhat. Next, the clotting power of the blood as percentage of normal is calculated by means of the following formula:

$$\frac{\text{Clotting time of normal control blood}}{\text{Clotting time of patient's blood}} \times 100 = \text{clotting power (in percentage of normal).}$$

The temperature of the room in which the test is conducted is not significant unless the room is rather chilly, in which case the tube and syringe should be warmed in the hand while the test is being conducted. If the values for prothrombin obtained are less than 80 per cent of normal, the decreased value for prothrombin is significant. Values less than 50 per cent of normal are considered to be in the potential bleeding zone.

It must be admitted that all the current methods for the estimation of prothrombin are of necessity indirect. However, certain of these methods of measuring prothrombin are the most nearly accurate methods available at present for estimation of a patient's tendency to bleed in the presence of a suspected deficiency of prothrombin. The information afforded by the measurement of prothrombin in the circulating blood is much more nearly accurate in the prediction of the tendency of a patient to bleed than is the measurement of the coagulation or bleeding time as formerly used in the consideration of such a tendency. The method described by Quick and his associates with some modifications and in skilled hands has proved in our experience to be the most useful method clinically.

DIAGNOSIS

Incidence and Manner of Bleeding.—*In Jaundice.*—The bleeding of patients who have jaundice occurs most frequently after surgical intervention which was calculated to relieve biliary obstruction. Hemorrhage usually is noted between the first and fourth postoperative days but it may appear as late as the twelfth to eighteenth day after operation. As is well known, cholemic bleeding ordinarily begins as a slow oozing from the operative incision, from the gums or nose, or from the gastro-intestinal tract. Often, however, the first evidence of hemorrhage is afforded by the appearance of severe hematemesis or melena. Such bleeding often is controlled temporarily by transfusions of whole blood, but all too frequently even repeated transfusions fail to control the hemorrhagic diathesis. Bleeding of this type is, in our experience and in the experience of many others, invariably associated with prolongation of the prothrombin clotting time.

As is well known, bleeding of patients suffering from jaundice occurs most often in the presence of those conditions in which bile is excluded completely from the gastro-intestinal tract. Those types of biliary obstruction in hepatic disease most commonly responsible for serious hemorrhage long have been familiar to the clinician and surgeon. Complete biliary obstruction produced by neoplasm of the pancreas, ampulla and gallbladder heads the list. Postoperative stricture of the common bile duct is accompanied perhaps by the second highest incidence of bleeding and intermittent obstruction caused by the presence of stones comes third. Complete external fistulas are relatively rare but often are associated with bleeding. Although bleeding is more likely to occur in those cases in which bile is excluded completely from the intestine, yet the physician must not overlook the fact that bleeding also can occur in the absence of jaundice if the liver has been injured considerably as the result of chronic cholecystic disease. Although the foregoing facts are somewhat useful for predicting whether or not a patient will bleed, yet the exceptions are so frequent that rigid clinical rules cannot be devised.

In Severe Hepatic Damage.—It has been well demonstrated experimentally that if the hepatic parenchyma is injured the amount of prothrombin in the circulating blood decreases. It has been further demonstrated by Warner and his associates and by Bollman and his associates that if the hepatic damage in these animals is too severe the level of prothrombin in the circulating blood does not rise after administration of vitamin K. It has been likewise well demonstrated clinically that patients who have severe hepatic damage have a decrease in the prothrombin in the circulating blood and that occasionally they will not respond to the administration of vitamin K.

These instances of severe hepatic damage can occur in any disease in which the liver might be involved but most frequently they are seen in cases of cirrhosis of the liver, in those in which obstruction or stricture of the common duct has existed over long periods and in those in which there is acute or subacute atrophy of the liver resulting from some primary disease or associated with acute cholecystitis. Although this group of cases is somewhat small, it is well to remember that it does exist. It is true that, frequently, repeated doses of vitamin K are necessary in order to produce the desired effect, but when one has doubled or tripled the usual therapeutic dose of vitamin K without producing desired effects one can be fairly certain that, regardless of the amounts of vitamin K administered, there will be little elevation of the prothrombin in the circulating blood.

In Various Intestinal Disorders.—A deficiency of prothrombin as the cause of bleeding in patients who have various intestinal disorders is something new in clinical medicine, and although instances of deficiency of prothrombin referable to the effects of intestinal absorption are not often encountered, yet they do comprise a rather distinct group and one which bears further investigation. The pathologic physiology concerned in such cases has been described under the section on pathology. When patients who have extensive disease of the intestine such as sprue, celiac disease, chronic ulcerative colitis, intestinal obstruction, multiple short-circuiting operations on the intestinal tract, ileitis, and so forth, experience hemorrhage, either before or after surgical treatment, deficiency in prothrombin should be recognized and corrected before other forms of treatment are instituted. The most important point in diagnosis of these conditions is for the surgeon and clinician to follow the prothrombin coagulation time closely in all cases of abnormalities of the intestinal mucosa or of interference with the continuity of the gastro-intestinal tract and in cases in which the postoperative condition requires continued aspiration of gas and secretions from the intestinal tract. This practice has solved the mystery of obscure intestinal bleeding, which occurs frequently in such cases, and definitely has reduced postoperative morbidity and mortality.

Of Infants.—The entire subject of bleeding in the newborn infant has been in a confused state chiefly because of the difficulty in a given situation of determining what is and what is not a real state of hemorrhagic diathesis. It is now well known that a deficiency of prothrombin in the circulating blood of infants is usually a physiologic occurrence. Many instances now have been reported of hemorrhagic disease of the newborn in which there was a deficiency of prothrombin and in which the bleeding was alleviated promptly by oral or parenteral administration of vitamin K. It also has been suggested that a deficiency of prothrombin existing at birth might account in many instances for those intracranial hemorrhages which frequently are associated with labor.

Value of the Prothrombin Clotting Time.—Obviously, knowledge of the conditions in which deficiency of prothrombin may occur is fundamental for correct diagnosis of possible deficiency of vitamin K. Although the possibility of hemorrhagic diathesis may be suspected in a particular case, the measurement of the prothrombin content of the circulating blood is necessary for accurate diagnosis as well as to evaluate proper treatment. It must be admitted that present methods for measurement of the content of prothrombin in the circulating blood of patients are subject to considerable error. The decrease in the concentration of prothrombin in the circulating blood of man seems to depend on certain unknown individual factors. Although in certain instances the concentration of prothrombin in the blood apparently depends on the degree of hepatic injury it certainly does not have any constant relationship to the type of hepatic or biliary disease present.

On the basis of the various studies of Smith and his associates it would appear that bleeding among animals in the experimental laboratory occurs when the value for prothrombin becomes less than 20 or 25 per cent of normal and that conversely so long as the value remains at about 20 or 25 per cent bleeding does not occur. If this conception is understood it is easy to see why in certain cases bleeding in man may occur postoperatively with little warning. Loss of blood, surgical trauma and the effects of anesthesia may reduce an already depleted supply of prothrombin to a dangerously low value; of these factors mechanical trauma is thought to be the most important. The prothrombin clotting time may and frequently does increase with no apparent reason within six to eight hours and with this increase free bleeding may occur without warning and apparently normal, coagulable blood may become virtually incoagulable.

Indication for Treatment with Vitamin K.—The prothrombin clotting time of the blood of patients who have *jaundice* usually increases to some extent for the first three or four days after surgical operation but it may increase rapidly even as late as the eighteenth postoperative day. For this reason the prothrombin clotting time should be determined daily for the first four days after operation and then every other day for at least eight or ten days longer. Any increase in the prothrombin clotting time should constitute an indication for the immediate oral or intravenous administration of vitamin K. To those patients the prothrombin clotting time of whose blood before surgical treatment has been high it is perhaps wise to administer the vitamin daily for several days after surgical operation regardless of the prothrombin clotting time. A patient whose blood gives a prothrombin clotting time of more than thirty seconds should be prepared with particular care and one whose blood gives a prothrombin clotting time of more than forty-five seconds must be considered to be a potential bleeder and treated as such.

The same important diagnostic points are also applicable to those cases of various intestinal lesions in which a deficiency of prothrombin in the circulating blood may develop.

It is equally important to follow if possible the prothrombin clotting time of newborn infants, although it is well known that during the first few days there is a physiologic deficiency of prothrombin. This caution is particularly important if any surgical procedure is contemplated during this period of life.

Unfortunately, the measure of prothrombin in the circulating blood does not always give the exact index of the tendency of the patient to bleed. Like any laboratory method this method may not give the clinical information which is always desirable. For these reasons prophylactic treatment is much better than treatment after bleeding once occurs.

13

TREATMENT

It is well to remember that no single specific remedy for the prevention and control of all instances of bleeding resulting from deficiency of prothrombin yet has been discovered. Proper administration of vitamin K or related compounds in most instances will be effective, but in addition, to obtain the best results all procedures which are known to be of value in the maintenance of adequate hepatic function must be employed. Obviously the *first objective* in treatment of the jaundiced patient who has a tendency to bleed is to restore continuity of the biliary passages and protection of the hepatic parenchyma. The latter objective still requires injections of glucose and a diet high in carbohydrates and nonmeat proteins, as has been necessary in the past.

Since the synthetic preparations which possess vitamin K activity have appeared on the market we have discontinued the use of naturally occurring concentrates of vitamin K. Details of the use of these concentrates can be found in the older work in the literature which appears in the references.

For purposes of routine *preoperative treatment*, patients who have jaundice are divided into three groups: (1) those whose blood gives a normal prothrombin clotting time; (2) those whose blood gives a prolonged prothrombin clotting time although active bleeding is not present and (3) those whose blood gives a prolonged prothrombin clotting time, active bleeding being present.

Those jaundiced patients of the first group, the prothrombin clotting time of whose blood is normal, receive prophylactic treatment for from two to five days before surgical intervention is undertaken. Usually 1 to 2 mg. daily of one of the synthetic products that have vitamin K activity given orally constitutes an adequate daily dose. This should be given together with from 1 to 3 gm. of animal bile salts. Almost any type of animal bile salts can be used; bile of man obtained from a biliary fistula or T tube can be employed.

Patients who have jaundice and the prothrombin time of whose blood is prolonged constitute a potential or real emergency. Patients whose blood gives a prothrombin clotting time of from thirty to forty-five seconds will respond well to the plan of prophylactic treatment for patients of the first group previously mentioned, but if the prothrombin clotting time is longer than forty-five or fifty seconds it has been thought advisable to administer vitamin K intramuscularly or intravenously. In such instances one of the water soluble synthetic compounds that have vitamin K activity is administered in doses of 1 to 2 mg. by the intramuscular or intravenous route. One such dose as a rule will bring the prothrombin clotting time to normal (Fig. 31) but in an exceptional instance it has been necessary to repeat this procedure once or more than once.

The problem of treating of patients who are bleeding actively (patients of group 3) is difficult, but not nearly so difficult since the availability of synthetic products with vitamin K activity which can be administered by the intravenous route. A transfusion of blood often is necessary to aid in combating the shock produced by hemorrhage and to provide a temporary supply of prothrombin. As a rule, transfusion will control bleeding only so long as the added supply of prothrombin lasts, a matter of from six to twelve hours. In such instances the intravenous administration of synthetic compounds possessing vitamin K activity in doses of 1 to 4 mg. often will control the hemorrhagic diathesis (Fig. 32), but not infrequently repeated doses

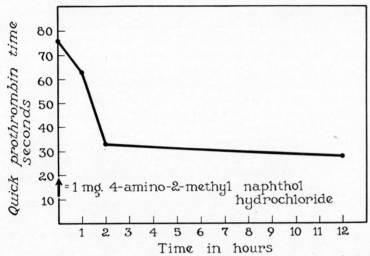

Fig. 31.–The effect of the intravenous injection of 1 mg. of 4-amino-2-methyl-1-naphthol hydrochloride on the elevated prothrombin clotting time of a patient who had obstructive jaundice. (Butt and Snell, *Vitamin K*, W. B. Saunders Company.)

of the same magnitude must be administered. The value of preoperative treatment cannot be overemphasized and when bleeding occurs which is the

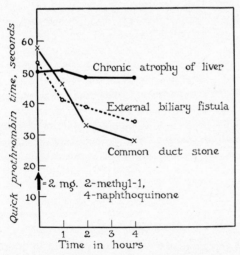

Fig. 32.–The effect and rapidity of action of the intravenous injection of 2 mg. of 2-methyl-1,4-naphthoquinone in a case of external biliary fistula and in one of calculus of the common duct. The figure also shows the failure of this compound to reduce the elevated prothrombin clotting time in a case of chronic atrophy of the liver. (Butt and Snell, *Vitamin K*, W. B. Saunders Company.)

result of hypoprothrombinemia the condition in most instances has not been well managed

Severe Hepatic Damage.—Although hepatic damage occasionally will not respond to the administration of vitamin K, this does not mean that vitamin K should not be administered to these patients. It has been our experience that although there is little or no response to vitamin K in such instances, yet the patient to whom vitamin K is administered, in spite of severe hepatic damage and an elevated prothrombin clotting time, rarely dies of hemorrhagic diathesis resulting from a deficiency of prothrombin

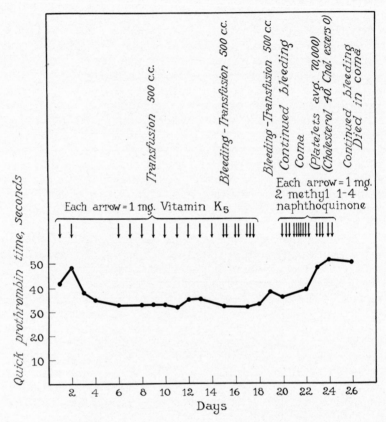

Fig. 33.—The prothrombin clotting time of a patient who had severe cirrhosis of the liver and who received over a long period various synthetic preparations possessing marked antihemorrhagic activity. In spite of these materials the prothrombin clotting time remained elevated. This type of case constitutes a failure of vitamin K to correct an elevated prothrombin clotting time. (Butt and Snell, *Vitamin K*, W. B. Saunders Company.)

(Fig. 33). In most instances we have administered as much as 3 to 5 mg. daily of one of the synthetic compounds exhibiting antihemorrhagic activity.

Intestinal Diseases.—In this group of cases treatment depends upon the fundamental facts already outlined for cases of obstructive jaundice and biliary fistula. Here again early recognition of possible instances in which hypoprothrombinemia may occur is all-important in treatment. The same dosage of the same compounds can also be employed here.

The Newborn Infant.—On the basis of work now available it appears that a dose of from 1 to 5 mg. of 2-methyl-1,4-naphthoquinone or any of the other synthetic quinone compounds available commercially is sufficient in most instances to control hemorrhagic disease of the newborn and that, if it is administered at the time of birth, it will prevent *transitory hypoprothrombinemia.* It must be remembered that failures also can occur in treatment of infants if sufficient hepatic damage has occurred. It has also been demonstrated that the same dose of vitamin K as given to the newborn infant, when administered to the mother twelve to twenty-four hours prior to delivery, results in the birth of a baby who has a higher value for prothrombin in the blood than is normally present. These synthetic compounds apparently are effective when administered either orally or parenterally. Toxic effects have not been noted in the examination of either the mother or the infant.

There would seem to be some surgical significance of these observations and it perhaps would be wise to administer vitamin K before any contemplated surgical operation is undertaken at this age. Such a simple precaution might greatly lessen the chance of unpleasant and serious bleeding at the time of and after operation. We would suggest that for the pregnant mother vitamin K be administered as 2-methyl-1,4-naphthoquinone, 2 mg. daily for one week prior to delivery and that, if necessity demands, the form of this compound prepared for intravenous use could be administered in the same dose at the time of labor. For the infant we suggest that 3.2 mg. of 2-methyl-1,4-naphthohydroquinone-3-sodium sulfonate or any other water soluble compound that has equal vitamin K activity be given intramuscularly immediately after birth. This, in almost all instances, will prevent the occurrence of hemorrhagic diathesis resulting from a deficiency of prothrombin.

Preparation of Vitamin K Available Commercially.—*Alfalfa.*—Alfalfa is a rich source of vitamin K and concentrates of this material have received extensive clinical application during the past few years. These concentrates are available commercially in capsules or in bulk form.* Two to six gelatin capsules of either of these products together with 1 to 4 gm. of animal bile salts seems to constitute an adequate daily dose for most patients.

Synthetic Compounds.—2-methyl-1,4-naphthoquinone possesses marked antihemorrhagic activity. It is available commercially for both oral and intravenous administration.†

Undoubtedly many more synthetic products possessing antihemorrhagic activity will appear commercially in the near future. Regardless, however, of the compounds employed for clinical use the important thing to remember still is the fundamental physiologic facts which underlie the production

---

* Klotogen, Abbott Laboratories and Vitamin K concentrate, Squibb.

† Kayquinone (Abbott Laboratories) is available in capsules of soft gelatin containing 1 mg. of 2-methyl-1,4-naphthoquinone and in tablets containing 1 mg. Proklot (Eli Lilly and Co.) is available in tablet form, each tablet containing 2 mg. of 2-methyl-1,4-naphthoquinone. Thyloquinone (Squibb) is available in capsules of soft gelatin containing 1 mg. of 2-methyl-1,4-naphthoquinone in corn oil.

Hykinone (Abbott Laboratories) is a product for intravenous or intramuscular use which contains 3.2 mg. of 2-methyl-1,4-naphthohydroquinone-3-sodium sulfonate per ampule which is equivalent to 2 mg. of 2-methyl-1,4-naphthoquinone. Synkamin (Parke, Davis & Co.) is available in ampules for intravenous use, each ampule containing 1 mg. of 4-amino-2-methyl-1-naphthol hydrochloride.

of deficiency of prothrombin for which vitamin K in most instances is specific.

REFERENCES

Brinkhous, K. M., Plasma Prothrombin—Vitamin K, Medicine, **19**: 329–416, 1940.
Butt, H. R. and Snell, A. M., Vitamin K, W. B. Saunders Company, Philadelphia, 1941.

VITAMIN A

Night Blindness, Keratomalacia, Xerophthalmia

It is difficult historically to trace the effects of deficiency of vitamin A but even as long as sixty or seventy years ago there were several definite medical reports about occurrence of grave epidemics of xerophthalmia and keratomalacia. It was noted then that this disease appeared chiefly in children whose food was principally of vegetable origin, whereas among the children of the coast, whose diets consisted principally of fish, the disease was rarely seen. It was noted also that this disease was eminently improved by ingestion of chicken liver, veal fat, or cod liver oil. These clinical observations were then followed by many experimental studies which suggested strongly that there was present in certain foodstuffs a fat soluble compound which was essential for normal growth. It was not, however, until 1913 that McCollum and Davis reported the occurrence in certain foods of a compound termed *"fat soluble A."* These authors later reported that severe spontaneous infection developed in rats suffering from deficiency of vitamin A, and although in this earlier work the diets used had been often deficient in vitamin D as well as in vitamin A, in 1922 it was shown clearly that the antiophthalmic factor in cod liver oil could be destroyed by oxidation without destroying the antirachitic factor.

In these early experiments it was noted that a swelling of the lids of one or both eyes developed in animals (rats) on a diet deficient in vitamin A following which there commonly developed an inflamed and catarrhal condition of the conjunctiva with a bloody or purulent discharge. It was noted that if this eye condition was not treated and the animal continued to live, the cornea became affected and blindness resulted. It was also significantly noted that without any local treatment, if the eye disease were not too far advanced, the symptoms disappeared rapidly following administration to the animal of food containing an adequate amount of vitamin A. This relation of disease of the eye to dietary deficiency was also demonstrated experimentally in other species as well as rats, and it was also shown in these studies that certain diseases of the eye of man might be the result of deficiency of vitamin A; and soon it was reported that xerophthalmia in man could be prevented or cured by the administration of food rich in the A vitamin.

Chemistry

Although vitamin A was the first vitamin to be described it was not until many years later that it was isolated and its definite function in the metabolism established. *Perhydrovitamin A*, the completely saturated compound, has been synthesized. The structural formula of vitamin A_1 is as follows:

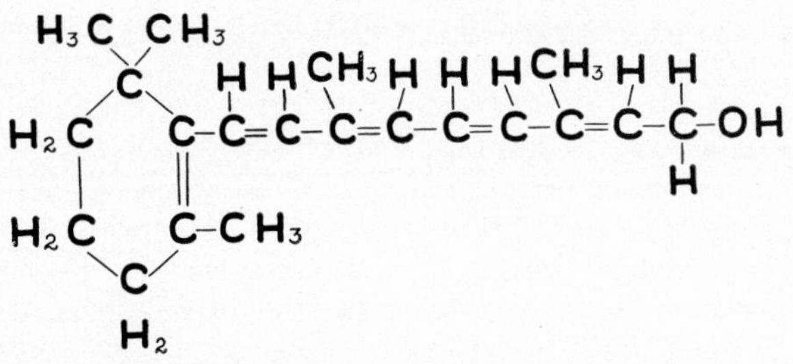

Fig. 34.–The structural formula of vitamin A_1.

This primary alcoholic structure of vitamin A is important in that it allows for esterification and therefore the formation of compounds of vitamin A with protein, bile acids, and fatty acids. These compounds of vitamin A are decomposed with liberation of the vitamin by such hydrolytic processes as occur in saponification; the vitamin is an alcohol, hence, it is not itself saponifiable. Vitamin A is a hydrogen acceptor probably because of its unsaturated form. There is some evidence to indicate that the substance readily absorbs oxygen in solution and is markedly pro-oxygenic when undergoing oxidation. However, highly oxidized vitamin A has no biologic activity. Vitamin A does not show any absorption band in the visible region of the spectrum but it does show a rather broad absorptive region in the ultraviolet. These properties form the basis for the spectrophotometric method for the quantitative estimation of vitamin A.

From recent reports it appears that there exists in addition to vitamin A a compound designated as vitamin A_2. In chemical structure vitamin A_1 is related very closely to vitamin A_2 and biologically the activity is the same. Rather extensive investigations of the distribution of these two forms of vitamin A have led definitely to the conclusion that vitamin A_1 predominates in the tissues of salt water fishes and vitamin A_2 predominates in the tissues of fresh water fishes. The absence of vitamin A_2 from the liver of mammals and other land animals probably can be explained by the absence of vitamin A_2 from their food.

Most of the vitamin A available to man in his diet is in the form of its precursors, the yellow and red carotenoid pigments (*provitamins*). For this reason the chemical properties of these compounds are rather important. Of this large group of pigments, only four substances are known at present from which animals can form vitamin A: alpha, beta, and gamma carotene and a related substance, cryptoxanthin, are all capable of yielding vitamin A. Of this group, however, the beta form yields two molecules of the vitamin, whereas each of the other produces only one molecule. This can be seen easily in the formula of beta carotene shown in figure 35. Theoretically, if the splitting occurs in the middle, one molecule may give rise to two molecules of vitamin A. It was the ingenious research of Karrer which first proved that beta carotene contains two beta-ionone rings. It was also shown by these investigations that the beta-ionone ring is an essential component of the molecular structure of vitamin A. All the carotenoids that yield vitamin A exhibit characteristic absorption bands in the visible region of the spectrum.

Although its exact function is unknown, *carotene* obviously is of great importance in the physiologic processes of plants. It is a family associated closely with chlorophyl although it is not lost when the chlorophyl disappears at the time of the yellowing of the leaves. However, it is destroyed completely in dry dead leaves. Rapid drying by artificial heat also destroys the provitamin. All these facts are important because carotene of green leaves is brought indirectly into human nutrition through milk and eggs.

The conversion of the precursors into vitamin A apparently takes place in the animal liver and it is of clinical significance that this transformation is retarded in phosphorus poisoning and in other forms of hepatic injury. It is

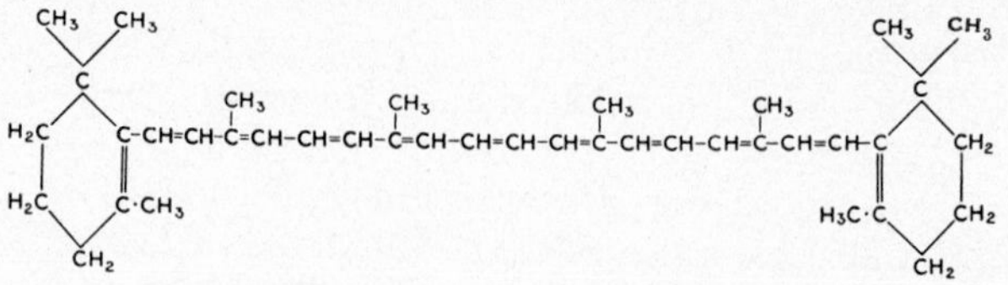

Fig. 35.—The structural formula of beta carotene, showing that, if the splitting occurs in the middle, one molecule may give rise to two molecules of vitamin A.

thought that the conversion of carotene into vitamin A takes place by the aid of an enzyme in the liver called *carotenase*.

PHYSIOLOGY

Absorption.—The absorption and utilization of vitamin A and carotene depend on many factors and because of the differences in absorption and utilization of these two compounds, they must be described separately.

Vitamin A is a fat soluble compound and its absorption apparently is facilitated greatly by the simultaneous absorption of a certain amount of fat. Most observers believe that the presence of bile is not necessary for proper absorption of vitamin A, although it is still perhaps good therapeutic medicine to administer bile salts with concentrates of vitamin A in the treatment of patients who have obstruction of the biliary tract. Absorption of the vitamin reaches the maximum in three to five hours after administration. Although there apparently is some loss of vitamin A in the stool, nothing is known of the degree of destruction of vitamin A in the gastro-intestinal tract under either normal or pathologic conditions. Studies on a person who had a fistula of the thoracic duct, following administration of vitamin A or carotene by mouth, revealed that very little of the carotene passes through the chylous fluid whereas nearly all of the vitamin A can be recovered.

Carotene is absorbed less readily than vitamin A and is subject to several more hazards. Proper absorption of carotene requires the presence of bile in the intestinal tract and, in those conditions in which bile is excluded completely or partially from the intestinal tract or in those instances in which bile salts of good quality are poorly excreted, bile must be given as a supplement to insure proper absorption. Chronic diarrhea, pancreatic dysfunction, celiac disease or sprue also may inhibit absorption of carotene. As with vitamin A, a certain amount of normal absorption of fat also seems necessary for proper transportation of carotene across the intestinal wall. It has been shown further that mineral oil may inhibit absorption of carotene seriously. For this reason, mineral oil should not be given soon after meals. Absorption of carotene reaches a maximal level in the blood in from seven to eight hours after administration, and the fecal excretion accounts for only a small portion of the unutilized excess. The rest of it apparently finds other channels of excretion or is destroyed in the intestine or elsewhere. The kidney apparently does not play any part in disposition of either vitamin A or its precursors, unless the body is flooded with either carotene or vitamin A.

Storage.—The capacity to store vitamin A varies widely in different species of animals. The rat has a remarkable capacity for the storage of vitamin A, whereas the rabbit and guinea-pig retain little of this substance even when on diets rich in carotene. In these particular animals a large part of the total vitamin A in the body is present in the liver, although small amounts appear in the lungs and kidneys. However, in other animals, for instance fish, greater amounts of vitamin A are deposited in the tunica propria of the mucosa of the intestine than in the liver.

After absorption, a greater portion of the carotene is held in the liver where it gradually disappears from the Kupffer cells as the concentration of vitamin A in the liver increases. Vitamin A itself also is stored properly in the liver in the Kupffer cells. In human beings, vitamin A content, as in all animals, is much lower in the liver at birth than in the liver of the normal adult, irrespective of the diet of the mother. The liver probably stores about 95 per cent of the vitamin A reserve of the body and the storage is as a rule lowest in the liver during childhood and increases gradually with advance in age. Examinations of livers of healthy persons who died suddenly from accidental causes show them to average 331 U.S.P. units of vitamin A per gram of liver.

The exact mechanism by which vitamin A is called forth from its reserve stores is not known but from several sources it appears that the distribution of vitamin A in the circulating blood and tissues is controlled in part of the nervous system.

Using fluorescence microscopy as a method of visualization of vitamin A in tissue cells, Poper and his associates found that the concentration of vitamin A in the human liver varies even under normal conditions. In young infants there was very little storage but in the embryo of about five months considerable amounts appeared although these depots of vitamin were reduced later and at birth only traces were distinct. The human adrenal and lactating breast tissues were found to be rich in vitamin A but the normal human kidney and inactive breast tissue, brain, cornea, bronchi and urinary tract were found free of the vitamin. It is interesting that by this method it was found that the retina of rats dying of avitaminosis A with ulceration of the cornea contained vitamin A.

Excretion.—Neither vitamin A nor carotene is excreted by the kidneys unless the organism is given an excessive dose of these substances. Under these circumstances the vitamin or its precursor is absorbed more rapidly than it can be stored or destroyed and there results some spilling over of these compounds into perhaps all the body fluids.

Only extremely small quantities of these compounds can be found in the feces and it is assumed for this reason that unutilized excesses find other channels of excretion or are destroyed in the intestine or elsewhere.

Human milk contains both carotene and vitamin A. The colostrum from the human breast has from two to three times the biologic vitamin A activity of early milk and early human milk has from five to ten times the biologic vitamin A activity of cow's milk. It is interesting that this biologic vitamin A activity of early human milk is not increased by feeding supplements of cod liver oil to the mother. Late human milk contains about the same amount of carotene and vitamin A as cow's milk.

Relation of Vitamin A to Specific Body Function and Specific Organs.— Relation to Infection.—Since McCollum in 1917 first pointed out that severe spontaneous infection develops in rats suffering from deficiency of vitamin A, there has been a bulk of literature on this subject and for many years it was believed that vitamin A did aid in some manner in combating the tendency to infection in man. It is believed by some that the frequency and high mortality of pneumonia in infants who suffer from vitamin A deficiency result from disturbance of function of the mucosa of all parts of the lung. Others believe that vitamin A in large amounts is beneficial in preventing the common cold, but this whole subject is in general very controversial. Undoubtedly, severe deficiency of vitamin A in man will lower the resistance to infection; yet administration of vitamin A during the course of an infection apparently does not have any beneficial effect on the outcome of the infection unless a severe deficiency of vitamin A also is present. Certainly there is enough evidence to indicate that there are many other factors of equal or greater influence on infection than is vitamin A and that there is no justification for calling vitamin A "the anti-infective vitamin."

Reproductive System.—Nothing is known of the effect of deficiency of vitamin A on the fertility of man. Nor is anything known concerning the importance of moderate deficiencies in either men or women.

Central Nervous System.—Deficiency of vitamin A apparently has a profound effect on the nervous system of animals but nothing definite in this direction ever has been shown in man. In young puppies, deafness results from diets deficient in vitamin A and in the labyrinths of these animals degeneration of the cochlear neurons is the most obvious pathologic change. It has been demonstrated also by some investigators that degeneration of the medulla oblongata is one of the fundamental lesions of vitamin A deficiency in rats.

Eye.—Decreased facility for *dark adaptation* is one of the earliest functional changes associated with deficiency of vitamin A. Evidence has been reported which suggests that the visual purple of the retina is a conjugated protein in which vitamin A is a prosthetic group. Exposure of the retina to light leads to a chemical change with bleaching of the visual purple and before sensitivity can be restored the pigment must be reconstructed. This process perhaps is reversible but it is not always efficient and therefore direct supplies of vitamin A must be constantly available. The selection of color and other visual functions depends on light of high intensity associated with the cones of the retina, whereas the rods are sensitive only to light and are especially adapted to function in dim light. Visual purple is found only in the rods and apparently serves to transform the energy of dim light into nerve impulses which within limits vary with intensity of the light. Although it was believed formerly that the cone played no part in vitamin A metabolism, it has been demonstrated recently that formation of visual violet or iodopsin in the cone takes place in much the same manner as does formation of visual purple in the rods.

EPITHELIUM.—Recently evidence has been reported which indicates that *vernix caseosa* is a manifestation of a vitamin A deficiency in the newborn infant and that it represents disturbances in cornification analogous to the dermal changes accompanying keratomalacia and other manifestations of vitamin A deficiency. In the particular work which supports this hypothesis, twenty-five mothers were given 50,000 to 100,000 units or more of vitamin A daily for six months or more. Twenty-one babies born to these twenty-five mothers were born with little or no vernix. Four babies were born with moderate or much vernix. To another group of twenty-nine mothers less than 50,000 units of vitamin A was administered daily for six months or more. Fourteen of the babies born to this group of mothers had little or no vernix and fifteen were born with moderate or much vernix.

Dryness and scaliness of the skin are perhaps among the earliest manifestations of involvement of the skin resulting from deficiency of vitamin A. Within the past few years several investigators have reported on patients who had cutaneous lesions which were considered to be the result of deficiency of vitamin A. One type of lesion is characterized by small pustules which appear around the hair follicles on the extensor surfaces of both upper and lower extremities, on the shoulders and on the lower part of the abdomen and buttocks. These pustules vary in diameter up to 5 mm., are hard and deeply pigmented, and have a surrounding area of depigmentation. In the center is an epithelial plug which when expressed leaves a crater. Other writers have described a type of lesion which resembles in many ways, but not in all respects, the acne pustule with the exception that pustulation is uncommon. It has been pointed out that it is important to remember that response of skin lesions to vitamin A is slow, depending as it does on anatomic repair, in contrast to the relief of night blindness in which the response depends on physiologic changes only and therefore occurs in a matter of hours or a few days.

URINARY SYSTEM.—Some experimental evidence seems to suggest that calculi of the urinary tract may result from a diet deficient in vitamin A, but this never has been definitely established in man and certainly further studies are required before the results can be applied to man.

THYROID.—It was reported a number of years ago that the milk from goats, which is normally pure white, is yellowish after thyroidectomy notwithstanding the fact that the diet is normal. The latter color apparently is due to failure to convert carotene into vitamin A. Later it was suggested that the thyroid hormone was essential for the conversion of carotene and also for the storage of vitamin A in the liver. Then carotenemia was observed in cases of hypothyroidism and striking general improvement of patients who had hypothyroidism was reported following administration of diets rich in vitamin A. Repeatedly it has been reported that the vitamin A in the blood of cretins is of decreased concentration or absent whereas the value for carotene usually is high. From this it was assumed that insufficiency of the thyroid hormone prohibits the conversion of carotene into vitamin A. It has been shown in clinical studies that *hyperthyroidism* depletes or destroys vitamin A reserves as evidenced by pathologic adaptations to darkness. All this work suggests that the thyroid hormone is essential for the conversion and storage of vitamin A, but this is not yet a well established fact. Certainly evidence is sufficient to indicate that vitamin A may be destroyed more rapidly by an organism in which the metabolic rate is increased from any cause including hyperthyroidism but it is not yet well established that vitamin A can decrease the activity of thyroxin.

LIVER.—It has been well established that the liver enacts a major rôle in the metabolism of vitamin A but the exact manner in which this is accomplished is still unknown. As early as 1895, Hori had made the clinical observation that frequently night blindness and keratomalacia accompany disease of the liver. Later it was shown that in patients who have alcoholic cirrhosis without jaundice there are subnormal powers of adaptation to darkness which improve on adequate administration of vitamin A. Others have demonstrated repeatedly that the vitamin A in the liver and in the blood of patients who have severe hepatic injury nearly always is decreased markedly. It has been suggested that since pathologic conditions of the liver result in incomplete transformation of carotene into vitamin A, *fish liver oil* should be given preference to carotene in treatment of hepatic disease.

PATHOLOGY

Effect of Deficiency of Vitamin A in Animals.—*Eye.*—In the experimental animal, as in man, pathologic changes in the eye occur late. Changes in both animals and man are essentially the same. Metaplasia of the epithelium of the conjunctiva and cornea is the earliest change, followed by vascularization of the cornea with edema and perhaps necrosis. Accumulation of keratin itself favors infection of the cornea which may ultimately lead to ulceration and hypopyon.

Epithelium.—In deficiency of vitamin A, certain specific pathologic changes are observed in many epithelial structures. There usually is atrophy of the epithelium concerned, as well as a gradual proliferation of basal cells and differentiation of the new product into a stratified keratinized epithelium. The replacement epithelium is identical with epidermis. Accumulation of keratinized epithelial cells may give rise to many striking gross pathologic features. This may lead to the occlusion of the bronchi and subsequent atelectasis. In the male, atrophy of the testis may occur and in the female retardation of growth and death of fetuses may occur.

Miscellaneous Organs.—Atrophy and metaplasia of the enamel organs take place in rats. Formation of enamel stops, and many deformities of the teeth result because of the defective formation of dentine.

No definite changes in the skin of experimental animals have been described following deficiency of vitamin A.

In the genito-urinary tract of rats, the ureters and renal tubules may be completely obstructed owing to accumulation of keratinized cells.

Lesions of the stomach and intestine of experimental animals resulting from deficiency of vitamin A are rare.

Mellanby reported the degeneration of cells of the superior ganglion and mild degeneration of the ophthalmic division of the fifth nerve in rabbits, dogs, and rats following administration of diets deficient in vitamin A but this work has not been confirmed completely. Most workers feel that deficiency of vitamin A in animals results in few if any definite nerve lesions.

Effect of Deficiency of Vitamin A in Man.—*Eye*.—The loss of visual acuity in dim light is one of the first symptoms of vitamin A deficiency in man. However, definite pathologic changes in the eye occur late in man on diets deficient in vitamin A. The early pathologic changes are the same as those described previously for animals. In this country xerophthalmia is an extremely rare disease. Although it is most common in infancy it may be seen at all ages. *Night blindness* usually develops in adults before any ophthalmias develop but usually the disease is ushered in by small triangular white patches on the outer and inner sides of the cornea covered by white, foam-like spots consisting of corneal epithelium, which has been shed and accumulates in this position (*Bitot's spots*). Photophobia and conjunctivitis appear early followed by a light brown pigmentation of the conjunctiva. The keratinization of the conjunctiva may extend to the cornea and lead to extreme softness and degeneration of the cornea and to ulceration, perforation, and total destruction of the eye (*keratomalacia*). This disease may destroy the eye rapidly and its prompt recognition therefore is very important.

For a number of years, Spies and associates have studied the ocular symptoms occurring from malnutrition in human beings. Ascher and Spies have observed that Bitot spots are frequent findings in these patients, and disappear soon after large doses of vitamin A. Follicular conjunctivitis is a frequent finding, particularly in children, and it also often disappears following the administration of large amounts of vitamin A.

Epithelium.—In the human infant, Wolbach and his associates have observed keratinizing metaplasia appearing earliest and most often in the trachea and bronchi and in the pelvis of the kidney. It was observed also in the conjunctiva, cornea, accessory sinuses, salivary glands, ureter, uterus and periurethral glands. In these cases no cutaneous condition which could be attributed solely to deficiency of vitamin A was observed. However, cutaneous lesions associated with deficiency of vitamin A and analogous to those occurring in other epithelial structures have been reported by several investigators. These changes have been discussed already under the heading "Relation of vitamin A to specific body functions and specific organs."

Toxicity.—If large amounts of vegetables containing carotene are ingested by normal persons and persons suffering from certain diseases such as diabetes, carotene may accumulate in the skin in amounts sufficient to cause a deep yellow color known as *carotenemia*. This syndrome, in so far as is known, is compatible with good health.

It is difficult to evaluate the reports concerning the injurious effects on man following ingestion of cod liver oil. Some observers, when administering large doses (80 cc.) of cod liver oil, have noticed the appearance of *dermatitis* of the face and scalp, and sensitivity to cod liver oil resulting in eczema also has been reported. However, from the general favorable clinical experiences in the use of cod liver oil and other preparations containing vitamin A, one must be extremely certain that it is harmful before discontinuing its use. Certainly with the average therapeutic dose no such toxic effect will be observed.

SOURCES AND HUMAN REQUIREMENTS

Food Sources.—Vitamin A is widespread in nature in the form of its precursors, the yellow and red carotenoid pigments (*provitamins*). These pigments are found in the plant world, being distributed from bacteria to garden fruits and vegetables. The pigments are found chiefly in association with chlorophyl and in the green leaves of plants but this is not invariably true, since carrots and sweet potatoes with their yellow color also are rich in these substances. Since most of our vitamin A is obtained in the form of its precursors, the plant pigments, the distribution of vitamin A will be discussed in terms of the distribution of the carotenoid pigments in nature.

There apparently is a direct parallel between greenness (chlorophyl content) and vitamin A activity in foods of plant origin. Among the best sources of vitamin A are thin green leaves. The exact relation between the degree of greenness and vitamin A activity is not understood but it is well known that the outer green leaves of iceberg lettuce or cabbage are much more potent in vitamin A than are the inner leaves. Peas, green beans, green peppers, parsley stocks, asparagus and green celery are all known to have a high vitamin A content. Carrots, sweet potatoes, apricots, yellow peaches, bananas, and yellow tomatoes, all of which possess a yellowish color, are rich sources of vitamin A. Nuts and cereal grains, with the exception of those having considerable green and yellow color, are very poor sources of vitamin A. Yellow corn is the most important vitamin A food in this group.

Whole milk, eggs, and milk products are perhaps the most important sources of vitamin A of animal origin.

Vitamin A is fairly stable to heat and not appreciably soluble in water; it is, however, destroyed by oxidation, and foods that are heated for long periods show appreciable loss of vitamin A potency. Since the vitamin activity is not affected at the temperature of boiling water, foods cooked in this manner retain their vitamin A potency. Canned foods have practically the same vitamin A value as the corresponding fresh foods, and foods that are stored in the frozen state maintain their maximal vitamin A value but dried and dehydrated foods show considerable loss of vitamin A content.

Requirements.—*Infants.*—It is believed that approximately 25 U.S.P. units of vitamin A per Kg. of body weight covers the minimal vitamin A requirement of most infants. The diets, however, of young infants usually contain more milk than the diets of adults and also their diets usually are supplemented with some kind of fish liver oil so that most infants obtain ten to twelve times as many units of vitamin A as those usually considered to be minimal requirements. It must be remembered that in the presence of diarrhea or jaundice larger doses of vitamin A must be administered. It may be necessary in such conditions to administer the material, if available, by the parenteral route.

Children.—For growing children between the ages of two and fourteen years, approximately 6,000 to 8,000 U.S.P. units of vitamin A daily is considered adequate. This is provided with about 1 quart (1 liter) of milk in addition to an egg, servings of green leafy vegetables and butter, and 3 gm. of cod liver oil daily as the main sources of protective foods rich in vitamin A. In growing children as well as infants, diarrhea and so forth may result in increased requirements of vitamin A which at times must be administered parenterally.

Pregnant and Nursing Women.—It has been recommended that a daily intake of at least 5,000 U.S.P. units of vitamin A be required for all nursing and pregnant women. This may be obtained by the ingestion of 1 quart (1 liter) of fresh whole milk, one egg, 1 ounce (28 gm.) of cheese, an average serving of a green leafy vegetable and a teaspoonful (5 cc.) of cod liver oil daily.

Working Adults.—A definite minimal vitamin A requirement of man is still unknown. This uncertainty of the requirement of man for this particular vitamin lies in the fact that there is wide variability in minimal and optimal requirements and in absorption, storage, utilization, and destruction, and finally that there is not complete agreement as to the standard which should be established as a measure of vitamin A sufficiency. It is believed generally that from 47 to 57 U.S.P. units of vitamin A per Kg. of body weight for adult man is required for the *prevention of night blindness.* Allowing a 50 per cent margin of safety for the maintenance of a moderate storage of vitamin A in the body, a total of about 3,000 U.S.P. units of vitamin A daily has been suggested by Booher for the normal adult. The average working adult who will take each day two eggs, two helpings of a leafy vegetable, the usual amount of butter, and frequent servings of liver probably will receive his optimal amount of vitamin A.

METHODS OF MEASURING DEFICIENCY OF VITAMIN A

Dark-adaptation Test.—The fact that night blindness is an early symptom of deficiency of vitamin A led to the development of visual adaptation in dim light as a method for the diagnosis of deficiency of vitamin A. However, attempts to produce pure vitamin A deficiency in man as measured by adaptation to dark continued to be very controversial. Some investigators contend that this method is satisfactory for measuring vitamin A deficiency in man; but others vigorously contend that, although some relation exists between the biophotometer reading and vitamin A nutrition, the relation is not close enough to warrant the use of the test as a means of diagnosing subclinical vitamin A deficiency. It has been pointed out that the method is time consuming and for this reason alone its routine clinical use is practically ruled out. Certainly minor fluctuations in dark adaptation in terms of vitamin A deficiency should receive little emphasis unless the physical methods are used to test the reliability of the differences. It is true that a majority of workers believe that the study of dark adaptation can be used as a test for vitamin A deficiency but until differences in technic and in interpretation of results have been resolved, it is impossible to be certain how far recorded observations represent physiologic facts.

No correlation between biophotometer readings and the vitamin A content of the blood has been observed and although it has been shown that the amount of vitamin A in the blood is dependent on the amount in the diet, evidence as to whether or not determination of the vitamin A in the blood is of value in judging the nutritional status is still contradictory.

Examination of Scrapings.—The same contradictory evidence is presented for measuring vitamin A by examination of scrapings from the eye and vagina. From all of these studies one would judge that the methods for measuring vitamin A deficiency in man are still somewhat unreliable and demand further study. Among some physicists and chemists there still is doubt whether one can measure, with the chemical methods now available, the small quantities of vitamin A present in the blood stream of man. There are others who feel that no satisfactory chemical method can be developed until one is capable of estimating in some degree the storage capacity of the body for vitamin A.

DIAGNOSIS

Undoubtedly the incidence of marked vitamin A deficiency in the United States is very small. Of course, the supposition that states of partial deficiency may be common has received repeated emphasis but as yet no definite methods have been developed by which these subnutritional states can be diagnosed.

Night Blindness.—The first symptom of this syndrome is a loss of visual acuity in dim light. This particular symptom may occur in various diseases

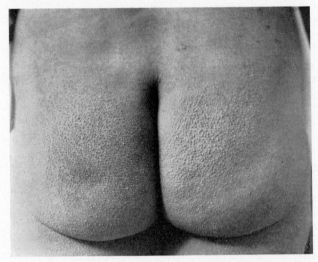

Fig. 36.—Photograph of the buttocks showing follicular hyperkeratosis which is associated with a deficiency of vitamin A. (Reproduced by courtesy of Section of Dermatology and Syphilology, Mayo Clinic.)

of the eye such as toxic amblyopia, detachment of the retina, or retinitis pigmentosa; but these conditions usually are excluded easily. The patient may complain of dancing lights before his eyes or similar visual disturbance and, of course, by means of dark adaptation he will show a pathologic condition. This condition must be suspected in cirrhosis of the liver, instances of severe and prolonged pyloric obstruction, severe chronic diarrhea, and any other condition which may produce a generalized nutritional deficiency.

Xerophthalmia.—The symptoms of xerophthalmia have been given already under the heading "Effect of deficiency of vitamin A in man.—Eyes."

Skin Lesions.—Within the past few years, several groups of investigators have reported patients who had cutaneous lesions which were considered to be the result of a deficiency of vitamin A. These lesions are shown best in figure 36. Many investigators believe that this manifestation of vitamin A deficiency is overlooked frequently.

Subclinical Form.—It is practically impossible to diagnose clinically subnutrition of vitamin A. However, the forms probably are frequent and must be considered under various conditions in which one would suspect inability for proper absorption or proper intake or utilization of vitamin A.

Differential Diagnosis.—Although various laboratory procedures such as measurement of vitamin A in the blood and urine and the measurement of dark adaptation may be in time very helpful in diagnosis of vitamin A deficiency, the best method of differential diagnosis still depends on close clinical observation. Night blindness, xerophthalmia and keratomalacia are not confused easily with any other conditions and should be recognized readily. Treatment should be instituted at once.

TREATMENT

The use of vitamin A in treatment is indicated in those syndromes which result from deficiency of vitamin A in the diet or from deficiency of vitamin A resulting from improper absorption or utilization. The best treatment with vitamin A still involves prophylactic therapy. In general, the response to treatment with vitamin A of specific syndromes resulting from the deficiency is prompt and effective.

Night Blindness.—Persons who possess normal powers of absorption of carotene and vitamin A and who have night blindness may be treated by diet alone or diet plus vitamin A supplement. Following the administration of 1,000 units of vitamin A in the form of potent fish liver oil, an improvement in dark adaptation may be demonstrable within normal limits. In those cases in which night blindness results from faulty absorption such as is caused by gastrocolic fistula, gastro-intestinal continuity first must be established before treatment unless the compounds are administered intramuscularly.

Xerophthalmia and Keratomalacia.—These conditions require the same treatment as night blindness but it is perhaps wise to give doses of from 50,000 to 100,000 units in the form of potent fish liver oil by the oral or parenteral route.

Skin Lesions.—In this condition the best results have been obtained from doses of 100,000 to 300,000 international units of vitamin A given daily over a period of from two to three months. It must be remembered that results from treatment of skin lesions require periods of from two to three months, and one should not become discouraged because there is not a dramatic response such as occurs in the treatment of night blindness resulting from deficiency of vitamin A.

Gastro-intestinal Diseases.—Patients who have chronic diarrhea require more vitamin A than is necessary for normal persons. Patients who have hepatic disease likewise require a rather large dose. In such instances from 10,000 to 20,000 international units of vitamin A daily is considered an adequate dose. A person from whose intestinal tract bile is excluded completely or partially should be given supplements of bile salts with vitamin A supplement.

Obviously in the treatment of any of these conditions, *diets* rich in vitamin A and its precursors should be prescribed in addition to the potent supplement containing vitamin A. Many preparations of vitamin A and its precursors are available, some of which are listed herewith:

1. *Carotene:* carotene in oil is on the market. It has a vitamin A content of not less than 7,500 units per gram. The potency of any preparation always appears on the label. Combinations of carotene with vitamin D concentrate are available in various brands. Fish liver oil is the most common form of prescribing vitamin A.

2. *Cod liver oil* (U.S.P.) has a minimum vitamin content of 600 A and 250 D. The U.S.P. dose is: infants 4 cc., adults 8 cc. There is little danger of overdosage, the main objection being taste. Many preparations of cod liver oil with malt have been put on the market but these have not contributed much toward increasing palatability.

3. *Cod liver oil obtainable in capsules* of 0.62 cc. (10 minims), 1.25 cc. (20 minims) or even larger.

4. *Cod liver oil reinforced with viosterol* is available in potency up to 60,000 A and 8,500 D per gram. This is also marketed in capsules containing more than 10,000 A and approximately 1,500 D each or in tablets containing more than 2,000 A and 300 D.

5. *Halibut liver oil* (N.N.R.) containing 44,800 A and 540 D per gram. It is obtainable in capsules containing 10,000 A and 170 D.

6. *Percomorph liver oil* (N.N.R.) has a maximal content of 60,000 A and 8,500 D per gram. In capsules as much as 13,300 A and 1,800 D are available.

REFERENCES

The Vitamins, published by the American Medical Association, under the auspices of the Council on Pharmacy and Chemistry and the Council on Foods, 1939.

Wolbach, S. B.: The Pathologic Changes Resulting from Vitamin Deficiency. J.A.M.A., **108:** 7–13, (Jan. 2) 1937.

Moore, Thomas: Vitamin A and Carotene: XIII. The Vitamin A Reserve of the Adult Human Being in Health and Disease. Biochem. J., **31:** 155–164, 1937.

DEFICIENCY OF VITAMIN D

(RICKETS)

INTRODUCTION

An attempt to trace the history of rickets through the ages is not a particularly satisfactory task. In ancient writings, medical historians have found many descriptions of a disease which they believed to be rickets. Such interpretations, however, are subject to doubt when one realizes that rickets is almost strictly a disease of the temperate zone whereas ancient civilization was cradled chiefly in tropical or subtropical areas. It is also true that Hippocrates is credited with a description of this disorder, but this has been the case with almost every other disease, and the description by Hippocrates would seem to fit more closely what is recognized today as tuberculous spondylitis. Since the birth of Christ, however, there have been numerous descriptions of undoubted rickets, and there can be no denying that it has been a very prevalent disorder for many centuries. Like many other diseases, its form has seemed to change as time advances, and even in the last few decades physicians have noted that the characteristic deformities are not so common as they were formerly. Physicians seem to be dealing today with a milder form than that with which their fathers were familiar, but equally serious since it has become more difficult to recognize.

The evolution of the etiology and specific treatment of rickets is more interesting than a chronological historical summary of the disorder. This is an outstanding example of the value of the basic sciences to clinical medicine, since there are few instances in which biology, inorganic and organic chemistry, and physics have made such useful contributions to the understanding of a disease.

In rickets, the pathogenesis lies in the condition of the Ca^{++} and PO_4^{---} in the blood serum. Further investigation led to the discovery of a relation between the sun's rays and the blood phosphate, namely, that the concentration of phosphate in the blood was higher in the summer than it was in the winter. It then followed for the physicist to segregate the rays of the solar spectrum and discover that the antirachitic properties of sunlight were attributable to the ultraviolet rays.

CHEMISTRY

McCollum in 1922 showed that vitamin D was distinct from vitamin A.

The work of the organic chemists on the isolation of the antirachitic sterols was a long and difficult task, and many pages could be devoted to a description of their investigations.

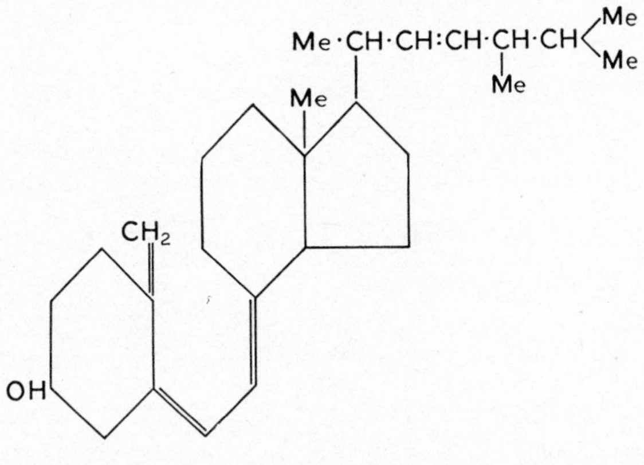

Fig. 37.—The structural formula for calciferol (vitamin D₂).

Ergosterol is the characteristic sterol of fungi and is prepared from yeasts and molds. The exposure of this substance to ultraviolet light sets in motion a series of photochemical changes, the end-product of which is *calciferol*, or vitamin D₂* (Fig. 37). This is the chief form of vitamin D present in viosterol, irradiated yeast, and "metabolized" or yeast milk. Fortunately, more radiant energy is required to produce calciferol than to decompose it, but even under the best controlled conditions calciferol will form only about 50 per cent of the total product. Overenthusiastic *irradiation* has been known to result in the formation of toxic substances, since with irradiation of ergosterol it is not true that "if a little is good, more is better." The changes produced in the ergosterol molecule by irradiation are

* To clear up any confusion that may exist in the reader's mind it might be well to point out that there is no vitamin D₁, this term having been pre-empted for a lumisterol-calciferol mixture originally mistaken for a pure vitamin. Vitamin D₄ is the name applied to activated 22-dihydro-ergosterol.

strictly of photochemical nature; there is no change in the structure of the molecule. The substance is insoluble in water and but slightly soluble in oils; it is completely soluble in the common fat solvents.

Most of the other antirachitic agents owe their virtue to activated *7-dehydrocholesterol*—vitamin D_3 (Fig. 38). The inactive form is the principal provitamin occurring with the cholesterol of animal fat. Ultraviolet irradiation of the skin, feathers and fur of animals therefore produces activated 7-dehydrocholesterol. For this reason the principal antirachitic agent present in natural fat oils, eggs, and irradiated milk is activated 7-dehydrocholesterol. Just as in the case of ergosterol, the changes produced by the activation of 7-dehydrocholesterol are entirely photochemical. The physical and chemical properties of 7-dehydrocholesterol resemble those of calciferol. Both of these substances have been isolated in crystalline form, but attempts at synthesis have been unsuccessful. Of the other sterols, only

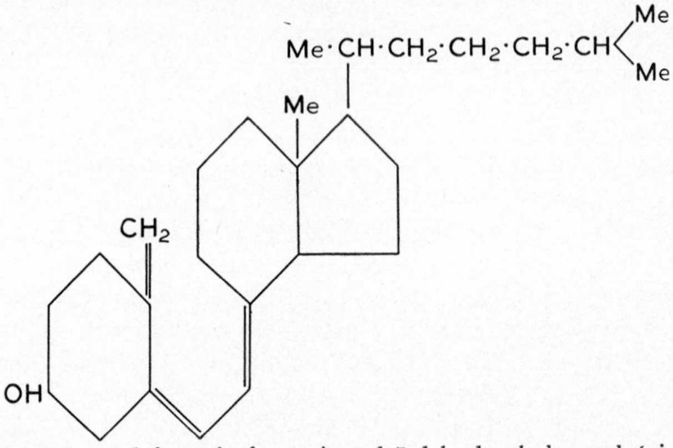

Fig. 38.—The structural formula for activated 7-dehydrocholesterol (vitamin D_3).

dehydrotachysterol is important enough to warrant mention. This substance is also known as *A.T. 10.*

Vitamin D is concerned chiefly with the regulation of the calcium and phosphorus in the body but the chemical nature of this mechanism is not understood. No one has demonstrated whether vitamin D enters directly into combination with these elements or their salts, or merely assumes the rôle of catalyst.

PHYSIOLOGY

Regarding the metabolism of vitamin D, knowledge is rather limited. The various forms of this vitamin are readily absorbed from the normal intestinal tract. Bile salts are necessary for this absorption, and recent investigations indicate that the salts of desoxycholic acid may be particularly concerned with the absorption of the liposoluble vitamins. Human beings have been found to store significant amounts of vitamin D in the skin and brain and smaller amounts in the lungs, spleen, and bones, but the liver is the chief warehouse for vitamin D. Failure of this storage mechanism coupled with defective secretion of bile salts may lead to secondary avitaminosis D in cases of hepatobiliary disease. This is not merely an academic observa-

* Like others, Spies, Browning and Lindblad have shown that infantile tetany can be relieved by A.T. 10 or by large doses of vitamin D. We prefer to administer to these persons a well-balanced diet and keep them free from tetany with adequate amounts of one or the other of these materials rather than to place them on a low phosphorus diet as is now done by some.

tion but a fact of importance which the clinician should keep in mind in the treatment of such disorders. This has been further emphasized by the observation that in animals normal liver function is necessary to promote the antirachitic action of vitamin D. The factor of absorption also enters into such diseases as celiac disease, sprue and other fatty diarrheas which are commonly attended by deficiency of vitamin D.

The body apparently has great powers for the conservation of vitamin D. Studies on excretion are lacking, but indirect evidence would seem to indicate that the tissues hold to their stores of vitamin D with great tenacity. It has been the experience of experimental workers that very small doses of this substance will exert an influence for several weeks. Large doses of vitamin D do not follow the course of the liposoluble vitamins in rapid destruction or excretion, but are carefully preserved for a long time. The concentration of vitamin D in the blood has been inadequately studied, and with the available methods such studies are impractical for even a well-equipped laboratory. Observations indicate that there is a wide zone of "normal" concentrations, as evidenced by one study which placed the limits at 66 to 165 U.S.P. units per 100 cc. of blood.

Calcium and Phosphorus Metabolism.—All the effects of vitamin D on the processes of the body are the result of its regulatory effect on the calcium and phosphorus content of the fluids of the body. In general, the concentrations of calcium and phosphorus in the blood serum reflect the amounts of these elements ingested. The ratio of these elements seems to be important in the rachitogenic diet since a high calcium and low phosphorus diet is associated with a low content of inorganic phosphate in the blood serum and vice versa. The absolute amount, as well as the ratio, determines the content of calcium and phosphorus in the body fluids and these values increase with increased amounts given. However, in the presence of an adequate amount of vitamin D, the values for calcium and phosphorus in the serum tend to become normal regardless of the type of diet.

Although secondary in importance to the calcium-phosphorus ratio, the *acid-base ratio* of the diet may be a factor in the production of rickets or tetany. There is some evidence to show that rickets is associated with an acid metabolism, and tetany with an alkaline one. In neither of these conditions, whether occurring clinically or produced experimentally in animals, is there a definite alteration of the acid-base equilibrium of the blood.

The action of vitamin D on calcium and phosphorus metabolism seems to be chiefly concerned with the absorption of the elements from the intestinal tract. The normal infant excretes about 90 per cent of his calcium intake in the feces and usually excretes a small amount in the urine. When vitamin D is not given, the calcium in the urine disappears. This is an attempt on the part of the body at mineral conservation. The concentration of calcium in the feces increases and the retention of calcium becomes subnormal. If the calcium intake is low or the deficiency severe, the fecal calcium may actually exceed the intake and the condition known as negative calcium balance ensues. A similar sequence of events occurs in the case of phosphorus, except that the amount of urinary phosphate is usually increased.

The effect of vitamin D in producing a reversal of these conditions is striking. The intestinal excretion of calcium and phosphorus is decreased, calcium appears in the urine, and the calcium balance is restored to normal. The changes in the concentration of calcium and phosphorus in the serum are reflectors of this calcium balance.

In recent years it has been shown that there exists in the body an enzyme, *phosphatase*, which is intimately related to phosphorus metabolism. The exact function of phosphatase in the serum is not known, but whatever it may be there is no question that in diseases of the bone, especially resorptive ones in which osteoblastic activity is increased, the concentration of phosphatase in the serum is increased. Such is the case in rickets. Its increase is perhaps the *first definite evidence* of development of the rachitic condition; it precedes roentgenologic changes and diminution of the serum phosphate. The concentration of serum phosphatase is high in cases of active rickets and the administration of vitamin D decreases the concentration toward normal, but more slowly than it decreases the concentration of calcium and phosphorus. The concentration of phosphatase may not reach normal for several months after there is evidence of healing. The increase of the concentration of serum phosphatase in cases of rickets acts apparently as a protective mechanism.

Vitamin D and Parathyroid Extract.—The difference in action of vitamin D and parathyroid extract is often the source of confusion, and it is important to the clinician that this distinction be clear. Although both preparations increase the concentrations of calcium and phosphorus in the serum, parathyroid extract acts specifically on the *serum calcium* and in parathyroid tetany it may even decrease the concentration of serum phosphate. In cases of rickets, the principal action of vitamin D is in raising the low concentration of serum phosphate; only when administered in very large doses does it raise the concentration of serum calcium above normal. Parathyroid extract increases the concentration of serum calcium by withdrawing the element from the bone; vitamin D exerts this effect by increasing the intestinal absorption of calcium or by diminishing its reexcretion from the intestinal mucosa. The distinction may be clearer if one remembers that the toxic effect of parathyroid extract is decalcification; that of vitamin D is hypercalcification.

Although the parathyroid glands have been shown to undergo hypertrophy in cases of rickets, this is a result, rather than the cause, of rickets. Indeed, injections of parathyroid extract have been shown to retard the healing of rickets, and removal of the parathyroid glands from animals makes the production of rickets more difficult.

THE HUMAN REQUIREMENT

There is remarkable variation in the requirement of vitamin D among persons of various ages and there exists a great difference in individual requirements even among persons of the same age group.

In Infancy.—The infant's requirement of vitamin D may be stated as that amount which insures sufficient retention of calcium and phosphorus (with an adequate intake of these minerals) to permit normal growth and mineralization of the teeth. This is a sound maxim, but it requires interpretation in terms of U.S.P. units. It is generally agreed that, in the ordinary quantities fed to babies, milk containing 135 units of vitamin D to the quart will furnish adequate vitamin D to prevent rickets in the majority of full-term infants. However, this amount is insufficient to prevent moderate or severe rickets in prematurely born or susceptible infants, and it seems unwise to furnish any baby with less than 300 to 400 units of vitamin D daily as cod liver oil. Milk containing 400 units to the quart furnishes sufficient vitamin D to prevent rickets of clinical significance in both full-term and premature infants.

Although the primary object in the administration of vitamin D is the prevention of rickets, one must not lose sight of an apparent growth-promoting effect of this substance. Infants receiving milk containing 135 units in a quart have been shown to grow at an average rate, whereas milk containing 400 units in a quart has produced growth somewhat faster than average. The requirement of breast fed infants for vitamin D is in general less than that of babies fed cow's milk. However, human milk is by no means antirachitic, and in order to insure optimal growth it is probably best to supplement this with the same amount used with cow's milk (300 to 400 units daily).

In Childhood.—The criteria of adequacy of intake of vitamin D are even fewer for children than for infants. The optimal quantity of vitamin D cannot be stated accurately, although there is no evidence that the total quantity needed is greater or less than the amount required for an infant. A daily allowance of at least 750 cc. of milk together with from 300 to 400 units of vitamin D seems to permit ample retention of calcium and phosphorus for proper development of bone and teeth.

In Adolescence.—Because of the rapid skeletal growth at this period of life, it would seem that the adolescent would require some vitamin D. However, studies on this subject are very scarce and knowledge of the vitamin D requirement at this age of life is entirely lacking. Apparently the variability and ability to utilize the calcium and phosphorus of the diet is a major factor in determining the quantity of these elements retained by adolescents as well as by young children. Vitamin D does not lower the minimal requirement for ingested calcium; therefore, no estimate can be made as to the optimal intake of either calcium or vitamin D.

In Adulthood.—The requirement of vitamin D during adult life remains to be determined. It appears strongly advisable to give vitamin D during pregnancy and lactation because of the fetal demand on the mother's tissues for calcium and phosphorus. The tendency of osteomalacia to develop among pregnant and lactating mothers in the Orient is well recognized. The optimal amount of vitamin D is not known. During lactation the requirement may be greater than at any other period of life and a daily dose of 800 units or more is suggested, together with an abundant intake of calcium and phosphorus.

SOURCES

The accepted standard unit for expressing the strength of vitamin D as adopted by the League of Nations Health Organization and by the United States Pharmacopeia is defined as "the vitamin D activity of 1 mg. of the international standard solution of irradiated ergosterol found equal to 0.025 micrograms of crystalline vitamin D." This is the international unit (I.U.) accepted as the U.S.P. unit. In administering antirachitic agents one should think in terms of units of vitamin D since this is the only way in which the doses of the various substances containing vitamin D, which differ greatly in volume, can be reduced to a common denominator. For example, 1 teaspoonful (4 cc.) of cod liver oil contains approximately 350 units; one quart of reinforced milk, 400 units; and 1 mg. of calciferol, 400,000 units.

Vitamin D in Food.—Vitamin D is contained in only a few of the foods in the average American diet. Some of these are herring, sardines, tuna and salmon, either fresh or canned. Eggs from all sources contain the vitamin. Hen's eggs are unreliable sources, however, since the amounts contained are variable. The diet of the average person is almost completely lacking in vitamin D since muscle meat, including the fat, kidneys and other glandular organs, fruit, sugar, cereal, and vegetable, contain none, or at the most, only traces. The amount in milk is negligible. Contrary to a popular misconception, butter, on the average, is estimated as containing only 80 units per 100 gm. Its potency, therefore, is about a thousandth of that of the average cod liver oil. Liver may contain a very small amount but not enough to be of any practical value. It may be concluded, therefore, that, although the diet occasionally may furnish appreciable amounts of vitamin D, in most instances it furnishes virtually none. For practical purposes it is best to regard the diet as being completely devoid of the vitamin.

Available Sources of Vitamin D.—*Cod Liver Oil.*—According to the United States Pharmacopeia (edition 11) cod liver oil must contain at least 100 units per gram. In all probability the cod liver oil sold in this country contains at least 100 units per gram, and some of the superior brands may contain two or even four times this official minimal standard. One teaspoonful (4 cc.) of cod liver oil, therefore, supplies at least 400 units. As already mentioned, the vitamin D in cod liver oil probably is chiefly activated 7-dehydrocholesterol.

Cod liver oil is effective in the prevention and treatment of any deficiency of vitamin D. It is universally obtainable; it also contains vitamin A (about 600 units per gram). Its single disadvantage is its fishy taste but its lack of concentration is regarded as a disadvantage by some physicians. This becomes of importance when large doses of vitamin D are required, since 1600 units (4 teaspoonfuls) represents the maximal practical daily dose. Cod liver oil is amply concentrated to prevent or cure rickets in almost all cases. Its unpleasant taste presents a real obstacle in its administration to older children and to adults, but infants do not seem to mind the taste provided the oil is given early and regularly. The refusal of a baby to take cod liver oil can usually be traced to the mother, who has communicated her severe dislike during its administration. Cod liver oil has been blamed by some as the cause of digestive disturbances. This is probably of rare occurrence and the practice of discontinuing its administration in hot weather has no sound basis. Hypersensitiveness to cod liver oil is very uncommon, but if this occurs another form of vitamin D must be used. Cod liver oil is best administered simply by a spoon, and attempts at disguise are not only unnecessary but usually futile.

Viosterol in Oil.—One gram of viosterol in oil contains "at least 10,000 units of vitamin D" to meet the requirements of the United States Pharmacopeia (edition 11). The special dropper accompanying commercial preparations is designed to deliver a drop containing 222 units. The vitamin D content of viosterol is 100 times that of standard cod liver oil. Viosterol owes its vitamin D activity to activated ergosterol.

Viosterol in oil is tasteless, which obviates the difficulty of administration encountered in the case of cod liver oil. The simplest method of administration is to drop the oil directly into the mouth, although it may be floated on orange juice. It is inadvisable to add viosterol to the feeding, since part of the viosterol may adhere to the bottle and thus be lost. Viosterol suffers one disadvantage as compared with cod liver oil and other fish oils; that is, it does not contain vitamin A. Its tastelessness makes it one of the best vehicles for administering vitamin D to adults and older children.

Fish Oils Naturally Concentrated in Vitamin D.—There is great variation in the concentration of vitamins A and D in the oils obtained from different species of fish. The oil of the Percomorphi exhibits the greatest concentration of vitamin D. Fish oils are prepared by the manufacturer by combining oils from various species in such a way that the final mixture has a concentration of vitamin D equal to that of viosterol in oil. These preparations have the merit of providing vitamins D and A in high concentrations so that both can be administered in doses measured in drops. The disadvantage of unpleasant taste is again encountered, but the quantity required is small, and this is not a serious disadvantage. Vitamin D in these preparations is chiefly in the form of activated 7-dehydrocholesterol.

Viosterol (Calciferol) in Propylene Glycol.—This preparation differs in no way from viosterol, save that it is in a different solvent.

Vitamin D Milk.—(*a*) IRRADIATED VITAMIN D MILK.—Vitamin D activity is added to milk of this type by exposure to active ultraviolet rays from artificial sources. The irradiation is accomplished in such a manner that standardization is at 135 international units per quart. It has been found impractical to irradiate the milk further because of the production of an unpleasant taste. In irradiated milk the vitamin is chiefly in the form of activated 7-dehydrocholesterol.

(*b*) METABOLIZED VITAMIN D (YEAST) MILK.—Activation is accomplished in this product by feeding irradiated yeast to cows. The criterion for standardization is 430 units per quart. The form of vitamin D is activated ergosterol.

(*c*) FORTIFIED VITAMIN D MILK.—This preparation depends for its vitamin D potency on the addition of vitamin D in the form of a concentrate derived from cod liver oil or the oils of other fishes or in the form of viosterol. Fortified vitamin D milk is standardized at 400 units per quart. The form of vitamin D in the milk obviously will depend on the supplement employed.

Vitamin D Bread.—This contains 460 units of the vitamin, viosterol, for a loaf weighing 24 ounces. The ingestion of six slices, or a quarter of a loaf, of bread daily would yield 115 units.

General Consideration of Sources.—The various sources of vitamin D vary in potency but may be substituted for each other on the basis of unitage. A good deal of work has been done to determine whether there is any difference in the antirachitic activity of the various chemical forms of vitamin D. The only conclusion that has been reached at present is that there is no essential difference.

In spite of the numerous claims for various preparations of vitamin D in oil, cod liver oil is still the most economical. It is interesting as well as practical to note that in terms of international units some of the more expensive brands of cod liver oil are more economical than some of the cheaper brands. For example, it requires only simple arithmetic to show that it is more expensive to use oil selling at fifty cents a pint, but containing only the required 85 units per gram than to use oil selling at ninety cents a pint and containing 350 units per gram. Oils depending on viosterol for the vitamin D are, in general, about twice as expensive, unit for unit, as the concentrated fish oils. The concentrated fish oils are as economical as many of the poorer brands of cod liver oil. Irradiated milk is about a third as economical as metabolized or reinforced milk. In any of these milks, however, the activation process adds about one cent per quart to the cost. These milks are considerably more expensive than cod liver oil or the concentrated fish oils. No extra charge is made for vitamin D in canned, evaporated milk, but the amount of the vitamin in the milk is very low, being only 135 units per reconstituted quart. Cod liver oil or the concentrated fish oils seem preferable to the preparations containing viosterol, if for no other reason than that it seems advisable to prescribe a preparation of vitamin D which is also rich in vitamin A rather than the one which contains only vitamin D.

The quartz mercury vapor lamp and the carbon arc lamp are expensive sources of vitamin D when compared with cod liver oil. The quartz mercury vapor lamp costs more initially but it is said it is less expensive to operate than the carbon arc lamp. However, these lamps are not necessarily expensive sources if large groups of children can be treated simultaneously as is possible in institutions. The carbon arc lamps are the ones best suited for this purpose.

ETIOLOGY OF RICKETS

In considering the cause of rickets we may accept vitamin D as specific in the prevention and cure. However, there exists a remarkable number of predisposing causes which must be mentioned in any complete consideration of this condition.

There is undoubtedly a *constitutional factor;* that is, all infants are not predisposed to rickets to the same degree. This individual variation in susceptibility is not understood. Heredity apparently plays no rôle in the cause of rickets, and congenital rickets is of such infrequent occurrence as to be almost disregarded. Prematurity assumes a position of great importance in the cause of rickets since this disorder occurs with exceptional frequency in an exaggerated degree among premature infants.

The rate of *growth* is one of the most important predisposing factors in the production of infantile rickets. Although experimental studies do not entirely substantiate this, the clinical dictum—"no growth, no rickets"— seems to hold true in general. It is a common observation that the extremely undernourished, marasmic infant practically never has rickets. Indeed, some authors feel that one of the greatest dangers of overfeeding is the possible development of rickets. This seems open to some question.

Age is one of the most important factors in the development of rickets. A review of age tables will show that rickets begins about the third month and ends about the eighteenth month of life. Sex appears to have no influence in the ordinary variety of rickets. This is notable since late rickets and infantile tetany are preponderantly disorders of male infants whereas osteomalacia is of very rare occurrence in this sex.

One of the dominant etiologic factors is *sunlight,* and, in general, a geographic or seasonal map of the incidence of rickets is the practical equivalent of a map of deficiency of sunlight. The important element in regard to the antirachitic activity of the solar rays is not so much the number of hours of sunshine as its quality and intensity. Winter sunlight has only a small amount of the effective rays as compared to that of the warmer months. The lack of fresh air and exercise apparently plays no rôle in the course of rickets.

Other than sunlight, *diet* is the only natural source of vitamin D available to the infant and obviously assumes a position of great importance. Breast milk stands preeminent in the prevention of rickets. The incidence of rickets is universally low among nursing infants. It must be remembered, however, that breast milk is not specific in the prevention of rickets as this disorder was rather widespread in the seventeenth century when all babies were breast fed. Experimental work has shown that human milk does not owe all of its antirachitic activity to its vitamin D content. There would seem to be some unidentified factor present which also exhibits this function. "Metabolized milk" and "irradiated milk" possess antirachitic activity about equal to human milk but are of value only in prevention and should not be depended on in treatment of active rickets. Of the other foods ordinarily included in an infant's diet during the age of greatest susceptibility, only eggs have any antirachitic properties. This is due to the vitamin D content of the yolk. Vegetables and fruits have absolutely no vitamin D content, as is erroneously thought. Butter is ineffective in the prevention of rickets. Obviously, in the prevention of rickets the calcium and phosphorus in the diet are of great importance, but since this is a discussion devoted primarily to vitamin D, this aspect of the diet will not be considered.

Pathology of Deficiency of Vitamin D

In order to afford a better understanding of the *bony changes* which occur in deficiency of vitamin D it might be advisable to review briefly the normal sequence of events in the growth of bones. Long bones increase in length by endochondral bone formation. The narrow place of epiphyseal cartilage is supported by bone on the epiphyseal surface and its diaphyseal side is uniformly penetrated by capillaries. During growth, a continuous proliferation of cartilage cells occurs on the epiphyseal side and there is degeneration of matured cells on the diaphyseal surface. These degenerating cells are replaced by capillaries and osteoblasts, which affect the deposition of bony matrix. Wolbach said that the growth of bone by endochondral bone formation is achieved "by a continuously retreating gap in the continuity of tissues maintained on the epiphyseal side by continuous renewal of cartilage cells and on the diaphyseal side repaired by vascular outgrowth comparable to repair of any defect of tissues by the process of organization or granulation tissue formation. In normal growth there presents on the diaphyseal side of the narrow cartilage a continuous layer of clear or empty cartilage cells forming an almost straight line."

In the development of rickets the first change is the cessation of this degenerative process in the mature cartilage cells and, consequently, no ingrowth of capillaries and osteoblasts. The epiphyseal cartilage increases in width because of continued proliferative activity and this thickening is irregular since the cessation of degeneration does not occur simultaneously in all portions of the plate.

In the absence of the ingrowth of capillaries and osteoblasts, there is a failure of calcification of the cartilaginous matrix, and newly formed bones during the active stage of the disease have an osteoid structure. The basic structural alteration in rickets is not the failure of formation of bone but the failure of calcification.

The disturbance manifests itself most markedly where the most rapid growth occurs, for example, at the lower epiphysis of the femur. Longitudinal sections of a rachitic bone will reveal a wide, irregular zone of ossification at the junction of the epiphysis and diaphysis. This region is known as the *rachitic zone*. Microscopically, a large amount of osteoid tissue is found adjacent to the shaft, and irregular columns of cartilage cells project into this osteoid tissue. Growth of the bone is delayed or stopped completely, in proportion to the severity of the process. On microscopic examination of sections of the shaft, osteoid lamellae are found under the periosteum, and lining the Haversian canals and marrow spaces. The structural changes in the bone are not identical in every case. In one type of the disease there is a large medullary cavity with a thin, porous cortex—a form approaching osteomalacia; in another type, the cortex is thick but porous and the medullary cavity is small.

The bony deformities resulting from these alterations vary with the amount of stress to which the individual bones are subjected. Before the infant walks there may be flattening of the occiput from the weight of the head, since the excess of osteoid tissue in the occipitoparietal bones makes them soft and yielding (*craniotabes*). There is enlargement of the costochondral junctions (rickety rosary), and alterations in the bony thorax may give rise to various deformities (Harrison's groove, pigeon breast, funnel breast). The weight of the body produces *deformities of the lower extremities* from bending of the bones in children who have assumed the erect posture. Growth of the long bones, particularly the femur, may be greatly delayed, and the adult may be of short stature as a result. The epiphyses are enlarged, and it is not uncommon for *genu valgum* or *genu varum* to develop. Occasional instances of dwarfism have a rachitic basis. Deformities of the spinal column are not common.

In *late rickets* the changes are similar to those of early rickets, except that the osteoid tissue develops in the subperiosteal and endosteal portions rather than at the epiphysis. Osteomalacia presents a similar picture.

The effect of vitamin D in reversing these changes has been clearly demonstrated with experimental animals. Following its administration the cartilage cells generally appear along the diaphyseal border at the end of twenty-four hours and extensive vascular penetration is visible within forty-eight hours; this permits the deposition of bone-forming salts. The mass of irregular cartilage cells becomes arranged into short, orderly columns of a few cells, and osteoid material is no longer formed. This is the basis of the "line test" used in assay of vitamin D.

It must be remembered that the fundamental defect in rickets is not in the bone. It has been shown that slices of rachitic bone and cartilage become calcified when placed in normal blood serum. The primary fault in rickets is in the body fluids, which do not make bone salts available to the bone. The action of vitamin D is to bring about alteration of the calcium and phosphorus in the body fluids so that they may be available to the bone.

PATHOLOGY OF HYPERVITAMINOSIS D

Whereas a lack of vitamin D can give rise to the striking changes which have just been described, certain pathologic changes also occur when excessive amounts of this vitamin are given. Actual changes have been observed only in animals that have received doses many times larger than ever have been administered to human beings. Hypervitaminosis D is an exaggerated form of the physiologic effect of the vitamin. The concentrations of calcium and phosphorus in the serum are increased. Calcification occurs at an increased rate, and the deposition of minerals at the provisional line of calcification is very dense. If the dose is increased to about 1000 times the therapeutic dose, calcification occurs in the epiphysis at the expense of the shaft. Negative calcium and phosphorus balances ensue and metastatic calcification takes place. This process most commonly affects the renal tubules, heart, blood vessels, bronchi, and stomach. These organs and the liver exhibit evidence of irritation and degeneration. The animals lose weight rapidly, an intense diarrhea develops, and death occurs in five to fourteen days. If smaller doses are given, the animal may survive and the described lesions will remain for at least six months. Diets low in calcium and phosphorus may prevent the calcification process but the degenerative changes occur.

Considerable experimental evidence has been presented by Agduhr which would indicate that prolonged overdosage of cod liver oil does produce definite organic changes in various organs of animals, particularly the heart. More recently, Jundell and Stenström have shown that cod liver oil given to children during the first twelve months of life produces alterations of the electrocardiogram presumably due to lesions of the conduction tissue and the myocardium. These alterations are of the same appearance as those obtained in experimental treatment of animals. Although these observations have not been extended to adult man, they must be considered before any extended overdosage of cod liver oil is given.

DIAGNOSIS OF DEFICIENCY OF VITAMIN D

In view of the repeated observations by students of nutrition, it seems superfluous to mention that deficiency diseases are still of rather common occurrence in the United States, but the importance of keeping the American physicians "vitamin conscious" becomes evident when one realizes that probably about 75 per cent of rickets escapes diagnosis and that deficiency of vitamin D is certainly the most common disorder of this type among infants of the temperate zone. The reason for this sad state of affairs is obvious. The great advance of modern pediatric clinics in the eradication of this disease has been so striking that it has produced a static state of mind among practising physicians. Further than this, some physicians have a faulty conception of rickets, having in mind only the severe affection. Their "diagnostic threshold" is reached only by the square-headed, pot-bellied baby with delayed teething and walking.

In general one may say that the ability of the individual clinician to diagnose rickets is in direct proportion to the care with which he elicits the story of the infant's nutrition, an essential part of any pediatric problem. With certain rare exceptions the possibility of deficiency of vitamin D can be promptly ruled out if the baby has been receiving cod liver oil but if such is not the case one should become suspicious and conduct a search for signs of rickets. Vague, indefinite symptoms, such as sweating, restlessness, and muscle flabbiness, are often described as early manifestations of the disease, but these are unimportant. The clinical diagnosis hinges on the finding of the various deformities described in the consideration of the pathologic changes. Among the more important of these are craniotabes and the rachitic rosary. The former is not difficult of recognition when the "box head" has developed with frontal bossing and occipital flattening. In the early or mild

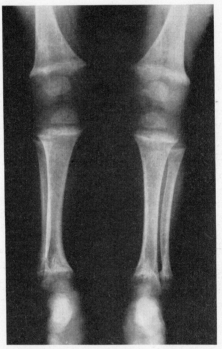

Fig. 39.—Generalized decalcification of the bones producing accentuation of visible trabeculations in a case of active rickets. At the ends of all the long bones there is marked flaring and the epiphyses have the characteristic moth-eaten appearance of rickets. (By courtesy of the Department of Radiology, The Mayo Clinic.)

stage the physician may encounter difficulty in distinguishing this condition from the normal softness of the baby's skull. It is well to remember that after the age of two or three months the infant's skull is rather firm and any increased softening revealed even by the unpracticed hand may be indicative of rickets. The rachitic rosary is one of the most constant signs of rickets but a good deal of skill is required to distinguish this from the normal enlargement of the costochondral junction. An enlarged fontanelle may be evidence of rickets but in many cases there is premature closure. Bowlegs and deformities of the thorax (chicken and funnel breasts, Harrison's groove) are of common occurrence but their presence alone is not pathognomonic since they occur in many other conditions.

To one acquainted with the intricacies of this sort of diagnosis the roent-genogram offers invaluable aid in the recognition of rickets, but there are many pitfalls in differential diagnosis. A description of the changes revealed by the roentgenogram (Figs. 39 and 40) is out of place here and the reader can find them in textbooks of radiology. Since rickets is not primarily a disease of bone, roentgenologic evidence may be lacking early in the course of the disease.

The concentrations of calcium and phosphorus in the serum are usually altered in rickets and determination of these concentrations may clinch the diagnosis. Although the concentration of inorganic phosphate is more con-

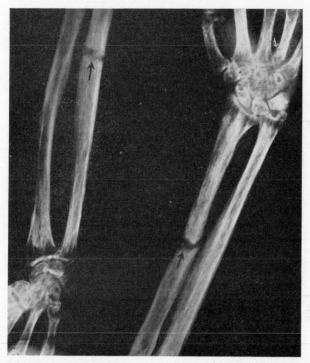

Fig. 40.—Avitaminosis with marked osteoporosis. There is a typical Looser zone in the middle of the shaft of the radius. (By courtesy of the Department of Radiology, The Mayo Clinic.)

stantly lower than that of calcium, the product of the concentration of these two minerals is of more constant value. By the methods used in most laboratories the product of concentrations of calcium and phosphorus is usually in the region of 40 but falls below 30 in the great majority of rachitic infants.

Differential Diagnosis.—This involves a number of conditions, most of which can be readily excluded. *Infantile scurvy* differs in the nature of the dietary deficiency, as noted in the history, the presence of hemorrhagic tendency and muscle tenderness, the roentgenologic changes in the bones and the concentrations of calcium and phosphorus in the serum, which are normal in cases of uncomplicated scurvy. *Congenital syphilis* presents no problem if the serologic reaction is positive. In the absence of a positive serologic reaction, other evidence of syphilis may be found in the patient or the parents. The infant's age may prove of some value in this situation since the symptoms of congenital syphilis are usually well developed by the age of three months. *Chondrodystrophy* usually affects older infants and is distinguished from rickets by the abnormal relationship between the length of the limbs and the body. *Osteogenesis imperfecta* is occasionally confused with rickets and a therapeutic test may be required for diagnosis. In cases of rickets, pathologic fractures heal rapidly with vitamin administration. *Cretinism* should not be confused if one is familiar with the typical characteristics of cretinism, namely, the typical facies, flat nose and large protruding tongue. *Congenital dislocation of the hip* has been mistaken for rickets, but roentgenologic examination will aid in making the diagnosis. In certain cases of *hydrocephalus* it may be necessary to await the results of the administration of vitamin D. *Anterior poliomyelitis* is rarely confused with rickets but may require careful neurologic examination as well as examination of the cerebrospinal fluid and a study of the blood chemistry.

Rachitic Tetany.—In one sense we may regard rickets and rachitic tetany as different manifestations of the same disorder—a derangement in calcium and phosphorus metabolism on the basis of a lack of the antirachitic vitamin. For a proper understanding of the two diseases it is not so important to recognize the obvious difference in the systems attacked by this deranged metabolism as it is to recognize that rachitic tetany is a disorder of calcium metabolism as contrasted with rickets, in which the metabolism of phosphorus or calcium may be altered. The importance of this distinction will be illustrated by the treatment of these conditions.

Two types of infantile tetany are encountered clinically, namely, the latent and manifest forms. In the former there are no apparent symptoms and the hyperirritability of the nervous system must be elicited by artificial excitation of the peripheral nerves. The manifest form gives rise to tonic states and generalized convulsions.

The most reliable and delicate sign in the diagnosis of latent tetany is *Erb's phenomenon.* A galvanic current is employed to distinguish irritability of the nervous system. The *Chvostek sign* is another rather reliable method of diagnosis. The *Trousseau phenomenon* is often described as diagnostic of infantile tetany but this sign probably is not as reliable as the other two mentioned. Among laboratory aids, the presence of low concentration of serum calcium is of extreme importance in the diagnosis of tetany. In latent tetany the value for the serum calcium is usually in the neighborhood of 7 to 8 mg. per 100 cc. and it may fall to 5 to 6 mg. in cases of manifest tetany.

The outstanding manifestations of tetany are the typical carpopedal spasms, the characteristic "tetany facies," laryngospasm, and, of course, the convulsive seizures. The diagnosis of manifest rachitic tetany is, as a rule, not difficult. In the differential diagnosis one must consider laryngitis, congenital laryngeal stridor, nervous holding of the breath, and meningitis.

Osteomalacia.—Although osteomalacia is a rare disease in the United States it is important enough to merit some mention. It is generally agreed that in cases of rickets or osteomalacia the essential abnormality is the same, namely, a deficient calcification of the osteoid tissue. The term "osteomalacia" is often erroneously used to designate the existence of any skeletal disease characterized by "bone softness."

There are usually numerous causative factors operative in any single case of osteomalacia, but in all cases there is a deficiency of vitamin D. In most of the cases of osteomalacia observed in the United States the condition is associated with chronic steatorrhea. As a result of the faulty digestion and absorption of fat, insoluble calcium salts are formed and the fat soluble vitamin D is excreted in the excess fat. This has been well demonstrated by various investigations carried out in cases of osteomalacia. The increased demands of pregnancy and lactation are another important cause of osteomalacia in this country.

The severity of the symptoms of osteomalacia is in direct proportion to the severity of the disease. In the mild form of osteomalacia the patient may complain only of weakness, pains in the bones of the legs or in the lower part of the back while standing or walking. In cases of severe osteomalacia the patient may seek medical aid because of the distressing symptoms of severe tetany. Another patient may suffer from a crushed vertebra resulting from moderate lifting or a minor fall. In cases of advanced disease, severe backache is the most common symptom. This pain is aching in character, often is generalized, and is worse in the winter when there is greater deficiency of vitamin D. Muscular weakness may be marked, and a waddling gait is not uncommon. There is often marked sensitivity of the bones to light pressure. The skeletal deformities are numerous. In the roentgenogram one finds generalized osteoporosis, thinning of the cortices, bowing, fractures, and deformities of various types.

The diagnosis of osteomalacia is not particularly difficult if one suspects its presence. Tetany occurring in association with chronic diarrhea or a calcium-phosphorus deficiency should always suggest osteomalacia. Any skeletal disease, characterized by generalized decalcification, such as the osteoporotic forms of hyperparathyroidism, senile osteoporosis, the osteoporosis of hyperthyroidism, basophilic adenoma of the pituitary body, suprarenal cortical tumor, occasionally multiple myeloma, and disuse atrophy, may be mistaken for osteomalacia. The treatment of osteomalacia is essentially the same as the treatment of rickets.

THE PREVENTION AND TREATMENT OF DEFICIENCY OF VITAMIN D

Prevention.—In the discussion of the etiology of rickets it was noted that age is an important factor and that rickets is primarily a disease of infants from three to eighteen months of age. For this reason it is of great importance that the administration of some form of vitamin D should be instituted at the beginning of the third week and that a full dose be administered by the end of the second month. It is best to begin with a dose of a half a teaspoonful (2 cc.) of cod liver oil (175 units); after a few days this may be increased to one teaspoonful (4 cc.—350 units) and in the next two weeks raised to two teaspoonfuls (8 cc.—700 units). This dose should be continued until the child is two years of age. If there is any reason to suspect that the child may be susceptible to rickets, the dose should be raised during the first year to supply 1000 units of vitamin D daily.

Most infants will take cod liver oil readily but in case difficulty of administration arises one of the concentrated preparations can be used. In such case the daily units of vitamin D should be the same as advised when cod liver oil is administered. Administration of cod liver oil to premature or

14

feeble infants is generally *contraindicated* because of the danger of lipid pneumonia from aspiration of the oil. Children who vomit frequently are particularly subject to such danger.

It seems advisable to continue the administration of antirachitic preparations even during the summer months, although it may be discontinued if the physician is sure that the child receives adequate sunlight. Aside from the question of prevention of deficiency of vitamin D, it must be remembered that the resumption of administration of cod liver oil may prove difficult or actually impossible when summer is over. The various activated milks which are now available form an important source of vitamin D in the infantile diet, but it is unwise to depend entirely on these for the prevention of rickets. Although metabolized and fortified milks are potent enough to prevent rickets in the average case, it is safer to provide a supplement of at least 350 units of vitamin D during the first six months of life. In the case of irradiated milk, the use of the supplement should be continued during the first year. In the second year it is a good precaution to continue supplementing irradiated milk whereas metabolized or fortified milk will probably supply sufficient vitamin D.

The activated milk does not exhibit sufficient potency in vitamin D for the prevention of rickets in cases in which a susceptibility exists. This refers particularly to premature infants and some full-term babies, particularly Negroes. If the irradiated milks are used they must be liberally supplemented and it is probably best to plan the amount of this supplement as though the milk were not activated. Susceptible children may require 5000 to 10,000 units daily. Unfortunately there is no didactic rule by which one can gauge the proper dose, and the unusual susceptibility often manifests itself only when the ordinary dose proves insufficient. The dose of vitamin D should be increased until the desired therapeutic effect is obtained. When large doses are to be given it will be necessary to utilize fish oil concentrates since the necessary quantity of cod liver oil would be too great.

Treatment.—In a case of *rickets* it is of prime importance that healing of the lesion be affected as rapidly as possible. For this reason the doses suggested as a preventive, although capable of effecting cure in a simple case, bring about this cure too slowly. Activated milk contains entirely too little vitamin D to be effective. If cod liver oil is used, 3 teaspoonfuls daily (12 cc.—1000 units) will bring advanced rickets under control within three to four weeks in a great majority of cases. If larger doses of vitamin D are desired it is best to use one of the concentrated preparations. In the case of premature infants it is often necessary to administer 10,000 to 20,000 units daily to effect a cure in a short period of time and in some cases the condition is so refractory as to require doses of 60,000 units daily. Once the disorder has been brought under control, as evidenced by blood calcium and phosphorus determinations, by roentgenologic or simply by clinical examinations, the dose of vitamin D may be reduced to a preventive level. In cases in which older children are hypersusceptible to rickets, it may be necessary to continue the administration of large doses; the increased requirements of the premature infant are usually transitory.

In the treatment of *rachitic tetany* it is important that the effects be produced rapidly. It has been pointed out that the primary derangement in tetany is in the concentration of serum calcium and it is necessary that this be rapidly remedied by the administration of calcium salts. The usual method is to administer 3 or 4 gm. of calcium chloride intravenously as an initial dose. This should be followed by a dose of 1 gm. four times daily for two or three days and then by 1 gm. twice a day for five to seven days. In the administration of vitamin D, a program similar to that described for the treatment of rickets may be followed.

In more recent years *Vitaminstoss* or shock therapy has gained popularity in some of the larger medical centers, particularly in Germany. This consists of the single, intramuscular injection of 500,000 to 600,000 units of vitamin D in a relatively pure solution of its crystalline form. Although this treatment has not gained widespread acceptance it appears to possess several advantages over present methods. Healing occurs more rapidly and, the physician being in direct control of the dose, the hazard of administration is eliminated. This last factor has assumed enough importance to cause Vollmer to devise a procedure for the prevention of rickets by the single injection method. In most cases shock therapy does not cause toxic reactions but in cases in which such reactions have been reported they usually could be assigned to impurities in the material employed. For this reason, any physician contemplating the use of this method should be warned to be sure of the purity of his preparation.

In occasional cases rickets is very refractory to vitamin D therapy. It is well to bear in mind that some of these cases are not cases of true rickets but cases of so-called *endogenous rickets* or *renal hypoparathyroidism.* Those cases of actual rickets in which the condition does not respond are a great problem and there is no satisfactory solution, although many preparations have received clinical trial. It is advisable to bear in mind the possibility of faulty absorption in these cases and not to pronounce a diagnosis of "refractory rickets" before administering the vitamin parenterally or using ultraviolet light.

Ultraviolet Light.—Sunlight may be relied on for the prevention of rickets in the summer months. Infants cannot receive too much ultraviolet light from the sun's rays, with the exception of blond children who burn easily. In the winter, the sun's rays may be regarded as devoid of antirachitic rays for all practical purposes. There is sufficient ultraviolet light in the rays of the summer sun to cure rickets, but this means should be condemned as too uncertain when compared to the administration of cod liver oil.

A few details of practical importance in the exposure of children to sunlight might be mentioned. During warm weather the child should be exposed outdoors. In the winter the exposure must be in the direct rays of the sun with the window open. Positions should be varied to prevent overexposure of the eyes. Large areas of the body may be exposed, a part at a time, without danger. If the sunlight is rich in ultraviolet rays, exposure of only a small part of the body for a short time is sufficient to produce a general antirachitic effect. It should be remembered that sky shine is as valuable as direct shine and is available on cloudy days. The rays of the winter sun in the temperate zone are active only in the noon period and then in very low degree.

The *artificial sources* of ultraviolet light are the quartz mercury vapor lamp and the carbon arc lamp. The former is more likely to cause burns than is the latter but the burns usually are very superficial. However, there is a danger from overirradiation from ultraviolet therapy. The reader is referred to books on physical therapy for description of the method of using these lamps. These forms of antirachitic treatment are particularly valuable for premature babies and for patients who cannot absorb cod liver oil properly. The use of these lamps is contraindicated only for blond persons who burn easily and never tan.

Evaluation and Results of Treatment.—Having made a diagnosis of rickets and having determined which method of treatment to pursue, the physician is now confronted with the problem of how to ascertain if this therapy is accomplishing the desired results. The best way to do this is to determine the concentration of calcium and phosphorus in the serum. If the concentration of calcium is within normal limits and the concentration of inorganic phosphate rises to 5 mg. per 100 cc., vitamin D therapy is succeeding. In ordinary cases in which the usual doses are administered, the concentration of the serum phosphates may be expected to reach normal on about the tenth day. Employing "shock" therapy will hasten this response, which may occur as early as the fifth or sixth day after the beginning of treatment. Roentgenographic evidence of healing may be noted in about three weeks in cases in which smaller doses are employed, whereas they may be expected about the fifth or sixth day in cases in which massive treatment is employed. In the absence of the chemical and roentgenologic examination, appraisal of treatment becomes very difficult; bony deformities disappear very slowly. Perhaps the best clinical indication that vitamin D is succeeding is improvement in muscle function, as evidenced by efforts on the part of the child to walk or sit up. He seems to gain strength and becomes more active. The bony deformities gradually disappear and the bones acquire an increased degree of rigidity.

TOXIC EFFECTS OF VITAMIN D

As observed in the consideration of hypervitaminosis D, pathologic changes were observed in animals only after doses many times the therapeutic dose were administered. No serious toxic effects have been reported in cases in which doses up to 1,000,000 units have been administered to rachitic children. However, physicians interested in this form of therapy should be cautioned to use a pure crystalline preparation of vitamin D, since many preparations have been shown to contain toxic by-products. Adults treated with large doses of vitamin D for arthritis have exhibited various manifestations of toxicity. It seems well established that the rachitic infant has much greater tolerance for vitamin D than the adult has. The symptoms of which adults complain are nausea, headache, diarrhea, loss of appetite, urinary frequency and nocturia and lassitude.

One need not fear toxicity from vitamin ·D unless *renal insufficiency* exists. The best danger signal is an increase in the concentration of serum calcium, and it is best to modify the dose if the concentration is more than 12 mg. per 100 cc. The value for the serum phosphate does not increase so rapidly, and it is thought that metastatic calcification may take place before the concentration increases. Repeated urinalyses should be conducted while vitamin D therapy is being employed. When excessive doses are administered, the concentration of calcium is greatly increased, and calcium casts may appear.

There is no treatment for *hypervitaminosis* D other than discontinuation of administration of the vitamin.

REFERENCES

The vitamins. A symposium arranged under the auspices of the Council on Pharmacy and Chemistry and the Council of Foods of the American Medical Association, Chicago, American Medical Association, 1939, 637 pp.

Park, E. A., The therapy of rickets, J.A.M.A., **115:** 370–379 (Aug. 3) 1940.

Hess, A. S., Rickets, including osteomalacia and tetany, Philadelphia, Lea & Febiger, 1929, 485 pp.

Bills, C. E., Physiology of the sterols, including vitamin D, Physiol. Rev., **15:** 1–97 (Jan.) 1935.

Spies, T. D., and Hanzal, Ramon F., Experimental Production of Hypercalcemia in Human Beings by Means of Irradiated Ergosterol, Proc. Soc. Exper. Biol. and Med., **31:** 747, 1934.

Agduhr, E., Post-natal development under different conditions of nutrition and circumstances of functioning. 1. The changes in the heart through the presence of cod-liver oil (Oleum jecoris Aselli) in the food. Acta Paediat., **5:** 319–410, 1925–1926.

Jundell, I., and Stenström, N.: A study of the electrocardiogram in infants of normal conditions and during treatment with cod liver oil and vigantol. Part I. The normal Ecg. of the child during the first year of life together with observations on the influence of infections on the Ecg. Part II. The appearance of electrocardiogram in infants treated with cod liver oil and Vigantol, with some observations on the influence of vitellus on the electrocardiogram. Acta Paediat., **12:** 113–151, 1931–1932.

THIAMINE DEFICIENCY

BERIBERI

The achievement of the Americans in the Philippines, of the English in India and the Malay States, of the Dutch in the East Indies, and of the Japanese in their own country, has inspired intense study of deficiency diseases throughout the western world. To mention the names of all who participated in the discovery and application of thiamine would be to list some fifty per cent of the mature biochemists of the world of today. It is doubtful if any substance ever isolated by biochemical means has cost so much in labor. The first gram of pure thiamine must have cost considerably more than several hundred thousand dollars. With quantity production now at hand, and with the ever-increasing knowledge of thiamine, a gift arising from a disease in the Orient is bringing relief to persons all over the world. For many it has banished ill health, making it possible for them to return to work; to others it has given rest and freedom from the pain that arises from nutritional neuritis. It has returned to normal persons with anxiety states that have been attended by unreasonable apprehension, fear, and rage.

The vast outlay of maintaining armies and missionaries in the Orient since the time of Columbus has been a heavy drain on the western world. It is regrettable that relatively insignificant expenditures have been devoted to scientific enterprise during this period. Certainly it is fair to say that the West and the East have profited little in the exchange of various infectious diseases with one another, but they have profited much from the benefits derived from the exchange of ideas. Throughout the scientific world, the names of Takaki, Eijkman, Funk, Vedder, Grijns, Williams, Peters, Cline, Westenbrink, Jansen, Seidell, Sinclair, Waterman, and many others are held in reverent esteem.

Thus, we can see that a disease affecting the teeming millions of the Orient incited and maintained the interest of scientists of the Occident until at last thiamine is relieving persons whose diet is deficient in this vitamin not only in the East but also in the western world.

BIOCHEMISTRY AND PHYSIOLOGY

Thiamine functions in a wide variety of micro-organisms, in lower and higher plants, in insects, and in all higher animals. In the higher forms of life it functions in a fundamental rôle in the physiology and chemistry of the cells. Thiamine is a colorless, basic organic compound, composed of a thiazole and a pyrimidine ring. The pyrimidine ring occurs in many physiologic substances, whereas the thiazole ring is rare in nature. The ease with which the connecting valence bond is broken between these two rings affects the stability of the compound. Any alkali cleaves it, and at room temperature sodium sulfite cleaves the bond so that the whole molecule is destroyed. The most widely used chemical test for thiamine depends upon the thiochrome reaction. It involves the use in acid solution of oxidizing agents, such as potassium ferricyanide, hydrogen peroxide and potassium permanganate. The amino group on the pyrimidine ring is oxidized and unites with the carbon in the thiazole ring. The resulting product, termed *thiochrome*, is an unsaturated three-ring structure. It has an intense blue fluorescence which can be measured quantitatively.

Any discussion of the physiology or biochemistry of thiamine must, for purposes of brevity, be limited to a survey of the present knowledge concerning its relationship to the various functions of the body. Although the final answer is not known, the volume of relevant literature thus far accumulated is so enormous as to make a thorough review of it impossible at this time.

Absorption.—Thiamine is readily absorbed from both the small and the large intestine, but individuals vary with respect to the efficiency of absorption. Thiamine is not readily eluted from a fuller's earth absorbate (such as the present international vitamin B_1 standard) in the large intestine. Such a product is therefore less effective than those which contain the vitamin already dissolved in a suitable aqueous medium. Dann and Cowgill found experimentally that diarrhea causes a failure of absorption of an appreciable fraction of the ingested vitamin; it does not cause an excretion of thiamine from the organism through the intestinal wall into the lumen of the intestine.

Storage and Excretion.—The various tissues of experimental animals contain thiamine in greater or lesser amounts, depending upon the thiamine content of the diets to which the animals have been subjected. The muscles, liver, heart, kidney, and brain are rich in thiamine; the blood, spleen, and lungs contain only traces. Westenbrink concluded that the liver and heart lose about four-fifths of their thiamine content during a single week of deficiency and that the loss thereafter proceeds more slowly. The brain is best able to conserve its thiamine supply. In general, the amounts stored decline rapidly at first, then more slowly, the last minimal amount being retained persistently. Of all tissues, the muscle is first and most nearly depleted. In birds and mammals a depletion period is necessary before thiamine deficiency becomes apparent. This is strong evidence of the capacity for temporary storage.

The chemical methods for the estimation of thiamine do not lend themselves to routine assays. In the case of the most widely used method thiamine is oxidized to thiochrome. The quantity of thiochrome is determined fluorophotometrically. The removal of interfering substances is tedious. The procedure involving the estimation of the reaction product between thiamine and alkaline diazotized para-aminoacetophenone is subject to the same limitations.

The fermentation method is comparatively simple. The method estimates the stimulating effect of thiamine on the rate of alcoholic fermentation. The response is quantitative only between narrow limits of concentration, and a correction must be made for pyrimidines. The method has been employed recently in clinical studies by Pollack and co-workers. Using this method, Emerson, Brownell and Spies found that a patient with manifest symptoms of several vitamin deficiencies who received supplements of nicotinic acid and riboflavin, excreted no measurable amount of thiamine in the urine. Following the daily administration of 50 mg. of thiamine hydrochloride, only 3 to 4 per cent was excreted daily during the first week of therapy.

Fecal excretion of thiamine is small and substantially constant over the usual range of intakes. The feces contain unabsorbed thiamine. Synthesis of thiamine by the intestinal flora does not take place in human beings. Thiamine is excreted mainly by the kidneys. The proportion that is excreted or destroyed by metabolic processes is not established, but changes in the intake are promptly reflected by the urinary output. It is clear that during periods of plentiful supply, the body stores thiamine; the excess is largely excreted. This limited capacity for storage requires that an adequate intake of thiamine be maintained.

Thiamine and Metabolism.—An increase in the total body metabolism raises the requirement for thiamine. The precise chemical processes in which the vitamin participates are not clearly understood, but it is known that thiamine is intimately concerned in intermediary carbohydrate metabolism and in biologic oxidative reactions.

One function has been fairly well established. Thiamine in its biologically active form, the pyrophosphate, is a coenzyme which, in combination with a specific protein, acts as a catalyst in the removal of pyruvic acid derived from lactic acid in normal carbohydrate metabolism. A secondary consequence of this removal is the dissipation of lactic acid, the dehydrogenation of which is inhibited by excess pyruvate. This phenomenon is accompanied by an increase in carbon dioxide and often by an increased oxygen uptake. The relative predominance of the two varies from one tissue to another.

In beriberi there is an accumulation of bisulfite-binding substances (chiefly pyruvic acid) in the blood, urine, and cerebrospinal fluid. Although a return to normal respiration and blood pyruvate concentration can be induced by thiamine or thiamine pyrophosphate, many investigators do not believe that the amount of bisulfite-binding substances in the blood is a specific test for thiamine deficiency. They point out that a similar increase occurs in other conditions, such as diabetes mellitus, in certain infectious diseases, and in severe congestive failure caused by organic heart disease. They state that any compound containing a carbonyl radical will give this reaction. There is much evidence to indicate that an accumulation of blood pyruvates does not cause the symptoms of beriberi.

It is conceded that thiamine pyrophosphate serves in the disposal of pyruvic acid, but the method of disposal is subject to much disagreement. Peters and his associates favor the pyruvate oxidase theory; Lohman believes that it acts as a cocarboxylase; others regard it as a coenzyme for a dehydrogenase-carboxylase; and it has been suggested that by its action pyruvic acid is used in the synthesis of fat.

Peters and his associates look upon the process as an oxidation of pyruvic acid with the formation of acetic acid and carbon dioxide, and it is a fact that a large increase in oxygen uptake accompanies the removal of pyruvic acid from the brain and other tissues. In 1937 Lohman and Schuster isolated from yeast a pyrophosphoric ester of thiamine which appears to act as part of a decarboxylating enzyme system. They attribute to it the power to dispose of pyruvic acid by a simple decarboxylation with the formation of acetaldehyde and carbon dioxide. They state that cocarboxylase is synthesized from free thiamine by brain tissues. A combined oxidative and decarboxylating effect is favored by Lipman, who believes that thiamine pyrophosphate functions as a coenzyme for a certain pyruvic acid dehydrogenase. He concludes that there is simultaneous loosening of hydrogen atoms as decarboxylation occurs in a single reaction:

$$CH_3COCOOH \longrightarrow CH_3COOH + CO_2$$

Cocarboxylase, when used to refer to thiamine pyrophosphate, is objectionable in that it emphasizes only one aspect of its physiologic activity.

A fourth rôle of thiamine has been suggested. McHenry has proposed the hypothesis that fat is synthesized in the presence of thiamine, utilizing pyruvic acid as the intermediate. This hypothesis offers a concrete idea of the mechanism of the thiamine-sparing action of fat. Minz has reported an entirely different function of thiamine. He concludes that thiamine intensifies the action of acetylcholine, and that phosphorylated thiamine acts as a coferment with acetylcholine in the humoral stimulation of the nervous system. Birch and Mapson state that thiamine causes the deaminization of adenine nucleotides.

All tissue respiration experiments, by virtue of their complicated nature, necessitate a great deal of interpretation by inference. We are compelled, by a consideration of the enzyme studies carried out to date, to suppose that thiamine has many functions as a coenzyme in nature. The best established ones are the two known reactions of its pyrophosphate which, in association with a protein of yeast, can bring about a pure decarboxylation of pyruvic acid, or, in association with other proteins, can act to promote a simultaneous dehydrogenation and decarboxylation of pyruvic acid to form acetic acid and carbon dioxide. The other functions mentioned are less thoroughly established. Some of these reactions may predominate in one tissue; others, in another tissue. It is not unreasonable to suppose that thiamine, in the form of its pyrophosphoric ester, acts as a coenzyme for several enzymic systems. The outstanding fact is that the metabolic processes concerned take place not in the individual organ as a whole or in specialized tissues, but in the cells themselves.

Thiamine and the Nervous System.—The exact rôle of thiamine in the nervous system is not known. It is known, however, that brain tissue depends predominantly upon combustion of carbohydrate. Himwich, Spies, Fazekas and Nesin found an average glucose utilization of 14.6 mg. per 100 cc. in normal persons; in contrast, pellagrins who also had beriberi had an average value of 6.4 mg. per 100 cc. and a subnormal oxygen utilization. The diminished cerebral metabolism offers an explanation for the mental changes observed in persons with thiamine deficiency.

Thiamine and the Heart.—Aalsmeer and Wenckebach stress that the cardiac enlargement of beriberi is due essentially to edema of the muscle tissue. Certainly the change is not a hypertrophy, because the administration of thiamine causes the edema to disappear rapidly. Hastings found that the auricle is more sensitive to thiamine shortage than the ventricle and therefore loses tone and becomes distended. It is difficult to state what part the peripheral dilation and increased capillary pressure may play in leading to right-sided dilatation of the heart. Weiss has reported that peripheral arteriolar dilation may predispose to circulatory shock and the formation of edema. Keefer emphasizes the fact that muscular exercise plays a tremendous rôle in the course of the disease: If the patient is not disabled by polyneuritis and is able to do muscular work, cardiac insufficiency tends to result; if painful polyneuritis prohibits muscular activity, the myocardium is protected and cardiac failure does not occur. The heart lesions and edema have not been produced experimentally as a result of increased blood pyruvate concentration. It is known that the carbohydrate metabolism of the heart tissues is affected by thiamine deprivation, but this does not explain the predominance of right-sided failure. Although thiamine deficiency may result in left-sided enlargement or enlargement of the entire heart, the prevalent opinion concerning Oriental beriberi is that the picture is chiefly one of right-sided enlargement. Further work is necessary to prove the mechanism and the chemical changes through which this is brought about.

Thiamine and the Gastro-intestinal Tract.—It is well known that animals and human beings with thiamine deficiency have symptoms arising from the gastro-intestinal tract. Loss of appetite has long been regarded as a prominent feature of this deficiency state, yet no specific cellular changes have been demonstrated to account for any of these symptoms. Our unpublished observations indicate that the symptoms of so-called "indigestion" and severe constipation in malnourished persons are frequently relieved by the administration of crystalline thiamine. Cowgill and his associates, and Fitts, have reported anorexia associated with gastric atony, spastic colon and hypochlorhydria in thiamine-deficient persons. It should be emphasized that thiamine plays a most important rôle in all the cells of the body and that alterations in the cells ultimately produce symptoms which disappear following therapy.

PATHOLOGY

Pertinent information with regard to the underlying pathologic changes of thiamine deficiency in human beings is more restricted than one would expect after many years of study. The ordinary methods of studying such changes have shown little concerning mild thiamine deficiency, yet one must assume that the minute biochemical changes have already occurred in the cells even though the crude methods of staining and microscopic examination do not detect them. The discussion which follows will deal with the findings of advanced thiamine deficiency, primarily with the accepted post-mortem studies of typical cases of Oriental beriberi. These findings vary tremendously from patient to patient; for convenience, they will be discussed under three major headings.

The Nervous System.—The most constant and striking findings of thiamine deficiency arise from chemical alterations which lead ultimately to degenerative changes in the nervous system. Many pathologists have reported congestion and edema of the brain and spinal cord in beriberi, but reports of microscopic studies of the central nervous system are relatively rare. Changes in the posterior spinal ganglion and anterior horn cells, as well as in the ganglion cells of the medulla and pons, have been noted. These cells may show chromatolysis and sometimes swollen and dislocated nuclei. These changes, in most instances, do not mean death of the cell, but indicate severe involvement. Degeneration of the medullary sheaths has been demonstrated in scattered fibers in all tracts of the cord, but especially in the posterior columns.

The pathological changes in the peripheral nerves resulting from protracted deficiency of thiamine are indistinguishable, whether the person had uncomplicated beriberi or thiamine deficiency associated with conditions such as chronic alcoholic addiction, Korsakoff's syndrome, pellagra, sprue, pernicious anemia, pregnancy, diabetes, tuberculosis, colitis, senility, malignancy, or cirrhosis of the liver. Hence, the authors regard the polyneuritis arising from a deficiency of thiamine as beriberi, irrespective of any other condition present.

Degeneration is most severe in the sciatic nerve and its branches, but degenerative changes may be found in any of the peripheral nerves. Characteristically, the distal portions of the nerves are first and most seriously affected. In the average case, early degeneration occurs in the brachial nerves at about the same time that late changes appear in the sciatic nerves. Changes often may be found in the phrenic, the recurrent laryngeal, and the cranial nerves, particularly the vagi. Degenerative changes of the branches of the cardiac plexus, the splanchnic nerves, and branches of the solar and renal plexuses have been described.

Degeneration of the myelin sheath is constant and affects the majority of the fibers. Observations from the Nutrition Clinic of the Hillman Hospital, Birmingham, Alabama, show that counts done on biopsies of terminal portions of the anterior tibial nerves of patients with thiamine deficiency show fewer myelin sheaths in a given area than are normally present. It has been stated that the axis cylinders may show fragmentation and atrophy, but except in more chronic and advanced beriberi, the majority of the axis cylinders appear normal. In the cases studied at the Nutrition Clinic, the axis cylinders were involved in the degenerative process usually in the same severity as the myelin sheaths (see Figs. 41 and 42).

The Heart.—In acute beriberi the heart is dilated and enlarged. Ellis found that the average weight of the hearts in 125 necropsies of beriberi was 379 gm. while the average weight of the hearts of 204 patients dying of other diseases was 255 gm. Japanese investigators also reported that the average weight of the hearts of patients with beriberi is above the maximum weight of the normal heart. In Oriental beriberi the enlargement is most pronounced in the right heart where the muscle is coarse and firm and the trabeculae and papillary muscles are especially prominent. The right auricle

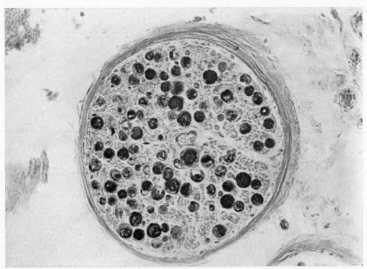

Fig. 41.—Cross section of the terminal portion of the internal branch of the anterior tibial nerve in neuritis due to thiamine deficiency, stained with osmic acid (× 350). The myelin sheath count in this nerve is 2674/sq. mm. There are many large sheaths whose centers are filled with black-stained material. (This may represent swelling in a degenerating nerve.)

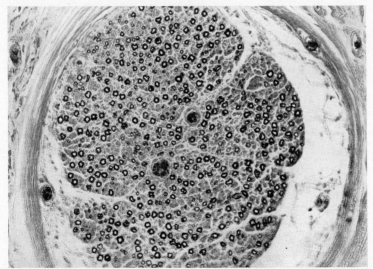

Fig. 42.—Cross section of a normal nerve (terminal portion of the internal branch of the anterior tibial nerve), stained with osmic acid (× 350). The myelin sheath count in this nerve is 6836/sq. mm. (normal 5000 to 10,000/sq. mm.). The myelin sheaths stain black with clear centers and are uniform in size.

may be huge, with a "paper-thin" wall, through which dark blood is visible. The valves are normal. Some cases with sudden circulatory collapse and death show hydropic degeneration of the cardiac musculature and pronounced edema (see Figs. 43 and 44).

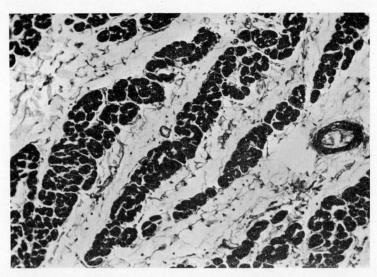

Fig. 43.–Microphotograph of a section taken from the heart of a patient with the clinical picture of wet beriberi. The interstitial spaces are widened by edema and a moderate increase of collagenous tissue. The muscle bundles are swollen and show vacuolization (× 175).

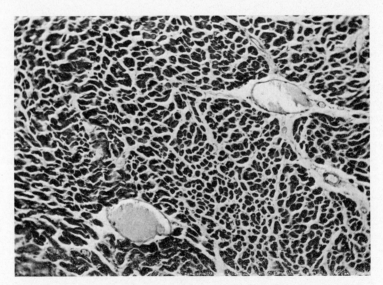

Fig. 44.–Microphotograph of a section of normal heart muscle (× 175).

Weiss and Wilkins have reported that persons with thiamine deficiency in the United States may have small hearts, less right- than left-sided failure, or left-sided failure alone. Since these findings differ strikingly from the classical picture of Oriental beriberi, could it not be that cases with small hearts also exist frequently in the Orient?

Edema and Serous Effusions.—Edema and serous effusions are common in adults or in infants with acute beriberi. The edema may be confined to the legs and thighs, or it may be generalized, but the tissues of the face are rarely involved. Following postmortem incision, large amounts of serous fluid pour from the subcutaneous tissue. This edema is frequently associated with serous effusions which occur most often in the following sequence: hydrops of the pericardium, pulmonary edema, hydrothorax and ascites. The fluid is clear and greenish-yellow in color and often occurs in quantities of 50 to 500 cc. in the pericardium and 50 to 2000 cc. in the pleural spaces. Ascites is seldom severe.

Other Pathological Observations.—There is a loss of the subcutaneous, retroperitoneal and epicardial fat in persons having chronic beriberi. The muscles supplied by the diseased nerves, particularly those of the leg and thigh, are atrophied. Histological studies show loss of cross striation and shrinkage of the sarcoplasm, often associated with cloudy swelling or fatty degeneration. Chronic passive congestion of the liver, spleen, kidneys, and intestines is usually present. Punctate hemorrhages are often found subpleurally and in the walls of the stomach and intestines.

Infantile Beriberi.—McLaughlin and Andrews have described postmortem findings in infantile beriberi similar to those found in adults dying of "acute cardiac beriberi." In their cases, the body appeared plump and well nourished; the skin was usually pale and anemic; and the flesh of the thighs and legs was often soft and flabby and, as a rule, pitted on pressure. The subcutaneous fat was grayish-white and moist; the edema tended to mask the actual loss of fat and the muscle atrophy. The changes in the heart were the same as those described in the adult. The hearts of the infants who died of beriberi had an average weight of 34.1 gm., while those of infants of comparable ages, who died of other conditions, weighed 20 gm. The lungs, abdominal organs, brain, and other tissues were congested and edematous, and frequently showed petechial hemorrhages. The central and peripheral nervous systems in infants are less severely affected by thiamine deficiency than are those of adults. Although much has been learned from animal experimentation concerning the etiology of beriberi, the pathology of human beriberi must not be confused with that of birds and animals. The histopathologic findings, however, are similar in experimental and human beriberi, and in both, the functional disturbances precede any anatomical changes.

SYMPTOMATOLOGY

Beriberi is characterized by multiple neuritis, often associated with congestive failure, generalized edema and serous effusions, and sudden death. Because these manifestations vary greatly in type, number, severity, and order of appearance, beriberi in the adult has been classified in three clinical types: 1. *Dry beriberi*, when degeneration of the nervous system, chiefly a multiple peripheral neuritis, is the chief manifestation. 2. *Wet beriberi*, when serous effusions and edema are the outstanding features. 3. *Fulminating*, acute or pernicious beriberi, when acute cardiovascular symptoms predominate. A combination of two or more of these types is often referred to as *mixed* beriberi.

Study of many persons developing beriberi shows that they have a long prodromal period of ill health. Observations by Spies, Bradley, Rosenbaum and Knott show that some impairment of intellectual and cognitive functions, exemplified by difficulties in concentration, attention and comprehension, and probably slight memory defects, may occur before any evidence of peripheral neuritis. These changes are usually accompanied by emotional disturbances, such as fear, apprehension, irritability, anger, hostility, depression, extreme sensitivity, and general emotional instability. Because these symptoms are relieved by the administration of thiamine, it seems evident that they constitute an important feature of thiamine deficiency disease.

Loss of weight, strength, and appetite precede diagnostic evidence of neuritis. For weeks or years the patient may complain of fatigue, of sensations of heaviness and a stiffness of the legs, and of inability to walk long distances. Other ill-defined disturbances, such as headache, insomnia, vertigo, dyspnea, dyspepsia, tachycardia, burning sensations in various parts of the body, and cramping and tenderness of the muscles, particularly in the lower extremities, may be present. If subclinical beriberi is not treated appropriately, eventually the full clinical syndrome will develop.

Nervous System.—The symptoms arising from involvement of the nervous system are predominantly those of an ascending symmetrical, peripheral neuritis, of which the initial symptoms are pain, weakness and cramps in the legs. Heaviness of the legs and tenderness to pressure of the calf muscles are noted. Weakness is often followed by burning and numbness of the ankles and feet, and impairment of dorsiflexion of the toes. The Achilles and patellar reflexes may be increased, later diminished, and finally absent. The weakness spreads upward, involving first the extensors and flexors of the leg; at this time toe and foot drop may be demonstrated. The muscles of the arms may be affected similarly, but motor symptoms do not usually appear in the muscles of the upper extremities until the symptoms of the lower extremities have become severe. The upper extremities, however, may be affected first, particularly in individuals who use their hands a great deal more than their legs.

Sensory disturbances may appear first and may be more prominent than the motor changes. Loss of sensation is greatest in the distal parts but there may be no sharp distinction between the areas containing normal and diminished sensation. Appreciation of vibration is diminished or lost. Hyperesthesia spreads over the lower extremities in a sock-like distribution, with anesthesia following in its wake.

Beriberi strikingly affects the vagi, and occasionally other cranial nerves. Phrenic or recurrent laryngeal nerve involvement may occur. In severe cases, the musculature of the trunk and abdomen is affected. In most instances, the sphincter muscles are not involved until the late stages of the disease. When muscular degeneration is severe, the gait usually becomes altered; there may be ataxia and incoordination. Contractures are common when paralysis is long standing. The patient may become bedridden, suffer pain from the pressure of the bedding, and tend to develop decubitus ulcers.

Cardiorespiratory System.—The cardiac type of adult beriberi is relatively infrequent in the western world. The manifestations most commonly seen are dyspnea and palpitation on exertion, tachycardia, and edema. In the case uncomplicated by failure, the arterial blood pressure is usually normal or low, often with an increased pulse pressure. On palpation of the larger arteries, a bounding quality is noted and "pistol shots" may be heard on auscultation. The venous pressure is generally increased but may be normal. Electrocardiographic changes, chiefly of the T wave and QT interval, have been reported. The skin is usually warm and of normal color. At any time during the course of the disease, more severe cardiac symptoms may develop. Without previous warning to the physician, acute cardiac failure may occur abruptly, with paroxysmal onset of dyspnea, cyanosis, increased venous pressure, tachycardia, precordial pain, and a small thready pulse. The heart generally shows striking enlargement, associated with pulmonary congestion. The speed of circulation is increased in the cardiovascular type of beriberi, whereas in other congestive failure, except that due to hyperthyroidism, there is usually a conspicuous slowing of the circulation.

Edema and Serous Effusions.—Edema, the most outstanding feature of "wet" beriberi, begins in the feet and legs, and may be mild or extreme. It frequently conceals the underlying muscular atrophy. Hydropericardium, hydrothorax, and ascites are frequently associated with a generalized edema. Edema of the lungs occurs in at least 50 per cent of the acute cases.

Observations on the children of several hundred families having pellagra, beriberi or riboflavin deficiency show that many develop early clinical signs of thiamine deficiency. The early symptoms are similar to those of pellagra, but these children, if untreated, eventually develop other evidence of beriberi.

Infantile Beriberi.—Three clinical forms of infantile beriberi have been described—the aphonic, the pseudomeningitic and the cardiac. The cardiac type is the most common and occurs most frequently during the first three months of life, although cases of 4, 5, 6 and even 10 months of age have been noted. It affects chiefly breast fed infants whose mothers have latent or manifest thiamine deficiency.

The onset of symptoms is insidious. The infant is nearly always plump, apparently well-nourished, good-natured and playful. The face is full, sometimes presenting a swollen appearance. Frequently edema of the lower extremities may be demonstrated. Somewhat later there is cyanosis, slight dyspnea, periodic restlessness and moaning, disturbed sleep, and occasional vomiting. There may be a slight cough and a peculiar shrill whining cry. Aphonia may be present for several weeks or it may occur only later in the disease. Constipation is the rule; diarrhea may occur, but in some cases the bowels are normal. Oliguria is a late symptom. The temperature tends to be subnormal. The skin is pale, soft and velvety. The pulse is normal or slightly increased in rate, irregular and of fair volume. The heart is grossly enlarged. The second pulmonic sound is accentuated. The apex beat may be clear or muffled. Later in the course of the disease, acute attacks of dyspnea appear. Eventually, if untreated, the infant dies of cardiac failure.

DIAGNOSIS

The physician must bear in mind that thiamine deficiency occurs particularly among the following groups:

1. The indigent and persons who have faulty dietary habits and idiosyncrasies. Such persons usually subsist on a diet abundant in overmilled rice, wheat, or corn. Their diets are high in carbohydrates and relatively low in protein, minerals and vitamins.

2. Patients who have organic diseases or other conditions which may affect their appetites or the assimilation and utilization of the essential food substances. Beriberi is associated particularly with functional and organic gastro-intestinal diseases, chronic debilitating diseases, pernicious vomiting of pregnancy, chronic alcoholic addiction, diabetes and pellagra.

3. Persons in whom the thiamine requirement is distinctly above the average because of rapid growth, the increased metabolic demands of pregnancy and lactation, febrile diseases, hyperthyroidism, or hard physical exertion.

The following procedures suggested by Vedder often aid in the diagnosis of mild cases of thiamine deficiency: Squeeze the muscles of the calf to detect *muscular hyperesthesia;* test the anterior surface of the leg with a pin for *anesthesia;* test the *ankle jerk* (any modification is to be suspected); have the patient perform the *squatting test,* squatting upon his heels in the Oriental manner of sitting (in the patient with beriberi this may cause pain and he may be unable to rise except by using his hands).

There is no satisfactory diagnostic test for thiamine deficiency suitable for the clinical laboratory or for the doctor in general practice, but the response to an adequately controlled therapeutic test is pathognomonic of thiamine deficiency. The patient should be given 50 milligrams of thiamine hydrochloride in physiological saline intravenously for several days. In making a diagnosis of uncomplicated beriberi, other causes of peripheral neuritis, organic heart disease and nephritis must be excluded. It is well to keep in mind, however, that beriberi may occur along with other organic diseases.

COURSE AND PROGNOSIS

Beriberi in the adult, whether endemic or associated with other diseases, is generally insidious in onset and chronic in course, except in cases of acute cardiac beriberi. Since most patients suffer from a partial deficiency of the vitamin, they may continue for long periods without further progression of their disease. Acute attacks may be precipitated by infections or excessive physical activity.

A favorable course depends upon an early diagnosis and intensive and persistent therapy. In acute beriberi of infants or adults, recovery is nearly always prompt and complete if proper treatment is given; chronic beriberi responds less rapidly and completely.

TREATMENT WITH THIAMINE

Chemical Description.—Thiamine is a white crystalline compound which is prepared synthetically as the hydrochloride. It is a combination of a pyrimidine and a thiazole ring (see Figs. 45 and 46). Because it contains sulfur, it is unique among the vitamins. The properties of the natural and the synthetic compounds are identical. The hydrochloride melts at 248–250° C. and is extremely soluble in water. It is stable at 100° C. in acid solution but is destroyed at 100° C. in neutral or alkaline solution.

Method of Administration.—Oral administration is the procedure of choice for the average ambulatory patient, although its effect is slower and much less certain. For the severely ill person with neuritis, edema or cardiovascular involvement, the use of the parenteral route is imperative. This method is also indicated in persons with intrinsic disease of the gastro-intestinal tract or in those recovering from major abdominal operations. Excretion is very rapid following parenteral administration, making frequent injections necessary to maintain a high blood thiamine concentration. The authors prefer the intravenous to the intramuscular route, since the devitalized tissues of persons with nutritional deficiency diseases are prone to infection and

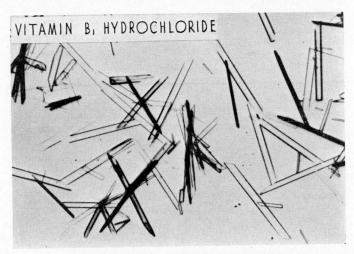

Fig. 45.—Microphotograph showing the structure of thiamine chloride hydrochloride crystals. (Courtesy of Merck and Company.)

abscess formation following repeated intramuscular injections. Thiamine, dissolved in physiological salt solution or in 5 per cent glucose in physiological saline, may be given by slow infusion. Since this vitamin is heat-labile, it cannot be autoclaved for sterilization.

In adults, mild thiamine deficiency may be treated by the oral administration of 10 mg. t.i.d.; for more severe cases, 25 mg. b.i.d. should be given

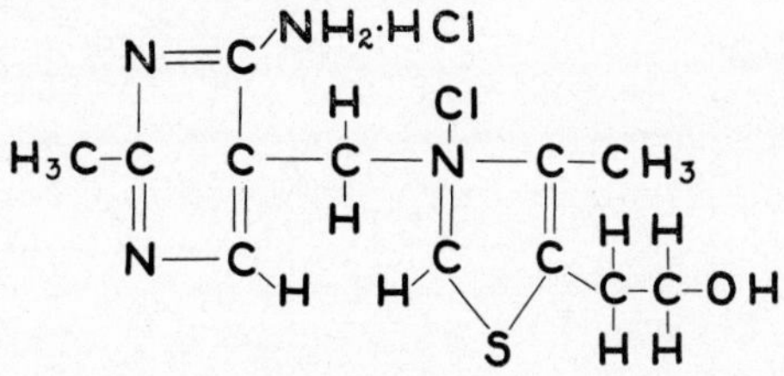

Fig. 46.—Thiamine chloride hydrochloride.

parenterally. Mild cases in children respond to 5 mg. orally; for severely ill infants and children, the intravenous administration of 10 mg. b.i.d. is recommended. Thiamine administered to the nursing mother will increase the amount contained in the milk, and thus the breast-fed infant will benefit indirectly.

No toxic symptoms in man follow the ingestion of 25,000 times the maintenance dose of thiamine, and no untoward results complicate the intravenous therapy of deficient persons with massive doses of the vitamin (500 mg.).

Response to Thiamine.—The parenteral administration of 50 mg. of thiamine to persons with thiamine deficiency is followed by rapid improvement of the initial nervous syndrome of thiamine deficiency; relief of pain and paresthesia due to peripheral neuritis, within twenty-four hours; disappearance of cardiac signs and symptoms, within twenty-four to thirty-six hours; and decrease or loss of edema, within twenty-four to forty-eight hours. Spies, Knott and Hamilton, in some carefully selected cases with thiamine deficiency, observed a striking change in the electroencephalogram soon after the intravenous administration of 50 mg. thiamine hydrochloride. Motor weakness and other manifestations of neuritis improve less dramatically, and two or three months of continuous thiamine administration may be required before any motor power returns. A person with thiamine deficiency should be treated with the idea of improving his general nutritive state, as described under Treatment of Dietary Deficiency Diseases (p. 490).

NICOTINIC ACID AMIDE DEFICIENCY: PELLAGRA

Millions of persons have died from the lack of nicotinic acid while bottles containing it have gathered dust on the shelves of chemical laboratories and warehouses. But how could Huber, the German chemist who first derived it from nicotine in 1867, understand that this laboratory product was a vitamin essential to life? Seventy years were to pass before it was shown to be a specific therapeutic agent in the relief of canine blacktongue and pellagra in human beings. These observations gave a focal point for more vigorous investigation in the fields of biology, chemistry, physiology, pharmacology, and medicine. The rapid advances are astounding, and often an article on vitamins becomes obsolete between the day of writing and the day of printing. Accordingly, it seems wise to limit this discussion to that which is fully accepted and to accentuate the underlying principles concerned, with special emphasis on practical application to the health and vigor of human beings.

Many studies indicate that nicotinic acid or its amide is an essential factor in promoting certain physiological processes in a great variety of living organisms. Since the authors are concerned chiefly with the early symptoms that arise in human beings from a deficiency of this material in their diet, let us consider the clinical findings after a discussion of the underlying physiology and chemistry.

PATHOLOGICAL PHYSIOLOGY

The antiquity of pellagra is a subject of considerable dispute, but any theory which attempts to explain the pathogenesis of this disease must harmonize some apparently contradictory facts and explain the complicated interrelationship of symptoms. Perhaps no single factor has so retarded the comprehension of this syndrome as the overemphasis placed upon the skin lesions. To the naked eye, the resulting changes appear to be only skin deep (see Fig. 47). It is now agreed that pellagra is a systemic or general disease, affecting all the cells of the body. We must look to a disturbance in the cells and the fluids of the body for an understanding of the symptoms arising from a deficiency of nicotinic acid. This will be more fully dis-

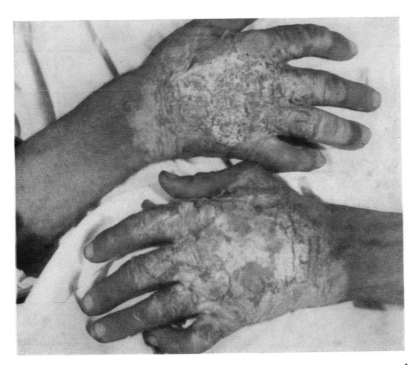

Fig. 47.–Moist type of pellagrous dermatitis. Note the bilateral symmetry of the lesions; the sharp line of demarcation from the normal tissue; and the striking swelling of the tissues of the wrist, dorsum of the hands, and fingers. The centers of the lesions are beginning to desquamate, revealing underneath a highly vascular, reddish, new growth of skin. Note the extensive ulcerated edges, particularly over the dorsum of the hands.

cussed in considering the relationship between coenzymes and nicotinic acid amide deficiency.

Relationship Between Coenzymes I and II and Nicotinic Acid Amide Deficiency Disease.—The spectacular clinical improvement following the administration of nicotinic acid or nicotinic acid amide to pellagrins has led to increased interest in the respiratory coenzymes I and II, cozymase and coferment, respectively, which are known to contain nicotinic acid amide. By definition these coenzymes are relatively heat-stable, dialyzable organic catalysts which retain activity even when separated from the living cell. They are necessary for the function of specific protein enzymes. Each is produced by living cells from a combination of nicotinic acid amide, ribose, adenylic acid, and phosphoric acid. The present knowledge of the chemical constitution of coenzymes I and II indicates that they are similar in that both are pyridine nucleotides, differing only in their content of phosphoric acid. The authors consider that the formation of enzymes governing respiration and growth of cells involves the synthesis of complex substances from simple compounds.

The methods for studying these enzymes are not satisfactory for the practicing physician, but nevertheless they offer important information concerning certain aspects of the pathogenesis of pellagra and other diseases. The concentration of coenzymes I and II in the whole blood of persons with deficiency diseases is lower than in normal persons on optimal diets. Low values for the coenzyme concentration of whole blood may be observed also in persons with diabetes mellitus, roentgen sickness, leukemia, and pneumococcal pneumonia. Infections, fever, and excessive physical exercise tend to lower the concentration in the blood, whereas the rest in bed and increased intake of nicotinic acid or related pyridine compounds tend to increase the concentration.

The coenzyme I content of the erythrocyte does not decrease as much in human pellagra as does the content of striated muscle. The very ill pellagrin may have only 60 per cent of the normal concentration of coenzyme I in his muscles. This offers a marvelous explanation of the long lingering weakness which characterizes the period of development of dietary deficiency. Spies, von Euler, Vilter, Bean and Schlenk, in unpublished observations, have shown that the intravenous injection of from 10 to 50 mg. of coenzyme I of the highest activity is followed by dramatic clinical improvement in acute pellagrous manifestations. This amount when distributed throughout the body is not detectable by our highly sensitive laboratory methods.

These observations lead to an *hypothesis* which may be stated as follows: When the available nicotinic acid amide or compounds with similar functions is not adequate to supply the needs of the body for reasons of decreased supply, inadequate assimilation, increased demand, or increased loss, a disorder in respiratory enzyme systems occurs. As a result a state of generalized reduction in normal cellular respiration supervenes. When this biochemical lesion is severe enough, or has existed long enough, it is translated into functional disturbances in various organ systems of the body. Vasomotor instability in the skin, functional disorders of the alimentary canal, the nervous system, and the circulatory system may occur. It is probable that the most readily affected systems are those weakened by hereditary predisposition or trauma in the wear and tear of everyday life. This may explain the infinite variety of the clinical picture. Finally, severe or persisting alterations in physiology lead to structural changes in various tissues which ultimately present the diagnostic lesions of pellagra.

That such an hypothesis is not established is indicated by the fact that pyrazine monocarboxylic acid and the diethyl amide of nicotinic acid (coramine) may relieve the symptoms of pellagra without any observable changes in the coenzyme factors so far studied. It may be that there are many respiratory ferments not yet known and some of these may explain apparent gaps in the chain of evidence pointing to a disorder of the pyridine coenzyme system as the basis of the pathogenesis of pellagra.

Pigment Metabolism.—It was recognized at an early date (1909–10) that an increased excretion of indican and certain porphyrins was frequently found in pellagra. Myers and Fine (1913) observed that indicanuria was most pronounced in the presence of a low gastric hydrochloric acid. Hunter (1916) observed that the previous diet was important in determining the fate of additional ingested tryptophane, and reported the finding of urorosein in the urine of pellagrins.

In a study of porphyrin excretion in alcoholic pellagrins, Beckh, Ellinger and Spies described a simple *colorimetric method* for detecting small quantities of abnormal pigments in the urine.* The procedure is as follows:

"A measured amount of urine (3–10 cc.) is acidified with glacial acetic acid to a pH of about 4.0 and shaken with 5–20 cc. of ether until no more red pigments can be extracted. The ether is then washed repeatedly with water. A complete separation of the two layers is allowed to take place. To a measured fraction of the ether is added one-fifth of that amount of 25 per cent hydrochloric acid. On shaking, the pigments contained in the ether fraction are completely transferred to the hydrochloric acid which becomes stained purple or pink, the intensity of the color depending on the pigment concentration. The colorimetric estimation is made either in a colorimeter of the Dubosq type against a standard solution of porphyrin, or by comparison with porphyrin solutions of known concentration. The time necessary for the complete transfer of the porphyrins from the urine into the ether and from the ether into hydrochloric acid differs in various specimens, being determined by the nature of the substance present. In most specimens, the process is completed in half an hour, but as a check the colorimetric estimations may be repeated after three hours and after twenty-four hours."

These authors believed the purple color was an indication of the presence of porphyrin, and that the intensity of the color was a roughly quantitative estimate of the amount present.

Soon after the use of nicotinic acid as a specific therapeutic agent for human pellagra, it was found that following such therapy the B.E.S. test, formerly positive, became negative. Studies revealed a positive B.E.S. test in a variety of abnormal conditions other than pellagra. It was observed that the test usually changed from positive to negative after nicotinic acid had been given in these conditions also. Spies and Bean have shown that large doses of roentgen ray over the upper abdomen are followed in many instances by excretion of urine giving a positive B.E.S. test. Recently, they

* Hereafter this test will be referred to as the B.E.S. test.

have shown that persons on a deficient diet are much more severely affected by x-ray exposure and become clinically ill on doses which do not disturb controls on a normal diet. Studies by Watson and Dobriner indicated that the B.E.S. test was not specific for porphyrin, since it also was positive in the presence of other urinary pigments, particularly urorosein.

The B.E.S. test is of value in appraising the nutritional status of an individual, particularly when he is suffering from certain chronic diseases before diagnostic signs of secondary deficiency diseases appear. Because of the positive B.E.S. test in many patients with pellagra, Bean and Spies investigated the urinary pigments in a variety of abnormal conditions which might be followed by faulty nutrition. Positive tests were noted in the urine from patients with the conditions outlined in Table 1

TABLE 1

CLINICAL CONDITIONS WITHOUT DIAGNOSTIC LESIONS OF PELLAGRA
IN WHICH POSITIVE B.E.S. TESTS HAVE BEEN FOUND

1. *Infections:* Tuberculosis, pyelonephritis, subacute bacterial endocarditis, bronchiectasis, chronic gonococcal pelvic diseases, gonococcal arthritis, liver abscesses, staphylococcal septicemia, chronic arthritis.
2. *Mechanical intestinal tract obstruction:* Carcinoma of the stomach, rectum, colon, and uterus (with rectal stricture); Hodgkin's disease with esophageal obstruction; rectal fistula; rectal stricture; obstruction from adhesions.
3. *Operations:* Resection of stomach, rectum, part of colon; pulmonary lobectomy; prostatic resection.
4. *Disordered metabolism:* Hyperthyroidism, diabetic acidosis, uremia.
5. *Myocardial failure:* Acute rheumatic pancarditis, syphilitic aortitis.
6. *Acute and chronic alcoholism* without signs of pellagra or cirrhosis.
7. *Liver disease:* Cirrhosis, catarrhal jaundice, carcinoma (primary).
8. *Dietary restrictions:* Gastric ulcer, gastric neurosis, food fads, diabetes, hypertension, mental diseases.

Following the suggestion by Watson, further studies on the B.E.S. test by Swain, Bean and Spies, have shown that among the substances which may give rise to pigments in the urine is indole acetic acid, the chromogen of urorosein. When an aqueous solution of indole acetic acid is tested by the B.E.S. technique, no color appears unless a trace of nitrite ion is also present but an excess of nitrite bleaches the color to a pale yellow. Since there is considerable variation in excretion of nitrites in normal individuals, we have made it a routine to add nitrites in performing the test. This may be done by adding two drops of a 0.5 per cent solution of sodium nitrite to the hydrochloric extract at the end of the customary period allowed for full color development. The solution should be mixed and observed after ten minutes for further color development. In testing the urine after administering indole acetic acid, either orally or intravenously, it is found that there is usually little or no color when a simple B.E.S. test is used, but a vivid red color is observed when nitrites are added. Tryptophane administered under identical conditions did not result in the excretion of pigments. Although it is impossible to demonstrate that abnormal tryptophane metabolism produces this indole acetic acid, it is probable that this reflects a disturbance either in gastro-intestinal function or in the metabolism within the body. In a few cases, indole acetic acid injections were followed by headache, nausea, vomiting, and a febrile reaction, though no such episodes followed the administration of the same amount of tryptophane.

Careful clinical studies have revealed that the B.E.S. test is not an exclusive test for porphyrins which are excreted by some pellagrins. Porphyrinuria appears to be related to liver damage rather than to pellagra *per se*. Urorosein may be excreted in large amounts, as may indican, by individuals with subclinical or clinical pellagra. Because the B.E.S. test may be positive before diagnostic evidence of deficiency disease appears, it is valuable as a warning signal of malnutrition. Nicotinic acid is of value in therapy where the test is positive but the exact nature of the change in pigment excretion in pellagra following therapy must be studied with more specific tests before the relationship of vitamin B complex substances to this aspect of pigment metabolism becomes clear.

GENERAL CLINICAL CONSIDERATIONS

Pellagra is a noncontagious, nonhereditary clinical syndrome which may occur in persons of any age, of either sex, and of every stratum of society. It occurs most commonly among the poorer classes, following a prolonged dietary inadequacy of nicotinic acid and substances physiologically similar. The lack of nicotinic acid affects every cell in the body, though the diagnostic signs and symptoms arise predominantly from involvement of the skin, alimentary tract, and nervous system. The incidence of the disease is greatest during the spring and summer, and it characteristically recurs at those times unless proper measures are rigidly and persistently applied.

The accumulated clinical information indicates that pellagra is caused primarily by a nutritional deficiency. The factors that operate to produce a nutritional deficiency are an inadequate intake, increased requirement, diminished absorption or utilization, or increased destruction or excretion of essential nutritional substances.

Pellagra is an extremely common disease. Sebrell of the United States Public Health Service recently stated: "In 1930 in North Carolina there were 1037 deaths from pellagra, or six times as many as from diphtheria, twenty times as many as from malaria, and about two and one-half times as many as from these diseases combined." Statistics furnished by the United States Public Health Service are misleading as to the actual incidence of the disease. Many cases are not recognized even in the terminal stages, and most cases recognized are not reported. The following points contribute to failure in diagnosis: (*a*) Many physicians do not think of pellagra or may be reluctant to consider the diagnosis unless the classic three D's—dermatitis, diarrhea and dementia—are present. As a matter of fact, this combination is rather infrequent and appears only during the advanced stages of the disease. (*b*) The early stages of pellagra are characterized by many vague symptoms which apparently arise from disturbances in all parts of the body. Such symptoms appear before the development of diagnostic lesions, and vary tremendously from one patient to another, even in the same family. They are often mistakenly called neurasthenia. (*c*) The syndrome is frequently superimposed upon some well-recognized organic disease. (*d*) Pellagra is prone to occur in association with a deficiency of many essential nutrients, many of which give a symptomatology of their own. An early diagnosis of pellagra is made by a careful interpretation of an accurate history and physical examination. It can be confirmed by characteristic response to therapy.

Diathesis.—Pellagra like most deficiency states is particularly prevalent among the following groups:

1. The poor and ignorant who live on an unbalanced diet, usually rich in carbohydrates and fats but low in proteins, minerals and vitamins. This is called *endemic pellagra.*

2. Persons who, because of organic disease, have difficulty in ingesting, assimilating or utilizing nicotinic acid compounds. Within this group we include persons who have lost teeth, those with disorders and diseases of the alimentary tract, those who have surgical operations, *etc.* This type is frequently called *pellagra secondary to organic disease.*

3. Persons with alcohol addiction who subsist mainly on calories derived from alcohol and whose appetites have decreased to such an extent that they eat little. These persons do not ingest sufficient nicotinic acid or substances acting similarly, and when they develop pellagra it is frequently called *alcoholic pellagra* or "pseudopellagra."

4. Food faddists and other persons with capricious appetites who tend to eat little food containing antipellagric materials. Some of these patients are on diets prescribed by physicians for the treatment of certain diseases and develop pellagra because the prescribed diet contains little of the antipellagric factor.

5. Persons whose requirements for antipellagric substances are greatly increased. Pregnancy, lactation, unusual growth, hyperthyroidism, infections, increased physical exercise all greatly increase the daily requirement for nicotinic acid.

Prodromal Symptoms.—This period may be of long duration with insidiously advancing symptoms, trivial in nature but gaining importance by their persistence rather than by their severity. Before diagnostic lesions of the mucous membranes or skin appear, there is loss of appetite which is at least in part responsible for weight loss. Ill defined disturbances of the alimentary tract, including "indigestion," and changes in bowel function, occur. General muscular weakness, lassitude, irritability, depression, memory loss, headache and insomnia develop without obvious reason. Inability to work, abdominal pain, burning sensations in various parts of the body, vertigo, numbness, nervousness, palpitation, distractability, flights of ideas, apprehension, morbid fears, mental confusion, and forgetfulness frequently occur. There may be intermittent diarrhea and constipation. There is much that obviously is abnormal at this stage, but nothing that is pathognomonic. Since the entire syndrome often appears without objective cause, a diagnosis of neurasthenia, anxiety state, malingering or neurosis is usually entertained.

After a long period of ill health which might properly be termed the deficiency development time, outstanding clinical lesions may arise in the skin, alimentary tract, or the nervous system. These symptoms are not invariably involved nor are they affected in any regular order, nor with the same degree of severity from case to case. Out of many thousands of cases studied, we have not seen two which are identical. The individual case, however, usually repeats with each recurrence the same order of development of symptoms.

Pellagra in Infancy and Childhood.—Spies, Walker and Woods have shown that early clinical signs of endemic pellagra are prone to develop in infants and children in "pellagra families." The identity of pellagra in the infant and in the adult is thoroughly established, but differences between the symptoms found in the two age groups make it advisable to consider them separately. These distinctions are due largely to the fact that in the adult deficiencies affect mature tissues, whereas in the infant or child they are engrafted upon tissues which are in the process of rapid growth and development. The symptomatology is also influenced by the striking difference in environment, the infant leading a sheltered existence compared with the active and exposed life of the adult. For purposes of clarity, infantile pellagra will be considered separately, but it should be borne in mind that from an etiological and pathological point of view such a distinction is artificial.

A careful history usually shows that the diet of the mother during pregnancy and lactation was inadequate, and that her breast milk was therefore lacking in quantity and quality. The infant was accordingly weaned soon after birth and was given a type of food which was inadequate for good nutrition. At a very early age, these children show poor appetites and usually eat irregularly. Most of them prefer carbohydrate foods and refuse most of the other foods offered. The parents seldom make any attempt to correct the food habits of such children even if a good diet becomes available.

The parents state that these children are irritable, easily frightened, apprehensive, and fretful. They cry a great deal, and are listless, apathetic, and tired. They do not show the normal interests of childhood, and if they have developed special interests before the onset of their illness, they soon lose them again. They are too tired to play and too fretful to rest; they sleep poorly and frequently awake crying. They gain weight slowly, or if they have been more robust before their illness, often lose weight rapidly. Most of these children complain of soreness of the tongue or lips, and of burning and pain in the abdomen, or of cramps and burning sensations in the legs. Vomiting and "indigestion" are common. Frequently they suffer from constipation, but occasionally they have bouts of diarrhea, especially during the spring and summer months. Their symptoms wax and wane, but tend to increase in severity with advancing years if adequate treatment is not instituted. As time passes, such children become increasingly subnormal in height and weight; they find it difficult to concentrate, and make poor progress in school.

Physical examination shows that these children are undernourished and underdeveloped for their age. They obviously are in ill health. Their skin is dry and atrophic, and they look like nothing so much as sad little old men and women. They may or may not have the typical dermal and alimentary tract lesions described in adult pellagrins; indeed, such diagnostic lesions frequently do not appear, but very ill children showing none of the typical lesions have been brought from the verge of death by prompt and intensive treatment with nicotinic acid or nicotinic acid amide.

A history of prolonged subsistence on an inadequate diet, plus the presence of pellagra in one or more members of the family, should lead one to suspect the diagnosis of pellagra in ill infants and children even in the absence of pathognomonic lesions. When there is doubt, the patient should be given the benefit of a controlled therapeutic test, since it is known that such children will show rapid improvement following specific therapy if early pellagra is present.

<h3 style="text-align:center">DIAGNOSIS</h3>

The clinical diagnosis of pellagra in adults or children depends upon identifying typical dermal lesions or characteristic mucous membrane lesions, or both. Typical dermal lesions are pathognomonic, and it is from them that the disease derived its name (*pelle* meaning skin, and *agra* meaning rough). Characteristic *skin lesions* may appear symmetrically placed on any part of the body. They are most frequently observed over sites of irritation, such as the dorsum of the hands, wrists, elbows, face, neck, knees, feet, under the breasts, and in the perineal region (see Fig. 48). In most instances, the

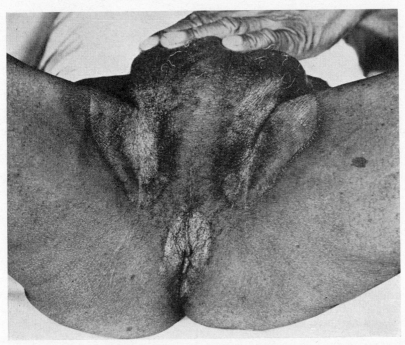

Fig. 48.—Typical perineal lesions in a 47-year-old colored male pellagrin. There was also dermatitis of the hands and feet. The symmetry, lines of demarcation, and general distribution are typical. Severe vomiting, diarrhea, glossitis, fever, tachycardia, and psychosis promptly improved following the exhibition of nicotinic acid.

area of dermatitis is separated sharply from the normal skin. The lesions are never static; they either advance or regress. Typical changes are well portrayed in figures 47, 49, 50 and 51. Bean and Spies have found that a considerable number of patients have skin lesions in atypical distribution, particularly around areas of old scars or on sites where the irritation is greatest. It should be emphasized that in many cases skin lesions never appear; these cases are termed "pellagra sine pellagra." The mucous membrane lesions affecting the tongue, oral cavity (see Fig. 52) and vagina are usually the earliest lesions diagnostic of the disease. The central nervous system frequently is affected, and the *mental symptoms* have been emphasized as a part of the pellagra syndrome for years. The patient may present a train of symptoms characteristic of neurasthenia, anxiety state, or other neuroses. In later stages, there is loss of memory, excitement, mania, delirium, hallucinations, and dementia. Even in the absence of diagnostic lesions of pellagra, a positive B.E.S. test on the urine from a malnourished person, irrespective of

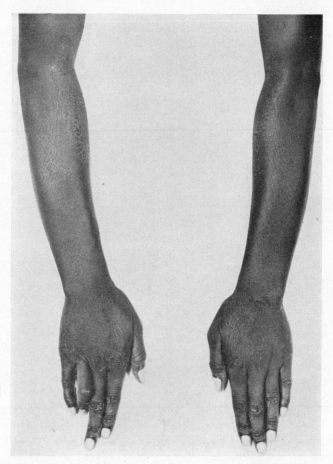

Fig. 49.—Stages in dermatitis of pellagra. I. Early phase showing changes a few days after the erythema has faded, leaving pigmented, roughened skin and early desquamation. The hands show only very slight changes. Note the line of demarcation above the elbow, and wrinkling of the skin of the hands.

whether he ate an unbalanced diet, or had infections, intestinal tract diseases, increased metabolism, alcoholic addiction, dietary restrictions, suggests that the person has latent pellagra.

In the past, many cases of pellagra were designated "pseudopellagra," "pellagra sine pellagra," "postalcoholic dermatitis," "secondary pellagra," or "alcoholic pellagra." Such terms are confusing and should be abandoned. The disease is or is not pellagra and should be so designated and treated.

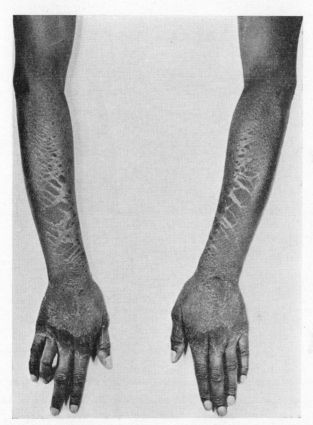

Fig. 50.—Stages in dermatitis of pellagra. II. Stage of desquamation. Large flakes may be pulled from dark areas over the surface, leaving tender new skin. There is relatively little involvement of the fingers. (Taken ten days after the first picture.)

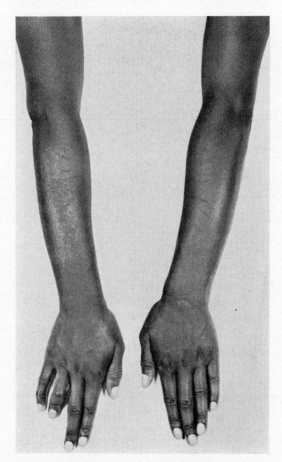

Fig. 51.—Stages of dermatitis of pellagra. III. Stage of healing. The process of desquamation is complete and new tender skin has replaced that involved in the dermatitis. It is smooth, not wrinkled. Streaks of pigmentation remain. (Taken thirty days after the first picture.)

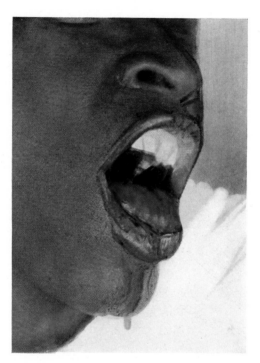

Fig. 52.—Pellagrous glossitis and stomatitis. Note the swelling and intense redness of the tongue and oral mucous membranes, and the thick mucoid saliva sticking to the teeth and drooling over the chin. (This patient drooled about one quart of saliva per day prior to treatment. The abnormal salivary secretion ceased within six hours following the administration of 500 mg. nicotinic acid. Within twenty-four hours the mucous membranes were normal and the patient could eat any type food.)

TREATMENT WITH NICOTINIC ACID

Nicotinic acid may be prepared in several ways, one of which is the strong acid oxidation of nicotine. It was from this method of preparation that the acid received its name, but its properties differ widely from those of the parent compound. Nicotinic acid is a white, crystalline compound (see Figs. 53, 54 and 55) which melts at 230–232° C. and is moderately solu-

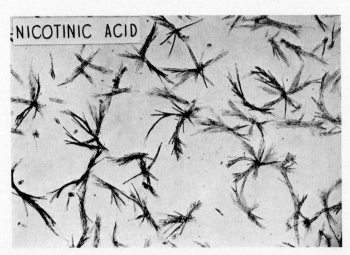

Fig. 53.—Microphotograph showing the crystalline structure of nicotinic acid. (Courtesy of Merck and Company.)

ble in hot water but only slightly soluble in cold water. The sodium salt and the amide are more soluble; hence, some commercial concerns prepare these in sterile physiological solution of sodium chloride for intravenous or intramuscular use. For parenteral administration, the amide (see Fig. 56) is preferable since it does not cause the flushing produced by nicotinic acid.

Clinical Pharmacology.—1. *Absorption.*—Observations on skin temperature have shown that following oral administration, nicotinic acid is ab-

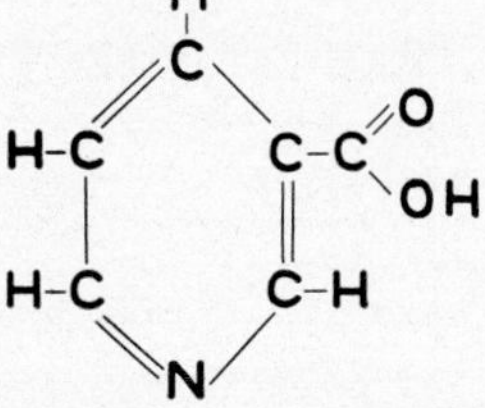

Fig 54.—Nicotinic acid (3-pyridine carboxylic acid).

sorbed fairly rapidly from the stomach and small intestine. Absorption is more rapid from an empty stomach than it is after meals (see Fig. 57).

Unpublished observations by Bean, Dexter and Spies, using skin temperature studies and bacteriological assays of nicotinic acid concentration in the blood, reveal that nicotinic acid is absorbed from the small and large bowel, as well as from the lower sigmoid and rectum.

	Structural Formula	Melting Point Centigrade	BLACKTONGUE Dose Milligrams	BLACKTONGUE Change in Symptoms	PELLAGRA Dose Milligrams	PELLAGRA Change in Symptoms	Staph. Aureus Concentration	Staph. Aureus Change in Growth	Dysentery B. Concentration	Dysentery B. Change in Growth	Flushing	Dinitrochlorobenzene Test Color
Nicotinic Acid	⬡COOH (N)	230°	60	Rapid Improvement		R.I.		+	$MX10^{-7}$	+	+	+
Sodium Nicotinate	COONa					R.I.		+			+	
Ammonium Nicotinate	COONH4											
Methyl Nicotinate	COOCH3							+	$MX10^{-7}$	+		
Ethyl Nicotinate	COOC2H5	129						0	$MX10^{-6}$	+		
Nicotinic Acid Amide	CONH2					R.I.		+	$MX10^{-7}$	+	0	+
Nicotinamide HCl	CONH2 · HCl	121	50	R.I.								
Nicotinamide Methochloride	CONH2 CH3 Cl	235										
Nicotinamide Glucosido-Iodide	O-CH(CHOH)3CH2OH CONHCH3		334	R.I.								
Nicotinic Acid N-Methyl Amide	CONHCH3	104.5	110	R.I.					$MX10^{-5}$	+		
Nicotinic Acid N-Diethyl Amide	CON(C2H5)2	liquid	140	R.I.		R.I.		0			0	+
Nicotinuric Acid	CONHCH2COOH	ca240	147	R.I.				0	$MX10^{-6}$	+		
Trigonellin Chloride	COOH CH3 Cl	258				No I.						0
Trigonellin Methyl Sulfate	COOH SO4CH3											0
Trigonellin Amide	CONH2 CH3 OH								$MX10^{-6}$	+		
6-Methyl Nicotinic Acid	COOH CH3 N	206-7	168	No Improvement							0	0
β-Acetyl Pyridine HCl	COCH3 HCl	174	193	Worse							0	0
Isonicotinic Acid	COOH	310-3	100	W.				0		0	0	0

Compound	Structural Formula	Melting Point Centigrade	Blacktongue—Dogs Dose Milligrams	Blacktongue Change in Symptoms	Pellagra Dose Milligrams	Pellagra Change in Symptoms	Staph. Aureus Concentration	Staph. Aureus Change in Growth	Dysentery B. Concentration	Dysentery B. Change in Growth	Flushing	Dinitrochlorobenzene Test Color
Picolinic Acid	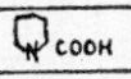 (structure)					Toxic		O	$MX10^{-4}$	Some		O
Picolinic Acid HCl	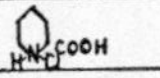 (structure)	214	260	W.								+
Quinolinic Acid	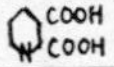 (structure)		50	W.				O	$MX10^{-4}$	Some		O
Dinicotinic Acid	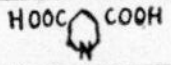 (structure)					R.I.		O				
2,4 Dimethyl Pyridine 3,5 Dicarboxylic A.	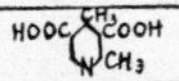 (structure)											
2,6 Dimethyl Pyridine 3,5 Dicarboxylic A.	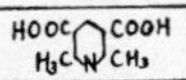 (structure)							O			O	+
2,4,6 Trimethyl Pyridine 3,5 Dicarboxylic A.	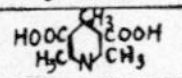 (structure)							O				
Pyridine	(structure)	liquid	100	W						O		+
β-Picoline	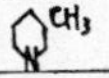 (structure)	140.3	50 / 200	R.I.		±		O		O		+
α-Picoline	(structure)											
Nicotinonitrile	(structure)	50	150	NoI.				O	$MX10^{-4}$	+		
3-Amino Pyridine	(structure)									O	O	
Pyridine β-Sulfonic Acid	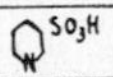 (structure)		200	Dogs died 2-3 days						O		
Nipicotic Acid HCl	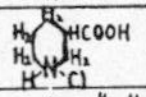 (structure)	237-9	130	NoI.				O				
Nicotine	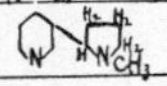 (structure)	liquid										+

Fig. 55.—This figure indicates some chemical, physiologic, and bacteriologic attributes of various pyridine compounds which bear some relation to nicotinic acid.

2. *Storage and Excretion.*—Excretion is more rapid when the material is administered parenterally than when it is given orally but regardless of the mode of administration, a large part of the total dose is soon excreted. A considerable amount appears in the urine as trigonellin, some as free nicotinic acid or its salts, and some in unidentified form.

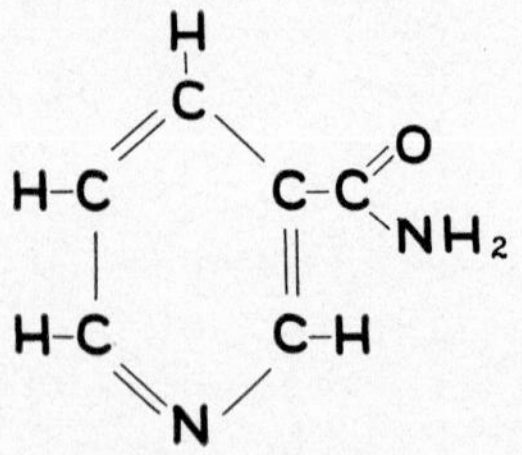

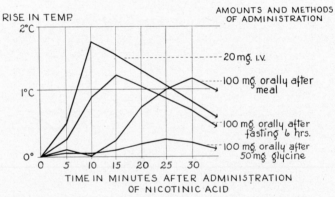

Fig. 56.—Nicotinic acid amide (3-pyridine carboxylic acid amide).

Nicotinic acid compounds have been found in all animal tissue. In general, the concentration is highest in tissues in which the metabolism is high. In human beings with severe nicotinic acid deficiency, the content of the nicotinic-acid-amide-containing substance, coenzyme I, is decreased as much as 60 per cent in striated muscle and may be somewhat decreased

SKIN TEMPERATURE RISE AFTER NICOTINIC ACID

Fig. 57.—This figure gives the changes in skin temperature obtained on an individual who had been kept in a constant temperature room (20° C.) for one hour before the various tests were made with nicotinic acid. Skin temperature was measured on fifteen spots on the head and neck using the Taylor Dermatherm. It can be seen that intravenous injection produces much more rapid rise in temperature than oral ingestion and that in addition the material is absorbed much more slowly in an individual when it is administered after a meal. In some instances, glycine prevents the rise in skin temperature when given shortly before an oral dose of nicotinic acid.

in the erythrocytes. Likewise, in this deficiency, the content of the nicotinic acid derivatives is below normal in whole blood and urine. When such patients are treated with nicotinic acid, the content of the nicotinic-acid-containing compounds in the muscle, blood and urine increases.

A knowledge of the level of nicotinic acid in the body tissues and excretions of pellagrins sometimes contributes valuable information concerning the degree of nicotinic acid deficiency. It is also useful in following the rate of recovery after nicotinic acid therapy has been initiated. Several methods, both chemical and microbiological, for the determination of nicotinic acid in micro quantities have therefore been introduced. We are using the microbiological technics in the study of biologically derived specimens since they possess extreme sensitivity, permitting the determination of nicotinic acid in amounts as small as a few hundredths of a microgram, and may be used in analyzing for nicotinic acid in the presence of large amounts of foreign material even if this be pigmented or in a solid state.

The microbiological method of Snell and Wright depends upon the estimation of the amount of growth of *Lactobacillus arabinosus* in a synthetic medium containing all of the essential nutrients for this organism with the exception of nicotinic acid. Any nicotinic acid supplied to the organisms therefore comes from the specimen being tested, which is added to the culture in known small amount. Since this amount of growth of the organisms in the lower range is proportional to the limiting nutrient, nicotinic acid, the measurement of the extent of growth by titration of the lactic acid produced by the Lactobacillus also affords an estimate of the amount of nicotinic acid present. Absolute values for nicotinic acid in samples may then be determined by reference to the amount of growth produced in a set of standards containing graduated amounts of nicotinic acid. This method has been used successfully in determining minute quantities of nicotinic acid in blood, urine, feces, saliva, fresh tissues and foods.

Using the above method, Gross, Swain and Spies have found that the average person with pellagra retains more of a 100-mg. test dose of nicotinic acid than the average person of similar size, injected under the same conditions, but having no evidence of pellagra.

3. *Toxicity.*—Nicotinic acid, in the amounts recommended for therapy, is not toxic although it and all related compounds containing the free

radical produce vasodilation in the skin and an increase in skin temperatures. Over 80 per cent of the persons to whom 100 to 300 mg. of nicotinic acid is administered orally feel temporary prickly or burning sensations. A few persons complain of nausea and cramping pains in the stomach. These symptoms are transient and are not associated with changes in general body temperature, pulse, respiration, or blood pressure. All persons to whom 20 mg. of nicotinic acid is administered intravenously have transitory vasodilation. It should be remembered, however, that nicotinic acid amide, which is also antipellagric, is the physiologic form of the compound and does not produce these vasodilating reactions.

The administration of quinine nicotinate (New York Quinine and Chemical Works) in sufficient amounts is followed by the vasodilator reaction.

15

Quinine nicotinate is very effective in treating persons with malaria, as would be expected, and it is also effective in the treatment of persons with pellagra. Our experience is too small to warrant saying that it is better in the cerebral type of malaria than quinine per se, but we have seen spectacular results. On theoretical grounds, it might be said that quinine nicotinate dilates the blood vessels of the brain, thus allowing freer passage of blood and quinine.

Further studies on ferrous nicotinate, quinine nicotinate, glutamine nicotinate all produce the same vasodilatation as that which occurs from other sources of nicotinate.

Indications for Oral Administration.—Oral administration of nicotinic acid is preferable to other methods because it is absorbed more slowly and an elevated blood concentration is maintained over a longer period of time. The amount of nicotinic acid or similar compounds necessary for a therapeutic response in pellagra varies tremendously from patient to patient. No arbitrary dosage can be set. The amount necessary depends upon the

EFFECT OF NICOTINIC ACID ON A
PELLAGRIN IN RELAPSE

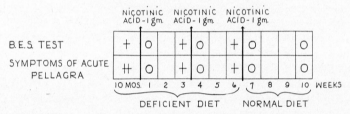

Fig. 58.—This figure indicates, first of all, that the symptoms of pellagra do not necessarily parallel the degree of abnormal pigment excretion. It shows very clearly the effect of nicotinic acid on the pigment excretion and on the acute symptoms of the disease in an individual who was allowed to relapse upon two occasions after treatment with nicotinic acid and who finally was placed on a good diet and showed no further relapse.

severity of the disease, the nature and severity of complications, and the condition of the alimentary tract. We have observed one person with long-standing pellagra who failed to respond to oral doses of nicotinic acid as high as 1500 mg. per day, but who improved rapidly following the intravenous administration of 50 mg. of nicotinic acid six times a day. For the average pellagrin, we recommend 50 mg. nicotinic acid, orally, ten times a day. Figure 58 shows the effect of nicotinic acid on a pellagrin in relapse and indicates that it or substances acting similarly must be continued for long periods of time if relapses are to be avoided.

Indications for Parenteral Administration.—Parenteral therapy should be used wherever a high blood concentration is desired within a short space of time and wherever gastro-intestinal absorption is inadequate. For *intravenous* administration, nicotinic acid amide is preferred because it is not attended by a flushing reaction. In most cases, 100 mg. per day is sufficient. As in oral administration, small doses at frequent intervals are desirable in order to keep the blood concentration at a high level. It should be administered in 25-mg. doses q.i.d., and injected slowly. In acutely ill patients where parenteral administration of saline or glucose is indicated, the vitamin can be dissolved in a physiological solution of saline or 5 per cent glucose and administered by slow drip.

Nicotinic acid can be given *intramuscularly* in the same dosage as that suggested for intravenous injection. However, intramuscular therapy in persons with deficiency diseases is *not recommended* because it is attended by some risk of abscess formation in devitalized tissues.

Administration to Infants and Children.—For infants a satisfactory daily dose is 50 to 100 mg. of nicotinic acid amide dissolved in the feeding. For parenteral administration, we suggest 5 mg. three to four times a day. Nicotinic acid or nicotinic acid amide given to a nursing mother increases the nicotinic acid which the breast-fed infant receives in the milk. For children, two or three times the dose for infants is suggested.

Response to Nicotinic Acid and Substances with Similar Physiological Action.—The administration of adequate doses of nicotinic acid or similar substances to a pellagrin will: cause fading of the fiery redness of the mucous membrane lesions and disappearance of the associated Vincent's organisms; cause disappearance of the acute mental symptoms of pellagra, such as delirium, hallucinations and mental confusion; relieve him of symptoms such as diarrhea, vomiting, and cramping which arise from alterations in alimentary function; cause fading of the dermal erythema; increase his strength and feeling of well-being; cause the disappearance of ether soluble red pigments from the urine; increase the coenzymes I and II concentration in whole blood and urine and, when therapy is prolonged, increase the coenzyme content of the muscle. The pellagrin and *not his disease* should be treated, as outlined in the section on general management (p. 491).

RIBOFLAVIN DEFICIENCY

Little could Blythe, the brilliant English chemist who first obtained a yellow-green pigment from milk in 1879, have realized that he possessed a chemical compound necessary for the health and well-being of animals and human beings. The world paid scant attention to his discovery for the time was not yet ripe for its significance to be appreciated. The undernourished millions of the East had no thought that chemistry might ever benefit them. America was busy healing the scars of the Civil War and extending the western frontier. Even the scientists of Europe were but slightly interested in his announcement, for they were engaged in heated argument concerning the germ theory of disease. Sixty years later we see that there has been a slow evolution of the scientist's thinking about his great natural enemies, pathogenic micro-organisms. Today, the germ theory is fully accepted and its application has been of immeasurable benefit to mankind. Yellow fever, smallpox, diphtheria, plague and many other infectious diseases are no longer rampant. Man is much concerned with the wide variety of maladies which threaten his health and life, and during the past twenty years the science of nutrition has developed vigorously. Studies in nutrition are steadily aiding in advancing the scientific aspects of medicine, with the result that certainty is replacing the art of speculation in the diagnosis and treatment of diseases of nutritional origin. During recent years, the science of nutrition has threatened to outstrip the worthwhile contributions to the well-being of the human race which resulted from the application of the germ theory of disease. It seems to be leading the scientific medicine of the future to heights as yet undreamed. What price we have paid in lives and funds for our existing knowledge concerning nutrition no one could or would venture to guess. That this knowledge has advanced our civilization and restored the health and well-being of countless numbers, we cannot gainsay. Each year, more tools are becoming available for work. Blythe's insignificant appearing yellow-green pigment has recently come into its own. Its isolation and synthesis were contributions of far-reaching importance for they made possible studies on plants, animals and human beings which show that it is practically indispensable for all forms of life. It is becoming increasingly evident that riboflavin will be an important aid in building a stronger and more vigorous civilization. Before proceeding to the incidence, diagnosis, and therapy of the syndrome resulting from a deficiency of riboflavin in the diet of human beings, we shall discuss those aspects of biochemistry and physiology which have a practical application to medicine and to the science of nutrition.

BIOCHEMISTRY AND PHYSIOLOGY

Riboflavin was considered of no biological importance until Warburg and Christian discovered it to be an important constituent of a cellular

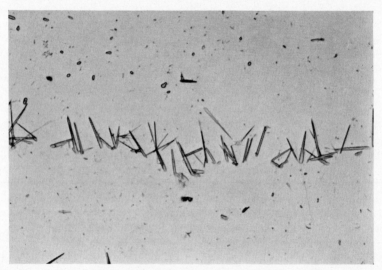

Fig. 59.—Microphotograph showing the structure of crystalline riboflavin. (Courtesy of Merck and Company.)

respiratory enzyme system. It was first isolated in 1933 and artificially synthesized in 1935. The crystalline appearance and structural formula are shown in figures 59 and 60. It is now identified as a combination of d-ribose and isoalloxazine. It is a freely dialyzable, intensely yellow, water soluble pigment which exhibits a characteristic green fluorescence under ultraviolet rays. It is irreversibly inactivated by either visible or ultraviolet light in acid or alkaline solutions. The phosphoric acid ester of riboflavin, believed to have the structure shown in Fig. 61, unites with a specific nonactive bearer protein to form the yellow enzyme.

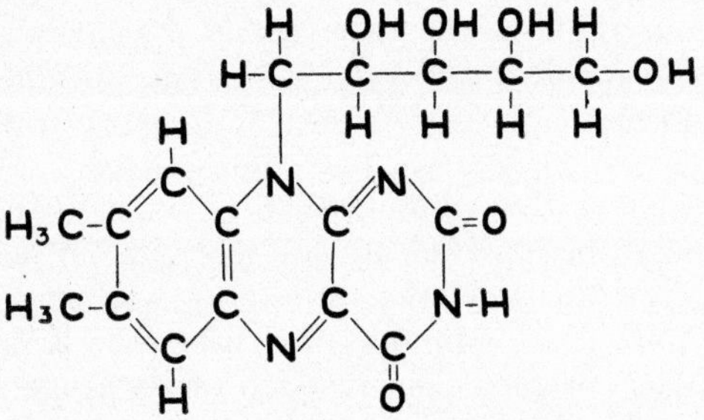

Fig. 60.—d-Riboflavin (6,7-dimethyl-9-(1'-d-ribityl)-isoalloxazine).

In the presence of an "activating enzyme" from yeast (*Zwischenferment*) and a thermostable coenzyme (since identified as coenzyme II—triphosphopyridine nucleotide), the yellow enzyme is capable of oxidizing

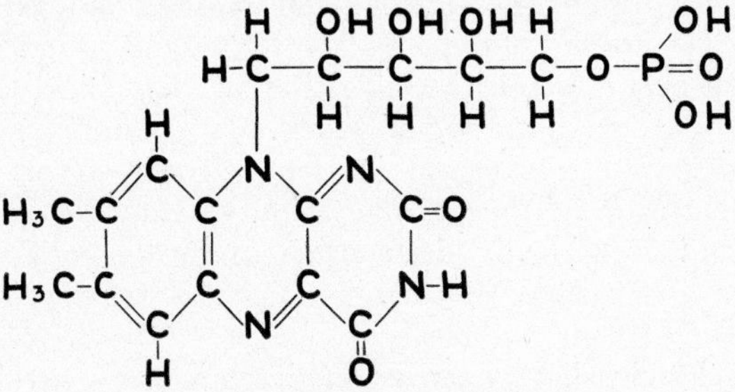

Fig. 61.—Riboflavin (5'-phosphoric acid ester—6,7-dimethyl-9-(1'-d-ribityl)-isoalloxazine-5'-phosphoric acid).

Robison's hexose monophosphoric ester. The following scheme has been postulated for the action of this system:

$$\textit{Zwischenferment}$$

(1) coenzyme + hexose monophosphoric acid ⟶ reduced coenzyme + phosphohexonic acid.

(2) reduced coenzyme + yellow enzyme ⟶ coenzyme + reduced yellow enzyme.

(3) reduced yellow enzyme + molecular oxygen ⟶ H_2O_2 + yellow enzyme.

This system, in contrast to other well-known oxidation-reduction systems, is not poisoned by hydrocyanic acid or carbon monoxide. Since the coenzyme is alternately reduced and oxidized by the yellow enzyme and the yellow enzyme itself is reversibly oxidized and reduced, only a very small amount of both these substances is required for the reaction to proceed.

Studies on similar enzyme systems have shown that there exists in nature a whole class of similar compounds (alloxazine proteids) differing in the constitution of the prosthetic group and in the structure of the bearer protein. Among such flavoproteins are d-amino acid oxidase, xanthine oxidase, and a flavoprotein recently isolated from heart muscle.

The yellow enzyme is present in all types of living cells, where it functions as an oxygen carrier between molecular oxygen and the substrate in association with other oxidative systems. The indispensability of riboflavin in the diet probably is due to the fact that it is an essential constituent of this yellow enzyme. When the identity of riboflavin and vitamin B_2 (G) was established, a rational approach to certain problems in vitamin research was possible.

Riboflavin has been demonstrated to be essential in the diet of the rat, chick, dog, pig, and man. A deficiency of this vitamin in the rat produces dermatitis, a marked decrease in the rate of growth, and cataract. If daily supplements of riboflavin are added to the diet when the first signs of lens opacity are noted, the cataract can be cured or its progress arrested. Riboflavin deficiency in the dog gives rise to vomiting and diarrhea, marked spasticity and muscular weakness with fatal termination, preceded by coma, fall in temperature and respiratory rate, and collapse. Death apparently is caused by cellular asphyxiation brought about by the lack of the oxidation catalyst.

Several investigators have reported the yellow color and fatty appearance of livers of riboflavin-deficient dogs, fowls, and rats. The experimental work of Lepkovsky, Jukes, Norris, Engel and others has shown that riboflavin is indispensable for the nutrition of the chick, and is required for a normal rate of hatching and viability.

Nerve degeneration was found in dogs suffering from riboflavin deficiency. Demyelination of the peripheral nerves and degeneration of their axis cylinders, and occasionally destruction of the medullary sheaths, have been found. Rats maintained on a similar diet did not develop neurological symptoms and showed no abnormalities.

Occurrence.—Flavins have been isolated from many natural sources, including egg white, milk, liver, kidney, barley malt, dandelion blossoms, grasses, egg yolk, yeast, the retina of fish eyes, and urine. (It should be emphasized that riboflavin deteriorates when exposed to sunlight, so that milk and other natural sources exposed even for relatively short periods of time may lose a high percentage of their initial store.) It was formerly believed that these compounds were different chemical substances, but further study has indicated that all are identical with riboflavin.

Absorption.—Riboflavin is readily absorbed from the alimentary canal. Phosphorylation occurs in the intestinal wall and other tissues throughout the body. Thus, it exerts its normal effect regardless of the way in which it is administered.

Storage and Excretion.—The flavin content of the body organs cannot be increased above a certain level even by forced feeding. The heart, liver, and kidneys of rats which have died of riboflavin deficiency contain one-third of their normal riboflavin content. Sherman demonstrated that the optimum intake of riboflavin in the rat is much greater than the minimum requirement. He concluded that the enrichment with riboflavin of an already adequate diet produced a healthier race. The blood content of riboflavin may range from 0.28 to 0.55 gamma per cc. of whole blood. There appears to be little correlation between the amount of riboflavin in the blood and the clinical symptoms of riboflavin deficiency.

Riboflavin is a normal constituent of the urine. Although assays in persons suffering from clinical riboflavin deficiency have shown that there is no significant alteration of the blood riboflavin, a decreased urinary excretion is generally the rule. When the dietary intake is very low, the excretion may for a time exceed the intake and, conversely, when the intake is high, the excretion may lag behind. The daily urinary loss of the normal adult on an adequate diet varies from 750 to 1250 gamma. Saturation tests, similar to those used to detect thiamine deficiency, have not proved effective for the diagnosis of riboflavin deficiency. The rate of destruction of riboflavin in the body is not known, but adults need about 3 mg. per day.

An increased consumption of riboflavin causes an increase in the flavin content of the breast milk of lactating women.

Toxicity.—Riboflavin is nontoxic in amounts which far exceed therapeutic dosage.

GENERAL CLINICAL CONSIDERATIONS

Riboflavin deficiency is a noncontagious, nonhereditary clinical syndrome. It occurs in any race and affects both males and females at any time from infancy to old age. It is more common in women than in men. The incidence tends to be higher in the spring and summer than at any other season of the year. Unless the diet becomes adequate or riboflavin or substances containing it are administered, relapses are likely to occur from time to time throughout the year.

Three years ago the clinical syndrome of riboflavin deficiency was not recognized in human beings. From the observations of Sebrell, Spies, Sydenstricker, and their associates, certain symptoms and signs have been pieced together and correlated, and we now have sufficient knowledge of the disease to be able to diagnose and treat it. Studies of the authors have led them to conclude that it is the most common vitamin deficiency disease in the United States. It probably affects several million people in this country, and reaches even into the very highest stratum of society. Although it occurs in association with a variety of conditions, it is very common among persons with pellagra, beriberi, or other deficiency diseases, and may appear before, during or after the development of diagnostic lesions of these diseases. The concurrence of riboflavin deficiency and deficiencies of other B-complex vitamins is due to the impossibility of eating a diet of natural foods deficient in only one of these vitamins. Diagnosis depends not only on the recognition of the usual clinical manifestations of the disease, but also on watching carefully for them under circumstances in which they are likely to appear. Only by these means can early changes be detected and early therapy initiated. The available laboratory tests, although precise, are not suitable for the use of the practitioner. Accordingly, diagnosis must depend upon the recognition of characteristic lesions and therapeutic tests with riboflavin.

Etiologic Factors.—The many factors which either singly or in combination give rise to or precipitate the appearance of clinical symptoms of the disease will be discussed briefly.

1. *Inadequate Food Intake.*—Among all strata of society there are persons who consume inadequate diets, but among the indigent and poor this is the most common cause of riboflavin deficiency. Others whose diets are frequently inadequate are food faddists, persons with idiosyncrasies of taste and appetite, and those who follow overconscientiously dietary regimens

prescribed for allergy, diabetes, peptic ulcer, obesity, hypertension, and many other conditions. Such diets often fail to supply adequate amounts of riboflavin. Riboflavin deficiency is found frequently in nursing infants whose mothers during pregnancy and lactation have had clinical or sub-clinical riboflavin deficiency. Lack of milk in the daily diet leaves many people on the borderline of a deficiency state.

2. *Faulty Absorption or Utilization of Food.*—Interference with the absorption of food predisposes to the development of riboflavin deficiency. Disorders of the alimentary canal, congestive heart failure, cirrhosis, and nephritis frequently interfere with proper absorption or utilization.

3. *Increased Requirement.*—Several factors may increase the requirement for vitamins. During periods of rapid growth in children, the amount of riboflavin required increases and if it is not met, riboflavin deficiency develops. The requirement during pregnancy and lactation is increased, and the clinical syndrome frequently appears in the later months of pregnancy. Hyperthyroidism and fevers increase metabolic needs and lead to a disparity between the intake and the need. In infections, especially chronic ones, there often is a combination of increased need to satisfy accelerated metabolism and loss of appetite which precludes filling this need. In diabetes mellitus, abrupt increments in carbohydrate intake and insulin may precipitate the deficiency syndrome.

4. *Increased Excretion.*—Although it is not known that an increased loss of riboflavin may occur in conditions in which there is an abnormally high excretion in the urine, this possibility should be kept in mind as a complicating factor in patients with diabetes insipidus or in persons undergoing diuresis of any sort.

5. *Chronic Alcoholic Addiction.*—Persons who regularly consume large amounts of alcohol usually fail to eat sufficient food to satisfy their nutritional requirements. In addition, alcoholic gastritis probably interferes with proper alimentation, and a certain number of persons addicted to alcohol develop liver disease which may interfere with the intermediary metabolism of riboflavin.

Prodromal Symptoms.—It is important to emphasize that a long period of ill health with symptoms of a vague, nondescriptive character usually precedes the appearance of diagnostic lesions. Because deficiencies of the B-complex vitamins tend to occur as complexities rather than as single entities, it is impossible to separate the premonitory symptoms of spontaneous riboflavin deficiency from those of pellagra or beriberi. Prominent among such symptoms are anorexia, weight loss, weakness, and inability to perform mental work. Digestive disturbances, nervousness, vague pains in various parts of the body, burning sensations of the skin, eyes and corners of the mouth, as well as soreness at the corners of the mouth, pain in the eyes and visual disturbances, headaches, dizziness, mental depression, insomnia, forgetfulness and mild states of confusion are common complaints. Frequently none of the symptoms are objective, and there are no signs indicating that any specific system in the body is primarily affected. Such symptoms may persist for a long time after diagnostic lesions appear, and in some persons they remain constant while the specific lesions wax and wane. The physician who is unfamiliar with deficiency diseases may interpret these prodromal symptoms as being functional in origin. They should, however, lead him to consider the possibility of an inadequate food intake or the faulty utilization of food playing a rôle in their development. Even though persons with such symptoms have no diagnostic signs of a deficiency disease, they should be observed repeatedly over a long period of time for, in many cases, diagnostic lesions eventually appear. From the knowledge gained from such retrospective studies, it is now possible to recognize many early cases and institute treatment when it is most valuable.

Special Lesions.—A. *Cheilosis.*—The most characteristic clinical sign in riboflavin deficiency is an angular stomatitis and an involvement of the lips in a process that is variously called cheilosis or cheilitis. Such lesions had long been observed in association with pellagra and it was known that they responded to treatment with yeast. Not until Sebrell and Butler reported

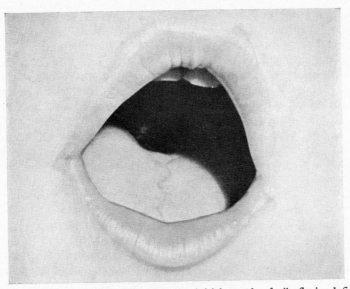

Fig. 62.—Very early changes found in an initial attack of riboflavin deficiency in a child. Early loss of specific tissue is seen at both angles, with slight maceration and piling up of crusts. The epithelium of the lip shows an increase in the transverse markings, a tendency to slight puckering and in areas wrinkling of the surface which gives the appearance of a skim as on boiled milk.

the results of their classical investigations on riboflavin deficiency, however, was the significance of these lesions appreciated. The earlier changes occur as a paleness in the lips, particularly at the angles, but not the moist area of the buccal mucosa. The pallor usually continues for days and is followed by maceration and piling up of whitish tissue on a pink background. Superficial fissures may invade the site of natural wrinkles at the corners of the mouth. These fissures may be single or multiple and usually appear on both sides. Subsequently the macerated lesions become dry, and a yellowish crust which forms at the angles may be removed without bleeding. The lips are usually red and there is likely to be an increase in the transverse markings, particularly on the lower lip (Figs. 62 and 63). Inspection of the tongue indicates that there are changes in the superficial epithelium, in the capillaries, or distortion of the normal papillae. In some cases, the tongue has a magenta hue which is similar to, but can be distinguished from that seen in cyanosis. As the disease progresses, the fissures in the corners of the mouth tend to become deeper and extend on to the cheek. They may extend within the mouth so that the constantly irritated angles become raw, bleeding areas with crusts or scabs. Such lesions are sometimes very painful in the acute stage, and occasionally are painful throughout the course of the disease. If the lesions recur frequently a cicatrix may be formed, giving the affected area an atrophic appearance (see Fig. 63). Hemolytic streptococci, hemolytic staphylococci and, in some cases, various yeasts and fungi have been obtained in cultures from acute lesions. Presumably these are secondary infections since the organisms disappear following adequate treatment with riboflavin. It is possible that the morphology of the lesions is altered to some extent by these secondary invaders.

B. *Ocular Symptoms.*—Spies and his associates first showed that riboflavin is an important factor in the relief of certain ocular disturbances. These disturbances disappear after riboflavin is given and return when therapy is discontinued. In many persons with ocular symptoms, vitamin A also is of specific value in relieving certain symptoms which persist after riboflavin therapy. Conversely, it has been found that when vitamin A is given before treatment with riboflavin, the addition of the latter produces further improvement. The disturbances include conjunctivitis (particularly of the lower palpebral and bulbar conjunctiva), itching, burning, photophobia, and the sensation of having sand or cinders in the eyes. Important observations by Sydenstricker, Sebrell, Cleckley and Kruse with the slit lamp indicate that many of these symptoms are associated with a superficial and interstitial keratitis. The earlier changes are described as an invasion of the cornea by the capillaries arising from the circumcorneal region. Anastomoses of the capillaries from different areas occur and from these, small branching capillaries appear to invade the cornea in the centripetal direction. Circumcorneal injection is usually obvious to the naked eye at such a stage. Later, interstitial infiltration with exudation may give rise to opacities either punctate or generalized. In some cases, there is also involvement of the iris. The characteristic changes occurring in such conditions as well as their treatment have been described in detail by Sydenstricker and his coworkers. Similar findings in rosacea keratitis have been reported by Johnson and Eckhardt.

C. *Unilateral Lesions.*—It should be emphasized that lesions sometimes occur on one side of the mouth only, and occasionally only one eye is involved (see Fig. 64). Furthermore, there are frequently differences in the severity of the lesions at the two angles of the mouth, and we have seen patients in whom the lesions at one angle progressed while the other regressed. We have seen at least one woman in whom the lesion appeared only at the right angle of the mouth, through four periods of relapse and remission. Some of the remissions were induced and others occurred spontaneously.

D. *The Skin.*—There may be a fine, scaly, slightly crusty desquamation on a mildly erythematous base in the nasolabial folds, on the alae nasi, within the nostrils, and on and about the ears. Very firm filiform excrescences may occur in a butterfly distribution across the nose and cheeks. A fine, scaly dermatitis of the hands, and areas of dermatitis around the vulva, anus, and

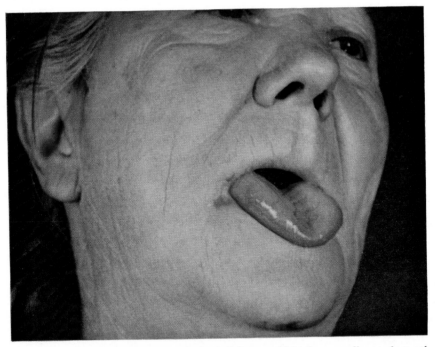

Fig. 63.—Chronic untreated riboflavin deficiency which shows scaling and atrophy at the angles of the mouth with an increase of vascularization and chronic, low grade infection. The edema and abnormal redness of the tongue, together with the fissures, responded following treatment with nicotinic acid and riboflavin. The lesions in the angles did not heal completely but left white, glazed, atrophic scars.

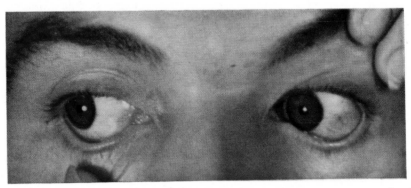

Fig. 64.—This photograph reveals the type of conjunctivitis seen among people with marked B complex deficiency diseases which is often relieved by the use of riboflavin. It should be noted that the lower lid is more involved than the upper lid and in this case the lateral rather than the medial aspect of the bulbar conjunctiva is involved. This case also represents asymmetrical involvement, where one eye is much more seriously changed than the other. (Spies in *Am. J. Med. Sc.*, Nov., 1940, Lea & Febiger.)

perineum have been observed to heal along with the remission of the mouth lesions following the administration of riboflavin.

We are at a loss to explain the irregular sequence in which the lesions of the mouth, skin, and eyes occur in different persons. In some there is a tendency for the conjunctival and corneal lesions to appear first and to be followed by the development of the oral and skin lesions. In others, lesions at the angles of the mouth occur before any of the specific eye symptoms appear. Changes in the skin, particularly over the bridge of the nose, over the cheek bones, and in the area where the nose joins the upper lip or cheek, in some cases, appear before the oral or ocular lesions. In still others, the mouth, eyes and skin are affected at approximately the same time and to the same degree of severity.

Riboflavin Deficiency in Infants and Children.—In our experience we have found that riboflavin deficiency is particularly common among children and that diagnostic lesions frequently appear even when there is no evidence of a deficiency of any other factor of the vitamin B complex. From the study of a large number of children we have learned that long periods of ill health associated with poor nutrition precede the appearance of diagnostic lesions. The lesions in children are similar to those seen in the adult. We have noticed particularly that the younger children in a large family are more likely to develop the disease. One possible explanation for this is that in large families in which the mother has had an almost continuous round of pregnancies alternating with lactation, or occasionally the two simultaneously, these children may begin vitamin deficiencies while still in utero. In many children general ill health and inability to make normal progress in school or to take part in the activities of childhood, have been considered characteristic of poor racial stock. We believe that often they may be caused by a deficiency of vitamins rather than a deficiency in germ plasm. The evidence for this rests in the fact that children in families in which any of the members have riboflavin deficiency often are benefited spectacularly by dietary supplements of riboflavin even though they have no diagnostic evidence of riboflavin deficiency.

Recurrence.—Manifestations of riboflavin deficiency, particularly the changes that occur in the lips, at the angles of the mouth and in the eyes, tend to undergo irregular cyclic variations in that the lesions wax and wane, sometimes clearing up completely, sometimes advancing to extreme severity over periods of weeks or months. The severity of the disease tends to be greatest during the spring and occasionally in the fall. Furthermore, in some patients these relapses occur without obvious relation to season. Usually, the feeling of ill health among persons with riboflavin deficiency is most intense during the time the lesions are increasing in severity and as they clear up, general health improves. This is especially true when the lesions heal in association with the administration of riboflavin. There is evidence that infections are sometimes associated with a relapse of the lesions and that periods of improved diet tend to be followed by remission.

DIAGNOSIS

The diagnosis of riboflavin deficiency is not difficult when lesions characteristic of the disease are present. During the prodromal period, it is not easy. The physician should suspect riboflavin deficiency in persons who subsist on poorly balanced diets containing little milk, meat, and green vegetables, in those who have diseases which interfere with the utilization and absorption of food, and in those whose requirements might for any reason be increased.

The diagnosis of riboflavin deficiency depends upon the observation of one or more of the following: Angular stomatitis and cheilosis; ocular disturbances with inflammation of the conjunctival vessels, and growth of vessels into the cornea; seborrheic changes in the skin of the face, particularly of the nose and adjacent regions; "magenta tongue," which includes changes in the papillae and in the capillaries. The beneficial response of the patient to the administration of riboflavin is the most important criterion for establishing a diagnosis in subclinical cases. If the patients improve regularly following the administration of riboflavin and relapse when it is discontinued, it is likely that they have a deficiency of this substance. There is no satisfactory clinical-laboratory test for the diagnosis of riboflavin deficiency. When such a deficiency is suspected, the diagnosis can best be made by careful interpretation of an accurate history and physical examination, aided by a well-controlled therapeutic test.

CHEMISTRY OF RIBOFLAVIN

Riboflavin is an orange crystalline compound which is sparingly soluble in water. The crystals have no sharp melting point but darken at 240° C. and decompose between 274–282° C. It possesses a characteristic yellow-green fluorescence in aqueous solution. Riboflavin is stable to heat and acids, but is readily destroyed by strong alkali and by exposure to ultraviolet or visible light. It is a complex organic molecule composed of isoalloxazine and d-ribose, and is identical with the naturally occurring flavins.

MODE OF ADMINISTRATION

Riboflavin is well tolerated when administered orally, intravenously, or intramuscularly. Oral administration is the method of choice, since riboflavin is readily absorbed from the normal gastro-intestinal tract. Some difficulty is encountered in preparing solutions of the vitamin for intravenous administration due to its low solubility in water, physiological saline or glucose. Sterile solutions of riboflavin can be obtained from reputable pharmaceutical concerns, or can be prepared and autoclaved with safety. In treating nearly a thousand cases of riboflavin deficiency, we have encountered no acute emergencies requiring parenteral therapy to save life.

The dose of riboflavin for adults is 2 mg. t.i.d. for several weeks. Children showing signs of riboflavin deficiency should be given 1 mg. t.i.d. for a similar period. Riboflavin may be administered to infants by adding 0.5 mg. b.i.d. in the prepared food. If the infant is being nursed, riboflavin administered to the mother in sufficient amounts will relieve the child's symptoms.

In order to avoid any anxiety on the part of the patient taking riboflavin, he should be informed that the compound will color the urine bright yellow. Intravenous or intramuscular administration may be used in all persons who for any reason cannot take the vitamin by mouth. The dose is 2 mg., dissolved in 10 cc. of sterile physiological saline, three times a day. Following the intravenous administration, a considerable portion is excreted in the urine. Persons receiving frequent intravenous injections of physiological salt solution may be given the vitamin dissolved in this solution.

A new preparation of riboflavin which has been lyophilized so that it is very soluble is now on the market. It is readily used in parenteral therapy.

Response to Riboflavin.—The administration of sufficient amounts of riboflavin or substances acting similarly to persons with clinical evidence of riboflavin deficiency induces a prompt increase in the amount excreted in the urine and a gradual rise in the blood content; striking increase in strength and sense of well-being within twelve to twenty-four hours; and gradual healing of the cheilosis, conjunctivitis and keratitis so characteristic of the disease. Just as we have seen pellagrins restricted to a deficient diet relapse while receiving large doses of nicotinic acid, so have we seen persons with riboflavin deficiency eating a restricted diet relapse in the face of taking large doses of riboflavin. Thus, the administration of a well-balanced diet is indicated. Patients with riboflavin deficiency should be considered as having a general nutritive failure, and the application of the principles outlined in the section on general management is recommended.

ASCORBIC ACID DEFICIENCY

The British Empire might have disintegrated long ago if scurvy had been allowed to go uncontrolled in the English Navy as it did among some other seafaring folk. In the eighteenth century James Lind, a famous surgeon in the British Navy, demonstrated that citrus fruit juices will prevent and cure scurvy. Unfortunately, Lind did not live to see scurvy disappear from the British Navy, as the Admiralty waited until the year after his death to apply his findings rigidly and stamp out the disease. Sailors in other countries taunted the British tar by calling him "limey," an epithet which is inaccurate because the citrus fruit which was used to prevent scurvy was not the lime, which actually contains little ascorbic acid, but the lemon.

The authors are unable to explain the great interest of western scientists of this period in the beriberi of the far-off Orient, in contrast with their meager attention to scurvy, which they recognized in their midst. Perhaps they were troubled by the apparent incongruity of deficiency diseases existing in a land of plenty and chose to think of them as affecting people in distant places. No country is free of scurvy, although it is usually most prevalent where vegetation is scarce. For hundreds of years there were epidemics in Europe among soldiers, sailors, and inmates of prisons, insane asylums, and poorhouses. Infantile scurvy was described in England in 1668, but it was almost entirely overlooked for two hundred years. Eventually, however, it was recognized that the disease affects many children in England and in America, where there was extensive use of artificial and processed foods.

It is one thing to know that citrus fruit juice will prevent or cure scurvy and another to identify the constituent responsible for this remarkable property. To Theobald Smith we owe the first description of experimentally induced scurvy. Some forty-five years ago, according to Sibyl L. Smith, Theobald Smith wrote as follows: "The death of No. 254 was undoubtedly due to the absence of such (green) food as the attendant had neglected to provide it after the disappearance of grass in the fall of the year. . . . When guinea pigs are fed with cereals (bran and oats mixed) without any grass, clover or succulent vegetables such as cabbage a peculiar disease, chiefly recognizable by subcutaneous extravasation of blood (that is, hemorrhages under the skin), carries them off in four to eight weeks." Smith did not associate this disease of improperly fed guinea pigs with human scurvy as his work was concerned primarily with the study of poultry, swine and cattle. More than a decade later, Holst and Frölich demonstrated that the symptoms of scurvy induced in guinea pigs are identical with those of scurvy in man. Twenty-five years were to pass before the substance responsible for its prevention and cure was identified and synthesized and even now, nine years after this discovery, there is much uncertainty as to human requirements for ascorbic acid and its mode of action in the body.

BIOCHEMISTRY AND PHYSIOLOGY

The isolation and identification of vitamin C by King and others in 1932 was followed by its synthesis in 1933 by Reichstein, Grussner, and Oppenauer. Ascorbic acid is related to the sugars, being an enediol-lactone of an acid similar in configuration to l-gulose. The formula for it appears below with that of the vitamin.

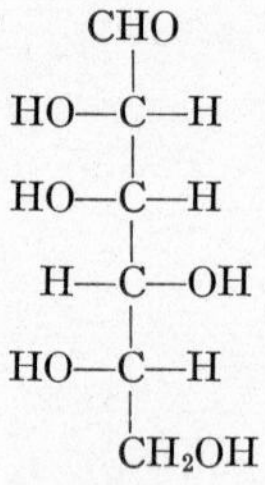

l-gulose 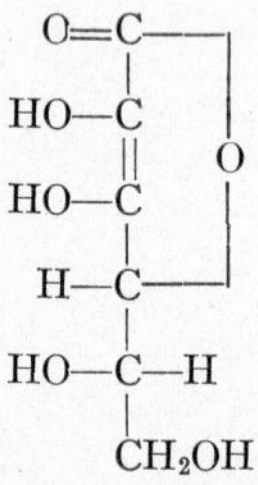   Vitamin C (l-ascorbic acid)

Several other synthetic substances have antiscorbutic activity, but to a lesser degree. d-Ascorbic acid will not protect against scurvy. Below a pH of 7.6 the vitamin in solution is not oxidized by exposure to air unless traces of copper or other catalysts are present. Methylene blue, quinones, and certain other organic compounds have the ability to bring about the oxidation, which is reversible below pH 4. At more alkaline reactions the process becomes irreversible, the first product, dehydroascorbic acid, giving rise to another strongly reducing substance of unknown structure which is in turn oxidized to oxalic and l-threonic acids.

Dry crystals of the vitamin do not decompose even when exposed to air and sunlight at room temperature for several years. The rate of aerobic oxidation in aqueous solution is greatly increased by exposure to light, especially in the presence of flavin.

Of the large number of species which have been examined, only man, the other primates, and guinea pigs lack the ability to synthesize ascorbic acid. The evidence which is frequently cited to prove its synthesis in infants, placental tissues, or any of the tissues of the animals named can better be interpreted as a selective conservation of vitamin in vital organs. The concentration of vitamin C in the tissues parallels roughly their metabolic activity. The following list approximates the concentration of ascorbic acid in descending order: the pituitary body, corpus luteum, adrenal cortex, young thymus, liver, brain, testes, ovaries, spleen, thyroid, pancreas, salivary glands, lung, kidney, intestinal wall, heart, muscle, spinal fluid and blood.

Normal human *blood plasma* contains about 1.2 mg. ascorbic acid per 100 cc. When there is no dietary intake this value rapidly falls to zero, but apparently there is no direct correlation between plasma levels and the state of nutrition. While a plasma concentration below 0.5 mg. per 100 cc. may not be dangerously low, such a finding is suspicious of a dietary paucity of vitamin C. A recent study of experimental human scurvy by Crandon and Lund shows that the vitamin C content of the plasma may remain at zero for as long as three months before the appearance of clinical scurvy. They suggest that the concentration in the white cell-platelet layer of centrifuged blood is a much better index of a vitamin C deficiency since this value fell to zero shortly before the subject developed typical scorbutic lesions.

Normal *human milk* contains four to five times as much vitamin C as cow's milk. If the mother's diet is deficient in antiscorbutic foods, the vitamin C concentration in the milk may fall below that of cow's milk; when the dietary deficiency is corrected the amount rises to normal levels.

Vitamin C is normally found in the urine but when there is no dietary intake the excretion gradually diminishes as the tissues become depleted. Restoration of a normal ascorbic acid intake replenishes the tissues and is followed by a resumption of excretion. In the normal state of saturation, the amount taken in exceeds that excreted by 50 mg. or more daily. The amount of the vitamin required to induce saturation appears to be a very rough measure of the state of vitamin C nutrition.

Ascorbic acid is essential for the maintenance of normal intercellular material of connective tissue, bones, teeth and perhaps blood vessels. The fibrils in loose connective tissue normally are cemented together by a translucent matrix of collagen, but in vitamin C deficient animals fibrils and collagen are absent. The formation of osteoid tissue and dentin is similarly dependent upon a supply of vitamin C. It is not known whether lack of vitamin C directly affects the intercellular colloids or the fibroblasts.

Sensitivity to injections of bacterial toxins, lowered metabolic activity, and lowered resistance to infection are some of the early changes in vitamin C deficient animals. A close relationship exists between vitamin C and guinea-pig blood complement. Normal activity of complement is dependent upon its being in the reduced state, and ascorbic acid was found to be the most important reducing agent in blood plasma in this connection. No positive identification of vitamin C with enzymic processes in normal animal tissues has been made, but many in vitro experiments suggest such a relation. The catalyst often called "ascorbic acid oxidase" is a protein combined with copper but is probably not specific for vitamin C as a substrate. The cytochrome-indophenol oxidase system has been shown to act as a catalyst for the aerobic oxidation of ascorbic acid, and the reducing power of plasma on dichlorophenolindophenol has been used in the clinical laboratory as a test for vitamin C.

PATHOLOGICAL PHYSIOLOGY

The primary effect of vitamin C deficiency is reflected in the intercellular substance of the connective tissue. Eventually this results in weakening of the periosteum, diminished muscular power, defective osteoid and dentin formation, and hemorrhage.

The changes in the *long bones* constitute one of the most uniform findings in vitamin C deficiency. Lesions are widely distributed throughout the skeleton but are most pronounced where growth is normally most rapid. The costochondral junction, the distal end of the femur, the proximal end of the humerus, both ends of the tibia and fibula, and the distal end of the radius and ulna are involved in approximately the order given.

In the affected regions enchondral bone growth ceases and the existing osseous bone becomes rarefied, widened and conical. Microscopic sections of the cartilage-shaft junction show a collection of columns, larger and less numerous than in normal bone, separated by an irregular mass of matrix. The calcified matrix contains numerous fractures. In severe scurvy, no conversion of matrix into bone occurs. Trabeculae previously formed are separated from the calcified matrix by a zone devoid of newly formed trabeculae—the "zone of destruction" or "zone of rarefaction" visible in the roentgenogram. Throughout the entire bone the osseous framework becomes attenuated. The carpal and tarsal bones, and the centers of the ossification of the long bones show changes of a similar nature but less pronounced degree.

Normal marrow at the epiphyseal ends of the bone is replaced by loose fibrous tissue, the so-called framework marrow or "*Gerüstmark*" which occupies the width of the shaft, forming a band which includes the zone of destruction. This abnormal marrow extends into the shaft for a variable distance, depending upon the duration and severity of the deficiency. The periosteum strips readily from the underlying bone, but invariably remains adherent at its junction with the perichondrium. Subperiosteal hemorrhages are common, and may be confined to the ends of the shaft, or may elevate the entire length of the periosteum.

In the *teeth* of adults with scurvy the dentin is resorbed and porotic, and the little replacement dentin that is formed is of inferior quality. In the pulp, chiefly around the vessels, atrophy, hyperemia, degeneration of odontoblasts and the formation of small cysts and foci of calcification occur. Few studies have been made of the dental lesions in infantile scurvy, but in the rapidly growing teeth of the guinea pig early and extensive changes occur in the dentin, enamel and cementum. Involvement of the gingiva is most frequent and severe when the teeth are erupted, particularly if they are deformed and broken. The lesions begin on the papillae as a hyperemia; destruction of epithelium follows. Infection, with ulceration, granulation, and even gangrene may occur. Rarefaction of the alveolar bone results in loosening of the teeth.

The *skin* commonly shows petechiae of various sizes, particularly on the trunk and lower extremities. In adults they are often perifollicular. Ecchymoses are common and are most frequent about the knees and ankles but may appear anywhere. In severe scurvy, particularly in adults, changes occur in the muscles: fragmentation of the striated fibers, multiplication of the sarcolemma, and, in prolonged cases, replacement by connective tissue poor in collagen. Moderate effusions, often blood-tinged, may occur in the pericardial, pleural and peritoneal cavities. Hemorrhage may be found anywhere in the body.

SYMPTOMATOLOGY

Because the tissues of the infant are in the process of rapid growth and development, there are certain differences in the symptomatology of scurvy in the adult and in the infant. For the purpose of clarity, the two conditions will be discussed separately, although from the viewpoint of etiology and general pathology this distinction is arbitrary.

Infantile Scurvy.—This disease occurs most commonly in artificially-fed infants; it develops in breast-fed infants only when the mother's diet is unusually limited in vitamin C. Restriction of the mother's diet during pregnancy seems to lead more often to deficiency in the mother than to deprivation of the fetus. The ability of the human breast to excrete milk with a higher concentration of ascorbic acid than is found in the maternal blood is a protection for the breast-fed infant.

In the majority of cases, symptoms of manifest scurvy appear between the ages of eight and thirteen months. Symptoms of mild vitamin C deficiency begin insidiously. The patient may show vague digestive disturbances—loss of appetite, irregular diarrhea and failure to gain weight—associated with pallor, apathy, irritability and possibly an increased susceptibility to infection. These symptoms disappear following adequate treatment with vitamin C, but if no therapy is given the full syndrome of manifest scurvy (severe vitamin C deficiency) develops, often with alarming abruptness.

Manifest scurvy is not rare among infants and, like the subclinical form of the disease, occurs more frequently than is recognized. The infant appears pale, listless and unhappy. He may have a peculiarly alert and worried expression, and cries when approached. He makes no effort to kick or play. Growth may be mildly retarded; weight is usually even more abnormal, often 10 to 20 per cent below average, but it may be spuriously high due to the presence of edema. The soft tissues are flabby and muscle tone is decreased.

Swelling of the extremities, due to subperiosteal hemorrhage, is a common finding. It appears suddenly, frequently at the lower end of the femur, and is produced by trauma which is often so mild as to be unrecognized. Pain and tenderness may be localized at the swelling or may extend over the entire extremity. The position assumed by the infant often bears a close relationship to the site involved: infants with subperiosteal hemorrhages in both thighs and legs generally assume the "pithed frog" position, with thighs semiflexed and externally rotated, and the legs semiflexed at the knee joints. The fingers, wrists, toes and, less often, the ankles may be moved spontaneously even when the rest of the extremity exhibits a pseudo-paralysis. At the costochondral junctions scurvy produces a chain of tender enlargements. These swellings may be rounded, or they may exhibit a sharp ridge where the cartilage and bone meet. In extreme cases, the entire sterno-chondral plate is often displaced posteriorly. Submetaphyseal infractions, the so-called "epiphyseal separations," are common in severe cases. They may be shown by crepitus or by roentgen examination, but should be suspected clinically by the persistence of localized tenderness after treatment has relieved the generalized tenderness.

Lesions of the gums are characteristic of scurvy. They are more severe when teeth are present. The gum appears swollen, congested and dark red or purple. With moderate swelling the surface is smooth and glistening, but later it becomes irregular and friable and hemorrhage occurs readily. In some cases, the swelling is so extensive as to bury the teeth. The breath is fetid and Vincent's infection is common.

Hemorrhage may occur anywhere in the body, giving rise to epistaxis, vomiting of blood, bloody stools, or when it occurs in the brain or abdominal organs, very alarming and confusing symptoms. Orbital hemorrhage, usually unilateral but occasionally bilateral, may cause proptosis. Ecchymoses of the eyelids are common and may be associated with edema. Subconjunctival hemorrhage is rare; the eyeball is usually not affected.

Petechiae and *ecchymoses* of varying size may appear anywhere in the skin, but they are most common where the hydrostatic pressure of the capillaries is elevated or where trauma has been inflicted: the lower extremities, the lower half of the trunk, forearms, face and neck. The miliaria seen in vitamin C deficiency is not specific and its pathogenesis is not known. Although some of the macules are hemorrhagic, the majority are not.

Fever and *increased pulse and respiratory rates* are common in infants with manifest scurvy. Rapid, shallow breathing, out of proportion to the fever and pulse rate, may be due to painfulness of the ribs and costochondral junctions. Hypochromic anemia, unassociated with blood loss, is a common finding. In uncomplicated scurvy the leukocyte and differential counts are normal. The number of platelets is not decreased; bleeding and coagulation times are usually normal, but in severe cases prolongation of either or both may occur. There may be changes in the serum calcium and inorganic phosphorus, but these changes are not constant. Hematuria occurs with great frequency; oliguria is common. Hyalin or granular casts, sometimes blood casts, and pyuria may be found.

Adult Scurvy.—The scurvy of the clipper ship era so vividly described by Hakluyt and Lind is now an infrequent disease. Even now, however, a large general hospital will admit some cases each year and the disease may be endemic in prison camps and homes for the indigent.

Characteristic is the long period (perhaps three months) during which total lack of vitamin C may produce no symptoms other than lassitude, weakness, irritability and an insidious loss of weight. During this time, intercurrent infections or metabolic disorders may precipitate the classic picture, the largest part of which is the result of capillary hemorrhage and anemia. Signs first seen are a sallow complexion and bloating of the face, especially a swelling of the pinnae which may extend into the scalp. Aching pains appear in the muscles at points of stress (usually the calves) and may be followed by painful swelling of the knees and edema of the ankles. Changes in the gums, similar to those seen in severe infantile scurvy, take place, particularly around broken and carious teeth.

Hemorrhages predominate in the general picture, appearing at points of mild trauma and sites of stress. Those in the muscles cause brawny induration and tenderness. Hemorrhages into the muscles are more common in adults than in infants, and may extend into the skin causing wide areas of lividity. Petechiae and ecchymoses occur as in infantile scurvy (see Figs. 65 and 66). Less frequently there are epistaxis, conjunctival, retinal and cerebral hemorrhages. Convulsions and paralyses may result from intracranial extravasation of blood. Bleeding from the gastro-intestinal and genito-urinary tracts is rare except in severe cases. Palpitation, dyspnea and cardiac

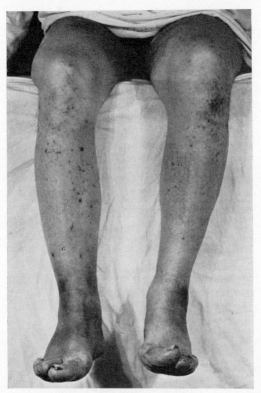

Fig. 65.—Adult scurvy, showing typical distribution of hemorrhagic skin lesions. The purpuric areas vary greatly in size and large ecchymoses are present over sites particularly subject to trauma.

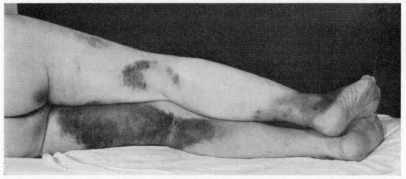

Fig. 66.—Same patient as shown in figure 65. Note extensive ecchymoses over the lower extremities and buttocks.

dilatation may be noted. Vasomotor collapse has been described. Changes in the blood and urine do not differ significantly from those seen in infantile scurvy.

It should be emphasized that scurvy in the infant and in the adult is not a self-limiting disease. If untreated, it will progress to a fatal outcome.

DIAGNOSIS

The diagnosis of manifest scurvy is not difficult. A careful physical examination and a history of inadequate intake of vitamin C may be helpful in making the diagnosis of mild deficiency. Characteristic roentgenologic changes add confirmatory evidence. A positive capillary resistance test suggests depletion of vitamin C, but false positives frequently occur in the presence of severe anemia or blood dyscrasia. Even in severe scurvy, a negative capillary test often occurs. It was thought that plasma levels of ascorbic acid below 0.3 mg. per cent give presumptive evidence of scurvy. Recently, however, it has been indicated that the ascorbic acid content of the white cell-platelet layer of centrifuged blood is much more accurate. When depletion has been severe or long-continued, very little vitamin C is eliminated in the urine and most of a test dose is retained. If the diagnosis is in doubt a therapeutic test is recommended: 250 mg. of ascorbic acid should be given parenterally; the patient should be kept on his usual routine, and should be watched carefully for alteration of symptoms.

TREATMENT WITH ASCORBIC ACID

Chemistry.—Ascorbic acid is a crystalline, colorless, water-soluble compound which melts at 192° C. Its crystalline form is shown in figure 67,

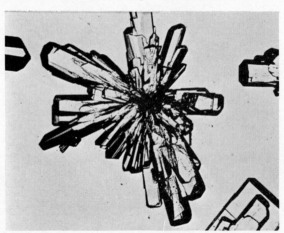

Fig. 67.—Microphotograph showing the structure of crystalline ascorbic acid. (Courtesy of Merck and Company.)

and its structural formula in figure 68. The substance is fairly stable in acidic water solutions which are not exposed to air or contaminating metallic radicals.

Methods of Administration.—Ascorbic acid may be administered orally, intravenously or intramuscularly. Parenteral injection is about twice as effective as oral administration. No difficulty is experienced in bringing ascorbic acid into solution in physiological saline or 5 per cent glucose. Since the solution is strongly acid, the suggestion has been made that it be partially neutralized with sterile sodium bicarbonate for parenteral injection.

In Prevention.—Beginning in the second or third week of life, the infant should be given 1 to 2 teaspoonfuls of fresh orange juice daily. The amount should be increased to 2 ounces by three months of age and to 3 ounces by five months. Other citrus fruit juices may be substituted, but when tomato juice is used, larger amounts must be given. If fruit juices are not tolerated, 25 to 50 mg. of ascorbic acid should be given daily. At least 3

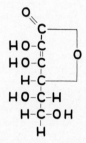

Fig. 68.—Ascorbic acid (*l*-2,3-enediol-gulonic acid lactone).

ounces of orange juice, or comparable amounts of citrus fruit or tomato juice, should be taken daily by the average adult (or 50 to 100 mg. of ascorbic acid). Larger amounts are indicated during pregnancy and lactation.

In Treatment.—For infants, 50 mg. of ascorbic acid q.i.d. orally or 25 mg. b.i.d. intravenously or intramuscularly should be given. For older chil-

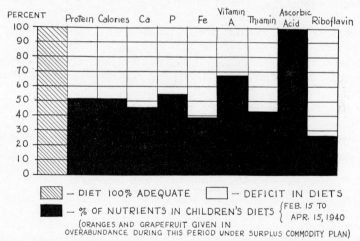

Fig. 69.—The dietaries of fifty children with deficiency diseases compared with an adequate diet.

dren or adults, the recommended amount is 100 mg. three to five times a day orally, or 100 mg. twice a day parenterally. In all cases ascorbic acid therapy should be supplemented by the addition of orange juice, other citrus fruits or tomato juice.

Ascorbic acid has a very low toxicity. Six grams have been given orally, and massive doses of 500 to 1000 mg. have been given intravenously without ill effects. (Vagotonic effects, such as bradycardia, increased peristalsis and erythema, have been described in children but are attributed to idiosyncrasy to ascorbic acid and not to hypervitaminosis.)

It should be emphasized that the present knowledge is so meager that a precise statement of what constitutes proper dosage is not practicable. Since vitamin C deficiency is frequently a part of mixed deficiency diseases, it is not enough to insure an adequate intake of vitamin C alone. Figure 69 illustrates the degree of deficiency of other essential nutrients which may remain after vitamin C deficiency is corrected.

Response to Adequate Therapy with Ascorbic Acid.—Bone tenderness decreases, purpura begins to fade, gums improve, appetite increases, and loss of apprehension occurs within twenty-four hours after adequate parenteral injection of ascorbic acid is given. The general treatment should aim at restoring the patient to a state of perfect nutrition (see section XI).

CLINICALLY LESS WELL-KNOWN VITAMINS

Throughout the vast literature on biology, organic substances are described as being essential to certain species. We know that vitamins are concerned not only with the nutrition of human beings but also with that of lower animals, birds, and many other species. One can neither argue a priori that a deficiency of vitamins will produce certain effects in human beings merely because such a deficiency has produced an effect in animals, nor can one say that organic compounds which are necessary for some lower animal will not prove to be of great importance in understanding the physiology of the higher species. Nevertheless, studies of animals, plants, insects, and bacteria are adding to our understanding of the various factors concerned with human nutrition. The science of nutrition is on the march, and it is likely that many substances important to some form of life are still to be found.

The literature is so filled with ill-defined, often still unnamed vitamins that we cannot list them. Considering the difficult technic used in the isolation of new factors, the progress is rapid indeed. Conservative investigators are of the opinion that the chemical structure of most, if not all vitamins soon will be known and that many, if not all, will be synthesized. Many investigators are concentrating their efforts on the isolation, identification, and synthesis of the various members of the vitamin B complex, and it is in this field that we may expect the most rapid strides in the immediate future. Perhaps the simplest definition of the vitamin B complex is a composite of all the water-soluble vitamins found in yeast and liver, exclusive of ascorbic acid. They are concerned with oxidation and reduction in the cells and with many other biochemical processes. Vitamin B_1 (thiamine), vitamin B_2 (riboflavin), and nicotinic acid have been discussed in preceding sections. Other members of the vitamin B complex may be described as follows: *Vitamin B_3* is a factor necessary for rapid gain in weight and proper nutrition of pigeons. *Vitamin B_4* is necessary for the prevention of a specific paralysis in rats and chicks. *Vitamin B_5* is a factor which is important for maintaining of weight in pigeons. Indications of the existence of many others are too numerous to list. The components of the vitamin B complex have been studied recently and are of considerable interest at this time.

PYRIDOXINE (VITAMIN B₆)

Pyridoxine is crystallized usually as the hydrochloride (see Fig. 70). This compound melts at 204–206° C., is extremely soluble in water and, when so dissolved, has a pH of 2.3. For the formula, see figure 71.

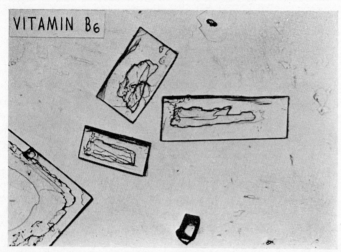

Fig. 70.—Microphotograph showing the structure of crystalline vitamin B₆. (Courtesy of Merck and Company.)

Little work has been done on the site of absorption of pyridoxine. Urine is the only physiological material which has been assayed extensively for this vitamin. Following a test dose of 50 mg., given intravenously to a normal adult, 6 to 10 per cent is excreted during the first hour.

Flexner has recently shown that patients with postencephalitic Parkinson's syndrome showed a subnormal output of pyridoxine following the

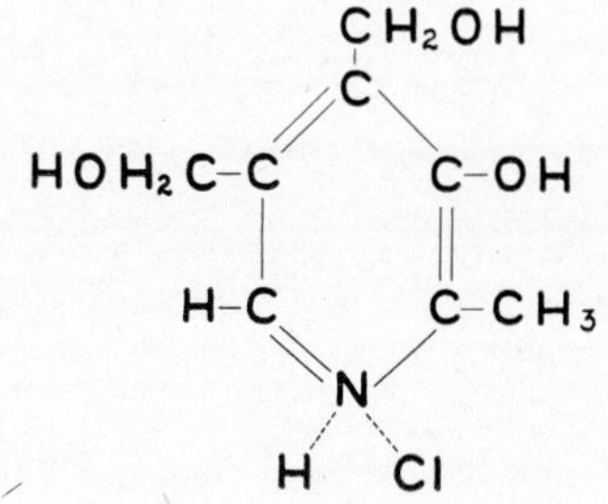

$$C H_2 O H$$
$$C$$
$$H O H_2 C - C \quad C - O H$$
$$H - C \quad C - C H_3$$
$$N$$
$$H \quad Cl$$

Fig. 71.—Pyridoxine (2-methyl-3-hydroxy-4,5-di(hydroxymethyl)pyridinehydrochloride).

intravenous administration of a test dose. Preliminary studies on patients with Parkinson's syndrome by Bean, Emerson and Spies have shown that most of them have reduced excretion of a 50-mg. test dose of pyridoxine.

The toxicity of this substance for human beings is very low; 50 to 100 mg. are commonly given without untoward effect. In some cases, sleepiness or actual sleep follows such an injection. Unna, Sampson, Antopol and

Molitor have shown that rats tolerate 1 gm. per kilogram of body weight without harmful effect; twenty-four hours after a dose of 3.7 gm. per kilo, periodic tonic convulsions occurred and in a few animals continued as long as three weeks.

Spies, Bean and Ashe have described in persons with deficiency diseases a syndrome characterized by nervousness, insomnia, irritability, abdominal pain, weakness, and difficulty in walking, which disappears dramatically following the intravenous administration of pyridoxine. These symptoms were not relieved by therapy with nicotinic acid, thiamine and riboflavin. Our studies on the urinary excretion of pyridoxine show that such persons excrete less than 0.5 per cent of the test dose, whereas the excretion in normal subjects averages 7.9 per cent. Dosage, so far, has been on an empirical basis, and the large amounts given are probably more than is necessary in this type of deficiency. In people with mixed deficiencies who have been treated with other B complex vitamins, it is important to remember that when weakness, lethargy, abdominal pain and ataxia occur, pyridoxine deficiency must be suspected and a therapeutic trial is indicated.

ADENYLIC ACID

Adenylic acid is a purine derived from plant and animal nuclear material. Yeast adenylic acid or adenosine 3-phosphoric acid is a cream-colored amorphous solid which is sparingly soluble in water. It does not melt

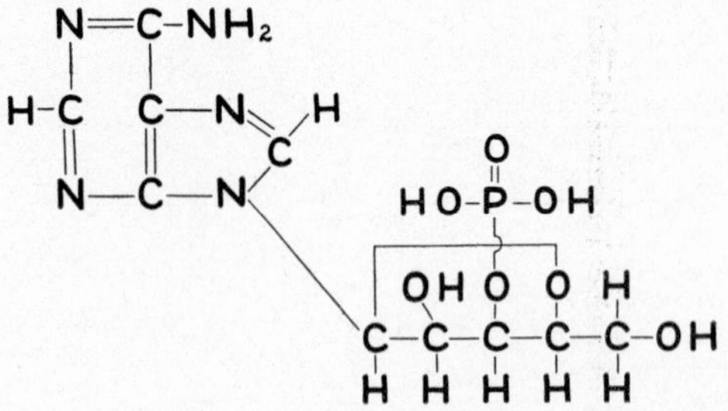

Fig. 72.—Yeast adenylic acid (adenosine 3-phosphoric acid).

sharply but browns and decomposes. The formula is found in figure 72. Muscle adenylic acid (adenosine 5-phosphoric acid) has similar properties.

The tests for adenylic acid are not sufficiently selective to study its absorption from the alimentary tract. The adenylic acid content of the tissues and blood is much higher than that of most vitamin derivatives. It is excreted from the body in various combinations. Adenylic acid is associated with many physiological catalysts and is one of the important structural links in nuclear material.

Adenylic acid prepared from different sources may have the same pharmacological properties in man. Given intravenously, the material has a very striking and unpleasant effect. As little as 3 to 10 mg. may cause a sudden gasp and a deepening of inspiration within ten to twenty seconds after the material is introduced into the vein. Some patients feel a momentary constriction in the chest and epigastrium which is alarming. The sensations subside within two to three minutes. Some persons can tolerate more intravenous adenylic acid than others, for as much as 75 mg. of the substance have been introduced slowly over a period of thirty minutes without ill effect. Prolonged toxicity has never been observed. Doses of 500 to 1000 mg. of adenylic acid, when given orally over a period of several days, do not usually cause toxic symptoms in adults, although a few persons complain of headaches.

It is probable that absorption of adenylic acid from the alimentary tract is poor since a person may have only a very slight response following the oral administration of 200 mg., whereas a very sharp reaction is observed after a small (10-mg.) parenteral dose. Preliminary in vitro studies by Browning, Vilter, Lindblad and Spies have shown that some constituent of gastric juice and duodenal juice splits phosphoric acid from muscle and yeast adenylic acids at pH 8.6. Whether this alters the pharmacological or therapeutic effect is being investigated.

Therapeutic Response.—Following the administration of adenylic acid to a selected series of pellagrins, these observations were made: Ulcerations of the mucous membranes and tongue healed within two to five days; burning sensations of the tongue were relieved within twenty-four hours; body vigor and strength improved within twenty-four hours; peripheral neuritis which had been refractory to therapy with thiamine hydrochloride for several months was improved within ten days to two weeks. After single doses of 50 mg. of adenylic acid, relapses were observed within two to three weeks. Remissions were induced by another injection of adenylic acid.

Yeast adenylic acid (Anheuser-Busch and Fleischmann Laboratories) and muscle adenylic acid (Ernst Bischoff Company, and prepared by Dr. Fritz Schlenk) have similar properties, though recent studies show that the latter may be more effective clinically.

We have observed that adenylic acid has brought about improvement in ulcers of mucous membranes which did not respond to adequate therapy with thiamine hydrochloride, nicotinic acid, and a high protein, high caloric diet. Due to its relatively high toxicity we do not recommend the use of adenylic acid at the present time.

PANTOTHENIC ACID

d-Pantothenic acid is a pale yellow viscous oil that is difficult to purify. The active material is prepared for commercial use in the form of the water soluble calcium salt (see Fig. 73), which is stable in solution and has a pH of approximately 8. The formula of the d-acid is seen in figure 74. Pantothenic acid is present in all plant and animal tissue, and it was from its universal occurrence that it received its name.

Although pantothenic acid has proved essential for the normal development of the rat and chick, little is known of its physiology or function in human beings. It is a normal constituent of the blood and urine. Studies by Spies, Stanbery, Williams, Jukes and Babcock on pantothenic acid in the blood of patients with multiple B complex deficiencies reveal a 25 to 50 per cent reduction from normal. These patients also show a lower urinary excretion. The excretion of pantothenic acid is increased temporarily after parenteral injection or oral administration of the vitamin. The increased concentration in the blood is not sustained for long, except in persons whose initial concentration is low. We have given a large series of persons from 50 to 100 mg. of pantothenic acid daily for more than a month without any evidence of toxicity.

Unpublished observations by Stanbery and Spies show that under similar conditions of study, normal persons excrete a higher percentage of a standard dose of dextrorotatory calcium pantothenate than do persons having typical lesions of nicotinic acid deficiency, thiamine deficiency or riboflavin deficiency. The procedure on the normals and persons with

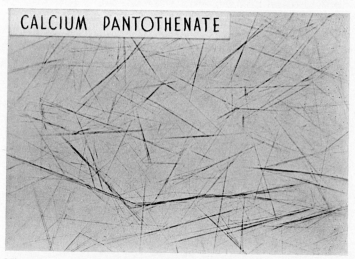

Fig. 73.—Microphotograph showing the structure of crystalline calcium pantothenate. (Courtesy of Merck and Company.)

deficient diets was as follows: A one-hour urine specimen was taken following which 50 mg. of dextrorotatory calcium pantothenate (Merck), dissolved in 5 cc. of sterile distilled water, were injected intravenously. The entire urinary output for the following four hours was collected. These urine specimens were assayed for pantothenic acid by means of the microbiological method. (The error in this method is approximately 10 per cent.)

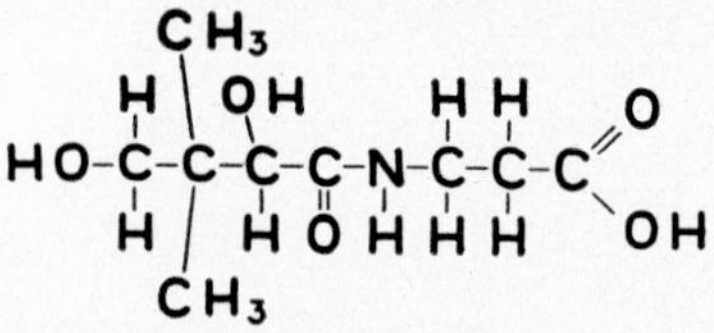

Fig. 74.—Pantothenic acid (N-(α,γ-dihydroxy-β,β-dimethylbutyryl)-β-alanine).

Since the hour-to-hour variation in pantothenic acid excretion has not been determined, we arbitrarily multiplied the amount excreted in the preinjection sample by four and subtracted this quantity from the amount found in the four-hour postinjection sample. The result was expressed as per cent of the 50 mg. which were excreted. The average excretion of persons with vitamin deficiency was 19 per cent, whereas the average excretion of controls was 102 per cent.

Pantothenic acid has been reported as the anti-gray hair factor* for certain animals under experimental conditions. Stanbery and Spies have administered it over a period of four to six months to six persons with gray hair. In no case did the hair change to its original color. Occasionally, in giving liver extract or yeast, or one of the specific chemical vitamins, such as nicotinic acid, along with an improved diet, we have noticed a great change in the hair. It has appeared younger in texture and in rare instances has returned to its original pigment content. Such cases showing changes, however, are extremely rare; we have seen only a few among several hundred treated and observed. It would seem unwarranted to allow claims for any of these substances as being a specific therapeutic agent for the treatment of gray hair.

INOSITOL

Inositol is a colorless, water-soluble crystalline solid that melts at 247° C. It is a saturated cyclic compound with some carbohydrate properties, but without the reducing power of a sugar. Its formula is found in figure 75.

The different tests for inositol have not had wide application, and therefore very little is known of its place in plant and animal physiology. The

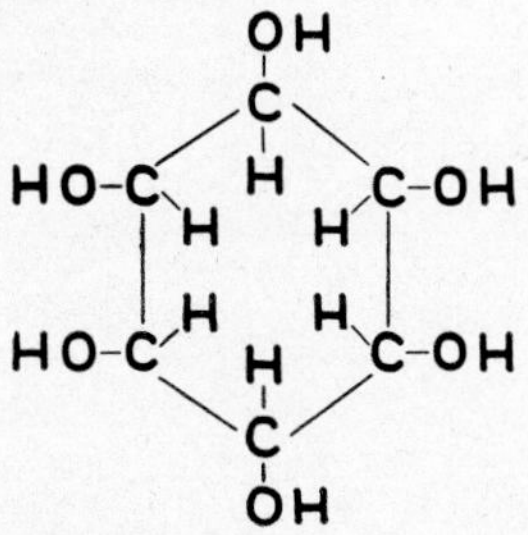

Fig. 75.—Inositol (hexahydroxycyclohexane).

content of inositol and its phosphoric acid ester, phytin, is high in the average diet, but normally most of it is oxidized or otherwise destroyed in the body and only a small part is excreted in the kidneys. Inositol is present in blood, muscle, heart and liver, and probably in other tissues. Its toxicity is apparently very low, since it has been reported that no harmful effects followed the ingestion of a dose as large as 50 gm. Woolley has recently found this substance curative in mouse alopecia. Its rôle in human physiology is not known. We have given 50 mg. inositol a day for a week to normal adults and pellagrins without evidence of toxic symptoms. We have not as yet tested it for physiologic properties in man.

BIOTIN

Biotin, a growth-stimulating substance, has been separated from the bios complex of vitamin-like growth factors. Its physiological activity has been investigated in lower forms of plant and animal life, and its occurrence in mammalian tissue forecasts wide importance. Recently, biotin has been shown to possess the biological activity previously ascribed to vitamin H (the egg-white injury factor), and coenzyme R.

* See Addendum, p. 502, second item.

The chemical properties of biotin were first described by Kögl who crystallized small quantities of it from egg yolk. According to this investigator, it has a basic nitrogen, a carboxyl group, and is amphoteric. Analysis of the compound has given the following empirical formula, $C_{11}H_{18}O_3N_2S$. The methyl ester crystallizes readily (see Fig. 76), melts at 148° C. and is physiologically active. Biotin is destroyed by benzoylation and acetylation, but not by methylation or by boiling with acid or alkali. Nitrous acid destroys the compound at the same rate as it does alpha amino acids.

When rats are kept on diets containing uncooked egg-white, they develop a characteristic syndrome known as *egg-white injury*. Continued feeding of this diet ultimately results in the death of the animal. It has been demonstrated that the injuries produced by such diets are not due to any direct toxic action of the egg-white, but result from an interaction of a specific protein, avidin, present in the egg-white with the biotin of the diet.

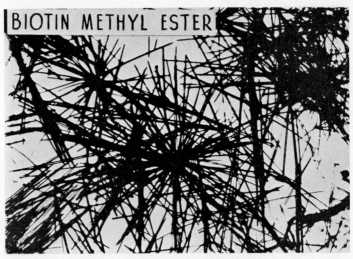

Fig. 76.—Microphotograph showing the structure of crystalline methyl ester of biotin. (Courtesy of Dr. Vincent duVigneaud, Dr. Klaus Hofmann and Dr. D. B. Melville.)

As a result, the biotin is rendered unavailable to the animal and a biotin deficiency develops, producing the typical "egg-white injury" syndrome. Highly concentrated preparations of avidin are just as effective as the original egg-white in producing the biotin deficiency.

In unpublished observations, Spies and Eakin have found subnormal biotin levels for the bloods of some patients who have been living on diets very poor in the B vitamins, but no clinical symptoms have been found which can definitely be associated with these low biotin values. They have also found that the urinary biotin excretion drops when patients are placed on diets containing raw egg-white. The biotin output of one patient who was kept on such a diet for a month was less than one-tenth the base-line value.

Biotin is a normal component of human tissue and excretory products. It is present in beef liver in a combined form from which it can be released by hydrolysis. Its function in human nutrition is unknown.

CHOLINE

Choline is a colorless base (see Fig. 77) which is usually crystallized as the hydrochloride. It is water soluble and stable in acid solution, but is split by strong alkali. The free base is strongly alkaline, absorbing carbon dioxide readily from the air. Choline is present in large quantities in the animal body as a constituent of the phospholipid, lecithin, and of acetylcholine.

The pharmacological actions of choline and its more powerful derivative, acetylcholine, have been exhaustively investigated. These compounds are vasodilators; they cause a fall in blood pressure and have a profound secretagogue effect. This effect does not seem to be exhausted by continuous functioning, because choline can be perfused through an isolated stomach and will stimulate steady secretion.

There is no evidence of toxic symptoms following the administration of 50 mg. choline daily for a week. We have not as yet tested it for physiologic properties in man.

In dogs and rats, choline deficiency causes the development of fatty livers, and choline is said to prevent the excessive deposition of neutral

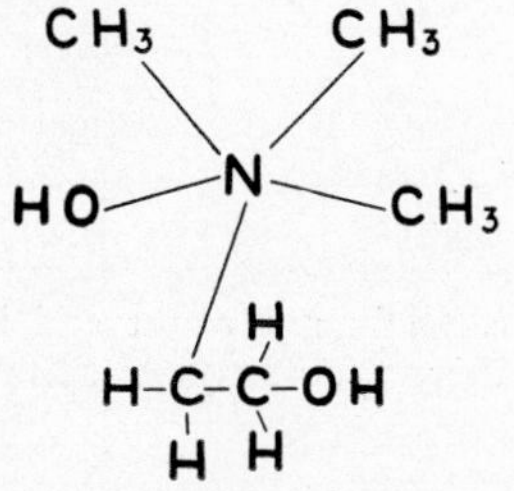

Fig. 77.—Choline (trimethyl-β-hydroxyethyl ammonium hydroxide).

fats and to aid in the synthesis of the phosphatides in the livers of these animals. A comparable deficiency has not been described in man.

"EXTRINSIC FACTOR"

Prolonged deficiencies of B complex vitamins which affect other organs and systems so dramatically often leave characteristic changes in the cellular elements of bone marrow and blood. Castle's classic experiments on the etiology of macrocytic anemia showed that an extrinsic factor (the food factor) and an intrinsic factor (the stomach factor) were essential to proper maturation of erythrocytes. Without the erythrocyte maturation factor, formed from the intrinsic and extrinsic factors and stored in the liver, the red cells in the bone marrow are arrested at the megaloblast stage and a macrocytic anemia occurs. It was considered probable that a deficiency of either the extrinsic or the intrinsic factor could bring about macrocytic anemia, and Castle concluded from his studies that Addisonian pernicious anemia was due to intrinsic deficiency.

Several observers have noted and reported isolated cases of macrocytic anemia occurring in persons on grossly deficient diets. Spies and Chinn were able to produce such an anemia in two epileptics who were maintained on a diet deficient in B complex vitamins for several months (see Fig. 78). A high protein diet restored the red blood cells to normal. Spies and Payne, and Sydenstricker, Schmidt, Geeslin and Weaver recognized the frequent association of macrocytic anemia and pellagra, and independently demonstrated the presence of intrinsic factor in the gastric juice of these pellagrins

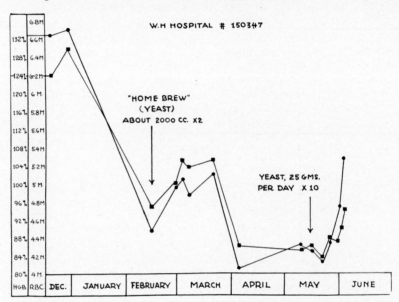

Fig. 78.—Figure shows the fall in red count and hemoglobin in an epileptic on a vitamin B deficient diet, and the response to the administration of yeast on two occasions.

(see Fig. 79). These demonstrations eliminated intrinsic factor deficiency as the cause of these macrocytic anemias. The investigations of Wills have indicated that a food factor other than the "extrinsic factor" may also be

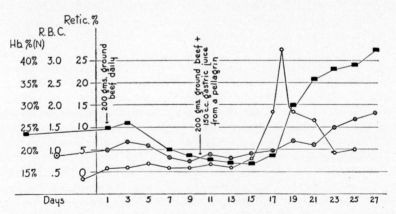

Fig. 79.—Hematopoietic response of patient with pernicious anemia to beef incubated with gastric juice from a pellagrin.

necessary for the maturation of red blood cells. She demonstrated that persons with nutritional macrocytic anemia in India did not respond to treatment with highly concentrated liver extracts which contained large amounts of the erythrocyte maturation factor, but did respond with characteristic reticulocytosis when given crude liver extract or yeast products.

Moore, Vilter and Spies analyzed the cellular elements of the blood and bone marrow in ten persons with severe macrocytic anemias, coexisting with nicotinic acid, thiamine or riboflavin deficiency states. These studies showed that macrocytic anemia of all degrees may be encountered in persons who subsist on grossly deficient diets. It may rival neglected pernicious anemia in severity. They found erythrocyte counts as low as 1,000,000, with the hemoglobin high in comparison and a color index above 1. The mean corpuscular volume, mean corpuscular hemoglobin, and mean corpuscular hemoglobin concentration per unit of cell indicated that the cells were large and well-filled with hemoglobin. Blood smears showed variations in size and shape of red cells with the large cells predominating. The white blood counts were usually low or low normal; the platelets were reduced in number; a relative lymphocytosis was present frequently; and the polymorphonuclear leukocytes were hypersegmented. The degree of reticulocytosis (less than 1 per cent to 10 per cent) seemed to depend upon whether or not the diet of the patient had improved recently.

The bone marrow biopsies taken from these patients were indistinguishable from those found in Addisonian pernicious anemia. Megaloblasts and early erythroblasts predominated and there was a general decrease in activity of the myeloid series of cells and of the megakaryocytes.

The gastric juice contained small amounts of free hydrochloric acid following histamine, except in two cases where there was a total achlorhydria. Intrinsic factor was present as was demonstrated by incubation of the gastric juice with raw ground beef and feeding the mixture to known cases of pernicious anemia with subsequent characteristic reticulocytosis.

These patients responded with a significant reticulocytosis and RBC rise when one-half pound of raw beef was added to their deficient diets for ten days, or when reticulogen (concentrated liver extract) was administered intravenously. The studies suggest that an extrinsic factor deficiency was responsible for the anemia which did not improve following the administration of nicotinic acid, thiamine, riboflavin, pyridoxine or pantothenic acid.

Unpublished observations by Moore, Vilter, Minnich and Spies show that the oral administration of a 70 per cent alcoholic solution of beef, in amounts of a few cubic centimeters each day for ten days, to persons with nutritional macrocytic anemia results in an increase in reticulocytes up to 25 per cent, followed by a rise of hemoglobin and red cells. These unpublished observations also strongly suggest that we are dealing with a pure extrinsic type of macrocytic anemia.

In summary, mild or severe macrocytic anemia occurs rather frequently in persons with nicotinic acid deficiency (see Fig. 80), thiamine deficiency, riboflavin deficiency, or pyridoxine deficiency. The anemia is morphologically similar to pernicious anemia, but the gastric juice of these persons contains intrinsic factor and usually small amounts of free hydrochloric acid. Malnourished persons with macrocytic anemia show no improvement in peripheral blood or bone marrow when they remain on their deficient diets and receive supplements of nicotinic acid, thiamine, riboflavin, pyridoxine, or pantothenic acid. The administration of one-half pound of ground raw beef or 0.5 cc. of concentrated liver extract ($7\frac{1}{2}$ U.S.P. units) intravenously daily for ten days will produce reticulocytosis and the red blood cell count will rise. A high protein diet or 2 ounces of dried brewers' yeast powder or liver extract per day for several months will induce a remission. The available evidence suggests that the anemia is caused by a deficiency of extrinsic factor.

THE HUMAN DIET AND MIXED DEFICIENCY DISEASES

For the student who would understand some of the problems facing the physician who must treat patients with mixed deficiency diseases, it is essential that he think in terms of a new field of medicine, the science of nutrition. It is a field concerned primarily with the proper nourishment of the individual cells. Because it is growing rapidly, information is often sketchy and uncertain; it lacks stability in nomenclature, and many of the problems concerned are still in dispute. Accordingly, we shall not touch on the alarming number of conflicting hypotheses, but will discuss the problems which invite the physician's study because of their practical value.

The respiration and growth of cells involve the synthesis of complex substances from simpler chemical compounds. By means of substances called *enzymes*, the cells are able to perform these functions without increased temperature and pressure. Enzymes are catalysts produced by living cells from combinations of organic substances, including the vitamins. These enzymes retain activity even when separated from the living cell. When a dietary deficiency of vitamins has existed over a long period of time, a biochemical lesion develops in the cell, often severe enough to cause functional disturbances. If the deficiency is not corrected, these disturbances become more widespread and eventually give rise to an infinite variety of symptoms forming a complex clinical picture. Finally, severe or persistent alterations lead to structural changes in the tissue, and ultimately the diagnostic lesions of a deficiency disease are likely to appear. The complexity of the subject is greatly increased by the fact that the several groups of the various vitamins usually occur together in nature, and the failure to provide one usually results in failure to provide many. Then, one has arising from a dietary fault innumerable vague, indefinite symptoms coming from cells affected because a number of catalysts are not working efficiently.

Often isolation and synthesis of a new vitamin shake the whole structure of medical theory to its foundation, and usually brings new hope to the sick and afflicted. Unfortunately, the application of these findings with vigor and enthusiasm has led to thinking too much in terms of isolated vitamin deficiencies, although *every method of study has indicated the predominance of mixed rather than single deficiency* of elements essential for life and well-being. So great has been the interest aroused by the recent discoveries among the laity and physicians alike that today everyone knows something about the vitamins. Investigation of the diets of large groups of people correlated with laboratory studies and direct experimentation has led to the startling observation that the margin of safety against deficiency disease is narrow rather than broad, that the presence of nutritional inadequacy is widespread and not limited to the lower economic group. As information is increasing, it is found that relatively few people in the United States consistently eat diets that are adequate in all respects.

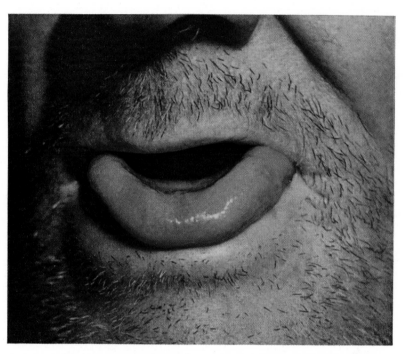

Fig. 80.—Tongue of an individual with mixed pernicious anemia and nicotinic acid amide deficiency. Note the erythema of the papillae with flattening, and the slick, almost gelatinous surface. There are several areas (pellagrous) of distinct hyperemia with a localized increased redness in the tongue. These red areas blanched shortly after nicotinic acid therapy, although there was no change in the papillae or the rest of the tongue.

PRIMARY ETIOLOGY

Studies of the food consumed by families in various sections of the country show that the chief difference between the better diets and the poor diets lies in the amount of milk, lean meat, fresh vegetables and fruit included. Table 2, showing the results of an analysis of diets eaten by per-

TABLE 2

FOODS CONSUMED BY PERSONS ON DEFICIENT DIETS IN CONTRAST TO RECOMMENDED
LOW COST DIET

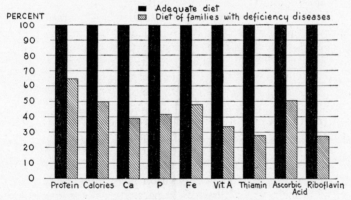

*Adequate diet: Stiebeling, Hazel K., and Clark, Faith: Good Diets at Low and Moderate Costs. Food and Life, Yearbook of Agriculture, 1939, p. 332.

■■■ — In the low cost diet, this represents the amount of each food recommended. In the diets of persons with deficiency diseases it represents the fractions of these amounts actually consumed.

☐ — This represents the difference between the food theoretically needed and that actually consumed by persons with deficiency diseases.

sons with varying degrees of deficiency diseases, indicates how truly serious the deficiency states may be in some areas of the country. Table 3 impresses

TABLE 3

AVERAGE DIETARIES OF FAMILIES WITH DEFICIENCY DISEASES COMPARED WITH AN
ADEQUATE DIET

The degree of nicotinic acid deficiency in the dietaries cannot be evaluated from the data on the nicotinic acid content of food available at the present time.

The majority of persons in these twenty families had clinical symptoms of pellagra, beriberi, scurvy, riboflavin deficiency, or vitamin A deficiency.

one even more with a comparison of the amounts of nutrients supplied to the same individuals and the estimated normal adequate diet. As reflected in table 2, we have analyzed the diets of a group of persons with deficiency diseases who have come under our observation. It is obvious that although these people may have had one outstanding deficiency disease syndrome, they actually were suffering from mixed deficiency diseases operating simultaneously. The average dietary of this group, classed as consuming poor

16

diets, furnished only 50 per cent of their estimated energy requirement. Assuming 0.5 gm. protein per kilo per day to be the maintenance requirement, their intake was only 35 per cent of this amount. Although the average person received 0.68 gm. protein per kilo of body weight, an amount above the theoretical maintenance requirement, only 5 per cent of the group had an optimum intake of 1 gm. per kilo. The total protein intake in at least 35 per cent of the cases studied was too low to maintain nitrogen equilibrium. Whether this results in a specific or general amino acid deficiency is uncertain, but it should be corrected if health is to be restored. Nearly all of these persons received substandard amounts of calcium, phosphorus and iron, and none obtained adequate amounts of all three elements.

The vitamin deficiencies in these dietaries were, on the whole, greater than those of other nutrients and the degree of the deficiency in the B complex vitamins was greater than that of any other vitamins. The thiamine and riboflavin intakes were only 28 per cent and 27 per cent, respectively, of the suggested standards. The nicotinic acid and pyridoxine content of a dietary cannot be estimated from the data available and man's requirement for them is not definitely known. Since the factors of the B complex are closely associated in natural foodstuffs, it is reasonable to assume that they, too, were present in amounts considerably below those required. The vitamin A content of the dietaries was 33 per cent of the requirement suggested for this vitamin. The deficiency of vitamin C, which was 53 per cent of standard, appears to be less severe than in the case of the other vitamins. It is to be noted, however, that these figures represent the average intake of a group of fifty patients. Several persons consumed diets in which there were no vitamin C-containing foods.

Why should this country, called by poets and statesmen "a land of plenty" provide a daily fare that is often inadequate for poor and rich alike? The average individual fails to appreciate the relation of food to health. Some diets become deficient through habit. In many instances, the knowledge of food values in relation to food cost is erroneous and the nutritive return on the money spent is paltry. On the other hand, the pauper's income, if any, provides the pauper's diet which, no matter how carefully it may be chosen, cannot supply the minimum food requirements. We are convinced that this last factor is an important cause of deficiency diseases among persons living in areas in which these diseases are endemic.

To take the passive stand that these people must continue to have deficiency diseases until there is a revolution in economic affairs is of course a counsel of despair—a socialist's nightmare. It is not too much to expect, however, that changes in the processing of foodstuffs or even the addition of essential elements as a nutritional subsidy may do much toward alleviating this burden of civilization. A noteworthy paper by Baker, Wright and Drummond traces the increasing use of white flour to the introduction of silk bolting cloth in 1840 and of roller mills in 1870 to satisfy greater demand. They estimate that "the best fed members of the population today are getting twice as much vitamin B_1 as people on a low income level, yet consume less vitamin B_1 than the parish poor of the eighteenth and early nineteenth centuries." We are realizing more and more that decortification of grain is dangerous, that there must be some change in milling methods. Greater care in guarding against loss of vitamins and minerals through processing, marketing and storing of foods would undoubtedly improve the quality of many diets. Among low income groups especially, education is necessary in respect to the use of evaporated and dried milk, and in the use of larger quantities of the less expensive green and yellow vege-

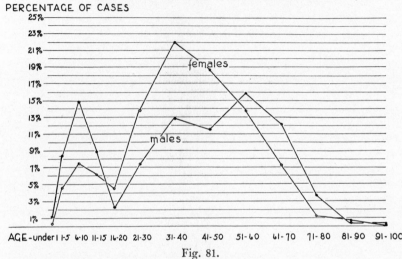

AGE INCIDENCE OF DEFICIENCY DISEASES IN MALES AND FEMALES
(IN THE SERIES OF 2187 CASES OF DEFICIENCY DISEASE THERE WERE 741 MALES AND 1446 FEMALES)

Fig. 81.

tables, fruits, tomatoes, potatoes, legumes and nuts—foods that yield excellent nutritive returns at a relatively low cost.

SECONDARY ETIOLOGY

The primary etiology of deficiency states occurring in the average person has already been discussed. This is to be modified by the knowledge that individual requirements for vitamins and minerals vary greatly. It is known that under altered environment or increased activity there may be increased need and more rapid destruction, diminished absorption and impaired utilization of the protective materials. Thus, a period of rest in bed without change in diet has caused the remission of symptoms in many pellagrins, symptoms which recur with resumption of normal activity.

A consideration of the changes in requirements wrought by altered environment introduces the secondary causes of nutritional deficiency. Because of the narrow margin of safety these may appear rapidly under the burden of acute or chronic infection, not only through infection per se but also as a result of the regimen to which the patient is subjected. Observations by Bean and Spies have shown that in an area where pellagra is endemic, approximately 10 per cent of the patients with clinical evidence of deficiency disease had some form of chronic diarrhea, including cases with partial intestinal obstruction, carcinoma of the rectum, colon, stomach, stricture of lymphopathia, bacillary dysentery, sprue, ulcerative colitis, intestinal tuberculosis, and gastrocolic fistula.

Extensive studies during the past eleven years of nonalcoholic and non-endemic cases of pellagra in Cleveland and Cincinnati have indicated that many diseases predispose to or precipitate this syndrome. This isolated observation merely confirms the long-established belief that a number of factors are usually involved in the production of clinical vitamin deficiency diseases. In 85 such cases in which alcoholism and deficient diets were excluded as the primary factors leading to pellagra, we found 28 cases secondary to acute or chronic infection with organic lesions of the alimentary canal, 18 associated with congestive heart failure, 10 with hyperthyroidism, diabetes mel-

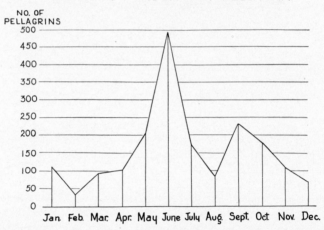

Fig. 82.—This figure shows the monthly incidence of pellagra. This curve is essentially the same for all deficiency diseases arising from lack of the water-soluble vitamins. Note the high peak in the summer and the secondary peak in the fall. Early symptoms of deficiency disease appear months before the average patient seeks a doctor. If the doctor would treat malnourished persons throughout the year rather than await the appearance of the full-blown clinical syndrome in the summer and fall, such peaks would tend to disappear.

litus, and other metabolic disorders, and 10 with miscellaneous diseases. We have not included patients in whom lactation and pregnancy were possible factors.

Therapeutic diets, like many drugs, are fine for the disease, faulty for the patient. Reducing diets, diets given to patients with alimentary tract disease, allergy, hypertension, nephritis, or heart disease frequently tend insidiously to produce deficiency diseases. Too often the patient is told what he must not eat but not what he may eat and, as a result, he chooses a grossly inadequate diet.

In summary, pellagra or other vitamin deficiency states may follow those conditions which prevent the normal intake, digestion, absorption, storage, or utilization of vitamins. On the other hand, these states may succeed conditions associated with an elevated metabolic level and an unsatisfied increase in the vitamin requirements of the body. These factors may operate singly or in combination, and may be enhanced by the restricted regimen prescribed by the physician for the patient.

CLINICAL FEATURES

The clinical picture presented by deficiency diseases is extremely complex. The ill informed might contend that persons who do not have pellagra, beriberi or scurvy have an adequate amount of nicotinic acid, thiamine and ascorbic acid. However, investigators in the field of nutrition have incontrovertible evidence that there is a wide gap between the amount of these substances needed to prevent the well-defined, usually terminal clinical signs of deficiency, and the optimum amount necessary to insure full health and vigor. It may well be said that subnormal or borderline nutritional states are those which occur most frequently and are least frequently recognized.

These early symptoms and signs are not well-defined and have been constantly attributed to a deficiency of one or another of the individual vitamins. Deficiency symptoms may not appear for several months or years after deprivation has started or they may appear after only a few weeks, particularly if some precipitating factor arises. The intensity of each likewise is variable. The *prodromal symptoms* common to many of the vitamin deficiencies, and hence to mixed deficiency, are loss of weight and strength, insomnia, depressed mental states and lassitude, nervousness and irritability, headaches, diarrhea, abdominal cramps, anorexia, indigestion, heartburn, vague paresthesias. It is to be noted that these symptoms have been ascribed individually at various times to a deficiency of vitamin B_1, nicotinic acid, vitamin B_6, riboflavin, vitamin C and vitamin E.

A most important aid in discovering mixed deficiency is the constant suspicion that where there are clear evidences of one deficiency there must certainly be some signs, perhaps veiled, of other specific deficiency states. It must be stated repeatedly that pure clinical pictures produced by the lack of a single vitamin rarely exist (except perhaps vitamins D and K). The classical pictures of beriberi, of pellagra, of scurvy have always been described as separate entities for the purposes of recognition and of specific therapy.

DIAGNOSIS

Because deficiency diseases are progressive rather than self-limited, and because we possess specific remedies for their prevention, the importance of early diagnosis and therapy cannot be overemphasized. Recognition generally is not difficult for those who have seen cases, but it is not easy for one who has gleaned the symptomatology from textbooks. It is our experience that the physician conversant with the literature from a theoretical standpoint frequently fails to diagnose a case, even a typical case, presented to him in the clinic. Where the classic signs are absent and the diagnosis uncertain, the most important aid is a precise knowledge of previous diet, accurate history and physical examinations, and observation of the response of the patient to specific therapy. These diagnostic points of necessity must be kept in mind in relation to the discussions which follow.

Deficiency diseases in adults and *infants and children* are similar, but naturally differ in the interpretation of subjective symptoms according to the mental age of the individual. An adult with scurvy complains of pains in various parts of the body, and bleeding gums. The infant is irritable, refuses to eat, and cries when touched at the tender areas over the bones. The dermatitis, diarrhea, and dementia of the adult pellagrin are characteristic, but the listless infant with enteritis who has failed to gain weight is a familiar problem to the pediatrician and may represent many conditions other than nicotinic acid deficiency. Once again, only a careful dietary analysis of the nursing mother, including knowledge of the diet prior to and during pregnancy, will give a hint as to the nature of the disease. In addition, should her diet be inadequate, one should suspect an iron deficiency anemia and deficiency of the entire B complex. The fact that rickets and vitamin A deficiency and scurvy are less frequently seen even in areas where B deficiency diseases are endemic bears testimony to the benefits derived from the education of parents to the use of cod liver oil and orange juice in infants' diets.

All possible combinations of vitamin and mineral deficiency cannot be described, for they are innumerable and vary with the individual. We have seen patients suspected of having only two or three deficiencies who showed improvement only up to a certain point when given the two or three specific vitamins. In such cases, residual burning of the mouth or paresthesias of the extremities may be relieved by adenylic acid; or refractory nervousness, abdominal cramps, and muscular rigidity may respond to vitamin B_6; again, insomnia, tinnitus and neuromuscular symptoms may cease only upon the administration of alpha-tocopherol.

The following representative history of Mr. and Mrs. Z. and family with clinically associated deficiency diseases is rather typical of affected families living in the rural areas in which these diseases are endemic. The studies extended through the calendar years of 1939 and 1940.

METHOD OF STUDY

Since all members of a family living together tend to eat a similar diet, a number of years ago we adopted the policy of studying an entire family. All members of the family were asked to report to the hospital at least once a month, and those in ill health were urged to come more frequently. Repeated clinical and laboratory examinations were made both in the home and in the clinic or, when the patient was severely ill, on the hospital ward. The dietary surveys included visits to the home, where the methods of food preparation and the types of food used were observed. A record of the actual food intake of each member of the family was kept for a period of one week. Special chemical, physiological, and bacteriological tests were done on the blood and urine, and sometimes nerves and muscles were biopsied before, during and after therapy. Even though we had excellent laboratory facilities available and experts in various fields collaborated with us to aid in interpreting our findings, we placed ourselves in the position of the general practitioner and studied our patients as they came to us. Whenever a diagnosis of a deficiency disease was made on any one patient, our studies were extended to include his family as a whole.

The physicians contributing to the study were: Dr. T. D. Spies, Dr. R. W. Vilter, Dr. W. B. Bean, Dr. C. D. Aring, Dr. K. Ascher, Dr. Milton Rosenbaum, Dr. C. V. Moore, Dr. S. T. Wright, Dr. R. A. Moore, Dr. J. W. MacQueen, Dr. J. B. McLester, Dr. T. S. Booser, Dr. F. A. Dowdy, Dr. B. Morris, Dr. H. H. Henderson, Dr. E. D. Warner, Dr. J. R. Knott, Dr. H. E. Himwich, Dr. F. H. Lewy, and Dr. John Bradley. The chemists included S. P. Vilter, A. E. Axelrod, S. R. Stanbery, A. P. Swain, Y. Sasaki, R. K. Ladisch, and E. K. Browning. Bacteriologists: M. B. Koch, J. W. Riddle, and Gordon Morey. Dentist: A. W. Mann. Social worker: Nelwyn Huff. Dietitian: J. M. Grant. Nurses: Verna Moore, Monette Springer, and Jane M. Mann. Technical scientific assistance was rendered by V. Minnich, J. Martin, C. A. Owen, J. F. Fazekas, S. Nesin, and T. S. Magruder. We are indebted for expert advice in various aspects of our study to Dr. C. A. Elvehjem, Dr. R. J. Williams, Dr. N. P. Hudson, Dr. Gladys Emerson, Dr. Harry Goldblatt, Dr. Zola Cooper, Dr. Leon Jonas.

ECONOMIC STATUS

Mr. Z., a thirty-year-old white man, his wife, twenty-eight years old, and four children, one, three, four, and five years of age, lived on a ten-acre farm which he owned. Approximately one-half the land was planted in cotton, two acres in corn, and the rest in pasture and garden. They had one cow, one mule, two hogs, two dogs, and a cat. Their cash income for the year was seldom more than $12 from their cotton crop. They lived in a two-room cabin. In the kitchen a small wood stove used for cooking was the only source of heat. Fuel was scarce. In the winter the walls were covered with newspapers to keep out the wind. In the room used as a bedroom the three oldest children slept in a single bed and the parents and baby in a double bed. A dilapidated table and three old chairs were the only other pieces of furniture in the two rooms.

DIETARY HISTORY

As nearly as could be ascertained this dietary history is typical of their habits for at least the past six years: During the summer they ate green vegetables from the garden, but before fall the garden was usually "burned out." Mrs. Z. canned about two dozen quart jars of vegetables each year but could not can more as she had no more jars and could not afford to buy more. The supply of canned vegetables never lasted beyond Christmas. During the winter they lived on black-eyed peas and dried beans which they grew, cornmeal, wheat flour, part of the meat from one hog they slaughtered, and sorghum syrup for which they traded the rest of their meat. The cow went dry a month or so after the calf was born, and the family had no milk the rest of the year. The two dogs and cat ate scraps from the family meals and rustled what they could. The children were very fond of candy and ate as much of it as possible. The parents dipped snuff whenever they could get a few pennies to buy it.

HISTORY OF ILLNESS (MRS. Z.)

One of the neighbors, who had been insane from pellagra and had returned home from a mental hospital after we treated her with nicotinic acid, told Mrs. Z. that she too had pellagra, and suggested that she come to us for treatment. At first, she was afraid to come. She was ashamed to think she might have a disease which in her neighborhood was considered a disgrace. Finally, early in April, her husband persuaded her to come to us. By this time, she said she was crazy and that she would "kill the kids if she could find them." She could not remember where they were.

In January or February of each year for several years, Mrs. Z. began to feel bad and each year felt a little worse than the previous year. By March, she began to have trouble with her stomach. Everything she ate caused pain and burning. She felt that she could drink milk, but they had no milk and could not afford to buy it. She lost all desire for food and could "scarcely stand to smell it cooking." Her tongue began to "burn" and became increasingly worse until it felt as if it had been scalded with boiling water and "nearly killed her" when she tried to eat. She lost weight and strength. Although she felt tired all the time, she could not rest. She worried constantly about her husband and children, and was afraid something was going to happen to them. She was irritable and cross, and although she loved her husband and children they "got on her nerves" and she felt as if she would have to run away. She could not stand having people around, yet when she was alone she wished she was dead. Her head ached terribly all day, and she felt dizzy and confused. It seemed to her that the harder she worked, the less she accomplished. Often when she tried to make bread she could not remember whether or not she had included all the ingredients. Even when it was cold she could not keep the bed covers on her feet because they "burned like fire." She had to get up and walk around frequently, trying to get the cramps out of her feet and legs, but most of the time she just lay in bed and cried with pain.

By March her tongue was red and sore, and the corners of her mouth began to macerate, crack, itch and burn. Some time before, the light began to hurt her eyes so much that she had to keep the shades down all day. When the light first struck her eyes as she walked outdoors, she cried out with pain. The skin on her whole body itched and burned, and she felt as though insects were crawling over it continuously. The skin on her forearms, neck, and ankles became red and sore "like sunburn," although she seldom exposed herself to the sun because she thought it made her worse. During all these months, she had been constipated but by the middle of March began having diarrhea, her bowels moving every hour or so. The soreness of her mouth and tongue became so severe that she could eat very little food. Finally, she became so weak she could scarcely get out of bed.

LABORATORY FINDINGS

Myriads of hemolytic streptococci and staphylococci, and Vincent's organisms were identified in the smears taken from the mucous membrane lesions in the oral cavity and in the vagina of this patient. Streptococcus hemolyticus and hemolytic strains of Staphylococcus aureus were isolated in pure culture from the cheilotic lesions and from some of the ocular lesions. Following the administration of nicotinic acid which healed the mucous membrane lesions, and the administration of riboflavin which healed the cheilosis and ocular lesions, the organisms disappeared rapidly.

Red cell and white cell counts, hemoglobin, and *hematocrit* determinations showed that this patient had a macrocytic anemia. The red cell count was 2.8 million; white cell count, 4200; hemoglobin, 11.6 grams (75 per cent); hematocrit, 34. Sedimentation was faster than normal. Blood smears showed variations in the size and shape of the erythrocytes. This type of macrocytic nutritional anemia, which is not unusual in pellagra, has been studied extensively by the authors. It responds to long-continued dietary treatment, to persistent yeast or liver therapy, or to the oral administration of beef. Apparently it is due to a lack of the extrinsic factor from the diet.

The concentration of *coenzymes* I and II in whole blood was determined, using the biological method of Vilter, Vilter and Spies, which depends upon the specific requirement of H. influenzae for these coenzymes. The coenzymes I and II concentration of the whole blood of this patient, in terms of cozymase equivalents, was 14 gamma/cc. of blood which is lower than the normal average of 31 gamma/cc. Following bed rest and the administration of nicotinic acid, the blood coenzyme values become normal. The coenzyme I content of the erythrocytes was determined, using the Barcroft apparatus. There was a tendency for the coenzyme I content to be slightly lower than the normal, but not strikingly so.

The *plasma prothrombin* level in this patient was normal, whereas in an occasional patient in the clinic, particularly one who has inadequate absorption from the intestine because of diarrhea, there is a slight lowering of the plasma prothrombin level.

Comparative determinations for *oxygen, glucose,* and *lactic acid* were made on the blood from the femoral artery and from the internal jugular vein. The average A:V difference for oxygen was 5.8 per cent, compared with 7.43 per cent in normal subjects. The average difference in the glucose content of the blood from artery and vein was 7.6 mg. per 100 cc. compared to the arterial-venous difference of 14.6 mg. of glucose per 100 cc. in normal persons. There was no difference in the lactic acid content of the arterial and venous blood. These findings suggest a diminished cerebral carbohydrate metabolism and might offer a partial explanation for the mental changes observed.

The concentration of *nicotinic acid* in the blood was studied, using Koch's modification of the Koser and Saunders method, which depends upon the fact that the dysentery bacillus requires for growth nicotinic acid or a compound which acts similarly. At the time this patient had pellagra, repeated daily tests showed that her blood supported growth for the Hiss dysentery bacillus in dilutions of 1:160, which is equivalent to a content of about 0.48 mg. per cent of nicotinic acid or compounds which are physiologically similar. The blood concentration of nicotinic acid in normal persons is about 2 to 3 mg. per cent. Within twenty-four hours following the oral administration of 1000 mg. nicotinic acid, in divided doses, her blood supported growth of the Hiss dysentery in dilutions of 1:320, which is equivalent to about 0.96 mg. per cent of nicotinic acid. After seven days of nicotinic acid therapy, her blood contained 1.92 mg. per cent nicotinic acid. She remained on her usual deficient diet and one month later, the nicotinic acid content of her blood had dropped to 0.96 mg. per cent. This test is not of diagnostic value, but it does give some idea as to the blood level of nicotinic acid in pellagra during relapse and subsequent to nicotinic acid therapy.

The blood concentration of *riboflavin* was determined by a biological method, using the growth of the Lactobacillus casei as an indicator. This patient had a value of 0.48 gamma riboflavin per cc. of whole blood. This method is very accurate, but the test is of no diagnostic value so far as the clinician is concerned, for the blood concentration of riboflavin in persons with a deficiency of this substance shows no significant variation from normal. Pantothenic acid was determined with a modified procedure, for the same strain of L. casei requires both pantothenic acid and riboflavin for growth. The method has been reported in detail by Pennington, Snell and Williams, and we have modified it so that it can be used in the clinic as a test for the blood pantothenic acid concentration. We have found that a high percentage of persons with beriberi, pellagra, or riboflavin deficiency have a low level of pantothenic acid in the blood. The blood *pantothenic acid* for this patient was 0.19 gamma/cc., whereas that of a normal person is 0.23 gamma/cc. Tests were done for *biotin*, but the results were inconclusive.

The whole blood and plasma *ascorbic acid* concentrations were studied, and were found to be considerably lower than normal; in fact, so low as to suggest that the depletion was advanced.

Repeated blood samples showed values within the normal range for calcium, phosphorus and phosphatase.

Serum protein determinations showed a 30 per cent reduction from normal. Many patients in the clinic used as controls did not show this degree of low serum protein. Serum iron determinations were slightly lower than normal. The serum colloid osmotic pressure was variable but appeared to be less than one would anticipate from the serum protein level.

Tests for *albumin and sugar in the urine* were negative. The specific gravity was 1.020. Studies of urinary pigments by the B.E.S. technique revealed ether-soluble red pigments both before and after the addition of nitrites. There was an increase over the normal amount of indican excreted in the urine. These abnormal pigments disappeared or returned to normal levels following treatment with nicotinic acid. Determination of the coenzyme content of the urine revealed an excretion of 0.0 to 3.0 gamma/hour (normal, 3 to 10 gamma/hr.).

Nicotinic acid was excreted in considerably less than normal amounts, when tested by either bacteriological or biochemical methods, although the exact amount is difficult to determine. Thiamine excretion revealed a figure slightly lower than normal for the 24-hour period. The urinary excretion of riboflavin amounted to approximately 1 gamma per hour (normal, 2 to 5 gamma/hr.), and of pantothenic acid, 0.5 gamma per hour which was considerably lower than the normal excretion of 25 gamma per hour. Pyridoxine (vitamin B_6) was excreted in small quantities for the 24-hour period. (Within the first hour following the injection of 50 mg. pyridoxine, only 0.5 per cent was excreted, whereas in normal persons between 6 and 10 per cent is excreted.) The urinary excretion of each of the vitamins was lower than normal before treatment but increased following therapy with each specific crystalline vitamin.

Biopsy sections of muscle are being studied for such evidence of *vitamin E* deficiency as defective striation, swelling of the fibers, and infiltration. The coenzyme I content of muscle was decreased 30 per cent.

Neurologic examination, including chronaximetric determinations, showed that there was considerable polyneuropathy of the motor and sensory nerves. Within 1 to 4 hours following the injection of 50 mg. thiamine, there was quantitative improvement in the electrical excitability of the muscles and in sensitivity to touch and pin prick. This improvement was maintained from one to five days, but the patient slowly regressed and eventually returned to the condition preceding thiamine therapy. Microscopic examination of biopsied peripheral nerves in this patient revealed a marked degeneration and loss of myelin sheaths. The axis cylinders were involved in the degenerative process, to the same degree of severity as the myelin sheaths.

Skin biopsies showed advanced hyperkeratosis with formation of verrucae (see Figs. 83 and 84). There was a focal atrophy of the epidermis, edema of the upper part of the corium, and atrophy of the sebaceous glands. Hyalinization and mucoid degeneration were present in the connective tissue of the deeper corium. The skin all over the body, irrespective of whether it is in the lesion, shows changes.

Gastric analyses were done before and after histamine injections. No free HCl, pepsinogen or rennin was found. The presence of the intrinsic factor of Castle was demonstrated by incubating raw beef with the gastric juice from this patient and giving the mixture for ten consecutive days to a patient with pernicious anemia. (The patient with pernicious anemia had a characteristic reticulocyte response, indicating that the intrinsic factor was present in the gastric juice of the pellagrin.)

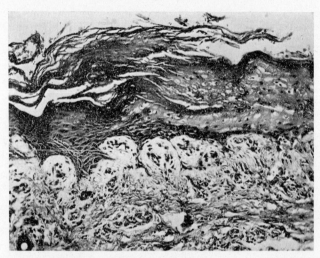

Fig. 83.—Figure shows area in skin in which desquamation has taken place, with the separation of the superficial layer of the epidermis from the underlying tissue. The horny layer of the skin shows marked hyperkeratosis. There is deformity of the papillary layer of the skin.

The *eyes* were examined by the physicians who made the routine examinations in the clinic, and since abnormalities were found, further studies were made, with particu-

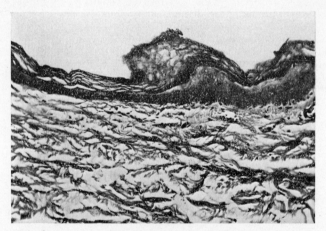

Fig. 84.—This figure shows the same changes as in Fig. 83 in the superficial layer of the skin, with areas of hyperkeratosis and formation of verrucae. The superficial layer in this area has not yet become detached from the underlying skin. There is extensive atrophy of all layers in the skin, with the exception of the superficial horny area. Edema may be seen in the interstitial areas of the subcutaneous tissue, and there is atrophy of the glandular elements.

lar reference to the lesions of the conjunctiva. In addition, ophthalmoscopic studies were made, and the corneal lesions were followed by repeated examination under the slit lamp. Biophotometer and adaptometer tests for vitamin A deficiency were not made.

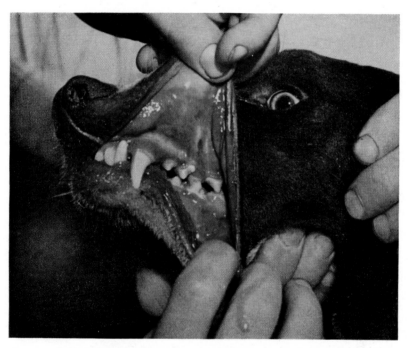

Fig. 85.—This is canine blacktongue. Note the widespread erythema and the local hemorrhages in the mucous membranes of the mouth and gums. Myriads of Vincent's organisms were seen in a smear that was taken from a small ulceration. These Vincent's "patches" disappeared and the erythema healed within 3 days after nicotinic acid therapy.

HOME HISTORY

When Mr. Z. brought his wife to the Nutrition Clinic he, too, was examined. For some time he had been unable to do much work. He complained of loss of appetite, weakness, indigestion, headache and insomnia. He was worried, apprehensive, and depressed. When asked about the children, he said he knew they were not well because they were cross, irritable, ate very little food, and refused to play. Both he and the mother noticed that the nursing infant and the three-year-old child had cracking at the corners of their mouths which their mother thought had been "caught" from her. We suggested that they bring all the children in for examination, but Mrs. Z. refused to let them come because she thought we might "experiment on them." A few days later we visited the home to obtain a dietary history and find out something of the family background. While there, we noticed an emaciated, dejected looking dog, its head hanging low, saliva drooling from its mouth, and so weak that it could not stand up. Mr. Z. said it had been having diarrhea for several days. Examination of the mouth showed redness along the gum margins and the back of the tongue, and ulcerated areas which were sharply demarcated from the surrounding zones of healthy tissue (see Fig. 85). The ulcers were filled with Vincent's organisms. The cat also appeared sluggish and apathetic. It made no effort to move when touched and offered no resistance when an examination of the oral cavity was made. Thick, foul smelling saliva drooled from its mouth; there was an ulcerated reddish margin in the upper part of the palate close to the midline, and the tongue was very red over the terminal portion. Mr. Z. said both animals "got to feeling bad like that every year." They both lived on scraps from the family's meals. The dog was given 50 mg. nicotinic acid t.i.d., and the cat, 40 mg. t.i.d. for two days. At the end of forty-eight hours, they had both improved remarkably.

Mrs. Z. was so impressed by what seemed to her the magic recovery of the dog and cat that she agreed to let Mr. Z. bring the children to the clinic. Examination showed that the two youngest children had cheilosis and injection of the conjunctivae, lesions characteristic of riboflavin deficiency. Pellagrous glossitis and stomatitis were present in all the children but were most severe in the oldest child who also had the typical erythematous dermal lesions of pellagra on her hands and ankles. The father said they had had intermittent diarrhea for the past month. All the children cried when one touched their legs, but the four-year-old child's legs hurt her so much that she cried almost constantly and screamed when she thought anyone was going to touch them.

RESPONSE TO ORAL TREATMENT

We gave Mrs. Z. 2 mg. riboflavin t.i.d. which, in a few days, healed not only her lesions but those of the breast-fed infant. We then gave her nicotinic acid, in doses of 50 mg. ten times daily, and her diarrhea as well as the diarrhea of the infant ceased. Within two days following the administration of 1000 mg. nicotinic acid, her mental symptoms had disappeared, her appetite improved, and she became strong enough to stay up most of the day. The burning in her feet and cramping in her legs and feet continued until she was given intravenous injections, 10 mg. each, of thiamine daily for three days.

Mr. Z. was given 50 mg. of nicotinic acid q.i.d., and the following day he felt strong enough to do his farm work again. Soon after this, he obtained part-time work in a nearby mine and was able to provide a better diet for the family.

The children were treated individually, each child being given specific vitamin therapy for his outstanding deficiency disease. The oldest child who had the dermal lesions, stomatitis and glossitis of pellagra was given nicotinic acid amide, 50 mg. t.i.d., for four days. The four-year-old, who had the severe thiamine deficiency, was given thiamine, 5 mg. t.i.d., for a week, and the two-year-old, in whom the riboflavin deficiency was most severe, was given riboflavin, 2 mg. b.i.d., for a week. As has been pointed out, the breast-fed infant was treated by giving the mother appropriate therapy. In each case, the symptoms for which these substances are specific improved rapidly. After the father was able to provide an improved diet, all their other symptoms disappeared slowly.

In all the members of the family who were given nicotinic acid, the B.E.S. test on their urine, which had been positive before treatment, became negative following therapy with nicotinic acid. An interesting observation was that while pellagra in man and blacktongue in animals respond to the same therapy, urine from the dog with blacktongue did not give a positive B.E.S. test.

Mrs. Z. improved remarkably following treatment and soon began to do her own housework again. Her diet did not improve, however, for although Mr. Z. was earning a little money she gave the additional food it provided to her husband and children while she continued to eat much the same food she had had all winter, except that her appetite improved and she ate more. She was kept under observation by weekly visits to the clinic and frequent visits to her home. Three weeks from the time treatment was discontinued, she began to complain of extreme nervousness, insomnia, irritability, difficulty in walking and pain in her abdomen. She became progressively worse until, at the end of four weeks, she was so weak she was unable to take more than a few steps. We had observed these symptoms in other patients who had been treated with nicotinic acid, riboflavin and thiamine, but who continued to eat their customary inadequate diets and had obtained a beneficial response to pyridoxine. Accordingly, Mrs. Z. was given 50 mg. of pyridoxine, in sterile physiological solution of sodium chloride, intravenously, and within twenty-four hours her symptoms had disappeared and her strength had increased so much that she walked well. She was urged to eat a more varied and liberal diet and has, to a certain extent, done so. When she was last seen, two months after treatment, she felt well.

SUMMARY OF FAMILY AND CASE HISTORY

Observations of such persons over a long period of time has convinced the authors that the onset of various deficiency diseases is slow, insidious, and difficult to recognize. Long before nutritional failure has developed to a degree where one can diagnose beriberi, pellagra, riboflavin deficiency, scurvy, or other well-defined syndromes, the persons have had months and years of ill health characterized by many vague symptoms and inability to work. The rapidity of the response to therapy is astounding, and leaves no doubt that the tissues which contain insufficient amounts of these chemical substances are allowed to function at a higher and more normal level as soon as they are supplied. This case and others like it indicate that such persons, when studied over a long period of time, have malnutrition with many vitamin deficiency diseases rather than a single clinical entity. The whole matter is very complex, and the presentation of today must be greatly altered because of the extraordinary speed with which new discoveries are being made. The most notable advances are resulting from the collaboration of biologists, chemists, physiologists and clinicians, and as can be seen in this attempt at study, we have tried to intensify this cooperative effort. With all this available information coming from a large group of recognized specialists and advisors in the field, we suspect there is much more to learn than we have learned about Mrs. Z. and her family. Yet Mrs. Z. and her family are representative of a large group of persons who present themselves to the practising physician, and he with all his manifold duties and lack of trained specialists to assist him is expected to understand the numerous ramifications of their disease.

THE TREATMENT OF DIETARY DEFICIENCY DISEASES

In the preceding sections we have seen that the common dietary deficiency diseases arise from a simultaneous deficiency of many factors. We have described patients with mixed deficiencies and the resultant complex clinical manifestations. We have pointed out that improper diet is not the sole cause of dietary deficiency diseases, but that impaired absorption from the alimentary tract, failure of utilization by the tissues, and inadequate storage may be contributing factors. Frequently, increased metabolism due to rapid growth, hyperthyroidism, exercise, infectious diseases, and pregnancy and lactation, may predispose to the development of clinical deficiency states. We have stressed particularly that the problems presented by patients with deficiency diseases vary greatly from one to another, and that it is essential for the physician to give careful consideration to the problems presented by each patient and to prescribe the type of therapy best suited to his needs. The following general principles of therapy, however, are applicable for all deficiency diseases: 1. The administration of a well-balanced, high protein diet. 2. The administration of specific therapeutic agents as supplements to the diet. 3. The elimination of coexisting conditions causing excess requirement for the vitamins. 4. Symptomatic treatment.

General Management

The object of treatment is to restore the patient to health as quickly as possible and to prevent recurrences. Whether the most prominent clinical syndrome arises from a lack of the water-soluble or fat-soluble vitamins, or both, a deficiency of many of the essential nutrients is likely to exist, even though symptoms are not apparent. The therapeutic agents prescribed depend upon the symptoms presented by each case under consideration, but of prime importance in every case is the ingestion and retention of a diet which will meet the body's requirements for calories, protein, minerals and vitamins. The diet must be one that the patient can eat, digest and assimilate. It must be remembered, however, that complete reliance on dietary therapy is inadvisable as well as impractical. In the first place, deprivation of these substances may have existed for years and consequently the deficiency is advanced. Many of the nutrients are present in foods in only trivial amounts and it is impossible for the patient to eat enough food to supply the amount necessary to restore his health quickly. Even the most carefully planned diets offer only slightly above the daily maintenance requirement of certain vitamins, and recovery from a nutritional deficiency is usually retarded if one depends only upon the vitamins supplied in food. The indications and limitations of dietetic measures in general will be discussed in detail under the section on dietotherapy. Suffice it to say here that the advances in our knowledge of dietary therapy during the past few years have been spectacular and far-reaching in their importance to human nutrition.

The more accurate the initial diagnosis of a deficiency of one or more of the water-soluble or fat-soluble vitamins, or any combination of them, the more likely is the physician to avoid futile treatment with unnecessary preparations. Where the diagnosis is clearcut, the problem is one of administering adequate amounts of the deficient substance or substances in a way that will insure satisfactory utilization. The amount necessary varies considerably from one patient to another and even in the same patient at different times. Since the minimal, maximal and optimal doses of the specific therapeutic agents are not known, no definite routine of treatment can be followed satisfactorily. It is better to prescribe too much than too little, too soon rather than too late. Irrespective of whether the manifestations of deficiency disease are mild or severe, the patient should have rest until convalescence is well established. It is advisable to hospitalize the more severely ill patients in order that they be under constant supervision of a physician, nurse and dietitian. Every possible effort must be made to eliminate the conditions which gave rise to the disease. Where there is defective absorption or poor utilization, therapeutic substances should be administered parenterally to assure immediate availability in the systemic circulation. Patients with increased requirement should be given additional amounts of the materials to meet the increased demand. In all cases, the proper utilization of the required amount of the essential vitamin or vitamins is necessary for the cure of deficiency diseases. Failing in that, all therapy fails.

DIETOTHERAPY

Dr. J. S. McLester has recently remarked in the *Journal of the American Medical Association* as follows: "Man's place in future history will depend

TABLE 4

CHART OF RECOMMENDED DAILY ALLOWANCES FOR SPECIFIC NUTRIENTS[1]

(From the Committee on Foods and Nutrition, National Research Council)

	Calories	Protein	Calcium	Iron	A[3]	Thiamine (B₁)[2]	Ascorbic Acid (C)[2]	Riboflavin	Nicotinic Acid	D
Man (70 Kg.)		gm.	gm.	mg.	I.U.	mg.	mg.	mg.	mg.	I.U.
Moderately active......	3000	70	0.8	12	5000	1.8	75	2.7	18	
Very active...........	4500					2.3		3.3	23	5
Sedentary............	2500					1.5		2.2	15	
Woman (56 Kg.)										
Moderately active......	2500	60	0.8	12	5000	1.5	70	2.2	15	
Very active...........	3000					1.8		2.7	18	
Sedentary............	2100					1.2		1.8	12	
Pregnancy (latter half)..	2500	85	1.5	15	6000	1.8	100	2.5	18	400–800
Lactation.............	3000	100	2.0		8000	2.3	150	3.0	23	400–800
Children up to 12 years										
Under 1 year[4]........	100 per Kg.	3–4 per Kg.	1.0	6	1500	0.4	30	0.6	4	400–800
1– 3 years...........	1200	40	1.0	7	2000	0.6	35	0.9	6	
4– 6 years[6]..........	1600	50	1.0	8	2500	0.8	50	1.2	8	
7– 9 years...........	2000	60	1.0	10	3500	1.0	60	1.5	10	5
10–12 years..........	2500	70	1.2	12	4500	1.2	75	1.8	12	
Children over 12 years										
Girls: 13–15 years.......	2800	80	1.3	15	5000	1.4	80	2.0	14	
16–20 years.......	2400	75	1.0	15	5000	1.2	80	1.8	12	
Boys: 13–15 years.......	3200	85	1.4	15	5000	1.6	90	2.4	16	
16–20 years.......	3800	100	1.4	15	6000	2.0	100	3.0	20	5

Note: The figures on this chart are essentially the same as those which have been approved by the Council on Foods of the American Medical Association.

[1] These are tentative allowances toward which to aim in planning practical dietaries. These allowances can be met by a good diet of natural foods; this will also provide other minerals and vitamins, the requirements for which are less well known.

[2] One mg. thiamine equals 333 International Units; 1 mg. ascorbic acid equals 20 International Units (1 International Unit equals 1 U.S.P. unit).

[3] Requirements may be less than these amounts if provided as vitamin A, greater if chiefly as the provitamin carotene.

[4] Needs of infants increase from month to month. The amounts given are for approximately 6–18 months. The amounts of protein and calcium needed are less if from breast milk.

[5] Vitamin D is undoubtedly necessary for older children and adults. When not available from sunshine, it should be provided probably up to the minimal amounts recommended for infants.

[6] Allowances are based on the middle age for each group (as 2, 5, 8, etc.), and for moderate activity.

in no small degree on the food he eats. The truth of this was foreshadowed about two decades ago when it was discovered that an animal's processes may be profoundly disrupted by the omission from its food of any one of a number of substances, each of them ridiculously small in the amount required. Today there has been added the further, highly significant observation that under certain circumstances an animal's life may be greatly improved by the addition of appropriate foods to a diet that previously had been regarded as entirely satisfactory. Through this knowledge, physiologists have been able to influence to a surprising degree the life history of their experimental animals and in some instances so to improve the stock as apparently to produce a new series. Can this be applied to man? Can man, by giving thought to the food he eats, influence the destiny of his race? There is reason to believe that he can."

In our experience with hundreds of persons with deficiency diseases, we have yet to observe two patients in whom the clinical manifestations were identical. Invariably, diets that fail to supply one nutrient in adequate amounts are deficient in others, and persons subsisting on such diets may develop a number of diseases simultaneously. Accordingly, the essential basis of treatment is a diet that supplies sufficient amounts of all essential nutrients—calories, proteins, fats, carbohydrates, minerals, vitamins, and water. In addition, the cost of food in relation to the patient's financial resources, its suitability to the patient's condition, food idiosyncrasies, food fads or prejudices must be considered. By including in the dietary sufficient amounts of certain foods, the nutritive requirement of the normal person can be supplied. A person who is severely ill, however, or whose requirement is greatly increased, can rarely consume a sufficient quantity of food to meet his need and the factor or factors in which he is deficient should be given as supplements to the diet. It may be imperative to use large amounts of crystalline substances or concentrates.

Diet therapy consists essentially in having the patient eat and retain a liberal and well-balanced diet. The type of food, mode of administration and frequency of feedings are determined by the patient's condition and his ability to tolerate food. Three diets are suggested (Table 5). Diet No. I and Diet No. II are intended for the severely ill patient who usually tolerates best either liquid or soft-solid foods. The foods suggested may be combined in any way desired. For example, the milk and cream may be combined with eggs in eggnog or thin puddings, with strained vegetables for soup, and with strained cereals as gruels. Vanilla, chocolate, and other flavorings can be added. Likewise, the time of feeding and the amount given at each feeding will vary with the patient's condition and his ability to tolerate food. Most patients feel better during the early hours of the morning and are willing to take more food then than at any other time of the day. Therefore, every effort should be made to give as much as possible between six and nine o'clock in the morning. When only small amounts of food can be tolerated at one time it may be necessary to give night feedings to insure an adequate intake. If, for any reason, sufficient food cannot be taken by mouth, tube feedings should be given. Food lost from vomiting or diarrhea should be made up by giving additional feedings. It must be kept in mind that the severely ill person is not interested in eating, and it takes much patience and personal attention to get him to take food.

Solid food should be added as early as possible, particularly if diarrhea is present. Diet No. III should be given as soon as the patient's appetite improves, if he can tolerate it. In most cases, it is best to divide the food for the day into three meals with feedings between meals and in the evening.

Each of these diets supplies between 2600 and 2800 calories. Additional calories should be supplied whenever it is practical by including other foods

TABLE 5

Food	Diet No. I (Liquid Diet)	Diet No. II (Soft Solid Diet)	Diet No. III (Solid Diet)
	Daily amount	Daily amount	Daily amount
Milk....................	1½ quarts	1½ quarts	1 quart
Cream..................	8 ounces	As desired	As desired
Butter..................	3 tablespoons	6 tablespoons—may be used in soups and milk toast	6 tablespoons
Eggs....................	4 used in eggnog or thin custard	4 soft cooked or in eggnogs or dessert	3
Cheese..................	....	Cottage or cream cheese if desired	As desired
Meat....................	....	....	Large serving of lean meat, chicken or fish daily. Liver at least twice a week if possible.
Fruit and fruit juices.......	2 glasses orange, grapefruit or tomato (if patient has sore mouth substitute non-acid fruit)	1 glass orange, grapefruit or tomato juice (if patient has sore mouth substitute non-acid fruit juice)	1 glass tomato, orange or grapefruit juice
		1 serving pureed canned or stewed fruit	1 serving other fruit
Green or yellow vegetable...	1 serving (pureed and used in soup)	2 servings—pureed (may be used in soup if desired)	2 servings
Potato...................	....	1 serving	1 serving
Dried vegetables, nuts......	....	....	As desired
Bread (preferably whole grain).................	....	3 slices (may be used as bread and milk or milk toast)	6 slices
Cereal (preferably whole grain).................	2 servings	2 servings	1 serving
Desserts.................	1 or 2 servings ice cream, jello, thin custard or cornstarch pudding	1 or 2 servings ice cream, jello or soft pudding	2 servings
Sugar...................	As desired	As desired	As desired

which the patient desires or by increasing the amounts of the foods suggested so that the patient receives 4000 calories per day.

YEAST, LIVER EXTRACT, WHEAT GERM, AND RICE POLISHINGS AS SPECIAL THERAPEUTIC AGENTS

The value of yeast, liver extract, wheat germ, and rice polishings has been stressed in the treatment of various deficiency diseases. The chief value of these therapeutic agents probably depends upon the vitamin B complex components which they contain. Perhaps the simplest working definition of the B complex is a composite of the water-soluble vitamins, excluding ascorbic acid, found in yeast and liver. No one knows the distribution of the various components of vitamin B in foods. The authors know too little about wheat germ and tikitiki to recommend them for general vitamin B deficiency, though we have had experience with them in treating persons with neural involvement arising from deficiency diseases. Yeast, liver extract, wheat germ, and rice polishings, when administered by mouth are less effective when the patient has severe vomiting or intractable diarrhea. At times it is difficult to get the patient to take them but, in general, they are more acceptable when mixed with a liquid.

Yeast.—The therapeutic value of yeast was recognized by the Egyptians hundreds of years before the time of Christ. It was employed as a curative agent by Hippocrates, and was mentioned in the writings of Pliny the Elder. Renewed interest was aroused by Pasteur's discoveries leading to new concepts of fermentation. In recent years, the true value of yeast as a therapeutic agent has become more and more apparent. A yeast cell is a minute organism capable of reproduction. It contains substances essential for its own growth and nourishment. The same substances are invaluable for the proper nutrition of many forms of life. Yeast was used first for the treatment of pellagra by Goldberger and Tanner in 1925. These investigators were of the opinion that 1 gm. per kilogram of body weight was adequate for a therapeutic dose, but Spies, Chinn and McLester more recently have found that much larger doses produce more rapid and lasting improvement. We have administered as much as 6 ounces of dried brewers' yeast per day for many weeks with no evidence of deleterious effect. Yeast is limited in its value as a curative or preventive agent because the taste is so disagreeable to some people that they refuse to take it, or will take it for too short a time. Persons with prodromal manifestations of deficiency disease have notoriously fickle appetites. Even with some of the most capricious, however, it can be used as a therapeutic agent by coaxing or by using a suitable method of administration. The unpleasant taste of yeast can be partially disguised by stirring it into milk or tomato juice, or by mixing it with water and adding tomato catsup. It can be added to bouillon, sprinkled over cooked cereals, or added to eggnogs. Some people consider that mixing it with food merely ruins what otherwise would be a palatable food and prefer having it mixed with water and taking it as a medication.

Dried brewers' yeast is not generally considered a staple food, and needy persons too often in the past have not liked its taste and have refrained from taking it in adequate amounts even when it was available. It seemed desirable to blend it with some well-liked and widely distributed food of high nutritional value and low cost. After experimenting for some time, we found that a mixture of 20 per cent dried brewers' yeast by weight and 80 per cent peanut butter was acceptable to most persons. Anheuser-Busch personnel have succeeded in producing a new type of dried brewers' yeast which is remarkably palatable and is a rich source of the natural vitamins of the B complex, as well as a good source of protein, fat and calories. A mixture of this yeast and peanut butter is practical and economically sound. Proteins, fats, and vitamins are by far the most expensive part of the human diet. The diets of the people we study so frequently show a greater deficiency of these substances than of carbohydrate. The mixture of yeast and peanut butter is stable, low in water content, palatable to taste, and can be widely distributed at low cost. It would go a long way toward correcting the deficiencies of proteins, fats and vitamins in the diets of many persons.

Unpublished observations by Spies, Huff and Malone show some striking results. Children selected from families each member of which had deficiency diseases then, and had had them for a number of years, were given the yeast-peanut butter mixture (Anheuser-Busch), while others in the same family were not given this mixture; the diets otherwise were identical. The children receiving the supplement showed varying types of improvement. Nearly all gained in weight. In most instances, they did not develop diagnostic lesions of deficiency diseases whereas nearly all the controls did. Those persons taking the yeasted peanut butter who did develop lesions invariably had infections of various types which preceded the development of deficiency diseases. The most striking improvement in the children was in their general dispositions. They tended to cry less easily, became more talkative, more alert, and interested in playing.

R. R. Sealock and J. R. Murlin, in determining the values for vitamins of the B complex in a whole wheat bread made from Earle process flour, have found that there are 2.73 micrograms of thiamine, 2.45 micrograms of riboflavin, and 3.14 micrograms of pyridoxin per gram of fresh bread. They state, "the values per slice of bread are 88, 79.0, and 101.0, respectively (average slice 32.2 gm.)." When several slices of this bread are included in the day's dietary, it is obvious that a rather considerable portion of the daily requirement of these factors is supplied.

It is therefore evident that the substitution of whole wheat bread for highly milled bread is an important prophylaxis against deficiency disease. A personal communication from J. R. Murlin and R. R. Sealock, of the University of Rochester, indicates that by eating whole wheat bread instead of white bread one obtains not only more calcium, phosphorus, and iron, and more vitamins, but protein of a significantly higher biological value.

Unpublished observations by Spies, Huff and Malone show that children with mild deficiency diseases who have received whole wheat bread instead of white bread or corn bread in their daily diet have gained weight and felt better. In some instances, lesions of pellagra and riboflavin deficiency have cleared following the substitution of this whole wheat bread for the ordinary corn bread or hot biscuit without any other form of therapy. Where the diets were extremely deficient in the group of B vitamins, we have combined this type of bread with the yeasted peanut butter with gratifying results.

Numerous varieties of brewers' yeast are available commercially, some of which are specially cultured under conditions which preclude contamination. There is extreme variation in the therapeutic potency between different brands, and often no effort is made to determine it. Many manufacturers make unwarranted claims which cannot be substantiated by laboratory or clinical investigation. It behooves the physician to prescribe a yeast of stated potency made by a reliable concern, for in this way alone can he be sure that the material will be beneficial. Concentrates of yeast are valuable under many circumstances, but since all the essential vitamin B complex factors are not known there is a possibility that some essential material may have been removed in the process of extraction and refinement. Irradiated yeast is a good source of vitamin D. The relationship of yeast to the anti-anemia factor of pernicious anemia is not clearly established, but a number of investigators have shown that yeast is effective in certain types of macrocytic anemia (see Fig. 80). In addition to being a rich source of the B complex vitamins, yeast has a high content of protein of excellent biological value, both important factors in the treatment of persons with deficiency diseases.

The Council on Food and Nutrition of the American Medical Association allows the following claims for yeast:

"The Council on Foods regards compressed fresh yeast, dried yeast and yeast extracts as foods with usefulness restricted to special purposes. These products are useful for increasing the vitamin B_1 (thiamine) and G (riboflavin) content of the diet. Fresh yeast and dried yeast if taken in sufficient quantity have a mild laxative effect on many persons. Special claims for yeast products must have the approval of the Council before use in advertising.

"Labels and advertising of yeast products should list the ingredients other than yeast substances and state the percentage composition in close proximity to the name of the product. The vitamin B_1 (thiamine) and G (riboflavin) content of the product as determined by biologic assay should be expressed in appropriate units."

The authors support those claims and, in addition, recommend that yeast may be used in the treatment of all the mixed deficiencies of the B complex, including pellagra, beriberi, riboflavin deficiency, vitamin B_6 deficiency and pantothenic acid deficiency.

Liver Extract.—Hundreds of years ago liver was used by the Egyptians and Chinese as a therapeutic agent. It was recommended in the treatment of pellagra, on empirical grounds, by Voegtlin in 1914. Following Minot's and Murphy's discovery that liver contained an anti-anemic substance specific for the relief of pernicious anemia, Goldberger and Sebrell demonstrated that liver extract was curative and preventive for experimental canine black tongue. Ramsdell and Magness, Spies and associates, and others have shown that it is specific in the relief of human pellagra.

From liver extract, Elvehjem and his associates isolated nicotinic acid amide, a substance which has proved to be a valuable therapeutic agent in pellagra. Crude liver extract, like yeast, is an especially good source of the B complex vitamins, and the more crude the product, the more effective it is in relieving deficiencies of these vitamins.

The dosage is dependent upon the potency of the extract, but in general it is similar to that of dried brewers' yeast. It usually is most acceptable to the patient when administered in water, broth or tomato juice.

Wheat Germ.—The germ or wheat embryo is that portion of the grain in which germination takes place. As obtained from the miller, it usually contains some bran. For human use, most of the bran and endosperm are removed, and it is treated to improve its keeping qualities. Despite the treatment to prevent spoilage, it is likely to become rancid if not kept in a refrigerator. The thiamine content of wheat germ is particularly high, the commercial preparations containing from 3 to 6 mg. of thiamine per gram. It also contains riboflavin, nicotinic acid or its amide, vitamin B_6, pantothenic acid, and biotin. From 150 to 300 gm. or more of wheat germ daily must be taken in order to prevent the development of pellagra in persons who are subsisting on poor diets. The therapeutic dose is extremely variable, but it may be said in general that the anti-pellagric effect is about one-third that of a good grade dried brewers' yeast powder. Wheat germ preparations contain vitamin E unless the fat is removed. It may be eaten as cereal or with cereal, or mixed with milk, water, fruit juice, tomato juice, or meat broth.

The allowable claims for wheat germ are as follows:

"The Council on Foods recognizes that in the amount of wheat germ ordinarily consumed (manufacturers suggest one-half to one ounce a day) there is sufficient vitamin B_1, vitamin G and phosphorus to warrant recognizing the following claims:

1. Wheat germ is a rich source of vitamin B_1
2. Wheat germ is a rich source of phosphorus
3. Wheat germ contains some vitamin G (riboflavin).

"Wheat germ in general will not be recognized as a good source of vitamin G unless the firm furnishes evidence that its particular product does furnish a suitable proportion of the "daily allowance" for this factor. Although wheat germ contains some vitamin B_6 no claim for this factor is recognized at the present time because the exact rôle of this substance in human nutrition and the daily requirements are not established. Wheat germ, when given in large quantities—200 gm.—contains sufficient nicotinic acid to cure pellagra, but in the amounts ordinarily consumed there is some doubt about there being sufficient nicotinic acid to be useful. For this reason the claim that a wheat germ preparation is a rich source of the P-P factor cannot be recognized until more substantial evidence of an acceptable nature is made available to the Council. There is no objection to the statement of composition of wheat germ on labels or in advertising or the statement that the product contains a definite amount of oil natural to the germ, but the phrase 'Wheat germ contains — per cent of natural wheat germ oil' is objectionable because 'wheat germ oil' practically means 'vitamin E.' No claim for vitamin E is recognized and wheat germ oil is not acceptable to the Council on Pharmacy and Chemistry.

"Accepted products of refined wheat germ, because of their low crude fiber content, may be given to children and to persons who have sensitive digestive tracts. In addition to contributing unique food values, wheat germ preparations are an appetizing addition to salads, vegetable dishes, biscuits, breads, cakes, meats, desserts and other dishes of the American table."

The authors are in agreement with these statements. In our experience, wheat germ is not as effective in treating B complex deficiencies as liver extract or a good grade of dried brewers' yeast.

Rice Polishings.—Rice is Asiatic in its origin and is the backbone of the diet of persons in most tropical countries. Only a small quantity of rice is marketed in its undecorticated form, and in this form it is known as brown rice. Rice polishings, because of different methods of milling, vary from one mill to another. The preparation of the rice for market is done by removing the husk. The decorticated grain is then polished and made white by the removal of the pericarp layer. Rice polishings or tikitiki are composed of the pericarp layer. Rice polishings are concentrated by extraction in a solution of 25 per cent alcohol for a period of forty-eight hours. The alcohol is then distilled, and the extraction is repeated until a clear syrup is produced. The process is often continued until 1 cc. of tikitiki extract represents 20 gm. of rice polishings. This material if stored too long is liable to become infested with insects and to develop high acidity, making it somewhat unpalatable.

Williams has shown that rice polishings have about 40 to 50 parts thiamine per million, of which only a small part can be removed by chemical methods. Tikitiki is useful as a curative and preventive material in the treatment of beriberi. Although the dosage varies greatly from case to case, the average dosage is about 3 ounces daily. Vitamins other than thiamine have not been studied in tikitiki.

The better known vitamins included in these preparations are discussed in detail in the preceding sections.

The Proper Use of Vitamins in Mixtures

It is apparent from the previous chapters that prolonged deprivation of vitamins produces a variety of diseases. The symptoms associated with these diseases are seldom well-defined and rarely appear uncomplicated. The resulting clinical picture is a complex one, and the physician frequently recognizes a number of distinct deficiency diseases in the same patient. While the functions of the individual vitamins, whether members of the fat-soluble or the water-soluble group, vary, they do tend to occur together in nature to some extent, and they are used customarily for therapeutic purposes as mixtures in the form of such preparations as cod liver oil, oleum percomorphum, yeast, liver extract, wheat germ, *etc*. Vitamin mixtures, whether natural or artificial, should not supplant all preventive and therapeutic measures but should supplement them.

We all deplore polypharmacy and the so-called "shotgun" prescriptions, given in the hope that if one ingredient doesn't hit, another will. Our studies have shown that there is considerable logic, however, in including some of the vitamins together. The patients fare much better when diseases are treated simultaneously, and the physician is not confused by the necessity of prescribing six or seven different preparations. Our clinical experience during the past three years in the treatment of over three thousand patients with deficiency diseases has shown that convalescence is delayed when one gives only one vitamin at a time in contrast to giving a number at once. The ideal mixture of vitamins for therapeutic use should be so calculated that the therapeutic dose would either be a fraction or a multiple of the estimated daily requirement. In that way, the physician can estimate how much to use for prophylactic purposes and how much to prescribe for particular clinical conditions.

Summary of Treatment

We owe much of our freedom from infectious diseases to those who have applied effective control measures on a wide scale. Unfortunately, many of those working in the interest of public health attempt to apply the same formula to the problem of eradicating deficiency diseases as they apply to preventing infectious diseases. It is hoped that they will soon reach the point of view that vitamins are necessary to the body and that they tend gradually to be lost from it, whereas pathogenic micro-organisms are foreign to the body and tend to multiply in it. It is vain to hope that attempts to prevent and treat deficiency diseases will be very successful until the general health of the people is considered rather than the eradication of a single deficiency disease.

The problem of increasing the well-being of all people by means of better diet depends upon the continued collaborative effort of physicians, nutritionists and groups concerned primarily with public health. Each must share in the responsibility of teaching the public the importance of good nutrition and the simple dietary rules for achieving it. The physician and nutritionist can aid by supporting important changes, such as the enrichment of flour with vitamins, fortification of oleomargarine with vitamin A, and the dissemination of a good grade of yeast and peanut butter mixture where indicated.

Without the full support of the physician, prevention and treatment of deficiency diseases are impossible. He not only is of aid in supporting the measures directed toward improving the nutrition of the whole population and in making specific recommendations in his own community, but he, more than any other, can assess the dietaries of persons in general. By recognizing malnutrition in the early stages, he can prevent years of illness. He and he alone can tell in any specific case whether a deficiency disease is likely to develop because of an inadequate diet or because of the presence of a disease which may interfere with proper nutrition.

The means of treating deficiency diseases at the disposal of the physician today are so great that all the therapeutic preparations available cannot even be catalogued. The physician and the patient naturally wish to use the simplest, cheapest, most effective, and most easily administered therapy, but the wealth of effective compounds makes it impossible to be didactic in the choice of a therapeutic agent. Treatment must be adapted to the individual case. Accordingly, we have indicated only in general the principles of treatment, the management of the patient, the indications for the various types of therapy, and the judicious use of vitamin mixtures.

Diagnosis must be stressed as the foundation upon which to build proper vitamin therapy. It is not uncommon for a patient with ill-defined symptoms arising from a deficiency of vitamins to undergo many tests and to seek advice from many physicians before a diagnosis is made and effective treatment is applied. Such cases are often said to be atypical and rare, whereas our experience has shown that they are far more common than the "textbook picture." From the study of many hundreds of cases of mixed deficiency diseases we have found it wise to make a tentative diagnosis based on careful study of the patient and to verify or disprove it by subsequent effort. The reduction in morbidity and mortality among persons with deficiency diseases proves that modern therapy is effective in saving lives, but it is also altering and improving the practice of medicine and nursing, as well as reducing the time the patient spends in the hospital, the cost of his treatment, the length of his convalescence and, thus, the time he loses from work.

RECAPITULATION

In the preceding chapters an effort has been made to describe a scientific basis for coordinating action in effecting better nutrition of the people. In order to have good health, the factors which operate to disturb the balance of the vitamins in the tissues must be equalized or overcome by factors which operate to maintain it. The most frequent cause of nutritional deficiency disease is a decreased intake of vitamins, though many persons develop deficiency diseases because of faulty assimilation or because of an abnormally high requirement. Excessive exercise precipitates clinical manifestations of deficiency diseases, and acute infections and fever place a still greater demand for vitamins upon the body. The homeostatic equilibrium is preserved in many ways. Long before the etiology of deficiency diseases was in any way understood, rest was advocated as a good method of treatment for the disease. The processes carry on for the benefit of some organs at the expense of others, but the maintenance of equilibrium becomes more and more difficult as the stores of these substances are depleted so that eventually they must be replenished. We have seen how these various deficiency diseases are characterized by a great diversity of disturbances. It is clear now that scientists in the past have placed too narrow significance on the rôle of the vitamins in the general physiologic processes. It would be far wiser to consider that all tissues need the vitamins for performance of their natural functions and that certain tissues, perhaps because they are more highly organized and more delicately balanced so far as specific requirement is concerned, become sufficiently altered after long deprivation as to give rise to clinical signs. For reasons which we do not fully comprehend at present, these clinical signs, which are most conspicuous in the late stages of deficiency diseases, arise predominantly from certain systems of the body.

The confusing and contradictory state of our present knowledge is due in the main to the fact that what we once supposed to be a single substance and glibly termed vitamin B, has turned out to be some fifteen separate entities. It would be stupid to suppose that we have safely passed all these pitfalls. The self-respecting physician will justifiably extend his clinical experimentation with the vitamins, for they appear harmless, but he should wisely exercise the greatest skepticism regarding how much may be attributed to their therapeutic effect. We have noted particularly that clinical deficiency diseases can be corrected by therapy directed along three lines: 1. The administration of the substances in adequate amounts to correct the deficiencies. 2. The elimination of conditions requiring excess requirement for the vitamins. 3. The treatment of coexisting diseases. Although a dramatic therapeutic response follows the administration of synthetic vitamins, they cannot replace a well-balanced diet and should be recommended as supplements to the diet of persons with nutritional deficiency diseases only until an adequate and well-balanced diet can be procured.

We have stressed that human beings and animals have fundamentally the same vitamin needs. It seems apparent that some 50 per cent of the people in the United States do not eat sufficient amounts of meat, milk, fruits and vegetables to enable them to enjoy full vigor and health. The vitamins are vital to the health of all human beings. The protracted absence of sufficient amounts of vitamin A leads to disastrous alteration of the epithelial lining protecting the various organs of the body. The protracted absence of sufficient quantities of ascorbic acid leads to failure in functions of the intercellular substances so that teeth, bone, and capillaries are affected. Protracted absence of sufficient amounts of thiamine is followed by unreasonable emotion, apprehension, fear, rage and hypersensitivity, and still later there is degeneration of the peripheral nerves and disturbance of the cardiovascular system. Protracted lack of vitamin D in children results in rickets with all the associated deformities of the bones. Protracted lack of riboflavin is followed by cheilosis, keratitis, and inability to read or to endure bright lights. Protracted lack of vitamin K in the tissues leads to failure of prothrombin formation and inability for proper blood clotting.

Above are a few of the manifestations of the deficiency states, but long before they develop, an individual goes through a period of months and years characterized by weakness, ill health, and general irritability.

Some nations some time will have the wisdom to apply the thoughts so poetically described by Dr. J. S. McLester: "In the past, science has conferred on those people who availed themselves of the newer knowledge of infectious diseases, better health, and a greater average length of life. In the future, it promises to those races who will take advantage of the newer knowledge of nutrition, a larger stature, greater vigor, increased longevity, and a higher level of cultural attainment. To a measurable degree, man is now master of his own destiny where once he was subject only to the grim hand of Fate."

The science of nutrition is making advances each year. Vitamins should not be regarded as curiosities of long-haired research workers but should be considered matters of life and death to every individual and to all nations. The life-giving substances come, directly or indirectly, from the soil. Primitive man had the advantage of natural whole foods, whereas comparatively few people today live on natural foods. The vitamins are often lessened or lost in the harvesting, the distribution, the processing, and the cooking; hence, tradition and food habits are not safe guides to the selection of foods.

People must be properly fed if the best is to be expected of them. Through plant and animal life the vitamins come from the soil and on decay they or their constituents must return to the soil, with the result, it seems, that the vitamin content of the soil might affect the vitamin content of the growing plant, which in turn would affect the animal or man feeding on the plant. It is appalling that agricultural people who should "feast on the fruits of the earth" should be suffering from protracted vitamin deficiencies.

BIBLIOGRAPHY

Annual Review of Biochemistry, Vol. IX, 1940.
Annual Review of Physiology, Vol. II, 1940.
Cowgill, G. R., The Vitamin B Requirement of Man. Yale University Press, 1934.
Food and Life (Yearbook of Agriculture), United States Department of Agriculture, 1939.
McLester, J. S., Nutrition and Diet in Health and Disease, W. B. Saunders Company, Philadelphia, Ed. 3, 1939.
Williams, R. R. and Spies, T. D.: Vitamin B_1 and Its Use in Medicine. The Macmillan Company, 1938.
Modern Medical Therapy in General Practice (Edited by Dr. D. P. Barr), Section on Deficiency Diseases. The Williams and Wilkins Company, 1940.
The Vitamins, Published by the American Medical Association, under the auspices of the Council on Pharmacy and Chemistry and the Council on Foods, 1939.
Mathews, A. P., Physiological Chemistry, The Williams and Wilkins Company, Baltimore, 1939.

ADDENDUM

Meyer, Bingham and Pohle of the University of Wisconsin, and Barker, Butt, Allen and Bollman of the Mayo Clinic, independently have shown that Dicoumarin 3,3'-Methylinebis (4-hydroxycoumarin), which has recently been isolated from "spoiled sweet clover" by Link and his associates, when administered by mouth to animals and man, results in an increase in the Quick prothrombin time and the coagulation time of the blood. It was shown that these alterations in the coagulation factors can be corrected temporarily by the transfusion of whole blood. Vitamin K is not effective in correcting these factors.

Para-aminobenzoic acid is another vitamin of the B complex. It is a constituent of yeast and of liver, and is a growth factor for chicks and certain organisms. It appears to nullify the bacteriostatic effect of chemotherapeutic agents of the sulfanilamide group. It has some anti-gray hair potency in the nutritional achromotrichia of the mouse and rat, and there is one report that the human is affected by the oral administration of this substance.

CHAPTER IX

UNDERNUTRITION

By L. H. Newburgh

GENERAL CONSIDERATIONS

Undernutrition is not merely the opposite of obesity. When the organism is deficient in any of the essential constituents of food, it is in a state of undernutrition. The deficiency may be brought about by insufficient ingestion of a substance, by lessened absorption of it, or by increased destruction of it. The items which the organism must ingest in adequate amounts are potential energy, the vitamins, a number of minerals, protein, and certain fatty acids. Even though in America we live in a land of plenty and are the richest nation on earth, we have not yet learned to select from our abundance a national diet which will give us the greatest possible degree of vigor. Our tendency to emphasize lean meat, refined cereals, white bread, potatoes, pie, and sugar, results in our getting marginal or submarginal amounts of calcium and the B vitamins at the very least. There is a particular need to teach children and pregnant and lactating women that milk is the best source of calcium.

Calcium.—A quart of milk contains about 1 gm. of calcium, whereas the other common foods, in particular meat and cereals, are so poor in it that the organism is not likely to obtain an adequate amount of calcium unless more milk is included in the diet. It is especially important for the female to be well supplied with calcium during the last three months of pregnancy, for during this period the fetus deposits calcium in its skeleton. The infant is unable to absorb enough of it from the digestive tract to build bone at the rapid pace which characterizes other growth in the early months of extrauterine existence; accordingly, it calls upon its own store of calcium acquired during the last months of fetal life. Present knowledge indicates that the mother's diet needs to contain at least 1.5 gm. of calcium at this time in order to prevent a deficiency of it in either herself or her baby. It is thus self-evident that the lactating woman will need large supplies of calcium to replace the losses through the milk.

Iron.—Exactly the same reasoning applies to iron. Anemia is very common in late pregnancy, because the dietary supply is not great enough to provide completely for the large fetal deposition of it.

The recent studies of the iron requirements are very enlightening. It has been shown that the urine is practically iron free, that there is no excretion of iron by the bowel, and accordingly that the fecal iron is simply that which has not been absorbed from the food. The normal adult male suffers no loss of iron, hence he may ignore the food content of it. However, the female does lose some iron with each menstrual flow and the amount may be much larger than is suspected. *Hypochromic anemia* may develop in women whose menstruation appears to be normal superficially but who can be shown to be losing unusually large amounts of iron. The few milligrams of iron contained in the usual diet are not sufficient under these circumstances. The dietary iron of the infant and young child also needs consideration, since the normal organism increases its iron content rapidly during these years.

Vitamin B Complex.—The isolation of the several members of the vitamin B complex has given investigators the opportunity of determining the dietary requirements of these substances as well as their sources. They point out that much of the vague ill health of our people is caused by inadequate ingestion of these vitamins. They are plentiful in the coverings and the germs of the seeds and in green leaves, but the refined cereals that we eat for breakfast, the white bread, the pie and cake, which form such a large part of our diet, are almost devoid of the B complex. Since the thiamine requirement is roughly proportional to the carbohydrate content of the diet, and since our national food habits emphasize the carbohydrates, our needs for this vitamin are large and our intake is small.

General Deficiency.—When an individual for any reason eats abnormally small amounts of food, he not only lessens his energy intake but he may also be curtailing the inflow of any of the substances which his body must have in sufficient amounts to remain healthy and which can be secured solely by adequate ingestion of them. Thus the obese individual who desires to lose weight, may, through lack of knowledge, place himself on a low calorie diet which is also low enough in some essential foodstuff to produce a deficiency of it. When this occurs he will be undernourished even though still obese.

Illnesses of all sorts lessen appetite and cause distaste for foods of various types. When the illness is prolonged it may require the most expert dietary manipulation to avoid the development of a deficiency disease.

Diseases accompanied by *diarrhea* cause wastage of all the essential dietary substances, and *infections* increase the requirements for them. The physician should scrutinize his patients' diet under any of these circumstances and assure himself that the patient is receiving a sufficient amount of each essential. It may be necessary to administer some of them as medication by mouth or subcutaneously.

ENERGY REQUIREMENTS

Since other chapters of this book contain detailed information about the requirements of protein, the minerals, and the vitamins, no more needs to be recorded about them here. It remains for this chapter to deal with energy requirements.

Body Weight.—The simplest way to form an opinion about the adequacy of the energy intake is by recording the weight of the individual. He should be weighed daily at the same time without clothes, before a meal and after urination. It is assumed that change in weight is a measure of gain or loss of adipose tissue. But this assumption is justified only when it is known that the individual is in nitrogen balance and water balance. Final information about the protein status may be obtained by quantitative analysis of the diet and the excreta for nitrogen. In children and in convalescents, retention of nitrogen should be taking place and recourse must be had to the laboratory to measure its extent. The retention of 1 gm. of nitrogen causes the organism to add 25 gm. of weight because 6.25 gm. of protein will be formed from the gram of nitrogen and the protein will acquire and hold three times its weight of water.

Much greater shifts in body weight may be caused by losses or additions of *water*. Patients who are undernourished may be seriously dehydrated also. This is especially true in diarrheal diseases. Inanition may cause lesser degrees of acidosis with its attendant dehydration. A continued gain of weight after the patient is placed on an optimal diet may mean only that dehydration is being corrected. Other diseases, for example beriberi and the anemias, often cause the organism to hold more than the normal amount of water. Since 10 or 15 pounds of water may be added to the body before edema is obvious, the physician may have no suspicion that the body of his patient contains too much water. A loss of weight by an emaciated patient following correction of diet may be a good sign since it may indicate merely that extra water is being released. The massive edema of the chronic nephritic may conceal the great wasting that becomes all too apparent after 30 or 40 pounds of the edema fluid have been removed.

Clearly the course of the body weight by itself is an unreliable means of judging whether a patient is receiving an adequate amount of energy in his diet. The shorter the period of observation, the greater is the difficulty of interpreting changes in weight.

Computation of Energy Requirement.—When it is known how many calories are expended by the individual the diet may be constructed to contain more energy than is dissipated and then the difference will be deposited as adipose tissue. Several methods are available for estimating expenditure of energy. The simplest procedure is to record the basal metabolism and then add a value to it according to the activity of the subject. It is often said that the twenty-four-hourly heat production of persons continuously in bed amounts to the basal metabolism plus 20 per cent of it; that patients given the freedom of the hospital ward expend 150 per cent of the basal metabolism; and that fully active persons, other than those who support themselves by mechanical work, dissipate twice the basal metabolism in the twenty-four hours.

Individual Differences.—While predictions of total expenditure of energy derived from the basal metabolism have some general value, they may be far from the truth when applied to the individual. Some of our own experiences in this field show how disappointing these predictions may be. We obtained the basal metabolism in the standard manner and measured the twenty-four-hourly heat production from the insensible loss of weight of three boys, one aged fifteen, the others eighteen years, who had been continuously in bed for six months because they were originally suspected of having minimal pulmonary tuberculosis. However, the diagnosis could never be established. They were well when we studied them. The basal heat production for twenty-four hours was 1550, 1580, and 1550 calories respectively. Since they were confined to bed, the predicted total heat was 20 per cent more than the basal value; that is, 1860, 1896, and 1860 calories. But the actual expenditure of energy was far greater, namely 2325, 2350, and 2558 calories. This was an actual increase of 50, 49 and 65 per cent respectively.

In another instance we compared the actual with the predicted heat production in the case of two men who were leading their usual lives. The first was a middle-aged insurance agent whose basal metabolism was 1640 calories. According to the prediction it would require 3280 calories per day, that is, twice the basal heat production to maintain him in energy balance, but the actual twenty-four-hourly expenditure of energy was only 2500 calories. He needed only an addition of half the basal value to maintain him.

The other subject, a young man, was a graduate student in biochemistry. With a basal heat production of 1600 calories, it took 3570 calories to maintain him. Accordingly, he needed considerably more than twice the basal value to keep him in energy balance.

In 1918, Lusk suggested a plan for calculating the energy requirements of various classes of persons. He began with hypothetical individuals thirty-five years of age whose height and weight were normal. The theoretical basal metabolism was then obtained by reference to the appropriate tables. An allowance of 10 per cent of this basal heat production for sixteen hours was then made to provide for sitting and standing. Next the extra calories required for various occupations as determined by earlier observations, were added. It seemed necessary to Lusk to add another 300 to 400 calories for movements not included in the allowance for occupation, such as walking to and from work.

The totals arrived at are exemplified in the following table.

TABLE 1

HYPOTHETICAL ENERGY REQUIREMENTS FOR SEVERAL TRADES

Men: Weight, 164 pounds. Height, 5 ft., 8 in. Age, 35 years

Trade	Calories
Tailor	2287
Bookbinder	2500
Shoemaker	2655
Metal worker	3050
Carpenter	3250
Stone mason	4340
Man sawing wood	5000

These hypothetical values are probably far below the actual energy requirements of most tailors, bookbinders, and shoemakers. Our own actual

TABLE 2

ACTUAL ENERGY REQUIREMENTS OF STUDENTS

Age, Years	Height, Inches	Weight, Pounds	Actual Heat Production 24 Hours		Predicted Heat Production 24 Hours (Twice the basal value) Calories
			Basal Calories	Total Calories	
30	70	123	1560	2975	3120
28	73	125	1454	2920	2908
25	70	147	1694	3425	3388
23	66	141	1622	3570	3244
24	70	145	1685	3550	3370

measurements of the caloric output by several young men occupied as laboratory workers or medical students yielded the information found in table 2.

It will be noted that the total heat production is within 10 per cent of twice the basal value for each of these active young men none of whom is engaged in a manual occupation. Such actual measurements throw a good deal of doubt on the prediction that the hypothetical tailor can maintain himself by adding only 33 per cent to his basal requirement and that the shoemaker needs only 57 per cent more than his basal caloric output. Careful records of the quantities of food of known composition, eaten for many consecutive days by persons in the various occupations are greatly needed.

In the case of children such information has been obtained for girls from the seventh to the thirteenth year by Koehne and Morrell[1] and by Wait and Roberts[2] for girls from the tenth to the sixteenth year. It was found that the average intake of girls, seven to eight years old, was seventy-three calories per kilogram of body weight. With increasing age the intake diminished about five calories a year, so that girls of sixteen took only thirty-seven calories per kilogram. No satisfactory data have been published for boys or for infants. It is estimated that 100 calories per kilogram of body weight are required during the first year of life. These various estimations and predictions are always concerned with average values for a group and even if they do yield accurate mean values, they may miss the mark widely in the case of any individual. This must be so because of the large individual variation in activity.

It is, however, possible to determine the actual energy requirement of the individual while he is leading his usual life. The measurement is based upon the insensible loss of weight. The amount of this loss is derived from the body weight at the beginning and end of a period of time, and the weights of the ingesta, urine and feces by means of the following equation: I.L. = (First body weight + ingesta) — (Second body weight + urine + feces) where I.L. is insensible loss of weight. The composition of the insensible loss is accurately expressed by the equation: $I.L. = I.W. + CO_2 - O_2$ where I.W. is the weight of the water evaporated from skin and lungs. I.W. is a means of removing heat from the body at the rate of 0.58 calorie per gram, and it has been shown that one-fourth of all the heat is removed in this way under a wide variety of conditions. The application of these principles has been developed into a method for measuring total expenditure of energy by Newburgh and his associates.[3]

TREATMENT

After the physician has decided how many calories he would like to feed his undernourished patient he may still be facing his most difficult task, for a number of interfering factors may stand in the way of success. First of all, he must gain the cooperation of the patient so that the food will be eaten. This will be exceedingly difficult or impossible in *anorexia nervosa* and in some of the psychoses. As a last resort tube feeding will have to be tried. This condition is illustrated by the following case:

Case 1.—The patient was an unmarried female, forty-two years of age. She sought relief for weakness, obscure transient pains and discomfort, and headache of twenty years' duration. She was a school teacher who was anxious to increase her knowledge and was interested in her profession. She had been studying higher mathematics recently. She had been a frail child but advanced in school and college at the normal rate. At the end of the first year of teaching she weighed 135 pounds. This was twenty years ago and it marked the beginning of an illness which was accompanied by a loss of twenty-five pounds during the next year. Her first symptom was headache and this has continued to the present. A slight cough and a reported positive roentgenogram of the lungs gave rise to the diagnosis of pulmonary tuberculosis for which she was kept in bed for six months. Her symptoms have continued since and her weight has gradually declined to ninety-seven pounds. During the past year she has experienced occasional night sweats and her afternoon temperature has sometimes reached 100° F. Menstruation has been irregular for ten years. On two occasions, she has failed to menstruate for as long as two years. She has been constipated all her life. Recently she has had numerous attacks of burning epigastric pains relieved by alkali.

The *physical examination* revealed marked emaciation, atrophic breasts, and widespread dental caries. There were no other abnormalities. Hair was abundant and healthy. The uterus was not atrophic. Blood, urine, blood cholesterol, and serum proteins were normal. The Kahn test was negative. Blood pressure was 130/70. The following basal metabolic rates on successive days were obtained: +33, +15, +2, −17, −18. x-Ray examinations of the chest, gastro-intestinal tract, and gallbladder revealed no abnormality.

Gradually, over a period of twenty years, she has come to loathe food. When food is being prepared for guests she is repelled by the sight of it. She avoids parties and never eats between meals. She would rather not discuss food. She dislikes and avoids fats, cheese, nuts, meat, and fish, and wheat because she was told that she is sensitized to it. She apparently eats no whole grain cereals, no green vegetables, no fruits other than citrus, and only about one-half glass of milk daily. She may have an egg once a week.

She was urged to eat the high calorie, high vitamin diet that was offered to her but she took only 300 to 500 calories daily during the first week. Even though there was no evidence of vitamin deficiency, 2000 International Units of thiamine were presently administered intravenously for several days without improvement in appetite. Tube feeding was tried next and the mixture contained 80 gm. of dried yeast. The patient removed the tube on the third day, stating that she would rather die than continue the use of the tube. After these failures, she was asked to select her food as she desired and to take six meals daily. She never exceeded 600 calories on any day.

During this period she frequently questioned whether her difficulties were not caused by an ovarian tumor. The depression and conviction that nothing could be done for her caused her to leave the hospital after twenty-three days having lost eight pounds.

The psychiatric consultant had nothing to offer.

This patient has been a semi-invalid since early adult life. Her debility may have begun as a part of pulmonary tuberculosis, but there was no clear evidence that she had ever had active tuberculosis; and it certainly was not active when we saw her. Her present resistance to food could not be attributed to it. No organic disease capable of causing the anorexia was discovered, nor could it be demonstrated that her difficulties were the result of inadequate intake of vitamins. The moderately low basal metabolism was merely what would be anticipated as a feature of inanition, and it had no special diagnostic value. The presence of abundant hair, the nearly normal menstruation, the normal blood pressure, the lively interest in teaching, the slightly elevated body temperature, and the absence of a serious lowering of the basal metabolism rate, all militated against the diagnosis of Simmonds' disease.

Her attitude towards food was thought to be characteristic of anorexia nervosa. Patients of this type, if amenable to treatment, can be helped only by psychotherapeutic measures. The outlook for most of them is extremely discouraging.

Other patients will swallow all that is offered, though grudgingly, only to vomit it because of obstruction, organic or functional, at the cardia or the pylorus. In other instances, absorption of the fat will be impeded because the pancreas fails to secrete a sufficient amount of lipase to split all of the neutral fat or because biliary obstruction deprives the intestine of the bile without which the lipids are only poorly absorbed. In diarrheal diseases the food may be so hurried through the digestive tract that the feces contain great excesses of protein and fat.

The patient described below is an example of undernutrition dependent upon chronic diarrhea.

Case 2.—He was first seen in November, 1929. He was thirty-seven years of age, 5 feet 6 inches tall, and weighed 105 pounds. During the past four years he has suffered from increasing shortness of breath, progressive weakness of legs associated with numbness, coldness, paresthesias and swelling. More recently he has been troubled by blurring of vision and by sores on his hands. A slowly increasing diarrhea has existed for several years. The feces are very soft and contain no blood. He has lost fifty pounds in weight. Four years ago he began treatment for diabetes mellitus. He went to many physicians because none of them prevented the progression of the debility.

The physical examination revealed marked emaciation, scaphoid abdomen, slow pulse, hypotension (blood pressure was 108/70). Reflexes were obtained with difficulty.

He was able to take a diet that yielded 120 gm. of glucose without glycosuria.

He had ten or more stools daily that contained no gross blood, pus, parasites, or ova. Stool cultures were negative for dysentery bacilli. *x*-Ray examinations revealed no lesions of the digestive tract. The rectal examination revealed no abnormalities and no amoebae could be found in the feces. The basal metabolic rate was —22 per cent.

To control the diarrhea, he was given bismuth subcarbonate, atropine, and tincture of opium, but the frequent soft movements continued.

In April, 1932, he was readmitted to the hospital for further study of the diarrhea, which was gradually becoming worse. The feces were watery, greenish brown, and contained mucus but no blood. The stomach contents following a test meal contained a normal amount of free and combined acid. *x*-Ray examination of the biliary tract revealed no stones and the gallbladder was well filled with the dye.

Since it was impossible to attribute the diarrhea to any of the dysenteries, to lues, tuberculosis, or malignancy of the bowel, to disease of the biliary tract, or to achylia gastrica, a provisional diagnosis of steatorrhea was made. The fact that the patient was a diabetic suggested that he might be suffering from a fibrous lesion of the pancreas which involved the acinar tissue as well as the islets. If this were the case, the pancreas might be able to produce only small amounts of the fat-splitting enzyme. To test this idea, the fat in the diet was reduced to the smallest possible amounts and sufficient calories were obtained by increasing the protein and carbohydrate. Utilization was effected by means of sufficient amounts of insulin. When he was fed 20 gm. of fat, 140 gm. of protein and 400 gm. of carbohydrate, the diarrhea ceased abruptly and he continued to have one or two formed stools daily during the next three weeks. The dietary fat was then increased stepwise and when it reached 75 gm., frequent loose movements occurred again. Only 50 gm. of dietary fat could be managed without diarrhea. Accordingly, his subsequent diet was arranged to contain not more than that amount of fat. There have been no recurrences of diarrhea.

Psychologic and Other Factors.—Even in the absence of all of these difficulties the physician will be dealing with a patient who has lost interest in food, who has strong dislikes for certain foods, or who suffers from nausea or a sense of fullness on slight provocation. It should not be forgotten that a distaste for food is often caused by the opium derivatives, the salicylates, and many other drugs. While it is quite true that pain usually causes anorexia the attempt to build up the nutrition of the patient suffering from rheumatoid arthritis cannot succeed if the drugs administered to relieve

TABLE 3

CAUSES AND EFFECTS OF UNDERNUTRITION

Causes	Effects
Inadequate Diet	
Inadequate energy (calories).	Abnormal leanness. Debility.
Inadequate protein.	Low plasma proteins resulting in edema. Microcytic anemia. Wasted muscles.
Inadequate vitamin A.	Keratoses of mucous membranes. Night blindness.
Inadequate vitamin B_1 (thiamine).	Polyneuritis. Beriberi.
Inadequate nicotinic acid amide.	Pellagra.
Inadequate vitamin B_2 (G) (riboflavin).	Debility, cheilosis, stomatitis, ocular symptoms, skin lesions. Details await further study.
Inadequacy of other members of vitamin B complex.	Effects in man not well defined.
Inadequacy of whole vitamin B complex.	Existence of any of the syndromes caused by deficiency of any members of the vitamin B family, implies deficiencies of the other members to varying degrees.
Inadequacy of vitamin C (ascorbic acid).	Fragility of capillaries. Scurvy.
Inadequacy of vitamin D (calciferol).	Rickets. Osteoporosis.
Inadequacy of vitamin E (tocopherol).	Sterility?
Inadequacy of vitamin K.	Increased bleeding time. Delayed clotting.
Inadequacy of calcium.	Rickets in infants. Osteoporosis, especially in women who have borne and nursed many babies.
Inadequacy of iodine.	Goiter.
Inadequacy of iron.	Hypochromic anemia, especially in children. In women during child-bearing period and after hemorrhage.

Prolonged semi-starvation may cause a confused and complicated clinical picture due to many deficiencies of varying extent. Anemia, edema, skin lesions, neuritis, purpura and ocular defects may all be found in a single patient.

Increased Metabolism	
Growth. If large requirement of energy, protein, calcium and iron not met.	Rickets, osteoporosis. Anemia. Stunting.
Pregnancy. Lactation.	Infant. Rickets. Anemia. Retarded growth.
Same.	Mother. Anemia. Osteoporosis. Debility.
Fever. Thyrotoxicosis. Leukemias.	Amounts adequate for normal state now inadequate because total metabolism is increased.

Diminished Absorption	

Most foods must be split into small units by *enzymes* before they can be absorbed.

Too little pancreatic lipase reaches the duodenum because (1) production lessened by chronic pancreatitis or (2) ducts obstructed by neoplasm of head of pancreas. Body deprived of chief source of energy. Fat-soluble vitamins poorly absorbed.	Steatorrhea. Chronic inanition.
Chronic diarrhea. Wastage of Fat, Protein, Vitamins, Calcium, Iron.	Anemia, osteoporosis, tetany, edema. Polyneuritis. Pellagra. Inanition.

the pain are causing nausea. Heat and immobilization may relieve the pain and not interfere with the appetite.

After the many disturbing factors have been sought out and set aside where possible, we come to the diet itself and here success will depend upon skill. Bulky meals must be avoided. The sight of a great mass of food may be expected to cause a revulsion for it. Everyone is aware that the gustatory sense is stimulated by certain odors associated with food. The ones that act favorably on the patient in hand must be discovered and emphasized. Colors have a similar effect. Care must be taken that food which is intended to be hot *is* hot. Pleasant companionship during the feeding periods will usually make it easier for patients to dispose of the food. Patients who are

SAMPLE HIGH CALORIC DIET

The following list of foods may serve as a basic adequate diet yielding 3000 calories. Additional calories may be secured from sugar, desserts, candy, sauces or any other foods which the patient may care to add.

Meat, fish, eggs or cheese	2 servings
Half milk and half coffee cream	3 glasses
Bacon	2 or 3 rashers
Potato	1 serving
Vegetables	2 servings (one raw)
Fruits	2 servings (one raw)
Whole grain cereal	1 serving
Whole grain bread	5 slices
*Butter	8 pats
Nuts	1 oz.

* One tablespoon of mayonnaise or French dressing may be substituted for one pat of butter

The list may be divided into meals as follows:

Breakfast:

Fresh fruit	1 serving
Bacon	2 or 3 rashers
Cereal	1 serving
Toast	2 slices
Milk and cream	1 glass
Butter	2 pats

Luncheon:

Meat or substitute	2-oz. serving or 2 eggs
Vegetable salad with mayonnaise	
Bread	2 slices
Fruits, stewed or canned	1 serving
Butter	2 pats
Milk and cream	1 glass

Dinner:

Meat or substitutes	4 oz.
Potato	1 serving
Vegetable	1 serving
Bread	2 slices
Butter	3 pats
Milk and cream	1 glass

The nuts may be eaten between meals.

so weak that they find it exhausting to sit up and those who are hampered by apparatus should be fed by an attendant who is not in a hurry. Increases in the quantity and variety of the diet should be undertaken gradually. The patient who is abruptly compelled or induced to eat a high vitamin, 3000-calorie diet is liable to suffer from increased nausea and distention that culminates in vomiting. A better plan is to begin with five or six small, concentrated feedings in the twenty-four hours, care being taken to avoid excessive sweetness and strong flavors.

17

Since undernutrition may appear under so many guises and disguises, and since it may jeopardize the recovery from scores of illnesses unless it is suspected, disclosed, and vigorously attacked, its causes and their most characteristic effects are summarized in table 3.

BIBLIOGRAPHY

1. Koehne and Morrell, Am. J. Dis. Child., **7:** 548, 1934.
2. Wait and Roberts, J. Am. Dietet. Assoc., **8:** 209, 1932.
3. Newburgh, Johnston, Lashmet and Sheldon, J. Nutrition, **13:** 203, 1937.

CHAPTER X

OBESITY

By Frank A. Evans

DEFINITION

An addition to weight occurs normally during the growth period of life, and with pregnancy. Some endocrine disturbances increase body weight by skeletal overgrowth and water retention. Increase in body weight due to water retention is also seen in other disorders, especially of the heart, kidneys, and liver. A weight increase greater than normal other than from these causes results only from the laying on of fat. With the exception of the negligible weight increase due to lipomata, and that of certain lipo-dystrophies which are more a variation in contour than in gross mass, this constitutes obesity.

Normal weight needs definition. Reference to average weights at all ages is not satisfactory. Such figures are too greatly influenced by the inclusion of those of the large majority of persons who put on fat during middle life. The ideal weight should at no age be considered greater than that for a normally built person of the same height and sex at age thirty to thirty-five years. Reference to average tables is acceptable for this. Furthermore, there is a progressive loss of muscle mass during the third decade, or at least the latter half of it, and subsequent years. Accordingly a weight maintained at that of the peak of physical development, to say nothing of additional weight, must be by the accumulation of fat. The body weight should for this reason be a little less at age fifty, and after, than the normal weight for age thirty to thirty-five. A maximum allowance of 10 per cent variation over or under ideal weight, depending on body build, is permissible for a very few patients. If these criteria are not fulfilled, the storage in the body of inert fat is present—the subject is obese.

CLASSIFICATION

Obesity has for many years been classified in degree as enviable, laughable, and pitiable. The menace to continued good health with the passing years of appreciable grades of obesity has been proved to be such that this classification must be revised. Different grades of obesity can now be described only as unfortunate, more unfortunate, and disastrous. Obesity must be considered a disease, dangerous in its implications and meriting the serious attention of the physician, the same as given, for example, to beginning high blood pressure.

No classification of obesity is possible on the basis of etiology. It is all alimentary. Obesity wherever seen results from ingestion of more energy units than are expended, that is, from overeating.

Obesity, differentiated as to types, has been classified as 1, alimentary; 2, metabolic; and 3, endocrine. The following designation of McLester[1] serves capitally as an outline for discussion:

A. Simple obesity.
    1. Alimentary (exogenous)
    2. Constitutional (endogenous)
B. The obesity which accompanies other disorders.
    1. Pituitary
    2. Gonad
    3. Adrenal cortex
    4. Thyroid

That designated as *alimentary* obesity is fat storage causing a weight in excess of normal, present without other recognizable disorder, often but not always easily demonstrable as due to excess eating, and sometimes admitted by the patient to be thus caused. The overeating in many patients results from simple carelessness, in others from lack of understanding. Others with good-humored enthusiasm consciously overindulge in gustatory delights, in the fun of eating. This betokens not only a good digestion but a hearty appetite.

A "hearty appetite" cannot be taken for granted without discussion. One which leads to gourmandizing sufficient to cause obesity is more than just exuberant good health and sense of well-being. It must be *constitutional*. Possible physiological backgrounds for the suggested constitutional difference between those who overeat and those who do not are presented below. The line of division between "alimentary" and "constitutional" obesity is, however, so indefinite in almost all causes of obesity that it can for practical purposes of diagnosis, and especially of treatment, be said not to exist.

It is noteworthy that McLester in listing so-called pituitary, gonad, adrenal cortex, and thyroid obesity writes, "The obesity which accompanies. . . ." This phraseology is used to indicate that the obesity, per se, is not caused by the endocrine disorders. These disturb only the level of energy output as related to the energy supply, either by lowered physical activity or increased calorie intake, by one of several possible mechanisms. It can be stated positively that the obesity associated with all endocrine disorders, as to its acquisition as well as in consideration of treatment, relates to calculations of energy intake and output balance, or lack of balance, exactly as the frankly alimentary types. Strang and Evans,[2] while studying the oxygen exchange of obese patients undergoing reduction by limited diets alone, found no difference in the response of the so-called "endocrine obesity" patients and those who overate. Freyberg and Newburgh,[3] in a study of the energy exchange of a verified case of pituitary basophilism, observed no variation from that known for alimentary cases. The output of energy of this patient was determined accurately. The energy intake was kept at 890 calories daily by a controlled diet. Balancing these figures of energy intake and energy output the expected weight loss was computed as 8376 gm. The actual weight loss observed was 8398 gm.

The designation "endocrine obesity" is useful only when describing the location of the excess fat in such patients. Pituitary obesity, Fröhlich's, and those closely related syndromes, gonadal and adrenal cortical disturbances, show the fat characteristically central in distribution. The abdomen, upper arms, and thighs may show great accumulations of fatty tissue while the face remains thin and the calves and ankles, feet, forearms, and hands, maintain trim lines. Fat in the face and neck also is seen in disorders associated with pituitary basophilism of Cushing.[4] These features supply only one physical finding among others of diagnostic importance in endocrine disorders. Detailed description of them and the others are better found in treatises on endocrine diseases. In a discussion of obesity it is necessary only to indicate the inaccuracy of the term "endocrine obesity." Rather one must think of "obesity in endocrine disease" and consider it as any other obesity, brought on by a breakdown of the regulating mechanism of energy intake to energy output, resulting in a plus energy balance. The mechanism of this breakdown is not proven. Possibilities are discussed below.

The manner of the breakdown of balance between energy intake and output in the excess weight accumulation seen with hypothyroidism can be stated with some assurance. An appreciable portion of this excess weight is due to water accumulation. That which is due to storage of fat tissue is brought about by a plus energy balance dependent upon a lowered energy output. The low basal level of oxygen exchange and the smaller basal plus work-fraction associated with the apathy, and the attendant diminished physical activity in hypothyroid states, are well-known features of this disorder. The excess fatty tissue in hypothyroid states is not characteristically located in any region of the body, but is general in its distribution. It is possibly worthy of repetition, specifically in relation to the obesity accompanying hypothyroid states, that it results from a plus energy balance, from eating more than the body uses, and is, therefore, alimentary.

All obesity is alimentary.

INCIDENCE

It is not possible to establish the true incidence of obesity in the general population, nor to relate it with completeness to age groups, sex, racial origins, or geographical areas.

Dublin and Lotka[5] state that 2.66 per cent of a sample of 60,000 applicants for ordinary life insurance were rejected because of obesity. The ratio was 2.1 per 100 for males, and 4.0 per 100 for females. According to age groups it was:

	Males	Females
Age	Ratio per 100	
Under 35	1.2	2.1
35 to 54	4.0	10.5
55 and over	4.8	10.4

Age.—The above classification by age groups is slightly misleading because although 20 per cent excess weight was the upper limit allowable for adults, greater variation was accepted in the young. Dublin, Fisk, and Kopf[6] report that the Life Extension Institute found 12.9 per cent of 17,000 male white policy holders of the Metropolitan Life Insurance Company to be 20 per cent or more above average weight. Their distribution by ages was:

Age	Per cent
All ages	12.9
Under 25	4.9
25–34	8.1
35–44	14.4
45–54	18.9
55 and over	19.8

Preble[7] recorded the frequency according to sex and at different age groups of 1000 cases of obesity. This tabulation appears in table 1. Preble

TABLE 1

Obesity by Age Groups. 1000 Cases*

Age	0–20	21–30	31–40	41–50	51–60	61–70	71 and over	Total
Men....................	1	11	53	85	68	18	8	244
Women.................	7	65	178	238	196	62	10	756
Total.............	8	76	231	323	264	80	18	1000

* From Preble, Wm. E., Boston Med. and Surg. J., **188**: 617, 1923.

commented on the fact that up to thirty years of age and after sixty there were comparatively few cases of obesity. The small number of cases after the age of sixty years is, he suggests, because few of them live that long. The greatest number in this group of obese were women between thirty and sixty years of age. This study was published in 1923, and it might well be that changing styles and improved knowledge of hygiene has changed this ratio. An analysis by the Metropolitan Life Insurance Company[8] of women examined for life insurance observed that for almost every height and age they weighed less in 1933–34 than in 1922–23. The findings are presented in table 2. This study showed in addition that women of the

TABLE 2

Gains with Age in Average Weights of Women*

Increases Recorded Between Specified Age Groups in 1922–1923 and Corresponding Age Groups (10 Years Older) in 1932–1934, Compared with Increase Expected According to Standard Weight Table†

Age Group		Increase in Average Weight (in Pounds) at Specified Height								
		5 Feet, 0 Inches		5 Feet, 2 Inches		5 Feet, 4 Inches		5 Feet, 6 Inches		5 Feet, 8 Inches	
1922 to 1923	1932 to 1934	Re-corded	Ex-pected	Re-corded	Ex-pected	Re-corded	Ex-pected	Re-corded	Ex-pected	Re-corded	Ex-pected
20–24	30–34	6	6	7	5	7	6	9	7	7	7
25–29	35–39	4	6	6	7	7	7	6	8	6	8
30–34	40–44	5	7	4	8	5	7	6	7	5	7
35–39	45–49	1	7	4	7	2	6	2	7	3	7
40–44	50–54	0	5	−2‡	5	−3‡	5	1	6	−1‡	8
45–49	55 and over	−1‡	2	−2‡	2	−2‡	2	−4‡	2	0	4

* From *American Women Getting Thinner*, Statistical Bulletin, Metropolitan Life Ins. Co., Ordinary Department **20**: 1, 1939.
† Medico-Acturial Mortality Investigation, 1912.
‡ Decrease.

average height of 64 inches and who in 1933–34 were fifty to fifty-four years old weighed slightly less than the women forty to forty-four years old, ten years younger, in the group examined 1922–23, ten years earlier.

Sex and Civil State.—Spencer[9] classified a series of 252 cases of obesity according to sex and civil state. These data appear in table 3. He cautions that these figures cannot be taken to indicate accurately the sex distribution

TABLE 3

SEX AND CIVIL STATE OF 252 OBESE PATIENTS*

			Per cent
Females:	Married	163	64.7
	Widowed	26	10.3
	Separated	6	2.4
		195	77.4
	Single	40	15.9
	Total	235	93.3
Males:	Married	12	4.8
	Single	5	1.9
	Total	17	6.7
	Grand total	252	100.0

* From Spencer, H., Med. Clin. No. Amer., **12:** 604, 1928–1929.

of obesity. The patients came from 186 families in which, including them, there were 325 brothers (42 per cent) and 445 sisters (58 per cent). There

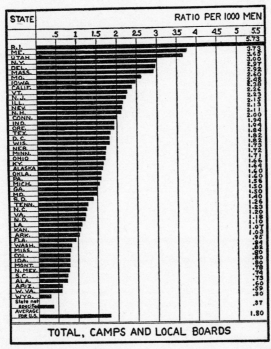

Fig. 86.—Incidence of obesity by states of men examined for the army in 1917–18. (Ireland, Love, and Davenport, "Defects Found in Drafted Men," Statistical Information by Government Printing Office, 1920.)

were 174 brothers (53.5 percent) who were obese, and 334 sisters (75 per cent). Thus, 22.6 per cent of the total 770 were obese males, and 34.3 per cent were obese females. The 508 of the total 770 who were obese were accounted for by 34.4 per cent males and 65.7 per cent females.

Geographical and Racial Incidence.—Some idea of the incidence of obesity in young men according to geographical areas and racial stocks may be obtained from the analysis of statistics compiled by examining boards for service in our army during 1917 and 1918.[10] The study involves an analysis of defects and diseases found in half a million men rejected by local examiners and two lots of approximately a million men in each who were examined at mobilization camps. These groups include about 80 per cent of all men examined and are characteristic of all. The men were

TABLE 4

SECTION DISTRIBUTION OF DEFECTS*

Obesity

Groups	Total Cases	Ratio per 1000	Ratio per 1000 Cases in Groups
Agricultural, native white, North, 73 per cent plus.	428	2.12	4.00
Agricultural, foreign and native white.	476	1.62	3.08
Agricultural, native white, South.	668	1.56	3.01
Agricultural, negro, 45 per cent plus.	176	0.98	1.77
Eastern manufacturing.	588	2.64	4.44
Commuters.	176	2.37	4.41
Mining.	108	1.13	1.98
Sparsely settled, 3 or less per square mile.	71	1.57	2.74
Desert.	14	1.16	1.73
Maritime.	39	1.94	2.83
Mountain.	83	1.57	2.75
Mountain whites.	85	1.17	2.06
Indian, sparsely settled.	47	1.48	2.78
Mexican, sparsely settled.	28	1.01	2.14
Native white, Scotch origin.	99	1.82	3.86
Russian, 10 per cent plus.	60	1.58	2.67
Scandinavian, 10 per cent.	265	1.69	3.11
Finns, 10 per cent.	26	1.91	3.67
French Canadians, 10 per cent plus.	344	3.72	5.44
German and Scandinavian, each 10 per cent plus.	157	1.59	3.08
German and Austrian, 20 per cent plus.	164	1.65	3.23
German and Austrian, 15 cent plus.	672	1.91	3.54

* From Ireland, M. W., Love, A. G., and Davenport, C. B., *Defects Found in Drafted Men, Statistical Information*, U. S. Govt. Printing Office, Washington, D. C., 1920.

eighteen to thirty years old, but relatively a larger proportion were twenty-one to thirty years inclusive.

The standards for classification of obesity in these examinations were very general and much individual variation between examiners must have occurred. A weight of 24 pounds in excess of the average was permitted for enlistment, and even a greater amount in vigorous and healthy men, who in the opinion of the examiners were not sufficiently handicapped by their obesity to preclude military service. Of these young men 4967 were, by these loose standard standards, classified as obese. Of this number, 2323 were from urban and 2644 from rural districts. It must be left to conjecture how much these numbers were influenced by the different opinions of the examiners in these cities as to what constituted obesity. The incidence of obesity analyzed according to states is shown graphically in figure 86. Analyzed according to mode and manner of life, and to racial stocks, the ratios showed interesting but confusing relationships. These and comparable data for another group classification appear in table 4.

MENACE TO GOOD HEALTH

The menace of obesity to continued good health and vigor with advancing years has been well demonstrated by analyses of insurance mortality statistics. It might be safe to assume that the mortality of the obese as a class would be greater than that of the obese among life insurance policy holders who are chosen as good risks after examination. These statistics have to do only with mortality rates. They afford no estimate of the increased number of minor and major disabilities suffered by the obese during life. No statistical study of this important point has been made.

Preble[7] gives the results of an investigation prior to 1923 of a committee for thirty of the larger insurance companies. The report presents data on 213,000 men and 50,000 women who were overweight. Table 5 gives the

TABLE 5

ACTUAL DEATH RATE BY DECADES OF OBESE MEN AND WOMEN EXPRESSED IN PER CENT OF EXPECTED DEATH RATE*

Variation from Average Weight	Ratio to Normal Death Rate
Men	
+10 Lbs.	97
+15–20 "	104
+25–30 "	113
+35–45 "	131
+50–60 "	144
+65–80 "	165
+85 and more Lbs.	223
Women	
+ 5–10 Lbs.	101
+15–20 "	114
+25–30 "	109
+35–45 "	122
+50–60 "	120
+65–80 "	157
+85 and more Lbs.	...

* From Preble, Wm. E., Boston Med. and Surg. J., **188**: 617, 1923.

ratio of expected to actual death rate, by decades of men and women. It may be noted in this series that for ten pounds overweight there is no increase in death rate for men, and a negligible increase for women. With greater excess weights there is a marked increase over the expected mortality, somewhat less in women than in men, possibly because women in the middle and later decades of life are not on the average so active as men.

This committee also gives the relative mortality both by age groups and by weight groups. In the data of Preble (table 6), it is reported that

TABLE 6

ACTUAL DEATH RATE ACCORDING TO AGE AND DEGREE OF OBESITY EXPRESSED IN PER CENT OF EXPECTED DEATH RATE*

Ages at Entry	Variation from Average Weight in Pounds			
	5–10 Lbs. Overweight	15–20 Lbs. Overweight	25–45 Lbs. Overweight	50–80 Lbs. Overweight
20–24 years.........................	96	96	101	103
25–29 years.........................	93	90	112	117
30–34 years.........................	99	86	119	134
35–39 years.........................	100	101	131	155
40–44 years.........................	94	110	140	175
45–49 years.........................	103	109	131	151
50–56 years.........................	102	121	124	149
57–62 years.........................	102	125	112	138

* From Preble, Wm. E., Boston Med. and Surg. J., **188**: 617, 1923.

TABLE 7

STANDARDIZED DEATH RATES PER 100,000 FOR SPECIFIED CAUSES OF DEATH, ALL AGES COMBINED, BY WEIGHT CLASSES—BASED ON THE MORTALITY EXPERIENCE ON ABOUT 200,000 INSURED LIVES*

Cause of Death	Standardized Death Rate per 100,000							
	Underweight			Normal Weight	Overweight			
	Total	15–34%	5–14%		5–14%	15–24%	25% +	Total
All causes............	848	913	833	844	1027	1215	1472	1111
Organic heart diseases.	65	63	66	80	115	135	129	121
Angina pectoris.......	14	12	14	16	32	39	37	35
Disease of the arteries.	17	15	17	23	34	46	41	38
Acute and chronic nephritis...........	63	56	64	82	108	202	224	141
Cerebral hemorrhage and apoplexy.......	49	46	50	70	101	115	170	110
Cancer..............	62	54	64	61	64	73	86	68
Diabetes.............	9	9	9	14	22	45	117	36
Pulmonary tuberculosis..............	115	166	103	57	28	21	†	26
Pneumonia (lobar and unspecified)........	70	90	66	63	56	64	72	59
Influenza............	20	29	18	20	29	24	†	28
Accidents............	55	44	58	60	65	65	87	67
Suicides.............	27	33	25	24	31	29	42	31

* Dublin, L. I., and Marks, H. H., Mortality of Women according to Build, The Assoc. of Life Ins. Medical Directors of America, Oct. 20, 1928.
† Not significant.

the increased mortality is negligible up to age twenty-five, but that it is very rapid after that until age fifty. The rate declines after age fifty possibly because these people represent the survival, not of the fittest, but of the outstanding exceptions culled out of the crowd by the careful

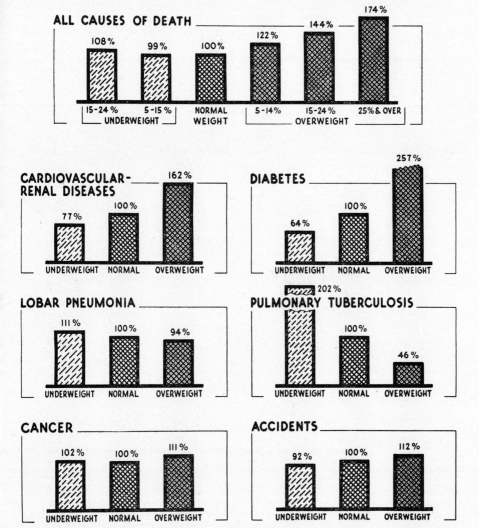

Analysis by Metropolitan Life Insurance Company of Union Central Life Insurance Company Records, 1887-1921

Fig. 87.—Influence of body weight on mortality. Subsequent mortality among men, according to build classes, expressed as percentage of death rate of normal weight men.

scrutiny given overweights after that age by the insurance medical examiners.

The increased mortality rate of insured obese patients is due principally to degenerative diseases. This is to be expected because of the increased resting work fraction of the total metabolism of the obese (see below, section on Oxygen Exchange), the cardiovascular and renal overstrain (see p. 578, section on Signs, Symptoms, and Results of Treatment), and the frequent occurrences of glycosuria (see p. 557, section on Glucose Tolerance and Glycosuria). The menace of obesity to recovery from needed surgical procedures is well known and should also be mentioned. Dublin and Marks[11] classified the different causes of death among persons of different grades of obesity and compared them with the number of deaths from these same causes in people of normal weight. Their findings are recorded in table 7. The rate was greater in the obese not only in the degenerative diseases but also even in accidents and suicides. The greater number of deaths due to accidents may be the result of less agility in the obese. The greater number of suicides does not check with the generally held opinion that the fat man is a jolly one. These data are recorded graphically in the following chart (Fig. 87). Dublin and Marks state that the mortality rate for different grades of obesity at different ages is about the same for women as for men, and occur from the same causes, in approximately the same proportion.

The increased death rate in the obese from diabetes is the most striking of all. It is two and one-half times greater than among persons who are underweight. Moreover the margin between that of the obese and that of normal people widens rapidly as the degree of overweight rises. The death rate from diabetes of those who are 25 per cent or more overweight is more than eight times that of people of normal weight, and thirteen times greater than of those who are underweight.

The increased death rate of the obese from diabetes merits special emphasis, because although it is the greatest menace of their obesity, it is also possibly the most amenable to treatment by reduction of weight (see below, sections on Glycosuria and Glucose Tolerance Tests). Many of these deaths are preventable. Indeed, it may be said with some reason that the greatest advance possible in preventive medicine at present would result from the prevention, or early cure, of obesity with the attendant lower death rate from diabetes alone.

NATURE AND CAUSES

Any energy intake in health in excess of the needs of the body is converted into and stored as fat. Undernutrition is a general food deficiency and during its cure there is a storage of useful materials. When a normal weight is attained this storage of useful materials ceases. Increase in weight above the ideal does not result from a building up of vital tissues. This is proven by studies of nitrogen exchange and creatinine excretion on obese patients on maintenance diets, and while undergoing reduction cure by diet alone. Strang, McClugage, and Evans[13] showed that obese patients have the same daily urinary nitrogen as people of normal weight and that while losing weight rapidly on a total daily caloric intake of 350 to 450 remain indefinitely in nitrogen balance if a protein intake of 1 gm. per kilogram of ideal weight was maintained. McClugage, Booth, and Evans[14] demonstrated also that the creatinine excretion of obese patients was the same as that of people of normal weight, and that during reduction by diet alone it did not change. These observations mean, in regard to muscle mass at least, that it is not built up by the attainment of weight above normal, and that an obese person can attain a normal weight by a severely limited food intake which, however, includes an adequate protein intake, without loss of muscle substance.

The degree of obesity is a measure, therefore, of the amount of overeating in which the patient has indulged. The material thus converted into fat has not been inhaled, has not been absorbed through the skin, cannot be blamed on any gland, endocrine or otherwise, for there is none with an aperture through which it could have been inserted. This material got under the skin by only one portal of entry, the mouth; it was eaten. Attempted compromises with this indisputable fact have seriously clouded thinking as to the nature and causes of obesity.

Individual Energy Needs.—The energy needs of the body vary greatly among individuals and, consequently, the number of calories which may be ingested without becoming obese is variable. A six-foot young man of normal weight (82 Kg.—180 lbs.) doing hard labor in a cold climate may expend 4000 to 5000 calories daily and can eat relatively enormous amounts of food without becoming obese. A seventy-two-year old lady, five feet tall, living as she should, a sedentary life, might get fat on a 1200-calorie daily intake. In her case one is hardly justified in saying that she became obese, not from overeating, but because she was elderly and only five feet tall. She became obese as a result of taking more calories than her need, however few they may be, in other words from overeating. The prevention of obesity consists simply in balancing the energy intake with the energy output at whatever level it may be, and from whatever cause. This is always possible.

A more efficient digestion and absorption of the food ingested has been suggested as one reason for the plus energy balance of the obese. Such has been shown to be not the case. Neuenschwander and Lemmer, quoted by Wilder[15] determined the caloric value of the feces and their content of nitrogen and fat for three obese and three control subjects. The subjects were confined to bed and the diet fed was below estimated requirements to maintain weight. The findings corresponded closely with those of Atwater. They showed absorption efficiency the same in normals and obese of ±90 per cent. These figures for obese and normal people may be compared to those for food utilization by undernourished people gaining rapidly on a forced high caloric intake. Strang, McClugage, and Brownlee[16] reported for nine such patients that the fecal solids averaged 5.8 per cent of the food solids; and the fecal nitrogen 11.8 per cent of the nitrogen intake. These investigators emphasized the slight variation in these figures between the patients and different periods of observation on all patients. Such variation as appeared indicated that there was, if anything, better food absorption with higher caloric intake than with lower (see table 8). These results for undernourished patients even when the diet taken might well be expected to put a strain on their digestive and absorptive powers, corresponded so closely to those above for obese and normal people that only one conclusion can be drawn. The excess energy intake of the obese is not due to increased efficiency of digestion and absorption of the food eaten.

When obese people say they do not eat much they usually refer to bulk rather than food value and may in that sense often be correct. Accurate investigation of the food value of the intake, however, will prove the contrary. One hundred grams of lettuce affords five grams of carbohydrate, or 20 calories. One hundred grams of olive oil, of less bulk than the equivalent weight of lettuce, affords 100 grams of fat, or 900 calories. A hypothetical case history will illustrate this point.

Twin sisters, twenty-one years old, 5 feet tall, weigh 110 pounds each. One sister balances her energy intake with her energy output. She, therefore, maintains her weight without change. The other sister has an average daily plus energy balance of 100 calories. This might well not be noticed by the untrained observer. A little deeper cut in the pat of butter, an extra shake of the salad dressing spoon, a soup cup emptied rather than left with one-fourth inch or less of soup at the bottom, one or two fewer trips upstairs during

TABLE 8

PERCENTAGE OF EFFICIENCY OF DIGESTION IN NORMAL AND OBESE PEOPLE

	Neuenschwander and Lemmer		Atwater
	Obese	Normal	Normal
Calories, per cent..............	87	88.0	88.3–97.4
Nitrogen, per cent............	84	85.5	88.3–96.2
Fat, per cent.................	83	85.5	87.3–98.3

UNDERNUTRITION PATIENTS
Strang, McClugage, and Brownlee

Diet (Calories)	Weeks	Absorption (per cent)
2000..	2	92
2500..	2	94
3000..	18	94
3500..	7	95
4500..	2	94
5000..	10	95

the day, would bring this about. One hundred calories a day excess intake means a weight gain in fat of 10 pounds a year. At age twenty-six, one sister weighs 110 pounds, and the other 160 pounds. Five years later, at the age of thirty-one, when the physician is consulted the comparative weights are 110 and 210 pounds. The obese sister may state that she does not overeat, and the twin sister will insist that this is true, saying with conviction that they have eaten all these years at the same table, the same food, and in equal amounts.

Strang, McClugage and Evans[17] made an attempt to evaluate the statement of some obese patients that they eat little or nothing yet coninue to gain. They told eight obese patients to eat, for three or four days after admission to the metabolic pavilion of the hospital, what they ordinarily ate at home. Careful account was kept of the intakes. These patients ate an average of 2570 calories a day for four days (maximum 3690; minimum 1450). This does not represent a small intake. But what is more significant, these patients lost an average of 2 pounds apiece during the four days of this food intake. In view of this one wonders what must have been the intake at home on which the patients gained weight. The patient with the maximum intake of 3690 calories, who weighed 359 pounds, lost 5 pounds in four days; the one on the minimum intake of 1450 calories, weighed 207 pounds, and lost 4 pounds in five days. Another series of six obese women on a caloric intake of 2510 calories for a total of eighty-eight days showed an average weight loss of 0.15 kilograms a day, 2.3 pounds a week.

Most young people and some older ones, enjoy an *automatic mechanism* for the balancing of intake to needs. They eat more when they are more active, and take a correspondingly smaller amount of food without giving the matter any attention when less active. This regulating mechanism, when functioning adequately, is amazingly efficient. The wonder is that with the genuine delight of eating being so freely offered to everyone there is not more obesity than there is.

What happens when this regulating mechanism breaks down? A simple explanation of increasing weight with age is that, as one grows older, he exercises less and may continue to eat the same amount. As weight increases the tendency to less and less exercise develops, and, as will be shown later, the more food it takes to satisfy, or rather the more can be taken without discomfort. Thus is a vicious circle initiated.

Appetite.—This intangible component can in many instances be attributed to family habits of eating. In a family where a groaning table is regularly set before healthy children, overeating, a delightful occupation, is likely to become a habit. Differences in types as well as in quantities of food served are encountered in households. The family which prefers to begin with thin soup and end with fruit or light desserts will ingest fewer calories by far than the one addicted to cream soups and heavy pastries. When the habit of overeating is well established more food is necessary to give a feeling of satiety, which is more important in children than in adults, as an indication to stop eating. Thus also is a vicious circle established. Preble[7] concluded from a study of 1000 cases of obesity that the cause in the overwhelming majority of cases lies in their habits of eating and states that "obesity is a habit, and a dangerous habit at that."

Cultivated habits of eating will not suffice to explain the obesity of many patients. It has been said that the trouble with the obese is purely one of *temperament*, that they lack ambition, are less aggressive, physically lazy, thus accounting for a lowered energy expenditure. It has been further said in regard to increased intake that they are primarily sensualists, people in whom far too great a proportion of their enjoyment of life comes from sensual indulgences, in their cases gustatory delights. But this, if true, must have a physiologic background. A colleague, interested in the causation of obesity, describes two families of his acquaintance. There are four children in each family. In one family one child is musical, while the other three are uninterested in music. No one will deny some organization of, shall we say, the central nervous system—in the musical child different from that of his nonmusical brothers and sisters. In the second family one child is definitely obese, while the three others are of normal build. Is it not possible that the obese child has an organization, shall we say again, of the central nervous system—different from the spare children? It would seem reasonable. Perhaps in families where all members are fat, this obesity is not always due to faulty habits of eating, but as suggested by Wilder,[18] to *hereditary disposition*, an increased activity of centers of the diencephalon controlling feelings of hunger and satiety. Gurney[19] noted a pronounced familial incidence of obesity and an hereditary factor in its causation.

It is inexpedient and unnecessary to discuss all the suggestions of possible mechanisms of control of hunger and satiety in the obese as compared to normals. Allusion will be made only to a few of the many interesting studies bearing on this point. In general the suggested possible differences fall into three groups: (1) an increased tendency because of some metabolic anomaly for the conversion of carbohydrate into fat; (2) fat not easily burned because of some metabolic disturbance in its handling; and (3) fat not available as fuel because it is diverted to depots by special chemotoxins.

Hagedorn, Holten, and Johansen[20] presented the hypothesis that obesity is due to a *qualitative anomaly in metabolism*, an abnormally increased transformation of carbohydrate into fat. They determined the respiratory quotients on obese and normal persons to whom they had given for two days a diet consisting chiefly of carbohydrates. They found that the respiratory quotients in the obese were lower than in normals, and that there was a relation between the respiratory quotient and degree of obesity. The lowest were found in the most obese, and in the slightly obese a minimal lowering approaching normal. This same possibility has been suggested by Mason.[21] The diets, chiefly carbohydrate, ingested for two days by the subjects of Hagedorn and his collaborators would seem to have afforded maintenance calories. They were not recorded quantitatively, however, nor were the weights of the patients reported before and after the two days' dieting. It is true that weights of patients over such a short period would be, because of water swings, of little value without intake and output figures. It is to be considered, however, that Hagedorn's diets were of caloric maintenance value for his subjects of normal weight, but in view of the increased level of oxygen exchange in the obese, were not of maintenance value for these subjects. Consequently, the obese were compelled to oxidize fat. This suggested explanation conforms to the findings in this study that the lowest respiratory quotients were found in the most obese.

Specific Dynamic Action.—Strouse, *et al.*,[22] suggested not only that obesity could be independent of amount of food intake but also that there was a difference in specific dynamic action of *protein, carbohydrate, and fat*, in the obese. Some observations[23] on the respiratory quotient would seem to indicate that in the obese, fat is burned with greater difficulty than in normal people and, therefore, is not utilized when carbohydrate and protein are available. This in no way contradicts the known fact that carbohydrate is more easily burned than fat, or that if no excess of energy intake is available, none will be laid down as fat. Waldvogel[24] felt that the obese burned fat with difficulty. He injected beta-oxybutyric acid subcutaneously and found a greater amount of acetone excreted in the urine and expired air of obese patients than in those of normal weight. One should also mention in this connection the finding of McKay and Sherrill[25] that there was less ketonuria in some obese persons during fasting than in normal people, thus indicating that less fat was burned. Although the fasting period was four and five days this variation might, because these patients had no preliminary period on a controlled diet, have resulted not from diminished availability of fat for oxidation in some of the obese, but because they began the fast with greater —even supersaturated—nonfat fuel stores. This suggestion is supported by the fact that some of the obese patients in this series had more ketosis than the normal controls. McKay and Sherrill suggested a classification of obesity on this difference; endocrine for those who had less, and alimentary for those who had more ketosis than the normal controls. These observations are not in agreement with those of Folin and Denis[26] that obese persons lose less body nitrogen during starvation than normals. This means that the additional protein sparing fuel available in the fat stores was being used. The periods of fasting to which the cases of Folin and Denis submitted were five and six days. Similar conclusions were drawn by Deuel and Gulick[27] from observations made on ten obese persons, five men and five women, during a seven-day fast. Also in accord with these observations are the negligible nitrogen losses observed by Strang, McClugage and Evans[17] in obese patients maintained, some for months, on diets affording an average of 58 gm. of protein, 14 gm. of carbohydrate, 8 gm. of fat, and 360 calories, an average of not more than three calories per day per kilogram of actual weight, on which they lost an average of almost 0.6 pounds per day.

A tendency of the obese for *fat fixation* (the *lipophilia* of Bergman) has also been suggested as the mechanism of a possible difference in control of hunger and satiety in the obese as compared to persons who maintain normal weights. Hetenyi[28] reported interesting observations supporting this hypothesis. The blood lipid level in obese patients on submaintenance diets fell 18 to 43 per cent and remained unchanged in those of normal weight. The lipid level of the blood tested hourly for five hours after the ingestion of 60 gm. of fat on a fasting stomach increased very much less in obese subjects than in normals. Similar findings were obtained when olive oil was injected subcutaneously. One cannot say, of course, that these results did not come from changed physiological activity attendant upon a long period of overeating, were secondary rather than a primary disorder. More weight could be given to the proposed lipophilia in people who become obese if the changes could be shown to persist after reduction, or better yet were found in a normal person who afterward became obese. However, Hetenyi injected olive oil subcutaneously in patients with lipodystrophy. The absorption was that of normal persons when injected into the thin upper extremities. The obese reaction resulted when the oil was put in the fat lower extremities. These observations, if confirmed, are very suggestive that in the obese there is a tendency to fat fixation and therefore, it is less available for oxidation. It is well known that the fat of lipomas, and of lipodystrophy persists despite starvation. One must also consider in this connection the observation of Best and Campbell[29] that anterior pituitary extract promotes the transportation of fat from body store to the liver, and the lipotrophic effect of choline and certain dietary proteins.[30] A different level of activity of this function might influence appetite. And finally one must mention Dragstedt's[31] lipocaic, a product of the pancreas concerned with fat metabolism. It has been pointed out by Wilder[15] that the effect after meals of withdrawing from the circulation even a little more fat than usual might well account both for the delayed sense of satiety and for the frequently abnormal taste for carbohydrate encountered in obese persons. Energy requirements must be satisfied one way or another, and if part of the food is made less available for metabolism, the result would inevitably be hunger. A very slight tendency of this kind might have significant results in the course of time. This hypothesis would explain also the characteristic distribution of fat in patients with endocrine disorders.

Energy requirements must, however, be satisfied first. This means that despite a possible tendency of the tissues to fat fixation, if no excess energy intake is available to be fixed, all ingested will be consumed by the primary demand of energy requirement. Adequate evidence has been brought by studies of oxygen exchange, nitrogen balance, and creatinine excretion that when an obese person is fed a diet affording the known essential foodstuffs but deficient in calories none of it is diverted to fat depots. Thus not only in the acquisition of obesity but during the much more exacting test of its removal there is no deprivation of vital tissues in favor of fat depots.

Once obesity, for whatever reason—carelessness, habits of eating either cultivated or due to hereditary tendency, a physiological variance in fat handling—has become established, a mechanism contributory to its continuance is set up. Strang, McClugage and Brownlee,[32] in a study of the *specific dynamic action of a fixed meal* in normal, thin, and obese people, found no quantitative variation between the groups (table 19) but demonstrated for each qualitative responses of significance in this connection.

Appetite is a subjective phenomenon and the suggestion of a possible relationship between satiety and the physiological stress resulting from the specific dynamic action of food is, of course, difficult to analyze. It is probable if such relationship may be assumed that when the existing rate of heat production changes at a certain rate, for example, 15 per cent per hour, the body as a whole experiences a feeling of well-being and comfort; but when the rate of change is appreciably increased, perhaps to 20 per cent per hour, the body rebels against the physiological strain and automatically prevents further insult by interrupting intake. Thus may complete satiety have been brought about. The application of this point of view to the findings of Strang, McClugage and Brownlee shows that the assumed satiety point, 20 per cent per hour rate of increase in heat production above the predetermined basal corresponded in normal people to the peak of the heat curve developed by eight hourly readings after ingestion of the fixed meal. In the thin, the assumed satiety point of 20 per cent per hour rate of increase, was passed long before the peak was reached. The curves of the obese failed to reach the satiety level by 25 per cent, and in fact coincided with the level of optimum sensation, 15 per cent of increase per hour. A comparable interpretation of this fact would suggest that the test meal, with its fixed total calories and specific dynamic action, would quite fail to satisfy these patients. In other words, if we assume that the test meal, with its 40 gm. of protein and 610 calories completely satisfied the normal group, the thin patients would, if permitted free selection of food, have been satisfied with much less, whereas the obese group would require a far greater intake. The selection of the values, 15 and 20 per cent for the critical points was quite arbitrary, and more careful investigation might have revealed entirely different true levels. However, regardless of the levels selected, the fundamental difference between the three groups would persist. Furthermore it might appear, by more frequent determination than Strang, McClugage and Brownlee employed, that the peaks of the curves of rate of change of heat production fell earlier than mentioned in the thin people, and later in the obese, as compared to normals. If, for example, the peaks were found to be at twenty minutes, forty minutes, and sixty minutes in the thin, normal, and obese groups the resultant effects upon their relative total food intakes would be accentuations of tendencies described above.

It will, therefore, be seen that the same factors which operate to produce the fixed eating habits and fixed body weights of normal individuals may become perverted in two directions. The resultant extreme in one case is the apparently healthy person who persistently holds a weight 20 to 25 per cent below normal. He functions at a low metabolic level and receives his optimal specific dynamic action stimulus from a small food intake which maintains his subnormal weight by a caloric intake equivalent to his output. The other extreme is the likewise apparently healthy person who maintains a weight 50 to 200 per cent above normal. This person operates at a very high level of oxygen exchange. He holds his weight, or as usually appears, slightly increases it, because of the correspondingly large caloric intake which is required to produce the requisite rate of change of heat production for optimum sensation of satiety. It may be emphasized that no pathologic factor in metabolism exists in either case. The thin person stays thin because, at his low metabolic level, the food intake which produces dynamic action giving him the optimum sensation of comfort amounts to 1500 to 1800 calories. The fat person stays fat because with his high metabolic level, a 3000- to 3500-calorie intake is required to give him the same optimum sensation.

In a scholarly discussion of the several different kinds of adipose tissue and their functions as organs, Wells[33] states that the fat of acquired obesity is stored in the cells of the reticulo-endothelial system. These are phagocytic cells. The nature of obesity acquired by overeating can, therefore in this sense, be said to be that of a foreign body.

We must not cloud the issue in discussing proposed physiological backgrounds for the fat of obese people by saying that they are, or may be, the cause of obesity. They are the cause of lowered physical activity, or more often, of increased appetite. Furthermore, when evidence of endocrine dysfunction and obesity appear together, the former is not necessarily primary. The endocrine disorder may be, as the obesity certainly is, due to overeating, to the ingestion of a faulty metabolic mixture, this in turn resulting from faulty habits of eating, or an uncontrolled hereditary abnormal appetite. The law of conservation of energy always holds true and must be respected. The abnormal appetite leading to overeating, which can be the only cause of obesity, although increasing the difficulty of dieting, does not, whatever its background (even if this be a hereditary tendency) justify the continuation of an unwholesome practice.

PHYSIOLOGICAL CONSIDERATIONS

Nitrogen Balance.—The level of nitrogen exchange in the obese on their customary diets is the same as for normal people, and is influenced by the same factors and in the same degree. Denis and Borgstrom[34] reported the average daily urinary nitrogen on a long series of students at Tulane University over several years to be 11.07 gm. as related to a 70-Kg. man. A similar study at Western Reserve University by Beard[35] produced almost identical figures: 11.16 gr. of urinary nitrogen daily for a 70-Kg. man. Strang, McClugage and Evans[13] determined the daily urinary nitrogen on obese patients who had an average weight of 168.5 Kg., which related to their average ideal weight of 65.9 Kg. represented the great excess of 155 per cent. These patients were on diets, submaintenance for their actual weight, averaging 2403 calories, but containing adequate protein—approximately 1 gm. per Kg. of ideal weight. Their daily urinary nitrogen was 11.1 gm., 0.16 gm. per Kg. of ideal weight, or 11.2 gm. as related to a 70-Kg. man. The almost exact correspondence of these figures for persons so gravely overweight with those for the two series on normal persons is noteworthy.

Strang, McClugage and Evans further studied the nitrogen exchange on these obese patients while undergoing reduction by dietary measures alone. Two diets were employed. The first, taken for an average of 39 days, afforded an average of 336 calories, 59 gm. of protein, 10 gm. of carbohydrate, 7 gm. of fat. The second, eaten for an average of 101 days, afforded 444 calories, 61 gm. of protein, 29 gm. of carbohydrate, 9 gm. of fat. The results are shown in table 9.

There was a negative nitrogen balance with the first diet. This resulted from a lowered protein intake as well as an increased nitrogen excretion. These patients were not hungry, and the lowered intake was caused by the monotony of the diet despite efforts to maintain the protein intake at 1 gm. per Kg. of ideal weight. The cause of the increased nitrogen output was questionable. The possibility that a portion of the protein was being burned as fuel because of the lowered availability of stored fat for fuel in the obese, seemed unlikely. If this were so the restoration of nitrogen equilibrium which occurred with the second diet employed would not have occurred. This diet supplied only 108 more calories than the first, a total of 444, and still left a caloric deficit of well over 2000. A call on the body fat to supplement a caloric deficit diminished by this small amount, less than 5 per cent, would not be expected to exert a protein-sparing influence. Possibly some protein was oxidized at first in an effort of the body to attain a physiologically more comfortable ketogenic-antiketogenic ratio. These patients, deriving such a great proportion of their fuel needs from stored fat, were operating at high theoretical ketogenic-antiketogenic ratios (see below, section on K-AK ratio). Folin and Denis[26] have pointed out that the body increases with practice its capacity to burn stored fat with a diminished formation of ketone bodies and additional protein sparing effect. It seems likely that some such mechanism as this was operative to bring about the smaller nitrogen loss of the second diet as compared to the first.

The average loss of body nitrogen in Evans and Strang's patients on the 336-calorie diet was 2.0 gm. per patient per day, or 78 gm. per patient for the period. Since the patients who were studied lost an average of 15.7 Kg. of body weight in the thirty-nine days, this 78 gm. of total nitrogen lost for the same period indicates a small loss of body nitrogen. That this amount was of little practical significance was suggested by a comparison with the nitrogen loss of the undernutrition patients of Benedict as analyzed by

of nitrogen metabolism. This work has been repeatedly confirmed. The independence of creatinine excretion from the other elements of nitrogen metabolism was shown by McClugage, Booth and Evans[14] to be true also for the obese. They found in these patients that there was no relation between creatinine excretion and the total urine volume, that it was independent of the total nitrogen excretion, and the presence of a positive or negative nitrogen balance.

Variations in amount of urinary creatinine among individuals of approximately normal weight are dependent largely, but not wholly, on variations in body mass. Repeated observations have shown the creatinine excretion is at a low level during the early weeks of life and increases to reach a constant level at about the time of puberty. In general, the excretion of women is lower than that of men. The average of the coefficients found by a group of investigators was nine for men and six for women. This lower figure for women was considered by Shaffer[38] to be an effect not of sex itself but

TABLE 10

NITROGEN AND WEIGHT LOSS IN UNDERNOURISHED AND IN REDUCTION PATIENTS*

	Undernourished†	Period II	Period III
Duration, weeks..........................	3	5½	14½
Diet, calories............................	1375.0	336.0	444.0
Daily nitrogen output, gm.................	11.3	11.4	9.8
Daily nitrogen loss, gm...................	3.1	2.0	0.1
Total nitrogen loss, gm...................	65.0	78.0	10.0
Estimated initial body nitrogen content, gm..	2037.0	1970.0	1980.0
Reduction body nitrogen, per cent..........	3.2	3.9	0.5
Initial body weight, kilo....	67.9	159.2	143.8
Ideal body weight, kilo....................	....	65.9	65.9
Body weight loss, kilo....................	4.5	15.7	21.6
Weight loss (initial body weight), per cent....	6.5	9.8	15.0
Weight loss (ideal body weight), per cent....	......	24.0	32.0

* Strang, J. M., McClugage, H. B., and Evans, F. A., Am. J. Med. Sci., Lea & Febiger, Publishers, 181: 3, 336, 1931.
† Lusk.[5]

rather of a greater proportion of adipose tissue and of a lower muscular development. This view is supported by the work of Tracy and Clark,[39] and of Hodgson and Lewis[40] showing that the creatinine coefficients of women trained in physical education correspond to those of men. McClugage, Booth, and Evans state in regard to the normal, obese, and undernourished subjects they studied that without exception those exhibiting a high creatinine coefficient were well muscled individuals whereas those exhibiting a low coefficient, as figured on their actual weight, were either poorly muscled or excessively obese. Meyers and Fine[41] and Palladin[42] have shown a direct relationship between the creatinine secretion and the total body creatine in the individual and in the species. Since muscle creatine comprises fully 98 per cent of the total body creatine[43] urinary creatinine becomes, for practical purposes, an index of muscle creatine or of muscle mass. To demonstrate this relationship Folin calculated the number of milligrams of creatinine eliminated per kilogram of body weight. Shaffer called this expression the "creatinine coefficient" and substituted in the expression, the number of milligrams of creatinine nitrogen for the number of milligrams of creatinine. It is in these terms that it is usually expressed.

Keeping in mind the variations in creatinine nitrogen excretion between people of different muscular complement and between the sexes, but disregarding the influence of food intake as negligible, McClugage, Booth, and Evans determined the creatinine nitrogen on a series of obese and normal people. The findings are presented in table 11. No variation between obese and normal people was demonstrated in the creatinine nitrogen excretion. Furthermore, this level remains the same during reduction by diets severely restricted to 400 to 600 calories, although containing an adequate amount of protein and other essential foodstuffs. Observations made on one patient reduced 36 Kg. in body weight are shown in table 12. This is in striking contrast to the findings of Cathcart and Benedict[44] in starvation presented in the same table for comparison. Such figures for creatinine nitrogen excretion when related to the actual weight give low creatinine coefficients for the obese. This is obviously incorrect because the fat stored in obesity is inert tissue, certainly not concerned in any way with total nitrogen ex-

TABLE 11

CREATININE NITROGEN EXCRETION*

	Gm. Daily	Observed Weight, Kg.
Obese....................................	0.42	137.0
Normal...................................	0.49	64.6
Variation................................	0.07	72.4

* McClugage, H. B., Booth, Geo., and Evans, F. A., Am. J. Med. Sci., Lea & Febiger, Publishers, **181**: 3, 349, 1931.

change or any fraction of it. Reference to the data in table 13 affords additional evidence of this fact. When the level of creatinine nitrogen excretion in the obese is related to ideal, not actual weight, the creatinine coefficient is seen to be the same as in people of normal weight, and to remain unchanged during dietary correction (Table 12). This fact proves that no muscle mass is lost by the obese when reducing on diets even of only 400 to 600 calories, if they also contain an adequate amount of essential foodstuffs.

Oxygen Exchange.—The popular prejudice that fat people are frequently small eaters and, therefore, have some mystic power of handling energy units more economically than normal people persists in spite of many studies demonstrating the reverse. The fact that the fat person actually consumes more energy than he would if he were not obese has been emphasized by Labbé and Stevenin[45] and by Lauter.[46] Observations have been made repeatedly that the basal calories per day for the obese lie between 2000 and 2200 instead of the normal 1400 and 1600.

Basal heat production is referred to the surface area of the body to arrive at the so-called basal metabolic rate which expresses the per cent deviation of the basal calories per unit of body surface from the average values for normal persons. An increase in surface area in the obese proportional to their greater basal oxygen exchange has been demonstrated by Means[47] who

TABLE 12

CREATININE EXCRETION OF OBESE PATIENT DURING REDUCTION BY DIETARY MEASURES ALONE*

Period of Observation, Weeks	Creatinine N Excretion, Daily (Gm.)	Creatinine N Excretion (Gm.), Cathcart, 1907	Creatinine N Excretion (Gm.), Benedict, 1915
First..........................	0.39	0.45	0.50
Second......................	0.52	0.38	0.48
Third........................	0.42	....	0.38
Fourth.......................	0.46	....	0.34
Fifth.........................	0.46	....	0.33
Sixth........................	0.48		
Seventh......................	0.47		
Eighth.......................	0.43		
Ninth........................	0.39		
Tenth........................	0.35		
Eleventh.....................	0.37		
Twelfth......................	0.46		
Thirteenth...................	0.35		
Fourteenth...................	0.44		
Fifteenth.....................	0.44		
Sixteenth....................	0.44		
Seventeenth..................	0.40		
Eighteenth...................	0.44		
Nineteenth...................	0.44		

The figures in this table are those of a patient reduced 36 Kg., and are typical of the entire group. The figures of Cathcart and of Benedict are converted to weekly averages for purposes of comparison.

* McClugage, H. B., Booth, Geo., and Evans, F. A., Am. J. Med. Sci., Lea & Febiger, Publishers, 181: 3, 349, 1931.

showed that the basal metabolic rates in obese people determined in this way were normal despite the higher level of oxygen exchange. Similar studies by Strouse and Wang,[48] and citations by them from earlier studies

TABLE 13

CREATININE COEFFICIENT IN OBESE AS RELATED TO IDEAL WEIGHT AND TO NORMAL AND UNDER-NOURISHED PEOPLE*

	Obese	Normal	Undernourished
Average theoretical ideal weight (kg.)........	65.4	62.2	63.4
Average observed weight (kg.)..............	137.0	64.6	47.6
Average creatinine coefficient ideal weight	6.7	7.9	4.4
Average creatinine coefficient observed weight	3.4	7.7	5.8

* McClugage, H. B., Booth, Geo., and Evans, F. A., Am. J. Med. Sci., Lea & Febiger, Publishers, 181: 3, 349, 1931.

confirmed Means' report. Additional evidence was brought by Preble,[7] Mason,[21] and Hagedorn and collaborators.[20] DuBois[49] stated that the basal metabolic rates of obese fall within normal limits.

It is, therefore, established that a pudgy woman of forty-nine years, five feet tall, weighing 294 pounds has only 6 per cent less energy exchange in the resting state than a man of the same age, 6 feet 3 inches tall, weighing 205 pounds. The surface is the same in the two cases, 2.22 square meters. There is, however, a fundamental difference in the two cases. The measure of the physiological status in the obese might better be stated by comparing the metabolism of the obese woman not with that of a normal person having the same surface—a veritable giant—but with that of a person comparable to her in all respects other than weight and surface. The reasonable basis of comparison is, therefore, the caloric requirements which she herself might have had if only she were of normal weight.

Strang and Evans[2] while studying oxygen exchange in obese patients undergoing reduction by diet alone found in agreement with investigators quoted above that the basal metabolic rate is normal in the obese. Relating the oxygen consumption to the ideal, not the actual, weight and surface area showed a high level of oxygen exchange in relation to the active, vital

TABLE 14

EXCESS OF WEIGHT, SURFACE, AND ENERGY IN THE OBESE*

	Number of Cases	Age	Weight			Surface			Total Basal Calories per Hour		
			Ideal	Observed	Excess	Ideal	Observed	Excess	Ideal	Observed	Excess
					per cent			per cent			per cent
Means......	10	37	140	253	80	1.69	2.17	28	62	81	30
Strouse and Wang.....	10	27	125	207	66	1.57	1.95	24	59	74	25
Strang and Evans....	7	37	129	238	83	1.59	2.06	29	58	73	26

* Strang, J. A., and Evans, F. A., J. Clin. Invest., 6: 277, 1928.

body tissues of the obese as represented by that ideal weight. Their figures for seven cases with normal metabolic rates actually showed an increase in calories of 26 per cent above normal for them if of ideal weight. A recalculation in this way by Strang and Evans of ten cases reported by Strouse and Wang showed an average increase of 25 per cent. They used only the cases studied by the Tissot method. A similar recomputation of the data published by Means[47] in 1916 gave an average increase of 30 per cent for ten cases. In order to afford a fair comparison, Means' data were recast in accordance with the present standards for weight, surface, and basal calories (Table 14). It will be noted that the increase in the energy exchange was not proportional to the increase in weight but was, as mentioned, of the same order of magnitude as the increase in surface.

The close approximation of the results of these three studies may be emphasized. However, in reviewing these data, the limits of normal variation of metabolism must be kept in mind. Harris and Benedict[50] published data in 1921 showing the extreme variations of metabolism in a given person, as much as 14 per cent over a period of two years. Du Bois thought that variations in metabolism were smaller than the possible errors of the determination. Variations in figures for basal metabolic rates in the obese greater than those for normal people almost surely occur. This is so because the obese probably never attain a true basal metabolic level.

A person of normal weight with the level of basal oxygen exchange shown by the obese, representing a rate of $+25$ to $+30$ per cent, would display thyrotoxic symptoms. The obese are not thyrotoxic as a result of this elevation of rate. This probably is because their so-called basal metabolic rate represents their basal rate plus the addition of an ever present work, and non-work, fraction. The level of oxygen exchange of the obese in excess of that which would be normal for them if of ideal weight can, therefore, be considered a measure of the physiological strain of their excess weight, a work fraction and nonwork fraction from which they can make no escape, even in their quietest moments of relaxation. Proof of this point of view is afforded by the fact that obese patients attaining, by diet restriction alone, a weight even entirely normal for them were not thyrotoxic. They were not thyrotoxic because with reduction in weight

TABLE 15

CHANGES IN THE LEVEL OF BASAL OXYGEN EXCHANGE RECORDED AS CALORIES PER HOUR SHOWN BY OBESE PATIENTS REDUCING RAPIDLY BY DIETS SEVERELY RESTRICTED IN CALORIES, BUT SUPPLYING ADEQUATE AMOUNTS OF ALL KNOWN ESSENTIAL FOODSTUFFS*

Case Number	Outset	First Month	Second Month	Third Month	Fourth Month	Fifth Month
1.	69	65	63	62	53	52
2.	70	68	63	64	63	
3.	72	75	73	76	72	69
4.	74	69	64	65	62	62
5.	70	66	58	60		
Average	71	66	64	65	62	61

* Strang, J. A., and Evans, F. A., J. Clin. Invest., 8: 277, 1928.

there was a concomitant lowering of the level of oxygen exchange measured under the usual conditions of a basal metabolism test, presumably by removal of the added work and nonwork fraction. Details of this adjustment from the report of Strang and Evans who recorded the levels of oxygen exchange under basal conditions of obese patients reducing rapidly on a severely restricted caloric intake but adequate supplies of all known essential foodstuffs appear in table 15. In table 16 are presented the initial and final findings set down with the figures for surface area and other pertinent data.

Despite these considerations, determinations of the level of oxygen exchange in the obese with the customary precautions to attain a basal level will be referred to as "basal."

The initial average surface of 2.0 square meters shown by these patients (maximum 2.16; minimum 1.88) was reduced to 1.83 (maximum 2.01; minimum 1.63). This represented a surface change of 8.5 per cent. The initial surface was, however, 26 per cent greater than the ideal, the final only 15 per cent greater, thus giving a drop of 45 per cent of the excess

TABLE 16

INFLUENCE OF WEIGHT REDUCTION ON ENERGY EXCHANGE*

Case Number	Age	Before Reduction									After Reduction										
		Weight			Surface Area			Total Basal Calories per Hour			Duration of Reduction	Number of Observations	Weight			Surface Area			Total Basal Calories per Hour		
		Ideal	Observed	Excess	Ideal	Observed	Excess	Ideal	Observed	Excess			Observed	Excess	Percentile Decrease in Excess	Observed	Excess	Percentile Decrease in Excess	Observed	Excess	Percentile Decrease in Excess
		lbs.	lbs.	per cent	m.	m.	per cent	cal.	cal.	per cent	wks.	number	lbs.	per cent	per cent	m.	per cent	per cent	cal.	per cent	per cent
1	50	131	206	57	1.56	1.88	20	55	69	25	20	12	145	10	82	1.63	5	75	53	−3	112
2	29	133	236	77	1.68	2.16	28	62	70	12	17	11	203	52	32	2.01	19	32	61	−1	108
3	32	125	251	100	1.56	2.11	35	57	72	26	20	11	216	72	28	1.95	25	28	69	+21	19
4	41	133	216	62	1.61	1.98	23	58	74	27	19	12	167	25	59	1.79	11	52	62	+7	74
5	28	121	202	66	1.52	1.90	25	56	70	24	9	7	173	43	33	1.77	16	36	60	+6	75
6	28	130	262	101	1.63	2.21	35	59	79	30											
7	49	133	294	121	1.57	2.20	40	57	77	37											
Average 1–7	37	129	238	83	1.59	2.06	29	58	73	26	17	10	181	40	47	1.83	15	45	61	+6	77
Average 1–5	36	128	222	72	1.58	2.00	26	58	71	23											

* Strang, J. A., and Evans, F. A., J. Clin. Invest., **8**: 277, 1928.

surface. It was noted above that in the initial state, the increase in the level of basal oxygen exchange in the obese ran parallel with the increase in surface, thus resulting in normal figures for their basal metabolic rate. The data in table 17 show, however, that there was a loss of but 8.5 per cent in surface area. Or, it may be said that the calories dropped 77 per cent of the excess as the excess surface area was reduced 45 per cent.

These cases showed a sharp drop in energy exchange under basal conditions immediately after dieting was begun and before an appreciable weight change had occurred. This probably, in part, measured the energy requirements of handling different amounts of food.

The 77 per cent drop in excess basal oxygen exchange and the 45 per cent reduction in surface area was to be compared to the 47 per cent of the excess weight that was lost. It is worthy of emphasis that before dieting the increase in basal calories consumed was proportional to surface area, rather than to weight increase; and that after dieting, the reduction in excess calories was out of proportion to that of both weight and surface area. The rate of drop in basal calories was more than one and one-half

TABLE 17

RATES OF CHANGE OF WEIGHT, SURFACE, AND ENERGY*

Group	Type	I Weight Loss	II Surface Loss	III Basal Calories Loss	IV Ratio Calorie Loss Weight Loss	V Ratio Calorie Loss Surface Loss
		per cent	*per cent*	*per cent*		
I.......	Acute	6.5	<1.0	32.0	4.9	32.0+
II.......	Starvation	17.0	5.0	30.0	1.7	6.0
III.......	Chronic	8.5	3.3	19.0	2.2	5.9
IV.......	Obese	18.0	8.5	14.0	0.77	1.6

* Strang, J. A., and Evans, F. A., J. Clin. Invest., **8**: 277, 1928.

times as great as the change in either weight or surface area. Strang and Evans, however, stated in this connection that in no instance in this series did the observed calories fall lower than minus 5 per cent of the theoretically normal level.

An understanding of the altered physiology of the obese is aided by noting that the correlation of the percentage loss of excess area and elevated level of basal oxygen exchange to loss of excess weight is a peculiar property of the obese. This is shown by comparing these figures with those of Benedict's undernutrition studies (Table 18).

It is useful to distinguish three degrees of undernutrition; acute and chronic undernutrition, and starvation. For comparison with data of the obese patients one example of each type is taken from Benedict (see Tables 17 and 18). The figures for the chronic and acute undernutrition cases are taken from Lusk's review of Benedict's work, and in consequence certain values differ very slightly from the original data of Benedict.

In comparing the obese with Benedict's subjects it must be emphasized that his were healthy active males. They had at the outset a physiologically normal basal metabolism, while that of the obese, although normal as calculated on their actual weight and surface area, was elevated 23 per cent as related to their ideal weight and surface area, that is to their vital functioning body tissues. Furthermore, none of the undernutrition cases approached the magnitude of weight loss of the obese. On a percentage basis the starvation case lost a comparable amount.

Clinically the response in the two groups was entirely different. The undernourished groups became less ambitious, less energetic, tried to conserve all possible energy. They were depressed, irritable, and unstable. The obese patients, in contrast, showed consistently more initiative, had a desire to do things, and felt in all respects better than for years previously.

The acute undernutrition and starvation cases dropped 30 per cent of their basal calories in three weeks. The chronic undernutrition cases dropped 19 per cent in approximately the time in which obese patients reduced their basal energy exchange only 14 per cent. This disparity is given more significance when it is recalled that the energy drop in the three groups of undernourished normals represented a lowering of the ideal basal metabolic level, whereas the 14 per cent depression in the obese corresponded rather

TABLE 18

METABOLISM IN VARIOUS FORMS OF UNDERNUTRITION*

	Type	Basal Calories Before Diet	Basal Calories Ideal Weight	Duration of Diet	Calories of Diet	Weight Loss	Weight Loss	Basal Calories After Diet	Percentile Loss in Calories
						kg.	per cent	cal.	per cent
I†	Acute	1745	1745	3 weeks	1375 net	4.5	6.5	1293	32
II†	Starvation	1432	1432	3 weeks	0	10.1‡	17.0	1002	30
III†	Chronic	1686	1686	4 months	1400 (1900 net)	5.7 (Held weight)	8.5	1367	19
IV	Obese	1700	1380	17 weeks	620 gross	18.6	18.0	1460	14

* Strang, J. A., and Evans, F. A., J. Clin. Invest., 8: 277, 1928.
† Essential data from Lusk[36] and Dubois.[49]
‡ Estimated from graph.

to a 77 per cent return of an excessive metabolism toward normal. This difference is emphasized further when the marked disparity in diets is noted. The "acute undernutrition" subjects, on a diet 6 per cent greater than the basal needs, had a depression of 32 per cent in calories and a small loss of weight. The "starvation" subjects, at the time of the lowest metabolism, had a 30 per cent drop in calories while the weight loss was about one-half that of the obese patients. The "chronic undernutrition" subjects, after the initial weight loss, held weight on a diet 42 per cent above the basal needs while the drop in calories was only 19 per cent of the initial value. The obese patients, however, on a diet 57 per cent less than basal needs showed a depression of only 14 per cent of the initial metabolism, and lost weight consistently.

These differences between the "undernutrition" groups and the "obese" group may be restated with different emphasis. The ratio of the rate of reduction of basal energy exchange to the rate of weight loss for the undernutrition cases were more than twice that of the obese patients.

Obese patients on limited diets with sufficient protein thus have been shown not to require the protective depression of the energy exchange which Lusk described in connection with the above groups of under-nourished.

Specific Dynamic Action of Food.—A depression of the specific dynamic action of food takes a prominent place among the many factors presented as of importance in the development of obesity. It has been suggested that in the obese there is not only lowered specific dynamic action, but that obese states can be classified into various subgroupings on the basis of variations of reaction.

Von Noorden showed that a daily excess consumption of 200 calories would lead in the course of a year to a deposition of 17 pounds of fat, or 20 pounds of fat tissue. DuBois[49] calculated that an excess of 89 calories per day would add 8 pounds of weight per year. The excessively obese patient may gain weight at the rate of 20 pounds per year or faster, while the milder degrees approach more nearly the lower rate. The caloric excesses, therefore, vary from 90 to 200 calories per day during the period of weight gain. Benedict and Carpenter[51] stated that, on the average in normal people, 6 per cent of a mixed meal was used for its specific dynamic effect. Therefore, of an average caloric intake of 2500 calories per day, 6 per cent, or 150 calories, would approximate the extra specific dynamic heat. The development of obesity within ten to fifteen years would require a real drop in this 150-caloric factor, certainly to 100 or even 75 calories. This means a 33 to 50 per cent diminution of total heat effect in the mild cases and a total absence of specific dynamic action in the severe grades. Depression of these magnitudes should be readily demonstrable.

Correct *measurements of heat response in the body* demand the establishment of a true basal level to which the elevation observed is related. The difficulty of determination of this factor was pointed out by Benedict and Carpenter. Despite the obvious importance of establishing a true base line it appears that the correctness of the results of some observers studying specific dynamic reaction of food in the obese can be seriously questioned because of neglect of this consideration. Some papers imply no preliminary training of subjects in submitting to the technique of basal metabolic determinations. Some investigators relied on a single trial basal rate reading on the day preliminary to the experiment. It is a matter of common knowledge that many persons need repeated trials before learning to attain basal conditions during the test, even sufficient for the relatively inaccurate readings satisfactory for routine clinical work. Attention should be called also to the daily variation in basal calorie exchange which may occur normally, probably greater in the obese than in others (see Oxygen Exchange above). This variation despite the greatest care might well introduce a false value for basal calories. If it did, however, the error would result in calculations showing different specific dynamic reactions for obese, thin, and normal people. Computations indicating no difference between the three types could only result if this and other factors had been controlled so that true values for basal oxygen level were available. A depression of the level of heat production in the obese after a meal has been reported by Lauter[52] and Bernhardt.[53] None could be demonstrated by Wilder and his associates.[18] Could this apparent "negative phase" have resulted from a false basal value? Benedict and Carpenter, who took such great care to establish a true base line, and Strang and McClugage, who observed their precautions, were unable to demonstrate any "negative phase" except insofar as it obviously indicated a falsely high basal line.

Correct determinations of the specific dynamic action of food demand careful attention to the meal employed. The meals used by workers in this field have been extremely varied. This makes difficult a comparison of results. High protein meals consisting of 150 to 200 gm. of lean beef alone, or with bread, have in general been given, since the effect of protein alone was under consideration. Some investigators used meals of 400 to 600 gm. of lean beef which were satisfactory for the object in view, to determine the maximum effect on the metabolic rate which could be produced. Comparative quantitative results can, of course, be obtained only by ingestion of similar meals, and this factor has not been controlled by some who have studied the specific dynamic action in the obese. A meal exclusively protein, in reasonable or larger amounts, is not necessary in a comparative study of specific dynamic action of food in different states of nutrition. The point can be determined as well by a study of a fixed amount of different food elements. Nor is an exclusive protein meal desirable in this type of study. It is difficult to ingest, and this fact may indeed influence digestion and absorption.

The *determination of the total heat effect of a meal* presupposes the complete digestion and absorption of the meal in the period of observation. Hawk and his coworkers[54] have shown that the normal period of complete emptying of the stomach for 100 gm. of beef averages three hours, with a variation of two and one-half hours in the fast types to three and one-half hours in the slow. It seems reasonable to suppose, therefore, that many of the test meals which have been used were not completely out of the stomach in the two- to four-hour periods of observation. Kraus and Rettig[55] have critically discussed this point, and in their series were able to demonstrate by roentgen-ray examination the complete emptying of the stomach in four and one-half hours, using, however, only about 30 gm. of protein. Another factor of importance seems to be the appetizing quality of the meal. Although Hawk has shown that once food is ingested successfully it is probably entirely digested, the importance of the *psychic control of digestion*, especially with reference to the secretion of proteolytic digestive juices, is well established. Such psychic factors might appreciably influence the prompt handling of meals designedly high in protein.

In view of the above, prolonged studies of the effect of a meal are necessary to obtain true quantitative values. A period of eight hours would seem to be adequate, but is surely the minimum. Shorter periods of study reported by some observers might put in question the reliability of the results. One-third of the total heat production occurs within the period four to eight hours after the meal. Frequent determinations over the period are also necessary to demonstrate any differences in qualitative response.

Conclusions may be drawn, when the question is the presence or absence of different specific dynamic effects, only from total heat increase, not from percentage relationships. Any given total heat effect in response to a fixed meal, if presented as a percentage relationship to the basal line would be misleading. This percentage would, of course, be smaller in the obese with their high level of basal oxygen exchange and greater when referred to the lower level of normal people and to the depressed level of the undernourished. Thus a difference in specific dynamic action of food in the three classes of patients might erroneously appear to exist, but would not be an observed fact. This has been emphasized by Benedict and Carpenter, Lauter, and Kraus and Rettig. The precaution against using percentage increase over basal, rather than the total heat effect of a meal applies whether the observed data are related to basic calorie level, surface area, or are subjected to other methods of handling.

Different body shapes, in people of the same weight have been suggested as influencing the specific dynamic action of food. Various pathological conditions, especially those commonly associated with obesity, have also been mentioned as of importance in this connection. Gibbons[56] found different specific dynamic actions in two dogs of the same weight, but of different shapes. These factors do not seem to be important in human beings. Aub and DuBois[57] found normal metabolism reactions in individuals having artificially diminished surfaces. Strang and McClugage found the same specific dynamic reaction in their series of cases which included people of both sexes, old and young, a perfect example of so-called hypopituitary disease, a fully developed acromegalic, and one subject who lacked a leg, the result of a mid-thigh amputation years before. A heat response similar to all the others in this series was also shown by a patient, twenty-four years old, who had an advanced chronic nephritis. This one case, at least, showed that any anomaly of protein metabolism which may be present in nephritis was not manifested in him during those stages of protein utilization upon which specific dynamic action depends.

Strang and McClugage, giving strict attention to the necessity for, and measures to determine true values for basal calories as emphasized by Benedict and Carpenter, recorded total heat production after a fixed meal for a period of eight hours in a group of patients presenting the diverse types mentioned above. They gave an accurately calculated mixed meal easy to ingest and presumably easy to digest and absorb. It afforded 40 gm. of protein, 52 gm. of carbohydrate, 26 gm. of fat, and 610 calories, of which 160 (26 per cent) came from protein. The entire meal was eaten, each time, in less than twenty minutes. The activities of the subjects were restricted throughout the period. For the most part between tests they sat reading in bed or seated on a chair. A limited amount of walking around the room was permitted in the interest of comfort. However, a twenty-minute period of complete relaxation in bed was carried out before each metabolic determination.

The patients in this series, wholly disregarding body shapes, were classified as normal, obese, and thin. A variation of less than 15 per cent from ideal was considered a normal weight. The obese patients studied ranged from 18 to 160 per cent above normal, and the thin from 15 to 20 per cent below the normal weight.

The total heat production absorbed for the eight-hour period was, for the normal group 51 calories, for the obese 58 calories, and for the thin 67 calories. The total for the first four hours was in even closer agreement: 37 calories for the normal, 42 calories for the obese, and 43 calories for the thin. The total related to the 610 calories of the meal showed the cost of handling to be 8.4 per cent for the normal, 9.5 per cent for the obese, and 11 per cent for the thin. This was somewhat greater than the 6 per cent mentioned by Benedict and Carpenter for a 2500-calorie intake. The difference may be accounted for by the fact that 26 per cent of the calories of the meal employed by Strang and McClugage came from protein, much greater than any percentage possible from protein in the 2500-calorie diet employed by Benedict and Carpenter.

Admitting the technical difficulties and the probable unavoidable inaccuracy in many of the data used in the computations, these figures did not show any tendency in the obese to lowered specific dynamic reaction as compared to normal and thin people. This conclusion was made more emphatic by the observation that any error introduced would influence the calculations in a direction to show an apparently lowered specific dynamic action in the obese. This is so because any such error would, in view of the greater uncertainty in the obese of a fixed true basal line throughout the 8 hours of the test, be more likely to occur, and be of greater degree, in them than in people of normal weight and the thin.

The smaller specific dynamic action which has been recorded in the obese by some observers, if real and not the result of misleading computations with the observed data, could account for no more than a 3 per cent

TABLE 19

EXTRA CALORIES PRODUCED BY INGESTION OF A FIXED MEAL*

Test	Calories Produced						Total Calories	First Four Hours	Second Four Hours	Basal Calories for Eight Hours	Increase in Basal Calories, Per Cent
	First Hour	Second Hour	Third Hour	Fourth Hour	Sixth Hour	Eighth Hour					
Normal...	10	11	9	8	8	5	51	37	14	466	11
Obese....	8	12	12	10	13	4	58	42	17	571	10
Thin.....	11	14	10	9	16	7	67	43	23	449	15

* Strang, J. M., McClugage, H. B., and Brownlee, M. A., Am. J. Med. Sci., Lea & Febiger, Publishers, 182: 49, 1931.

reduction in the total daily metabolism. A contribution of this magnitude to a plus energy balance, if present, would contribute somewhat to the acquisition of obesity, but is wholly inadequate to account for the facts in most cases.

The absence of any quantitative difference in the specific dynamic effect of food in the obese, normal, and thin subjects, including even such diverse types as those in the series of Strang and McClugage, does not support the suggestion that obesity can be classified as to type on the basis of such difference.

The studies of Strang and McClugage demonstrating no quantitative difference in specific dynamic action in different nutritional states merit no special comment other than that they conform to, and confirm, those of other investigators who have been exacting in their controls and critical of their investigating technique.

The analysis of these data with regard to qualitative response illustrated, however, important variations between types, and established facts of interest and practical value. The point of greatest interest for different nutritional states is not the total heat production which they may show in response to a fixed meal, but the physiological strain of adjustment to it. The amount of

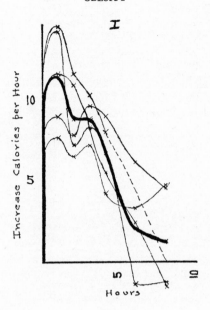

Normal

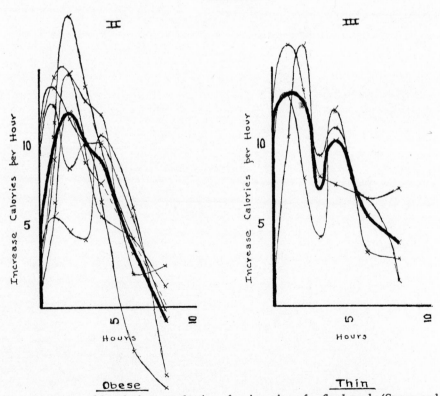

Obese

Thin

Fig. 88.—Curves of hourly heat production after ingestion of a fixed meal. (Strang and McClugage, Am. J. Med. Sci., **182**: 3, 1931. Lea & Febiger, Publisher.)

physiological strain results not only from the total load but is related also to the percentage increase, and to the time after the meal the peak of the load appears, which marks the time when the maximum physiological stress is in play.

A record of the hourly heat production data, table 19 showed that in the first half of the experimental period the heat production in all three groups was very closely comparable. The average figures for four hours were: normal group, 37; fat, 42; and thin, 43 calories. The major effects of the meal are to be expected in this period, and it was in this period that the observed heat values were practically identical. Much more variation occurred in the second four hours. The group figures were 14, 17, and 23 calories respectively. The bulk of the differences in the various groups fell, therefore, in the period of diminished food influence. Curves of hourly heat production for each subject and the composite curves appear in chart (Fig. 88). The contours show delayed secondary rises. These were more conspicuous in the normal and thin groups. The delayed rises in heat production were perhaps associated with extraneous factors such as fatigue which of themselves produced elevations above the basal calories. Benedict and Carpenter have discussed this point at length. It may be noted that there is no relation between the height of the peak and the total area of the curve of heat production, thus emphasizing the fallacy introduced by comparing maximum rate of heat production with the true specific dynamic action of a meal.

The basal calories of the patients in the series of Strang and McClugage determined before ingestion of the meal were, for the normal people 58.2, for the obese 71.4, and for the thin 56.1. Making the improbable assumption of constant base lines, the basal caloric exchange for the eight-hour period can be calculated, 466 for the normal group, 571 for the obese, and 449 for the undernourished. When the total observed calorie increases during the eight-hour period, 51 for the normal, 58 for the obese, and 67 for the thin, were related to the total basal calories thus arrived at, they showed percentage increases of 10 per cent for the obese, 11 per cent for the normal subjects, and 15 per cent for the thin. This represented for the thin people a 50 per cent greater percentage increase in absolute heat production than for the obese. Such percentage values, while not, as explained above, bearing upon the question of presence or absence of different specific dynamic effects, do afford a measure of the degree of physiological adjustment in the obese and thin to the ingestion of a similar amount of food. The observations made one hour after the ingestion of the meal, presented in the same manner, showed a 14 per cent increase for the obese, and 21 per cent for the undernourished, representing the same percentage relationship as for the total period. The data recorded two hours after showed an 18 per cent elevation above the accepted basal level for the obese, and still 21 per cent for the thin. Average figures for the entire period for the three groups appear in table 20.

The physiological strain after handling a meal depends not only on the percentage increase in heat production and the time of its appearance but also, and probably of more practical significance, on the speed of adjustment necessary. This brings into the problem questions of the rate of change. The average rate of change of heat production in the patients of Strang and McClugage appears in table 21. The individual curves of all the subjects and the composite curves derived from them appear in chart (Fig. 89). From the chart it will be seen that immediately following the ingestion of food the curves rose to a sharp peak at the first hour. It was quite probable that the true peak of this curve was obscured by the use of hourly observations rather than those at shorter intervals. For the second and third hours the rate of heat production did not change significantly, the low part of these curves

TABLE 20

CHANGES IN BASAL METABOLIC RATE BASED UPON ACTUAL SURFACE AFTER INGESTION OF A FIXED MEAL*

Test	Basal Metabolic Rate Per Cent	Increase Over Basal Metabolic Rate					
		First Hour Per Cent	Second Hour Per Cent	Third Hour Per Cent	Fourth Hour Per Cent	Sixth Hour Per Cent	Eighth Hour Per Cent
Normal....	−6.8	18.3	14.6	14.6	11.1	4.8	3.0
Obese......	−2.2	14.1	17.8	14.1	12.9	6.2	0.2
Thin.......	−9.0	21.1	21.0	12.2	16.9	9.4	6.8

* Strang, J. M., McClugage, H. B., and Brownlee, M. A., Am. J. Med. Sci., **182**: 49, 1931.

corresponding to the nearly flat tops of the curves of rates of heat production. The secondary short slow rise with the maximum in the sixth hour represented the period in which the heat effect of the meal was rapidly diminishing and the total metabolism returning to normal. This analysis showed clearly that following a meal the body was required to readjust itself within an hour to a change in heat production of 20 per cent. The

TABLE 21

RATE OF CHANGE OF RATE OF HEAT PRODUCTION AFTER THE INGESTION OF A FIXED MEAL*
(These figures are obtained by comparing the observation of each determination to the rate of heat production for the hour preceding. The numerical difference is then divided by the total heat production of the preceding hour, thus giving per cent of change)

Test	Basal Cal.	First Hour Per Cent	Second Hour Per Cent	Third Hour Per Cent	Fourth Hour Per Cent	Sixth Hour Per Cent	Eighth Hour Per Cent
Normal....	58.2	20.1	2.4	2.0	3.3	5.5	3.1
Obese......	71.4	15.3	4.6	2.9	3.3	7.1	5.7
Thin.......	56.1	24.7	6.4	7.5	5.1	7.0	3.1

* Strang, J. M., McClugage, H. B., and Brownlee, M. A., Am. J. Med. Sci., Lea & Febiger, Publishers, **182**: 49, 1931.

subsequent changes were small and comparatively unimportant. The important physiological strain, therefore, occurred in the latter part of the period of food ingestion and the period immediately succeeding it. Only a small fraction of the total extra heat was produced during this interval, but by the time the maximum rate of heat production had developed, the adaptations to this rate had become complete. It was, therefore, important to distinguish

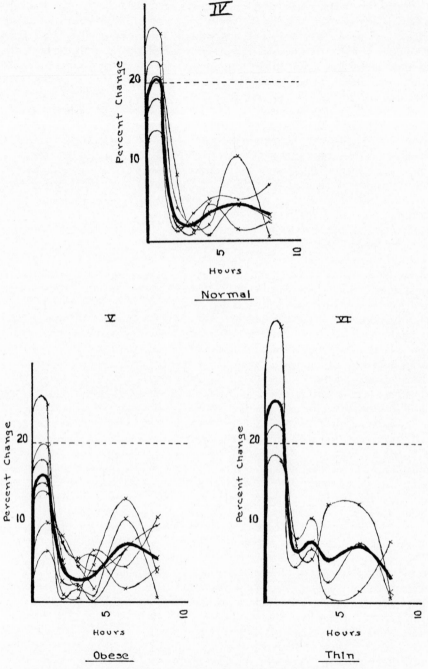

Fig. 89.—Rate of change of heat production after ingestion of a fixed meal. (Strang and McClugage, Am. J. Med. Sci., **182:** 3, 1931. Lea & Febiger, Publisher.)

sharply between the two phenomena, the rate of extra heat production, and the physiological response to this extra heat.

Rather important variations were revealed when the physiologic load which was thrown upon the obese and upon the thin by the specific dynamic action of food was approximated in the manner described above. The general form of the curve for the obese was quite comparable to that of the normal group. The significant point was that the maximum of the composite curve of the obese fell at 15 per cent, which was 25 per cent less than for the normals. The curve for the thin on the other hand reached its maximum at 25 per cent, which was 25 per cent higher than the normal group. Although identical meals produced the same total heat reaction in normal, thin, and obese persons, the physiologic load which this extra heat production threw upon the body was approximately one-fourth less in the obese and one-fourth greater in the thin than in normal subjects. In fact, the thin group bore a 66 per cent greater physiologic strain than the obese in the handling of a meal which was identical in protein, fat, and carbohydrate, but particularly in total calories. If it were possible to demonstrate a relationship between this physiologic load and the sensation of satiety which normally determines the limit of food ingestion, an important factor would be exhibited in the chain of causes which determine why fat people unwittingly eat large meals and stay fat, and thin people automatically eat small meals and remain thin. A very probable relationship of this kind exists and has been discussed above (see section on Nature and Causes).

The influence of specific dynamic action of food in the development and continuance of different nutritional states, is not the result of any quantitative factor. A qualitative factor, however, a different type of response to a fixed intake in timing and in percentage relation to the total metabolism, is of the greatest importance.

Skin Temperature.—The sensation of warmth after eating has been shown by Bazett[58] to be the result of the rate of change of the temperature around the nerve end-organs of the skin, rather than of changes in the actual temperature of the tissues. This is of interest in relation to the slower rate of change of the rate of heat production, and the delayed attainment of the maximum rate of change in response to food, in the obese as compared to normal people, which was suggested by Strang and McClugage[32] as a possible explanation of the greater amounts of food necessary for the obese to attain satiety.

Booth and Strang[59] gave to a series of obese and normal persons a meal of ground beefsteak with sufficient stewed tomatoes to render it palatable. The subjects were requested to eat as much as they could possibly consume, taking as long as they desired to do so. Changes in skin temperature were measured with a Tycos dermotherm every two minutes for an hour from the time of beginning of the eating, at the palm of the hand, the ball of the thumb, the sole of the foot, and the ball of the great toe. These points were chosen because in a preliminary observation of fifteen points described by Benedict[60] these four points showed the maximum variations in temperature. Each reading recorded was the average of four made, each within a minimal variation of the others, after adequate rest period before eating, and with the temperature, humidity, and motion of the surrounding air controlled. Repeated tests yielded results very close to the original in the normals. Later tests in the obese after reduction showed a response similar to the normals. This is illustrated by the data in table 22. These data, characteristic of the entire group of subjects studied, illustrate the size of the meals eaten, the extent of skin temperature elevation, and the timing of maximum change. Data for the entire series showed that ten obese women ate considerably more than ten women of normal weight; and that nine normal men ate more than four obese men, a group not large enough, however, to offer reliable comparable figures.

The subjects of normal weight showed a greater and more prompt elevation of skin temperature than the obese. The average of all observations is presented graphically in the following chart (Fig. 90). Normal men showed greater rise than normal women; and obese men a greater rise than obese women. This is shown graphically in chart (Fig. 91). Blood pressures throughout the periods showed a uniform reaction in the obese and normals

TABLE 22

ORIGINAL OBSERVATIONS OF SKIN TEMPERATURE AND THOSE MADE SEVERAL YEARS LATER*

Case	Date	Percentage of Ideal Weight	Surface Area, Sq. M.	Meat Meal, Gm.	Time of Initial Change in Skin Temperature, Minutes	Maximum Change in Skin Temperature, C.	Time of Maximum Change in Skin Temperature, Minutes
1	11/13/31	102.6	1.85	500	10	+2.6	44
	11/19/33	100.0	1.84	650	12	+2.6	38
2	11/18/31	96.6	1.75	600	18	+4.1	64
	11/19/33	98.0	1.76	600	12	+4.6	82
3	11/17/31	94.0	1.82	700	34	+0.7	54
	11/20/33	94.0	1.82	700	6	+1.9	38
4	11/24/31	171.7	2.04	400	2	−0.5	30
	11/27/33	178.6	2.09	550	28	−1.0	44
5	12/ 1/33	150.5	1.95	750	4	+3.6	46
	1/16/34	131.4	1.85	600	8	+1.1	72
6	12/ 1/31	110.7	1.72	750	46	−1.0	64
	12/13/33	104.9	1.67	900	4	+4.2	64
7	11/11/31	116.8	2.11	500	8	+0.5	22
	12/ 3/33	108.8	2.05	900	14	+1.3	50

* Booth, Geo., and Strang, J. M., Arch. Int. Med., 57: 533, 1936.

of both sexes. There was a rise immediately following the start of the meal with a return to the previous level immediately after completion of the meal.

Persons of normal weight were unable to continue eating with a rise in skin temperature of 0.9° C. in 22 minutes. The smaller rise in skin temperature of the obese prevented the attainment of the level at which the normal people could eat no more. This phenomenon might well be related to the slower rate of change of heat production of the obese in response to ingested food mentioned by Strang and McClugage. As such it demonstrated a physiological difference between the obese and others of importance in relation to satiety which may account for the consumption of food by the obese in excess of the actual physiological requirements.

Water Balance.—Wide daily variations in body weight occur normally in all persons. The immediate and greater swings are readily understood to be dependent upon ingestion and excretion. A pint of water weighs a pound. Two ordinary glasses of water drunk by a thirsty man would increase his weight as shown on the scales by one pound. Many ordinary meals weigh two to three or more pounds. Urinary bladders may hold, without undue discomfort, 500 cc., to be passed at one voiding with an immediate change

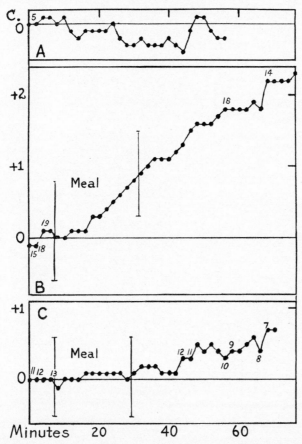

Fig. 90.—Composite curves of the temperature reactions of the skin during the control period with the meal omitted (*A*) and of persons of normal weight (*B*) and obese persons (*C*) before, during and after a meal of meat to the level of satiety. (Booth and Strang, Arch. Int. Med., Vol. 57, p. 533, 1936.)

in the scale reading one pound. A normal bowel movement may weigh one-half pound, and a purge with watery stool eliminating 1500 cc. will reduce the weight by three pounds of fluid alone.

Daily variations in weight wider than that in normals are commonly met with in the obese. They may be as much as four pounds. This results from greater variations in the amounts of water in the body at different times. The body heat regulating mechanism is disturbed under the conditions imposed by obesity, and water exchange becomes a more important factor of it than in normals. It thus occurs that with changes in environment, air temperature and humidity, and exercise, larger volumes of water exchange takes place. Furthermore, fat deposits have a variable capacity for water storage, said by Lauter[46] to be from 8 to 70 per cent.

The variable capacity of fat tissue for storage of water is of importance in relation to the observed weight changes in the obese while undergoing reduction which record wide water swings in addition to the fat loss. Yet other factors are operative. It has frequently been observed that obese patients treated by diet alone show a true weight loss due to the excretion of water. This effect may be due to the fact (1) that patients have a mild grade of congestive heart failure even when, in the presence of the obesity,

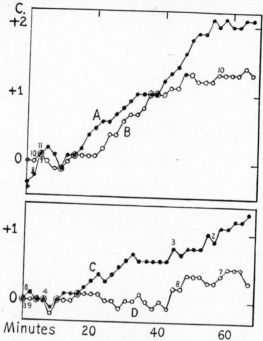

Fig. 91.—Composite curves showing the difference in the magnitude of the temperature reaction of the skin between the sexes. A is the curve for men of normal weight; B, for women of normal weight; C, for obese men, and D, for obese women. (Booth and Strang, Arch. Int. Med., Vol. 57, p. 533, 1936.)

no edema can be demonstrated with assurance, and (2) that the institution of the diet is followed, in many cases, with prompt reestablishment of cardiac competency and consequent pouring out of fluid. One case with demonstrable edema observed by Strang and Evans[61] accounted for thirteen pounds of weight loss by water excretion in the first week of dieting. Strang, McClugage and Evans[13] found also, that when employing reducing diets resulting in a negative nitrogen balance there was an increased water loss. The reduction of weight accounted for in part by water excretion with correction of the myxedematous state of hypothyroid patients by administration of thyroid is well known.

The obese, during *reduction by diet*, also show periods of water storage.

This, with the above, not only results in wide variations in the daily observed weight changes, but also in periods of constant weight, and seemingly of no fat loss, despite a markedly deficient caloric intake. These observations have been suggested as evidence of some mysterious metabolic anomaly in these patients, but they are to be explained simply by variation in water content of the body. A study by Newburgh and Johnston[62] proved this point definitely. These observers, confirming the statement of Benedict and Root[63] that the basal insensible perspiration bore a constant relation to the basal caloric exchange, were able to show that a similar relation existed for total insensible perspiration and total caloric exchange.[64] Thus was developed a method for calculating with accuracy the total caloric exchange and total insensible perspiration. Examples of the application of this method given by Newburgh and his collaborators appear in tables 23 and 24.

TABLE 23

DETERMINATION OF TOTAL OXYGEN EXCHANGE FOR TWENTY-FOUR HOURS

By noting weight lost as insensible perspiration and relating this to 30 grams = 1405 calories (Benedict). The weight lost as insensible perspiration is determined by subtracting body weight at end of period plus weight of urine and stools from body weight at beginning of period plus weight of food and water intake*

I		II	
	Grams		Grams
First body weight	62,260	Second body weight	61,900
Weight of food	1,599	Weight of urine	1,157
Weight of water	378	Weight of stool	0,000
	64,237		63,057
	63,057		
	1,180		

1180 grams is insensible loss for twenty-four hours

$$\frac{1180}{24} = 49.2 \text{ grams insensible loss per hour}$$

or

2000 Calories for the twenty-four-hour period.

* Newburgh, L. H., and Johnston, M. W., J. Clin. Invest., 8: 197, 1930.

Using this instrument they could state with confidence that the difference between weight loss expected from calculation, and that actually observed, is due to a plus or minus water balance. The data supplied by one case, a fourteen-year-old girl, 73 inches tall and weighing 244 pounds at the beginning are presented in table 25. The actual weight loss of 10 gm. in one period when 2896 gm. was the calculated expectancy, permitted a prediction of water retention of 2886 gm. The actual retention of water of 2672 gm. corresponded so closely to the prediction that it proves the lack of weight loss was due to storage of water. During another period when the weight loss was more rapid than the calculated prediction, it was shown to be due to an outpouring of water. The actual weight loss was 3995 gm. but the prediction was only 1629 gm. This permitted a prediction of water loss of 2366 gm. The actual negative water balance was 2266 gm.

Newburgh and his collaborators demonstrated equally accurate and conclusive data on patients with obesity which was frankly alimentary and with

TABLE 24

DETERMINATION OF WATER LOST INSENSIBLY*

I		II	
	Grams		Grams
First weight......................	57,790	Second weight....................	57,840
Weight of food...................	2,041	Weight of urine..................	1,108
Weight of water.................	75	Weight of stool..................	0,000
Weight of oxygen................	570	Weight of CO_2.................	628
	60,476		59,576

	Grams
I.....................	60,476
II.....................	59,576
	900 Water lost insensibly

* Newburgh, L. H., and Johnston, M. W., J. Clin. Invest., **8**: 197, 1930.

obesity associated with definite endocrine disorders. Among the latter was a middle-aged woman who began to gain weight after an operation upon the

TABLE 25

WATER BALANCE OF OBESE GIRL FOURTEEN YEARS OF AGE UNDERGOING REDUCTION*

Diet: Protein 65 Gm.; Fat 40 Gm.; Carbohydrate 74 Gm. (Calories 914)
Total N out (daily): 11.7 grams
Calories used each 24 hours: 2137
Metabolic mixture: Protein 73 Gm.; Fat 172 Gm.; Carbohydrate 74 Gm.
From body (daily): Protein 9 Gm.; Fat 132 Gm.; Water 40 Gm.

Period A. Plateau			
Loss of weight		Retention of water	
	Grams		Grams
Predicted........................	2,896	Predicted........................	2,886
Actual...........................	10	Actual...........................	2,672

Period B. Steep Fall			
Loss of weight		Loss of water	
	Grams		Grams
Predicted........................	1,629	Predicted........................	2,366
Actual...........................	3,995	Actual...........................	2,266

* Newburgh, L. H., and Johnston, M. W., J. Clin. Invest., **8**: 197, 1930.

pituitary gland eight years earlier, and who weighed 295 pounds; and one woman diagnosed as having Dercum's disease, and who was 62 inches tall and weighed 420 pounds.

Periods of no weight loss due to water retention, despite removal of the expected amount of fat, may be long. Newburgh and Johnston, in the reports cited above, mention one girl weighing 231 pounds who maintained her weight for eleven days on a caloric intake of 800; and another who demonstrated such a plateau for nine days. A patient, studied by Evans and Strang, who weighed 354 pounds at the beginning, lost 46 pounds in seventy days on a daily maximum caloric intake of 400. A 2-pound reduction was recorded during the next twenty days on the same diet. A more rapid rate of weight loss was then resumed amounting to 19 pounds in thirty-two days. The three periods added showed a total loss of 67 pounds in one hundred and twenty-two days. For the total period this constituted a reduction of 3.8 pounds per week, the calculated expectancy.

No doubt the wide variations in the capacity of fat tissue normally for water storage are exaggerated during its rapid removal. Wassermann, quoted by Wells,[33] found that the rim of cytoplasm of the distended fat cell can swell up with fluids, and the depleted fat cells can become hydropic. Common to all obese patients reducing by diet, these water swings are, in general, irregular in occurrence. Evans and Strang, however, noted some periodicity in their patients. Dumping of water occurred frequently in the early days of dieting, followed shortly by a period of retention. The cycles became more conspicuous as the period of dieting continued and were exaggerated after the third month. The extent and duration of the swings varied widely in different patients, and in the same patient at different times, and could not be predicted. As stated, they could be related only very roughly to the period of treatment and not at all to any other feature of the case. The up and down swings of water exchange balanced, however, over a long period and the scales showed the true weight loss due to removal of fat. Adding up the figures for two short periods of the case in table 25 presented by Newburgh and Johnston, it is seen that the difference between the predicted and the actual weight due to water is very small. The total predicted weight loss for the two periods, 4525 gm., differs from the actual loss of 4005 by only 520 gm. Again the conclusive accuracy of this method is demonstrated when the predicted water storage of 520 gm. is compared to the actual observed 314 gm.

It is important that these water swings be understood by patients undergoing treatment. Failure to do so often results in discouragement sufficient to interrupt the dieting.

Ketogenic-antiketogenic Ratio.—In considering this subject cognizance must be taken of the new and apparently sound hypothesis of the etiology of ketosis as postulated by Stadie[70] and his associates and which is presented in the chapter on Lipid Metabolism in this book. Shaffer[65] in 1921 showed that one molecule of fatty acid was burned completely only in the presence of the burning of one molecule of glucose. This point was made also by the brilliant clinical study of Woodyatt[66] who further stated the fact, of great importance in diabetes in pre-insulin days, that a diet affording a ketogenic-antiketogenic ratio of more than 1.5 to 1 was unsafe. The general physiological considerations are not, however, so simple as that because ketosis does not always result from diets of ketogenic-antiketogenic ratios higher than 1.5 to 1. Hubbard and Wright[67] demonstrated that subjects taking diets of higher ratios fell far short of the figure for acetone excretion expected from a 1.5 to 1 ratio calculation. Shaffer has shown that ketogenic-antiketogenic ratios as high as 3 to 1 are frequently not accompanied by pathological ketosis. This consideration is of importance in obesity because the obese are called upon during dietetic treatment to metabolize mixtures of high ketogenic-antiketogenic ratios, and seem to have excellent tolerance for them. McKay and Sherrill[25] found less ketosis in some obese persons during fasting than in normal controls. Folin and Denis[26] observed no increased ketosis in the obese during starvation. The periods of fasting to which their cases submitted were five and six days, long enough to eliminate the influence of any greater storage of nonfat fuel substances which the obese may have had. Folin and Denis stated that obesity is not a contributing, nor even a predisposing factor to the onset or severity of the acidosis of starvation. Deuel and Gulick[27] found no increased ketosis in the obese during fasting. Yet the obese, because of their higher level of oxygen exchange, burn more fuel during a fast, which after exhaustion of stored nonfat fuel substances, comes primarily from fat. This suggests, but much other evidence contradicts (Lusk[36]), that stored fat is a source of available glucose for combustion. A possible greater utilization of body protein in the obese for its antiketogenic properties does not supply the answer. Folin and Denis found in the obese during starvation no greater loss of body protein than in people of normal weight. Strang, McClugage, and Evans[13] suggested this as a possible explanation of a minimal nitrogen loss in patients maintained for long periods on diets affording adequate protein but only 14 gm. of carbohydrate. The prompt establishment of nitrogen equilibrium when the carbohydrate was increased only to 40 gm., and while patients were still deriving 80 per cent of their caloric needs from stored fat, proves that antiketogenic properties derived from greater utilization of body protein do not explain the high tolerance of the obese for metabolic mixtures of high ketogenic-antiketogenic ratios. The higher level of oxygen exchange in obesity may be of importance in this connection. Wilder, Boothby, and Beeler[68] showed that the limits of safety of the ketogenic-antiketogenic ratio varies with individuals, possibly directly with the level of oxygen exchange. Perhaps some improved mechanism for fat burning comes into play under these circumstances, related to secretion of the alpha cells of the Islets of Langerhans suggested by Bensley and Woerner, quoted by Wilder, Browne, and Butt[69] as of importance in the oxidation of fat; or to the pancreas-derived lipocaic studied by Dragstedt and his collaborators.[31]

Every obese patient taking a reducing diet which is sufficiently limited to attain results is handling a metabolic mixture of high ketogenic-antiketogenic ratio. This is especially true of the severely restricted diets employed by Strang and Evans. One such patient lost 0.36 kilograms daily over a four-week period of dieting. The diet consisted of 50.0 gm. of protein, 8 gm. of carbohydrate, and 7 gm. of fat. There was an average daily loss of 0.4 gm. of nitrogen, 12 gm. of protein tissue. The remaining 348 gm. of daily weight loss may be regarded as fatty tissue. The losses of protein tissue and fatty tissue represent the metabolism of 2.5 gm. of protein and 303 gm. of fat. This added to the food ingested gives for the metabolic mixture oxidized, protein 53 gm., carbohydrate 8 gm., and fat 310 gm., the ketogenic-antiketogenic ratio being 4.3 to 1. Hubbard[71] showed that when diets low in antiketogenic material are fed, the amounts of the acetone bodies excreted are the same whether the fat burned is derived from ingested or stored fat. Yet the patient above showed not only no evidence of acidosis but no ketonuria, and several plasma CO_2 determinations during the period were normal.

Everyone who has followed obese patients during reduction has observed acetonuria (sometimes pronounced) in an appreciable number during the first few days of dieting, but in every instance lasting only a few days. A lowered tendency to ketonuria was noticed by Folin and Denis[26] in the obese with repeated periods of fasting. Despite the ketonuria which one sees, however, acidosis has never appeared. This observation applies also to obese glycosurics. Strang and Evans have treated a number of obese patients with glycosuria, a high fasting blood sugar, and a diabetic glucose tolerance curve, by diets affording less than 500 calories, and having glucose equivalents of 75–80 gm., thus compelling the metabolism of mixtures of high ketogenic-antiketogenic ratios. Acidosis resulted in not one case, and a relatively frequent ketonuria of the first few days disappeared promptly in all.

The reason for the high tolerance of the obese for metabolic mixtures of high ketogenic-antiketogenic ratios is not available. (Of great interest in this connection is the evidence presented by Stadie[70] favoring the replacement of the successive beta oxidation hypothesis of fatty acids by the multiple alternate oxidation hypothesis. The subject needs further investigation.) This high tolerance has, however, been proved to exist. Acidosis is not a menace to the obese or a factor to be considered in planning treatment.

Glucose Tolerance and Glycosuria.—The observation that diabetes is more common in those who are, or who have been, obese has long been recognized. This statement is made with primary emphasis on the diabetes, already established. The relationship between diabetes and obesity may be presented in a different way, with primary reference to the obesity. It is generally known that an appreciable number of obese patients will frequently show glycosuria. Spencer[9] reporting on 252 obese patients found elevated fasting blood sugars in 24 per cent. It is also a fact many times proved that almost all obese glycosurics do not continue to show sugar in the urine when reduced by diet. This is to be expected because any diet sufficiently limited to result in weight loss must of necessity have a low glucose content; and a diabetic state in an obese person must be mild, else he would not maintain his obesity (see Chap. XVI).

Studies on glucose tolerance curves are of interest and great practical significance in this connection. Beeler and Fitz[72] made such a study on thirty-two patients who did not show glycosuria. The series included eight men and twenty-four women, some of whom were excessively obese. One man weighed 370 pounds, another 285 pounds, and another 253 pounds; one woman weighed 291 pounds, and several others more than 225 pounds. As a group these patients showed glucose tolerance curves between that characteristic of diabetes and that of normal persons, approaching the normal more closely. Four patients had elevated fasting blood sugar values, thus suggesting a prediabetic state. Two of these patients had normal glucose tolerance curves, but the other two showed curves typical of diabetes. Six other cases, although commencing with normal fasting blood sugar levels, had curves characteristic of mild diabetes. Thus, eight of thirty-two obese patients without glucosuria, 25 per cent, showed glucose tolerance curves typical of diabetes. The test employed for all patients regardless of weight was 100 gm. of glucose by mouth on a fasting stomach.

Paullin and Sauls[73] determined glucose tolerance curves in twenty-six obese patients, without glycosuria, ranging in age from sixteen to seventy-one years. High curves were found in 58 per cent; and in 75 per cent of those between the ages of thirty and fifty years. This is somewhat higher than the 25 per cent recorded by Beeler and Fitz. Likewise, a higher percentage of diabetic type glucose tolerance curves, corresponding closely to that of Paullin and Sauls was observed by John.[74] He found such curves

TABLE 26

EFFECT OF REDUCTION OF WEIGHT ON DISPOSAL OF DEXTROSE*

	When Obese				After Reduction of Weight			
	Fasting	1 Hr.	2 Hr.	3 Hr.	Fasting	1 Hr.	2 Hr.	3 Hr.
	105	236	256	152	78	126	107	52
	127	303	244	174	93	146	115	59
	168	290	370	302	104	113	90	74
	166	300	344	264	106	153	136	69
	99	212	216	164	82	156	105	70
	162	202	210	240	71	146	129	50
	124	294	125	99	86	154	93	60
	161	300	202	178	91	166	87	51
	148	234	282	176	93	156	136	113
	113	212	200	115	78	178	100	77
	73	188	200	97	93	147	110	94
	115	200	196	196	76	121	109	76
	133	300	236	164	112	149	50	68
	148	314	270	146	89	170	93	57
	113	234	200	164	98	109	88	59
	119	230	185	102	85	135	107	66
	121	172	192	107	89	117	96	96
	141	230	202	156	97	139	84	62
	106	270	252	222	83	154	119	63
	117	238	242	192	92	192	129	58
	300	504	508	428	111	192	76	59
Averages........	136	260	244	183	91	149	104	68
	124†	278	266	111	87	200	188	88

* Newburgh, L. H., and Conn, J. W., J.A.M.A., 112: 7, 1939.
† Only patient showing incomplete recovery after reduction of weight.

in 65.6 per cent of 172 obese patients without glucosuria, about equally distributed between men and women—46 per cent male, 54 per cent female. John also used for the test 100 gm. of glucose by mouth on a fasting stomach.

These studies certainly do not show any increased efficiency in the obese for utilization of sugar.

Newburgh and Conn[75] studied glucose tolerance curves on thirty-five obese middle-aged patients *with* glycosuria. Many of these patients displayed symptoms characteristic of diabetes, and some had been treated for diabetes for longer or shorter periods. The test used was 1.75 gm. of glucose per kilogram of ideal weight by mouth on a fasting stomach after three days of a standard diet affording 300 gm. of carbohydrate, 80 gm. of protein, and maintenance calories. All these patients, while obese and glycosuric, were shown to be able to oxidize an amount of glucose normal and adequate for their fuel needs, and those who were reduced, continued to oxidize this amount after reduction. Yet each patient showed a diabetic type of glucose tolerance curve in reaction to the test employed. Twenty-

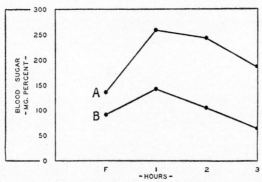

Fig. 92.—Composite dextrose tolerance curves for twenty-one patients before A and B after reduction of weight. (Newburgh and Conn, J.A.M.A., Jan. 7, 1939.)

one of these patients accepted reducing diets and continued them until the attainment of a normal, or near normal, weight. Glucose tolerance curves done during reduction showed an approach toward normal, and the establishment of an entirely normal curve by all patients except one when a near-ideal weight was reached. These data appear in table 26. Figure 92 shows graphically the composite dextrose tolerance curves of these patients

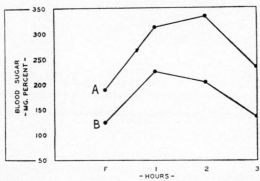

Fig. 93.—Composite dextrose tolerance curves for fourteen patients before A and B after partial reduction of weight. (Newburgh and Conn, J.A.M.A., Jan. 7, 1939.)

before and after reduction. In figure 93 appear the composite dextrose tolerance curves for fourteen patients before and after partial reduction in weight. One patient became mildly obese after reduction and showed again a diabetic type of curve, and a normal curve after reducing a second time. The data on this patient appear in table 27.

In view of these observations Newburgh and Conn consider, with reference to the ability shown by these patients to burn an adequate amount of glucose for fuel needs, the possible mechanism of glycosuria and diabetic curves when they occur in obesity. They suggest that, since there is no crippling impairment of sugar-burning mechanism in these cases as in true diabetes, the disturbance is one of conversion and storage of that in excess, or appreciably in excess, of fuel needs. They tentatively relate this to a diminished reserve insulin supply, but think that it is more likely the result of impaired glycogen storage function of the liver due to fat infiltration. This question merits further investigation. It should be emphasized that upon whatever impairment this phenomenon depends, it is of late occurrence.

Newburgh and Conn studied only middle-aged obese glycosurics. Ogilvie[76] observed that sugar tolerance in obese patients was increased in one third of the patients during the early states of obesity, but that it was diminished later. His findings justified the conclusion that impaired glucose tolerance was present in a high percentage of cases after eight or more years of obesity, and that the degree of impairment was related to the duration, but not the severity of the obesity. Ogilvie used 50 gm. of glucose by mouth on a fasting stomach, and the patients included sixty-three women

TABLE 27

EFFECT OF RECURRENT OBESITY ON DEXTROSE TOLERANCE CURVE

Overweight, Percentage	Fasting	1 Hr.	2 Hr.	3 Hr.
45................	128	314	322	202
0................	91	140	72	61
25................	119	230	185	102
0................	87	135	107	66

* Newburgh, L. H., and Conn, J. W., J.A.M.A., **112**: 7, 1939.

and two men, twenty-three to sixty-five years of age, who were 14 to 137 per cent overweight.

Newburgh and Conn, from their studies of glucose tolerance in obese glycosurics, drew inferences of practical significance. Forty-nine per cent of the 370 patients diagnosed as having diabetes at the University of Michigan Hospital during 1936 were obese. Seventy-two per cent of the total number of patients were in the age group thirty to sixty-five years, and 61 per cent were obese. These obese, middle-aged glycosurics represented 44 per cent of the total 370 patients diagnosed as having diabetes mellitus. If the ratio of 20 out of 21 who became not only sugar free, but attained normal glucose tolerance curves by reduction in the series of Newburgh and Conn held for diabetics everywhere, even in part, the results would be truly significant. It would mean that almost half of the diabetics extant could be removed from this category simply by the cure of their obesity (see Chapter XVI).

Preble[7] found glycosuria in fifty-three of 700 cases of obesity, a percentage of 7.57. He cites Joslin to the effect that one in every hundred of the population has or may develop diabetes, and observes that this is an incidence of glycosuria seven and one-half times Joslin's expected incidence of diabetes. With a prescience that is noteworthy in reference to the subsequent study of Newburgh and Conn, Preble does not say that his obese patients show seven and one-half times as many diabetics as Joslin predicted, but that they "show an incidence of glycosuria, and presumably of diabetes of over seven and one-half times the normal figure."

TREATMENT

Obesity is caused by a plus energy balance with resultant storage of this excess as fat. The cure of obesity, therefore, consists in creating a negative energy balance until the stored excess is consumed. It is hardly necessary to observe that any measure which is not based on this fact, such as massage, bath powders, and other fanciful suggestions, are of no value for the removal of fat.

A negative energy balance can be created by increasing the energy output. It is advisable, however, to accompany this by measures to prevent a corresponding, or greater, energy intake. A negative caloric balance can also be created by decreasing the energy intake, i.e., by limitation of diet. No other measure is needed if this can be employed. Restrictions of diet sufficient in degree to result in a negative energy balance, regardless of how limited the energy output may be, are possible, with complete safety. If dietary restriction is practiced it is not necessary to increase the energy output by added exercise or drugs, both of which are so often inadvisable.

INCREASED ENERGY OUTPUT

Exercise.—The most obvious and least unwholesome method of increasing energy output is by added exercise. Where this is possible with or without diet, it is worthwhile. One vigorous young man while dieting accurately played eighteen or more holes of golf every day and reduced from 229¼ to his ideal weight of 177 pounds—52¼ pounds in eleven weeks. The removal of this amount of fat without the exercise would have taken much longer. This patient was on a rigidly restricted diet. That amount of exercise taken by anyone young and vigorous enough to stand it without injury would so stimulate the appetite that, without control of intake, the additional food eaten would cancel the increased energy expenditure, and no caloric deficit to be supplied by his own fat would result.

One must keep in mind, when planning to increase energy output by exercise, what a tremendous amount of exercise is necessary. Bedroom calisthenics both morning and night do not suffice. A forty-year-old man of 70 kilograms ideal weight, living a wholly sedentary life, will maintain his weight by a daily calorie intake of 2600. This man, if he takes up golf and plays eighteen holes every day in the week will hold his weight with no more than 800 or 1000 calories additional. The reverse of this means that the fat man will lose no more than one and three-quarters pounds a week with this much exercise—provided he does not, as a result of it, eat any more than he did previously. Such exercise, if not impossible for several reasons, is unwise and dangerous for most obese people. All bodies are, with variations of minor importance, constructed proportionally in relation to ideal weight. The structures of the feet, knees, thighs, and lower back, are built to function for a body weight without added fat. The greater load thrown on these structures by the increased avoirdupois will, in many instances, result in functional insufficiency causing symptoms which, if not crippling, do prevent exercise in amounts necessary to produce an effective increase in energy output. Furthermore, the entire body economy is carrying an appreciable added work fraction because of the obesity alone. This is especially significant in relation to the disorganized heat-regulating mechanism and cardiovascular strain. It can be said for the obese that exercise in any but minimal amounts is difficult for most, is deleterious for almost all, and is dangerous to many. Exercise alone for the cure of obesity is impracticable, and for many patients is definitely contraindicated.

Physiotherapeutic Measures.—Physiotherapeutic measures which are not so severe that they put a strain on the circulatory system are not, in contrast to appreciable amounts of exercise, contraindicated for the obese. They do not, however, contribute anything to the removal of the accumulated fat. Systematic massage will, as in people of normal weight, tone up flabby muscles and give, for brief periods afterward, a feeling of physical well-being. The increased energy output by reason of stimulated metabolism is, if present at all, so slight as to be of no practical value. Massage may be of value in tightening up loose areas of skin rendered flabby by removal of the fat in the subcutaneous areas which have been distending it, if the flabbiness is not severe. If the looseness of the skin is of appreciable grade, massage will be of no value because this condition results not only from stretching of the skin, but also from hypertrophy of the subcutaneous supporting tissue. The hypertrophied subcutaneous supporting tissue, in younger persons at least, seems to contract and otherwise retrogress to some extent with resultant increase of firmness of the skin; but massage does not hasten it. Sweating procedures reduce weight by removal of water only. Any but the mildest are contraindicated because all others put a strain on the circulatory system which is already so burdened by the obesity. Furthermore, this strain in the obese because of the altered heat regulating mechanism in them, is greater than in people of normal weight.

Drugs.—*Thyroid.*—Thyroid products are the best known and most widely used drugs to increase energy output for removal of stored fat. Their use is justified when the excess weight is encountered in a myxedematous patient. A true low basal metabolism brought up to normal by thyroid medication, and the increased activity with added "work fraction" which usually follows, will increase the total energy output in amount sufficient to result in a slow removal of fat. The greater fraction of weight loss under these circumstances is, however, due to excretion of excess water. Thyroid medication may also be used safely and to advantage in the occasional obese person (perhaps 1 per cent of all) who with restriction of diet develops a basal metabolic rate of −20 or below. These patients, not myxedematous but with personality traits reminiscent of reptilian sluggishness, have also a minimal "work fraction" added to the low basal rate. The total oxygen exchange is so low that with the most severe restriction of diet a weight loss of only 1½ to 2 pounds a week can be accomplished. This can be brought up to the reasonable and more encouraging rate of 2½ to 3 pounds a week with thyroid. The amount of thyroid given such patients, or the truly myxedematous ones, should, however, never be more than enough to bring the basal metabolic rate to normal as related to ideal weight.

Thyroid products should never be given to that great majority of patients who have normal basal metabolic rates before dieting and who maintain them throughout the period of reduced intake. One must remember the high level of oxygen exchange of the obese despite a basal metabolic rate which is normal because of the increased surface area to which it is related; that this high level probably results in large part from an ever present increased work fraction; and that this related to the ideal weight shows an alarmingly high level of oxygen exchange for the active vital tissues of the body. A woman, aged fifty years, who weighed 206 pounds had a basal oxygen exchange of 69 calories. This made her basal metabolic rate +4 per cent. That caloric exchange when related to her ideal weight of 131 pounds gave a basal metabolic rate of +25 per cent. A normal basal rate for her ideal weight would have resulted from 55 calories per hour. One is certainly not justified in increasing still more a basal metabolic rate of +25 in any patient, and especially in one whose cardiovascular system is known to be, and to have been for some time, under serious strain.

Thyroid extracts, in addition to their effect on oxygen exchange, influence nitrogen metabolism. There is an increased elimination of nitrogen as long at least as any storage protein products remain, and probably even after. This nitrogen loss is unwholesome. So also is the tachycardia, the emotional instability, and the other well recognized effects of thyroid poisoning.

Thyroid administration increases the amount of food necessary for a sensation of satiety. Strang and McClugage and Brownlee[32] presented evidence that the feeling of satiation after food comes from the attainment of the optimum rate of change to heat production in response to it. This rate of change of metabolism with a meal of a given specific dynamic action is, of course, less in relation to a high basal metabolism than to a low one. In other words, it takes more food to give a feeling of satiation in a person with a high basal metabolic level than in one with a lower one; or conversely, the satiation from a fixed amount of food is greater with a low basal metabolic rate than with a higher.

Thyroid preparations, unphysiologic and dangerous in the treatment of obesity, are contraindicated also because they are relatively ineffective. If the basal exchange of 69 calories, already high, of the patient mentioned above could be raised 30 calories per hour to 99 it would give a basal metabolism of +55 for her active functioning body tissues. This high level of oxygen exchange could not be maintained for long without collapse, but until then it would result in an increased energy expenditure of 720 calories per day. Add, without commenting on the additional physiological strain, another 500 calories for the increased work fraction as a result of the nervous irritability instituted, and the total increase in calorie output is but 1220. This patient's total daily caloric exchange without thyroid medication would be not less than 2250. Given a diet supplying all the essential foodstuffs for her ideal weight but affording only 450 calories, a move in the direction of a negative caloric balance of 1800 calories is accomplished. This regimen, which can be continued indefinitely with improvement in the patient's general health, is 50 per cent more effective than the improbable outside limit of what can be accomplished for a short period by thyroid in the example given.

A *special warning* is necessary about the administration of thyroid to obese children. Many girls who are fat at the time of puberty, and especially those who have been obese for some years prior to that, have difficulty in establishing normal menstruation. Some of these girls and an occasional fat boy at puberty have basal metabolic rates in the minus twenties and thirties. This would seem to be an indication for thyroid medication, *but it is not.*

The attainment of a normal weight by diet will, in an appreciable number of these patients, be accompanied by a gradual increase of the metabolic rate to normal. If thyroid is given to these patients thyroid addiction may result.

This thyroid addiction, however, if taken in time may be cured. Several patients who for low metabolic rates at puberty had been taking thyroid for three or four years, were still fat. Interruption of the thyroid administration resulted in metabolic rates approaching minus forty and mild symptoms of hypothyroidism. Normal weights brought about by diet alone, a painfully slow process over many months, resulted also in normal basal metabolic rates and disappearance of symptoms of hypothyroidism.

Thyroid medication should not be employed in obese children especially at puberty, despite the apparent indication of a low metabolic rate, until they have shown no improvement after having been on a wholesome dietary regimen for the better part of one year at least.

Dinitrophenol.—Alpha-dinitrophenol (1–2–3) first studied and described by Cutting, Mehrtens, and Tainter,[77] has commanded much attention as an agent useful in the treatment of obesity by increasing energy expenditure. This and related drugs elevate the basal metabolic rate and do not, as thyroid products do, cause certain unpleasant side reactions such as tachycardia, palpitation, and tremor.

The study of the effects of dinitrophenol made by Strang and Evans[78] may be chosen from among several others to illustrate the effects produced by its use. These investigators employed this product in six young and middle-aged women varying from moderately to grossly obese. The observations were recorded for two periods. The first, that in which the patient received a diet estimated to be of approximately maintenance caloric value, was divided into a period of stabilization, a period with added dinitrophenol, and then a final period of the same diet after the drug had been discontinued. The second period, that in which a severely restricted reduction diet was given up, was also divided into alternate periods with and without dinitrophenol. The dosage employed was up to 300 mg. daily.

The same unpleasant side-effects discovered by others were noted in this study. The first to appear and seen in all patients was drenching sweats. Itching occurred in some patients, and in some pruritus and toxic dermatitis were seen. Nausea and epigastric pain were encountered, and a few patients reported dizziness and precordial distress. The latter might well have been, not a direct effect of the drug, but secondary to the altered metabolism resulting from it.

The data for all patients in the series of Strang and Evans for the entire period of study were surprisingly uniform. The findings on one patient, characteristic of the group, appear in figure 94. It will be seen that on the slightly submaintenance diet of over 2500 calories, and also on the reduction diet of less than 600 calories, the rate of weight loss was greater without than with the drug. This is paradoxical because the basal metabolic rate was increased 13 to 16.4 calories when dinitrophenol was taken. There was also without doubt an additional energy expenditure because of greater heat dissipation from the surface of the skin from the erythema caused by the drug, and from a direct stimulation of the sweat glands. Possibly there was no real increase in calorie exchange because the drug may have produced some irregular method of oxygen utilization that resulted in a qualitative alteration of relationship of heat production and oxygen consumption not correctly shown by the usual procedures. It seems probable, however, that there was a real elevation of total heat exchange with an increased rate of fat removal, and that the weight loss resulting was obscured by water

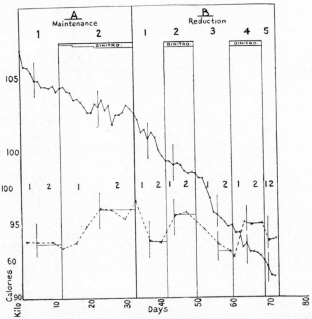

Fig. 94.—Daily weight and basal metabolism of a patient, characteristic of all by diet and by drug periods—dinitrophenol. Solid line—weight curve. Broken line—basal metabolism, calories per hour. (Strang and Evans, J.A.M.A., 104: 1957, 1935.)

storage. This is strongly indicated by the great outpouring of water in the patients of this series shortly after the drug was discontinued, with a greater weight loss during these days than when the drug was being taken, or on the same caloric intake before it was given. (Fig. 94.) Water storage might be caused by a toxic effect of dinitrophenol on the body cells, possibly with the production of cloudy swelling. Damage to body tissues must be slight, however, otherwise the outpouring of water seen in these patients would not have occurred so promptly.

One can say in regard to dinitrophenol, as to thyroid, that in addition to the contraindication of its toxicity, it is dangerous to increase further the already high level of energy exchange of the obese person. Furthermore, it is relatively ineffective even though, concurrent with its use, sufficient attention is given to diet to keep the intake constant. The total elevation of basal metabolic rate found by Strang and Evans in their patients averaged less than 16 calories per hour, 388 calories for twenty-four hours. Calculate a very generous 500 calories for a possible additional basal-plus fraction which may or may not result from the drug, and the total increased oxygen exchange which can be counted upon from its use is less than 900 calories. This will account for 110 gm. of fatty tissue a day, a loss of one and three-quarter pounds a week—if the diet remains constant. The 580 calories of the reducing diet subtracted from the 2510 calories of the slightly submaintenance diet give a diminished intake of 1930 calories. This will mean a loss of over 230 gm. of fatty tissue a day, more than twice that possible with dinitrophenol.

Use of dinitrophenol is now, happily, almost discontinued since understanding of its toxicity and the all too frequent development of cataracts following its use has become generally known.

DECREASED ENERGY INTAKE

Tape Worms and Regurgitation.—Attempts to diminish the energy intake without curtailing the food eaten have been made. Infestation with *Taenia saginata* by swallowing capsules containing scolices is a constantly recurring suggestion, but examples of its use have never been confirmed. Regurgitation of ingested materials, an old Roman custom, has not, in regard to food at least, become reestablished in modern times. Further discussion of these procedures will not be indulged in.

Drugs.—*Ipecac.*—Ipecac in doses too small to cause nausea but large enough to impair appetite has been used to bring about reduced energy intake in the treatment of obesity.

Digitalis.—Digitalis has been similarly employed.[79]

Benzedrine.—Benzedrine to reduce the appetite was used in conjunction with dietary measures by Lessees and Meyerson[80] in the treatment of obesity. The wide-spread physiological effects of this powerful drug need not be presented here. It suffices to say that they are such that its continued use is not possible. Friedenberg[81] recorded a patient treated by diet and benzedrine sulfate with some success who became addicted to the drug. After it was stopped the patient complained that she felt worn out and depressed, and that she could not get along without its stimulation. This effect presents another contraindication for the use of benzedrine sulfate in the treatment of obesity.

The objection to drugs such as these calculated to reduce energy intake by impairment of appetite is the same as to those employed to increase energy output. They are powerful drugs with diverse effects, and they cannot be taken continuously. Any reduction resulting will be temporary because such drugs can be taken only for short periods, and because no correction of faulty habits of eating has been accomplished. It is essential in the treatment of obesity, if the cure is to be permanent, to teach the patient to control his appetite and correct cultivated unwholesome tastes and habits of eating. This cannot be accomplished if any artificial measure is employed. For this reason any agent less toxic than the ones now available which may be subsequently presented to reduce body weight by increased energy expenditure, or decreased energy intake, will prove to be a disappointment.

Purges.—Reduction of energy intake through elimination of ingested calories by purging has been suggested as a treatment for obesity. Most of the agents recommended have been salines, some of them marketed under intriguing and foreign trade names. A purging sufficiently violent does no doubt result in a minimal calorie wastage for a very short time. This procedure can, however, never be continuous, and the occasional slight calorie elimination thus obtained would not be great enough to be of practical help. The real weight loss shown by the scales after purging is due to elimination of water. Three pounds or more from the elimination of three pints or more of fluid is frequently seen. Patients will often say, when this is pointed out to them, that they will maintain the weight reduction by drinking no water. Usually water is the only liquid mentioned for the proposed abstention. Patients do not realize that most of the food eaten contains much water and that with no fluid intake the body will retain from this supply all the water necessary to reestablish a normal fluid balance.

Diets.—Limitation of diet is the only way to obtain a practically effective reduction of energy intake, and is the only measure which can be carried on long enough to accomplish a weight reduction which is worthwhile and permanent. Furthermore, limitation of diet, alone of all suggestions, teaches the patient the principles of wholesome nutrition and tends to correct faulty habits of eating.

Several methods of dietary limitation have been used.

Folin and Denis[26] found repeated fast periods each of four to six days' duration which were both effective and safe for the removal of body fat. Although this regimen was accompanied by appreciable amounts of β-oxybutyric acid in the urine and minimal amounts of acetone in the breath, there was never any clinical acidosis. There was also no increased nitrogen loss. A smaller amount of β-oxybutyric acid and nitrogen in the urine was found during later periods of fasting than at first. This suggested that the body improved with practice its capacity to utilize a metabolic mixture high in fat.

Gordon and Nissler,[82] keeping in mind a theoretically possible hypoglycemia with restricted food intake devised a dietary regimen called "dextrose moderately low caloric diet." This regimen was presented for those who became obese seemingly because they could not tolerate a low calorie diet without symptoms of hypoglycemia. Gordon and Nissler suggested for those patients a vicious circle: increased carbohydrate intake, stimulation of increased insulin secretion, and need for more carbohydrate.

The patient recorded his customary food intake and exercise, and noted the time and type of symptoms for a period of three days. On the fourth day he was given 1200 to 1400 calories and activities and symptoms were again tabulated. On the fifth day 2 gm. of glucose were added in the form of candy or powder every half hour from 9:30 to 11 A.M.; and from 8:30 to 9:30 P.M. These were the periods of expected low blood sugar values. The starch portion of the diet was further reduced on the sixth day and the amount of glucose was increased from 2 to 4 gm. at 10:30 A.M., at 3 and 3:30 P.M., and at any other times when symptoms occurred. Dextrose candy of varying flavors was given on different days to reduce monotony. A good recipe for making dextrose candy is given by the authors.

This regimen resulted in satisfactory weight loss and was effective in relieving circulatory failure in the obese.

Harrop[83] devised a reducing diet of milk and bananas exclusively for periods of ten to fourteen days, or for two meals a day over longer periods. This diet was wholesome except for a too scant supply of protein and perhaps some other essential foodstuffs. It was effective despite a caloric content slightly greater than necessary. The banana was chosen because of its palatability, its high satiation value and low fat content, and with the idea that its carbohydrate would combat an expected tendency to ketosis. Milk was given to supply sufficient protein and for its vitamin content.

The strict diet consisted of six large ripe bananas and 1000 cc. of skimmed milk daily, spaced as the patient desired. To this may be added one-fourth of a medium sized head of lettuce or cabbage with mineral oil mayonnaise dressing. This diet afforded less than 1000 calories as follows:

	CHO	Pro.	Fat	Cal.
6 large bananas.............................	132	8	1	569
1000 cc. skimmed milk (4 ordinary glasses).....	50	36	3	371
Total.....................	182	44	4	940

The more liberal diet recommended by Harrop for prolonged use was made up of one or two large bananas and 250 cc. (one glass) of skimmed milk at breakfast and lunch. Dinner consisted of a clear soup, a moderate portion of lean meat, two or three portions of 5 per cent vegetables, a small slice of bread with a minimal amount of butter, and a portion of raw fruit. This diet was calculated by Harrop to afford from 1000 to 1200 calories.

Harrop commented on the simplicity and inexpensiveness of the milk and banana dietary regimen, points well worthy of emphasis.

General diets moderately limited in calories affording caloric deficits of 500 to 1000 per day and a weight loss of one to two pounds a week are employed by many physicians. They consider these diets preferable because they are thought to be easier for the patient, and the slow weight reduction safer. The objection to a moderately reduced diet, that it must be endured longer and patients may not persist, is not a valid one because the successful and permanent cure of obesity depends upon the willingness of the patient rigidly to control his appetite for the rest of his life. The menus below afford 60 and 75 gm. of protein, and 1200 and 1400 calories. One of them will be satisfactory for all patients, except the very small and elderly, if a slow reduction is desired. Specific instructions to each patient are necessary and individual recommendations are desirable. Specialization for separate patients, more detailed than are included in the four menus presented, is not necessary when so generous an intake is prescribed. These general diets permit such a wide choice of foodstuffs that the menu contains an adequate supply of vitamins, metals and electrolytes. Viosterol and compressed brewer's yeast in the customary doses should, perhaps, be added to the menu of adolescents, and since their caloric content is negligible for practical purposes, may be given also, if desired, to adults.

Calories 1200—Protein 60

	Grams	Carbohydrate	Protein	Fat
Oatmeal................	20	13	3	1
Milk—whole	500	25	17	20
Vegetable Group I.........	200	8	2	
Vegetable Group II........	100	8	2	
Bread....................	30	16	3	
Fruit Group II............	230	30	2	
Egg.....................	50	..	7	5
Meat Group I.............	60	..	12	15
Meat Group II............	60	..	12	9
Butter...................	13	..	..	11
	...	100	60	62

Breakfast   Grams

Oatmeal.. 20 (dry)
Milk—whole 100
Bread.. 20
Butter... 5
Egg... 50
Fruit Group II................................. 130

Dinner

Milk.. 200
Vegetable Group I............................. 150
Bread... 10
Meat Group II................................. 60
Butter.. 4
Fruit Group II................................ 50

Supper

Milk.. 200
Vegetable Group I............................. 50
Vegetable Group II............................ 100
Meat Group I.................................. 60
Butter.. 4
Fruit Group II................................ 50

Substitutions

1. In place of 100 gm. Vegetable Group I, you may substitute 50 gm. Vegetable Group II.
2. In place of 100 gm. Vegetable Group II, you may substitute:
   (a) 200 gm. Vegetable Group I or
   (b)   50 gm. Vegetable Group III.
3. In place of 60 gm. Meat Group II, you may substitute:
   (a) 60 gm. Meat Group III plus an additional 7 gm. of butter for that meal or
   (b) 75 gm. Meat Group IV plus an additional 9 gm. of butter for that meal or
   (c) 48 gm. Meat Group V plus an additional 10 gm. of butter for that meal.
4. In place of 60 gm. Meat Group I, you may substitute:
   (a) 60 gm. Meat Group II plus an additional 7 gm. of butter for that meal or
   (b) 43 gm. American Cheese.
5. In place of 50 gm. Fruit Group II, you may substitute 110 gm. Fruit Group I.

More rigid limitation of caloric intake is employed by some and much preferred by them to the moderate diets. Considerations other than caloric limitation are important in making up a severely restricted diet. Much care must be taken that it contains an adequate amount of all the known essential foodstuffs. Neglect of this fact is the most common fault of diets originating in beauty parlors, movie circles, and around tea tables. The essential foodstuffs need be supplied in amounts adequate only for the active vital

Calories 1400—Protein 60

	Grams	Carbohydrate	Protein	Fat
Oatmeal...................	20	13	3	1
Milk—whole	500	25	17	20
Vegetable Group I..........	200	8	2	
Vegetable Group II........	100	8	2	
Egg.......................	50	..	7	5
Bread.....................	60	32	5	1
Fruit Group II.............	270	35	3	
Meat Group I.............	50	..	10	13
Meat Group II............	55	..	11	8
Butter....................	32	..	..	27
	...	121	60	75

Breakfast   Grams
    Oatmeal... 20 (dry)
    Milk—whole 100
    Egg.. 50
    Bread.. 20
    Fruit Group II................................. 160
    Butter... 8

Dinner
    Milk... 200
    Vegetable Group I............................. 150
    Bread.. 20
    Meat Group II................................. 55
    Butter... 12
    Fruit Group II................................. 60

Supper
    Milk... 200
    Vegetable Group I............................. 50
    Vegetable Group II............................ 100
    Bread.. 20
    Meat Group I.................................. 50
    Butter... 12
    Fruit Group II................................. 50

Substitutions

1. In place of 100 gm. of Vegetable Group I, you may substitute 50 gm. Vegetable Group II.
2. In place of 100 gm. Vegetable Group II, you may substitute:
    (*a*) 200 gm. Vegetable Group I or
    (*b*) 50 gm. Vegetable Group III.
3. In place of 55 gm. Meat Group II, you may substitute:
    (*a*) 55 gm. Meat Group III plus an additional 6 gm. of butter for that meal or
    (*b*) 70 gm. Meat Group IV plus an additional 8 gm. of butter for that meal or
    (*c*) 45 gm. Meat Group V plus an additional 8 gm. of butter for that meal.
4. In place of 50 gm. Meat Group I, you may substitute:
    (*a*) 50 gm. Meat Group II plus an additional 6 gm. of butter for that meal or
    (*b*) 35 gm. American Cheese.
5. In place of 50 gm. Fruit Group II, you may substitute 110 gm. Fruit Group I.
6. In place of 60 gm. Fruit Group II, you may substitute 125 gm. Fruit Group I.

functioning tissue, that is, calculated on the basis of the ideal, not the actual, weight. If this is done wasting of vital tissues does not ensue, only fat is burned. This is proven by several facts. There is no negative nitrogen balance. The level of nitrogen exchange remains the same as before dieting, and the same as in people of normal weight. The creatinine coefficient is not altered. The level of basal oxygen exchange never falls below a rate normal

Calories 1200—Protein 75

	Grams	Carbohydrate	Protein	Fat
Oatmeal..................	20	13	3	1
Milk—whole	500	25	17	20
Vegetable Group II.........	100	8	2	
Vegetable Group I..........	200	8	2	
Bread.....................	30	16	3	
Fruit Group II.............	235	31	2	
Egg......................	50	...	7	5
Meat Group II.............	95	...	19	14
Meat Group II.............	100	...	20	15
	...	101	75	55

Breakfast   Grams
Oatmeal....................................... 20 (dry)
Milk—whole 100
Bread.. 20
Egg.. 50
Fruit Group II................................ 135

Dinner
Milk... 200
Vegetable Group I............................ 150
Bread.. 10
Meat Group II................................ 95
Fruit Group II................................ 50

Supper
Milk... 200
Vegetable Group I............................ 50
Vegetable Group II........................... 100
Meat Group II................................ 100
Fruit Group II................................ 50

Substitutions

1. In place of 100 gm. Vegetable Group I, you may substitute 50 gm. Vegetable Group II.
2. In place of 100 gm. Vegetable Group II, you may substitute:
   (a) 200 gm. Vegetable Group I or
   (b) 50 gm. Vegetable Group III.
3. In place of 95 gm. Meat Group II, you may substitute:
   (a) 95 gm. Meat Group III plus an additional 10 gm. of butter for that meal or
   (b) 120 gm. Meat Group IV plus an additional 15 gm. butter or
   (c) 75 gm. Meat Group V plus an additional 15 gm. butter.
4. In place of 100 gm. Meat Group II, you may substitute:
   (a) 100 gm. Meat Group III plus an additional 12 gm. of butter for that meal.

when referred to the ideal weight, in contrast to the low levels which are seen in starvation. The lassitude and depression of starvation are replaced by increased energy and a feeling of physical well-being (see sections on Nitrogen Exchange, Creatinine Coefficient, and Energy Exchange).

The first essential foodstuff, water, having no caloric content needs no consideration. Its intake may be left entirely to desire with the full assurance that as far as the obesity is concerned the body will maintain a wholesome balance. The next essential foodstuff is protein. An adequate intake, long ago insisted upon by Preble,[84] must be included in the menu if health and vigor are to be maintained. A deficient intake of nitrogenous food, with its resultant negative nitrogen balance, will be accompanied by a depression

Calories 1400—Protein 75

	Grams	Carbohydrate	Protein	Fat
Oatmeal..................	20	13	3	1
Milk-whole..............	500	25	17	20
Vegetable Group II.........	100	8	2	
Vegetable Group I..........	200	8	2	
Egg.....................	50	...	7	5
Bread...................	60	32	5	1
Fruit Group II............	260	34	3	
Meat Group I.............	90	...	18	23
Meat Group II............	90	...	18	14
Butter..................	6	...	..	5
	...	120	75	69

Breakfast   Grams

Oatmeal.................................... 20 (dry)
Milk-whole................................ 100
Egg....................................... 50
Bread..................................... 20
Butter.................................... 6
Fruit Group II............................ 160

Dinner

Milk...................................... 200
Vegetable Group I......................... 150
Bread..................................... 20
Meat Group I.............................. 90
Fruit Group II............................ 50

Supper

Milk...................................... 200
Vegetable Group I......................... 50
Vegetable Group II........................ 100
Bread..................................... 20
Meat Group II............................. 90
Fruit Group II............................ 50

Substitutions

1. In place of 100 gm. Vegetable Group I, you may substitute 50 gm. Vegetable Group II.
2. In place of 100 gm. Vegetable Group II, you may substitute:
    (a) 200 gm. Vegetable Group I or
    (b) 50 gm. Vegetable Group III.
3. In place of 90 gm. Meat Group I, you may substitute:
    (a) 90 gm. Meat Group II, plus an additional 10 gm. of butter for that meal or
    (b) 90 gm. Meat Group III, plus an additional 21 gm. of butter for that meal or
    (c) 63 gm. American Cheese.
4. In place of 90 gm. Meat Group II, you may substitute:
    (a) 90 gm. Meat Group III plus an additional 10 gm. butter or
    (b) 110 gm. of Meat Group IV plus an additional 15 gm. butter or
    (c) 70 gm. Meat Group V plus an additional 15 gm. butter.
5. In place of 50 gm. Fruit Group II, you may substitute 110 gm. Fruit Group I.

1. All meats are to be weighed or measured without bones or visible fat.
2. Roast meats are to be weighed or measured after they have been cooked.
3. Steaks, chops, cutlets, liver and fresh fish are to be weighed or measured before they are cooked.
4. Salad greens and vegetables are weighed or measured raw.
5. Cooked vegetables are to be weighed or measured after they are cooked.
6. All fruits are to be fresh or canned without any sugar.

Vegetables

Group I. C-4 P-1 F-0

Asparagus—fresh
Asparagus—canned
Brussels Sprouts
Broccoli
Cabbage
Celery
Cauliflower
Cucumber
Eggplant
Green Peppers
Lettuce
Pumpkin—fresh
Radish
Rhubarb
Sauerkraut
Spinach
Salad Greens
String Beans
White Squash
Tomatoes—fresh
Tomatoes—canned
Tomato Juice
Sauerkraut juice

Group II. C-8 P-2 F-0

Beets
Carrots
Mushrooms
Onions
Green Peas—canned
Rutabagas
String Beans—fresh
Squash—yellow
Turnips

Group III. C-16 P-4 F-0

Green Peas—fresh
Lima Beans—canned
Corn—fresh
Parsnips

Fruits

Group I. C-6 P-1 F-0

Muskmelon
Honeydew
Cantaloupe
Watermelon

Fruits (cont'd)

Group II. C-13 P-1 F-0

Apples
Apricots
Cherries
Grapes—as purchased
Grapefruit
Loganberries
Blackberries
Blueberries
Lemons
Oranges
Peaches
Pears
Pineapple
Plums
Red Raspberries
Black Raspberries
Strawberries

Group III. C-76 P-3 F-1

Dates
Figs
Prunes
Raisins

Meats

Group I. P-20 F-25

Roast Beef
Filet of Beef
Beef Tongue—canned
Ham
Lamb Chop
Salt Mackerel
Turkey
Tuna Fish

Group II. P-20 F-15

Beef Heart
Corned Beef
Bologna
Chicken
Frankfurts
Roast Lamb
Roast Pork
Pork Tenderloin
Sardines—canned
Sweetbreads

Meats (cont'd)

Salmon—fresh
Salmon—canned
Sirloin Steak
Veal Chop
Halibut—smoked

Group III. P-20 F-5

Bluefish
Duck
Herring
Heart—Chicken
    Veal
Liver—Beef
    Calves
    Chicken
    Pork
Kidney—Beef
    Veal
Mackerel—canned
Mackerel—fresh
Round Steak
Roast Veal
Shad
Smelts
White Perch
White Fish
Veal Tongue
Halibut—fresh

Group IV. P-16 F-1

Crabmeat—canned
Clams—hardshell
Cod
Frog's Legs
Flounder
Sturgeon
Lobster—fresh or canned
Haddock

Group V. P-25 F-1

Chicken Gizzard
Smoked Haddock
Shrimp—canned

of metabolism in all ways similar to the starvation patients of Benedict and Lusk. One gram of protein per kilogram of ideal body weight is the minimum for safety. An intake greater than this is helpful because of protein's high satiation effect, if the maximum possible restriction of calories is not desired. It is also necessary to make up the protein allowance from foods of high biological value. No amino acids may be omitted. A minimal supply of carbohydrate foods equal to two-thirds to three-fourths of a gram for each gram of protein is necessary to maintain the patient in nitrogen equilibrium despite an intake of 1 gm. of protein per kilo of ideal weight (see section on Nitrogen Exchange). The menus must include in addition to the food, extra anions and cations and some vitamins from sources supplying no calories.

Keeping the above points in mind it is possible to compile menus supplying all essential foodstuffs in adequate amounts and affording no more than 400 to 600 calories. Such diets are the only ones effective for inactive elderly people, especially if of small stature, who maintain an excess weight on an intake of 1100 to 1200 calories. Active young and middle-aged patients on this regimen obtain a caloric deficit of 1800 or more, permitting a removal of 2½ to 4 pounds a week. A special diet fitted to the ideal weight of each patient is necessary. The menus below were the ones employed in patients whose ideal weights were 55 and 70 kilograms respec-

REDUCING DIET

DIET FOR PATIENT—IDEAL WEIGHT—55 KILOGRAMS

Carbohydrate—40   Grams—73
Protein—55   Ratio—.45
Fat—low   Calories—461

Food	Grams	Carbohydrate	Protein	Fat
Egg white	80	..	10	
Orange	100	12	1	
Egg	50	..	7	5
Peas	35	6	2	
Round steak	140	..	32	4
Radishes	50	3	1	
Lettuce	80	2	1	
Celery	30	1		
Peaches	80	8		
Raspberries	60	8	1	
	...	40	55	9

Breakfast	Grams	Lunch	Grams	Dinner	Grams
Orange	100	Round steak	70	Round steak	70
Egg	50	Fresh peas	35	Radishes	50
Egg white	20	Lettuce	40	Lettuce	40
Brewer's yeast	3	Celery	30	Raspberries	60
Plus water	40	Egg white	60	1 Alkaline* Tablet with	
1 Alkaline* Tablet with		Egg white (hard cooked)	60	water	200
water	200	Peaches	80	Viosterol	℥vi
Viosterol	℥vi	1 Alkaline* Tablet with		Tea	150
Tea	150	water	200		
		Viosterol	℥vi		
		Tea	150		

* The alkaline tablet employed was Burroughs and Wellcome Effervescent Alkaline Tablet.

tively.* The basic features of these menus are the same for all patients. They can be modified to fit any patient by changing the protein to afford 1 gm. of protein per kilogram of ideal weight, and adding to, or subtracting from, the carbohydrate in them by two-thirds of a gram for each gram of protein added or subtracted.

It is very apparent that these menus make no concessions to gustatory sensualism. It is possible perhaps to compile menus somewhat more inviting, certainly more bulky. Evans and Strang[61] considered this an unwise

*Food values taken from Atwater, W. O. and Bryant, A. P., United States Department of Agriculture, Bulletin 28. "The Chemical Composition of American Food Materials."

practice. They found that the smaller the diet the less appetite there appeared to be, and felt that patients who would not be content with menus of limited bulk would not continue with one of greater bulk. They quote patients who asked why they were not hungry with this menu when with less severe limitations of caloric intake to 1200 or 1600 on previous attempts to reduce, they were hungry all the time. Furthermore, they found that the long period of this severe gustatory discipline reformed for many patients the abnormal appetite which caused the obesity so that when reduced

REDUCING DIET

DIET FOR PATIENT—IDEAL WEIGHT—70 KILOGRAMS

Carbohydrate—40 Grams—82
Protein—70 Ratio—.48
Fat—low Calories—521

Food	Grams	Carbohydrate	Protein	Fat
Milk	150	8	5	6
Gelatin	10	..	9	
Egg white	65	..	8	
Pineapple	90	9		
Orange	50	6		
Brussels sprouts	100	3	2	
Haddock	100	..	17	
Round steak	120	..	27	3
Carrots	80	7	1	
Raspberries	55	7	1	
...		40	70	9

Breakfast		*Lunch*		*Dinner*	
	Grams		Grams		Grams
Orange	50	Haddock	100	Round steak, ground	120
Milk	150	Brussels Sprouts	100	Egg white	65
1 Alkaline Tablet with		Pineapple	90	Raspberry juice	55
water	200	Gelatin	5	Gelatin	5
Brewer's yeast	3	Water	100	Water	100
Plus water	40	1 Alkaline Tablet with		Carrots	80
Viosterol	℞vi	water	200	1 Alkaline Tablet with	
Coffee	150	Viosterol	℞vi	water	200
		Tea	150	Viosterol	℞vi
				Tea	150

they were able to maintain their corrected weight with a minimum of self-denial and without apparent discontent. This most desirable result did not follow so regularly when the calories were not so strictly limited, or when to the minimum caloric diet they prescribed, artificial bulk was added or sensuality in appetite was indulged.

These diets have not been employed during pregnancy lest some as yet unknown vitamin essential to the development of the fetus, or health of the mother, had been inadvertently omitted. No patient with pulmonary tuberculosis has been treated with these diets. Evans and Strang recognized no other contraindication.

It is worthy of emphasis that the years of childhood, of puberty, and of advanced age are not contraindications to the employment of a low calorie reduction diet. Indeed, puberty is attained more wholesomely by girls who

19

are not obese than by those who are, and the increasing menace of obesity in later years of life makes a rapid reduction more important then than at other periods of life. One ten-year-old boy lost 31½ pounds in twelve weeks with nothing but improved general well-being. During the period of dieting he grew one-half inch. One twelve-year-old girl reduced from 208½ to 164½ pounds, 44 pounds in twenty weeks with marked improvement in her physical and mental equipment. At the other extreme of life, one patient, sixty-seven years old presented herself for treatment walking with difficulty. She was having 15 to 18 extrasystoles a minute and her blood pressure was 240 systolic, 110 diastolic. She reduced from 278 to 182 pounds, 96 pounds in twenty-four weeks, an average of 4 pounds a week. Her blood pressure after four weeks of dieting was 135 systolic, 80 diastolic, and she was marketing and doing some housework with ease and comfort.

Cardiac and renal decompensations, glycosuria, and hyperglycemia have been recognized as urgent indications for, rather than contraindications to, a radical reduction diet. Strang and Evans encountered no disasters, nor even minor mishaps, in the patients treated with the severely limited diets which they employed.

The treatment of endocrine disorders by special products where indicated, and when they are available, should be carried out in the obese as in other patients and may be expected to correct several abnormal factors encountered including, at times possibly, an abnormal appetite. Appetite may not yield to this therapy without reeducation because of the easily cultivated habit of overeating. The feature "obesity" itself can be corrected only by diet.

The obesity associated with *hypothyroidism* should, as all others, be treated by diet. However these patients have a low energy output and although a diet can be designed upon which they lose weight without medication, it is too slow to be endured. Furthermore, a weight reduction alone does not relieve the other distressing symptoms of hypothyroidism. Thyroid should be given to improve the hypothyroidism. Secondarily, the weight loss will be speeded up beyond that resulting from diet alone. Under no circumstances should thyroid be given beyond the point of normal true basal metabolic rates.

Constipation is a troublesome feature in many patients on reduction diets, especially the very restricted ones of Evans and Strang. The food bulk is smaller than that of the previous customary diet of the obese person, but the generous allowance of 3 and 6 per cent vegetables supplies sufficient indigestible residue to make it unlikely that this is the cause of the constipation. It seems more probable that it results from the lower intake of carbohydrate foods. This annoying feature must be met symptomatically, preferably with saline laxatives on arising in the morning. Mineral oil is usually not effective, and may have the added unfortunate property of preventing vitamin B absorption. Sometimes during the course of treatment, constipation disappears as though the colonic function had adjusted to the revised regimen. Otherwise, the resumption of a normal intake of fruit and starches when the desired weight is attained usually corrects the disorder. When it does not, the factors causing the constipation are as in other patients and are to be so treated.

Maintenance After Reduction.—A patient who has continued his diet until an acceptable weight has been attained should not be dismissed without further attention. He must be told that despite the reduction by physiological measures, he cannot resume the practice of careless eating without becoming obese. He is as any other person of his weight; if he eats correct amounts of food he will remain normal; if he overeats, he will become obese again. This should not come as a surprise to the patient because during his dieting he should have become educated in the principles of wholesome nutrition, and to have learned that he cannot, without penalty, indulge in uncontrolled gustatory licentiousness. This control is relatively easy for many patients after the long period of discipline they have achieved. An appreciable number will claim long after discharge that they get as much, or almost as much, pleasure from wholesome amounts of correct foods as they did previously from an unwholesome diet. One is surprised occasionally to hear the erstwhile confirmed pie eater enthuse over chilled sliced tomatoes and crisp lettuce with salt, and, at bedtime, several stalks of tender celery.

The comparative high calorie content of fat foods should be mentioned and the relative caloric values per gram of fat, carbohydrate, protein, and alcohol, reviewed again. Patients ordinarily expect to be warned about fats, but often do not realize the care necessary with concentrated carbohydrate foods. All patients should be cautioned once more not to be misled by certain fallacies. Reducing breads and candies do not reduce; honey and oleomargarine do have food value; citrus fruit juices and sauerkraut juice do not dissolve body fat. These examples will serve for the group of *fallacies*, always being contributed to in a manner beyond human ingenuity to anticipate.

Patients after reduction are relieved to be freed of the necessity for weighing or measuring the articles on the menu. They should be given a list of foods affording the essential foodstuffs in approximately the right amounts, but deficient in calories, which they must eat every day. This list, of course, resembles the reduction diet itself, if a severely limited one has been employed. Choice of food in addition to this necessary to bring the daily fuel value up to that which will maintain, not increase, the normal weight, may be left to the patient. This food constitutes "fun calories." Instead of estimating the number of them and weighing the foods it is more convenient for the patient to weigh himself and thus control the quantity to the correct amount. This is less irksome and tends to initiate the wholesome habit of stepping on the scales frequently. Concentration on the 3 and 6 per cent vegetables is desirable and a list of them should be supplied. A list of foods primarily carbohydrate is found useful by the patient.

Final instructions given to the patient embodying the above points may be presented as follows:

I—EAT EVERY DAY

1. One egg.
2. A glass of skimmed milk.
3. A portion of raw fruit.
4. A generous portion of any cut of lean fresh lamb, beef, poultry or fish.
5. Generous portions of each of three vegetables selected from those listed below, one of them raw at frequent intervals.

II—IN ADDITION

After having eaten each day everything listed in I, eat in addition anything you want and find you can while maintaining your weight between . . . and . . . pounds as determined by a weighing at the same time and on the same day of each week. The weight is most accurately recorded when taken undressed on arising, after having voided, and before taking anything to eat or to drink.

III—ACCEPTABLE VEGETABLES

(referred to in No. 5 of I)

Artichokes	Celery	Leeks
Asparagus	Carrots	Mushrooms
Broccoli	Chard	Okra
Beet Greens	Dandelions	Onions
Brussels Sprouts	Eggplant	Pumpkin
Cabbage	Endive	Parsnips
Cauliflower	Kohlrabi	Peppers
Cucumbers	Lettuce	Radishes
Spinach	Squash	String Beans
Sauerkraut	Turnips	Turnip Greens
Tomatoes	Tomato Juice	Water Cress

IV—BE SPARING WITH

1. Fats, oils, and alcohol.
2. Concentrated carbohydrate foods:
   (a) Sugars which are:
       Sweeteners
       Candies
       Fruits
       Preserves
   (b) Starches which are:
       Breads
       Pastries
       Cereals
       Mealy vegetables which are:
           Potatoes
           Beans
           Peas
           Cereals used as vegetables which are { Macaroni Spaghetti Rice Corn

It is necessary to add to the list of essential foodstuffs for adolescents one or more glasses of milk, and additional meat.

The patient should be asked to report once a month for six months for a check-up. He rarely will do this because if he is maintaining a normal weight he sees no need for it; if he has relapsed he is reluctant to do so, at least until he is ready to diet again.

SIGNS, SYMPTOMS, AND RESULTS OF TREATMENT

Weight Loss.—The result of treatment of obesity by measures to increase energy output, such as drugs and exercise, is, if attention is also given to diet, a reduction in weight. This comes primarily, but not always exclusively, from removal of fat. The weight reduction attendant upon the use of some drugs results in part also from a loss of body nitrogen, always unfortunate, and that of others merely from a depletion of water. Weight reduction attained in this way will not persist, and the rate of reduction cannot be predicted.

Treatment of obesity by reduction of energy intake with diets affording essential foodstuffs but deficient in calories results in weight loss exclusively by removal of fat except for temporary changes due to water swings. Any loss, however great, necessary to attain a normal weight is accomplished with safety by such dietary measures, and is maintained by a satisfactory percentage of patients.

The calculated and observed weight losses often are not the same over short periods of observation. This is accounted for by the variable water content of the body from time to time, the influence of which is discounted over long periods. Newburgh and Johnston proved this point in their study of water exchange in the obese during treatment (see section on Water Balance, p. 551). If the measures they devised for accurate estimation of the extent of these water swings are employed to correct the error introduced, the amount of fat removed can be shown to be that predicted by calculations for even short periods. Correct predictions of a schedule of weight loss from month to month are possible regardless of other features which may accompany the obesity, such as signs and symptoms of endocrine disease. The expected and observed losses always approach each other, over long periods, so closely as to be well within the limits of error of observation. A characteristic example is afforded by the calculation for one of their patients presented by Strang and Evans[2]

Basal calories per hour = 65 (derived from basal metabolic rate determination)
Basal calories per 24 hours = 1560
Daily energy requirement—basal plus 20 per cent = 1870 cal.
Average calories in reducing diet = 620
   1870 − 620 equals 1250 calories from body fat
1250/9.3 equals 134 grams of fat equals 134 × 75/65 or 155*
   grams of fatty tissue per day
Average duration = 17 weeks or 119 days

$$\frac{155 \times 119 \times 2.2}{1000} \text{ equals } 40.6 \text{ pounds}$$

Weight loss observed = 41 pounds

The modest caloric deficit, 1250, of the example given above removed about 2½ pounds of fat per week. Deficits of 2000 or more calories a day were often obtained by the limited diets employed by Evans and Strang, resulting in removal of about 4 pounds of fatty tissue a week. The first series reported by them showed results as follows[61]:

98 completed cases
98 patients in 858 weeks lost a total of 2590 pounds.
Average time of diet, 8.75 weeks.
Average loss per patient, 26.4 pounds.
Average loss per week, 3.02 pounds.

111 patients at end of first week
111 patients lost 714 pounds.
Average loss per patient, 6.43 pounds.

75 patients at end of four weeks
75 patients lost 1209 pounds in four weeks.
Average loss per patient in four weeks, 16.1 pounds.
Average loss per week, 4.03 pounds.

47 patients at end of eight weeks
47 patients lost 1265 pounds.
Average loss per patient, 26.9 pounds.
Average loss per week, 3.36 pounds.

*9.3 calories from each gram of fat oxidized. Each gram of fat oxidized = 75/65 of body fat tissue.

The second series[85] reported showed results as follows:

121 completed cases

121 patients in 964.5 weeks lost a total of 2627.75 pounds
Average time on diet, 8 weeks.
Average loss per patient, 21.7 pounds.
Average loss per week, 2.7 pounds.

108 patients at end of first week

108 patients lost 597¼ pounds.
Average loss per patient, 5.5 pounds.

92 patients at end of two weeks

92 patients lost 863¼ pounds.
Average loss per patient, 9.3 pounds.

59 patients at end of four weeks

59 patients lost 872¾ pounds.
Average loss per patient, 14.8 pounds.

34 patients at end of eight weeks

34 patients lost 823 pounds.
Average loss per patient, 24 pounds.
Average loss per week, 3 pounds.

The series of Evans and Strang include several patients reduced more than 100 pounds. One unemployed colored woman who remained in the hospital during the total period of dieting reduced from 389 to 169 pounds, a net reduction of 220 pounds. Thirteen pounds of this was accounted for by the removal of an abdominal apron of stretched skin and hypertrophied subcutaneous supporting tissue. She lived in the hospital for two periods of about a year each, with approximately a month's vacation between them. During this vacation she gained some 30 pounds which is to be added to the final net weight loss above. This patient during much of the period of dieting was ingesting less than 5 calories per Kg. of actual weight. For the whole period she was well, cheerful, and helpfully busy about the hospital pavilion; she remained in nitrogen equilibrium, and maintained a constant index of creatinine excretion, normal as related to her ideal weight. Short[86] maintained a patient with an initial weight of 402 pounds for a period of eighteen months on a diet planned to include all the essential foodstuffs but supplying only 700 calories. She lost 239 pounds and during the entire period remained in good health and spirits.

The number and diversity of symptoms during middle and later decades of life relieved by the cure of obesity are surprising. This discovery is one of the greater contributions accruing from the widespread interest of people during recent years in the attainment of a normal weight. Indeed it may be said with reason, that the cure of no symptom in the obese should be undertaken without at the same time instituting measures to correct the obesity. Such measures alone are often effective. The relief of these symptoms suggests that they are caused by the obesity. They are, rather, probably the result of the underlying disturbance of normal physiological activities attendant upon this unwholesome bodily state.

Blood Pressure.—Elevation of both systolic and diastolic blood pressure is a relatively common accompaniment. Robinson, Brucer and Mass[87] studied blood pressure levels in relation to weight in 7478 men and 3405 women who were well or suffering only from minor complaints. They classified these subjects into underweight, medium, and overweight groups on the basis of *ponderal index* which is the ratio of weight in pounds divided by height in inches. They found that systolic hypertension was almost three times, and diastolic hypertension four and one-half times, as frequent in obese as in undernourished men; and that systolic and diastolic hypertension was six times as frequent in obese women. The statistics also showed that in the obese men high systolic pressures are two and one-half times, and high diastolic three times, as frequent as low pressures; and in obese women high systolic and diastolic pressures were found three times as often as low pressures. These relationships are shown graphically in figure 95.

John[74] found the systolic pressure to be above 140 in 42.5 per cent of 120 cases. A normal level was obtained by reduction of weight more frequently in John's patients whose elevation was moderate. This presumably was because the duration and degree of assault had been less in relation to the resistance of the vessels so that the hypertension was still on a func-

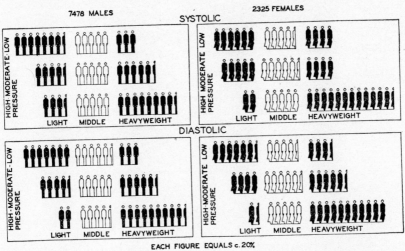

Fig. 95.—The relation of weight to blood pressure. Per cent of actual to expected incidence. (Robinson, Brucer and Mass, J. Lab. and Clin. Med., **25**: 807, 1940.)

tional basis rather than dependent upon organic damage. Lowered blood pressure with treatment occurred in about as many of these patients as one might reasonably expect had not acquired permanent organic lesions. A response more gratifying than that shown by the systolic was seen in the diastolic level. This may be related to diminished myocardial strain.

Table 28 shows the systolic and diastolic pressures recorded by Spencer[9] on admission to his clinic. He says in regard to these data: "The lower limit of the table of systolic pressures indicates the average increase in pressure of healthy adults as they grow older. The upper line is drawn in as worked out through the courtesy of the statistical department of the Metropolitan Life Insurance Company and is founded upon the mathematical theory of least squares." Spencer found that the blood pressure tended to fall and remain at a lower level as long as the patient did not resume his overeating. Improvement was least, as is to be expected, among those patients who had high diastolic pressures.

Preble[7] recorded the blood pressure by decades of age of 194 obese patients before treatment, and after reducing 10 pounds or more. These observations appear in table 29. The average drop for the entire group was 18 mm. Hg systolic, and 10 mm. Hg diastolic. Among the 1000 cases of obesity analyzed by Preble, sixty-two had a systolic blood pressure of 200 or above. Twenty-two of these were treated by reducing the weight 10

TABLE 28

SYSTOLIC AND DIASTOLIC PRESSURES OF THE OBESE*

Systolic Pressures

	10–14	15–19	20–24	25–29	30–34	35–39	40–44	45–49	50–54	55–59	60–64	65–69
200–						1	3		4	3		
190–199							2			2	1	
180–189						1	1	1	1	1	1	
170–179						1	1	2	1	1		
160–169				2	1	3	2	3	2	1	2	2
150–159				1	1	3	2	3	4	4	1	2
140–149			2	2	4	8	6	6	7	5	2	2
130–139		1	4	2	7	6	8	2	4	4	1	
120–129	1	1	4	9	6	4	5	8	6	2		
110–119		4	2	9	6	8	2	1		1		
100–109	1			2	2	3	1					
90– 99		1										
On or above mean	1	1	8	11	15	24	25	17	22	19	7	6
Below	1	6	5	16	12	14	8	9	7	5	1	

Diastolic Pressures

	10–14	15–19	20–24	25–29	30–34	35–39	40–44	45–49	50–54	55–59	60–64	65–69
On or above mean	1	2	6	11	12	13	18	16	10	10	5	3
Below	1	5	7	15	14	12	8	8	14	11	3	3

	10–14	15–19	20–24	25–29	30–34	35–39	40–44	45–49	50–54	55–59	60–64	65–69
130–							1		1			
120–129					1		1		1	1		
110–119						2	2		1	3		
100–109						2	1	1	1	1		
90– 99			2	4	6	3	5	7	7	5	4	3
80– 89		2	4	7	5	6	8	8	7	7	2	1
70– 79	1	1	5	10	10	9	6	6	6	3	1	1
60– 69	1	4	2	5	4	3	2	2	1	1		1

* Spencer, H. J., Med. Clin. No. Amer., 12: 604, 1928–29.

pounds or more, and in them the average systolic dropped from 219 to 176, or 43 mm. Hg, the diastolic from 129 to 108, or 21 mm. Hg.

Evans found the systolic blood pressures of 100 consecutive cases taken without regard to age, sex, and degree or duration of obesity, to be above 140 in 61 per cent. Eleven per cent of the total were above 180, and 10 per cent above 200. The diastolic pressures of these patients were above 100 in 36 per cent. Seven per cent of the total were above 110, and 8 per cent above 120. Treatment reduced the systolic pressure below 135 in 75 per cent of those whose level was from 140 to 180, in 50 per cent of those whose level was 180 to 200, but in only 20 per cent when the pressure was above 200. Many of the patients with the higher pressures, although not attaining normal levels did show an appreciable reduction. All but one of the patients with diastolic pressures of 100 to 110, and of 110 to 120 attained, with treatment, a diastolic pressure of below 90, but only 20 per cent of those whose diastolic level was above 120, reduced to normal.

Cardiovascular Strain.—Breathlessness on mild exertion is frequent in obesity. It is, in many instances, on a purely mechanical basis and improves promptly with reduction. Sometimes it is severe, with orthopnea and cyanosis, and associated with edema, enlarged liver, urinary albumin and casts. These frank symptoms of congestive heart failure are not only seen frequently, but are almost a constant accompaniment of appreciable grades of obesity in all but young people. Relief of these symptoms occurs so

TABLE 29

BLOOD PRESSURE BEFORE TREATMENT AND AFTER (194 Cases)*

Ages, years	Before treatment						
	0–20	21–30	31–40	41–50	51–60	61–70	71
Systolic..........	130	129	147	157	165	180	179
Diastolic.........	80	88	101	101	98	113	95
	After reducing 10 pounds or more						
Systolic..........	115	127	132	101	143	166	150
Diastolic..........	70	81	90	89	90	102	86
	Average: Before, 155/96; after, 133/86						

* Preble, Wm. E., Boston Med. and Surg. J., **188**: 617, 1923.

regularly with dietary treatment that it can almost be considered a specific. Gordon and Nissler,[82] with their diet of 1100 calories reinforced with glucose lozenges at the periods of expected low blood sugar values, reported prompt relief in eight ambulant patients. Two of these with edema showed a marked diuresis. Evans and Strang[61] obtained the same results. They did not, however, recognize the need for reinforcement at periods of low blood sugar. No cardiovascular lesion accompanied by congestive heart failure was considered by them a contraindication for dietary measures, even the severely restricted ones they employed. Evans and Strang have encountered no disasters as a result of this practice. On the contrary, prompt relief in the great majority of cases was obtained and, in the remainder, a marked relief limited in degree according to the grade of underlying permanent damage present.

Albuminuria and Cylindruria.—Albuminuria and cylindruria, even without congestive heart failure, are frequent findings in middle-aged and elderly obese patients. These findings are improved in every case, and in most are reduced to that to be expected at the patient's age if treatment is continued until a weight approximately normal is attained.

Glycosuria.—Glycosuria, high blood sugar values, and even diabetic-type glucose tolerance curves are encountered in some middle-aged obese persons. The patients, if neglected, may well become genuine diabetics. The estimated number of these, the results of reduction, and the possible significance are presented above (see section on Glucose Tolerance and Glycosuria). Glycosuria in an obese person is an urgent indication for reduction, and by diet alone. It is, if continued until a normal weight is attained, effective in correcting this abnormality in almost all patients.

Digestive Disorders.—One does not ordinarily think of digestive disorders in obese patients, but a surprising number have such disturbances. The symptoms are not mentioned frequently, but are sometimes admitted on direct questioning. More often attention is called to them by the observation of the patient after a short period of dieting that he no longer has dyspepsia. This improvement of digestion in many patients on the limited diets, compiled without regard to digestibility, indicates that the symptoms arose from mechanical features alone—from overloading the stomach. The relief from pain, eructation, and distention may be slight or absent in cases of cholecystitis and cholelithiasis, which frequently follow long periods of overeating and are common in the obese.

Dizziness and Headache.—Dizziness, an occasional complaint of the obese, rarely persists after relief of congestive heart failure and digestive disorders. Headaches are frequent complaints of the obese and occur without symptoms of circulatory or digestive strain. Complete disappearance of them with dieting may be expected with assurance after no more than two weeks' dieting, and occurs so regularly that, if the headache persists, some fundamental underlying cause must be sought.

Sleeplessness.—Most moderately obese persons do not think of themselves as poor sleepers. Indeed, many say they sleep quietly and lament that they have to sleep too much. Restlessness in sleep is a common complaint of the markedly obese. This probably comes from overloading the gastro-intestinal tract rather than from the mechanical handicap and discomfort of the fat. More restful sleep comes early in the period of dieting, too early to be the result of removal of the small amount of avoirdupois which has resulted in the short period. Nocturia in these patients, probably when associated with the restlessness rather than with a systemic disorder, is diminished appreciably. The improvement in nocturia in patients with glycosuria is explained on that basis.

Pains in Joints.—Pains in joints are frequent annoyances of the obese. Some relief can be promised to all patients if the pains are limited to the lumbosacral region, hips, knees, ankles, and arches. In many cases the discomfort results chiefly from the mechanical strain imposed by the added weight to be carried and, therefore, relief does not occur early in treatment. A gratifying number of patients will report complete relief of all joint symptoms of the lower extremities when the reducing diet has been continued long enough to accomplish a significant weight loss. Sometimes great relief results even when there is definite organic damage to the joint structures. Such joints seem to have sufficient functional capacity remaining to carry on a moderate amount of work without symptoms, but are unable to endure the overstrain imposed by the obesity.

Skin Disorders.—*Intertrigo* is very often a troublesome condition in the obese. Immediate local treatment is indicated. The tendency to recur will be found to be greatly diminished with the removal of the excess fat. Numerous other conditions such as *epidermophytosis, acne rosacea,* and *pityriasis* have been observed to yield promptly to dietary treatment of obesity. No direct relation between these conditions and obesity and their relief by its correction has been demonstrated. The benefit probably results from the improved general physical condition after correcting the improper eating habits.

Flabbiness of localized areas of skin after reduction in all but young patients is likely to persist. If an abdominal apron is large and annoying it can be removed surgically. Discomfort in the lipectomy scar if a panniculus begins to reappear has proved to be a salutary measure in a few patients for continued control of appetite. The appearance of wrinkles in the face and neck and a deepening of the nasolabial fold are to be expected in older patients and should be mentioned before dieting is begun. Although patients in the third decade of life are likely to look younger after reduction, those in the fourth and later decades may look older. This is discounted in some patients by an improved complexion, greater animation of expression, and a more youthful figure.

Hernias.—The effect of reduction in weight on hernias in the obese, especially when it is accomplished at a rapid rate, has been given much attention. The possibility was considered that removal of fat from the dilated inguinal or femoral canal might lead to unfortunate results. Just the opposite has been found to be the case. Many cases showed improvement of symptoms and decreased size of the sac. This suggests that the fat was a factor in the development of the dilatation and that correction of obesity in the early stages of weakening of the rings might prevent some hernias.

Varicose Veins.—The fear that varicose veins of the lower extremities might be made worse by removal of the support of the surrounding fat tissue has been shown to be groundless. Without exception, varicose veins in the legs of the obese improve with reduction in weight. Apparently subcutaneous fat, as is to be expected when one considers anatomical relations, affords no support for dilated veins. Rather it tends to obstruct the flow in all veins and thus influence adversely those already dilated.

Disturbances of Menstruation.—Various disturbances of menstruation occur with great frequency in obese young women. Pain and irregularity are the most common complaints. Accurate dieting for a period will alleviate the symptoms in most patients, and will relieve them completely in some. A few patients who have had no menstrual difficulties will develop irregularity for several months during the period of treatment but become regular again with adjustment to the new physiological status. Abnormalities of menstruation have been presented as evidence that the obesity was also a result of endocrine imbalance. The correction of menstrual disorders in the obese with dieting suggests rather that some endocrine troubles may be due to the ingestion of faulty metabolic mixtures at a physiologically impressionable period of the patient's life, such as puberty, and not that some metabolic dyscrasia is secondary to disturbed endocrine function. A striking case of improvement in menstrual function in response to diet is presented by the case of an unmarried woman, twenty-three years old. She weighed 150 pounds when eighteen years old. Menstruation began when she was fourteen years old and was normal for eight years until she was twenty-two. From eighteen until twenty-two years of age she gained 50 pounds, bringing her weight to 200 pounds. Menses then stopped. She presented herself for treatment a year later, weighing 259 pounds and not having menstruated for eleven months. Primary endocrine disturbance was suggested by a marked hypertrichosis of the upper lip, chest, forearms and legs, and a masculine distribution of the crines. This patient lost 86 pounds during twenty-eight weeks of dieting and in that period menstruated normally six times without discomfort.

Sterility.—A few women seek reduction in the hope that it will cure their sterility. Too many other causes may be, and usually are, operative to expect much from diet in this connection. Several young women after years of sterility and obesity have, after reduction, become pregnant and reported later with delight the birth of a full-term infant. One such patient thirty-one years old, referred by her obstetrician, had always been obese and had remained sterile through seven years of married life. She reduced from 187 pounds to 138¾ pounds, 48¼ pounds in twenty weeks. Twenty-one months after attaining normal weight she reported the completion of a normal pregnancy with the birth of a healthy son. One woman, unappealingly middle-aged at thirty-three years, when reduced from 168¾ pounds to 133¾ pounds was recreated as an attractive young woman. After two full-term pregnancies before becoming obese she had been sterile throughout four and one-half years of obesity. She reported that some of her friends blamed a miscarriage shortly after attaining a normal weight on dieting, of which they did not approve. The friends of some cured obese patients are inclined to credit or blame the dieting with anything that happens subsequently. One could not with this patient deny the suggested connection, at least insofar as the pregnancy was concerned.

Mental Attitude.—One of the most pleasing results of dieting by the obese, especially when diets of maximum possible limitation of calories are employed, is the improved mental attitude. No doubt this comes in part from the relief of symptoms. The general feeling of physical well-being is satisfying in every patient who can bring himself to continue with the dieting. Many report after a month or two of treatment that they had forgotten what it was to feel well. Some patients insist, however, that they are happy because of the discovery of their capacity for self-mastery, enabling them to give up the fun of eating, thus throwing off the shackles of their enslavement to gustatory sensualism. The happiness is most marked in young and adolescent girls, for many of whom their entire social attitude is materially changed for the better. This improved mental attitude is fortunate. Many persons instinctively respond to an obvious loss of weight in another as an evidence of serious disease, and with impulsive solicitude they tell the obese friend after cure that he "looks terrible" and inquire anxiously about the cause. The contentment of the patient in his accomplishment and condition should discount the distress of these contacts.

Permanence of Results.—Permanence of results after reduction in obesity is difficult to determine accurately. Relapses are, of course, relatively frequent. It seems, however, that the original weight rarely is fully regained. Many patients resume their reduction diets for short periods without medical supervision to correct slight weight increases. A number of patients report to the physician for reduction under guidance a second time. Most patients seem to have learned their lesson after correction of one relapse, and do not gain again, but there have been some who have reduced three times. A food addiction in some persons is too strong to resist. The colored patient mentioned on page 580, who reduced 220 pounds by diet alone, reported to the hospital some years later weighing 420 pounds, and with a cancer of the lung. Hypodermic administration of morphine given about noon one day a week before decease to control obvious pain elicited from her the request: "Doctor, can't you put that hypodermic off until after lunch?"

Removal of Menace.—The cure of the obese person, it is to be hoped, will eliminate the menace of obesity to continued good health and vigor mentioned above. No statistical study is available to show whether or not this is true. Immediate objective results in those not permanently damaged would indicate, however, that one can reasonably expect the cure of obesity to have removed its menace.

COOPERATION

The treatment of obesity is so prolonged that residence in hospital during the period is not feasible. It must be carried out by patients supervising their own diets at home. This demands a high degree of cooperation, which can be obtained from patients only if they are given an understanding of the nature and causes of obesity, of the metabolic principles concerned in its treatment, and of what constitutes proper eating. Few patients will continue to a successful conclusion if, without discussion, they are merely given a menu, or worse yet a long list of foodstuffs with articles to be eaten, or omitted, checked on it.

A correction of the attitude generally held toward *hunger* is probably the first point to be made. Most healthy persons during the middle decades who have a normal zest for the pleasant things of life must choose between being obese or hungry much of the time. It should be pointed out that to be hungry is a natural, wholesome state rather than a symptom to be treated, as soon as noticed, by an overabundant food intake. Patients must be told that eating should be interrupted far short of satiation instead of being continued beyond by the taking of desserts. Desserts are probably made tasty because if they were not so enticing no more would be eaten at that stage of the meal. Desserts have no place in the normal dietary. They should be reserved for a rare indulgence on holidays and birthdays, and for the celebration of other special occasions. Bread, and starches generally, readily oxidizable fuel foods, were the "staff of life" for the large energy expenditures of pioneers and those who labored before the machine age. The fuel value inseparably bound up in those foods which are necessary to supply the essential foodstuffs in adequate amounts so closely approaches the fuel needs of the body in these days of easy living that little is left for carbohydrates and sweets if an excess energy intake is avoided. Asceticism, necessary during treatment, is not desirable, and is not to be advised for prevention of obesity or after the cure is accomplished. It is necessary, however, to recognize enjoyment of gustatory delights as an indulgence. The attitude toward alcohol of those who do not abuse it, if applied to extra food will prevent the abuse of food also. One must not be a food drunk. Not many years ago the struggle for existence was so severe that a rotund figure was an evidence of health and prosperity, a spare one a social and business handicap. The age of machine-made plenty, when not only the most worthy but also the most inadequate can get not only enough but too much food, has changed this. The obese person now is not considered *per se* a successful member of the community. Rather he is looked at askance as one who has lived in a slovenly manner and who has not controlled his sensuality. All this must be pointed out to the patient.

Asceticism, so unfortunate in relation to many things of life, is essential in the successful treatment of obesity. Obese patients should be told that for relief they must give up gustatory sensualism for a time. Some obese patients are so uncomfortable or alarmed that they will carry through any measure which holds promise of relief. Some have few annoying symptoms, and an appreciable number are actually euphoric. It is necessary to point out to those in the last two classifications that there is no way other than rigid dieting by which they can be relieved. They must give up "the fun of eating." The contraindications for giving thyroid and the futility of an attempt at the excessive amount of exercise needed should be explained. These patients must be warned that their excess weight is an indication that gustatory delights form a great part of their enjoyment of life, and to give them up might make life too uninteresting to endure.

Occasionally it is wise to suggest that the grade of obesity is so severe that it indicates a food addiction too strong to resist, and to urge delay for further consideration of the sacrifice as explained. Some patients will withdraw and never return. Newburgh and Johnston have said of that type that "the combination of a weak will and a pleasure-seeking outlook on life, lays the background for the condition. The mental make-up of these people resembles that of the chronic alcoholics." Some patients return soon, or sometimes even a year later, prepared for the ordeal. Most protest that they are not sensualists in regard to food; that they merely did not know. And indeed this is true. Many people are not calorie conscious and eat carelessly. Often one sees a diner eat thoughtlessly and with little if any enjoyment, a roll and one or more portions of butter while waiting for the first course to be served. A few patients display scepticism born of repeated trials with ill-conceived diets which brought on, with weight reduction, depressing lassitude and weakness. It is easiest of all to obtain cooperation from these patients. They have a demonstrated capacity for accurate dieting. It is necessary to obtain from them only a promise of cooperation for two weeks or if they prefer, the much popularized period of eighteen days. By that time they will have discovered that they feel much better, not only than when dieting on earlier trials, but even than when not losing weight.

Many obese patients, because they sincerely believe that they are not large eaters, mention with hope and longing some gland trouble as the cause. No quarrel need arise on that score. It is possibly unwise at this time to discuss with the patient different unproved hypotheses of endocrine gland function in relation to appetite and fat deposition and distribution. It is better to refer to the law of conservation of energy and point out that the weight is made up of tangible material and that there is no gland with an aperture through which this material could have been introduced under the skin. The patient will agree that this material was not rubbed through the skin, did not enter through the eyes as views, nor through the ears as sound, and will admit it entered the body through one opening, the throat. It has been swallowed, so however little the patient may seem to be eating, if he is overweight he can be convinced that it is too much.

A simplified explanation of the nutritional principles involved in the contemplated treatment is usually understood by the patient and is much appreciated. Sometimes a hesitant patient is impelled toward cooperation by pointing out to her who weighs, for example, 190 pounds and should weigh 130, that she is made up of 130 pounds of her charming self and 60 pounds of dead inert fat. Fear of debility can often be removed by promising that it is the physician's great care in making up the menu to supply in adequate amounts all the known essential foodstuffs for the 130 pounds of the patient's true self. It may be difficult to convince the patient that this food will go where intended and not be diverted to making fat with the consequent deprivation of vital tissues. The firm conviction of the physician that this is true as shown by adequate experiments will go far toward giving the patient assurance on this point. Another fear, that of being unendurably hungry can be partly dissipated by the statement, which can be made with great assurance, that there will be little, certainly no more than normal hunger after the first two or three days, even with the limited diets of Evans and Strang presented above. One or two glasses of plain or charged water will remove temporarily the sensation of hunger in the dieting obese person, as it will for all others. Some gustatory sensualism will persist for a time in a few patients but they usually recognize, when it is pointed out to them, that this is "the memory of the fun of eating," not hunger, and take themselves in hand. No number of glasses of plain or charged water will effect this sensation.

The weight loss as water by obese patients with circulatory embarrassment who have carried through a dietary treatment accounts for a minimum per cent of the total. The nitrogen loss, when one gram of protein and two-thirds of a gram of carbohydrate per kilogram of ideal weight, is given, is negligible in amount. The total weight reduction in the patients in the two published series of Strang and Evans was 8286 pounds. When calculated as all fatty tissue this represents a collective dietary caloric deficit of thirty-three and one-half millions. Such a record of self-mastery is worthy of comment and proves that adequate cooperation even with the severely restricted diets they must employ, can be obtained from patients supervising their own diets at home.

BIBLIOGRAPHY

1. McLester, J. S., Nutrition and Diet in Health and Disease, W. B. Saunders, Phila., 3rd Ed., 1939, p. 434.
2. Strang, J. A., and Evans, F. A., J. Clin. Invest., **6:** 277, 1928.
3. Freyberg, R. H., and Newburgh, L. H., Arch. Int. Med., **58:** 229, 1936.
4. Cushing, H., Bull. Johns Hopkins Hosp., **50:** 137, 1932.
5. Dublin, L. I., and Lotka, A. J., Length of Life, The Ronald Press, New York, p. 200, 1936.
6. Dublin, L. I., Fisk, E. L., and Kopf, E. W., Am. J. Med. Sci., **170:** 576, 1925.
7. Preble, Wm. E., Boston Med. and Surg. J., **188:** 617, 1923.
8. American Women Getting Thinner, Statistical Bull. Metropolitan Life Ins. Co., **20:** 1, 1939.
9. Spencer, H. J., Med. Clin. No. Am., **12:** 604, 1928–29.
10. Ireland, M. W., Love, A. G., and Davenport, C. B., Defects Found in Drafted Men, Statistical Information, Gov. Printing Office, Washington, D. C., 1920.
11. Dublin, L. I., and Marks, H. H., Mortality of Women According to Build, The Asso. of Life Ins. Med. Directors of Am., Oct. 20, 1938.
12. Girth and Death, Statistical Bull. Metropolitan Life Ins. Co., **18:** 2, May, 1937.
13. Strang, J. M., McClugage, H. B., and Evans, F. A., Am. J. Med. Sci., **181:** 3, 336, 1931.
14. McClugage, H. B., Booth, Geo., and Evans, F. A., Am. J. Med. Sci., **181:** 3, 349, 1931.
15. Wilder, R. M., Arch. Int. Med., **61:** 297, 1938.
16. Strang, J. M., McClugage, H. B., and Brownlee, M. A., Arch. Int. Med., **55:** 958, 1935.
17. Strang, J. M., McClugage, H. B., and Evans, F. A., Am. J. Med. Sci., **179:** 687, 1930.
18. Wilder, R. M., Internat'l Clin., **1:** Series 42, 31, 1932.
19. Gurney, R., Arch. Int. Med., **57:** 557, 1936.
20. Hagedorn, H. C., Holten, C., Johansen, A. H., Arch. Int. Med., **40:** 30, 1927.
21. Mason, E. H., J. Clin. Invest., **4:** 93, 1927.
22. Strouse, S., and Dye, M., Arch. Int. Med., **34:** 267, 1924.
23. Wang, C. C., Strouse, S., and Saunders, A. D., Arch. Int. Med., **24:** 573, 1924.
24. Waldvogel, R., Deutsch. Arch. f. klin. Med., **89:** 342, 1907.
25. McKay, E. M., and Sherrill, J. W., Endocrinology, **21:** 677, 1937.
26. Folin, Otto, and Denis, W., J. Biol. Chem., **21:** 183, 1915.
27. Deuel, H. J., Jr., and Gulick, M., J. Biol. Chem., **96:** 25, 1932.
28. Hetenyi, G., Deutsch. Arch. f. klin. Med., **129:** 134, 1936.
29. Best, C. H., and Campbell, J., Am. J. Physiol., **86:** 190, 1936.
30. Best, C. H., Grant, R., and Ridant, J. H., Am. J. Physiol., **86:** 337, 1936.
31. Dragstedt, L. R., and collaborators, Arch. Int. Med., **64:** 1017, 1939.
32. Strang, J. M., McClugage, H. B., and Brownlee, M. A., Am. J. Med. Sci., **182:** 49, 1931.
33. Wells, H. G., J.A.M.A., **114:** 2177, 1940.
34. Denis, W., and Borgstrom, P., J. Biol. Chem., **61:** 109, 1924.
35. Beard, H. H., Am. J. Physiol., **82:** 577, 1927.
36. Lusk, G., Physiol. Rev., **1:** 523, 1921.
37. Folin, Otto, Am. J. Physiol., **13:** 66, 1905.
38. Shaffer, P. A., Am. J. Physiol., **23:** 1, 1908.
39. Tracy, M., and Clark, E. E., J. Biol. Chem., **19:** 115, 1914.
40. Hodgson, P., and Lewis, H. B., Am. J. Physiol., **87:** 288, 1928.
41. Meyers, V. C., and Fine, M. S., J. Biol. Chem., **14:** 9, 1913.
42. Palladin, A., Quoted by Hunter, A., in Ref. 43.
43. Hunter, A., Creatinine and Creatine, Longmans, Green and Co., New York, 1928.
44. Cathcart, E. P., and Benedict, F. G., Quoted by Hunter, A., Ref. 43.
45. Labbé, M., and Stévenin, H., Comptes rendus Soc. de biol., **88:** 9, 1923.
46. Lauter, S., Klin. Wchnschr., **5:** 1696, 1926.
47. Means, J. H., Arch. Int. Med., **17:** 704, 1916.
48. Strouse, S., and Wang, C. C., Arch. Int. Med., **34:** 275, 1924.
49. DuBois, E. F.: Basal Metabolism in Health and Disease, Lea and Febiger, Philadelphia, 1927.
50. Harris, J. A., and Benedict, F. G., J. Biol. Chem., **46:** 257, 1921.
51. Benedict, F. G., and Carpenter, T. M., Carnegie Inst. of Washington, Pub. No. 261, p. 1, 1918.

52. Lauter, S., Deutsch. Arch. f. klin. Med., **150:** 315, 1926.
53. Bernhardt, H., Ergebn. d. inn. Med. u. Kinderh., **36:** 1, 1929.
54. Hawk, P. B., Rehfuss, M. E., and Bergeim, O., Am. J. Med. Sci., **171:** 359, 1926.
55. Kraus, E., and Rettig, R., Deutsch. Arch. f. klin. Med., **163:** 337, 1929.
56. Gibbons, R., Am. J. Physiol., **70:** 26, 1924.
57. Aub, J. C., and DuBois, E. F., Arch. Int. Med., **19:** 840, 1917.
58. Bazett, H. C., Physiol. Rev., **7:** 531, 1927.
59. Booth, Geo., and Strang, J. M., Arch. Int. Med., **57:** 533, 1936.
60. Benedict, F. G., Leopoldina, **4:** 129, 1929.
61. Evans, F. A., and Strang, J. M., Am. J. Med. Sci., **177:** 339, 1929.
62. Newburgh, L. H., and Johnston, M. W., J. Clin. Invest., **8:** 197, 1930.
63. Benedict, F. G., and Root, H. F., Arch. Int. Med., **38:** 1, 1926.
64. Johnston, M. W., and Newburgh, L. H., J. Clin. Invest., **8:** 147, 1930.
65. Shaffer, P. A., J. Biol. Chem., **47, 49:** 433, 449, 143, 1921.
66. Woodyatt, R. F., Trans. Asso. Am. Phys., **36:** 269, 1921.
67. Hubbard, R. S., and Wright, F. R., J. Biol. Chem., **61:** 377, 1924.
68. Wilder, R. M., Boothby, W. M., and Beeler, C., J. Biol. Chem., **5:** 311, 1922.
69. Wilder, R. M., Browne, H. C., and Butt, H. R., Arch. Int. Med., **65:** 399, 1940.
70. Stadie, Wm. C., Trans. Asso. Am. Phys., p. 247, 1940. Published in J. Clin. Invest., **19:** 843, 1940.
71. Hubbard, R. S., J. Biol. Chem., **55:** 357, 1923.
72. Beeler, C., and Fitz, R., Arch. Int. Med., **28:** 804, 1921.
73. Paullin, J. E., and Sauls, H. C., South. Med. J., **15:** 249, 1922.
74. John, H. J., Endocrinology, **13:** 388, 1929.
75. Newburgh, L. H., and Conn, J. W., J.A.M.A., **112:** 7, 1939.
76. Ogilvie, R. F., Quart. J. Med., **28:** 345, 1935.
77. Cuttings, W. C., Mehrtens, H. G., and Tainter, M. L., J.A.M.A., **101:** 193, July 15, 1933.
78. Strang, J. M., and Evans, F. A., J.A.M.A., **104:** 1957, 1935.
79. Braun, I., Med. Record, **151:** 131, 1940.
80. Lessees, M. F., and Meyerson, A., New Eng. Med. J., **218:** 119, 1938.
81. Friedenberg, S., J.A.M.A., **114:** 956, 1940.
82. Gordon, B., and Nissler, C. W., Med. Clin. of No. Amer., **12:** 1167, 1929.
83. Harrop, Geo. A., J.A.M.A., **102:** 2003, 1934.
84. Preble, Wm. E., Boston Med. and Surg. J., **172:** 740, 1915.
85. Evans, F. A., Internat'l Clin., **3:** Series 48, p. 19, 1938.
86. Short, J. J., J.A.M.A., **111:** 2196, 1938.
87. Robinson, S. C., Brucer, M., and Mass, John, J. Lab. and Clin. Med., **25:** 807, 1940.

CHAPTER XI

XANTHOMATOSES, GLYCOGEN DISEASE, AND DISTURBANCES OF INTERMEDIARY METABOLISM

By Edward Mason

XANTHOMATOSES (LIPOIDOSES)

Classification.—The most satisfactory classification of these disturbances of lipid metabolism is based upon the type of lipid concerned, thus:

1. Gaucher's disease—the lipid is kerasin.
2. Niemann-Pick's disease—the lipid is phosphatide.
3. Generalized xanthomas (Schüller-Christian syndrome)—the lipid is mainly cholesterol and cholesterol esters.
4. Localized (cutaneous and visceral) xanthomas, which are both primary and secondary.

Characteristic of the syndromes of these conditions is an excess storage of the respective lipid in large cells of the reticulo-endothelial system. These cells may phagocytose the lipid from the blood stream or they may synthesize it; which process occurs is not known. The xanthomatoses, being diseases of childhood, are probably congenital errors of metabolism.

Gaucher's Disease.—*Definition.*—Gaucher's disease is a rare disease of childhood characterized by enlargement of the spleen due to excess storage of kerasin in large cells of the reticulo-endothelial system (Gaucher cells). The liver, lungs, and skeleton also show infiltrations of Gaucher cells.

Etiology.—Despite its general rarity Gaucher's disease is the commonest of the primary lipoidoses. It is essentially a constitutional abnormality with a strong family tendency. Though present during infancy it may not be recognized until childhood is reached.

Pathologic Anatomy.—The outstanding gross feature is the enlarged spleen with its smooth or granular surface. The cut surface shows an irregular yellow network which is due to foci of Gaucher cells filled with the cerebroside, kerasin. The liver is enlarged, cirrhotic and infiltrated with Gaucher cells. Similar infiltrations may involve the bone marrow, the lymph glands, and the skeleton. The last mentioned may lead to patchy osteoporosis and pathological fractures. Pigmentation of the skin occurs and is due to deposits of hemosiderin. Hemorrhages are common.

Symptoms.—The onset is insidious. Enlargement of the abdomen, with pain in the left upper quadrant, may be first observed. The spleen, the edge of which is firm, becomes tremendously enlarged. The liver is usually palpable. There is a tendency to secondary anemia and leukopenia. The skin, in long-standing cases, is pigmented with hemosiderin. The blood cholesterol concentration is not raised. Notwithstanding the associated cirrhosis of the liver, ascites is not usual.

Niemann-Pick's Disease.—*Etiology.*—This congenital abnormality is highly familial, and occurs mainly in the Hebrew race. It is six times more common in the female than in the male. It is closely related to the infantile type of amaurotic idiocy known as Tay-Sachs disease.

Pathologic Anatomy.—The enlargement of the liver and spleen is moderate and ascites is usual. The liver is yellowish and cirrhotic. Infiltration of the whole splenic pulp with "foam" cells containing the lipid phosphatide gives a yellowish color to the cut surface. The cytoplasm stains with the Sudan III dye. A similar infiltration of the liver and lymph nodes is present. Histologic changes in the brain may be very similar to those found in infantile amaurotic idiocy. The phosphatide content of the involved organs is high.

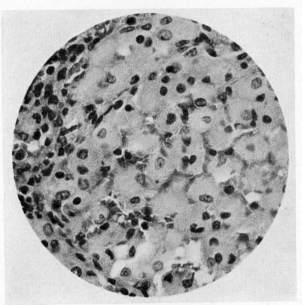

Fig. 96.—Microphotograph (high power) of the spleen in a case of Gaucher's disease. Note the infiltrations of the splenic pulp with large cells with eccentric, deeply staining nuclei, so-called Gaucher cells. These cells are filled with the lipid kerasin.

Clinical Manifestations.—The failure to grow in infancy or childhood may cause concern. The abdomen is enlarged, there is ascites, and the liver and spleen are palpable. The blood shows a moderate secondary anemia with a leukocytosis (15,000). The blood cholesterol level is raised. Mental sluggishness and retardation may be associated with either hypotonicity or spasticity. Involvement of the bones may lead to osteoporosis as seen by roentgen-ray examination. The findings on roentgen-ray examination of the lungs have been reported to simulate those found in miliary tuberculosis.

The course of the disease is rapid, ending fatally in infancy. There is no known effective treatment.

Generalized Xanthomas (Schüller-Christian Syndrome).—*Definition.*—Another rare disturbance of lipid metabolism is that which is characterized by deposition of xanthomatous material in the flat bones of the skeleton and is associated with exophthalmos, diabetes insipidus, and retardation of growth. The lipid material comprises cholesterol and cholesterol esters deposited in the typical "foam cells." The syndrome is that of a systemic xanthomatosis.

Etiology.—The onset occurs in early childhood. There is no racial or familial tendency. The syndrome may follow infection or trauma. The

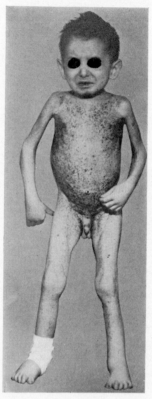

Fig. 97.—Photograph of a boy with Schüller-Christian syndrome. Note the large number of cutaneous lesions, some of which are hemorrhagic. (From Horsfall and Smith, Quart. Jour. Med., Jan., 1935.)

xanthomatous material is frequently deposited at the site of a previous trauma.

Pathologic Anatomy.—Prominent among the evidences of this syndrome are the xanthomatous deposits in the membranous bones of the skull. These deposits occur in a patchy distribution and tend to involve the base of the skull. Pressure upon or invasion of the hypothalamic hypophyseal area by xanthomatous deposits produces diabetes insipidus, and involvement of the orbit results in the exophthalmos, which may be unilateral. The vertebrae, pelvis, and other bones of the skeleton may be involved. More rarely the skin, liver, and spleen contain xanthomatous infiltrations. The characteristic cell of the infiltrations is the "foam cell," a storage cell with multiple nuclei derived from the reticulo-endothelial system and filled with cholesterol and cholesterol esters. As the disorder progresses there is a marked tendency for the xanthomatous areas to undergo fibrosis with cyst formation.

Clinical Manifestations.—The classical triad consists of: (1) defects in membranous bones, (2) diabetes insipidus, and (3) exophthalmos. Roentgen-ray examinations show distinctly the irregular areas of decalcification that affect both bony tables of the skull. A search of the skeleton will find other bones involved, especially those of the spine and pelvis. The osteoporosis may result in pathologic fractures.

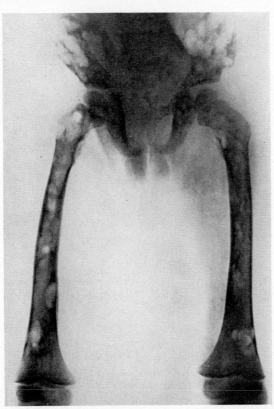

Fig. 98.—*x*-Rays of pelvis and femurs of same case as Fig. 97. The irregular bony defects due to lipid infiltrations are very numerous. (From Horsfall and Smith, Quart. Jour. Med., Jan., 1935.)

Retarded growth and muscular wasting are usual in this disease. Xanthomas may occur in the skin and the liver. The spleen and lymph glands may be enlarged. Severe anemia is usual in this disease. The cholesterol level in the blood is raised in about 50 per cent of the cases—a level of 1000 mg. per 100 cc. has been reported. A thrombocytopenia may be present, in which case hemorrhages are prone to occur.

The progress of the disease is slow, extending over a period of years unless death occurs as the result of an intercurrent infection.

Diagnosis.—Given the triad, defects in membranous bones, exophthalmos, and diabetes insipidus, the diagnosis is easily made. Confusion with multiple myelomata might occur but roentgenographic differentiation of them is not difficult. A biopsy of the xanthomatous material makes the diagnosis certain.

Treatment.—A diet with a low fat content will reduce the hypercholesterolemia, and deep roentgenotherapy will sometimes cause sufficient shrinkage of xanthomatous infiltrations to ameliorate the symptoms.

Localized Xanthomas.—*Definition.*—Localized xanthomas involving the skin and viscera in contradistinction to a generalized distribution are the characteristic feature. Xanthomas may be primary or secondary. As in the Schüller-Christian syndrome, the "foam cells" of the reticulo-endothelial system contain large amounts of cholesterol and cholesterol esters.

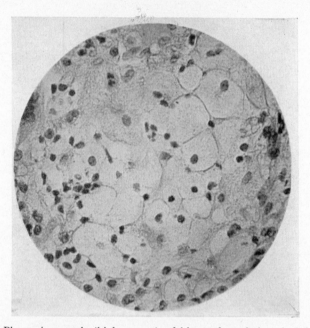

Fig. 99.—Photomicrograph (high power) of biopsy from lesions in left humerus of same case as Figs. 97 and 98. Note the large "foam cells" with clear cytoplasm filled with lipid (cholesterol and cholesterol esters). (From Horsfall and Smith, Quart. Jour. Med., Jan., 1935.)

Pathologic Anatomy.—Xanthomas are not true tumors, as they increase in size by addition of cells, not by cell division. The contained lipid gives them their yellowish color. Their histologic appearance is fundamentally the same as in Schüller-Christian syndrome already described. With healing they undergo fibrosis and scar formation.

Clinical Picture.—*Primary* xanthomas may invade the skin only or the viscera as well. Their involvement of the skin is especially characteristic; here they appear as small yellowish tubercles with predilection for the extensor surfaces, and termed *xanthoma tuberosum.* Similarly xanthoma tubercles may invade the vascular system, larynx, lungs, tendons, and synovial membranes. When the gall bladder is the site of xanthomatosis, it is known as the "strawberry" gall bladder. Complete obstruction of the common bile duct by xanthomas has been reported. Angina pectoris may follow involvement of the coronary arteries. The blood may or may not show an increased cholesterol content. As a rule, primary xanthomas are benign, but sometimes due to their location they may cause death.

Secondary xanthomas occur in the presence of other diseases where there is a disturbance of cholesterol metabolism. Xanthomas involving the skin of diabetic patients even in the pre-insulin days were uncommon. The tubercles of xanthoma diabeticorum are especially numerous upon the extensor surfaces and in some cases they involve the whole trunk. Their presence indicates poor control of the diabetes as shown by hyperglycemia, lipemia, and marked hypercholesterolemia. With control of the diabetes the

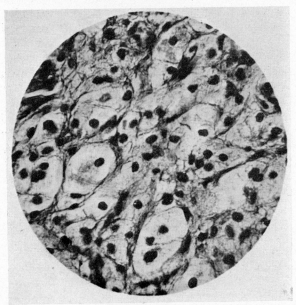

Fig. 100.—Photomicrograph (high power) of a biopsy of a skin xanthoma in a case of diabetes mellitus. Note the "foam cells" with multiple nuclei filled with the specific lipid.

yellowish tubercles disappear. In some cases whitish patches of scar tissue are left in the skin, but more often no evidence of the disorder remains. A less extensive xanthoma involvement of the skin is seen in obstructive jaundice, myxedema, hypertension, and nephrosis—all conditions associated with hypercholesterolemia.

GLYCOGEN DISEASE

Definition.—Glycogen disease is a rare congenital disorder of metabolism characterized by marked hepatomegaly due to glycogen stored within the liver cells. Other organs, especially the heart and the kidneys, may show similar excess glycogen storage. von Gierke[1] in 1929 described the first two cases of glycogen disease.

Biochemical Considerations.—The glycogen stored in the cells of the liver, heart, and kidneys, has not been shown to be abnormal chemically, but it possesses great stability, and the process of glycogenolysis with the maintenance of the normal blood sugar level is carried out with the greatest difficulty. Even after death from an acute febrile illness the glycogen largely persists in the liver.

Various hypotheses have been advanced as to the nature of the fundamental disturbance but little exact knowledge is available. It has been suggested that (1) the glycogen is abnormally stable due to chemical structure, (2) the glycogen is linked to protein making it immobile, and (3) glycogenolysis is defective due to lack of liver amylase. Experiments conducted by Schönheimer with autopsy material from one of von Gierke's cases, showed that the glycogen from the liver and kidney was rapidly broken down when mixed with normal liver. He concluded that there was a lack of liver amylase. In many respects the tissue glycogen in this disease reacts in a similar way to fetal glycogen that cannot be mobilized in the cold or by epinephrine. This suggests the persistence of a fetal state, glyconeogenesis being more easily carried out than glycogenolysis.

As a result of the immobility of the liver glycogen the systemic blood sugar borders on the level of hypoglycemia (60 mg. per 100 cc. or less) but hypoglycemic symptoms and convulsions are unusual even following exercise. After subcutaneous injection of 5 minims of 1:1000 solution of epinephrine there is very little or no increase in the blood sugar level. A glucose time curve shows a moderate delay in glycogen storage and a retarded return to a mild hypoglycemic level. There is a tendency toward acetonuria owing to incomplete fat oxidation. Prolonged mild hypoglycemia leads to slow tissue starvation and secondary retardation of growth.

Pathologic Anatomy.—From autopsy material available in some twenty-one cases, it has been determined that death usually follows from an intercurrent infection. The liver is greatly enlarged, smooth, and brownish in color. It may extend to the pelvis. In the case of a child of eight it weighed 2000 gm. (three times the normal). The spleen has not been found to be enlarged. The kidneys in some cases have been twice the normal size.

Quantitative analysis of the liver and kidney glycogen in one of von Gierke's cases gave 33.7 and 36.8 per cent dry weight respectively. The liver cells are tremendously distended with glycogen and the organ shows no cirrhosis. Heart muscle fibers may be similarly filled with glycogen. The glycogen in the kidneys is deposited in the tubular cells. No consistent abnormality of the endocrine system has been found, although one of von Gierke's patients had atrophic adrenal glands.

Clinical Manifestations.—Glycogen disease is usually diagnosed in childhood and it may be present at birth. Up to 1939, fifty-nine certain cases have been reported. A family history is important, as the disease has been reported in two brothers (Kimmelstiel) and in two sisters (Ellis), and Ellis has stated that the disease may be inherited as a mendelian recessive character.

The patient seeks medical help because of enlargement of the abdomen, the delayed growth, or because of hypoglycemic symptoms (rare). The liver is grossly enlarged, smooth, and firm. The spleen is not enlarged. There are no evidences of obstruction of the portal system. Growth and secondary sex characteristics may be delayed two to four years. These findings in an obese child and supported by the biochemical findings of a low fasting blood sugar level, acetonuria, and a raised blood cholesterol level (up to 400 mg. per cent) are suggestive. The epinephrine test fails to show the usual rise in the blood sugar level and the glucose time curve is abnormal. The blood glycogen concentration is raised. Examination of the blood microscopically is not especially helpful. A moderate leukocytosis is sometimes present. The basal metabolic rate is of no diagnostic value in this disease.

Differential Diagnosis.—Two conditions causing marked hepatomegaly have similar features, (1) hypertrophic steatosis and (2) hepatomegaly in diabetic children. In hypertrophic steatosis the liver is distended with fat

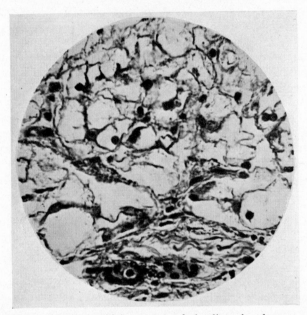

Fig. 101.—Photomicrograph (high power) of the liver in glycogen disease. Note the great distention of the liver cells with glycogen which has been removed in the process of preparation.

and there may be a low fasting blood sugar with moderate acetonuria. Hepatomegaly in diabetic children is probably due to excess fat storage and has occurred especially in those children receiving diets containing large amounts of fat. The findings of glycosuria and hyperglycemia are helpful in making a diagnosis.

Prognosis.—The prognosis is fairly good but there is a marked tendency for retardation of the skeletal growth and sex differentiation. Resistance to infections is definitely lowered. Sudden death may occur from severe hypoglycemia or from cardiac failure. The usual cause of death is from secondary infection.

Treatment.—There is no known treatment of permanent value. A diet rich in carbohydrates controls the hypoglycemic tendencies, and one poor in fats decreases the acetonuria. Thyroid therapy, preparations of the anterior lobe of the pituitary gland, and gonadotropic hormones have been tried without success. It is suggested that the more active suitable hormones of the pituitary gland, given hypodermically, be given a trial.

DISTURBANCES OF INTERMEDIARY METABOLISM

Alkaptonuria.—*Definition.*—Alkaptonuria is a rare disease referable to an inborn error of protein metabolism, resulting in the excretion of homogentisic acid in the urine. Our present knowledge would indicate that the two amino acids tyrosine and phenylalanine are the sources of the excreted homogentisic acid. The error in metabolism is usually complete and maximal, the amount of excreted homogentisic acid bearing a definite ratio to the total nitrogen in the urine.

Etiology.—The nature of the disturbance in the intermediary protein metabolism is still obscure, but a few observations have been reported which may lead the way to a clearer understanding of the anomaly. Gibson and Howard showed that the intramuscular injection of liver extract would free the urine of homogentisic acid for from eight to ten hours. Alkaptonuria has been produced in white rats and guinea pigs by feeding them phenylalanine and tyrosine. In the case of guinea pigs the alkaptone produced by *l*-tyrosine feeding was completely abolished by large doses of ascorbic acid. The alkaptone produced by *d*-tyrosine in guinea pigs was not so marked and the inhibiting influence of vitamin C was not so great. Using *l*-tyrosine, significant amounts of homogentisic acid have been produced in two normal humans, and with large dosage of crystalline vitamin C its excretion ceased.

Clinical Manifestations.—The clinical manifestations of alkaptonuria were described by Marcet (1823), but the nature of the reducing substance in the urine was recognized in 1887 by Marshall. It is a harmless anomaly, more frequent in the male than in the female, and usually congenital in origin. First cousin marriages have been a factor in yielding alkaptonuric offspring, as is well shown by Garrod's eleven cases in four families, where all parents were first cousins. However, many cases have now been reported where no congenital basis could be found. In 1929 Bagnal in a search of the world's literature found 126 cases, 17 having been reported from North America.

Symptoms and Diagnosis.—The patient with alkaptonuria has no subjective symptoms and the diagnosis is usually made in early life from the dark stains upon diapers or linen. Such urine, upon standing and becoming alkaline, gradually turns brown to black in color with oxidation of the homogentisic acid. *Homogentisic acid* reduces the alkaline copper solutions (Benedict's and Fehling's) and may thus, by being mistaken for glycosuria, lead to an error in diagnosis. It does not reduce an alkaline bismuth solution (Nylander's reagent). With the addition of 10 per cent sodium hydroxide solution to urine containing homogentisic acid a black precipitate is formed. Homogentisic acid does not ferment with yeast; it does not rotate polarized light, but with the addition of a dilute ferric chloride solution a transitory deep blue color appears until oxidation is complete.

In rare instances the cartilages of these patients turn black. This discoloration is most evident in the pinna of the ear. The blood may show a nonspecific fixation of complement, hence the results of the Wassermann test must be judged very critically in alkaptonuria.

Treatment.—Treatment may be directed to decreasing the output of homogentisic acid by decreasing the protein intake. High carbohydrate feeding will also decrease protein catabolism. The experimental observation that vitamin C in large dosage by mouth will decrease homogentisic acid excretion in man may lead to an improved method of therapy.

Ochronosis.—*Definition.*—Ochronosis is the name applied to the clinical state in which there is a varying degree of darkening of the cartilages, the ligaments, and the fibrous structures of the body. It is not a specific entity in that the discoloration has more than one cause.

Incidence.—To date about sixty cases of this pigmentary disorder have been published. It is more common in men than in women, and the pigmentation tends to become more marked with advancing years.

Pathologic Anatomy.—The characteristic anatomic evidence of ochronosis is the pigmentation of the cartilages of the ears, nose, ribs, and in later life of the intervertebral disks. The tendons of the hands and feet may be involved. The pigment is usually intracellular, and may be so extreme that the cartilaginous structures are coal black. In its chronic course there is a tendency for premature systemic arteriosclerosis to develop, and the involved cartilages show degenerative changes, osteoarthritic outgrowths and ultimately arthropathies with deformities.

Etiology.—The reported cases fall into the three groups: 1. A group that includes the majority of the cases and is characterized by the presence of alkaptonuria. This anomaly of protein catabolism is only occasionally associated with ochronosis. 2. Cases in which the tissue staining is due to the prolonged use of carbolic acid preparations, usually in the course of treatment of a chronic ulcer. 3. Cases in which there is an associated melanuria. The melanin that discolors the tissues is a derivative of the protein molecule.

Symptoms and Diagnosis.—In its early stages ochronosis causes no symptoms. As cartilage destruction and osteoarthritis occur, symptoms characteristic of the joint involvement are present. The discoloration of the cartilages, especially those of the ear and the nose, is of great diagnostic aid. Transmitted light is helpful in depicting the contrast in color. Examination of the urine will reveal the homogentisic acid if present (see *alkaptonuria* for special tests). A history of prolonged use of carbolic acid is suggestive. A biopsy of the skin for staining of the melanin pigment is sometimes helpful in establishing the diagnosis.

Treatment.—When ochronosis is associated with alkaptonuria treatment is usually of little avail. However, the use of large doses of vitamin C may help in arresting the discoloring process. When the condition is caused by carbolic acid therapy this drug must be discontinued. In the rare type associated with melanuria no helpful treatment is known.

Porphyria.—*Biochemical Considerations.*—Porphyrins are pigments which occur throughout the plant and animal worlds. In the plant world actioporphyrin is the pigment basis of chlorophyll. The porphyrin of blood pigment is protoporphyrin. Porphyrins can form compounds with metals.

Protoporphyrin combined with iron and globin is the basis of hemoglobin, the blood pigment of vertebrate life.

All porphyrins have a common chemical structure, namely four pyrrole rings bound by four additional carbon atoms. There are two porphyrins that are the most important in cases of porphyria, coproporphyrin which occurs in normal feces, and uroporphyrin which is found in small quantities in normal urine. These two porphyrins as they normally occur in excreta are probably derived from plant and animal tissues taken as food. Under unknown circumstances uroporphyrin and coproporphyrin are produced in excess and excreted in the urine and feces. It is thought that their over-production is a matter of reversion to an embryonic type of pigment metabolism, as the embryo's red cells contain uroporphyrin as well as hemoglobin. There is no satisfactory evidence that these porphyrins are derived from the breakdown of hemoglobin.

Tests for Porphyrins.—Uroporphyrin and coproporphyrin, and in a few cases Waldenström's porphyrin, are the commonest urinary porphyrins. Their concentration in normal urine is insufficient to affect its color and to produce absorption bands. When they occur in pathologic amounts the urine may vary from red to almost black. Coproporphyrin may be present as a colorless chromogen, porphyrinogen, which with sunlight is changed to coproporphyrin. This color change can be accelerated by an oxidizing agent such as potassium permanganate.

In addition to the color of the urine the spectroscopic bands are of specific diagnostic value, namely the four characteristic absorption bands for the alkaline porphyrin. Another diagnostic test of value is the exposure of urine to filtered ultraviolet rays. A pink fluorescence develops if porphyrins are present.

Classification.—Cases of porphyria may be best classified as (1) congenital, (2) acute, and (3) chronic.

1. CONGENITAL.—Congenital porphyria was first described by Günther (1911). This is a rare inborn error of metabolism and is probably present at birth and continues throughout life. It may be due to a persistence of a fetal pyrrole metabolism, and it is inherited as a recessive mendelian characteristic. It is characterized by (1) the excretion of large amounts of urinary porphyrin, (2) discoloration of the teeth and bones by uroporphyrin, and (3) sensitivity of the skin to light.

2. ACUTE.—Acute porphyria is almost a clinical and metabolic entity. The disease is more common in women than in men. It may be familial and has been observed in three generations. It is inherited as a mendelian dominant characteristic. The attack is associated with the urinary excretion of large amounts of porphyrin, and is characterized by abdominal, nervous, and mental symptoms. There is no light sensitivity. The mortality is high.

3. CHRONIC.—The chronic cases run a prolonged course and fail to fall into the two previous groups. They show a heavy urinary excretion of porphyrin and frequently light sensitivity. Intestinal tract symptoms may predominate. They may follow the prolonged administration of the barbituric acid compounds.

Symptoms.—1. CONGENITAL.—The main clinical features are (1) the color of the urine, (2) the pigmentation of the teeth and the bones, and

(3) the sensitivity of the skin to light. The urine varies from a pink to red or black color. It sometimes darkens after exposure to light (photo-oxidation), and the porphyrins present are copro- and uroporphyrin. The pigmentation of the enamel of the teeth varies from brown to pink, and in a case studied by Garrod the milk teeth upon eruption at nine months were stained pink. The bones of the hand may develop a brown pigmentation sufficiently deep to be visible upon transillumination. The sensitivity of the skin to ultraviolet light is the cause of the skin lesions. It is known that the different porphyrins vary in their photosensitizing action. In the congenital type there is probably a tendency for deposition of the porphyrins in the skin early because skin sensitivity is usually evident in childhood. The skin eruptions vary from simple erythema to vesicle formation and large bullae filled with a colorless or blood-stained fluid. The hands, neck, and face are usually affected. With healing permanent scars develop, and there is a tendency for brownish pigmentation of the skin in protracted cases. Other features are hirsutism, and in later life enlargement of the spleen and liver.

2. Acute.—Acute porphyria is characterized by (1) acute colicky pain in the lower abdomen, (2) neuritic pains radiating from the lower abdomen, and (3) the voiding of red urine. The abdominal pain is largely confined to the lower abdomen, is colicky in character, and has been mistaken for gall stone colic. Laparotomy showed vigorous intestinal peristalsis only. The neuritic pains tend to shoot down the legs, may be associated with foot-drop and wrist-drop and go on to a symmetrical progressive ascending paralysis with death from respiratory failure. The urine may be red upon voiding or become red after exposure to light. Its porphyrin content is especially high during the acute attack, and is a mixture of copro- and uroporphyrin. Light sensitivity is not present in acute porphyria. Varied types of psychic disturbance have been seen.

Mortality is high in acute porphyria. In patients who recover the porphyrin disappears from the urine in three to four weeks.

3. Chronic.—The chronic forms of the disease run a protracted course and may have acute exacerbations. Gastro-intestinal symptoms such as cramps, vomiting and constipation occur. Light sensitivity is usual. The urine is dark in color from an increased porphyrin excretion.

The chronic forms may follow the prolonged use of such drugs as sulfonal, trional, and possibly veronal, even in ordinary dosage. Nervous depression is often present.

Recovery is usually slow but the disorder may prove fatal.

Pathologic Anatomy.—In acute porphyria with severe ascending paralysis the nerves lose their myelin sheaths and the anterior horn cells in the cord show marked degenerative changes.

Treatment.—The cause of this disorder is unknown and there is no specific treatment of value. In the congenital type exposure to sunlight should be avoided. Skin lesions should be protected from secondary infection. Liver extract and large doses of vitamin C (ascorbic acid) have been reported to decrease the porphyrin excretion.

The manifestations of acute porphyria may be improved by the intravenous administration of calcium. In the chronic cases barbiturate drugs should be discontinued and supportive treatment carried out.

Cystinuria.—*Definition.*—Since Medes (1936) has shown that the amino-acid cystine occurs in small amounts in the urine of normal individuals, cystinuria as a disease entity should be confined to an excessive excretion of cystine in the urine.

Chemical Pathology.—The sulfur-containing amino-acid, cystine, is normally broken down into urea and inorganic sulfates. It occurs in its greatest concentration in the keratin-containing tissues such as hair and nails. Apparently the cystinuric patient is able to metabolize cystine when taken by mouth because only an excessive dose will cause an increased excretion in the urine. Under these circumstances the cystine is changed to inorganic sulfur. This observation would suggest that the cystinuric subject possesses the ability to break down cystine and that the cystinuria is dependent upon some other error of intermediary metabolism. It has been suggested that there is a break in the endogenous protein catabolism or that there might be a lowered threshold for cystine excretion in the kidney. Our present knowledge indicates that the parent substance of urinary cystine in the protein molecule is methionine.

Etiology.—Cystinuria affects both sexes and occurs at all ages. There is undoubtedly a congenital tendency which follows a recessive mendelian characteristic. It has been reported in three generations of a family. The most remarkable story of a cystinuric family has been told by Thin. It concerns two half-brothers; the elder, not a cystinuric, had twelve children of whom seven had cystinuria. The younger half-brother had ten children none of whom had cystinuria. Three of the younger brother's children married the older brother's children. Two of the latter had cystinuria. Two of the children of these three marriages had cystinuria and in one case both parents were not affected.

Symptoms and Diagnosis.—Simple cystinuria causes no symptoms. The urine shows the typical hexagonal plates, which are almost colorless. If the crystals are difficult to find the urine should be acidified with acetic acid and allowed to stand for a few hours. One may also dissolve the centrifuged sediment in ammonia and allow it to evaporate upon a glass slide. The crystals will precipitate out.

As a rule cystinuria is not diagnosed until calculi have formed in the genito-urinary tract. Cystine lithiasis is a disease of the young, and occurs in almost 2 per cent of cystinuric patients. Infection and stasis predispose to stone formation. The stones are frequently multiple and bilateral, cast x-ray shadows, and after removal tend to recur. Sharp colicky pain, hematuria, and albuminuria occur. The urine is acid and of a high specific gravity. If infection is present the risk of calculus pyonephrosis is great.

Treatment.—No known therapy will alter the inborn error of metabolism. A low protein diet, liberal fluid intake and the maintenance of a neutral urine by administering orally adequate amounts of soda bicarbonate, may prevent the formation of stones. Lavage of the renal pelvis with alkali has been reported to cause the disappearance of a cystine calculus, but surgical removal is usually required. Following removal of the calculus alkalinization of the urine is necessary to prevent recurrence.

Phosphaturia.—*Definition.*—Physiologically a normal person excretes 1 to 3 grams of phosphoric acid as an alkaline (Na, K) or earthy (Ca, Mg) salt in the urine each day. When this excretion is excessive or the phosphates are precipitated in the genito-urinary tract this condition is termed phosphaturia.

Biochemical Considerations.—Urinary phosphorus occurs in the main as an inorganic salt (95 to 99 per cent). The sodium and potassium phosphates are soluble in both acid and alkaline urine, while the calcium and magnesium salts are insoluble in alkaline urine. Therefore the phosphate deposit in phosphaturia depends upon the calcium and magnesium phosphates present.

Etiology.—The cause of phosphaturia may be due to (1) excess administration of an alkaline drug such as sodium bicarbonate, (2) excess ingestion of fruits and vegetables which have an alkaline ash, (3) infection of the genito-urinary tract by bacteria that convert urea into ammonium

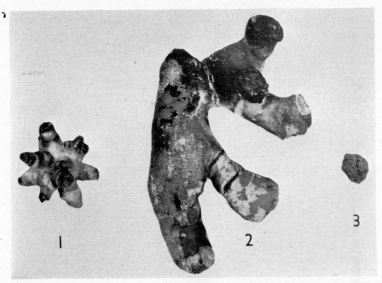

Fig. 102.—Photograph of urinary calculi: No. 1. Calcium oxalate calculus from the urinary bladder. Note "Jack-stone" shape. No. 2. Phosphate calculus from the pelvis of the kidney. No. 3. Calcium oxalate calculus from the pelvis of the kidney, "mulberry" type.

carbonate with the aid of the enzyme urease, and (4) in certain diseases affecting the bones, such as osteomalacia, rickets, and hyperparathyroidism, where there is an increased excretion of calcium.

Symptoms.—Other than a slight burning on micturition, the symptoms are related to the presence of calculi when present.

Diagnosis.—The turbidity of the urine due to phosphates occurs only in a neutral or alkaline medium. To be of significance the deposit must be heavy and occur in freshly voided alkaline urine. The phosphate cloud that appears upon heating clear urine is physiological and its disappearance with dilute acetic acid differentiates it from protein (albumin).

The history may reveal an excessive intake of alkali or an alkaline ash diet. Infection of the genito-urinary tract (cystitis, pyelitis) is diagnosed by the finding of pyuria and positive urine cultures. Diseases of the bones associated with an increased calcium excretion may be obscure. It is interesting that phosphaturia may also be found in neurasthenia. The calculi that sometimes occur in the genito-urinary tract are composed of ammonium magnesium phosphate crystals mixed with calcium phosphate, oxalates, and urates.

Treatment.—The cause, in the main, determines the nature of the treatment. Discontinuance of alkali administration or a change to an acid-forming diet may be indicated. If infection is present the urine should be made acid with acid sodium phosphate and ammonium chloride. Mandelic acid may be used. If calculi are present they may require surgical removal.

Oxaluria.—*Definition.*—The excretion of excessive amounts of oxalic acid as calcium oxalate in the urine is called oxaluria.

Chemical Pathology.—Oxalic acid normally occurs in the urine in three crystalline forms: the envelope, the dumbbell, or the ovoid form. These crystals may be found in acid, neutral, and alkaline urine. Their solubility is dependent upon the sodium acid phosphate as well as the calcium and magnesium chloride content of the urine.

The source of supply of oxalic acid to the body is our food. Urinary oxalic acid is partly dependent upon this exogenous source, but it also has been shown by Lommel (1899) that oxalic acid is present in the urine after twelve days of fasting. This fact is considered to be proof of its endogenous origin. The hydrochloric acid of the gastric juice favors oxalic acid absorption by breaking down the insoluble calcium oxalate in vegetables. The fermentation of carbohydrate in the stomach that occurs in achlorhydria results in the formation of oxalic acid in its free form which is readily absorbed. Likewise intestinal fermentation increases the absorption and excretion of oxalates.

Symptoms and Diagnosis.—Smarting at the end of micturition is the usual symptom referable to the passage of calcium oxalate crystals. If small stones have formed there may be colic, hematuria, and albuminuria. Calcium oxalate stones most frequently form in the pelvis of the kidney and are hard and rough. Bleeding is usual. Tenosynovitis referable to the precipitation of calcium oxalate crystals has been reported, and its cure was dependent upon controlling the oxaluria. Apparently there is some relationship between *glycosuria* and oxalic acid excretion. A heavy glycosuria is associated with a decreased oxalic acid output and vice versa.

Treatment.—The supply of exogenous oxalic acid should be limited by restricting those foodstuffs that contain the insoluble calcium oxalate in the greatest concentration, *i.e.*, rhubarb, figs, beets, strawberries, potatoes, plums, spinach, tomatoes, and the beverages tea, coffee, and cocoa. An increased urinary acidity, best produced by acid sodium phosphate, helps to keep the oxalates in solution, and an increased fluid intake is indicated. When calcium oxalate calculi are present their surgical removal is usually necessary.

Uraturia.—*Definition.*—Uraturia means an excess excretion of urates (salts of uric acid in the urine).

Etiology.—In man and the higher apes uric acid is an end product in purine metabolism and is excreted in the urine as sodium, potassium, and ammonium salts. This uric acid excretion amounts to 200 to 800 mg. in twenty-four hours. Most probably uric acid is excreted by filtration through the glomeruli and subsequently concentrated in the tubular system (Luekens). These urates remain in solution in the urine unless there is a sufficient concentration of acid phosphates present to fix the base and liberate the free uric acid. Under those circumstances uric acid crystals are precipitated out (cayenne pepper grains) and calculi may form.

In most diseases such as gout and leukemia, where there is increased uric acid excretion, no calculus formation occurs, because the organic acid is held in solution as a salt.

Symptoms and Diagnosis.—Uraturia itself produces no symptoms, but uric acid calculi cause irritation, bleeding and colic. Urates precipitate out from standing urine as a pinkish amorphous sediment which is readily dissolved by heat. Uric acid crystals are usually colored by the urinary pigments. When formed in the pelvis of the kidney they may cause colicky pain upon passing down the ureter and a burning, cutting pain in passing through the urethra. Pure uric acid calculi cast no roentgen-ray shadow, but if they contain calcium a shadow will be shown.

Treatment.—Uric acid excretion may be influenced by diet. Restriction of the purine-containing foodstuffs (*e.g.*, meat) lowers its excretion. A diet high in fat and low in carbohydrate reduces the excretion of uric acid in the urine. This is not a matter of an associated ketosis or of total calories, but depends directly upon the high fat content.

Alkali administration will help to keep uric acid in solution and a forced fluid intake is considered helpful. The use of drugs which accelerate uric acid excretion is not indicated unless one is dealing with a disease wherein the blood has a high uric acid content.

BIBLIOGRAPHY

XANTHOMATOSES

Gaucher's Disease
   Pick, L., Amer. Jour. Med. Sci., **185**: 453, 1933.

Niemann-Pick's Disease
   Niemann, A., Jahr. f. Kinderheilk., **79**: 1, 1914.
   Pick, L., Med. Klin., **20**: 1399, 1924.

Schüller-Christian Syndrome
   Schüller, A., Wien. Med. Wschr., **71**: 510, 1921.
   Christian, H. A., Contributions to Med. and Biol. Research, New York, **I**: 390, 1929.
   Horsfall, F. L., Jr., and Smith, W. R., Quart. Jour. Med., n.s. **4**: 37, 1935.

GLYCOGEN DISEASE

Ellis, R. W. B., and Payne, W. W., Quart. Jour. Med., n.s. **5**: 31, 1936.
van Creveld, S., Medicine, **18**: 1, 1939.
von Gierke, E., Beitr. Path. Anat., **82**: 497, 1929.

ALKAPTONURIA

Cuthbert, C. F., Lancet, **I**: 593, 1923.
Garrod, A. E., Inborn Errors of Metabolism, H. Froude, Hodder & Stoughton, London, 1909, p. 41.
Gibson, R. B., and Howard, C. P., Arch. Int. Med., **28**: 632, 1921.
Papageorge, E., and Lewis, H. B., Jour. Biol. Chem., **123**: 211, 1938.

   20

Ochronosis

Howard, C. P., and Mills, E. S., Oxford Medicine, **4**: 223, 1932.
Oppenheimer, B. S., and Kline, B. S., Arch. Int. Med., **29**: 732, 1922.

Porphyria

Dobriner, K., and Rhoads, C. P., Phys. Rev., **20**: 416, 1940.
Günther, H., Dtsch. Arch. Klin. Med., **105**: 89, 1911.
Mason, V. R., Courville, C., and Ziskind, E., Medicine, **12**: 355, 1933.
Waldenström, J., Acta Med. Scand., **83**: 281, 1934, and Acta Med. Scand., Supp. **82**, 1937.

Cystinuria

Garrod, A. E., Inborn Errors of Metabolism, 2nd Ed., H. Froude, Hodder & Stoughton, London, 1923.
Hammer, H. J., and Thompson, G. J., Urol. and Cut. Rev., **44**: 341, 1940.
Thin, R., Edin. Med. Jour., **36**: 490, 1929.

Oxaluria

Cohen, H., and Reed, J. B., Liverpool Med.-Chir. Jour., **43**: 193, 1935.

CHAPTER XII

GOUT

By Walter Bauer and Friedrich Klemperer

Definition.—Gout is a hereditary constitutional disease, preeminently of males, occurring at any age and in most instances characterized by recurrent, acute arthritis. The articular inflammation may become chronic and is caused by deposits of sodium urate (*tophi*) which may be found in many tissues. The clinical picture is one of extreme latitude, varying from asymptomatic hyperuricemia to severely crippling joint disease even in the same individual. Hyperuricemia and diminished renal excretion of uric acid, the outstanding laboratory findings, may be present long before the ailment assumes its striking articular form. While they strongly incriminate the mechanism of uric acid disposal as the fundamental metabolic defect, the exact etiology of the disease is unknown.

For centuries it was believed that a *noxa* falling drop by drop into a joint was the cause of gout, hence its derivation from the Latin *gutta*, a drop. The term "gout," introduced in the thirteenth century, continues to enjoy common usage and deserves to be retained until an etiological designation can be substituted. It is an admirable name in that it connotes no theory, has little nosological significance and implies no pathogenic scheme. It is preferable to the term *podagra* which refers to only one of the articular manifestations of gout, namely, pain in the foot. Similar objections might be raised against various other synonyms introduced in the past.

History.—To the historians of medicine, gout has an unusual appeal. Recordings of its ancestry are found in the earliest medical literature. Its pedigree is a most distinguished one, and no disease has enjoyed a more royal patronage. Descriptions of its dramatic appearance, the ensuing pathos and the whimsical aspects of the disease have been documented by the ablest authors in fiction and biography. Victims of the disease have been the favored subjects of caricatures.

The excellent clinical accounts of gout ascribed to Aretaeus of Cappadocia, Caelius Aurelianus, Hippocrates, and others testify to the intimate knowledge of its varied features possessed by the Greek and Roman physicians.[1] Aretaeus, for instance, mentioned that during the asymptomatic periods, a gouty subject was capable of winnning in the Olympic games. However, the earlier writers failed to differentiate gout from other joint disorders. Sydenham, the modern Hippocrates, was one of the first to make this distinction,[2] and his masterly clinical portrayal of the disease, based in part on his thirty-four years of personal affliction, remains unsurpassed and marks the beginning of the modern history of gout.

The relation of uric acid to gout was not established until the development of chemistry made available the necessary analytic methods. Shortly after Scheele (1776)[3] had discovered uric acid as one of the constituents of a kidney stone, Wollaston (1797)[4] and Pearson (1798)[5] succeeded in demonstrating the same substance in the "chalkstones" (*tophi*) of patients suffering from gout. Garrod's[6] discovery (1848) of increased amounts of uric acid in the blood of gouty patients (by the "thread test") finally established the key position of this substance in the pathogenesis of gout. Subsequently, differentiation of this disease from the other arthritides was made with growing frequency and accuracy. Evidence that uric acid is the end-product of human purine metabolism was provided by a series of independent investigations. Miescher[7] in 1871 showed that the chief constituents of cell nuclei are the nucleoproteins, which on hydrolysis yield nucleic acid. Kossel[8] later demonstrated that purines are essential building stones of nucleic acid. It remained for Emil Fischer[9] to prove the chemical constitution of uric acid and to establish its structural relationship to the purines. Since then the rôle of purine metabolism in the pathophysiology of gout has been accepted. The introduction by Folin[10] of a reliable method of determining the uric acid content of the blood (1913), and its improvement by Folin[11] and Benedict,[12] have aided greatly in the subsequent metabolic and clinical studies of gout.*

PURINE METABOLISM

Chemistry of the Nucleoproteins, the Precursors of Uric Acid.—Nucleoproteins are contained in the nuclei of all living tissue. On hydrolysis they are split into a protein and nucleic acid, a protein-free constituent. Nucleic acid can be further hydrolyzed into nitrogenous bases (purines and pyrimidines), sugar and phosphoric acid, as shown in the following scheme:

Nucleoproteins

Protein   Nucleic Acid

Purines and Pyrimidines   Sugar   Phosphoric Acid

The purines are derivatives of the following ring-compound called purine (*uricum purum*) by Fischer.[9]

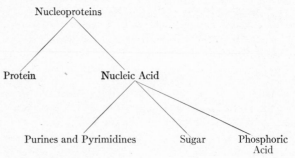

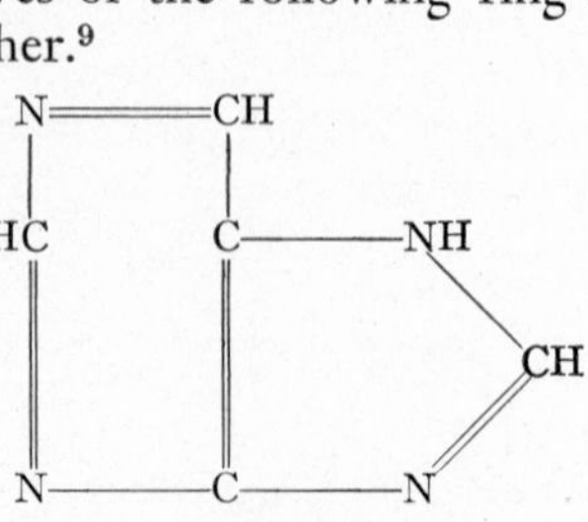

Purine

* Uric acid content is not determined specifically by these methods. Differences and defects in methods probably explain the divergency of values obtained in various laboratories and partially account for the formulation of conflicting theories of uric acid metabolism in health and disease.

Preformed in all nucleic acids are the aminopurines, adenine and guanine. These can be deaminized and oxidized to form hypoxanthine,
xanthine, and uric acid.

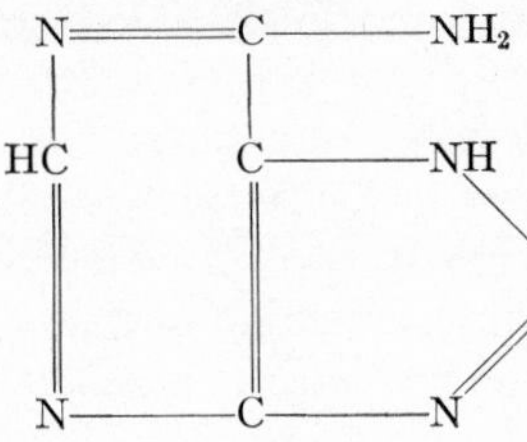

Adenine

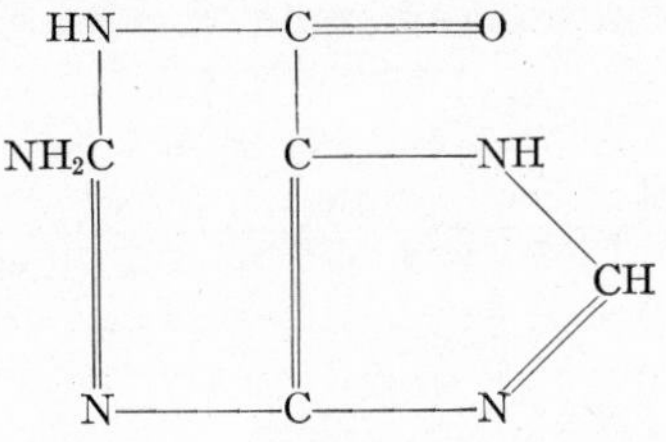

Guanine

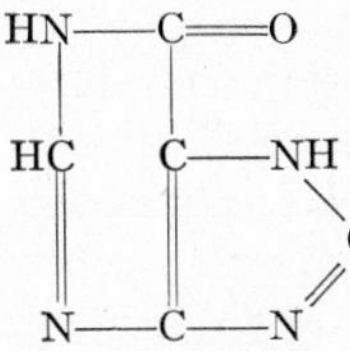

Hypoxanthine

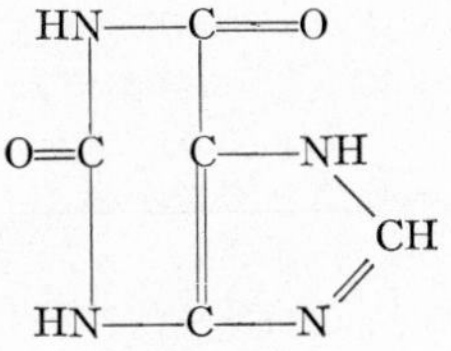

Xanthine

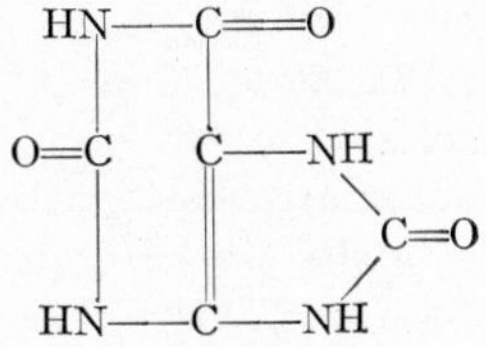

Uric acid

The pyrimidines which have been isolated from nuclear material are thymine, cytosine and uracil.

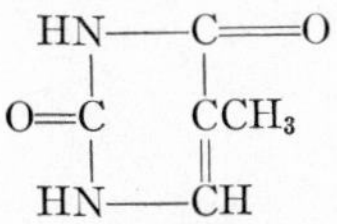

Thymine

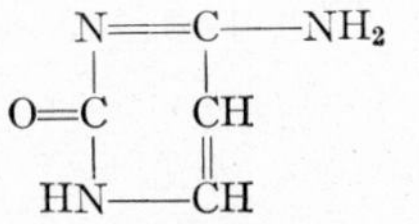

Cytosine

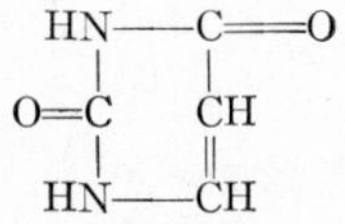

Uracil

In the body they are broken down to form urea and therefore have no
relation to purine metabolism. The sugar, d-ribose, can be isolated from
nucleic acids of plant origin (yeast-nucleic acids), whereas the animal-
nucleic acid (thymonucleic acid) yields the very unstable desoxyribose.[13]
Isolation of larger fragments of nucleic acid (nucleotides and nucleosides)
aided in elucidating the type of linkage connecting the bases, sugar and
phosphoric acid, as demonstrated by the following formula:

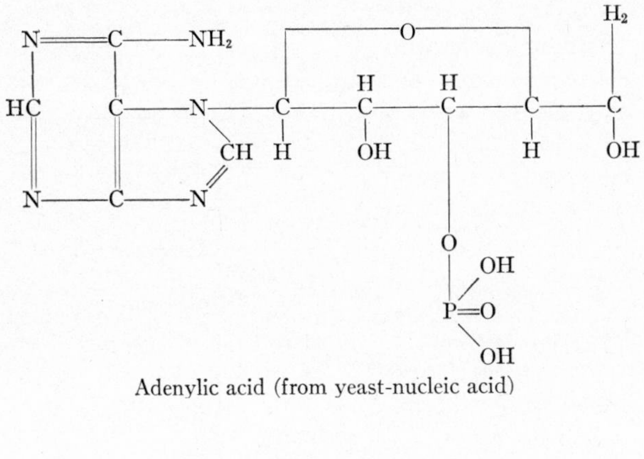

Adenylic acid (from yeast-nucleic acid)

Nucleosides are compounds which contain one molecule of base and one molecule of sugar, while nucleotides contain in addition one molecule of phosphoric acid. The purine nucleosides, adenosin (adenine-riboside) and guanosin (guanine-riboside) are derived from the nucleotides, adenylic acid (adenosine-phosphoric acid) and guanylic acid (guanosine-phosphoric acid). These compounds can be oxidized without breaking the nucleotide linkage to form inosinic acid (hypoxanthine-ribose-phosphoric acid) and xanthylic acid (xanthine-ribose-phosphoric acid). Upon further oxidation the bond between purine and sugar breaks. Thus it appears extremely unlikely that either a uric acid nucleotide or nucleoside exists.

The number of nucleotides contained in the nucleic acid molecule and their manner of linkage remain undetermined. On the basis of titration curves, Levene[14] postulated an ester linkage between the phosphoric acid and a hydroxyl group of ribose. Although this type of linkage is considered most likely, it fails to explain some of the chemical properties of nucleic acid.[15]

In animals as well as in plants, some nucleotides exist in a free form outside the cell nucleus. Their functions as co-enzymes are known in many instances. Methylated purines (caffeine, theobromine and others), present in certain plants, although pharmacologically important, are never transformed into uric acid in the human body. They are excreted unchanged or are partly demethylated.[16, 17]

$$CH_3—N—C=O$$
$$O=C\quad C—N<^{CH_3}_{CH}$$
$$CH_3—N—C—N$$

Caffeine

Metabolism of Ingested Nucleoproteins.—In the stomach and small intestine, the protein component of nucleoproteins is hydrolyzed by the successive action of pepsin and trypsin, with subsequent liberation of nucleic acids. These in turn are broken down into nucleotides by the action of duodenal secretions.[15] It has been suggested that the traces of adenylic acid and guanylic acid found in blood represent nucleotides absorbed from the gastro-intestinal tract.[18, 19] The remaining nucleotides are acted upon by intestinal phosphatase which splits them into phosphoric acid and nucleosides.[15, 20, 21] The latter are probably absorbed as such from the upper intestinal canal. The formation of inosinic acid and inosine (hypoxanthine-riboside) from nucleic acid by intestinal enzymes proves that deaminization of nucleotides and nucleosides can take place.[20, 21] Further hydrolysis with formation of purines has never been demonstrated in the intestines. Nucleotides and nucleosides which escape absorption, and the major portion of the purines are decomposed completely by the bacteria of the lower intestine, and ammonia is liberated.[22]

The ultimate fate of the absorbed nucleotides and nucleosides is one of hydrolysis and oxidation to uric acid. This was clearly shown by experiments in which these compounds were incubated with liver tissue[23] or injected into living organisms.[24] That this transformation can also take place in other than hepatic tissue was proved by liver-extirpation experiments[25] and by the demonstration in most organs of enzymes capable of hydrolyzing and oxidizing purine nucleotides. Whether nucleotides are first hydrolyzed and the resulting purines subsequently oxidized, or whether

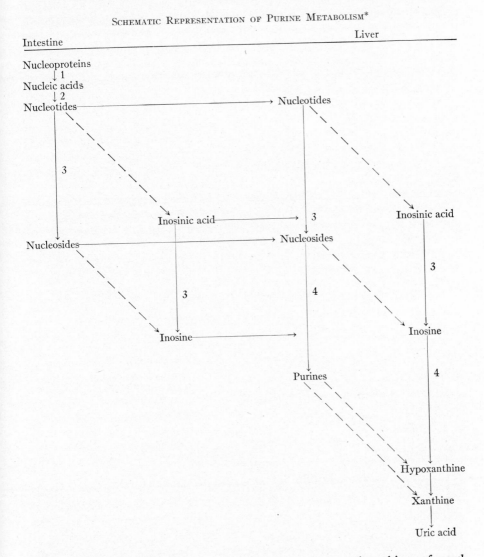

SCHEMATIC REPRESENTATION OF PURINE METABOLISM*

oxidation occurs on the intact nucleotide molecule, was the subject of much controversy following Benedict's claim[26] that a uric acid nucleotide existed in blood. In the light of Emil Fischer's work,[9] the existence of a uric acid

* In the intestine the protein part of nucleoprotein is digested by proteolytic enzymes (1). Nucleic acids are hydrolyzed by polynucleotidase (2) to nucleotides. These are split by phosphatase (3) into phosphoric acid and nucleosides. Oxidation of nucleotides and nucleosides, indicated by the broken arrows, occurs in the intestine. The horizontal arrows designate intestinal absorption of nucleotides and nucleosides. Hydrolysis (vertical arrows 3 and 4) and oxidation (broken arrows) occur simultaneously in the liver. The end-product, uric acid, is excreted in the urine.

nucleotide seems highly improbable. Although enzymatic studies have been of little aid in this dispute, failure to isolate compounds intermediary between nucleotides and uric acid suggests that hydrolysis and oxidation take place simultaneously.[23]

In most mammals, other than the human and ape, uric acid is subject to the action of an enzyme, uricase, which oxidizes uric acid to allantoin. The

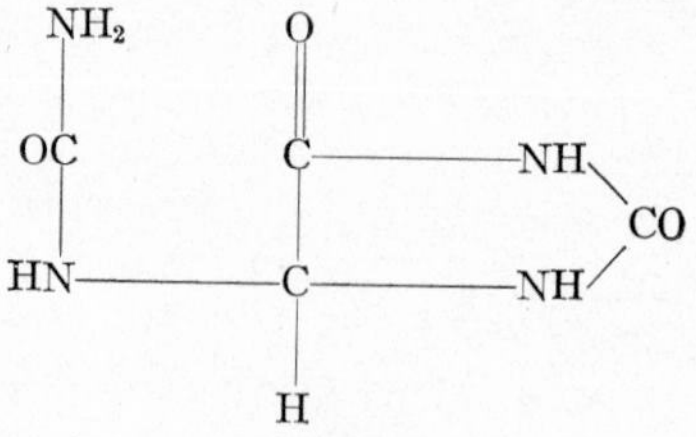

$$
\begin{array}{ccc}
NH_2 & O & \\
| & \| & \\
OC & C\!\!-\!\!-\!\!-\!\!-\!\!NH & \\
| & | & \quad CO \\
HN\!\!-\!\!-\!\!-\!\!-\!\!-\!\!C & C\!\!-\!\!-\!\!-\!\!-\!\!NH & \\
& | & \\
& H & \\
& \text{Allantoin} &
\end{array}
$$

latter is excreted as the end-product of purine metabolism. Uricase has never been demonstrated in human organs and the allantoin eliminated by humans amounts to only 5 to 35 mg. per day.[27, 28, 29] Its excretion is uninfluenced by feeding uric acid or its precursors, suggesting that the allantoin normally excreted is derived directly from traces of the substance present in ingested food. The fate of uric acid and its excretion will be discussed later.

Synthesis of Purines in the Body.—A considerable amount of data has been collected, indicating that purines are synthesized in the body. Miescher's[30] observation on the spawning salmon is the first study supporting this view. Salmon form large amounts of nucleoproteins at a time when they ingest no food. Later it was shown by Kossel that the purine content of hens' eggs increases during the period of incubation.[31] Burian and Schur[32] in their experiments on puppies, proved that mammals are likewise capable of performing this synthesis, and there is every reason to assume that the same process takes place in the growing infant on a milk diet. Our best evidence that it applies to the human adult dates from experiments[33, 34] in which subjects kept on a diet practically free of purine remained in good health and continued to excrete constant amounts of uric acid.

The path of synthesis and the material from which purines are built remain unknown. Akroyd and Hopkins[35] and Rose and Cook[36] suggested that the iminazol ring of histidine plays an important part in the synthesis.

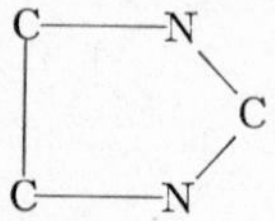

$$
\begin{array}{ccc}
C\!\!-\!\!-\!\!-\!\!N & \\
| & \!\!\diagdown \\
| & \quad C \\
| & \!\!\diagup \\
C\!\!-\!\!-\!\!-\!\!N &
\end{array}
$$

They demonstrated that the allantoin excretion of rats was diminished on a histidine-free diet. Gyorgy and Thannhauser,[37] however, were unable to influence the uric acid excretion of human infants by eliminating histidine from their diet. Although the body is able to synthesize the purine ring, there exists no evidence to suggest that a direct synthesis of uric acid from ammonia, carbon dioxide and a three-carbon compound is possible. The very fact that uric acid production is independent of the ingestion of nitrogenous material other than purines is evidence against this mechanism.

However, direct synthesis does take place in birds and reptiles, both of which excrete large amounts of uric acid. In these animals in contrast to mammals, uric acid represents an end-product of both amino-nitrogen and purine metabolism. That the nitrogenous waste is transformed to uric acid in the liver is readily shown in liver-extirpation experiments.[38] Under such experimental conditions, the uric acid excretion is diminished to a level corresponding to that of the purine catabolism, the remainder of the nitrogen being excreted as ammonium lactate.[38]

Endogenous Uric Acid Metabolism.—Humans on a purine-free diet continue to excrete uric acid, termed "endogenous uric acid" by Burian and Schur.[33] As can be seen from the following table (data collected by Rockwood[34]), the amount excreted under such conditions, although subject to

TABLE 1

URIC ACID EXCRETION

Time	Daily Averages	
	Urine Nitrogen Gm.	Uric Acid Gm.
Subject A		
December to January.................	11.99	0.308
January to February.................	11.58	0.305
March...........................	11.15	0.315
May.............................	12.63	0.321
July............................	12.68	0.313
November........................	9.99	0.298
Subject B		
January..........................	13.41	0.478
March...........................	13.92	0.452

daily fluctuations, remains remarkably constant from month to month. In experiments of this type it is extremely important to maintain an adequate caloric intake, otherwise the purines released from the increased breakdown of muscle tissue will enhance uric acid excretion. The nucleoproteins of the body, subject to constant and simultaneous processes of catabolism and replacement, are the chief source of endogenous uric acid. The amount contributed by the free nucleotides, present as co-enzymes in every cell, is probably insignificant. Proof of the breakdown of cellular nucleoproteins into uric acid was first presented by Horbaczewski[39] and later by Spitzer.[40] Both workers were able to show that the *in vitro* autolysis of liver and spleen in the presence of oxygen resulted in the formation of uric acid. As regards the living organism, we have ample evidence of increased uric acid excretion in those pathological states (leukemia, polycythemia, resolving pneumonia, etc.) in which an undue amount of nucleoprotein is destroyed. In such instances, the path of breakdown is probably the same as that of the nucleic acids derived from food, since nucleolytic enzymes are present in practically all mammalian organs.

The Problem of Uric Acid Destruction in the Human Body.—It was previously stated that all purine-containing material, exogenous and endogenous, is metabolized to uric acid and excreted as such. The question whether uricolysis ever occurs in humans warrants discussion because of its disputed rôle in the pathogenesis of gout. If it does occur, the mechanism involved must be entirely different from that operating in animals, because the formation of allantoin has never been demonstrated nor has uricase ever been isolated from human tissues. The only alternative, namely, the oxidation of uric acid resulting in the production of urea appears very unlikely, since repeated and diligent search has failed to reveal enzymes capable of catalyzing this reaction. In earlier studies designed to gain information on this point, individuals whose endogenous uric acid excretion had been established (by eliminating purines from the dietary) were fed uric acid or its precursors. These experiments, which resulted in incomplete recovery of uric acid, must be considered inconclusive since bacterial destruction of the ingested uric acid in the intestinal tract could not be ruled out.[22] In subsequent studies, uric acid, usually as the soluble lithium salt, was injected intravenously. The results were variable; occasionally recoveries of only 30 per cent were observed,[41] but other workers reported both complete recovery and an excretion of uric acid in excess of that administered. The latter was presumably due to the toxic action of the large doses of uric acid injected and the resulting destruction of tissue.[41] In experiments of this type, one is limited to the introduction of small amounts of uric acid, if unphysiological conditions are to be avoided. Furthermore, the daily endogenous uric acid excretion fluctuates sufficiently to make an accurate evaluation impossible, and to deprive the low recoveries reported of their theoretical significance. Thannhauser[24, 42] recovered 70 to 100 per cent of uric acid whether nucleotides or an equivalent amount of uric acid had been injected, indicating that destruction of the purine ring does not take place prior to hydrolysis of nucleotides. From the evidence quoted and other metabolic data,[43, 44, 45, 46, 47] most workers have concluded that in humans the purine ring remains intact and destruction of uric acid does not take place.

Uric Acid Excretion.—Uric acid is excreted preponderantly in the urine and only traces are found in intestinal secretions. In concentrations obtaining in body fluids, urates are freely diffusible, and therefore are equally distributed in plasma and glomerular urine.[48] They are subsequently concentrated in the tubules.[49] The fact that the clearance values for urates are always much lower than those of inulin and urea indicates that tubular excretion does not occur and that concentration in the tubules is limited.[49, 50, 51, 52] This characteristically low concentrating power accounts for the high serum uric acid levels of humans (3 to 6 mg. per cent) compared for instance to that of Dalmatian dogs,* which excrete several times more uric acid but rarely have plasma values exceeding 1 mg. per cent. In humans, neither the concentration ratio of urate in plasma and urine nor

---

* Benedict[53] was the first to show that Dalmatian coach hounds excrete large amounts of uric acid. However, they also eliminate considerable quantities of allantoin.[54] This fact and the presence of large amounts of uricase in their livers[55, 56] indicate a fundamental difference between their uric acid metabolism and that of man.

the urate clearance is constant. Large fluctuations occur even under basal conditions. It has been shown, however, that the blood urate concentration markedly influences not only the urine urate concentration but also the volume of blood cleared per minute. Brøchner-Mortensen found an average increase in clearance from 7.4 cc. per minute to 15.3 cc. per minute when the plasma uric acid concentration was raised from 6.6 to 10.7 mg.* per 100 cc. following the injection or ingestion of uric acid.[51] This excretory mechanism is similar to that for glucose and serves to maintain a relatively constant blood level in normal individuals. Brøchner-Mortensen further observed that uric acid excretion is a direct function of diuresis, since the urate clearance increased appreciably when the diuresis exceeded 1 cc. per minute. These factors have been overlooked by most investigators and may possibly explain the inconsistencies of some interpretations.

Starvation, a high-fat diet, exercise, and the injection of lactic acid are said to cause a diminished uric acid excretion.[57, 58] Most workers have considered this reduction the result of the acidosis accompanying these conditions.

It has been shown that certain drugs influence the elimination of uric acid. Berglund[50] and others[52] demonstrated that following the administration of salyrgan there occurred a rise in uric acid excretion greater than could be accounted for by diuresis alone. A similar but less pronounced effect was obtained with aminophyllin,[50] while caffeine was without influence, despite the fact that a diuresis resulted.[50] Epinephrine caused an increased urinary concentration,[59] whereas pituitrin,[50] ergotamine[50] and atropine had a depressing effect.[50] The most pronounced increase in urate excretion and clearance was observed following the ingestion of cinchophen[50, 52, 60, 61, 62]; salicylates gave a similar result.[63, 64] The action of these two drugs was abolished following denervation of the kidney.[65] In the intact animal, the cinchophen effect was counteracted by the simultaneous administration of ergotamine, but not of atropine. These latter experimental results and those observed following the administration of epinephrine, pituitrin, ergotamine and atropine prove that the autonomic nervous system has a regulatory function in uric acid excretion. They further show that some drugs influence its excretion not by direct action on the kidney cells but through the mediation of nerves.

ETIOLOGY

Urate Excretion.—Various theories have been advanced to explain the complex features of gout, but unfortunately they are neither compatible with all known facts nor supported by adequate experimental evidence. Claims referring to a disturbance of the enzymes involved in purine metabolism, dysfunction of the liver, altered alkalinity of the blood, infection, allergy, and other similarly vague hypotheses have found their way into the literature. The definition of gout to which we are forced on the basis of well established clinical observations makes it apparent that no scheme will be acceptable unless it accounts for the hyperuricemia and the precipitation of urates in tissues.

* In these studies a titration method was used which gives consistent but high values.

Theoretically, the elevation in the blood uric acid level might be the result of decreased destruction, increased formation or decreased elimination of uric acid. However, since evidence is entirely lacking that uricolysis ever occurs in humans, the hyperuricemia cannot be ascribed to the first-named mechanism. If it were due to enhanced uric acid formation, a relatively greater excretion should be demonstrable in all cases, as is the case with glucose in diabetes. If, on the other hand, the hyperuricemia were the result of impaired renal function, the uric acid excretion would be decreased, a finding actually observed by many workers. Most gouty subjects when kept on a low purine diet excrete less than 500 mg. per day, the average being lower than that found in normal individuals.[41, 66] However, instances of increased uric acid excretion are on record[41, 67] and have led certain workers[67] to postulate that an augmented production of uric acid is responsible for the hyperuricemia of gout.

According to our present knowledge of purine metabolism, increased formation of uric acid could be secondary only to accelerated nuclear metabolism, for which no evidence has been presented in these cases. On the other hand, if we assume that the increased output of uric acid recorded in some studies represents a temporary event, even though extended over a period of several months, the results are not incompatible with the known variability of urate excretion in gouty subjects. Under this premise the increase would constitute the partial elimination of urates retained during a preceding period of diminished renal function. Surely a mechanism of this sort must come into play to allow for disposal of urates derived from the resorption of tophaceous deposits, a not uncommon occurrence in gout.

A definitive answer to the question raised here will be possible only after further prolonged balance studies have been done. At present it seems more reasonable to explain the rare cases of gout with high uric acid excretion on this basis than to discard the mass of evidence showing that the daily uric acid excretion of gouty subjects is normal or reduced. In summary, it would appear that the intermediary purine metabolism of the gouty patient is normal and that his hyperuricemia is accounted for by a limitation of renal excretion of uric acid, which is the invariable end-product of purine metabolism.

Kidney Function.—Garrod[1] postulated that renal disease is the cause of gout. However, all proven kidney function tests such as the measurement of phenolsulfonphthalein excretion, concentration or clearance of creatinine, urea and inulin may be normal in gouty subjects with hyperuricemia even though they have suffered one or more attacks of acute arthritis.[52, 67, 68, 69] In a later stage, to be sure, the disease is frequently complicated by marked renal damage resulting in retention of nonprotein nitrogen and further rise of the blood uric acid level. Irrespective of these late developments data have been presented suggesting that specific impairment of the function to excrete uric acid may exist in gouty individuals without otherwise demonstrable kidney disease.[66, 68] This is readily shown by relating the uric acid excretion to its concentration in the plasma. For example, the concentration of uric acid in the urine of persons with normal kidneys having a hyperuricemia due to resolving pneumonia or leukemia is always fifteen to thirty times greater than that of the blood (Thann-hauser[66]). On the other hand, gouty subjects with equally high or higher blood uric acid levels never exhibit such high urinary urate concentrations.[52, 66, 68, 70] Urate clearance studies have yielded essentially the same results.[51, 52, 68] As stated previously, the uric acid clearance of normal individuals is increased considerably if the blood uric acid is raised to hyperuricemic levels, yet the gouty subjects, despite a high uric acid concentration in the blood, never shows a high uric acid clearance. Similar differences between normal and gouty individuals are observed following the injection of uric acid. In a normal person the clearance rises and the injected uric acid is excreted promptly, whereas in the gouty subject increased clearance is not observed and complete recovery of the injected uric acid is often impossible,[41] indicating its retention in the tissues. Failure in the past to compare the urate clearance of gouty subjects with that of other individuals having an elevated blood uric acid has led to the erroneous conclusion that the uric acid excreting mechanism is normal in gout. In fact, all pertinent evidence indicates that the urate clearance of the gouty subject with an elevated blood uric acid is considerably lower than that of normal individuals, providing the rate of urine excretion and blood uric acid concentration are comparable.

Various workers[46, 47, 68, 69, 71, 72] have reported normal blood uric acid values and normal ability to excrete uric acid in a few patients who had experienced one or more typical attacks of gouty arthritis. Some of these patients had on occasions shown transitory elevations of the blood uric acid levels. Unfortunately, data are not available confirming that in such cases coincident with hyperuricemia a temporary impairment of uric acid excretion takes place, although the previously cited experimental results strongly suggest that it does. If these observations can be further substantiated, one will be forced to assume that the specific impairment of renal function, which represents the chief physiological alteration of gout, is reversible in the early stages of the disease. Later, the disturbance may become more permanent and the blood uric acid remain elevated. If we were to be guided solely by our own experience, the first assumption would be unnecessary, since we have never observed an unequivocally normal fasting serum uric acid value during or after an initial attack of gouty arthritis.

Precipitation of Urates in Tissues.—Although the theory of functional inhibition of urate excretion explains the hyperuricemia of gout, the formation of tissue urate deposits remains an enigma. Considered as a purely physicochemical phenomenon, an increased uric acid concentration of the body fluids might result in the precipitation of urates. The solubility of urate is largely a function of the hydrogen and sodium ion concentrations and under physiological conditions, saturation is probably reached at a concentration of about 6.5 mg. per cent.[73] If this is correct, precipitation should never occur unless the urate content of body fluids is elevated, a fact borne out by clinical observation. However, urates do not precipitate readily from even a supersaturated solution. In plasma, probably because of the presence of colloids, much higher uric acid concentrations do not lead to precipitation.[70, 74] Folin[41] obtained values of 300 to 400 mg. per cent in birds following ureteral ligation without precipitation in the blood. It does not occur in the tissue fluids of humans who for months or years have had an elevated blood uric acid concentration due to conditions other than gout (chronic leukemia and Bright's disease). Therefore, we must conclude that hyperuricemia, although an essential feature of gout, is not the sole cause of urate deposition. Local trauma, very likely a contributing factor in many instances, by itself affords no etiologic explanation, since patients with hyperuricemia due to other disorders, unless these are complicated by gout, are not known to develop urate precipitates. The participation of infectious agents has often been claimed but never proved. It is a fact that tissues with poor vascular supply are the favored foci of urate crystals, but as will be shown later, circulatory impairment cannot be considered the cause of the precipitation. Umber[46] and later Gudzent,[47] without presenting adequate evidence, attempted to interpret gout as an allergic disease in which certain tissues acquire a specific affinity for uric acid. This theory fails to account for the high uric acid content of the blood and the associated low concentration in the urine, so often seen in gout. Rather, it would appear that two coexisting factors are necessary to explain the biochemical alterations observed in gout, first, a diminution of the uric acid concentrating power of the kidney and second, the presence of a local change in certain tissues which induces precipitation of sodium urate from a supersaturated solution.

Metabolic Alterations Observed During the Acute Attack.—Although diminished uric acid excretion is observed in most gouty subjects for several days prior to an attack,[46, 67, 75, 76] increased excretion has been noted occasionally.[67] Immediately preceding or at the peak of the seizure, the urate elimination is usually augmented, gradually returning to normal as the attack subsides. Associated with these fluctuations, there are alterations in the water and mineral metabolism.[77] Twenty-four to seventy-two hours before the onset of the attack the urinary output rises, falling to normal during the recovery period, as was first observed by Scudamore[78] and has frequently been confirmed. In this period of diuresis, a marked increase in sodium and chloride excretion and a slight diminution of the concentration of these ions in the serum are demonstrable. During the attack proper the urinary potassium, calcium, ammonia, and phosphate are elevated but their concentration in the serum remains unchanged except for potassium which may be raised.[77] It appears somewhat paradoxical that a gain in body weight occurs at the time of the diuresis. A simultaneous decrease in insensible perspiration has been offered as an explanation.[77]

The significance of these latter findings particularly in their application to the etiology of gout is unknown, but it is obvious that temporary urate retention is not the sole cause of an attack. Some workers[66, 79] have tried to explain the altered kidney function as well as other manifestations of the acute seizures on the basis of disturbed nervous regulation. Attractive as this theory may be, it has not been possible to prove it.

PATHOLOGY*

Although our knowledge of the pathogenesis of gout is incomplete, it appears well established that the pathological manifestations of the disease

* We are indebted to Dr. Granville A. Bennett, Department of Pathology, Harvard Medical School, for the photomicrographs contained in this section.

are dependent upon the deposition of sodium urate in various tissues and the inflammatory and degenerative changes resulting therefrom. The urate deposits surrounded by tissue exhibiting inflammatory and foreign-body reactions constitute the one pathognomonic lesion of the disease and are readily demonstrated providing the tissues to be examined are properly fixed and stained.*[80] For a long time this may be the only discernible lesion. Many of the anatomical alterations observed in the late stages of gout are the result of the ill-understood arterial and arteriolar sclerosis which frequently manifest themselves as the disease advances.

The local tissue changes which make possible the precipitation of uric acid, in the form of sodium urate, are unknown. It is much more prone to occur in relatively avascular structures. Ebstein[81] insisted that irrespective of the tissues affected, a previous injury or *tissue necrosis* was a prerequisite to urate deposition. Although this theory has a certain appeal, there is equally good reason for assuming that uric acid is deposited in normal tissues and that the necrosis seen is a secondary phenomenon. We think it logical to conclude as did Minkowski[82] that the acute inflammation observed during an attack of gout constitutes, in part, an unsuccessful attempt of the affected organ to rid itself of uric acid. The reaction of the tissues to urate deposition is, as might be expected, extremely variable. When it occurs in the soft tissues, an acute inflammatory reaction of the severest grade usually results, yet marked precipitation in the cartilaginous structures of joints, ears, and nose may take place unknown to the patient. Such a reaction is sometimes followed by the appearance of a visible *tophus;* in other cases, the offending urates may be completely absorbed. Again, we are without a satisfactory explanation for these differences although they are probably accounted for by the amount of uric acid set free in the tissue, the vascularity of the part affected and the ability of the tissue to eliminate the precipitated urate.

The Gouty Joint.—Urate deposits in the articular structures are the cause of the most frequent disability resulting from gout. The occasional failure to demonstrate them in the tissues of a joint which has been subjected to recurrent attacks of gouty arthritis suggests that urates may at times be completely absorbed.

No joint is exempt, although certain ones are more frequently involved,[78, 83, 84] for instance, the joints of the lower extremities as compared to those of the arms. The metatarsophalangeal joints of the great toes are most regularly involved and may be the only site. Next in order of frequency are the small joints of the feet, the ankles, hands and wrists. The knees, elbows, shoulders and hips are less commonly, the sacro-iliac, the sternoclavicular joints, and the articulations of the spine, jaw, and larynx most rarely foci of urate deposition.

Gross examination of a joint which has been the site of recurrent attacks of gouty arthritis may reveal no external changes and few or no intraarticular abnormalities other than urate precipitates in the articular cartilage. In chronic gout, the affected joints may be enlarged and grossly deformed because of extensive tophaceous deposits and bony destruction (see Figs. 113 and 114, p. 633). In such instances urates may be demonstrable in the

* The fresh tissue should be fixed immediately in absolute alcohol and later stained according to the technique of deGalantha.

articular cartilage, perichondrium, ligaments, synovialis, and such periarticular structures as tendons, bursae, bone marrow, subcutaneous tissues or
even the overlying skin. Practically all specimens in this phase show the
gross characteristics of degenerative joint disease, including marginal over-
growths or exostoses to a more marked degree than is ordinarily seen at a
corresponding age.[85] The synovial membrane usually presents only minimal
changes, although urate deposition may be sufficiently marked to cause extensive proliferation and fibrous tissue ankylosis. Even bony union may
ensue, but such severe changes are rare and generally confined to the smaller
articulations.

Postmortem studies have demonstrated that the *articular cartilages* are
the most common and at times the exclusive sites of urate deposition. The

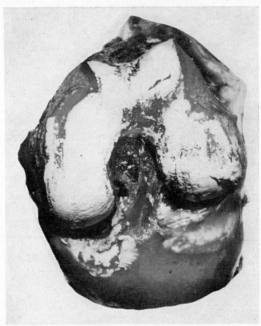

Fig. 103.—Extensive urate deposition in the articular cartilage of the femur and the
synovial membrane of the knee joint. One further notes degenerative changes of the
cartilage and secondary marginal overgrowth at the perichondrial margins. (This specimen was prepared by Dr. S. B. Wolbach for the Warren Museum, Harvard Medical
School.)

accumulations are always much more pronounced in the central avascular
part than in the more vascular joint margins. An affected joint surface appears as though it had been imperfectly coated with white lacquer or a
mortar-like material (Fig. 103). The extent of the articular surface deposit
varies greatly from joint to joint. In some it is confined to irregularly
placed, small white specks and streaks, in others, a considerable portion of
the articular cartilage is covered by large white plaques.

Microscopic examination discloses that the *urate deposits*, although
superficial, are actually embedded in the intercellular matrix. They are almost always confined to the upper layers of cartilage, although they

occasionally extend into bone. On the articular surface, the urate deposits appear as a coating of amorphous material (Fig. 104). This is densest near the joint cavity and grows progressively thinner as it penetrates into the

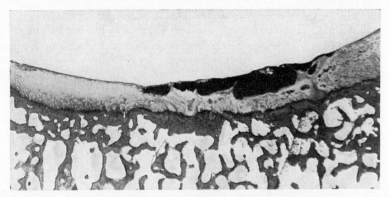

Fig. 104.—A photomicrograph (× 60) of the phalangeal side of a first metatarso-phalangeal joint. One observes a heavy deposit of urates in the upper half of the articular cartilage associated with marked degenerative changes.

middle or lower portion of the cartilage. Where the deposit is most sparse, the characteristic acicular crystals are seen most often (Fig. 105). The re-action of cartilage to the infiltration is directly proportional to the amount

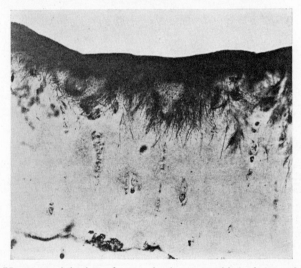

Fig. 105.—Heavy precipitation of urates in the upper third of the articular cartilage. In the deepest portion the characteristic sheaths of urate crystals are clearly shown. (A. M. Brogsitter's monograph, Histopathologie der Gelenk-Gicht, 1927, F. C. W. Vogel, Leipzig.)

of urate present. Microscopic examination of cartilage strips from which the urates have been digested shows profound alterations in those portions of the matrix where urate deposition had been heaviest. Little or no reaction is discernible in the areas which contained only minute foci. When urates are present in large amounts, one finds cartilage changes such as pits, depressions, fissures, crevices and thinning of a more severe grade than is compatible with the age of the subject.[85] In addition, one notes diminution in number, scattering, and clumping of the cartilage cells.

The striking predilection of urate deposits for articular cartilage rather than other body tissues remains unexplained. As stated previously, they occur most often in the avascular central area, which derives a portion if not all of its nourishment from synovial fluid. The latter normally, as well as in gout, contains the same amount of urate as the blood plasma. Urates, being freely diffusible, undoubtedly gain access to normal cartilage as do other synovial fluid constituents. In the gouty subject, whose hyperuricemia is reflected in the synovial fluid, an excess of urates is thus made

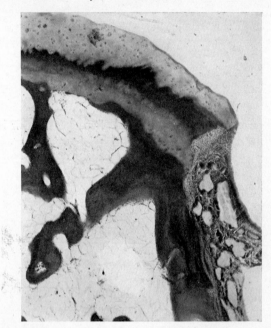

Fig. 106.—Characteristic foreign body reaction accompanying urate deposition in the synovial tissue at the perichondrial margin of a finger joint. It has resulted in pannus formation which has extended onto the articular cartilage surface. (× 60.)

available to cartilage. The prevalence of urate crystals in some joints and their complete absence in others cannot be explained adequately and indicates that factors other than an increased urate concentration must be operative.

Urate deposits in the synovial membrane and capsular tissue cause the nonspecific, *inflammatory reaction* which characterizes the acute stage of gouty arthritis. Failures, reported in the past, to demonstrate the foreign substance in the soft articular tissues may have been due to improper fixation and staining. In appropriately prepared material, obtained from a joint which has been subjected to repeated attacks, they are easily recognized microscopically. The lesion consists of a central mass of urates, often amorphous in appearance, embedded in vascular granulation tissue. Crystals,

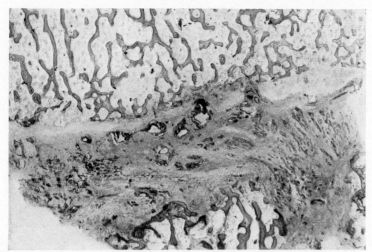

Fig. 107.—Fibrous ankylosis of the astragalotibial joint (low magnification, × 10). A few small strips of eroded articular cartilage adjacent to the astragalus remain. The numerous light areas in the connective tissue are deposits of monosodium urate, surrounded by zones of marked chronic inflammation.

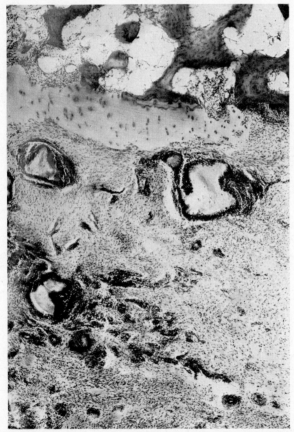

Fig. 108.—High power photomicrograph of an area of the section illustrated in Fig. 107, showing invasion and destruction of articular cartilage by urate-containing fibrous tissue which has extended into subchondral bone spaces.

enmeshed in interstitium, are more readily seen in the smaller foci. Older urate deposits may be surrounded by a relatively avascular fibrous tissue capsule. In their immediate neighborhood, one finds mononuclear phagocytes, giant cells, polymorphonuclear leukocytes, eosinophils and plasma cells. Focal areas of lymphocytes are numerous and vascular sclerosis is frequently seen.[84, 85] Heavy precipitates in the synovial lining and subsynovial tissues result in marked proliferative activity, and occasionally in the formation of a pannus which spreads onto the articular surfaces and may envelop them completely. In consequence, there results invasion and destruction of cartilage (Fig. 106) which in some instances leads to fibrous and bony ankylosis (Figs. 107, 108).

Abarticular Tophi.—The term, tophus (chalk stone or concretion), has through general usage come to denote urate deposits in tissues other than joints. They are most commonly seen in the helix or antihelix of the ears,

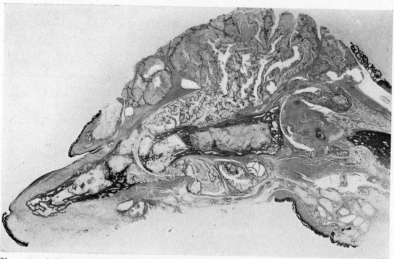

Fig. 109.—Microscopic section through an index finger, showing extensive tophaceous deposits which have largely replaced the bony structures and the adjacent subcutaneous tissue. In this instance protrusion of the chalky urate material had taken place.

the olecranon and patellar bursae, the tendons of fingers, hands, wrists, toes, feet, ankles, and heels (see Figs. 109 and 110). Less frequently they are met in the skin of the palms and soles, the tarsal plates of the eyelids, the nasal cartilages, the finger tips, the tendinous expansion of muscles, and in the cornea and sclerotic coats of the eye.[142] The kidneys may also be the seat of urate precipitates. Very rarely they have been found in the corpus cavernosum and prepuce of the penis,[76] the aorta, myocardium, and aortic valves, the tongue,[86] epiglottis, vocal cords, and the arytenoid cartilages. Occasionally the crystals have been recovered from the sputum of gouty subjects.[76] Isolated reports of urates in the central nervous system and its coverings have not been verified. Such abarticular deposits are followed by the foreign body inflammatory reaction previously described and varying in extent and degree with the vascularity of the affected tissue. When present in the bone marrow, they may represent a direct extension of articular pannus containing uric acid foci or a primary deposition of urate.[85] In either instance they result in lacunar absorption of adjacent trabeculae and replacement of the marrow by fibrous tissue (Fig. 111). These tophaceous deposits consist of sodium urate, the crystals of which are readily demonstrable (see Fig. 112).

Kidney Lesions.—The renal lesions observed in gout have been called *gouty nephritis, gouty form of Bright's disease, interstitial* or *arteriosclerotic nephritis,* and *renal impairment of gout.* This varied terminology in-

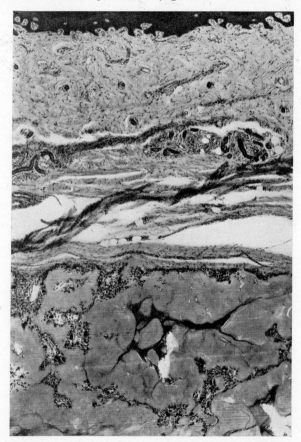

Fig. 110.—Section through the tophaceous deposit in the subcutaneous tissues of the finger illustrated in figure 109. The large masses of urates are surrounded by small connective tissue septa which contain foreign body giant cells and chronic inflammatory cells. (× 60.)

dicates that no unanimity of opinion has existed concerning the nature of these changes, but all authors are agreed that the incidence of kidney disease is higher in gout than in other chronic disorders (rheumatoid arthritis, diabetes mellitus, and pernicious anemia). However, few, if any, would argue that anatomical alterations of the kidney can be demonstrated as the primary cause of gout.

Grossly, the kidneys are reduced in size, their capsules being moderately adherent to an irregular surface.[46, 87] The cortex is diminished in thickness.

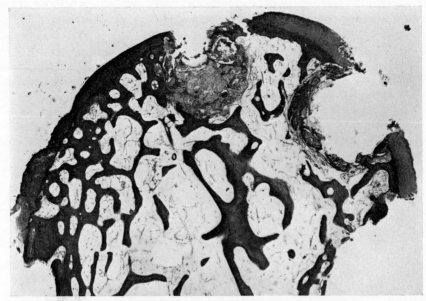

Fig. 111.—Proximal phalanx of a finger. The surface of the articular cartilage is frayed and uneven. There is cartilaginous and bony overgrowth (lipping) at the articular margins. The two large circular defects (punched-out areas) in the articular cartilage and subchondral bone were lined with fibrous tissue infiltrated with large numbers of inflammatory cells and studded with numerous masses of sodium urate crystals. Isolated urate deposits were seen in the bone marrow of this phalanx. (× 20.)

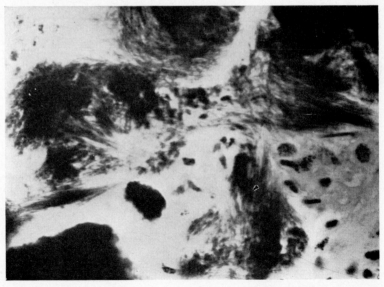

Fig. 112.—Showing acicular urate crystals in tophaceous deposits. This section was taken from a subcutaneous nodule and stained by the deGalantha method. (× 900.)

The extent of such changes is correlated to the severity and duration of gout. Urate deposits may be seen on the cut surface of the kidney. They appear most commonly as punctate foci in the cortex or as long white streaks in the interstitial tissue of the medulla. The glomeruli show varying grades of fibrosis and the collecting tubules may contain small urate calculi. Urate deposits call forth in the kidney the same type of inflammatory reaction as in other vascular tissues, but they are rarely present in sufficient amounts to cause serious renal damage. More recent studies[69] have shown that although glomerular nephritis may be present, it is probably unrelated to gout. We agree with contemporary students[69, 88] of the disease that the renal lesion incident to gout is primarily a vascular sclerosis similar to that seen in other portions of the vascular system. Indeed, arterial and arteriolar sclerosis can be readily seen.

Cardiovascular Lesions.—Since vascular sclerosis is the predominant trait of the pathology of the gouty kidney, one might anticipate a higher than average incidence of generalized vascular disease and hypertension. Some authors contend that "the gout is to the arteries as the rheumatism is to the heart." [89] Others opine that "gout has nothing to do with arteriosclerosis," [90] and hypertension is a chance finding. Actually, the incidence of *arteriosclerosis and hypertension* is higher in gouty subjects than in a control group of comparable age.[69, 91, 92, 93] The latter is usually a late manifestation. The triad of arteriosclerosis, nephrosclerosis, and increased arterial tension frequently leads to hypertrophy of the left ventricle. Marked arteriosclerotic degeneration of the aorta is not uncommon. Extensive coronary and cerebral vascular disease may be the immediate cause of death. Terminal pericarditis has been reported. Other pathological changes associated with the disease are similar in nature and extent to those found in any corresponding age group.

Comparative Pathology.—A condition resembling chronic tophaceous gout is known to occur spontaneously in birds[94, 95, 96, 97] and may be produced experimentally by prolonged and abundant feeding of protein,[94, 98] by ligation of the ureters, or by removing or poisoning the kidneys.[81, 99, 100] Under these conditions, urate deposition in the joint cartilages takes place and large tophi appear in the extremities. Urate precipitates may appear in practically all tissues. Although anatomically avian gout is similar to the human disease, the pathophysiology is not strictly comparable. In birds practically all nitrogenous waste is transformed to uric acid and interference with renal excretion may result in blood uric acid levels as high as 400 mg. per cent. Feeding of meat alone may elevate it to over 30 mg. per cent. Acute attacks simulating those in human gout have not been described.

A disorder occurring in hogs is of particular interest because it constitutes the only known disturbance in intermediary purine metabolism. Virchow,[101] and later Mendelson,[102] described crystalline deposits resembling guanine in muscle and joints of pigs. This finding was confirmed by chemical analysis.[103] Pecile[104] discovered guanine in the urine of a "gouty" pig. Since this substance is not normally present,[105] it appears that inability to oxidize guanine accounts for this rare disorder. Nothing is known about the clinical appearance of these animals, since the various observations were made postmortem in the course of inspection for Trichinella spiralis.

INCIDENCE

The incidence of gout is unknown. The statistics reported for various sections of the United States of America and other countries are difficult to evaluate.[71, 106, 107, 108, 109] They range from a small fraction of one per cent among meat-eating people[107] to seven per cent in natives of India who are largely vegetarians and teetotalers.[109] These astonishing variations are due partly to the differences in populations studied and in diagnostic standards applied and to the variable degree in which physicians are familiar with and aware of this disease. Undoubtedly many more cases are seen in private practice than in hospitals because acute gouty arthritis is, as a rule, self-limited and of short duration. Hench[71] estimates that five per cent of all patients with joint disease seen at the Mayo Clinic have gout. This is a much higher incidence than has been found in most other clinics. Perhaps the best available evidence is derived from pathological studies. Beitzke[140] who examined 200 unselected cadavers over twenty years of age found histological proof of gouty arthritis in ten cases. Heine[141] in postmortem studies on 1002 patients ranging from fifteen to ninety-five years old noted an incidence of 1.1 per cent. Considering such marked discrepancies and the lack of definite clinical data, the authors do not accept the view that gout is a rare or even declining disease.[110, 111] In our opinion the diagnosis frequently is not made because the patient does not exhibit the classical features of chronic gout. Alertness to its early manifestations and application of modern diagnostic means will enable us to gain more reliable knowledge concerning the incidence of the disease.

Heredity.—From the time the first clinical observations on gout were made, medical writers have stressed its hereditary nature. More recent specific reports vary greatly, some[112, 113, 114] showing a low, others[78, 115, 116] a significantly high familial incidence. There can be little doubt that the frequency with which one obtains affirmative information on this point depends upon the thoroughness with which the inquiry is pursued. Circumspect questioning on repeated visits and interviews with the patient's relatives have often procured a positive family history where it had been denied previously. The propensity of the disease to pass over one generation is an additional hindrance to the investigator gathering genealogical data. It is commonly stated that women, although infrequent victims of gout, are very likely to transmit it to their children.[76] Thus a patient may have inherited his maternal grandfather's gout although his mother never experienced any clinical manifestations of the disease. A familial incidence as high as 75 per cent has been observed.[78, 117] Similar well-authenticated reports and the frequent finding of hyperuricemia in the patient's kin, who do not exhibit other signs of gout,[118, 119, 120] lead us to consider that gout is always an inherited disease. Those workers who are of the opinion that the disease can be acquired believe that this acquired characteristic can be transmitted, a genetic possibility which most biologists would seriously question.

Sex.—Slightly over 95 per cent of all individuals afflicted with the disease are males. It is stated that women are less prone to develop tophi.[71, 76, 121] The explanation for this strikingly different incidence of gout in the two sexes is unknown.

Age.—Since gout is an inherited disease, its potentialities are assumed to be present at birth. The finding of hyperuricemia in apparently normal young relatives of gouty patients and its presence with or without tophi in adults for years prior to the onset of articular complaints indicate that the disease antedates the appearance of symptoms. It very rarely manifests itself in infancy or the teens. Acute arthritis occurs with increasing frequency from the second to the sixth decade, being most common in the forties. However, the first evidence of the disease may not appear until late in life; cases are on record demonstrating the initiation of symptoms in the sixties, seventies, and eighties. In such instances, the attacks as well as the subsequent course tend to be mild. The converse is likewise true, onset at an early age frequently portends severe seizures, often polyarticular in distribution, and may lead to extensive crippling and severe vascular nephritis before middle life.

Race and Climate.—There is at present no accurate information concerning the relevance to gout of either race or climate. Allegedly a disease of the temperate zones, it is known to occur in the tropics, and does affect Negroes, Chinese, and East Indians. Until we have more comprehensive analyses, further discussion will be baseless.

Habits and Occupation.—Those who believe that gout is the nemesis of high living quote a higher incidence among people whose occupation is conducive to overindulgence in food and drink. Until more conclusive statistical information concerning the occupational incidence of the disease is available, it is impossible to evaluate past statements or to make further comment. The incidence of gout among lead workers will be discussed later.

CLINICAL MANIFESTATIONS AND COURSE

The symptomatic or articular manifestations of gout have been designated by various terms. The acute attacks, which are followed by complete remissions, have been called *acute gout,* and *regular* and *acute recurrent gouty arthritis,* in distinction from chronic gout, signifying chronic gouty arthritis with or without tophi. Hench[71] has proposed a somewhat arbitrary classification, dividing the disease into two phases, each including two stages, based on degrees of clinical severity and the presence or absence of hyperuricemia. Because this suggests an obligatory clinical course, which indeed this disease with its extremely diversified and irregular manifestations does not follow, and since hyperuricemia is almost invariably associated with the first attacks of gouty arthritis, we prefer the simpler, and equally satisfactory classification of acute and chronic gouty arthritis.

The *onset* of the first attack of *acute gouty arthritis* is, as a rule, dramatic. The individual, usually a healthy appearing, middle-aged man, is suddenly seized with severe, sometimes excruciating pain, often in one of the metatarsophalangeal joints. Although such attacks frequently begin at night, they may occur at any time. Within a few hours of the onset, the afflicted joint is swollen, red, hot, and exquisitely tender. The swelling may appear so rapidly that within a few hours the patient may be unable to remove his shoe without cutting it. The inflammatory edema is much more marked than in other acute arthritides and often extends some distance beyond the joint margins. Effusions into the larger joints are not uncommon. At the peak of the attack, the intense swelling of the foot accompanied by redness and increased heat resembles septic inflammation or an extensive cellulitis. There may be an associated lymphangitis. The skin is red, tense, and shiny. The superficial veins are distended. The *pain,* often described as "crushing," usually worse at night, generally confines the patient to his bed or room because weight-bearing is intolerable.

As tenderness and redness subside, pitting edema is demonstrable. With the disappearance of the swelling, the overlying skin appears loose and thin, and desquamation of the cutis and itching may follow. The combination of these findings is rarely encountered in other types of acute arthritis, and therefore of singular diagnostic significance. The attack subsides spontaneously, within ten days to a few weeks, with complete restoration of normal joint function and health.

Approximately 50 per cent of the initial attacks are confined to the first metatarsophalangeal joint, but not infrequently other joints are affected at the same time. The neighboring metatarsal and tarsal joints or those of the opposite foot may be involved simultaneously or in rapid succession. A bursa, more commonly that over the olecranon or patella, may be the site of an attack. The younger the individual, the more likely is the attack to be polyarticular and migratory in nature. *Fever,* again more prominent in young patients, is usually mild, rarely lasts for more than a few days and may be entirely absent. The severity of the initial attack varies greatly. In some individuals the acute illness is extremely mild and lasts only a few days. Occasionally one sees abortive attacks.

Physical examination at the time of the first attack of gouty arthritis is usually negative except for the articular findings. Maximal joint tenderness is usually present on the mesial aspects of the involved joint. A tophus, unknown to the patient, may be found in the helix of the ear, indicating that the disease has been present for some time.

The *clinical course subsequent to the initial attack,* although usually conforming to a distinct pattern, may vary considerably. Very rarely the patient remains symptom-free altogether or for an interval of many years as exemplified by one instance in which the initial seizure at twenty-seven years of age was succeeded by the second one sixty-two years later.[121] In the benign form, two to six attacks may be scattered over a period of thirty to fifty years or concentrated in one of the middle decades of life.

The *recurrent attacks* of acute arthritis are commonly followed by remissions during which the patient experiences no articular symptoms whatever. These latent periods tend to become progressively shorter until acute episodes occur once or twice yearly, often with a certain regularity. Some patients, for unexplained reasons, are taken ill each spring and fall. At this stage of the disease, the patient is less likely to experience complete remissions and his illness is approaching or has entered upon the phase of chronic gouty arthritis or chronic gout. In very few instances, most of which belong to the juvenile form, the disease is chronic from the onset. More frequently a period of five to forty years separates the initial attack from the chronic phase.

In the *advanced stages* of the disease, an increasing number of joints are affected, particularly those of the feet, hands, ankles and wrists and the knees and elbows. Subcutaneous tophi, representing infiltrations of urates into periarticular and bursal tissues are then frequently found and are

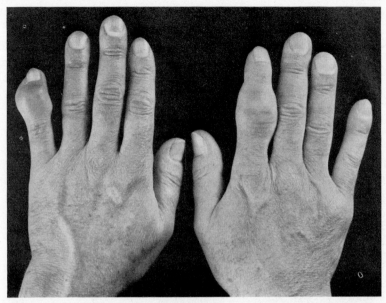

Fig. 113.—Knob-like deformities of a terminal and a midphalangeal joint due to tophaceous deposits.

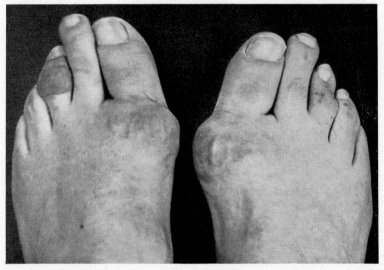

Fig. 114.—Deformities of the first metatarsophalangeal joints caused by bony and soft tissue urate deposits. Tophi are present in both third toes. On the right, the tophaceous deposit is considerably reduced in size because of previous extrusion of the chalklike material.

responsible for the knobby deformities of the knuckles and the interphalangeal joints (Figs. 113 and 114). They may also be seen about the knee and elbow and along the tendons of the fingers, toes, ankles, and wrists. Tophaceous deposits occur in nonarticular cartilage; indeed their most common site in chronic gout is the helix of the ear (Fig. 115). They vary in size from a barely palpable nodule to deposits measuring as much as 5 cm. in diameter. Their presence in cartilage may be unattended by any symptoms, but in subcutaneous tissue visible inflammatory reaction usually results. Here, the deposits appear first as slightly reddened elevations which gradually develop into white, cream-colored or yellow nodules of varying size (Fig. 116, *A*). The skin overlying a tophus may ulcerate (Fig. 116, *B*) and discharge a white, chalky material which on microscopic examination shows the characteristic acicular crystals of sodium urate. Such ulcerating lesions may occur anywhere on the body surface but are more common in hands and feet. They rarely become infected.

Tophi are found in about 50 per cent of all cases of gout. In some they antedate the acute joint disease, while in others they are not found until

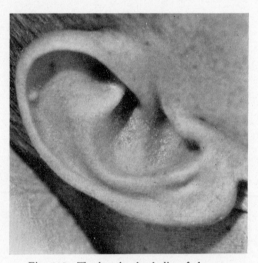

Fig. 115.—Tophus in the helix of the ear.

ten to thirty years after the initial attack. They should not be confused with the subcutaneous nodules of rheumatic fever and rheumatoid arthritis. Because they constitute the one pathognomonic lesion of gout, they should always be searched for. Regardless of whether a nodule has the characteristic clinical appearance of a tophus, it is unwise to accept it as such until it has been needled and the monosodium urate crystals (Fig. 112) have been demonstrated or a positive murexide test has been obtained.

The term, *irregular gout*, still used by some writers, designated a group of nondescript symptoms which in the past has also been referred to as *lithemia* or as a *uric acid, lithic acid,* or *gouty diathesis*. The clinical markings of irregular gout were most varied and it apparently incorporated all the inexplicable complaints which occurred in the gouty subject. Some of these were probably the result of medication with impure colchicum preparations. However, the term was also applied to the indefinite ailments of members of gouty families who had never suffered an attack of gouty arthritis. In these latter cases the symptoms were often ascribed to "an excess of uric acid" proved by the finding of urate sediments in the urine! We do not recognize this or an irregular type of articular gout postulated by some current writers.[122, 123] The patients described, usually women, exhibit none of the characteristic findings of symptomatic gout. Their arthritis is insidious in onset, slowly progressive without remissions or associated tophi. As a rule, these individuals are advanced in years and show only a slightly higher than normal blood uric acid value. In a few cases, hyperuricemia, probably due to nephritis, and rarely a family history of gout were found. If such variations of gout occur, they should be suscep-

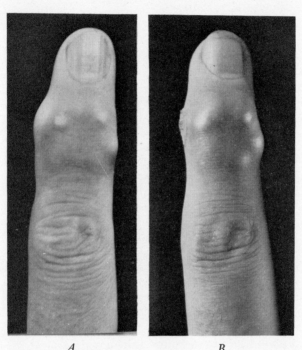

A   *B*

Fig. 116.—Tophaceous deposits about the terminal phalangeal joint of an index finger (*A*), which subsequently increased in size causing breakdown of the overlying skin and discharge of urates (*B*).

tible to pathological proof and when present, generally show favorable response to the therapy administered for acute gouty arthritis. We are equally dubious of the propriety of using such terms as visceral or abarticular gout.

PREMONITORY SYMPTOMS

The specific changes which presumably take place in the gouty subject between birth and the onset of the clinical illness have not been studied, but hyperuricemia has been demonstrated at an early age.[118, 119, 120] Whether it is ever present at birth, we do not know, nor do we understand the bodily alterations immediately preceding the gouty seizure, the so-called *larval state*. Many patients experience no premonition of the impending attack; some even claim to feel their best at that time. Others complain

of anorexia, nausea, indigestion, melancholia, stiffness, aching, polyuria, and
nocturia. The diuresis may be taken as an expression of the altered mineral
metabolism, while the other prodromata remain unexplained.

PRECIPITATING FACTORS

Considerable importance is generally attached to a number of factors
said to precipitate attacks of arthritis in a patient with latent gout. Their
true significance in relation to the disease has not been determined, and it
is difficult to evaluate how often they are chance associations.

Trauma.—Minor or major trauma has long been considered the most
common precipitating factor. Tissue necrosis was postulated by Ebstein[81]
as a prerequisite to urate deposition which can be induced in this manner.
The prevalent involvement of the joints of the large toes has been attributed
to chronic strain on these articulations sustained in walking or from pressure of ill-fitting shoes. Many similar examples of injury as an antecedent to
gouty arthritis can be cited. The rôle of trauma in gouty arthritis is susceptible to and should be determined by exact experimental studies.

Food.—The belief that certain foods are promotive of gout is one of
the oldest medical traditions and is still accepted by a majority of competent clinicians. It recently received succor from European physicians who
claimed to have observed a reduced incidence of gout during the first
World War in countries suffering from a shortage of food in general and
particularly of meat. The proponents of this theory contend that the ingestion of purine-rich articles by the gouty subject results in an accumulation
of uric acid in the blood, thus inducing an acute attack of gout. Habitual
dietary excesses are considered predisposing factors, whereas periodic
indulgence supposedly serves as a precipitating force.[71] It is a most regrettable circumstance that these teachings, which are shrouded in the semi-
sanctity of a long and venerable heritage, have never been tested by either
adequate experimentation or comprehensive statistical analysis of clinical
data. A careful survey of the past and current literature reveals the astonishing fact that conclusive evidence pertaining to the effect of dietary
regulation on clinical gout is entirely lacking.

Because of the far-reaching practical importance of this question, we
recommend the consideration of the relevant basic facts. Since predisposition to gout is inherited, it follows that dietary factors cannot be the cause
of the disease. While it is well proved that a high *purine intake* will raise
the blood uric acid content of the gouty subject, it has likewise been shown
that neither hyperuricemia nor an elevated uric acid concentration in tissue
fluids is by itself always sufficient to produce an attack of gouty arthritis
even in a predisposed individual. High purine diets do not provoke the
acute illness in latent gout with any regularity and no correlation has been
possible between the degree of hyperuricemia and the frequency, severity
and duration of arthritis in gouty patients. It has been found that most
gouty subjects do not show an adverse response to occasional excess purine
feedings and that in well-controlled studies covering an extended period,
the frequency of seizures does not vary in alternating intervals of high and
low purine intake. The incidence of gout among vegetarians is much higher
than is generally assumed.[109]

The natural course of the disease is characterized by very sudden changes in an erratic, unpredictable pattern. The temptation to both patient and physician to fasten the responsibility for these to some tangible factor is great, but the evidence quoted here should caution us against accepting as verified the influence of dietary habits on the development and progress of gout.

It has also been stated that certain foods, regardless of their purine content, are capable of producing attacks regularly in some gouty patients, supposedly as an allergic manifestation. A specific brand of cheese or wine or a particular kind of fruit or vegetable has been held responsible. We have not made similar observations.

Attacks have been observed subsequent to the institution of a keto-genic[124] or high fat diet. Lockie[125] proposed that the latter be used as a provocative test. Others[126, 127] have not found it successful as such.

Alcohol.—Some clinicians consider ingestion of alcohol the most important of all precipitating factors. Fermented beverages are thought to be much more provocative than distilled liquors. Attempts have even been made to relate the incidence of gout in a given community to the type of alcoholic beverage prevalently consumed. Others hold the mode of use a significant circumstance, considering that individuals who overindulge in meat habitually partake of red wine and malt liquors, and therefore sustain the combined effect of two inciting agents. All are agreed that certain gouty individuals fare sumptuously with some regularity and that some of their attacks follow dietary and alcoholic indiscretions. However, this sequence more often does not exist even in the same patient. One subject experienced but two attacks in twenty years, although his debaucheries continued throughout the symptom-free interval, another suffered ten attacks in ten years during middle life and none during the subsequent fifteen years, while his habits of eating and drinking remained unchanged. Instances of this description are by no means exceptional and serve to emphasize that the instrumentality of alcohol in precipitating gouty arthritis is unproved. Actually chronic alcoholics[121] have been said to show no higher and teetotalers no lower than the average incidence. Only the collection of accurate data from a significant number of cases will give us the final answer.

Medicinal Preparations.—Attacks of gouty arthritis are said to have followed the administration of liver extract intramuscularly, of salyrgan, ergotamine tartrate, insulin, decholin, thiamine chloride and other medicinal agents. The case reports are too sparse to allow a conclusion as to cause and effect.

Operations.—Hench[128] has repeatedly stressed that gout should be suspected when arthritis occurs during the first seven days following a surgical procedure. The exact incidence of postoperative gout is unknown.

Miscellaneous Factors.—Coincidental diseases such as leukemia, polycythemia, and chronic glomerular nephritis, as well as marked blood loss and transfusions are said to have activated latent gout. Severe purgation, foreign protein therapy, exposure to cold and dampness, and emotional upsets have been accused of producing attacks.

DIAGNOSIS

Clinical Diagnosis.—The diagnosis of joint diseases is relatively easy, in most instances, when based upon a detailed medical history and a complete physical examination. A few well-chosen laboratory tests or a therapeutic trial with specific medication are often valuable adjuncts. Biopsy may be necessary. The passage of time and further observation are indispensable.

A history of recurrent attacks of acute arthritis spaced by completely asymptomatic intervals should always suggest a diagnosis of gout, particularly in a middle-aged male. Provided the presence of the disease is suspected, confirmation in most instances is relatively simple. The abrupt onset of severe articular pain, usually without known cause, followed rapidly by a red, hot swelling of the joint, extending beyond the articular margins, is of great diagnostic significance especially in a first attack. Additional aids are a positive family history, positive identification of tophi and the occurrence of cuticular desquamation as the edema subsides, a finding highly characteristic of gouty arthritis. The dramatic response to full doses of colchicine, rarely observed in any other types of arthritis, is of real diagnostic significance.

Laboratory Findings.—Our experience with gout has led us to conclude that hyperuricemia is an almost invariable if not constant feature of the disease. Its presence, therefore, if not attributable to other causes, constitutes evidence of prime importance. We have rarely found serum uric-acid values lower than 6 mg. per cent. In the few exceptions (less than 2 per cent), they varied between 5.2 and 5.8 mg. per cent.

For the determination of uric acid, we use either one of the two most commonly employed methods, that of Folin[11] or that of Benedict.[12] Both depend upon reduction of complex tungstate reagents to colored compounds. This reaction is not strictly specific for uric acid and may be enhanced or inhibited by unrelated substances present in the blood. While neither test offers undue technical difficulties, only the greatest care in preparing the reagents and frequent control determinations assure reliable results. The use of *serum* is preferable to that of whole blood. Since the distribution of urates between plasma and cells is a function of the bicarbonate, specimens should be collected and centrifuged under oil if the greatest accuracy is desired. Folin's[129] method for unlaked whole blood is free from the objections to other whole blood methods, but since it is doubtful whether diffusion of urates from the cells is ever complete, the method should not be used if sufficient blood can be obtained for a determination on serum. Recently, Blauch and Kloch[130] determined the uric acid content of normal whole blood directly with the aid of the specific enzyme, uricase, and found values ranging from 1.04 to 3.83 mg. per cent. From these considerations it will be immediately apparent that one cannot interpret blood uric acid values correctly unless the standard for each method used has been established by a sufficient number of determinations on normals. Comparison of the values obtained in different laboratories has shown wide discrepancies which may partially be accounted for in this manner.

No characteristic change in *serum uric acid* occurs immediately prior to an acute attack of gouty arthritis. In some instances, it remains unchanged, in others it may be increased or decreased. In order to avoid erroneous interpretations, particularly of response to therapy, it is extremely important to appreciate that the blood uric acid level is inconstant, cyclic changes occurring at irregular intervals. In one case, variations between 7.4 and 14.5 mg. per cent were observed[85] which could not be attributed to any known cause and were in no way related to the incidence of arthritis. Various tests[68] designed to measure the urate-concentrating power of the kidney are neither entirely satisfactory nor necessarily of diagnostic value in gout.

We have had an opportunity to analyze the synovial fluid from five effusions in gouty arthritis. The detailed findings compared to normal values[131] are given in table 2. Urate crystals were never observed in these fluids, but have been seen in synovial fluid obtained post mortem from cases of chronic gouty arthritis.

Patients with acute gouty arthritis generally have a mild to moderate *leukocytosis*. The mononuclear count is frequently increased. The sedi-

TABLE 2

SYNOVIAL FLUID IN GOUTY ARTHRITIS

	Normal			Gout		
	Average	Low	High	Average	Low	High
Leukocytes, per cu. mm.......	63	13	180	13,800	1,000	31,400
Polymorphonuclears, per cu. mm...................	6.5	0	25	83	48	94
Relative viscosity............	150	51	403	4.8	3.6	5.9
Protein, gm. per 100 cc.......	1.72	1.31	2.13	4.30	3.10	4.97
Globulin, gm. per 100 cc......	.05	......	....	1.39	1.08	1.79
Mucin N, gm. per 100 cc.	.105	.068	.135	.065	.034	.098
Sugar.....................	Essentially same as in serum			Essentially same as in serum		
Uric acid.................	" " " " "			" " " " "		

mentation rate may be elevated. In several cases, we have seen rates as high as 2.0 mm. per minute (the upper limit of normal being .40 mm. per minute[132]). Evidence of mild renal impairment is commonly met. Achlorhydria occurs no more frequently in gouty patients than in other individuals. An abnormal sugar tolerance curve, occasionally present, is of no diagnostic significance.

Roentgenologic Findings.—The roentgenographic findings most suggestive of gout are well-defined, *punched-out areas*, usually 5 mm. or more in diameter. They are commonly observed in the subchondral bone at the bases or heads of the phalanges (Figs. 117 and 118). The feet are more apt to show these lesions even in cases in which they have never been affected clinically. Such changes may appear late in the disease, as demonstrated in 19 per cent of one series.[133] The nineteen patients had had gout for twenty-eight years or longer, exhibited tophi and hyperuricemia in every instance, yet failed to show subchondral lesions roentgenographically. The frequency with which these defects, the result of urate deposition in bone, are found is

21

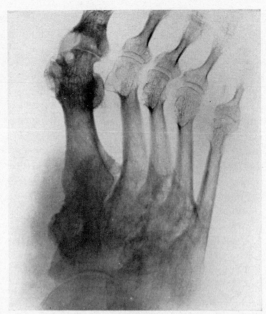

Fig. 117.—Characteristic punched-out areas seen in the bones of the first metatarso-phalangeal joint.

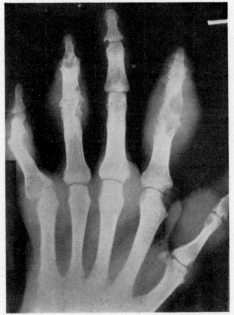

Fig. 118.—Extensive destruction of the phalangeal and metacarpophalangeal joints of a patient suffering from chronic gouty arthritis.

directly related to the severity of the disease. They may be demonstrable in the region of joints not commonly affected, for instance, in the neighborhood of the sacro-iliac (Fig. 119). They should be distinguished from

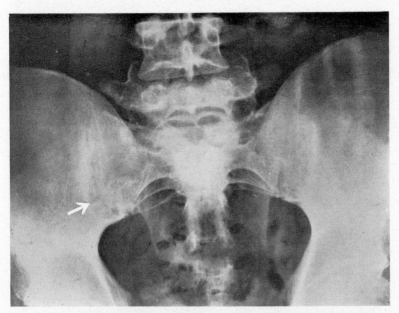

Fig. 119.—The punched-out areas in the region of the sacro-iliac joints of this roentgenogram, indicated by the arrow, are due to urate deposition.

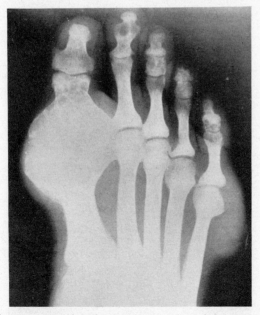

Fig. 120.—In this instance urate deposits caused expansion of the bones of the first metatarsophalangeal joint, thus giving the appearance of a bone tumor.

the circumscribed areas of rarefaction seen in degenerative joint disease and rheumatoid arthritis. Similar findings may be produced by the gummata of syphilis, by leprosy and yaws, as well as by tuberculosis and Boeck's sarcoid. Occasionally, tophaceous deposits result in bone expansion (Fig. 120)

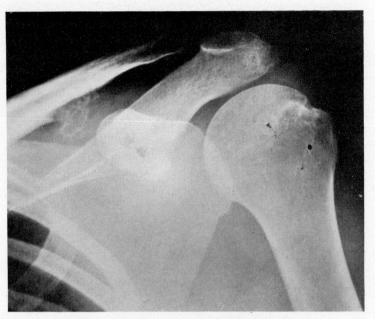

Fig. 121.—Destruction of the cortex of the clavicle due to urate deposition. The mass of extruded material is clearly illustrated.

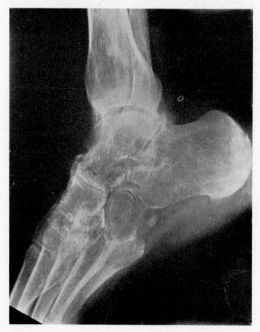

Fig. 122.—Lateral view of a foot, showing marked decalcification, destruction of the joint spaces and ankylosis. This patient had widespread ankylosis at the age of twenty-eight years.

or bone expansion and destruction (Fig. 121), thus simulating, roentgen-ographically, a bone tumor. In addition to such abnormalities, one may find soft tissue thickening, joint narrowing, conspicuous marginal overgrowth, and marked destruction of the articulating surfaces.

Decalcification is rarely seen except in patients who have suffered pro-longed severe attacks involving the small joints of the feet and wrists. In these exceptional instances, the marked decalcification, joint destruction and obvious ankylosis closely approximate the changes seen in specific infec-tious or rheumatoid arthritis (Figs. 122 and 123). Premature arteriosclerosis is frequently demonstrable in the vessels of the legs and feet.

Although the *x*-ray findings in gouty arthritis are characteristic and consistent, they cannot be considered specific. The roentgenologist's im-

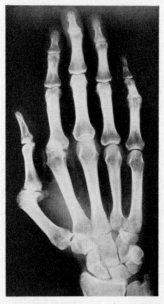

Fig. 123.—Hand of the patient referred to in the legend of figure 122. The phalan-geal joints are narrowed. The midphalangeal joint of the little finger is fused. There is obvious destruction of the metacarpophalangeal joints of the first and second fingers.

pression should therefore be taken only as corroboration of a clinical diagnosis.

Provocative Tests.—Our experience with provocative tests has been most disappointing whether they were applied immediately after an attack or during a remission. This has been true of a high-purine (2.5 to 3 gm.) or a high-fat (250 to 300 gm.) diet, or of large amounts of port wine admin-istered singly or in combination with the others. Failure to precipitate at-tacks with any regularity has caused us to abandon these tests as of no diagnostic aid.

Differential Diagnosis.—Occasionally gouty arthritis may be confused with traumatic joint disease, cellulitis, rheumatic fever, one of the specific infectious arthritides, rheumatoid arthritis, Heberden's nodes and acute bursitis, particularly when the latter is associated with a hallux valgus deformity.

Traumatic arthritis is as a rule readily diagnosed. Articular pain and swelling follow almost immediately upon a known injury. Marked inflammatory reaction of the periarticular tissue is not discernible and the symptoms always remain confined to the affected joint. The patient exhibits none of the characteristics of the gouty individual and his arthritis never responds to colchicine therapy. However, it should be remembered that trauma may mark the onset of acute gout as well as of infectious arthritis. In such cases differentiation is greatly aided by aspiration and analysis of the joint fluid. An acute traumatic effusion contains rarely more than 1000 leukocytes per cubic millimeter and polymorphonuclears ranging from 0 to 20 per cent, in contrast to the higher values usually found in the other acute arthritides.[117]

Cellulitis or septic inflammation is frequently suspected; in fact, sometimes it is diagnosed before it becomes evident that one is actually dealing with acute gouty arthritis. Occasionally, the affected joints have been incised and drained. One can readily appreciate the diagnostic difficulties offered by a patient who presents himself with a painful, red, hot swelling of the dorsum of the hand or foot with or without lymphangitis and fever. Failure to find a skin abrasion or other portal of entry for an invading organism and careful elucidation of the past history will generally lead to the correct diagnosis.

Rheumatic fever, especially in younger individuals, can be simulated by recurrent attacks of gouty arthritis as in the following case history. A young man of nineteen years entered the hospital with a provisional diagnosis of rheumatic fever. At the age of nine he suffered from a hip affliction which was considered tuberculous in origin and treated by immobilization in plaster casts. Between the ages of fourteen and nineteen he experienced numerous attacks of polyarthritis, migratory in nature and accompanied by fever. They were always followed by complete recovery and diagnosed rheumatic fever, although he did not develop endocarditis. When first seen by us, he had a blood uric acid level of 9.2 mg. per cent. Since then the fasting serum values have varied between 12.3 and 14.8 mg. per cent and he has developed tophi. Undoubtedly a good many similar cases of juvenile gout are mislabeled rheumatic fever. The clinical differentiation, however, should not be difficult. The arthritis of rheumatic fever usually follows an upper respiratory infection or other precipitating factor by seven to fourteen days. Patients frequently exhibit weight loss, nose bleeds, skin eruptions, subcutaneous nodules, tachycardia and precordial pain. The electrocardiogram often shows a prolonged P-R interval and other alterations. The ultimate development of valvular heart disease is of the utmost diagnostic importance.

Specific infectious arthritis, due to a pyogenic organism, in the acute phase more nearly resembles acute gouty arthritis than does any other type of joint disease, particularly since it may occasionally be recurrent in nature. In such instances, usually caused by the gonococcus, the clinical picture may show some similarity to that of gout, as in the case of a patient who entered the hospital suffering from his eighth attack of arthritis. He stated that recovery from the previous seven seizures had been complete. Differentiation was facilitated by a history of genito-urinary infection and such constitutional symptoms as chills and fever preceding in close parallelism every exacerbation of arthritis. Although the inflammatory swelling of specific infectious arthritis may be severe, it rarely is as marked or occurs as precipitously as in gouty arthritis. Particularly with the aid of synovial fluid findings, one should not encounter serious diagnostic difficulties.

Typical *rheumatoid arthritis*, ushered in by constitutional, vasomotor, and neurological symptoms, of insidious onset and characterized by symmetrical joint involvement, should rarely if ever be mistaken for gouty arthritis. However, in 18 per cent of all cases rheumatoid arthritis is marked by an atypical onset and in 7 per cent it may remain atypical for a long time. In this form, an apparently healthy individual experiences an acute attack of arthritis without prodromata, preceding acute illness, or obvious focus of infection. The joint involvement may be polyarticular, migratory or occasionally monarticular. Recovery from the first attack is often complete and the remission may last for a few months or even years. The patient may have a number of attacks before the disease becomes chronic. Careful clinical observation and determination of the blood uric acid concentration will facilitate the distinction between the two diseases.

The clinical features of chronic gout with ankylosis may resemble those of rheumatoid arthritis even more closely. We have seen two such cases in a relatively early stage of the disease, and others have been reported.[84, 134] In one[85] the onset of gout at twenty-one years of age was followed by chronic arthritis within five years. Widespread ankylosis was demonstrable at the age of twenty-eight. The diagnosis of gout was confirmed by the identification of sodium urate crystals in tophi of the ear, in the finger, the olecranon bursa and the tissues of four joints examined. Of particular interest were the findings in the astragalotibial joint. Extensive pannus formation, responsible for complete fibrous ankylosis, simulated strikingly the gross pathological changes of rheumatoid arthritis. Even the microscopic appearance of the synovial tissues might have been difficult to distinguish definitely from the chronic inflammatory lesions of rheumatoid arthritis except for innumerable small urate foci (see figures 107 and 108). Such unusual forms of gouty arthritis are admittedly rare. They should not be confused with rheumatoid arthritis. Clinical differentiation is greatly aided by painstaking inquiry into the past and family histories. Biopsies of nodules, tophi, and synovial tissue will often ascertain the correct diagnosis. Synovial fluid analysis may or may not help to distinguish one from the other. Association of the two diseases is extremely scarce. A few cases have been reported, but we know of no authenticated instance.

Bursitis, particularly as a manifestation of a hallux valgus deformity, has probably been mislabeled gouty arthritis on innumerable occasions. This diagnostic error can be avoided if the affected part is carefully examined. The swelling is limited to the bursa and the immediately adjacent tissue, and the distended sac may be easily palpated. The metatarsophalangeal joint motions are painless within a limited range.

Heberden's nodes, classical stigmata of degenerative joint disease, consist of hypertrophic osseous changes, at the articular margins of the terminal interphalangeal joints. They are insidious in development, not usually productive of severe symptoms, and may be readily differentiated from tophaceous deposits in the skin and deeper tissues surrounding these joints. Occasionally, however, Heberden's nodes are acute in onset and have then frequently been confused with gouty arthritis. The distal finger joints may be painful, reddened, bulbous, fluctuant and extremely tender. Numbness and tingling of the involved fingers may also be complained of. Heberden's nodes occur predominantly in women and affect the index and middle fingers more often than the other phalanges. Tophi are much more common in males and are discernible by their yellowish color. It is well known, of course, that the two disorders may be associated coincidentally or causally.

COMPLICATIONS

Cardiovascular Lesions.—As stated in the section on pathology, premature vascular disease and the anatomical and physiological alterations resulting therefrom constitute the important complications of gout. Some of the older writers[76, 121] have stressed the high incidence of venous thrombosis, a finding which has been rare in our observation.

Renal Disease.—The appearance of persistent albuminuria and casts usually marks the beginning of a vascular nephritis which may ultimately be fatal. The majority of gouty patients die from uremia. Because of the frequency with which nephritis occurs in gout, Hench states, "Chronic arthritis associated with distinct renal impairment suggests gout until proven otherwise."[133] Some writers speak of secondary gout caused by chronic nephritis, other renal disease, or leukemia. From our experience, we have concluded that such instances represent latent gout complicated by other diseases associated with hyperuricemia. Under these conditions, it is important to obtain a detailed family history and if possible blood uric acid determinations on the patient's relatives.

Urinary Calculi.—The incidence of urinary calculi in gouty subjects is relatively high, amounting to 12 per cent in Hench's series.[133] An occasional patient may experience one or more bouts of renal colic prior to the first gouty seizure. Arthritis in connection with urinary lithiasis should always suggest the diagnosis of gout. No sound theoretical explanation for the frequent association of the two conditions is known. The incidence of urate stones has not been determined.

Saturnine Gout.—Previously gout was assumed to be prevalent among lead workers, hence the term, *saturnine gout.* It, too, was considered an example of secondary gout due, in this instance, to the vascular nephritis of plumbism. While gout is more rarely a complication of lead poisoning than was previously assumed,[135] it may of course be associated by chance with the vascular nephritis of plumbism. Other types of arthritis occurring in an individual with hyperuricemia due to renal damage from lead poisoning may in the past also have been erroneously diagnosed gout.

Miscellaneous Complications.—Episcleritis due to urate deposits occurs rarely.[117, 142] Eczema, psoriasis, and various complications reported are no more frequent than in other individuals of comparable age and are probably unrelated to gout.

TREATMENT

In the current literature on gout it is commonly stated that treatment should be aimed at the *prevention* of the disease. While there can be little disagreement with the ideal goal of therapy, its pursuit in the case of gout would entail a formidable eugenic policy imposing measures of birth control on all gouty subjects and their relatives. The disease could, no doubt, eventually be eradicated in this manner, but the physician should not be encouraged in the unfounded belief that he can prevent gout by the prescription of certain food and drink restraints.

ACUTE ATTACK

Colchicine.—The treatment of the acute attacks of gouty arthritis is extremely satisfactory. Colchicum obtained from the seeds of *Colchicum autumnale* (fall crocus), was first recommended by Alexander of Tralles (525–605)[136] and, as colchicine, remains the drug of choice. Its mode of action in gout is unknown beyond the fact that it does not affect the hyperuricemia nor the renal excretion of uric acid. We have never seen it fail to give relief when administered properly, and it is practically a specific therapeutic agent for the acute illness. It has fallen into disrepute in times past, due undoubtedly to the use of impure or impotent preparations, in the form of the wine or tincture. Therapeutic failures will be avoided if the drug is always administered as crystalline colchicine. The preliminary use of a saline cathartic is recommended by some.[71] We prescribe $\frac{1}{120}$ grain (0.5 mg.) every one or two hours until relief from pain is obtained or until diarrhea or nausea and vomiting result. The drug is then discontinued. Provided the patient is kept at bed rest, pain and swelling usually subside within twenty-four to seventy-two hours after the first loose bowel movement. Rarely do the articular symptoms disappear sooner. The ensuing diarrhea is frequently severe enough to require treatment with paregoric; 4 cc. is given following each loose stool until the diarrhea is checked. Bismuth subcarbonate may be used instead of or in conjunction with paregoric.

Once the amount of colchicine necessary to produce such symptoms has been established for the individual patient, the total dose may be reduced by one or two tablets ($\frac{1}{120}$ or $\frac{1}{60}$ grain) to avoid severe gastrointestinal symptoms without curtailing the desired effect. The total amount required to alleviate the acute attack varies from 8 to 16 tablets ($\frac{1}{15}$ to $\frac{2}{15}$ grain) or granules of colchicine and rarely exceeds this quantity. We have never observed any other untoward effects from crystalline colchicine. Hypersensitivity to the drug is unknown, nor does it lose its efficacy with repeated administrations. The patient should always carry colchicine. The appearance of any prodromal symptoms or the first twinges of articular pain call for immediate institution of therapy. If these rules are followed, the patient will be spared many prolonged and incapacitating seizures. Some object unwisely, but sufficiently, to the side action of colchicine as to delay therapy until the attack has fully developed.

Other Drugs.—We can find no indications for the use of cinchophen and substances closely related to it, either alone or in conjunction with colchicine. To be sure, the risk attendant upon their administration, primarily that of acute liver necrosis, is statistically small, although minor symptoms of toxicity are a more frequent annoyance to the patient and as a warning signal call for immediate cessation of therapy. In omitting these drugs, we are guided by the fact that colchicine, when given properly, is not only entirely safe but also much more effective. Morphine or codeine may be needed to insure comfort before the colchicine effect is secured. At the time of the seizure, no other dietary measures than those given for any painful illness of short duration are required. Patients rarely desire anything more than liquids and soft foods, and a daily fluid intake of 3000 to 4000 cc. should be encouraged.

Rest.—Absolute bed rest is always indicated for the duration of the attacks, whether or not weight-bearing joints are involved. Premature resumption of normal activity not infrequently precipitates an exacerbation. Avoidance of even normal joint use prevents minor trauma, thereby shortening the period of incapacitation. Protection of the affected part by a cradle eliminates the pressure from bed clothing and lessens the chance of accidental jolting. Hot compresses every three hours are a useful adjunct, although an occasional patient derives greater relief from cold *packs*. Moist heat is always preferable to dry heat. *Diathermy* as a rule is not tolerated well.

INTERVAL TREATMENT

It is unfortunate for both patient and physician that interval therapy effective in the prevention of future attacks does not exist.

The few measures which are of positive help are directed against the complications of the disease. The likelihood of urate stone formation is lessened by a liberal daily fluid intake (3000 cc.) and alkalinization of the urine. The latter can be accomplished by administering two to four drams of sodium citrate each day. The pH of the urine can be determined by nitrazine paper. The body weight of the *obese* gouty patient should be reduced in order to avoid the complications of obesity and to minimize traumatization of joints.

Diet.—In accord with a widely disseminated belief that adherence to a rigorous, usually "purine-free" dietary will reduce or eliminate acute seizures and will sufficiently alter the course of the disease as to prevent chronic arthritis and the complications of gout, countless gouty patients have been subjected to undue and sometimes serious nutritional restrictions. In a previous section (p. 636) we have indicated the lack of clinical, statistical and experimental data to justify this particular form of treatment. Nowhere could we find any validly controlled studies in which a significant number of subjects had been observed on a constant metabolic regimen and in which the physiological variations in blood uric acid level were taken into consideration. We also adduced considerable evidence suggesting that dietary regulation, more specifically the addition or omission of purine-containing foods, is probably ineffective in changing the clinical course of gout. Without more convincing proof, we do not consider warranted the imposition of a strict alimentary rule, which the patient usually disobeys because of its monotony and which favors a deficiency in certain amino acids, iron, and vitamin B.

The orthodox diet for gout, low in fat which is said to inhibit urate excretion, and low in purines (100 to 150 mg. as compared to a normal intake of 500 to 800 mg.), is poorly balanced and necessitates a large intake of such protein foods as milk, cheese, and eggs. In contrast, we prescribe a diet appropriate in caloric value, satisfying the usual protein, fat, carbohydrate, mineral, and vitamin requirements, which is well tolerated by gouty patients and has caused no untoward effects. Specifically, we allow any meat, fish, or other sea food once a day. On the other hand, we compromise with current medical practice by excluding from the dietary the foods listed below which contain very large amounts of purine:

PURINE CONTENT PER 100 GRAMS

Sweetbreads	825 mg.
Anchovies	360 mg.
Sardines	300 mg.
Liver	230 mg.
Kidneys	200 mg.
Brains	195 mg.
Meat extracts	160–400 mg.

Although there is no pertinent evidence to indicate that we can thereby lessen the number and severity of attacks or otherwise influence the course of gout, we do so because of the proved difficulty which gouty patients have in disposing of large quantities of uric acid and because as long as the exact etiology of gout is unknown, we have to concede at least the possibility that some patients may be harmfully affected by excessive purine feeding. There is very little meaning in further tabulating individual food articles since different analyses have shown wholly incongruous results. Suffice it to say that meats, fish, and sea food contain 75 to 150 mg. of purine per 100 gm., and that vegetables, fruits, and dairy products contain small or negligible amounts. For reasons previously stated, there is no need to exclude tea, coffee, chocolate and cocoa. Those who adhere to the allergic theory of causation delete from the dietary of the gouty patient all foods to which he is supposedly sensitive (determined by "provocative" effect). Such dietary restrictions have not been successful in our experience. Unqualified abstinence from alcoholic beverages is almost uniformly advocated, although there is no proof of its therapeutic value. We allow small amounts of *alcohol* and in reverence to the dictates of the past, whiskey rather than beer.

Cinchophen has been employed extensively in the interval treatment of gouty arthritis. Its use is advocated in doses of 7.5 grains (0.5 gm.) three times daily for three consecutive days each week. As a precautionary measure against toxic effects, a daily fluid intake of 2 liters, a high carbohydrate diet, and maintenance of an alkaline urine are usually recommended. The theoretical considerations for the use of cinchophen, beyond its well-known analgesic action, warrant a short analysis. It is said to influence gout favorably by promoting urate diuresis, thus lowering the blood uric acid level. Granting this effect on urate elimination, which lasts only two or three days, previously quoted evidence indicates that the course of gout cannot be influenced, at any stage, by a transitory decrease of blood uric acid. Equally enhanced urate diuresis and a similarly effective analgesia can, moreover, be obtained without resorting to a potentially dangerous drug by the administration of 5.3 to 6.6 gm. (80 to 100 grains) of sodium salicylate on three consecutive days each week.[137]

Some authors[138, 139] advise *glycine* 10 gm. daily for three days out of each week in conjunction with salicylates as another means of augmenting the output of urates. We have never employed this combination, but our experience with glycine alone has been disappointing. We have seen no beneficial effects from the administration of thiamin chloride.

Rapidly recurring attacks and chronic gouty arthritis are least amenable to treatment. Some of our patients feel certain that colchicine, grains $\frac{1}{120}$ three times a day, provides a measure of relief. Regular rations of salicylates are often necessary until a relatively asymptomatic period ensues. Wisely chosen physiotherapy, joint aspirations, immobilization of joints, correction of deformities, application of foot pads, special shoes and operative procedures may be indicated in selected cases. Excellent foot care particularly should always be insisted upon. Troublesome tophi can usually be excised safely and without precipitating an attack of gout. We know of no special benefit derived from spa therapy. The complications of gout must be treated according to their specific requirements.

PROGNOSIS

The physician caring for gouty patients must be endowed with a sympathetic understanding of their changing moods and unstable humors. The victims of this disease but mirror the nature of their affliction, the progress of which is punctuated by capricious attacks striking when least expected and abating for an unpredictable period of time. The vicissitudes of gout are part of its natural history and must be considered when therapeutic benefits are to be evaluated or future developments presaged. Characteristically symptomless for years, its first articular manifestation may remain its only one or may at once initiate an unrelentingly advancing ailment. Typically, it leads to recurrent attacks of acute arthritis at decreasing intervals. The fulminating episode, if promptly treated, usually subsides in two to three days, but the chronic seizure may take an intractable course, defying all therapeutic efforts. Actuarial tables show that most gouty patients die five years before their natural *life expectancy*, but the prospect of longevity depends largely upon the presence or absence of complications. If the kidneys escape injury and the attacks are not too frequent or extended, the state of general health may not be significantly affected. Even in the presence of albuminuria, usually taken as an ominous sign, some patients may live for years and reach old age without showing evidence of marked nephritis.

SUMMARY

A modern treatise cannot, perhaps, add substantially to our medical ancestors' knowledge of gout but it can define somewhat more clearly the specific problems requiring investigation. It is for this reason that the inadequacies of both our understanding and treatment of gout have been freely emphasized. We have seen that at two principal junctures the pathogenesis cannot be traced with any degree of certainty. Given a subject predisposed to gout, is his hereditary disorder in effect at any time during life and can it be demonstrated, or what are the circumstances actuating the inhibition of uric acid excretion? An equally stimulating and no better understood problem is offered by the local tissue changes through which asymptomatic hyperuricemia is transformed into a most painful and ofttimes chronic illness. Possibly a better comprehension of these etiologic elements will pave the way to more satisfactory therapy. Colchicine, to be sure, is a safe and highly effective weapon against the acute seizure but the so-called preventive treatment, in so far as it prohibits most of the gratifying and some of the essential dietary articles, is predicated upon unsound theoretical and dubious clinical reasons. A disease, like gout, which has been within the orbit of medicine for many centuries, inevitably carries not only a rich tradition of masterly clinical observation but also certain prejudices and superstitions. It is our obvious duty to reexamine transmitted concepts, including those now accepted by us, from time to time in the light of newly gained experience.

BIBLIOGRAPHY

1. Garrod, A. B., The Nature and Treatment of Gout and Rheumatic Gout, Walton and Maberly, London, 1859.
2. Sydenham, T., Tractatus de podagra et hydrope, G. Kettilby, London, 1683.
3. Scheele, K. W., Examen chemicum calculi urinarii, Opuscula II, p. 73, 1776. Cited from Levene and Bass (see reference number 15).
4. Wollaston, Phil. Tr. London, **87**: 386, 1797.
5. Pearson, G., Phil. Tr. London, **88**: 15, 1798.
6. Garrod, A. B., Medico-Chir. Tr. London, **31**: 83, 1848.
7. Miescher, F. Hoppe Seyler, Medizinisch-Chemische Untersuchungen, p. 441, 1871.
8. Kossel, A., Ztschr. f. physiol. Chem., **3**: 284, 1879; **4**: 290, 1880; **5**: 152, 1881; **10**: 248, 1886; **12**: 241, 1888; Arch. Anat. Physiol., 181, 1891.
9. Fischer, E., Untersuchungen in der Puringruppe. Julius Springer, Berlin, 1907.
10. Folin, O. and Denis, W., J. Biol. Chem., **13**: 469, 1912–1913.
11. Folin, O., J. Biol. Chem., **106**: 311, 1934.
12. Benedict, S. R., and Behre, J. A., J. Biol. Chem., **92**: 161, 1931.
13. Levene, P. A., and Jacobs, W. A., Ber., **42**: 1198, 2102, 2469, 2474, 3247, 1909. Levene, P. A., and London, E. S., J. Biol. Chem., **81**: 711, 1929; **83**: 793, 1929.
14. Levene, P. A., and Simms, H. S., J. Biol. Chem., **65**: 519, 1925; **70**: 327, 1926.
15. Levene, P. A., and Bass, L. W., Nucleic Acids, Chemical Catalog Company, New York, 1931.
16. Krüger, M., Ber., **32**: 2818, 3336, 1899.
    Krüger, M., and Schmid, J., Arch. f. exper. Path. u. Pharmakol., **45**: 259, 1901.
    Krüger, M., and Schmid, J., Ber., **32**: 2677, 1899.
    Krüger, M., and Schmid, J., Ztschr. f. physiol. Chem., **32**: 104, 1901; **36**: 1, 1902.
17. Minkowski, O., Arch. f. exper. Path. u. Pharmakol., **41**: 375, 1898.
18. Thannhauser, S. J., and Czoniczer, G., Ztschr. f. physiol. Chem., **110**: 307, 1920.
19. Jackson, H., Jr., J. Biol. Chem., **59**: 529, 1924.
20. Bielschowsky, F. and Klein, W., Ztschr. f. physiol. Chem., **207**: 202, 1932.
21. Bielschowsky, F., and Klemperer, F., Ztschr. f. physiol. Chem., **211**: 69, 1932.
22. Thannhauser, S. J., and Dorfmüller, G., Ztschr. f. physiol. Chem., **102**: 148, 1918.
23. Thannhauser, S. J., and Ottenstein, B., Ztschr. f. physiol. Chem., **114**: 17, 1921.
24. Thannhauser, S. J., and Bommes, A., Ztschr. f. physiol. Chem., **91**: 336, 1914.
25. Bollman, J. L., Mann, F. C., and Magath, T. B., Am. J. Physiol., **72**: 629, 1925.
    Bollman, J. L., and Mann, F. C., Am. J. Physiol., **104**: 242, 1933.
26. Benedict, S. R., J. Biol. Chem., **20**: 633, 1915.
27. Wiechowski, W., Biochem. Ztschr., **25**: 432, 1910.
28. Fosse, R., Brunel, A., and Thomas, P. E., Compt. rend., **192**: 1615, 1931.
29. Larsen, H. W., J. Biol. Chem., **94**: 727, 1931–1932.
30. Miescher, F., Verhandl. d. Naturforsch. Ges. in Basel, **6**: 138, 1874.
31. Kossel, A., Ztschr. f. physiol. Chem., **10**: 248, 1886.

32. Burian, R., and Schur, H., Ztschr. f. physiol. Chem., **23:** 55, 1897.
33. Burian, R., and Schur, H., Arch. f. d. ges. Physiol., **80:** 241, 1900; **87:** 239, 1901.
34. Rockwood, E. W., Am. J. Physiol., **12:** 38, 1904–1905.
35. Akroyd, H., and Hopkins, F. G., Biochem. J., **10:** 551, 1916.
36. Rose, W. C., and Cook, K. G., J. Biol. Chem., **64:** 325, 1925.
37. György, P., and Thannhauser, S. J., Ztschr. f. physiol. Chem., **180:** 286, 1929.
38. Minkowski, O., Arch. f. exper. Path. u. Pharmakol., **20:** 41, 1886.
39. Horbaczewski, J., Monatsh. d. Chem., **10:** 624, 1889.
40. Spitzer, W., Arch. f. d. ges. Physiol., **76:** 192, 1899.
41. Folin, O., Berglund, H., and Derrick, C., J. Biol. Chem., **60:** 361, 1924.
42. Thannhauser, S. J., and Weinschenk, M., Deutsch. Arch. f. klin. Med., **139:** 100, 1922.
43. Soetbeer, F., and Ibrahim, J., Ztschr. f. physiol. Chem., **35:** 1, 1902.
44. Wiechowski, W., Beitr. z. chem. Phys. u. Path., **11:** 109, 1908.
45. Dohrn, M., Ztschr. f. klin. Med., **74:** 445, 1912.
46. Umber, F., Ernährung und Stoffwechselkrankheiten, Urban und Schwarzenberg, Berlin, 1925.
47. Gudzent, F., Gicht und Rheumatismus, Julius Springer, Berlin, 1928.
48. Bordley, J., III, and Richards, A. N., J. Biol. Chem., **101:** 193, 1933.
49. Smith, H. W., The Physiology of the Kidney, Oxford University Press, New York, 1937.
50. Berglund, H., and Frisk, A. R., Acta Med. Scand., **86:** 233, 1935.
51. Brøchner-Mortensen, K., Acta Med. Scand., Supp. 84, 1938; **99:** 525, 1939.
52. Coombs, F. S., Pecora, L. J., Thorogood, E., Consolazio, W. V., and Talbott, J. H., J. Clin. Investigation, **19:** 525, 1940.
53. Benedict, S. R., J. Lab. & Clin. Med., **2:** 1, 1916–1917.
54. Trimble, H. C.: Personal communication.
55. Wells, H. G., J. Biol. Chem., **35:** 221, 1918.
56. Klemperer, F. W., Trimble, H. C., and Hastings, A. B., J. Biol. Chem., **125:** 445, 1938.
57. Lennox, W. G., J. Biol. Chem., **66:** 521, 1925.
58. Quick, A. J., J. Biol. Chem., **110:** 107, 1935.
59. Harpuder, K., Ztschr. f. d. ges. exper. Med., **42:** 1, 1924.
60. Nicolaier, A., and Dohrn, M., Deutsch. Arch. f. klin. Med., **93:** 331, 1908.
61. Starkenstein, E., Biochem. Ztschr., **106:** 139, 1920.
62. Grabfield, G. P., and Pratt, J. H., J. Pharmacol. and Exper. Therap., **42:** 407, 1931.
63. Sée, G., Bull. de l'Acad. de méd., **6:** 689, 1877 (cited by Grabfield, see reference number 64).
64. Grabfield, G. P., and Knapp, E., J. Pharmacol. and Exper. Therap., **32:** 341, 1928.
65. Grabfield, G. P., and Gray, M. G., J. Pharmacol. and Exper. Therap., **50:** 123, 1934.
    Gray, M. G., and Grabfield, G. P., J. Pharmacol. and Exper. Therap., **52:** 383, 1934.
    Grabfield, G. P., Prescott, B., and Swann, W. K., J. Pharmacol. and Exper. Therap., **61:** 293, 1937.
    Grabfield, G. P., and Swanson, D., J. Pharmacol. and Exper. Therap., **66:** 60, 1939.
66. Thannhauser, S. J., Lehrbuch des Stoffwechsels und der Stoffwechselkrankheiten, J. F. Bergmann, Munich, 1929.
67. Talbott, J. H., and Coombs, F. S., J.A.M.A., **110:** 1977, 1938.
68. Brøchner-Mortensen, K., Acta Med. Scand., **99:** 538, 1939.
69. Schnitker, M. A., and Richter, A. B., Am. J. Med. Sci., **192:** 241, 1936.
70. Lichtwitz, L., and Steinitz, E., Handbuch d. inneren Med., **4:** 830, 1926.
71. Hench, P. S., Modern Medical Therapy in General Practice, p. 3395, Williams and Wilkins Company, Baltimore, 1940.
72. Gibson, H. J., and Kersley, G. D., Med. Press, **196:** 353, 1938.
73. Peters, J. P., and Van Slyke, D. D., Quantitative Clinical Chemistry, Volume 1, p. 415, Williams and Wilkins Company, Baltimore, 1935.
74. Klemperer, G., Verhandl. d. Cong. f. inn. Med., **20:** 219, 1902.
75. His, W., Deutsch. Arch. f. klin. Med., **65:** 156, 1899.
76. Futcher, T. B., in Osler, Sir William, and McCrae, Thomas, Modern Medicine, Volume I, edition 1, Lea Brothers, Philadelphia and New York, 1907.
77. Talbott, J. H., Jacobson, B. M., and Oberg, S. A., J. Clin. Investigation, **14:** 411, 1935.

78. Scudamore, C., A Treatise on the Nature and Cure of Gout, Longman, Hurst. Rees, Orme, and Brown, London, 4th edition, 1823.
79. Grabfield, G. P., Ann. Int. Med., **11:** 651, 1937.
80. deGalantha, E., Am. J. Clin. Path., **5:** 165, 1935.
81. Ebstein, W., Die Natur u. Behandlung der Gicht, J. F. Bergmann, Wiesbaden. 1882.
82. Minkowski, O.: E. von Leyden's Handbuch der Ernährungstherapie und Diätetik. Volume 2, p. 217, G. Thieme, Leipzig, 1904.
83. Moore, H., Trans. Path. Soc. London, **33:** 271, 1881–1882.
84. Brogsitter, M., Histopathologie der Gelenk-Gicht, F. C. W. Vogel, Leipzig, 1927.
85. Ludwig, A. O., Bennett, G. A., and Bauer, W., Ann. Int. Med., **11:** 1248, 1938.
86. Schlesinger, M. J., Unpublished data, Beth Israel Hospital, Boston, Massachusetts.
87. Levison, F., Ztschr. f. klin. Med., **26:** 293, 1894.
88. Brogsitter, A. M., and Wodarz, H., Deutsch. Arch. f. klin. Med., **139:** 129, 1922.
89. Huchard, H., Traité clinique des maladies du coeur et de l'aorte. O. Doin, Paris, 1st edition, p. 174, 1899.
90. Aschoff, L.: E. V. Cowdry, ed., Arteriosclerosis, The Macmillan Company, New York, p. 10, 1933.
91. Mathieu, L., Collesson, L., and Choltus, R., Ann. de méd., **35:** 124, 1934.
92. Sydenstricker, E.: E. V. Cowdry, ed., Arteriosclerosis, The Macmillan Company, New York, p. 131, 1933.
93. Alvarez, W. C., and Stanley, L. L., Arch. Int. Med., **46:** 17, 1930.
94. Kionka, H., Arch. f. exper. Path. u. Pharmakol., **44:** 186, 1900.
95. Fox, H., Diseases in Captive Wild Mammals and Birds: Incidence, Description, Comparison, J. B. Lippincott Company, Philadelphia, 1923.
96. Kaupp, B. F., Poultry Diseases, Including Diseases of Other Domesticated Birds, Alexander Eger, Chicago, 1923.
97. Schlottenhauer, C. F., and Bollman, J. L., J. Am. Vet. Med. Assn., **85:** 98, 1934.
98. Schlottenhauer, C. F., and Bollman, J. L., Am. J. Digestive Dis. and Nutrition, **3:** 483, 1936.
99. Galvani, 1766. Cited from Ebstein (see reference number 81).
100. Schröder, W., Arch. f. Physiol., Supp., p. 113, 1880.
101. Virchow, R., Virchow's Arch. f. path. Anat. u. Physiol., **35:** 358, 1866; **36:** 147, 1866.
102. Mendelson, W., Am. J. Med. Sci., **95:** 109, 1888.
103. Salomon, G., Virchow's Arch. f. path. Anat. u. Physiol., **97:** 360, 1884.
104. Pecile, D., Ann. der Chem., **183:** 141, 1876.
105. Schittenhelm, A., and Bendix, E., Ztschr. f. physiol. Chem., **48:** 140, 1906.
     Schittenhelm, A., Ztschr. f. physiol. Chem., **66:** 53, 1910.
106. Cohen, A., Pennsylvania Med. J., **41:** 1100, 1938.
107. Van Breeman, J., Proceedings of the International Congress on Rheumatism and Hydrology and the Bicentenary Congress on Chronic Rheumatism, p. 302, Headly Brothers, London, 1938.
108. Kahlmeter, G., Proceedings of the International Congress on Rheumatism and Hydrology and the Bicentenary Congress on Chronic Rheumatism, p. 298, Headly Brothers, London, 1938.
109. Das Gupta, S. C., Indian Med. Rec., **55:** 97, 1935.
110. Thomson, F. G., Brit. J. Rheumatism, **1:** 25, 1938.
111. Aldred-Brown, G. R. P., J. Roy. Inst. Pub. Health and Hygiene, **1:** 298, 1938.
112. Cohen, A., Am. J. Med. Sci., **192:** 488, 1936.
113. Monroe, R. T., The Detection of Gout, Med. Clin. N. Amer., **18:** 999, 1935.
114. Futcher, T. B., J.A.M.A., **39:** 1046, 1902.
115. Hutchinson, J., M. Times and Gaz., **1:** 543, 1876.
116. Luff, A. P., Gout: Its Pathology, Forms, Diagnosis and Treatment, Cassell and Company, London, 1907.
117. Unpublished data.
118. Jacobson, B. M., Ann. Int. Med., **11:** 1277, 1938.
119. Folin, O., and Denis, W., Arch. Int. Med., **16:** 33, 1915.
120. Talbott, J. H., J. Clin. Investigation, **19:** 645, 1940.
121. Roberts, W., Allbutt's System of Medicine, Volume 3, p. 155, The Macmillan Company, New York, 1900.
122. Buckley, C. W., Med. Press, **197:** 482, 1938.

123. Kersley, G. D., Clin. J., **65:** 367, 1936.
124. Hench, P. S., J. Lab. and Clin. Med., **22:** 48, 1936.
125. Lockie, L. M., and Hubbard, R. S., J.A.M.A., **104:** 2072, 1935.
126. Hench, P. S., J.A.M.A., **113:** 1064, 1939.
127. Bauer, W., J.A.M.A., **113:** 1065, 1939.
128. Hench, P. S., M. Clin. N. Amer., **19:** 551, 1935.
129. Folin, O., J. Biol. Chem., **101:** 111, 1933.
130. Blauch, M. B., and Koch, F. C., J. Biol. Chem., **130:** 443, 1939.
131. Ropes, M. W., Rossmeisl, E. C., and Bauer, W., J. Clin. Investigation, **19:** 795, 1940.
132. Rourke, M. D., and Ernstene, A. C., J. Clin. Investigation, **8:** 545, 1930.
133. Hench, P. S., Vanzant, F. R., and Nomland, R., Trans. Assn. Am. Phys., **43:** 217, 1928.
134. Pommer, G., Mikroskopische Untersuchung über Gelenkgicht, Gustav Fischer, Jena, 1929.
135. Aub, J. C., Fairhall, L. T., Minot, A. S., and Reznikoff, P., Lead Poisoning, Williams and Wilkins Company, Baltimore, 1926.
136. Garrison, F. H., History of Medicine, 4th edition, W. B. Saunders Company, Philadelphia, p. 124, 1929.
137. Jennings, G. H., Reports on Chronic Rheumatic Diseases, Volume 3, p. 106, H. K. Lewis and Company, Ltd., London, 1937.
138. Quick, A. J., J. Biol. Chem., **101:** 475, 1933.
139. Rutledge, D. I., and Bedard, R. E., Proc. Staff Meet. Mayo Clinic, **12:** 149, 1937.
140. Beitzke, H., Ztschr. f. klin. Med., **74:** 215, 1912.
141. Heine, J., Virchows Arch. f. path. Anat., **260:** 521, 1926.
142. Weve, H. J. M., Aver Keratitis Urica en andere Vormen van Jichtig Ooglijden, W. J. Van Hengel, Rotterdam, 1924.

CHAPTER XIII

HYPERINSULINISM

By Garfield G. Duncan

**Relationship between Hyperinsulinism and Spontaneous Hypogly-
cemia.**—Hyperinsulinism and spontaneous hypoglycemia are not synony-
mous. Hyperinsulinism is a definite clinical entity. Spontaneous hypoglycemia
is not a clinical entity but rather an indication of one of several disturbances
in the exceedingly complex mechanism which has to do with the carbohydrate economy of the organism. It is an objective evidence or sign of
functional or organic disease. Altered insulin production is only one consideration in its production. The liver, endocrines, nervous system, and to a
less extent the diet and exercise exert profound influences on carbohydrate metabolism and hence are significant factors in the regulation of the
level of the blood sugar. It is not surprising, therefore, that spontaneous
hypoglycemia occurs in a number of conditions presenting a varied and
bizarre symptomatology.

The most important of the disorders in which spontaneous hypoglycemia is observed and in which symptoms attributable to abnormally low
blood sugar levels occur are presented below. Between 80 and 90 per
cent of all cases of spontaneous hypoglycemia are due to disturbances of the
nervous system, to diseases of the liver, and to hyperinsulinism, organic and
functional.

The main object in this chapter is the consideration of hyperinsulinism.
This can be done with clarity only by presenting clear-cut evidences of
this condition as distinct from other disorders in which low blood sugar
values are also found. Spontaneous hypoglycemia is not uncommon, in
contrast to hyperinsulinism, which is rare, but which has as one of its
characteristics attacks of spontaneous hypoglycemia.

CAUSES OF SPONTANEOUS HYPOGLYCEMIA

A. *Disease of the Endocrine Glands*
- (a) Hyperinsulinism
  - (1) Tumors, benign or malignant, of the islets of Langerhans
  - (2) Functional hypertrophy with hyperplasia of the islets of Langerhans
- (b) Adrenal cortex insufficiency (Addison's disease)
- (c) Hypophyseal disorders
  - (1) Simmonds' disease
  - (2) Tumor (pituitary)
- (d) Hypothyroidism

B. *Disease of the Liver*
- (a) Extensive hepatic disease such as is observed in acute yellow atrophy,
  primary or metastatic carcinoma, cirrhosis, arsphenamine and other poisonings, and Von Gierke's disease
- (b) Chronic infectious hepatitis (ascending cholangeitis)

C. Disturbances of the Nervous System

(a) Functional disturbance of the sympathetic nervous system
(b) Organic disease of the nervous system

D. Miscellaneous

Exercise, undernutrition, afebrile cachexia, diarrhea, progressive muscular dystrophy, status thymicolymphaticus, lactation and renal glycosuria.

E. Unknown Etiology

HYPERINSULINISM

Hyperinsulinism is a disease originating in the pancreas. It is the antithesis of diabetes mellitus in that, lacking normal regulation, there are excessive amounts of insulin produced as well as excessive activity of insulin. The entire symptom complex, including the spontaneous hypoglycemia, of hyperinsulinism is due to excessive insulin action. This is in contrast with the faulty glycogenesis and glycogenolysis in infectious hepatitis and to disturbances in the nervous regulation of glycogen depots in certain disorders of the nervous system and to different opposing hormones in certain diseases of the endocrine glands to be discussed in the following pages.

Pathogenesis.—The clinical complex of hyperinsulinism is due to functionally overactive islet cells, a hyperplasia of the islet cells, or to tumors, benign or malignant, of the islets of Langerhans. The present conception of hyperinsulinism is based on a series of observations dating from the discovery of the islet tissue in the pancreas by Langerhans in 1869. The observations made by Banting and his co-workers[1] on the hypoglycemic effects of large doses of insulin (1921) were especially important. Recognition of signs and symptoms identical with those of insulin reactions, but in patients who had not received insulin, were correctly interpreted by Gibson and Larimer, and later prompted Harris[2] (1924) to postulate a new clinical entity, "hyperinsulinism."

Low blood sugar values and an abnormal tolerance for carbohydrate were recognized in patients suffering from this disease. Wilder[3] (1927) and his co-workers removed any doubt that remained as to the genuineness of hyperinsulinism when they recovered large amounts of insulin from an islet-cell carcinoma and from the metastatic growths in the liver. Howland[4] (1929) reported the first cure of a case of hyperinsulinism following the removal of an adenoma of the islets of Langerhans, and Whipple[5] collected seventy-four cases of tumors of the islets of Langerhans, fifty-six of them found at operation and eighteen at autopsy, which were reported prior to 1938. It is of interest that Whipple's first six patients with this disease were referred to him from the Neurological Institute.

Adenomas of the islets of Langerhans are insulin-containing, encapsulated, and highly vascularized. They have an average diameter of 4 mm. to 2 cm. They are comprised of islet cells which are packed with specific islet-cell granules. These adenomata have been called nesidioblastomas by Laidlaw.[6] They occur most frequently in the tail of the pancreas where islet-cell tissue predominates, but occasionally they are found in the head of this organ. As a rule they appear singly, but two or more separate adenomas have been found in the same pancreas. They may be buried in the pancreas or stand out as lilac colored, highly vascularized masses on its surface (Fig. 124).

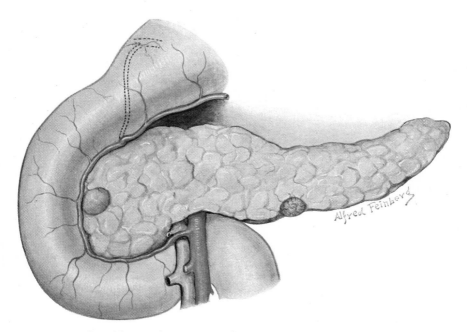

Fig. 124.—The difference in appearance between an adenoma and an enlarged lymph node. Note the richer capillary network over the lilac colored adenoma at the junction of the body and tail of the pancreas. (After Whipple and Frantz, Annals of Surgery, **101**: 1299, 1935, J. B. Lippincott Co.)

Active mitosis of the tumor cells, invasion of the capsule of the adenoma and of the surrounding pancreatic tissue with metastasis to the lymph nodes or to the liver by islet cells are evidences of malignant changes. The tumor cells resemble those of normal islets, but differ in cell arrangement and pattern. They occur as gigantic islets in rosettes about capillaries, in sheets, and in tubular or ribbon formations. Hyaline fibrous tissue, calcification, and degenerative changes predominate in some cases. Pathologic changes in hyperinsulinism have been largely restricted to the pancreas and to the brain. Cerebral edema, perivascular infiltration of the meninges and brain, atrophy of the cerebral cortex, and minute scattered hemorrhages have been noted. In clinically severe cases of hyperinsulinism with convulsions, psychotic manifestations, and organic dementia, a correlated advancing destruction of the cerebral cortex and basal ganglia have been observed. A review of the cerebral changes in hyperinsulinism to which the reader is referred has been presented by Malamud and Grosh.[7]

The pathological changes in functional hyperinsulinism characteristically seen in the newborn babies of diabetic mothers are hypertrophy and hyperplasia of the islets of Langerhans. Similar changes have been observed in adults.

Symptomatology.—Hyperinsulinism is a chronic disease punctuated at varying intervals by episodes of hypoglycemia and the clinical disturbances which result.

The onset of symptoms may be sudden, as in Case I (see p. 662), but it is usually gradual with mild manifestations for weeks, months and even years before an attack sufficiently severe to cause loss of consciousness occurs. The disorder may reach a certain degree of severity and remain apparently unchanged for many years. On the other hand it may become progressively worse, and, if malignant changes occur, it may defy all measures ordinarily employed for its control.

The symptomatology of hyperinsulinism is closely related to the *nervous system*. In fact the subjective and objective signs of this disease are almost entirely attributable to the effect which the hypoglycemia exerts on the central and sympathetic nervous systems. In the early and usually milder attacks evidences of disturbances in the sympathetic nervous system predominate. These are sweating, flushing, pallor, numbness of the circumoral region, nausea, chilliness, hunger, epigastric pains, trembling, dizziness, weakness, elevation of the blood pressure, cardiac palpitation, and syncope. These symptoms may be due entirely to a secondary discharge of epinephrine.

Evidences of disturbances of the central nervous system are noted, for the most part, in severe attacks and attributed to the hypoglycemia *per se* and are as follows: restlessness, thick speech, diplopia, tonic or clonic muscle spasms, convulsions and, in the extreme cases, coma and death.

Psychiatric manifestations of the hypoglycemic complex of hyperinsulinism are observed in mild, moderately severe and severe attacks. These are: emotional instability, apprehension, difficulty in concentration, disorientation, amnesia, negativism, mania, and unconsciousness.

Attacks or "spells" are prone to occur before breakfast. There may be difficulty in arousing the patient. Attacks are precipitated during the daytime if a meal is unusually delayed and especially if the patient has had vigorous physical exercise. It is significant that the symptoms are increased in severity by a reduction in the food intake and by a loss of weight. Furthermore, attacks are likely to be more frequent and more severe during menstruation. They tend to be less severe, reduced in number, or absent if the diet is increased, if frequent nourishments are taken, if a gain in weight occurs, and during the course of an acute infection.

As the hypoglycemic feature of the disorder progresses a variety of combinations of symptoms appear. Headache, difficulty in concentration, emotional disturbances, difficult speech, disorientation and mental confusion appear and increase in severity. Vertigo, faintness, diplopia, cardiac palpitation and coldness of the extremities occur. The patient has a staring expression during attacks. He may be unable to walk and he may be melancholic or restless and maniacal. Unless recognized and treated the condition causes, in the severe cases, loss of consciousness, muscle twitching, generalized convulsions, following which there is a retrograde amnesia. Patients may indeed be amnesic as a result of mild attacks of hypoglycemia. During severe attacks the normal color of the mucous membranes is maintained but there may be pallor or flushing of the skin; the blood pressure is elevated and the pulse is full and bounding; tendon reflexes are usually exaggerated and a Babinski sign is almost invariably present. A subnormal blood pressure and a weak pulse occur in patients who are *in extremis* and so are to be looked upon as ominous signs.

In *bona fide* cases of hyperinsulinism the *blood sugar level* during attacks is invariably below 50 mg. per 100 cc. and usually it is below 35 mg.

Complete, sudden and dramatic relief from these symptoms and signs is the rule upon the administration of dextrose by vein. However, residual disturbances of the nervous system may remain in isolated cases.

Diagnosis.—There is a widespread tendency to designate hypoglycemic values and "flat" or "plateau" glucose tolerance curves as being due to hyperinsulinism. Hyperinsulinism, *per se*, is a relatively rare condition. Only one instance of this disease was recognized in 18,000 admissions to one of the large Veterans' Administration Hospitals up to 1934. Only twelve cases of hyperinsulinism were identified as such at the Mayo Clinic over a period of twelve years.[8] Whereas abnormally low blood sugar values and "plateau" dextrose tolerance curves are frequently observed. The latter unless secured under standardized conditions, as described later, lose much of their diagnostic value. As hyperglycemia occurs in a number of disorders besides diabetes mellitus, so do hypoglycemia and an apparent increased tolerance for carbohydrate occur in a number of conditions other than hyperinsulinism. The hypoglycemic state warrants a careful investigation because the various etiological conditions require widely divergent methods of treatment. The diagnosis of hyperinsulinism must not be assumed until extrapancreatic causes of the hypoglycemia are eliminated.

It is obvious that the diagnosis of hyperinsulinism is not to be made loosely on the basis of a hypoglycemia alone, but upon a general appraisal of the patient's condition, the symptoms of hypoglycemia occurring especially at the end of the longest periods without food, the low postabsorptive (fasting) blood sugar values and the prompt correction of symptoms and a resulting improvement of the blood sugar concentration after the ingestion of food.

The following outline of the criteria for making a diagnosis of hyperinsulinism is the same, except for minor modifications and additions, as Whipple's and Wilder's.[9] It is as follows:

I. An abnormally low postabsorptive (fasting) blood sugar level—below 60 mg. per 100 cc.

II. Symptoms of a hypoglycemia with the confirmatory evidence of a blood sugar level below 50 mg. per 100 cc. during the attack. The blood sugar concentration may be reduced and an attack precipitated by omitting the patient's breakfast and by having the patient exercise in moderation. This is a valuable test when it is indicated but need be employed only in case of doubt regarding the diagnosis.

III. The dramatic and immediate relief from the symptoms of hypoglycemia following the administration of glucose (dextrose) by vein.

IV. Glucose Tolerance Tests. A reliable diagnosis of hyperinsulinism can not be made on the basis of these tests alone. They are to be interpreted in the light of the foregoing considerations. The value of glucose tolerance tests has been discredited because of the variety of types of curves obtainable in any one patient. This objection is overcome, as Conn[10] has shown, by conducting the test under standard conditions. The test is then of confirmatory value in the differential diagnosis of hyperinsulinism.

It is well known that diets aimed at undernutrition and diets low in carbohydrate content depress, whereas diets with liberal or high carbohydrate quotas increase the carbohydrate tolerance. Hence curves that are to be compared should be secured under the same dietary circumstances. The features which I consider requisite to give tolerance curves of greatest diagnostic value are (1) the avoidance of undernutrition and (2) the ingestion of 250 gm. of carbohydrate daily for three days before the tolerance test is made. An illustrative diet prescription for this purpose is as follows: protein 1 gm. per Kg. of body weight, carbohydrate 250 gm. and fat sufficient to bring the total calories to 35 calories per Kg. of body weight.

The results of the glucose tolerance test under these conditions reveal, in *hyperinsulinism*, (*a*) a subnormal postabsorptive (fasting) blood sugar level, (*b*) the highest peak of the blood sugar concentration rarely exceeding 120 mg. of sugar per 100 cc., and (*c*) restoration of subnormal values within two hours. These values are usually maintained throughout the third, fourth, fifth and sixth hours.

The characteristics of these glucose tolerance tests are presented in figure 125 and are contrasted with that found in spontaneous hypoglycemia due to infectious hepatitis and that found in functional conditions of the nervous system.

Glucose tolerance curves in *functional nervous disorders* reveal: (*a*) the fasting blood sugar at the lower border of, but not below normal, (*b*) one hour after the glucose is given, blood sugar characteristically slightly higher but within the normal *post cibal* range, and, (*c*) at the second and third hours hypoglycemic values with a tendency to spontaneous restoration to a normal concentration at the fourth, fifth, and sixth hours.

In *infectious hepatitis* (ascending cholangeitis) the glucose tolerance curve commences with a subnormal value, as low as 18 mg. of sugar per 100 cc. in Conn's cases, but rapidly rises to hyperglycemic levels, followed by a slow return to normal during the day time and to subnormal levels after a fast of more than twelve hours.

V. Evidence of a remarkable increase above the normal rate at which glucose is removed from the blood should be demonstrable in every case of hyperinsulinism. A test illustrating this feature as applied in Case 1 is presented in figure 126.

Other Diagnostic Considerations.—In the review of the psychiatric aspect of the subject of hyperinsulinism, Kepler and Moersch[11] recorded the various early diagnoses made in twenty-one cases of spontaneous hypoglycemia. Among these are hysteria, acute confusional states, intoxication with alcohol, tumor of the brain, acute delirium, epilepsy, and encephalitis. The epigastric pain, the fatigue and hunger which are relieved by taking

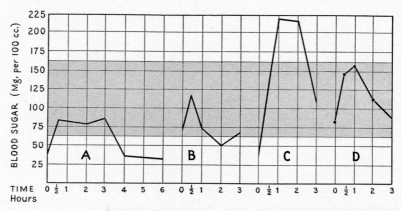

Fig. 125.—The types of glucose tolerance curves observed in: *A*, Hyperinsulinism; *B*, disturbances of the vegetative nervous system, especially vagotonia, and, *C*, infectious hepatitis (ascending cholangeitis) as contrasted with the normal curve. *D*, The shaded zone represents the extent of normal fluctuations of the blood sugar level during this test.

food as is observed in patients suffering from hyperinsulinism may be confused with the symptoms of a duodenal ulcer, neurosis (anxiety and gastrointestinal) and vagotonia. Chronic idiopathic hypoparathyroidism may be confused with hyperinsulinism until a careful "metabolic investigation" is made. When the symptomatology is considered it is easy to understand why these patients find their way to psychiatrists and neurologists before reaching the internists.

The fulfilment of the five requirements outlined above with no evidence of extra pancreatic causes of the hypoglycemia, justifies the diagnosis of hyperinsulinism.

A relentless progress of the disorder until clinical attacks of hypoglycemia are severe, until they occur with increasing frequency, and are more difficult to correct, is strong evidence of a tumor of the islets of Langerhans. It is evidence that the insulin producing and exporting mechanisms are out of control.

Adenomas of the islets tend to undergo malignant changes early and because of this they should be removed as soon as the diagnosis is reasonably well established.

The diagnosis of hyperinsulinism is extremely difficult in some cases. It is recommended that, when extrapancreatic causes of attacks of spontaneous hypoglycemia are excluded, the pancreas should be explored surgically. The finding of a tumor of the islets of Langerhans at operation is indisputable evidence of hyperinsulinism.

Tumors of the Islets of Langerhans.—These may be (1) benign adenomas, or (2) carcinomas, with or without metastases. It may be impossible to distinguish between the two clinically. The benign adenomas usually cause less severe clinical manifestations and the tendency to progressiveness is not so marked as when the tumor is malignant. I believe it is significant

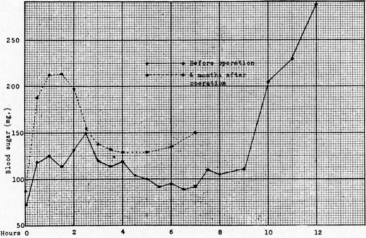

Fig. 126.—The abnormally great ability to remove dextrose from the blood in spite of increases in the rate of dextrose administration by venoclysis, from 28 gm. per hour at the end of five hours, to 36 gm. per hour at seven hours, to 44 gm. per hour and at nine hours to 54 gm. per hour before operation, is contrasted with the normal blood sugar level response when dextrose in a 15 per cent solution was given continuously at the rate of 28 gm. of dextrose per hour after operation (Case 1).

that patients with adenomas of the islets have distinct phases of extreme sensitiveness to exercise, fasting, menstruation, diarrhea and loss of weight, which tend to precipitate hypoglycemic reactions with longer intervals between in which it is difficult to provoke an attack of hypoglycemia. Furthermore, the cycles of increased sensitiveness are most pronounced during some, but not during all, menstrual periods. The malignant tumors are more apt to cause more extreme degrees of hypoglycemia which are more difficult to correct. The attacks tend to be more frequent and are precipitated with greater ease by merely withholding food, and they also tend to increase in intensity. Malignant tumors occur in young as well as in middle-aged patients of either sex. Federoff's patient, referred to by Whipple, was a male, sixteen years of age, and Judd reported a case of carcinoma of the islets of Langerhans in a girl aged eighteen years.

ILLUSTRATIVE CASE

Case 1.* A white girl, aged nineteen years, weighing 108 pounds (49 Kg.) and measuring 62 inches (155 cm.), was admitted to the Pennsylvania Hospital on March 27, 1938, complaining of attacks of vertigo, headaches and unconsciousness. These attacks began in March, 1937, with sudden loss of consciousness one afternoon, although subsequent attacks occurred, for the most part, in the morning before breakfast. She was roused with difficulty but was able to resume her duties. In September (1937) she had spells of weakness on rising in the morning and a feeling that she was going to faint.

One morning in November (1937) she felt weak and dizzy. She dressed, went downstairs, and while preparing breakfast became emotionally upset and shortly lost consciousness. She was seen by Dr. W. B. Turner, who admitted her to the Carlisle Hospital. A blood sugar level of 23 mg. per 100 cc. was found. A high carbohydrate diet was prescribed, but the blood sugar values remained low, between 35 and 45 mg. per 100 cc. Two weeks after discharge she was readmitted in a stuporous condition but responded readily to intravenous glucose (dextrose). The blood sugar level varied from 30 to 50 mg. per 100 cc. There were no convulsive seizures.

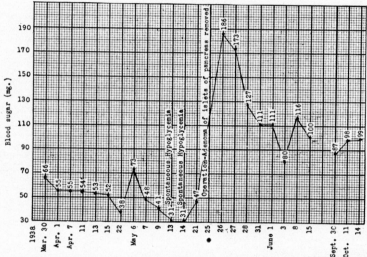

Fig. 127.—The hypoglycemic values before, the transitory hyperglycemia immediately following, and the normal blood sugar levels from three days to four months after, the removal of an adenoma of the islets of Langerhans are presented (Case 1).

A glucose tolerance test at that time revealed the following values for blood sugar: fasting, 28 mg.; one-half hour, 90; one hour, 97; and at two hours, 100 mg. per 100 cc. A postprandial blood sugar value was found to be 57 mg. per 100 cc.

The patient continued to suffer from spells of weakness and vertigo on two or three consecutive days at three- to five-week intervals. The attacks were more severe during menstruation, though during some menses there seemed to be no increase in the susceptibility to attacks. She had had no attacks for three weeks prior to her admission to the Pennsylvania Hospital.

Examination on admission (March 27, 1938) revealed considerable flushing about the neck and at times of the face, hair and skin oily, some acne, complete edentia, some reddening of the anterior tonsillar pillars and diseased tonsils. There was an unusually great separation of the nails from the matrix of fingers and toes, and there was moderate proximodistal tilting of the nails. The hands and feet were moist. There was a slight tendency to masculine distribution of suprapubic hair and there was a considerable growth of hair on the extremities.

* This and the following case has been reported in greater detail by Duncan, G. G., Hayward, G., and Flick, J., elsewhere; Med. Clin. N. Amer., vol. 23: 1481, 1939.

Laboratory Data.—The fasting level of the blood sugar (March 28) was 58 mg. per 100 cc. and the results of a six-hour glucose tolerance test (100 gm. glucose) on March 30 were as follows: fasting blood sugar level, 66 mg.; one-half hour, 106; one hour, 107; two hours, 100; three hours, 123; four hours, 93; five hours, 88; and six hours, 62 mg. per 100 cc.

The blood urea nitrogen level and the urea clearance were normal as was also the levulose tolerance test for liver function. An analysis of the fractional gastric contents showed a low free and total acid.

Diet.—Throughout the following studies a weighed diet containing 65 gm. of protein, 200 gm. of carbohydrate, and 93 gm. of fat (2400 calories) divided into three meals and three nourishments were allowed.

The preoperative blood sugar values (fasting) were all below normal (70 mg. per 100 cc.) and during spontaneous attacks of unconsciousness they were as low as 31 mg. per 100 cc. (Fig. 127).

The patient appeared well and for several weeks it seemed that the inactivity of ward life was sufficient to counteract the tendency to spontaneous attacks of hypoglycemia. Moderate exercise did not precipitate an attack.

Attempts were made to determine the ease or difficulty with which attacks might be provoked and also to learn if the susceptibility to attacks altered from time to time. The following studies made this clear:

Provocative Tests.—Omission of breakfast, while the gastric contents were being extracted for examination (April 5), was followed at 11 A.M. by vertigo and headache, and the patient complained of feeling cold. Prompt relief was secured by giving orange juice. Though low values for blood sugar were obtained no spontaneous attacks (usually considered characteristic of hypoglycemic reactions) occurred during a twenty-four-hour fast.

The effect of *exercise* was next tried. On April 8 the usual breakfast was given at 8:15 A.M. and the patient spent three twenty-minute periods exercising on a rowing machine between 9:30 and 11:30 A.M. At 11:30 she complained of hunger and of slight headache but was well otherwise. The blood sugar values were: 8 A.M. (fasting), 52 mg.; 10 A.M., 57; 12 noon, 51; and 2 P.M., 50 mg. per 100 cc. The patient was not allowed any breakfast (no food after 8 o'clock the previous evening) and the exercise test was repeated on April 11. The blood sugar value at 8 A.M. was 54 mg. per 100 cc.

TABLE 1

EFFECT OF FASTING PLUS EXERCISE ON THE BLOOD SUGAR VALUES (MG. PER 100 CC.)

The effect of fasting and exercise on the blood sugar before, is compared with that obtained four months after operation (Case I).

Time	8 A.M.	10 A.M.	12 N.	2 P.M.
Preoperative blood sugar............	54	31	40	46
Postoperative blood sugar............	99	92	85	92

Periods of exercise (twenty minutes each) were begun at 8 A.M. and repeated at hourly intervals.

and 31 mg. at 10 A.M. (Table 1), when there was muscle twitching and the patient was pale but did not perspire. She felt tired and when returned to bed she promptly slept, but could be aroused easily. She had fully recovered by 11:15 A.M. In spite of continued exercise and lack of food the blood sugar had increased to 40 mg. per 100 cc. at 12 noon and to 46 mg. at 2 P.M. This increase, though slight, was attributed to spontaneous epinephrine response to the low blood sugar level.

In an attempt to determine the approximate rate of withdrawal of sugar from the blood before operation a *continuous intravenous administration of glucose* (dextrose) was begun on May 6 at 7 A.M. Blood sugar values were obtained at one-half hour intervals. Twenty-eight gm. of glucose (in 15 per cent solution) in distilled water were given each hour, from 7 A.M. until noon (five hours). An early increase in the blood sugar concentration was soon overcome (Fig. 126) and it appeared obvious that this rate of glucose administration would not cause a hyperglycemia. The rate was increased to 35 gm. per hour, and after seven hours to 44 gm. and at nine hours to 52 gm. per hour. No pronounced increase in blood sugar values were found until 5:00 P.M. (after ten hours of continuous dextrose administration). A rapid elevation of the blood sugar ensued: 203 mg. per 100 cc. after ten hours (5 P.M.), 230 mg. at eleven hours, and 286 mg. at twelve hours. Glycosuria increased from 1.3 per cent at 4 P.M. to 10 per cent at 6:30 P.M., and was 9.9 per cent at 8:10 P.M.

The patient felt unusually well during the test. The total glucose given in twelve hours was 3700 cc. of a 15 per cent solution, or 555 gm. The amount lost in the urine was 182 gm. and the amount retained 373 gm.

The daily total sodium chloride excretion in the urine varied from 2 to 5 gm. in twenty-four hours and an increase to 8.6 gm. occurred on one day when the intake was increased by 15 gm. The plasma chloride was 612 mg. per 100 cc.

On May 13, the patient began to menstruate. At 8 A.M. (May 13) she had a spontaneous attack of clinical hypoglycemia just before breakfast. Rapidly deepening unconsciousness followed. By 8:25 A.M. she was very pale, with pupils widely dilated, and there were frequent muscle twitchings of the limbs and body. Her blood pressure was 110 mm. systolic and 74 mm. diastolic and the blood sugar level was 31 mg. per 100 cc. Epinephrine, 1 cc. (1:1000 solution) was given subcutaneously (no glucose or other nourishment) at 8:25 A.M. and by 8:35 consciousness was restored; at 9 A.M. she complained of being nervous and was emotionally unstable but conscious and cooperative. Her blood pressure was 154 mm. systolic and 74 mm. diastolic.

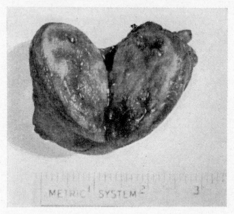

Fig. 128.–The incised adenoma in Case 1.

Another spontaneous attack occurred on May 14 at 3:45 A.M. The patient's face was flushed and she tossed about in her bed and could not be aroused. The blood sugar level at 3:52 was 31 mg. per 100 cc. Epinephrine was given at this time and was repeated at 3:58. Within five minutes of the second dose the restlessness subsided and she could be aroused and was cooperative. She was given 6 ounces of orange juice.

Spontaneous attacks occurred on May 15 and May 22. On each occasion orange juice was given and consciousness was quickly regained.

The acute onset, the chronic course, the hypoglycemia with symptoms especially prominent at the time of the menstrual period and at the end of the longest period in the day without food, the relief of symptoms by taking food and on receiving epinephrine, the type of glucose tolerance curve and the remarkable rapidity with which glucose was removed from the blood stream, all favored the diagnosis of hyperinsulinism.

The severity of the disorder and the rhythm with which great susceptibility to spontaneous attacks occurred with intervening periods during which, unlike cases of functional hyperinsulinism, it was difficult to precipitate an attack, led to a preoperative diagnosis of adenoma of the islets of Langerhans.

Operation.–For twenty-four hours prior to operation liberal amounts of carbohydrate were given by mouth. The fasting blood sugar value on the day of operation

(May 25) was 63 mg. At 11 A.M., 500 cc. of a 10 per cent solution of glucose (dextrose) was given in normal saline by venoclysis.

At 11 A.M. the patient was given morphine sulfate, 0.011 gm. (⅙ grain), and atropine sulfate, 0.0004 gm. (¹⁄₁₅₀ grain). One hour and forty-five minutes later spinal anesthesia was induced with 200 mg. of primocaine. A transverse incision was made 4 cm. above the umbilicus, dividing both recti muscles. The lesser peritoneal cavity was entered through the gastrocolic omentum and the pancreas was exposed. No tumor was visible, but a round hard mass, approximately 1.5 cm. in diameter, was palpated in the tail of the pancreas near the distal end. Careful palpation of the pancreas elsewhere failed to reveal any other area suggestive of tumor. The indurated mass of tissue (Figs. 128 and 129) was excised. Several small vessels were ligated with fine silk and the defect in the pancreas was closed with interrupted fine silk sutures. The gallbladder and liver appeared normal. The abdominal incision was closed anatomically, using interrupted sutures of silk in all the layers. The peritoneal cavity was not drained.

Following operation there was a slight febrile reaction, the patient's temperature reaching a peak of 101° F. on the third postoperative day and gradually receding, to reach normal on the thirteenth postoperative day. During this period the patient at

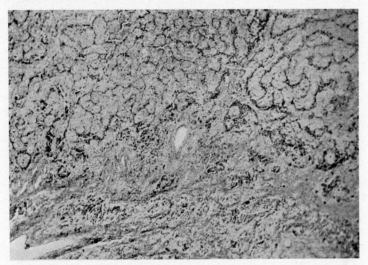

Fig. 129.—A section of the adenoma reveals a fibrocellular structure with thin cords and rosette cell arrangements, hyaline fibrous tissue and degenerative changes. No mitotic figures were seen (Case 1).

times complained of pain in the left flank and was slightly tender below the twelfth rib on the left side. Convalescence otherwise was undisturbed.

Postoperative Course.—Four hours after operation the blood sugar level was 186 mg. per 100 cc. The following morning it was 173 mg. and subsequent values were normal. There was a practically normal response to the glucose tolerance test three days after operation, in contrast to the low curve obtained preoperatively (Table 2).

A prompt hyperglycemic response followed the continuous administration of dextrose on the second day after operation. The dextrose was given at the same initial rate as on the previous similar test, but without the increases which were necessary to provoke a hyperglycemia pre-operatively.

Examination on Readmission.—The patient was readmitted on September 17, 1938, in order that comparative metabolic studies might be made. She had enjoyed excellent health in the interim. There were no changes observed on physical examination with the exception that she had gained 7 pounds (3.1 Kg.).

The patient's diet was unlimited in the interim but, on readmission, for the sake of uniformity, the diet employed on her previous admission (65 gm. of protein, 200 gm. of carbohydrate and sufficient fat to make a total of 2400 calories) was resumed.

TABLE 2

DEXTROSE TOLERANCE TESTS (6 HOUR)

The low type of curve obtained in response to 100 gm. of dextrose before operation is contrasted with normal responses two weeks and four months after the removal of the adenoma of the islets of Langerhans (Case 1).

	Fasting	½ hr.	1 hr.	2 hrs.	3 hrs.	4 hrs.	5 hrs.	6 hrs.
	Preoperative test (April 1, 1938)							
Blood sugar (mg. per 100 cc.).	66	106	107	100	123	93	88	62
	Postoperative test (June 8, 1938)							
	116	154	173	139	94	92	102	102
	Postoperative test (October 11, 1938)							
	87	117	171	90	102	114	97	97

After ten days the various tests done before operation were repeated.

The glucose tolerance test was normal (Table 2). A normal response to intravenous glucose (dextrose) was obtained (Fig. 126). The low total sodium chloride excretion in the urine and the poor response to added sodium chloride in the diet before operation were in contrast to the normal excretion and a good response to added sodium chloride four months after operation (Table 3). This patient was enjoying excellent health in October, 1941.

TABLE 3

SODIUM CHLORIDE OUTPUT IN URINE

The low sodium chloride excretion before, is contrasted with the normal values obtained after operation (Case 1).

	Preoperative			Postoperative	
Date, 1938	Volume of Urine (Cc.) per Diem	Urine Chlorides, Gm. per Diem	Date, 1938	Volume of Urine (Cc.) per Diem	Urine Chlorides, Gm. per Diem
June 6	865	2.0	Sept. 21	1500	6.9
14	1380	4.6	22	1550	6.8
17	1240	3.3	23	1510	9.6
18	1175	3.7	24	1100	7.3
19	1090	3.1	25	1640	7.6
20	2010	5.0	26	1370	8.5
22	(15 Gm. NaCl added to intake)		27	1460	7.8
	1420	8.6	28	1600	7.3
24	1620	4.1	29	1480	4.1
			30	1580	9.8
			Oct. 1	(15 Gm. NaCl added to intake)	
				1320	14.7

Fasting plus exercise produced marked hypoglycemic values when fasting alone failed to produce symptoms before operation. The observations repeated four months after the operation revealed but a slight reduction in the blood sugar level.

Case 2. A white youth, aged eighteen years, weighing 133 pounds (60 Kg.) and measuring 68 inches (160 cm.), was admitted to Dr. Hobart Reimann's Service at the Jefferson Hospital on June 22, 1939. He complained of having had about twelve attacks of unconsciousness associated with convulsions. The first attack occurred in November, 1936. A hypoglycemia had been found by his attending physician in 1937.

The patient's physical condition was good, though he had lost 13 pounds (6 Kg.) in the two months preceding admission. He had several spontaneous attacks of unconsciousness with convulsions while in the hospital. These were promptly relieved by epinephrine alone and by glucose (dextrose) given intravenously. The blood sugar levels were 19 mg., 23 mg., 18 mg., and 26 mg. per 100 cc. during different attacks and there was a continuous hypoglycemia, the blood sugar values (fasting) varying from 31 to 42 mg. per 100 cc.

A six-hour glucose tolerance test (100 gm. glucose) revealed capillary and venous blood sugar and phosphorus values as follows:

	Capillary Blood Sugar, Mg. per 100 Cc.	Venous Blood Sugar, Mg. per 100 Cc.	Blood Phosphorous Mg. per 100 Cc.
Fasting	42	39	2.5
1 hour	99	81	1.78
2 hour	108	79	1.1
3 hour	93	86	2.1
4 hour	40	36	1.4
5 hour	36	35	1.5
6 hour	35	34	1.4

The blood cholesterol was 118 mg. per 100 cc. (free cholesterol 38 mg. and cholesterol esters 80 mg.).

The blood count, basal metabolic rate, ophthalmoscopic and neurologic examinations, roentgen examination of the sella turcica, cholecystogram, electrocardiogram,

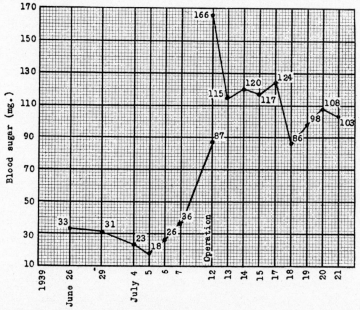

Fig. 130.—The chronic hypoglycemia before, and the transitory hyperglycemia following promptly after removal of the tumor of the islets are illustrated. The return of the blood sugar level to the normal zone is also shown (Case 2).

and liver function studies were negative. The sodium chloride excretion was low (7.7 gm. in 2200 cc. of urine), but was within the normal range.

The chronic hypoglycemia, the attacks of unconsciousness and convulsions which were promptly relieved by glucose (dextrose) therapy, the long periods without symptoms, and the phase during which the attacks were spontaneous warranted a preoperative diagnosis of a tumor of the islets of Langerhans.

An adenoma, the size of a small English walnut, was removed from the tail of the pancreas by Dr. G. P. Muller on July 12, 1939.

Immediately after operation, the patient having had no glucose (dextrose) therapy, the blood sugar was 87 mg. per 100 cc. Subsequent values were normal, with the exception of a level of 166 mg. found on the evening of July 12 (six hours after operation). A glucose tolerance test on July 24 revealed: Fasting, 82 mg. of sugar per 100 cc.; one hour, 120 mg.; two hours, 86 mg.; three hours, 76 mg.; four hours, 91 mg.; five hours, 90 mg.; and six hours, 89 mg. per 100 cc. The postoperative convalescence was complicated by a mild but continuous fever for eight days. The patient had considerable abdominal pain which was troublesome for three weeks after the operation.

The tumor was encapsulated, but histologic examination revealed active hyperplasia of the epithelial cells, mitosis and the presence of acini and islet cells. The *diagnosis* was: Adenoma of the islets of Langerhans which was probably undergoing malignant changes.

FUNCTIONAL HYPERINSULINISM

The subjective and objective evidences of this clinical condition are due to the liberation of abnormally large amounts of insulin by overactive islet cells of the pancreas. In primary hyperfunction of insular tissue the export of insulin is badly adjusted to the need for insulin (Wilder). Though the insulin released may be continually in excess of postabsorptive needs, it may be inadequate to prevent a hyperglycemia and even glycosuria after meals. This disturbance in the regulatory mechanism of the release of insulin explains the apparent diabetes mellitus and hyperinsulinism occasionally occurring in the same individual.

In functional hyperinsulinism the fasting blood sugar concentration is usually not below normal. There is little or no tendency of the disorder to progress; attacks occur during the daytime, after the patient has had one meal and especially if the next meal is delayed; attacks occur between three and four hours after food is taken but are not likely to occur after midnight when the patient is at rest. Spontaneous recovery from an attack is usual but rapid relief is afforded by giving food; the blood sugar during the attack is lower than the fasting level which is attributed to the insulinogenic effect of the carbohydrate content of the preceding meal. Increases in the carbohydrate intake increase the likelihood and severity of attacks. One patient lost consciousness three hours after taking 100 gm. of glucose orally. At the time of the attack the blood sugar concentration was 55 mg. per 100 cc. The postabsorptive value was 82 mg. Glucose taken orally promptly corrects attacks of hypoglycemia but at the same time, because of its stimulation of the production of insulin, predisposes to another attack which may follow the first within three or four hours.

It is my belief that functional hyperinsulinism is a rare condition and that most disorders considered as such are in reality extrapancreatic in origin, notably disturbances in the sympathetic nervous system, and less frequently disturbances in the liver and rarely some endocrine dysfunction.

A true and serious form of functional hyperinsulinism occurs *in infants* born of mothers who have uncontrolled diabetes. Unless anticipated and prevented these attacks may prove fatal. Hartmann and Jaudon[12] have reviewed this subject, and they attach importance to the hypoglycemia occurring in infants of diabetic mothers. Duncan and Fetter[13] regard an otherwise unexplained gain in the diabetic mother's tolerance for carbohydrates in the last trimester of pregnancy as unfavorable for the child as it is due in all probability to hyperinsulinism in the fetus.

In a summary of the pathologic changes observed in infants born of diabetic mothers Bauer and Royster[14] observed that the pancreas was grossly enlarged in six of thirteen cases; that in those cases in which estimations of the number of islets were made it was found to be greater than normal and that hypoglycemia is associated with hypertrophy and hyperplasia of the islets of Langerhans and with no observable histologic changes in the islet cells or other endocrine organs. Bauer and Royster state "It is striking that in the cases reported there was a lack of adequate control of the diabetes in the mother during the period of pregnancy."

The hypothesis which has stood the test of clinical observations and experiments with animals is that unusual demands are made upon the infant's pancreas as a result of the mother's uncontrolled diabetes. Insular hypertrophy and hyperplasia ensue, the mothers' diabetes is improved by the hyperinsulinism of the fetus, and, following delivery, the infant possesses an insulin-producing mechanism out of all proportion to its need. The export of insulin is not adjusted to the need. As a result, unless adequate measures are taken to prevent hypoglycemia during the first three days of life—the period essential to readjustment to the altered circumstances—there is danger of a fatal outcome for the newborn child.

THE CONSIDERATION OF OTHER CAUSES OF SPONTANEOUS HYPOGLYCEMIA

Disease of the Liver.—There is no difficulty in recognizing the cause of the hypoglycemia in patients who have acute yellow atrophy or other extensive disease of the liver. These patients are gravely ill and have other signs of hepatic disease which are more obvious than the hypoglycemia. Rabinowitz[15] has presented the salient clinical features as well as the hypoglycemic tendencies in these cases and Sprague (1934) has demonstrated that animals in which the liver has been damaged or partially extirpated have an increased sensitivity to insulin. Mann (1927) produced profound hypoglycemia in dogs by hepatectomy and mild hypoglycemia by partial hepatectomy. Any disease causing extensive damage to the liver is likely to cause a mild hypoglycemia, especially after fasting or after attacks of diarrhea.

A greater diagnostic problem is presented by patients who are not acutely ill but who, on careful investigation, are found to have disease of the biliary tract. Every patient found to have a chronic hypoglycemia should be investigated for a possible infectious hepatitis. The following tests are of value in revealing disturbances in the function of liver which might otherwise escape detection:

(1) The hippuric acid test (Quick).
(2) Glucose tolerance test, for further details see pp. 659, 744.
(3) Bromsulfalein test.
(4) The serum or plasma albumin-globulin ratio; the ratio is usually reversed in cases of infectious hepatitis in which the damage is sufficiently widespread to cause hypoglycemic levels.

(5) The bilirubin content of the blood. (Van den Bergh or icteric index.)
(6) Cholecystography.
(7) Macrocytosis has been found in cases of hepatogenous hypoglycemia.

Conn and his associates[16] have reported six cases of chronic hypoglycemia due to an ascending cholangeitis. In one patient (Case 1), attacks of unconsciousness occurred from nine to twelve hours after the evening meal and the blood sugar values, while the patient was fasting, ranged from 14 to 18 mg. per 100 cc. Symptoms which were typical of a severe hypoglycemia were promptly corrected by giving glucose (dextrose) intravenously. Glucose tolerance tests showed subnormal fasting blood sugar levels and an impaired ability to remove absorbed dextrose from the blood stream, allowing glycosuria to occur in some cases and yielding a curve, during the first two or three hours after the ingestion of this glucose, similar to that obtained in diabetes and not like the one seen in hyperinsulinism due to a functional disturbance or to a tumor of the islets. The test, carried over four and one-half hours, revealed a return to hypoglycemic levels. This type of curve (see curve C, Fig. 125) in the presence of low fasting values for blood sugar strongly suggests hepatic injury.

Retention of the bromsulfalein dye, an abnormally low serum protein with a reversal of the albumin-globin ratio, hyperbilirubinemia (2.5 mg. per 100 cc.), and an impaired galactose tolerance, gave further evidence of hepatic disease. A cholecystogram revealed but slight visualization of the gallbladder.

A gallbladder containing a calculus and 2 or 3 ounces (60 to 90 cc.) of pus was removed. A biopsy of the liver revealed an active chronic cholangeitis, biliary cirrhosis, cloudy swelling, and fatty infiltration. After operation the level of the blood sugar became normal as the evidences of hepatic damage gradually disappeared and there were no recurrences of the spontaneous attacks of hypoglycemia.

Unlike hyperinsulinism, a high carbohydrate intake (400 to 500 gm.) during the preoperative period benefits these patients and a reduction of the carbohydrate intensifies the hypoglycemia. A liberal protein intake (1.0 to 1.5 gm. per Kg. of body weight) fortifies against further damage to the liver and enhances recovery after operation in cases of ascending cholangeitis.

In Von Gierke's disease (glycogenosis) hypoglycemic values are found, but curiously enough the symptoms usually associated with such values are absent.

Diseases of Other Endocrine Glands.—(a) *Adrenal Insufficiency* (Addison's Disease).—Deficiency of the adrenal cortex may cause a hypoglycemia which may be readily mistaken for hyperinsulinism. Welty[17] reports two such cases. One patient was seen in coma at which time the blood sugar level was 40 mg. per 100 cc. Consciousness was promptly regained following glucose (dextrose) therapy. A six-hour glucose tolerance test revealed progressively lower blood sugar levels, below 60 mg. per 100 cc., at the fifth and sixth hours. A later attack was fatal, there being no apparent response to glucose and the administration of adrenal cortical hormone. Fibrocaseous tuberculosis of the adrenal glands and a healed primary pulmonary tuberculosis were found at autopsy.

The *clinical features* of Addison's disease should remove the danger of confusing this disease with hyperinsulinism in most cases. In Addison's disease there is muscle weakness and languor; hypotension, bradycardia, and anorexia; and hypochlorhydria and vomiting. The pigmentation of the skin and mucous membranes is characteristic of Addison's disease. There is an intensification of the dark color in normally pigmented areas, especially about the nipples. Black "freckles," cutaneous and in the mucous membranes of the mouth, and the bronzing, tanning, or dirty brown coloring of the skin are classical signs of this disease. Also, the basal metabolic rate is low and the body temperature is subnormal. There is an increased loss of sodium, a rise in the serum potassium, general dehydration, and depression of sexual functions. Hypoglycemia, though uncommon in these cases, may occur and be the immediate cause of death. (For further consideration of Addison's disease, see Chapters V and VI.)

Hypophyseal Disorders.—(*a*) *Hypophyseal Cachexia* (Simmonds' Disease).—This rare disease is due to destruction by atrophy or degeneration of the anterior lobe of the pituitary gland. It is not surprising that with removal of such a potent insulin-opposing gland, hypoglycemic values should result. This is a relatively unimportant feature of the disease, however, when contrasted with the symptoms characteristic of senile decay, *i.e.*, falling out of hair, loss of teeth, wrinkling of skin, emaciation and an appearance of rapid aging. Anemia develops, the metabolic rate and the blood sugar level are subnormal and there is atrophy of the gonads with suppression of sex characteristics, with mental deterioration and muscle weakness. These disturbances are relentlessly progressive, eventually causing coma and death. The patient suffering from hyperinsulinism, in contrast, appears normal between attacks and if the general nutrition is disturbed it is usually toward that of overweight.

(*b*) *Tumors.*—Extensive destruction of the anterior lobe of the pituitary gland by a tumor growth may result in disturbances in the regulation of the blood sugar level. Cushing in 1912 reported an instance of this kind caused by a chromophobe adenoma. The blood sugar concentration was reduced to 39 mg. per 100 cc. Wilder observed a similar case.

The symptoms produced by a tumor of the pituitary gland are diagnostic and it would appear hypoglycemia is but a small part of the disturbance, the identification of which should offer little difficulty.

Hypothyroidism.—Hypoglycemia, even of a mild degree, is an uncommon finding in patients suffering from hypothyroidism. It is rarely of sufficient severity to cause spontaneous clinical manifestations of hypoglycemia. There should be no difficulty in recognizing such attacks as complications of the general and characteristic manifestations of hypothyroidism which in brief are: apathy with slow cerebration, thick puffiness and dryness of the skin, dry, brittle and sparse hair, mild obesity, low blood pressure and a subnormal metabolic rate. Patients suffering from hypothyroidism complain of fatigue, unusual sensitiveness to low temperatures, loss of hair, and, constipation. Restoration of a normal or nearly normal metabolic rate by

22

thyroid therapy provides relief from symptoms and corrects the hypoglycemia.

Disorders of the Nervous System.—A. *Functional Disturbances of the Sympathetic Nervous System.*—Increased carbohydrate tolerance with, at times, actual hypoglycemia accompany certain disturbances of the sympathetic nervous system, especially vagotonia, neurocirculatory asthenia and various neuroses. Glucose tolerance tests reveal "plateau curves" with mild degrees of hypoglycemia, 50 to 70 mg. per 100 cc., five and six hours after the administration of the glucose. These disturbances of the nervous system are likely to be confused with hyperinsulinism. In fact some authors, notably Conn,[18] designate the hypoglycemia of neurosis as functional hyperinsulinism. I cannot agree that the pancreas should be maligned when the disturbance actually lies in the nervous regulation of the blood sugar level.

A patient recently observed and at first suspected of having hyperinsulinism was found to be suffering from neurocirculatory asthenia. He was twenty-one years of age and complained of periods of depression, of "spells" of weakness, fatigue and palpitation on mild exercise. Because of the latter he feared all kinds of physical exertion. He also had attacks of discomfort in the epigastric region. His pupils were widely dilated, there were marked vasomotor disturbances, dermographia, cold clammy hands and feet, tachycardia with sinus arrythmia and a spastic palpable colon. His blood pressure was 92 mm. Hg systolic and 60 mm. diastolic, and his temperature was subnormal. Though some signs of sympathicotonia were present those of vagotonia predominated. A six-hour glucose tolerance test (100 gm. of glucose) revealed the following blood sugar values: fasting, 99 mg. per 100 cc.; one-half hour, 123 mg.; one hour, 104 mg.; two hours, 101 mg.; three hours, 69 mg.; four hours, 80 mg.; five hours, 89 mg. and six hours, 90 mg. In contradistinction to hyperinsulinism, a hypoglycemia did not exist during a "spell" of weakness; food failed at times to provide relief from symptoms; recovery was spontaneous; "spells" occurred without apparent relationship to meals, and (what was considered of great diagnostic importance) neither "spells" nor a hypoglycemia was provoked by fasting plus vigorous physical exercise (on a rowing machine). Furthermore fasting blood sugar values were not subnormal.

Patients of this type are seen very much more frequently than are cases of hyperinsulinism. The fact that the treatment for one is psychiatric and the other dietetic or surgical makes the importance of arriving at the correct diagnosis apparent.

B. *Organic Diseases of the Nervous System.*—Hypoglycemia complicates several disturbances of the central nervous system. Though hyperglycemia is more common when the base of the brain is involved, low blood sugar values are sporadically seen in *various psychoses* (*e.g., schizophrenia*), in *subdural hemorrhage*, and in *general paralysis*, as pointed out by Wilder.[19] The hypoglycemia is apparently due to disturbed nervous control of the glycogen depots.

Attacks of *epilepsy* may be and are confused with those of hyperinsulinism. Epilepsy does not fulfill the criteria necessary for a diagnosis of the latter (p. 659). The attacks bear no relationship to meals, they are not precipitated by fasting or exercise, and the blood sugar is within the normal range during the attack.

Careful observation of the psychiatric aspect, the clinical phenomena and the blood sugar level should remove any confusion which may exist regarding the diagnoses of disturbance of the nervous system and hyperinsulinism.

Miscellaneous Causes of Hypoglycemia.—*Exercise*, if prolonged (as in marathon races), causes low blood sugar levels. The degree of hypoglycemia is not severe. It is due to the rapid depletion of the sugar in circulation and to the unusual reduction of the glycogen reserves. Symptomatic attacks of hypoglycemia occurring as a result of exercise are most frequently seen in individuals with an unstable autonomic nervous system.

Lactation and *renal glycosuria*, and severe degrees of *undernutrition* such as observed in *anorexia nervosa* also may be complicated by hypoglycemia. In each instance the underlying cause is a deprivation of nourishment to the organism. Increased food intake in frequent feedings correct the disturbance.

TREATMENT OF HYPERINSULINISM

The management of patients suffering from hyperinsulinism falls logically under three headings: (*a*) treatment of the acute attack, (*b*) conservative treatment in general and the prevention of acute attacks, and (*c*) surgical measures.

Treatment of the Acute Attack of Hypoglycemia.—The method correcting the hypoglycemic attack as seen in hyperinsulinism and the symptoms which it causes is identical with that employed in the treatment of a hypoglycemia induced by an overdose of insulin (see p. 781). Briefly the treatment comprises the giving of fruit juice, a meal, or glucose lozenges if the symptoms are mild. Patients are instructed to ward off attacks by taking food immediately upon the onset of symptoms. Should the attack be severe glucose (dextrose), 20 cc. or more, of a 50 per cent solution, is given by vein. Twenty grams of glucose or corn syrup dissolved in eight ounces of warm water given slowly by rectum has served well in emergencies when sterile solutions were not available for intravenous therapy, and when oral feeding was impractical. Epinephrine, 0.5 to 1 cc. of a 1:1000 solution, given subcutaneously may revive a patient sufficiently to take carbohydrate by mouth.

Conservative Treatment in General and the Prevention of Attacks of Hypoglycemia.—*Diet.*—Special diet is effective in bringing relief to the majority of patients suffering from functional hyperinsulinism. It is futile in cases of islet-cell tumors and should be abandoned in favor of surgery as soon as this diagnosis is made. The quickly absorbable carbohydrate foods are of utmost value in the correction of the acute attack of hypoglycemia, but because of the stimulating effect which they have on the elaboration of insulin and because of the increased insulin sensitivity which follows their use they are to be avoided in the general conduct of the treatment.

CARBOHYDRATE.—The carbohydrate content of the diet should not exceed 150 gm. (the normal diet for the average adult contains between 300 and 400 gm. of carbohydrate), and is best provided in a form which is slowly absorbed, such as cereals, bread, some fruits such as bananas and apples, and vegetables.

PROTEIN.—A liberal protein quota (120 to 140 gm. in the average diet) is desirable, as advocated by Conn.[10] The glucose derived from protein (approximately 58 per cent of the protein is utilized as carbohydrate) is released slowly and has no apparent stimulating effect on the production of insulin.

TABLE 4

ILLUSTRATIVE DIET FOR THE TREATMENT OF FUNCTIONAL HYPERINSULINISM

120 Gm. Protein, 191 Gm. Fat, 125 Gm. Carbohydrate
2700 Calories—Six Feedings

Food	Weight Grams	Household Measure	Protein	Fat	Carbohydrate
Breakfast:					
Cereal..............	20	½ cup	3	...	16
Bacon, crisp.........	15	2 slices	3	8	
Egg................	100	2	14	10	
12% fruit..........	100	1 serving	.....	...	12
20% cream..........	60	¼ cup	2	12	2
Mid-morning:					
Egg................	50	1	7	5	
20% cream..........	60	¼ cup	2	12	2
Milk...............	120	½ cup	3.5	5	6
Crackers...........	8	3 small	1.5	1.5	6
Noon Meal:					
Meat, fish or fowl.....	90	3 ounces	21	15	
3% vegetable........	100	1 serving	2	...	3
9% vegetable........	100	1 serving	3	...	9
Bread..............	30	1 slice	3	...	16
20% cream..........	60	¼ cup	2	12	2
Butter.............	20	4 teaspoonfuls	......	17	
Mid-afternoon:					
20% cream..........	60	¼ cup	2	12	2
Milk...............	120	½ cup	3.5	5	6
Crackers...........	12	4 small	2	2	8
Cheese.............	30	1 ounce	9	11	
Evening Meal:					
Meat, fish or fowl.....	90	3 ounces	21	15	
3% vegetable........	100	1 serving	2	...	3
6% vegetable........	100	1 serving	2	...	6
18% vegetable.......	100	1 serving	5	1	18
Butter.............	25	5 teaspoonfuls	.....	21	
Oil................	15	1 tablespoon	.....	15	
Bedtime:					
Cheese.............	15	½ ounce	4.5	5.5	
Crackers...........	12	4 small	2	2	8
Butter.............	5	1 teaspoonful	.....	4	
Total...............			119	191	125

FAT.—Fat in liberal quantities is allowed and the total diet should have a high caloric value, 35 or 40 calories per Kg. of the normal body weight.

The diet may be divided, as illustrated in table 4 into three meals and three nourishments, the latter being taken midway between breakfast and lunch, between lunch and supper, and before retiring. Undernutrition should be avoided. A loss in weight exaggerates symptoms in true cases of hyperinsulinism. A sample diet which has proved useful in the treatment of this disorder is presented in table 4.

Physical exercise, because of its blood sugar lowering effect, should be restricted. It is well to instruct the patient to take extra food and in this way fortify his carbohydrate reserve preceding unavoidable exercise. For this purpose starchy foods, such as bread, crackers, apples, bananas and cereals serve admirably.

Drugs.—Drugs, with the exception of epinephrine (which has but a fleeting effect and is employed for relief from the acute attack), are of little value in the treatment of hyperinsulinism. Epinephrine in oil, it might be expected, would have a more lasting hyperglycemic effect. This drug increases the amount of sugar in circulation without increasing its combustion (Conn). Its effect is closely related to the glycogen reserve which in these cases may be small or not available. The subcutaneous administration of epinephrine is recommended for trial in the treatment of functional hyperinsulinism and in cases of tumors of the islets if operation is refused or fails to cure. A dose of 1 mg., in oil, may be given two or three times in twenty-four hours. Thyroid substance, if it is to have any appreciable effect, must be given in doses sufficiently large to elevate the basal metabolism considerably above normal. This procedure does not seem to be justified. Pituitrin gives little evidence of its reputed insulin-resistant qualities in the treatment of this disease. Theoretically preparations from the anterior pituitary gland might be useful in the treatment of this disease. Because of the danger of provoking a "total diabetes" their use might be justified only when operation is refused or fails to cure. Through their aid in reducing physical activity, sedatives may be of some value. Phenobarbital in doses of 0.065 gm. (1 grain) given night and morning has been suggested for this purpose. John[20] (1933) has suggested giving small doses of insulin before meals to prevent the postprandial increase in the blood sugar which has an insulinogenic effect. This treatment has been effective in cases of functional hyperinsulinism. It is well to remember, however, that these patients, especially those who are thin, are extremely sensitive to insulin. This sensitiveness is doubtless increased by the great amounts of carbohydrate which these patients have been in the habit of taking before seeking treatment.

Surgical Measures.—Surgery is indicated in the treatment of hyperinsulinism when a thorough trial of conservative treatment as outlined above fails to prevent attacks of hypoglycemia and when hepatic, adrenal and hypophyseal lesions are excluded as causes of the hypoglycemia.

It is beyond the scope of this book to present in detail the surgical aspect of this problem. This aspect of the subject has been well reviewed by Whipple.[5] It is permissible and important, however, to point out that the object in resorting to surgery is to cure the disease by the removal of a tumor or *tumors of the islets of Langerhans* or, failing to find a neoplasm, by the partial resection of the pancreas. The search for tumors should be thorough. The islet tumors are discrete nodules and are firmer than the surrounding pancreatic tissue. Whipple and others have had the experience of removing one tumor without alleviating the disease until at a second operation another tumor was found and removed. It may be impossible to identify a small islet-cell tumor, especially one embedded in the head of the pancreas.

Failing to find a tumor the surgeon is confronted with the difficult problem of deciding whether he should remove a portion of the pancreas and face the possibility of allowing a small undetectable tumor to remain in the head of the pancreas on one hand and the possibility of provoking a diabetes on the other.

Pancreatectomy.—Until recently the partial resection of an apparently normal pancreas did not provide sufficient improvement to warrant the risk of such a procedure. Evidence is accumulating that this is no longer so. Early failures may be attributable to the failure to remove an adequate amount of the pancreas. In support of subtotal pancreatectomies in selected cases Wilder quotes the case, reported by Graham and Hartmann, of a twelve months old child having convulsions due to hypoglycemia, the sugar content of the capillary blood being 18 mg. per 100 cc. The pancreas, at operation, appeared normal. As much of the organ as could be resected was removed, leaving a remnant estimated to be one eighth of the whole gland. No abnormalities were found in the section removed yet the blood sugar level returned to normal. Two years later the child appeared to be in normal health.

The likelihood of producing diabetes by removing a large portion of a normal pancreas must be faced. I agree that the risk of causing a disease so readily controlled as diabetes is excusable because the risk is less than that attending hyperinsulinism of the degree which fails to be controlled by conservative measures.

Preparation for Operation.—Liberal amounts of slowly absorbable carbohydrate and of protein are allowed at frequent intervals, every three or four hours, throughout the twenty-four hours preceding the operation. One hour before operation 500 cc. of a 10 per cent solution of glucose (dextrose) is given slowly in normal saline by vein.

The selection of the anesthetic and the general postoperative care is the same as that usually adopted for an abdominal section. Ether is preferred by some surgeons and hyperinsulinism *per se* is no contraindication to its use.

A transitory hyperglycemia usually follows the removal of an adenoma of the islets. It is a favorable sign as it usually signifies that no adenoma has escaped detection. It may be advisable to administer small amounts of insulin for two or three days, though in our experience this has not been necessary (see illustrative cases).

BIBLIOGRAPHY

1. Banting, F. G., Best, C. H., Collip, J. B., Campbell, W. R., and Fletcher, A. A., Canad. Med. Assoc. Jour., **12**: 141, 1922.
2. Harris, S., J.A.M.A., **83**: 729, 1924.
3. Wilder, R. M., Allan, F. N., Power, M. H., and Robertson, H. E., J.A.M.A., **89**: 348, 1927.
4. Howland, G., Campbell, W. R., Maltby, E. J., and Robinson, W. L., J.A.M.A., **93**: 674, 1929.
5. Whipple, A. O., Jour. Internat. Chirurgie, **3**: 237, 1938.
6. Laidlaw, G. F., Amer. Jour. Path., **14**: 125, 1938.
7. Malamud, N., and Grosh, L. C., Jr., Arch. Int. Med., **61**: 579, 1938.
8. Wilder, R. M., Clinical Diabetes Mellitus and Hyperinsulinism, W. B. Saunders Co., Philadelphia, p. 349, 1940.

9. Wilder, R. M., Ibid., p. 358.
10. Conn, J. W., J.A.M.A., **115:** 1669, 1940.
11. Kepler, E. J., and Moersch, F. P., Amer. Jour. Psychiat., **94:** 105, 1937.
12. Hartman, A. F., and Jaudon, J. C., Jour. Pediatrics, **11:** 1, 1937.
13. Duncan, G. G., and Fetter, F., Amer. Jour. Med. Sc., **187:** 347, 1934.
14. Bauer, J. T., and Royster, A. R., Bull. Ayer Clin. Lab. of Pennsylvania Hospital, **3:** 109, 1937.
15. Rabinowitz, I. M., J. Biol. Chem., **83:** 333, 1929.
16. Conn, J. W., Newburgh, L. H., Johnston, M. W., and Sheldon, J. M., Arch. Int. Med., **62:** 765, 1938.
17. Welty, J. W., and Robertson, A. F., Amer. Jour. Med. Sc., **192:** 760, 1936.
18. Conn, J. W., J. Clin. Invest., **15:** 673, 1936.
19. Wilder, R. M., Ibid., p. 403.
20. John, H. J., Endocrinology, **17:** 583, 1933.

CHAPTER XIV

DIABETES INSIPIDUS

By Garfield G. Duncan

Definition.—Diabetes insipidus is an uncommon and chronic disturbance in the water balance of the body. It is characterized by the frequent passing of excessive quantities of pale urine of low chloride content, free from sugar, and having an unusually low specific gravity, varying between 1.001 and 1.005. As a result of the uncontrolled diuresis, tissue dehydration and an intense thirst develop. The thirst becomes intolerable should the fluid intake be reduced to normal amounts.

PATHOGENESIS

Diabetes insipidus is a deficiency disease, there being, presumably, an insufficiency of the secretion of the posterior or neural lobe (also designated as the pars nervosa) of the pituitary gland, or a failure of functional response to this hormone. The normal production of the antidiuretic factor by the posterior lobe of the pituitary gland is dependent upon the integrity of a functional unit comprising: the gland itself, the paraventricular and supraoptic nuclei in the hypothalamus, and the supraopticohypophyseal tract of nerve fibers. This tract of nerve fibers, discovered independently by Pines[1] and Greving[2] (1926), arises in the nucleus supraopticus and the nucleus paraventricularis, and pursues a course down through the hypothalamus near the tuber cinereum, through the infundibular stalk to end in the posterior lobe of the pituitary gland. (See Fig. 131.)

It is believed that the nucleus supraopticus in the floor of the third ventricle is a center which, through a neural mechanism, influences the posterior lobe of the pituitary gland. *Water metabolism* is regulated by a continuous exchange of neural and hormonal stimuli between the posterior lobe of the pituitary and the diencephalon. In the presence of an intact anterior lobe of the pituitary gland, a bilateral injury to the supraopticohypophyseal tract disturbs this function and causes diabetes insipidus. Fisher and his associates[3] repeatedly induced diabetes insipidus in cats by interrupting the supraopticohypophyseal tract. Furthermore they found that atrophic changes took place in the supraoptic and paraventricular nuclei and in the posterior or neural lobe of the pituitary gland as a result of these injuries. It is clear that the functional capacity of this supraopticohypophyseal unit is dependent upon the integrity of each part. Destruction of the nuclei is followed by atrophy of the posterior lobe. Furthermore, destruction or enucleation of the posterior lobe leads to atrophy of these nuclei. A sharply defined lesion, transection of the hypophyseal stalk, without trauma to the base of the brain or to the hypophysis produced permanent (eleven years) polyuria and polydipsia in a human (Dandy[4]).

Total removal or destruction of the pituitary gland fails to produce diabetes insipidus because, according to von Hann's generally accepted theory, the diuretic principle of the anterior lobe has been removed. However, the antidiuretic principle found, and possibly produced, in the tuberal region of the hypothalamus could account for the failure of diabetes insipidus to occur after total hypophysectomy. There is convincing evidence that the amount of urine is normally regulated by a sensitive balance of the normally present diuretic principle in the anterior and the antidiuretic factor in the posterior lobe of the pituitary gland. It follows that when the production of the antidiuretic principle is reduced or stopped without disturbing the diuretic principle, this finely adjusted balance is upset and the polyuria of diabetes insipidus is precipitated. Reabsorption of water by the renal tubules seems to be almost specifically inhibited.

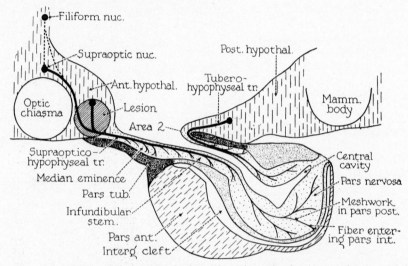

Fig. 131.—Diagram of a midsagittal section through the hypothalamus and hypophysis of the cat, showing the two divisions of the hypothalamicohypophyseal tract, the supraopticohypophyseal and the tuberohypophyseal tracts. The broken lines indicate proposed filiform-supraoptic connections and the tractus paraventricularis-cinereus of Greving. The obliquely striped circle indicates the position of a typical lesion designed to produce diabetes insipidus. (Fisher, Ingram and Ranson, "Diabetes Insipidus," Edwards Bros., 1938.)

The foregoing hypothesis regarding the cause of diabetes insipidus, though being the most attractive is by no means accepted by all authorities. There are prominent workers in this field who believe that the cause lies in disturbances in the hypothalamus and that the pituitary gland has no part in it. The antidiuretic action of extracts of the posterior pituitary gland is the outstanding obstacle to this hypothesis.

The part played by the thyroid gland in causing and preventing diabetes insipidus is controversial. Keller[5] believes the presence of the thyroid gland is essential to the production of diabetes insipidus. Fisher and his co-workers[3] refute this with convincing evidence.

Diabetes insipidus occurring as a result of disturbances in the areas already referred to is revealed clinically by an inability on the part of the kidneys to retain water. Polyuria ensues. Excessive thirst is compensatory and appears secondary to the uncontrolled diuresis.

TYPES OF DIABETES INSIPIDUS

(*a*) A **primary idiopathic form,** in which no organic cause is demonstrable. It may be hereditary or the result of a predisposition by heredity. If hereditary, it may be transmitted as a simple mendelian dominant characteristic. On the other hand, in one family of 220 members, reported by Weil,[6] there were, in five generations, 35 who had diabetes insipidus. Males are more often affected than females. Idiopathic diabetes insipidus usually appears in infancy and *persists throughout life* without affecting the patient's general health or longevity. In some cases the disorder appears and disappears and in others it may subside entirely. It may be associated with other congenital physical and mental defects, however, among which is the Laurence-Moon Biedl syndrome. The basis of the pathological changes of hereditary diabetes insipidus is unknown.

(*b*) A **secondary** or **symptomatic form,** in which etiological organic changes in the hypothalamic area have occurred. In this type signs and symptoms other than those of diabetes insipidus may be latent for a long period but eventually they become prominent. In some cases of diabetes insipidus the polydipsia and polyuria, which are readily corrected and the concentrating power of the kidneys restored by injection of the antidiuretic hormone of the posterior lobe of the hypophysis, may be the only symptoms. In another group the polyuria is accompanied by the permanent loss of renal ability to concentrate chlorides, bicarbonate, and basic elements, though the normal urine volume is restored by hormonal therapy. In some cases the diuresis is largely overcome, being reduced to two liters or thereabouts in twenty-four hours but without restoration of the ability of the kidneys to concentrate the urine.

Clinical evidence of the symptomatic or secondary form tends to confirm experimental observations concerning the etiology of diabetes insipidus. Frank[7] in 1912 reported an injury, in which a bullet lodged in the sella turcica and precipitated diabetes insipidus. The disease has been attributed to *developmental abnormalities;* it has followed *trauma* due to a fracture at the base of the skull; it has followed *acute infections*, notably measles, diphtheria, pertussis, scarlet fever, chicken pox, mumps, erysipelas, influenza, and encephalitis; it has been seen as a sequel to postvaccinal encephalitis; and it may follow *chronic infections*, such as syphilis (congenital or acquired), tuberculosis, and actinomycosis. *Neoplasms*, either primary or metastatic, or benign cysts in the base of the brain may be the cause. Warkany and Mitchell[8] recorded as causes of diabetes insipidus, different types of *tumors* occurring at the base of the pons, in the pineal body, and in the regions of the sella turcica, optic chiasm, third ventricle, infundibulum, and in the interpeduncular region. In short, tumors of the diencephalo-pituitary region are apt to cause diabetes insipidus. *Infiltrations* such as occur in syphilis (notably gummata), leukemia, sarcoidosis, lymphoblastoma or lymphadenoma (Hodgkin's disease), and in xanthomatoses, and which are part of the Hand-Schüller-Christian syndrome and involves the hypothalamic area, are known causes of diabetes insipidus.

Xanthomatosis is among the more frequent causes of diabetes insipidus in early childhood. Of 103 cases of xanthomatosis in children reported by Atkinson[9] symptoms of diabetes insipidus were observed in sixty-one. *Pellagra* is also a cause of diabetes insipidus. Rassuleo has estimated that 25 per cent of patients with pellagra present symptoms of diabetes insipidus. The foregoing agents produce diabetes insipidus either by direct destruction of the tissues in the diencephalopituitary area, or by pressure exercised directly, or by an internal hydrocephalus.

The *morbid anatomy* seen in nonidiopathic or secondary diabetes insipidus comprises the evidences of trauma, infection, new growths, or abnormal infiltrations in the hypothalamic and hypophyseal areas. There is a scarcity of records of studies of anatomic changes in the hypothalamus and in the pituitary gland in cases of idiopathic diabetes insipidus. In both the secondary and idiopathic types of this disease it is common to find enlarged hyperemic kidneys and a dilated bladder with hypertrophied walls. The ureters and the pelves of the kidneys may be dilated.

SYMPTOMATOLOGY

The untreated patient suffers from *polyuria* and an *intense thirst*. Five to 15 liters (quarts) of colorless urine are excreted daily. Amounts up to 43 liters are recorded (Trousseau). The polyuria may be reduced during febrile disturbances and is less while the patient is at rest than while he is active. An *excessive appetite* for food is not infrequent. The caloric intake is considerably in excess of that ordinarily estimated as necessary to maintain a constant body weight. It seems likely that this is a compensatory response to neutralize a heat debt incurred by drinking large quantities of water, the temperature of which is below that of the body. Fatigue and mental depression, resulting from disturbed rest necessitated by the frequent need of urinating, are common. There is a *dryness of the mouth* with the formation of thick tenacious mucus in the mouth and pharynx. The *skin* is dry, being a manifestation of a general dehydration, and there is an abnormal sensitiveness to cold. The *body temperature* tends to be subnormal unless some complication intervenes. *Obstinate constipation* is common. The disorder usually develops gradually, though it may appear abruptly, and it may be transitory or, as is often the case, it may remain stationary without serious impairment of health throughout life with thirst and polyuria the only symptoms. The latter is usually the case in idiopathic diabetes insipidus. Bed wetting may be the first symptom of the disease in children. The symptoms may be alleviated or intensified during pregnancy.

In those patients in whom the disorder is secondary to other disease processes the outcome is dictated by the behavior of the underlying abnormality.

The symptoms may change from those of an apparent functional derangement to those of increased intracranial pressure. This is especially prone to occur in cases of neoplasm in the diencephalo-pituitary area. In some cases the field and acuity of *vision* are gradually reduced. Edema of the optic disks, ocular palsies, especially of the sixth nerve, with one-sided, bitemporal or homonymous hemianopsia, strabismus with inequality of pupils, tremor, and convulsions also develop as a result of tumor growth. Intense frontal *headache,* nausea, vomiting, dizziness, pains in back and legs, transitory hemiplegias, mental deterioration, and infantilism also occur. These are the general symptoms of increased *intracranial pressure* and localizing signs, depending on the site of the lesion. Precocious sexual development is an unusual complication in these cases, occurring when the tumor involves the pineal body. *Loss of weight* to the degree of extreme cachexia may occur, though obesity associated with endocrine disorders is not an unusual complication. Edema of the extremities may follow if the disturbances in nutrition are marked. The profound emaciation and exhaustion with disturbed function of the anterior lobe of the hypophysis predispose to impotence, cessation of menses, and rarely to acromegaly. *Dystrophia adiposogenitalis* also occurs as a result of involvement of the anterior lobe of the pituitary gland. Intractable diarrhea and a terminal pneumonia with drowsiness progressing to coma and death are not uncommon in cachectic patients with increased intracranial pressure.

Diabetes insipidus is easily recognized as a symptomatic entity but it may be difficult to ascertain the underlying etiologic process.

LABORATORY FINDINGS

The *positive* laboratory data in cases of diabetes insipidus are: (1) the great volume of colorless urine with a low specific gravity, varying from 1.001 to 1.005; (2) traces of albumin and inosite may be found in the urine; (3) the reduction of chloride excretion below the normal daily value of 8–13 gm.; and (4) approximately normal total daily excretion of solids.

Correction of the diuresis and the increase in the specific gravity of the urine which follow the administration of the hormone of the posterior lobe of the pituitary gland, are diagnostic criteria. Furthermore an increase in specific gravity of the blood and an increase in the red blood cell count occur if the untreated patient is deprived of water. The chloride content of the blood is sometimes high; rarely is it low. These findings have served to classify diabetes insipidus into the *hyperchloremic* and the *hypochloremic* types.

Important *negative* findings in diabetes insipidus are: the absence of sugar in the urine; the normal ability of the kidneys to excrete nitrogen; a normal response to dye excretion tests with unchanged urea and creatinine clearances, and the absence of any appreciable disturbance in the basal metabolism.

PROGNOSIS

Idiopathic diabetes insipidus is relatively benign. It may cause little, if any, emaciation. Indeed the patient may experience no ill effect except for the thirst and polyuria. In these cases life is not shortened by the disease. The prognosis is not related to the degree of polyuria.

The outcome when diabetes insipidus is secondary to some other disturbance, be it infection, trauma, new growth, abnormal infiltrations, or congenital defect, depends upon the nature of the underlying lesion. In the secondary group cachexia is common and there is a predisposition to terminal intercurrent infections.

SUGGESTIVE SIGNS OF PATHOLOGIC CONDITIONS ASSOCIATED WITH DIABETES INSIPIDUS
(After Warkany and Mitchell)

SYMPTOMS AND SIGNS WHICH AID IN DIFFERENTIAL DIAGNOSIS	ASSOCIATED PATHOLOGIC CONDITIONS	COMMENT
Familial occurrence	Idiopathic-hereditary form	More frequent in males; general health and development usually normal
Polydactylism, syndactylism, retinitis pigmentosa, obesity, hypogenitalism, retarded mentality	Laurence-Moon-Biedl syndrome or other defect or lesion of diencephalon	
History of abortion or miscarriage	Syphilitic involvement of pituitary gland or diencephalon	
Trauma of head (usually basal skull fracture)	Injury (hemorrhage or scar formation) of pituitary gland or diencephalon	Diabetes insipidus may follow quickly or after interval of several months; in some cases obesity, failure of sexual development, involvement of cranial nerves
Age period	Congenital (hereditary type); early childhood (xanthomatosis); later childhood (tumors, postencephalitic conditions)	
General health	With hereditary type, unaffected; with other types, dependent on underlying condition	
Body temperature	With inflammatory lesions, elevated; with involvement of hypothalamus, elevated or subnormal	
Sexual precocity	Pineal tumor	
Retardation of growth	Tumor of brain; xanthomatosis; postencephalitic lesions of diencephalon	
Generalized lymphadenitis	Leukemia; xanthomatosis; syphilis; lymphogranulomatosis	
Harelip or cleft palate	Developmental defect of diencephalon	
Beefy red tongue	Pellagra	
Gingivitis, loss of teeth	Xanthomatosis	
Necrotic exudate on tonsils	Leukemia	
Roentgenograms of lungs	May show characteristic changes in case of tuberculosis, xanthomatosis, sarcoids, leukemia	
Cardiac enlargement	Chronic nephritis	Absent with idiopathic-hereditary form
Bradycardia	Tumor of brain; hydrocephalus; pellagra	
Hepatosplenomegaly	Xanthomatosis; leukemia; chronic nephritis (from cardiorenal disease)	
Anemia and hemorrhagic manifestations	Leukemia; xanthomatosis	
Roentgencgram of bones	With pineal tumor, advanced epiphysial closure; with Laurence-Moon-Biedl syndrome or other defect or lesion of diencephalon, delayed epiphysial closure; with syphilis or xanthomatosis, characteristic changes	
Pseudo spina ventosa	Schaumann-Besnier-Boeck disease (sarcoids)	Other sarcoids in skin, lungs or bones
Increased intracranial pressure (nausea, vomiting, headache)	Tumor of brain, xanthomatosis, etc.	Nausea, vomiting and headache occur also in cases of water intoxication
Enlargement of head	Tumor cf brain, xanthomatosis, etc.	
Mental deficiency	Laurence-Moon-Biedl syndrome; encephalitis and other lesions of brain	Intelligence usually normal with idiopathic-hereditary type, but behavior may be capricious or "neurasthenic"
Exophthalmos	Xanthomatosis; also perhaps with tumors and hydrocephalus	
Loss of vision (atrophy of optic nerves, choked disk)	Tumor of brain, xanthomatosis, etc.	Retinitis pigmentosa with Laurence-Moon-Biedl syndrome
Deafness	Trauma (basal fractures); xanthomatosis	
Cutaneous lesions	With all forms, day skin and acrocyanosis; with xanthomatosis, bronzing, xanthomas; with pellagra, typically distributed pigmentation, etc.; with leukemia, infiltrative skin lesions and later purpura; with Schaumann-Besnier-Boeck disease, sarcoids	
Basal metabolism	Decreased in many forms	Has been reported as normal with idiopathic-hereditary type
Hypercholesterolemia	Xanthomatosis	Not always present
Roentgenograms of skull	With trauma, fracture; with hydrocephalus, increased convolutional markings, separation of sutures, enlargement of ventricles (encephalograms); with xanthomatosis, typical changes; with tumor, distortion of sella turcica, etc.	

DIAGNOSIS

Though several disorders may be confused with diabetes insipidus the therapeutic test, using the hormone of the posterior lobe of the pituitary gland, is diagnostic. Only in diabetes insipidus does improvement follow this therapy. The diagnosis may be made clear by giving 1 cc. of beta-hypophamine (N. N. R.) (pitressin) or pituitrin hypodermically and observing in patients with diabetes insipidus that the thirst and polyuria disappear only to recur when the effect of the drug is exhausted.

The intense thirst, headache, fatigue, loss of weight, hypothermia, tachycardia, and prostration which follow when the untreated patient is deprived of water is not duplicated in any other disease. Diabetes insipidus must be *differentiated* from:

(1) **Temporary Polyuria.**—The polyuria which results when normal persons habitually drink large quantities of water, alcoholic beverages or those which contain caffeine may be confused with that of diabetes insipidus. Unlike the reaction in diabetes insipidus, the withdrawal of these liquids fails to provoke an abnormal thirst. Evidences of dehydration are also lacking in these individuals and furthermore a reduced fluid intake causes a prompt diminution in the amount of urine and an increase in its specific gravity to exceed 1.020, unless prevented from doing so by a co-existing nephritis.

(2) **Chronic Glomerular Nephritis and Polycystic Disease of the Kidneys.**—In these diseases quantities of urine having a low specific gravity may be passed. Small amounts of albumin are usually present. In freshly voided specimens hyaline casts are also frequently found. Elevation of the blood pressure and evidences of vascular involvement are usual. Impaired kidney function is revealed by tests of renal function (phenolsulfonephthalein dye excretion, impaired urea and creatinine clearances) and by the retention of nitrogen in the blood (azotemia). These features and the absence of great thirst should establish the identity of the underlying disease.

(3) **Hysteria.**—Polyuria due to hysteria is likely to be intermittent and accompanied by other evidences of psychic or nervous disorders. Furthermore a reduction in the fluid intake is not attended by the distressing thirst experienced by patients suffering from diabetes insipidus.

(4) **Diabetes Mellitus.**—In contradistinction to diabetes insipidus there occurs in diabetes mellitus glycosuria, a urine with a high specific gravity—above 1.030, usually—and hyperglycemia. Furthermore, in diabetes mellitus the objective and subjective evidences of the diseases, including excessive thirst and polyuria, yield promptly to treatment with suitable diet and insulin, but not to injections of pituitrin or pitressin. It should be noted, however, that diabetes insipidus and diabetes mellitus do occasionally co-exist in the same patient.

TREATMENT

The treatment of diabetes insipidus comprises substitution therapy, either alone or combined with the management of an underlying disorder if such a disorder is detected and identified.

Substitution Therapy.—Schafer in 1906 revealed a definite relationship between the action of the posterior lobe of the pituitary gland and urinary excretion, but it was Von den Veldon[10] and Farini[11] (1913) who independently observed that preparations from the posterior lobe of the pituitary gland alleviated the polyuria and thirst of diabetes insipidus. Though the mechanism is not clearly understood it is known that most of the patients having this disease experience temporary alleviation of these symptoms following the administration of this hormone and that retention of water in the body is made possible. The thirst subsides, the polyuria is reduced, and in most cases the ability of the kidney to concentrate the urine is restored until the effect of the drug is dissipated. This substitution therapy is harmless and may be continued for many years without ill effect. It is effective in the alleviation of the symptoms in approximately 90 per cent of the cases of diabetes insipidus.

Substitution therapy by means of the antidiuretic hormone is, and should be considered, a palliative measure, although occasional and unexplained remissions do occur. This therapy must be continued for the remainder of the patient's life, except in the rare case in which the cause is identified and successfully removed or when unexplained recovery occurs spontaneously.

Beta-hypophamine (*N. N. R.*) (*pitressin*) is an effective posterior lobe preparation and is commonly employed. Administered hypodermically in doses of 0.5 to 3.0 cc. daily, the amount depending upon the severity of the condition and the individual reaction to the drug, pitressin affords the patient relief from symptoms for four to eight and occasionally as long as forty-eight hours. When a single daily injection suffices it is best given in the evening in order to secure the greatest freedom from symptoms during the night. In this manner one of the most distressing features of the disease, namely, the necessity for frequent urination during the night is overcome. In the milder cases 0.5 cc. once daily may suffice, but usually two administrations daily, one in the morning and one in the evening, are needed. Although the antidiuretic effect lasts on the average between four and twelve hours, occasionally treatments every six hours are needed. Pitressin is also effective when administered by a nasal spray or a nasal tampon.

Recently Greene and January,[12] using *pitressin tannate in peanut oil** secured a prolonged pitressin effect. An intramuscular injection of 1 cc. (equivalent to 5 pressor units of pitressin) of this preparation controlled the manifestations of diabetes insipidus for thirty to eighty-two hours without untoward side effects. The dose need be repeated only as often as is necessary to control the symptoms. This appears to be the therapy of choice.

Obstetrical pituitrin, administered subcutaneously, may be employed in doses of 0.5 to 1 cc., with the same effect as pitressin in alleviating the symptoms of diabetes insipidus. *Surgical pituitrin*, double the U.S.P. potency and twice as potent as obstetrical pituitrin may be given, hypodermically, 0.5 cc. or 1 cc. each evening. The stimulating action which both of these preparations have on peristalsis may cause looseness of the bowels. It is well to give either drug early in the evening in order that this effect will have had time to subside before the patient retires. The minimum amount of any one of these preparations which yields satisfactory results

* Supplied by Parke, Davis and Company.

should be established and administered as frequently or as rarely as necessary.

A great reduction in the polyuria from 10 liters or more to a normal or nearly normal output with a higher specific gravity and with an attendant alleviation of the thirst and dehydration, occurs as a result of this treatment in nearly all patients with this disease. Overdosage does not cause oliguria. Patients receiving this substitution therapy are instructed to take only enough water to satisfy their thirst. Should this counsel be ignored symptoms of "water intoxication" as described by Snell and Rowntree[13] may be precipitated. Patients with postencephalitic mental changes must be carefully supervised in this respect. This complication of treatment—water intoxication—is due to a large fluid intake after the polyuria is controlled. It should be suspected if otherwise unexplained restlessness, mental confusion, poor muscle coordination, hypothermia, headache, nausea, and vomiting are encountered at such times. Convulsions, coma, and death may ensue.

A few patients derive no benefit from the pituitary extract and others, while relieved of the thirst and polyuria, become pale and experience nausea, intestinal cramps, diarrhea, and cardiac palpitation shortly after the injection. In this event smaller doses may be given at more frequent intervals. Latent anaphylactoid reactions to the pituitary preparations have been reported and atrophy of the subcutaneous fat at the site of the injection sometimes follows repeated injections in the same area.

Intranasal Application of Aqueous Solution of Pituitrin.—An alternative treatment and one that is being more widely used is that described by Blumgart,[14] namely the use of a nasal spray of 1 cc. of surgical pituitrin in 30 cc. (1 ounce) of normal salt solution. This method is not always effective and is expensive. A nasal tampon soaked with 0.5 to 1.0 cc. of the "surgical pituitrin" placed against the roof of the nasopharynx preferably in one side at a time has proved of value. This procedure may be repeated two or three times daily.

Nasal Insufflations of Powdered Posterior Lobe of the Pituitary Gland.—A powdered posterior lobe preparation now generally available, when applied to the nasal membranes in doses of 40 to 50 mg. is efficacious in alleviating the symptoms of this disease.[15, 16] The powder is snuffed up or is blown into the upper portion of the nasal chamber at three- or four-hour intervals during the day and once during the night. When properly applied it gives rise to a slight stinging sensation between the eyes. The powder may be mixed with a bland nasal jelly to facilitate and ensure its application to the nasal mucus membrane. It may be administered on the finger tip or by a suitable nozzle.

This form of therapy is gaining in popularity and may be recommended because it is effective; it can be conducted without hypodermic injections; the technique is simple, convenient and without danger; and not the least consideration is the greatly reduced cost, being approximately 4 to 10 cents daily in contrast to 35 to 70 cents for the aqueous injectable solutions. Furthermore there are no untoward symptoms produced by it with the exception of the mild stinging sensation when the powder comes in contact with the nasal mucous membrane. Intranasal administration of the hormone is less effective during attacks of coryza. At such times the hypodermic administration of pitressin or pituitrin is desirable.

Preparations from the posterior pituitary gland are ineffective when given orally or by rectum.

Intermedin,* an extract of the pars intermedia of the pituitary gland, was found by Zondek and Krohn[17] to be effective in controlling the symptoms of diabetes insipidus. It does not affect the smooth musculature of the intestines nor does it raise the blood pressure, and because of these qualities it has been recommended for trial in patients who have vasomotor and gastro-intestinal disturbances following the administration of extracts of the posterior lobe. Intermedin is said to check only the water output, in contrast to pitressin which reduces both water and sodium chloride excretion. The beneficial effects of intermedin have been observed in this country by Sulzberger, in the management of two patients.

Lumbar puncture.—Recovery from diabetes insipidus has occurred following a reduction of the intracranial pressure. The slow removal of 8 to 15 cc. of the spinal fluid may be of particular value in cases of increased intraventricular pressure. The relief secured is likely to be temporary. Herrick[18] records benefit from this measure and Rowntree advocates its trial with the usual precautions which surround this procedure and unless it is contraindicated by the pressure of an intracranial neoplasm. The withdrawal of spinal fluid should be very slow if the intraspinal pressure is above normal or if there is edema of the optic disks. The alleviation of diabetes insipidus has been observed to follow encephalographic examinations; the modus operandi is not known.

Treatment of Associated Diseases Having a Probable Etiologic Basis.— Complicating syphilis should be actively treated by antisyphilitic measures. A combination of such treatment with preparations from the posterior pituitary gland is indicated. Basilar syphilitic meningitis or gummatous changes may be of etiological significance and their correction offers some hope of a cure. Four of Futcher's nine patients who had diabetes insipidus also had syphilis.

If xanthomata are detected, roentgen-ray therapy over the hypophyseal area offers a possibility of benefit.

Diet.—The hypercholesterolemia, associated with xanthomatosis, may be corrected by means of a diet rich in carbohydrate (400 to 500 grams), poor in fat (40 grams or less), and having a low cholesterol content. Such a diet carries possibilities of preventing a progressiveness of the disorder, and improvement may ensue.

A diet poor in salt with a restricted protein content has been advocated by Allen[19] as a palliative measure in dealing with diabetes insipidus. I have observed several patients who were benefited by the withdrawal of salt from the diet but whose improvement fell far short of that which may be secured by suitable hormone therapy. Beverages, notably tea, coffee, and certain "soft drinks" are curtailed because of their caffeine content. Liquids should be reasonably restricted after 6 o'clock in the evening. Diets of a high caloric value and high in vitamin content, fortified by the vita-

---

* This preparation and a similar one, pitmelanin, are not available for general clinical use and have indeed been little used in clinical practice.

min B complex, riboflavin, and nicotinic acid, should be given to those patients who have symptoms of pellagra. (See p. 437.)

Surgery.—Diabetes insipidus due to a tumor of the hypophysis may be cured by successful enucleation of the growth, if the removal is accomplished without destroying the posterior lobe or dividing the infundibular stalk. Operative intervention for a tumor of the brain must be decided upon criteria other than the associated diabetes insipidus. The removal of an adenoma from the thyroid gland has been reported to have alleviated the symptoms of diabetes insipidus. Such an operation should be done when a patient who has both conditions is encountered.

Miscellaneous.*—Various empirical methods of no lasting value have been recommended from time to time. Sedatives belong to this group.

Amidopyrin in doses of 2 gm. (30 grains) daily for five days has been advocated by Scherf and found effective in reducing nocturia in cases of chronic mesencephalitis by Lichtwitz.[20] Amidopyrin should in no way be considered a substitute for hormonal therapy and considering the possibility of its producing agranulocytosis its use is not devoid of risk. Fever reduces the polyuria but its artificial induction is not to be recommended as a form of therapy. *Estrin* (follicular hormone) has been reported as being helpful in a number of cases of diabetes insipidus. This result is attributed to the depressing effect which this hormone exerts on the anterior lobe of the pituitary gland. It is presumed that this permits the antidiuretic principle of the posterior lobe to exert a greater apparent effect.

Preparations from the anterior pituitary and thyroid gland preparations and diuretics are contraindicated in the management of this disease. *Thyroidectomy* should not be considered unless it is indicated irrespective of the diabetes insipidus.

* Many agents which have little to recommend them have been reported as having a favorable effect upon the symptoms of diabetes insipidus. Some are of temporary value, some are valueless, and none have been proved by the test of time to compare favorably with products from the posterior pituitary gland. References to the reports on these various preparations are included in Warkany and Mitchell's review,[8] to which the reader is referred. In isolated instances patients appear to have been benefited by treatment with gonadotropic substances from the urine of pregnant women (antuitrin S), estrogen, testicular extracts, corpus luteum extract, insulin, fluid extract of ergot, valerian, opium, parenteral injection of milk, hydrotherapy, short-wave therapy, transplantation of the posterior lobe of the pituitary gland from a person of the same blood group but of different sex into the rectus muscle of the patient, implantation of sheep's gland, and depot injection of tonephin.

BIBLIOGRAPHY

1. Pines, I. L., Ztschr. f. d. ges. Neurol. u. Psychiat., **100:** 123, 1926.
2. Greving, R., Deutsch. Ztschr. f. Nervenh., **89:** 179, 1926.
3. Fisher, D., Ingram, W. R., and Ranson, S. W., Diabetes Insipidus, Edwards Bros., 1938.
4. Dandy, E., J.A.M.A., **114:** 312, 1940.
5. Keller, A. D., Proc. Exp. Biol. Med., **36:** 787, 1937.
6. Weil, A., Deutsch. Arch. f. klin. Med., **93:** 180, 1908.
7. Frank, E., Berl. klin. Wchnschr., **49:** 393, 1912.
8. Warkany, J., nd Mitchell, A. G., Amer. Jour. of Child., **57:** 603, 1939.
9. Atkinson, F. R. B., Brit. J. Child. Dis., **34:** 28, 1937.
10. Von den Veldon, R., Berl. klin. Wchschr., **50:** 2083, 1913.
11. Farini, A., and Ceccaroni, B., Gass. d. osp. Milano, **34:** 879, 1913; also Clin. Med. Ital. Milano, **52:** 497, 1913.

12. Greene, J. A., and January, L. E., J.A.M.A., **115:** 1183, 1940.
13. Snell, A. M., and Rowntree, L. L., Endocrinology, **11:** 209, 1927.
14. Blumgart, H. L., Arch. Int. Med., **29:** 508, 1922.
15. Choay, A., and Choay, L., Rev. Neurol., **1:** 267, 1924.
16. Vigdoff, B., Endocrinology, **16:** 289, 1932.
17. Zondek, B., and Krohn, H., Klin. Wchnschr., **30:** 1293, 1932.
18. Herrick, J. B., Arch. Int. Med., **10:** 1, 1912.
19. Allen, F. M., and Sherrill, J. W., Jour. Metabolic Dis., **3:** 479, 1923.
20. Lichtwitz, L., Bull. New York Acad. Med., **15:** 773, 1939.

CHAPTER XV

MELITURIA

By Abraham Cantarow

NORMAL URINE SUGAR

In the normal individual, glucose is excreted by the renal glomeruli but, constituting one of the so-called "threshold bodies," it is largely reabsorbed into the blood stream through the tubular epithelium. A small amount, however, which escapes this conservation process, is eliminated in the urine. The amount of copper-reducing substance or substances in the normal urine varies considerably (0.5–1.5 gm. daily), and perhaps only a small portion is glucose.[1] Some investigators believe that the reducing substances in normal urine are made up of poorly assimilable or nonassimilable carbohydrates and of substances derived from the protein of the food and from endogenous sources.[2] The importance of the appreciation of the presence of *reducing substances* in normal urine is obvious. It is important, also, to distinguish between this so-called "glycuresis,"[3] a physiologic phenomenon, and glycosuria, usually a pathologic phenomenon. This distinction may be summarized according to the conception of Folin and Berglund[4] as follows: Glycuresis follows every ordinary carbohydrate meal, the increase in reducing substances being independent of the amount of sugar in the blood and being due largely to the excretion of foreign unassimilable carbohydrates and carbohydrate decomposition products produced during the preparation of food. A portion of these reducing substances is represented by glucose. Hassan[5] found glucose to be present (osazone test) in 20 to 30 per cent of cases after one to two hours, in 12 to 15 per cent after four to five hours, and in 7 per cent after twelve hours. On the other hand, the output of glucose is less after the ingestion of 50 gm. of pure glucose than following an ordinary mixed meal, and the administration of even as much as 200 gm. of glucose is not followed by glycosuria. After meals of bread, and particularly in concentrated urine specimens, the ordinary reduction tests may yield positive results. According to Sumner,[6] the urine of normal subjects contains reducing substances in concentrations varying from 0.05 to 0.15 per cent in terms of glucose; about 60 per cent of the reduction is due to sugar. Values of 0.25 per cent are to be considered with suspicion and 0.3 per cent as definitely pathologic, especially if the urine is not concentrated.

RENAL THRESHOLD

The concept of a threshold limit of renal "impermeability" to glucose has served as a convenient basis for the classification of various forms of glycosuria. The renal threshold may be defined as that concentration of sugar in the blood which must be reached before an excessive quantity of glucose is eliminated in the urine. This "threshold value" is generally assumed to be about 140 to 160 mg. per 100 cc. of whole blood and 170 mg. per 100 cc. of plasma.

There are two diametrically opposed schools of thought in this connection. The one affirms a belief in the existence of a renal threshold for glucose. Folin and Berglund,[4] who are among the proponents of this belief, state that hyperglycemia definitely below the threshold does not normally produce the slightest leakage of glucose through the kidneys and that normally not a trace of circulating glucose is lost. They admit, however, that there is apparently no such threshold for galactose and lactose, the elimination of which is independent of their concentration in the blood. On the other hand, Benedict and Osterberg[7] believe that the glucose threshold is wholly an artifact, and that whereas the causes leading to glucose excretion by the kidneys are usually the same as those leading to an increase in the blood sugar, the two latter phenomena need not be always causally related.

There can be no question that the term "renal threshold" is misleading from a physiological standpoint. As stated by Peters,[8] the concept of renal threshold appears to be that of a barrier or dam. As long as the concentration of glucose in the blood plasma remains below the top of the dam it does not appear in the urine; when it rises above this level it passes over the dam and continues to escape in the urine until the concentration in the blood has fallen below the critical level. This concept is inconsistent with established facts. Glucose passes freely into the glomerular filtrate from the blood, its concentration in the former being approximately the same as in the plasma.[9] Under normal conditions it undergoes practically complete reabsorption in the tubules, probably in the proximal convoluted tubules.[9] As stated by Peters,[8] when its concentration in the glomerular filtrate, and in the blood about the tubules, is unusually high, the tubular absorptive mechanism becomes inadequate, and some glucose escapes in the urine. The point at which this occurs is extremely variable, depending upon physiological conditions that are not well understood. Experimental evidence suggests that the total quantity of glucose which passes the glomerular filter is of greater significance in determining the occurrence of glycosuria than is the concentration of glucose in the blood. Nevertheless, it would appear that although the concept of a renal barrier to glucose excretion is untenable from physiological standpoints, from a practical standpoint the view may be accepted that the reabsorption of glucose in the tubules is checked when its concentration in the blood rises to an excessively high level.

The concept of such a threshold is useful from a clinical standpoint. It must be recognized, however, that the "threshold value," if such exists, is extremely variable, differing not only among individuals but also in the same individual at different times. This may be due to one or more of several causes:

(1) The "permeability" of the kidney for sugar is dependent not only on the level of blood sugar at that moment but also upon the duration of an existing hyperglycemia.

(2) Blood and urine (bladder) removed at the same time do not represent simultaneous specimens, for the rate of urine formation varies as does

the blood sugar concentration during and prior to the period of urine formation.

(3) The concentration of sugar in venous blood may not always be a true index of its concentration in the arterial blood supplying the kidney.

(4) The relationship between the level of sugar in the blood and its excretion in the urine varies with both rising and falling blood sugar values. It has been found that following the administration of glucose, its elimination in the urine began when the blood sugar concentration was 150 mg. per 100 cc. and continued until it had dropped to 60 mg. According to Folin,[4] this is due to the fact that, prior to the excretion of the sugar, the holding capacity of the tissues, including the kidneys, is exceeded, thus producing a local functional strain with the consequence that the glycosuria, once begun, does not stop when the blood sugar has fallen to the threshold value or even lower.

If one admits the practical value of the concept of a renal threshold for glucose, it must be realized that the threshold level possesses a wide individual variation and is capable of extreme variation in normal individuals under certain circumstances. Glycosuria has been observed in normal persons with a blood sugar concentration of 60 mg. per 100 cc. and, as in a patient with ether anesthesia reported by Mackay,[10] glycosuria may not occur in the presence of a blood sugar level of over 350 mg. per 100 cc. The renal threshold is believed to be lowered during pregnancy. It is frequently elevated in nephritis and arteriosclerosis, and in patients with diabetes after long periods of insulin therapy. In such cases of diabetes, blood sugar values as high as 425 mg. per 100 cc. have been reported without concomitant glycosuria. With these facts in mind, the statement may be made that glucose is excreted in the urine when the level of blood sugar has risen above the normal "threshold level" for that individual. If the commonly accepted threshold values of 140 to 160 mg. per 100 cc. are considered as normal, persons with glycosuria may be classed in two divisions: (1) with normal renal threshold and excessive hyperglycemia, and (2) with low renal threshold and normal blood sugar (renal glycosuria).

MELITURIA[11] *

The term "melituria" is properly employed to designate the presence, in the urine, of an abnormal amount of sugar. When the sugar is glucose the condition is termed "glycosuria"; when levulose, it is called "levulosuria"; when pentose, "pentosuria"; when lactose or galactose, "lactosuria" and "galactosuria." Since all meliturias are not glycosuria, the identification of the sugar becomes a matter of considerable moment.

Tests for the Detection of Sugars

Metallic Oxide Reduction Tests.—The most widely used routine method for the detection of sugar in the urine is one of the copper reduction tests of which the Benedict test is perhaps the most satisfactory. It yields positive results when glucose is present in as low a concentration as 0.1 per cent, and the Benedict reagent is less susceptible to reduction by nonsugar

* This section is taken largely from "Clinical Biochemistry," by Cantarow and Trumper, Second Edition, W. B. Saunders Company, Philadelphia, 1939.

substances than is the Fehling reagent. These substances include uric acid, nucleoprotein, conjugate glycuronates and chloroform, when present in sufficient concentration. Creatinine may, by dissolving cupric oxide, mask slight degrees of reduction caused by small amounts of sugar.

The following sugars are capable of reducing metallic oxides in alkaline solution: glucose, levulose, galactose, pentose, lactose and maltose.

Fermentation Test.—The fact that certain sugars are fermentable by yeast has been the basis for the widespread use of the fermentation test in the identification of urinary sugars. The statement is ordinarily made that glucose, levulose and galactose are fermentable by yeast and that maltose and sucrose are fermentable only after their inversion by the enzymes maltase and invertase present in the yeast. Lactose is said to be nonfermentable by ordinary bakers' yeast. One possible source of error has been indicated by Neuberg,[12] who demonstrated that yeast possesses the property of splitting off carbon dioxide from the carboxyl group of amino acids normally present in the urine. Another important observation has been made by Castellani and Taylor,[13] who found that ordinary bakers' yeast is not pure and usually consists of one or two species of saccharomyces with a contaminating gram-positive bacillus. They showed that most cultures of so-called "pure yeast" ferment glucose, levulose, galactose, sucrose, maltose and, in many instances (15 per cent), lactose. Obviously, positive differentiation of urinary sugars on the basis of this test is impossible.

Castellani[14] has elaborated a method of differentiating various sugars on the basis of fermentation by specific fungi and gas production by specific bacteria. For example, glucose alone is fermented by *Monilia balcanica;* glucose and levulose are fermented by *Monilia krusei; B. coli* forms gas with lactose, whereas *B. paratyphosus* does not. The combined use of reduction tests and gas production by specific fungi and bacteria is of great value in the positive identification of urinary sugars.

Phenylhydrazine Reaction.—This reaction depends upon the formation of a crystalline osazone, the structure of which is typical, to a certain degree, for various sugars. Glucose and levulose form osazone crystals of identical structure. The identification of lactose by this test is not practicable, for lactosazone crystals, although typical, are formed with difficulty in urine. At times the determination of the melting point of these crystals is utilized as a means of differentiating the sugars, but it is not a procedure of practical clinical value.

Specific Rotation.—The degree of rotation of polarized light, determined by means of a polariscope or polarizing saccharimeter, may be employed as an aid in the identification of urinary sugars. This procedure is not frequently resorted to clinically. Furthermore, glucose and lactose cannot be differentiated by this method.

Other tests which are of value in the positive identification of urinary sugars will be dealt with in discussing the various types of melituria.

GLYCOSURIA

The term "glycosuria" signifies the excretion in the urine of abnormal amounts of glucose. Glucose may be identified in the urine on the basis of the following tests:

1. Positive reduction test.
2. Fermentation with bakers' yeast.
3. Typical glucosazone crystals with phenylhydrazine.
4. Gas production with Monilia balcanica.[14]
5. Specific rotation of polarized light.

As has been indicated, the properties of reducing power and fermentation by yeast are shared by many sugars and are therefore not specific for glucose. The following criteria may be established for the positive *identification of glucose:*

1. Typical osazone crystals with phenylhydrazine in the presence of a negative Seliwanoff reaction (resorcinol-hydrochloric acid) to exclude levulose, or
2. Gas production with *Monilia balcanica,*[14] or
3. Specific rotation of polarized light ($-52.5°$) in the absence of a positive mucic acid test to exclude lactose.

The several forms of glycosuria may be conveniently classified clinically under two headings:

1. Glycosuria unassociated with hyperglycemia, or "nonhyperglycemic glycosuria."
2. Glycosuria associated with hyperglycemia, or "hyperglycemic glycosuria."

Nonhyperglycemic Glycosuria.—Glucose may appear in the urine in the presence of a normal concentration of sugar in the blood. This condition may be produced experimentally by the administration of phlorhizin. It is observed clinically in so-called "renal glycosuria" (renal diabetes), during pregnancy and, as some believe, in the condition commonly termed "alimentary glycosuria."

Phlorhizin Glycosuria.—The administration of phlorhizin is followed by glycosuria associated with a normal and, indeed, in many instances a subnormal blood sugar concentration. There appears to be little doubt that phlorhizin glycosuria is in the true sense of the term a renal glycosuria. There is rather convincing experimental evidence that this substance produces its glycosuric effect by inhibiting reabsorption of glucose from the renal tubules.

Renal Glycosuria.—The frequency of incidence of this condition, also known as "renal diabetes," "benign" glycosuria and "diabetes innocens," is perhaps not so great as is commonly supposed. When rigid diagnostic criteria were established, Marble[15] was able to find only sixteen cases in 9000 patients with glycosuria. He outlined the following standards for the diagnosis of true renal glycosuria:

(1) Fasting blood sugar within normal limits and a normal (or supernormal) glucose tolerance curve. (2) Glucose should be present in every specimen of urine, whether voided in the fasting state or after a meal. The quantity of sugar in the urine should be largely independent of the diet, although it may vary somewhat depending on the amount of carbohydrate ingested. (3) Carbohydrate utilization should be normal, as evidenced by determinations of respiratory quotient and serum inorganic phosphorus after glucose ingestion. (4) There should be no disturbance of fat metabolism, ketosis being more likely to develop when the patient fasts than

when he overeats. (5) Moderate doses of insulin should have little or no effect on the glycosuria.

The condition is believed by many to be hereditary and familial, and it seems likely that, once developed, it persists throughout the life of the individual. Folin and Berglund,[4] in contrast to Marble,[15] are of the opinion that it occurs comparatively frequently, existing in 1 to 2 per cent of otherwise normal students whom they have studied. They believe, likewise, that the majority of instances of so-called "alimentary glycosuria" are, in reality, cases of renal glycosuria. The importance of its recognition depends upon its apparent harmlessness; so far as can be determined, it never results in diabetes mellitus nor in any metabolic derangement whatsoever. As stated by Marble,[15] practical danger in making the diagnosis of renal glycosuria lies in the confusion of this condition with potential or mild diabetes mellitus. Care must be exercised also in the diagnosis of the glycosuria of pregnancy, which is not always of the benign type. He believes that the patient must be watched carefully over a period of at least three years before the diagnosis of renal glycosuria can be established definitely.

The essential cause of renal glycosuria is unknown. It is assumed that the "permeability" of the kidneys for glucose is increased, but the use of this term, except in its broadest sense, is obviously inaccurate, since the defect is probably one of inadequate reabsorption of glucose in the renal tubules.

Glycosuria of Pregnancy.—Glycosuria occurring during a normal, uncomplicated pregnancy, appears to be due to lowering of the "renal threshold," since it is associated with no elevation of blood sugar. It is observed in as many as 10 to 15 per cent of normal pregnant women, particularly in the late months, and more frequently in primigravidae than in multigravidae. Pregnancy glycosuria is ascribed by some observers to decreased carbohydrate tolerance resulting from the physiologic hypertrophy of the pituitary gland which occurs during that period. Lactose is not normally present in the urine during pregnancy under normal conditions of lactation, physiologic lactosuria occurring only during the period of lactation.

"Alimentary" Glycosuria.—Opinion is divided regarding the metabolic status of this condition. The term is employed to designate the urinary excretion of glucose by certain apparently normal subjects after ingestion of excessive amounts of cane sugar, glucose, or, at times, starch. It is evident that the occurrence of glycosuria under such circumstances must be due either to a "lowering of the renal threshold" for glucose or to absorption of glucose from the intestine at a rate too rapid to allow of its adequate removal from the circulation by the liver.

It has been shown that the *normal* individual can utilize glucose injected intravenously in amounts up to 0.8 gm. per Kg. of body weight per hour; when this rate is exceeded glycosuria occurs.[16] It has also been demonstrated that the absorption of glucose from the intestine proceeds normally at a maximum rate of 1.8 gm. per Kg. of body weight per hour, regardless, within wide limits, of the quantity of sugar ingested. Consequently, if the liver removes a minimum of 1.0 gm. per Kg. per hour, allowing 0.8 gm. to pass into the general circulation, glycosuria should not be expected to occur in normal individuals. In the absence of any abnormality of hepatic or tissue glycogenic function, alimentary glycosuria might be explained on the basis of increased permeability of the intestinal mucosa for glucose resulting in its absorption at a rate more rapid than can be adequately handled by the liver; it therefore reaches the tissues, including the kidneys, in excessive amount, with the result that a portion is eliminated in the urine. This hypothesis does not necessarily imply the existence of venous hyperglycemia for, tissue utilization being unimpaired, slight grades of arterial hyperglycemia may possibly be corrected and the concentration of glucose in the blood leaving the tissues may be within normal limits. This possibility has been supported by studies of capillary and venous blood sugar tolerance curves in benign glycosuria.[17]

Glycosuria in Nephritis and Nephrosis.—Glycosuria occurs at times in a considerable proportion of patients with glomerulonephritis, nephrosclerosis and nephrosis.[18] In a great majority of such individuals glucose is excreted in the urine in larger quantities than in normal subjects, gross glycosuria occurring in many (30 to 50 per cent in some reported series). In some cases of nephritis and nephrosclerosis this glycosuria is associated with fasting hyperglycemia or diminished glucose tolerance or both. However, in many instances the glycosuria appears to be dependent upon a decrease in the "renal threshold" for sugar. This increased elimination of glucose in the urine may be due possibly to failure of the renal tubular epithelium to reabsorb the sugar from the glomerular filtrate as efficiently as normally. In such cases the urine may contain more than 1 per cent of glucose after ingestion of a carbohydrate-rich meal.

Hyperglycemic Glycosuria.—The occurrence of glycosuria in association with hyperglycemia is readily understood. If one accepts the normal "renal threshold" value as being 140 to 160 mg. per 100 cc., the elimination of glucose in the urine may be expected in the presence of higher blood sugar levels. The fact must be kept in mind, however, that the renal threshold may exhibit rather wide variations in different individuals and under different conditions. Obviously, the causes of hyperglycemia are potential causes of glycosuria. These include the following: (1) Diabetes mellitus, (2) hyperthyroidism, (3) hyperpituitarism (acromegaly, basophilic adenoma), (4) hyperadrenalism (medullary tumor, excessive mental strain, emotional excitement, severe exercise, etc.), (5) increased intracranial pressure (brain tumor, cerebral hemorrhage, fractured skull, etc.), (6) arterial hypertension, (7) chronic hepatic disease, (8) ether anesthesia, (9) asphyxia, and (10) acidosis. These conditions are discussed elsewhere (p. 735).

LEVULOSURIA

Levulose (fructose) reduces metallic oxides in alkaline solution, is fermentable by bakers' yeast and yields an osazone with phenylhydrazine which is morphologically identical with gluocosazone. Levulose may be identified in the urine by the following methods:

(1) Gas production with *Monilia krusei* but not with *Monilia balcanica* to exclude glucose.

(2) Characteristic osazone crystals and positive Seliwanoff (resorcinol-hydrochloric acid) or Borchardt reactions, to exclude glucose. The presence of nitrites or indican in excess interferes with the development of the

characteristic yellow color of Borchardt's reaction. Glucose, in large amount (2 per cent) may yield a positive Seliwanoff reaction.

(3) Rotation of polarized light to the left in the absence of other levorotatory substances, such as conjugate glycuronates and betahydroxybutyric acid.

Levulose may appear in the urine under the following circumstances:

(a) In severe cases of diabetes mellitus, always in association with glucose.

(b) Alimentary levulosuria, following the ingestion of large quantities of levulose, particularly in patients with hepatic functional impairment. This has been used as a test of hepatic function, but is unsatisfactory for this purpose. Approximately 10 per cent of normal individuals eliminate levulose in the urine following the ingestion of 100 gm. of levulose.

(c) Essential levulosuria, implying the occurrence of levulosuria in the absence of the above-mentioned factors, is a rare condition. Silver[19] regards it as a specific, probably inborn error of metabolism, localized primarily in the liver where, he believes, a specific enzyme deficiency exists, resulting in impaired ability to fix fructose as glycogen. The metabolism of other carbohydrates is undisturbed. A few cases have been reported in which there was a total absence of tolerance for levulose, the sugar being eliminated if any whatsoever was ingested. Heeres and Vos[20] state that regardless of the amount ingested, about 14 per cent is eliminated. Insulin has no influence on this condition; no rise in the respiratory quotient follows the administration of levulose to such individuals, indicating failure of utilization of this sugar. It is said that rectal administration produces more severe levulosuria than does oral administration.

PENTOSURIA

Pentoses reduce metallic oxides in alkaline solution and are not fermentable by bakers' yeast. They may be identified in the urine by the following methods:

1. Positive Bial reaction (orcinol-hydrochloric acid).

2. Positive Benedict reaction and negative fermentation test with bakers' yeast in the absence of lactose and nonsugar reducing substances.

3. Characteristic pentosazone crystals with phenylhydrazine.

4. Positive Benedict reaction, gas production with Bacillus coli communis and B. paratyphosus B (to exclude lactose) and no fermentation with Monilia tropicalis (to exclude galactose).

Pentose may appear in the urine under the following circumstances:

(a) **Alimentary Pentosuria.**—This is a temporary condition, occurring in normal individuals after the ingestion of large quantities of fruits which have a high pentose content (prunes, cherries, grapes, plums). It is of no clinical significance apart from the fact that it may be mistaken for glycosuria because of a positive copper-reduction test.

(b) **Diabetes Mellitus** (some cases).

(c) **Essential Pentosuria (Chronic Pentosuria).**—This is a relatively rare and extremely interesting condition which is analogous to essential levulosuria. Pentoses, usually the optically inactive form of arabinose, are more or less constantly present in the urine, the quantity excreted bearing no relation to the amount ingested. It is of no known clinical significance, since the utilization of other carbohydrates is unimpaired. It appears to be familial and hereditary in nature. As in the case of alimentary pentosuria, its chief importance lies in the possibility of mistaking it for glycosuria.

LACTOSURIA

Lactose reduces metallic oxides in alkaline solution (Benedict, Fehling solutions, etc.) and, in about 15 per cent of cases, is fermented by bakers' yeast. It may be identified in the urine by the following methods:

1. Positive Benedict test, gas production with B. *coli communis* and no gas production with B. *paratyphosus* B (to exclude pentose).

2. Positive mucic acid test and negative phloroglucinol reaction (Tollens) to exclude galactose.

3. Characteristic lactosazone crystals with phenylhydrazine. This test is usually unsatisfactory.

4. If positive Benedict test and no fermentation with bakers' yeast, negative Bial test to exclude pentose.

Lactosuria occurs in a considerable proportion of women during the period of lactation. It does not occur normally during pregnancy under normal conditions of lactation. The lactosuria of lactation must be regarded as physiologic and has no apparent significance.

GALACTOSURIA

Galactose reduces metallic oxides in alkaline solution and is fermented by most samples of bakers' yeast, although usually not so actively as are glucose and fructose. It may be identified in the urine by the following methods:

1. Positive mucic acid test to exclude all other reducing substances except lactose, and positive phloroglucinol-hydrochloric acid reaction (Tollens) to exclude lactose.

2. Positive Tollens reaction and no absorption bands upon spectroscopic examination (to exclude pentose and glycuronic acid).

Galactosuria is not frequently observed except following the ingestion of supertolerance doses of galactose. It has been found to occur in nursing infants in association with derangements of gastro-intestinal function (from lactose). The excessive excretion of galactose in the urine following ingestion of this sugar has been utilized as indication of hepatic functional impairment. A similar phenomenon occurs in hyperthyroidism, due apparently to acceleration of the rate of absorption of sugar from the intestine.[21]

BIBLIOGRAPHY

1. Neuwirth, I., J. Biol. Chem., 51: 11, 1922.
2. Benedict, S. R., Osterberg, E., and Neuwirth, I., J. Biol. Chem., 34: 217, 1918.
3. Greenwald, I., Gross, J., and McGuire, G., J. Biol. Chem., 75: 491, 1927.
4. Folin, O., and Berglund, H., J. Biol. Chem., 51: 213, 1922.
5. Hassan, A., Biochem. J., 22: 1332, 1928.
6. Sumner, J. B., J. Biol. Chem., 62: 287, 1924–1925.
7. Benedict, S. R., and Osterberg, E., J. Biol. Chem., 55: 769, 1923.
8. Peters, J. P., Body Water, C. C. Thomas, Springfield, Ill., 1935, p. 268.

9. Richards, A. N., Am. J. Med. Sci., **190:** 727, 1935.
10. Mackay, R. L., Brit. Med. J., **1:** 892, 1928.
11. Cantarow, A., and Trumper, M., Clinical Biochemistry, W. B. Saunders Company, Philadelphia, 1939.
12. Neuberg, C., *et al.*, Biochem. Ztschr., **31:** 170, 1911; **32:** 323, 1911; **37:** 60, 68, 76, 1911.
13. Castellani, A., and Taylor, F. E., J.A.M.A., **78:** 651, 1926.
14. Castellani, A., J. State Med., **39:** 621, 1931.
15. Marble, A., Am. J. Med. Sci., **183:** 811, 1932.
16. Sansum, W. D., and Woodyatt, R. T., J. Biol. Chem., **30:** 155, 1917.
17. Friedenson, M., Rosenbaum, M. K., Thalheimer, E. J., and Peters, J. P., Arch. Int. Med., **43:** 633, 1929.
18. Hawkins, J. A., J. Clin. Invest., **8:** 107, 1929.
19. Silver, S., and Reiner, M., Arch. Int. Med., **54:** 412, 1934.
20. Heeres, P. A., and Vos, H., Arch. Int. Med., **44:** 47, 1929.
21. Althausen, T. L., Am. J. Med. Sci., **199:** 342, 1940.

CHAPTER XVI

DIABETES MELLITUS

By Garfield G. Duncan

INTRODUCTION

Definition.—Diabetes mellitus is a chronic disease of metabolism which develops as the result of an insufficient supply of endogenous insulin. It is readily controlled but rarely, if ever, cured. The greatest apparent disturbance caused by this disease is in the utilization of carbohydrate, though the metabolism of fat and of protein, and, indeed, the total food metabolism is affected. An insufficient secretion of insulin by the pancreatic islets of Langerhans, no matter what the cause, will precipitate the clinical syndrome of diabetes mellitus. Diabetes is not, however, as simple as this would make it appear. There is much convincing evidence that the reduction of insulin production is secondary to disturbances in other, but closely related, endocrine glands. Of these the diabetogenic influences of the anterior lobe of the hypophysis, and the adrenal glands are of outstanding importance. The extent of the effect of the thyroid gland on the pancreas is not yet determined but it is not considered to be great. In some instances it seems that the insulin insufficiency is relative and not absolute; that there actually may be a normal amount of insulin produced but that its effect is neutralized to a greater or lesser degree by some antagonist. There can be little or no doubt that an insulin antagonist possessing an opposing physiological action or a chemical neutralizing agent, exists in some instances.

Practically, whether the insulin inadequacy is relative or absolute the immediate result is the same. The metabolism of carbohydrate is reduced, yet large quantities of glucose are secreted by the liver. The concentration of sugar in the blood increases above normal (*hyperglycemia*), and when the renal threshold for glucose is exceeded sugar appears in the urine (*glycosuria*). Nourishment is thus lost.

As the amount of glycosuria increases polyuria develops, a great loss in body weight ensues, and other characteristic symptoms appear. Notable among these are excessive thirst (polydipsia), an excessive appetite (polyphagia), and general weakness. As the disease process progresses there develops in the patient (1) a predisposition to infections, especially staphylococcal and tuberculous infections, (2) chronic degenerative changes, notably arteriosclerosis, disease of the coronary arteries, diabetic retinitis, peripheral neuritis, and less frequently cataracts, and (3) a ketosis. The last mentioned is an acute disorder developing as a result of disturbed carbohydrate and fat metabolism. It is the specific complication of diabetes and unless curbed by appropriate treatment, progress of the disorder is hastened by such metabolic stimulants as infection, toxemia, and fever until coma and death ensue.

The fact that this march of events, which is especially relentless in the case of children, may be stopped, the disturbances corrected and controlled, and the clinical well being of the patient restored is one of the epochal chapters in the history of medicine made possible by the discovery of insulin (Banting and Best) in 1921.

History.—It is appropriate, in dealing with a disease the study of which has taught us so much about metabolism, that we review briefly a few of the important mileposts in its history. A better understanding of the modern conception of diabetes mellitus may be aided by such a summary.

Allen,* following Cantani, has divided the history of diabetes into four periods (a) the Ancient Period (to 1675 A.D.), (b) the Second or Diagnostic Period (1675–1796), (c) the Period of Empiric Treatment (1796–1840–50), and (d) the Modern or Experimental Period (1840–50 until the present time). Joslin has appropriately subdivided the Modern Period into four distinct eras, I the Naunyn, II the Allen, III the Banting, and IV the Hagedorn Eras.

The Ancient Period.—The passing of frequent and large quantities of urine was recorded in the papyrus Ebers, a copy of an Egyptian medical journal already old in the time of Moses (Saundby). That this may have been due to disease of the kidneys is not denied. Celsus (30 B.C.–50 A.D.) wrote concerning, "polyuria without pain but with emaciation and danger." Aretaeus (30–90 A.D.) described diabetes and gave to it the Ionic Greek name meaning "to run through a siphon." He wrote of its progressiveness and of the fatal prognosis.

Opium, emetics, bleeding, and purging were recommended treatments in 550 A.D. A Chinese physician, Tchang Tchong-king (200 A.D.) described diabetes as "the disease of thirst." He observed that a diabetic patient might drink ten liters of liquids per day, with an equal amount excreted as urine. Further Chinese medical writings of about 600 A.D. mention polyphagia, polydipsia and polyuria. Later furunculosis and (in the fifteenth century) tuberculosis were recognized complications of diabetes. The sweetness of the diabetic urine was first mentioned in the Ayur Veda of Susruta (Chunder Rose). It was noted also that ants flocked around the patient's urine. The weakness, emaciation, polyuria and carbuncles were recorded as being associated with diabetes. Avicenna (980–1037 A.D.) gave the first description of diabetic gangrene, and Paracelsus (1493–1541) was the first to evaporate the urine and recover "salt." Lipemia in the diabetic patient was first recorded by Helmont (1578–1644).

In the Second, or Diagnostic Period, Willis (died 1675) observed that the urine of the diabetic patient was "wonderfully sweet as if imbued with honey or sugar." Willis became the author of the first carbohydrate or undernutrition "cure." Morton (died 1698) was the first to make clear the hereditary characteristics of diabetes, though they were noted as early as the seventh century. Dobson in 1775 grasped the fact for the first time that the sweetness of the urine was due to sugar.

In 1788 Cawley gave the first description we have of a fatal case of

* The history of diabetes has been extracted largely from the writings of Allen, F. M., Stillman, E., and Fitz, R., Monographs of the Rockefeller Institute for Medical Research, **11:** 1, 1919.

diabetes with abnormal changes in the pancreas. There were multiple calculi and much destruction of pancreatic tissue. Cullen (1709–1790) added the adjective "mellitus" to the disease in order that it might be distinguished from diabetes insipidus. Francis Home isolated sugar from the urine and observed that on the addition of yeast the urine lost its sweetness, thus proving the fermentability of the sugar.

The *Third Period*, or *Period of Empiric Treatment*, saw Rollo's (1796) restriction of the diet to animal food and a few green vegetables of low food value, occasionally permitting some milk and a little bread. Drugs were given to decrease the appetite. Rollo (1796) was the first to note and record the significance of diabetic cataracts.

The odor of decaying apples—doubtless acetone—was noted on the breath of a young diabetic patient by Marshal (1798). Chevreul (1815) found that the sugar present in the urine of diabetic patients was identical with glucose and Gregory (1825) described the differences between diabetes mellitus and diabetes insipidus. Prout is credited by Naunyn (1820) as being the first to advocate restriction of protein in the treatment of diabetes. He also introduced washed bran in the treatment of this disease. Furthermore he was the first to mention coma as a typical termination of diabetes.

At the outset of the *Modern* or *Experimental Period*, M. Gregor demonstrated a fermentable sugar in the blood of diabetic patients. Trommer reported his qualitative test for sugar in the urine in 1841, and Fehling a quantitative test in 1850. Claude Bernard (1885) founded the theory of sugar formation from glycogen. He discovered glycogen and the glycogenic function of the liver and he postulated that the increased blood sugar concentration was an overproduction of sugar by the liver. Mialhe in 1845 recommended large doses of alkali in the treatment of diabetes. Bouchardat (1806–1886) revived the Rollo treatment but modified it by substituting fat and alcohol for carbohydrate; he individualized his patients' needs; advocated small diets and instituted occasional days of fasting; he devised the practice of cooking vegetables and discarding the water, in this manner reducing the starch content. This practice has been abandoned only since 1922. Bouchardat invented gluten bread and hence originated the idea of substitutes for bread; he noted the advantage of exercise in the treatment of diabetes and he advocated daily testing of the urine for sugar.

Petters (1857) obtained from the urine of a patient in diabetic coma positive reactions for acetone but it was Kussmaul in 1874 who gave the first detailed clinical description of diabetic coma. The characteristic breathing of "air hunger" still bears his name. Cantani (1837–1893) set a new standard of severity in diet. His patients were strictly isolated and allowed only lean meat and various fats. "Fast days" and exercise were employed and after two months without glycosuria, green vegetables and later a greater variety of foods were resumed. Cantani insisted on complete freedom from glycosuria.

Baumel was the first to set up the hypothesis that all diabetes is pancreatic in origin. Ehrlich called attention to the so-called glycogenic degeneration of the real tubules in diabetes, and Kutz (1845–1895) discovered oxybutyric acid in the urine of diabetic patients. Furthermore, he proved the negative results obtained in the treatment of diabetes with various drugs and the uselessness of various waters. He recognized the advantage of exercise for the patients having mild diabetes and the absence of benefit if the diabetes was severe. He tested individually the carbohydrate tolerance of each patient.

Langerhans, in 1869, discovered islet-cell formations in the pancreas which bear his name, von Mering and Minkowski in 1889 discovered diabetes in a dog following pancreatectomy. They established the doctrine of the *internal secretion of the pancreas*. Minkowski also discovered the low CO_2 content of the blood in diabetic coma. Naunyn introduced the term acidosis in stating: "With this name I designate the formation of beta-oxybutyric acid in metabolism." Naunyn recognized clinical renal glycosuria. He believed that diabetes was a uniglandular (pancreatic) disease, and that underlying everything in most cases was the diabetic "anlage" or inherited constitutional predisposition. His treatment consisted of a low carbohydrate, and, if necessary, a low protein intake with adequate fat to prevent undernutrition.

A number of carbohydrate "cures" for diabetes were advocated. Among these were Smart's "milk cure," von During's "rice cure," Dujardin-Beaumetz's "potato cure," and von Noorden's "oat cure." Blum (1911) established the fact that patients who did well on carbohydrate "cures" had essentially mild diabetes. It is obvious now that the benefit secured was from the undernutrition which was invariably associated with the "cures."

Hydropic degeneration of the islets of Langerhans was observed by Weichselbaum and Stangle, but it was Opie (1901) who put forward the hypothesis that diabetes is due to alterations in the islets of Langerhans.

Guelpa introduced a treatment of fasting, purging, and undernutrition until the patients could tolerate a diet rich in carbohydrate. Patients having mild diabetes could tolerate this treatment, but for those having severe diabetes it was inevitably disastrous. Foster (1915) supported Naunyn's treatment but employed stricter undernutrition with better results. Roulston and Woodyatt used "high fat" diets. Through the influence and example of Joslin the undernutrition treatment advocated by Allen received general adoption. Joslin found that by decreasing the fat content of the diet the patient's health was improved. The undernutrition regimen of Allen was suggested when (1) diabetes apparently disappeared in various forms of cachexia, (2) fasting alleviated the diabetes of depancreatized dogs and (3) Joslin observed that accompanying the rapid emaciation of tuberculosis there was in one carefully studied patient a diminution of both glycosuria and acidosis.

Allen investigated diabetic therapy by experiments on partially depancreatized dogs on the premises that diabetes is a disorder of the total metabolism and not of carbohydrate utilization alone and that the entire diet and the maintenance of the entire body mass constituted a load upon the internal secretion of the pancreas. Experimental and clinical proof that the diabetic patient's carbohydrate tolerance was affected by the total caloric value of the diet and that greater benefits could be obtained by restricting the total diet than could be obtained when carbohydrate alone was restricted promptly followed. This new doctrine was rapidly accepted. These principles are still employed by Allen,[1] Joslin and their pupils in the treatment of diabetes. It is gratifying that because of insulin the extremes of undernutrition, formerly essential, are no longer necessary.

Newburgh and Marsh, Woodyatt, Petren, Wilder and Shaffer used diets containing greater amounts of fat, of higher caloric values and lower in protein content than was allowed in the Allen regimen. Numerous formulae were devised by which carbohydrate, protein and fat quotas were calculated to provide the maximum number of calories with minimum carbohydrate without danger of acidosis.

The *Banting era* was introduced in 1921 with the discovery of insulin.[2] Enthusiasts for each dietetic regime found this new remedy of inestimable value in the routine treatment of diabetic patients and in the management of diabetes during complications. A trend to diets with higher carbohydrate and lower fat contents ensued.

A period of enlightening experimental work which has revolutionized our ideas concerning the etiology of diabetes was begun when Houssay and Magenta (1924) found that the removal of the pituitary gland from a dog increased the animal's sensitivity to insulin. In 1929 Houssay and Potick discovered that the insulin hypersensitiveness of the hypophysectomized toad was diminished by treatment with preparations from the *pars glandularis* of the hypophysis. Then Houssay and Biasotti (1930) found that in toads and dogs hypophysectomy diminished the severity of diabetes produced by pancreatectomy. A transitory diabetes was provoked by giving a normal animal an injection of anterior pituitary extract (Houssay, Biasotti and Rietti; Evans, et al.; Bauman and Marini, 1932) and diabetes was made more severe by treatment with anterior pituitary extracts (Houssay and Biasotti; Houssay, 1936). These brilliant observations were brought to a climax in 1937 when Young[3] produced permanent diabetes in dogs by injecting intraperitoneally increasing amounts of crude extract of the anterior lobe of the hypophysis. Long and Lukens (1936) attenuated the diabetes by removing the adrenal cortex from depancreatized cats. Lukens and Dohan (1938), by giving large doses of cortin, aggravated the diabetic state in depancreatized and adrenalectomized dogs. The full significance of these studies is to be found in the section on etiology (p. 711).

Clinically, insulin hydrochloride (unmodified), while of great value, had the distinct disadvantage that because of its short period of action, four to eight hours, multiple doses were usually necessary to secure a continuous effect. Hagedorn[4] succeeded in reducing the immediate effect and prolonging the action of insulin by adding protamine.

The resulting product, *protamine insulin,* was relatively unstable, but Scott and Fisher,[5] by adding small amounts of zinc, prolonged its activity and made the product more stable. Abel[6] obtained insulin in crystalline form in 1927. Zinc insulin crystals in solution were made commercially available in 1938 following the demonstration of its clinical value by Sahyun and Altschuler. This product is purer than unmodified insulin, contains less protein and is less apt to give rise to allergic reactions. Marble, Ricketts and Wilder, and Duncan in 1939, in independent studies, concluded that there was little if any difference in the therapeutic activity of zinc insulin crystals in solution and unmodified insulin. Hence, with the advantages of crystalline insulin it is not surprising that it is steadily replacing unmodified insulin in general use.

Lukens and Dohan[7] have shown experimentally that insulin therapy in the partially depancreatectomized animal may restore to normal hydropically degenerated islets of Langerhans (the degenerative changes having been brought about by injecting an extract of the anterior hypophysis), providing the treatment was conducted before these changes reached an irreversible state. This work confirms the observations of Allen, and of Copp and Barclay, who produced hydropic degeneration of the islets by functional overstrain of the remnant of pancreas remaining after partial pancreatectomy. Furthermore Haist, Campbell, and Best[8] have found that the production of diabetes by injection of the anterior pituitary extract is prevented if large doses of insulin are given at the same time as the pituitary extract. They also found it impossible to provoke diabetes by injection of the pituitary extract if the animal was on a starvation regimen or receiving a high carbohydrate diet.

Incidence.—It is estimated that there are approximately 660,000 cases of diabetes in the United States.* This information is obtained from the National Health Survey, based on a house to house canvass of some 800,000 families, including 2,800,000 persons in 83 cities and 23 rural areas in 19 states. It has been assumed on the basis of the general trend of increasing frequency of diabetes that 3,000,000 persons now living either have or will develop the disease. It is estimated that in the United Kingdom there are between 150,000 and 200,000 persons who have diabetes, in Canada 30,000 and in Germany before the present war, 300,000 (Joslin[9]).

It was predicted that following the discovery of insulin, with the removal of the stigma of death from the young diabetic patient and indeed from many older patients, there would be a gradual increase in the prevalence of diabetes for a considerable number of years. This has occurred in city, state, and country. Nowadays children do not need to die of diabetes. The fact is that they mature, marry, and procreate—a distinct contrast to the invalidism and early death of children suffering from this disease prior to 1922. Two new groups of individuals have appeared and are increasing in numbers. These are, first, the adults who have had diabetes since childhood and, second, the children of these patients.

The outlook is most favorable for the young diabetic patient who has had adequate treatment, yet the mortality rate from this disease is higher than it ever was. The United States census records a death toll from diabetes in the United States of 31,037 in 1938. This does not represent the total number of persons having diabetes at death but only those instances in which this disease was considered the primary cause of death during this period. Diabetes as a cause of death in the United States advanced from twenty-seventh place, in 1900, to ninth place, in 1938. A broad upward trend in the death rate has prevailed since 1900 with but two interruptions. These occurred during (1) the later stages of the World War (1914–1918)

* Dr. L. I. Dublin states in a personal communication, "according to a recent estimate we placed the number of diabetics in the country at between 500,000 and 600,000. This is slightly lower than the figure of 660,000 which is published in the preliminary report of the National Health Survey for 1933–1936."

when undernutrition was prevalent and (2) during the two years immediately following the commercial introduction of insulin (1922).

Diabetes is most prevalent when the *per capita income* is high. In all countries the same trend has been observed but in no principal country has the mortality from diabetes increased so rapidly as it has in the United States. This is in contrast with a reduction in the mortality rate from 15.7 to 11.2 per 1,000 due to all causes in the United States between 1906 and 1937. The mortality rate from diabetes, 31.3 per 100,000 of estimated population in Pennsylvania ranked sixth for all the states in 1937. The rates of Rhode Island, New York, Massachusetts, Connecticut, and New Hampshire being higher—from 42.0 to 31.4 per 100,000, with New Mexico the lowest, at 8.1 per 100,000 (Table 1). The increasing mortality rate from

TABLE 1

DIABETES DEATH RATE PER 100,000 ESTIMATED POPULATION, TAKEN FROM FIGURES PUBLISHED
BY THE BUREAU OF THE CENSUS, 1937

State	Rate	State	Rate
Rhode Island	42.0	South Dakota	19.1
New York	36.9	Nevada	18.8
Massachusetts	33.7	Utah	18.5
Connecticut	32.5	Colorado	17.9
New Hampshire	31.4	Wyoming	17.9
Pennsylvania	31.3	Florida	17.7
New Jersey	30.8	Louisiana	17.6
Delaware	28.4	North Dakota	17.1
District of Columbia	28.1	Virginia	17.0
Illinois	27.6	Idaho	15.4
Ohio	26.7	West Virginia	15.2
Wisconsin	26.6	Kentucky	13.9
Maryland	26.3	Georgia	12.6
Michigan	26.2	Mississippi	12.6
Nebraska	26.1	Texas	12.6
Oregon	25.9	Oklahoma	12.3
California	25.3	South Carolina	11.7
Indiana	24.6	Tennessee	11.4
Minnesota	24.5	North Carolina	11.1
Vermont	24.5	Alabama	10.6
Kansas	24.1	Arizona	10.0
Washington	23.5	Arkansas	9.2
Maine	23.4	New Mexico	8.1
Iowa	22.5		
Montana	21.9	United States	23.7
Missouri	20.6		

diabetes in the United States is contrasted with the decreasing general death rate from all causes in figure 132, compiled by Strome and Blaine.[10] The paradox of better means of diagnosis and treatment and yet a higher mortality rate needs explaining. Few communities have escaped the rising tide of fatalities from diabetes. The factors which enter into and explain this paradox are: 1. The population of the country is increasing and more people than ever before are reaching the "diabetic zone"—between forty and sixty years of age. 2. The methods of diagnosis are improved and many cases of diabetes which formerly would have escaped detection are now readily identified. 3. Both lay and professional interest in this disease have increased tremendously.

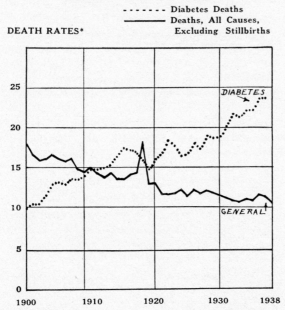

MORTALITY IN THE UNITED STATES
REGISTRATION AREA, 1900-1938

- - - - - - Diabetes Deaths
———— Deaths, All Causes,
Excluding Stillbirths

DEATH RATES*

DIABETES

GENERAL

Fig. 132.—General death rates are per 1000 population. Diabetes death rates are per 100,000 population. (After Strome and Blaine, Pennsylvania M. J., Vol. 43, 1940.)

MORTALITY IN PENNSYLVANIA, 1906 1938

- - - - - - Diabetes Deaths
———— Deaths, All Causes
Excluding Stillbirths

DEATH RATES*

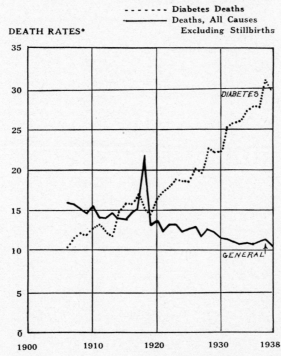

DIABETES

GENERAL

Fig. 133.—General death rates are per 1000 population. Diabetes death rates are per 100,000 population. (After Strome and Blaine, Pennsylvania M. J., Vol. 43, 1940.)

The relation which age, sex, color, occupation and race bear to the incidence and mortality rate of diabetes is important.

Age and Sex.—Improved treatment has noticeably reduced the mortality rate of diabetic children and young adults of both sexes. Diabetes, however, is characteristically a disease of middle life and in consequence an improvement in the treatment of young diabetic patients, who are, in contrast, few in number, influences but little the mortality rate for all ages.

The improved mortality rate carries through middle life for the male but not for the female. Here again the disease is less common in the males than in the females. Not until we succeed in reducing the death rate among the middle-aged female diabetic patients can we hope for an effective reduc-

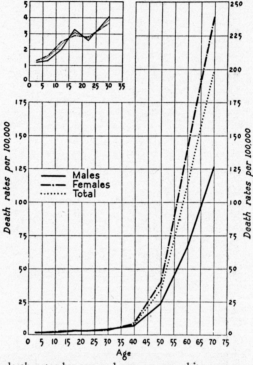

Fig. 134.—Diabetes death rates by sex and age among white persons. (Metropolitan Life Insurance Company, Industrial Department, 1926–1930.)

tion in the mortality rate for all ages and both sexes. The difficulty in changing the trend is apparent when it is realized that a greater number of persons are reaching this age group than ever before. Joslin, Dublin and Marks[9] (1933) have observed that diabetic death rates of both sexes are fairly equal up to forty years of age (Fig. 134). After forty—at and after the menopause—the mortality rate of the females increases much more rapidly than that of the males: Between thirty-five and forty-four years of age the rate for females exceeds that for males by 28.4 per cent; between forty-five and fifty-four by 68.9 per cent and between fifty-five and sixty-four by 108.4 per cent. Between sixty-five and seventy-four the difference is less, being reduced to 89.0 per cent. It is obvious that to reduce the mortality rate from diabetes the offensive must be directed in such a manner that the women at and past middle life will be benefited. It is of interest that the sharp rise of the mortality curve at middle life is more rapid in the United States than in any other principal country. This is doubtless a penalty for high standards of living—less manual work with ample food in contrast with other countries. The increasing electrical conveniences in the home with a corresponding reduction of physical effort by housewives has been suggested as an influence on the increasing prevalence of obesity and its too frequent penalty, diabetes.

TABLE 2

DIABETES AND OCCUPATION. OCCUPATIONS IN ORDER OF RANK OF MORTALITY FROM DIABETES.*
METROPOLITAN LIFE INSURANCE COMPANY, INDUSTRIAL DEPARTMENT, 1922–1924

(After Joslin, Dublin and Marks)

Occupation	Standardized relative index, ages 15 to 64†
HIGH DIABETES MORTALITY (INDEX 115 OR OVER)	
Merchants and storekeepers	204
Tailors and other clothing workers	185
Saloonkeepers and bartenders	157
Railway enginemen and trainmen	154
Electricians	140
Store clerks and salesmen	137
Watchmen and guards	125
Clerks, bookkeepers and office assistants	121
Stationary engineers and firemen	118
AVERAGE DIABETES MORTALITY (INDEX 86 TO 114)	
Machinists	107
Iron and steel-mill workers	107
ALL OCCUPATIONS (EXCLUDING RETIRED)	100
Railway track and yard workers	97
Plumbers, gasfitters, and steamfitters	96
Textile (except cordage, hemp, dyeing, and finishing) millworkers	91
LOW DIABETES MORTALITY (INDEX 85 OR LESS)	
Teamsters and drivers	84
Furniture and other woodworkers	81
Farmers and farm laborers	77
Laborers	68
Janitors and building employees	68
Painters, paperhangers, and varnishers	61
Carpenters	59
Coalminers (underground)	51

* Occupations with less than 15 deaths excluded except where the mortality is very high or low.

† For explanation of this term the reader is referred to Dublin, L. I., and Vane, R. J., Jr. Causes of Death by Occupation, Bull. U. S. Bureau of Labor Statistics, No. 507.

Occupation.—The diabetes mortality rate is consistently higher and is increasing more rapidly in urban than in rural communities, the former being between 60 and 70 per cent higher than the latter. This difference is doubtless due largely to the nature of the respective occupations in the two areas. The rural population is given to occupations requiring physical exercise and is not as likely to develop obesity as the urban population.

The incidence of diabetes is greatest among the employing and professional groups, and among those engaged in selling and serving food and drinks. The diabetic mortality rate of merchants and storekeepers is the highest of all occupations. That of tailors and other clothing workers, and saloonkeepers and bartenders come next in the order named, whereas laborers, farm workers, carpenters, and miners have a low mortality from diabetes. The mortality rate for diabetes affecting those of other occupations is presented in table 2. These observations repeatedly made simply mean that manual labor tends to prevent, while physical inactivity plus an abundance of food tends to cause or at least precipitate diabetes. Farm owners who on the average do less physical work and live more sumptuously than their hired help acquire diabetes twice as frequently as their laborers. The era of mechanized labor has reduced the amount of actual manual labor and has caused a flow of workers from arduous occupations to those requiring less expenditure of energy. The result is obvious, less physical exertion, more obesity and more diabetes.

Racial and National Differences.—Jews are prone to develop diabetes. Diabetes is one and one-half times to twice as common among the older Jews as in the average population. The unusual predisposition of the Jewish race to diabetes is true in all countries, though it is probably more clearly shown in Greater New York. (Jewish Commercial Survey, 1931.)

Great interest is attached to the excessive frequency with which Jews are afflicted with diabetes. Racial persecution which forbade them to own or till the land has made them by tradition sedentary workers; the tendency of the Jewess to become obese at middle life, and the unbalanced diet with inadequate exercise have all been offered as explanations for the peculiar predisposition of this race to the disease. Furthermore the Jewish, being an inbred race, is especially exposed to the influence which heredity exerts in predisposing to diabetes.

In general diabetes is common among the Teutonic races and uncommon among the Slavs and Latins. Joslin points out that there is a surprisingly high mortality rate from diabetes among the Irish in the United States but a low rate for the inhabitants of Ireland. Improved living conditions and the disproportionate number of Irish in the liquor business in the new world is offered as an explanation.

The Negro race was formerly and erroneously believed to be immune to diabetes. The mortality rate due to diabetes in the colored has increased more rapidly than it has in the white race, but as might be expected from the occupational differences the mortality from diabetes is still greater among the more prosperous white population. Approximately 25 per cent of the patients attending the clinic for diabetic patients at the Pennsylvania Hospital in Philadelphia are Negroes.

Diabetes is relatively infrequent among the Chinese and Japanese and when it does occur it is of a mild form.

REFERENCES

1. Allen, F. M., J.A.M.A., **63:** 939, 1914.
2. Banting, F. G., Best, C. H., Collip, J. B., Campbell, W. R., and Fletcher, A. A., Canad. Med. Assoc. J., **12:** 141, 1922.
3. Young, F. G., Lancet, **2:** 372, 1937.
4. Hagedorn, H. C., Jensen, B., Krarup, N. B., and Wodstrup, I., J.A.M.A., **106:** 177, 1936.
5. Scott, D. A., and Fisher, A. N., Proc. Am. Soc. Biol. Chem., **8:** 88, 1936.
6. Abel, J. J., Geiling, E. M. K., Rouiller, C. A., and Wintersteiner, O., J. Pharmacol. and Exper. Therap., **31:** 65, 1927.

7. Lukens, F. D. W., and Dohan, F. C., Science, **92**: 222, 1940.
8. Haist, R. E., Campbell, J., and Best, C. H., New Eng. J. Med., **223**: 607, 1940.
9. Joslin, E. P., Dublin, L. I., and Marks, H. H., Amer. J. Med. Sci., **86**: 753, 1933.
10. Strome, F. P., and Blaine, B. C., Pennsylvania M. J., **43**: 481, 1940.

ETIOLOGY

By C. N. H. Long

It is probably correct to say that the continuance of the disorder of metabolism known as diabetes mellitus rests on a disproportion between the requirement of the organism for insulin and the capacity of the islets of Langerhans to meet this demand. The various factors that initiate this disproportion appear at first sight to bear little relation to each other but as our knowledge of metabolism and the mechanism by which it is adjusted under normal conditions becomes clarified it will no doubt be possible to integrate the conditions associated with the appearance of diabetes in man into a more orderly pattern than is possible at present.

Before considering these conditions it is of advantage to recapitulate the effect of a total loss of insulin (pancreatectomy) upon the metabolism of the organism and to again emphasize that the disturbance in metabolism involves not only that of carbohydrates but also that of fat and protein as well as the electrolyte and water balance.

Effect of Pancreatectomy in Dog and Cat.—Following pancreatectomy, at least in dogs and cats, the sequence of events is:

(*a*) The blood glucose rises rapidly and such stores of liver glycogen as are present are soon depleted. When the blood glucose level exceeds the renal threshold glycosuria occurs and continues at a high level even though the animal is fasted. Approximately 3 gm. of sugar per Kg. of body weight are lost each day for the first few days after pancreatectomy by the fasting depancreatized animal.

(*b*) Since it is apparent that such a profuse glycosuria could not be sustained by the existing stores of carbohydrate, other substances must be contributing to this and only two of these (protein and fat) are present in the body in sufficient quantity for this purpose. The evidence that the former can form glucose is conclusive and in consequence of the accelerated conversion of protein to carbohydrate in depancreatized animals an excess of nitrogen is found in the urine. Indeed, during the first few days a reasonable proportionality is found in the urine between the glucose and nitrogen content provided the animal is fasted or fed a meat diet. The question of the conversion of fatty acids to glucose has been discussed elsewhere (Chapter II), and since it is the opinion of the writer that this does not occur the conclusion must be reached that the glycosuria is derived either from preformed carbohydrate or from protein.

(*c*) The administration of glucose, or of substances that form glucose, to depancreatized animals is followed by the excretion in the urine of the major part of such carbohydrate. The proportion excreted may be quantitative for the first few days after operation but if the animal survives and undergoes a great loss of weight a progressively larger quantity of the administered glucose may be retained.[1] The respiratory quotient of depancreatized animals does not rise after glucose feeding as in intact animals.

(*d*) Since the basal metabolism of a depancreatized animal is increased and since a large proportion of the energy of carbohydrates and proteins is lost in the urine, the requirements of the animal can be met only by an increased catabolism of fat. The acetone bodies that are the intermediary metabolites of fatty acid catabolism are utilized to supply a major part of this energy but in addition are produced in such quantities that often considerable amounts appear in the blood and urine giving rise to one of the most characteristic features of diabetic animals and men—ketosis. As was pointed out previously (Chapter III), the work of recent years has shown that contrary to previous opinion ketosis is not a consequence of the failure of carbohydrate utilization but is simply an expression of the high rate of fat catabolism.

(*e*) Now, while it is theoretically possible that an animal can survive under conditions in which carbohydrate utilization is at a minimum and the energy requirements are supported by fat, in practice the disordered metabolism of depancreatized animals soon evokes secondary consequences that prove fatal. In the first place, the profuse glycosuria removes from the body not only large quantities of water but also sodium chloride. This leads to dehydration and contraction of the volume of circulating fluids which is further aggravated by the fixation of base by the acids derived from fat catabolism as well as from those from tissue breakdown. The organism attempts to meet this loss of base by the excretion of large quantities of ammonia but the acidosis that develops in time is followed by the characteristic coma and death.

Effect of Pancreatectomy in Other Species.—Other species show certain differences following pancreatectomy from those described above for the dog and cat. The effect of this operation in pigs, goats and birds is summarized in table 3 and the observations on dogs and cats are included for comparison. It will be seen that pancreatectomy has the least effect in the bird where, after an initial period of hyperglycemia, the carbohydrate metabolism is only moderately if at all impaired. In the pig the glycosuria is much less but the acetonuria is intense; while in the goat glycosuria is very small indeed as is the degree of acetonuria. These differences may be explained in part by the different dietary and digestive habits of the different species and in part, as Lukens has suggested,[2] by different degrees of anterior pituitary activity.

The results of pancreatectomy in the monkey as reported by Collip, Selye and Neufeld[3] and by Chapman and Fulton[4] are surprising, but in this species the first effects of pancreatectomy are comparable to those seen in the dog and cat although after this first period as the animal loses weight a marked amelioration of the condition is found. Indeed, in all species if survival is prolonged and is accompanied by loss of weight an improvement in the carbohydrate tolerance will be found. Such an occurrence in dogs has been fully described by Barker, Chambers and Dann.[1]

Effect of Removal of Other Endocrine Glands on Pancreatic Diabetes.— In addition to the variation in the character of pancreatic diabetes in different species alterations can also be produced by interference with or removal of other members of the endocrine system. These effects have been discussed elsewhere (Chapter II), but it may again be pointed out that a striking amelioration both as regards survival and the character of the metabolism follows removal of the anterior pituitary or adrenal cortical tissue. Thyroidectomy although it reduces the degree of glucose and nitrogen excretion does not materially influence the survival of the depancreatized cat or dog.[5, 6] Removal of the gonads, posterior pituitary or adrenal medullary tissue has no effect on the course of events.

Induction of Diabetic State by Other Means than Pancreatectomy.— The presence of glycosuria and other symptoms of diabetes mellitus in persons suffering from tumors of the pituitary and adrenal cortex has been known for many years but it is only recently that it has been shown by animal experiment that disorders of carbohydrate, protein, and fat metabolism similar to those produced by pancreatectomy could be evoked in normal animals by the injection of suitable extracts of the anterior pituitary gland and adrenal cortex.

TABLE 3

EFFECT OF PANCREATECTOMY IN DIFFERENT SPECIES

Species	Number	Survival (days)	Blood Glucose mg. %	Urine			Notes
				Glucose g/k/d	Nitrogen g/k/d	Acetone mg/k/d	
Dog...................	4	10	310–345	2.8	1.0	Present	Fasting
Cat...................	10	5	212–788	3.2	1.4	133	Fasting
Pig*..................	5	9	30–232	0.2	0.5	179	Fasting
Goat†.................	4	Up to 44 days	124 (58–194)	0.1	0.4	10	Fasting
Duck‡.................	12	41–163	100–200				Fed
Monkey§ (1st period)....	12	7–305	14–410	2.5–4.0		Intense	Fasting
Monkey (2nd period)....				0		0	Fed

* Lukens, F. D. W., Amer. J. Physiol., **118**: 321, 1937.
† Lukens, F. D. W., Amer. J. Physiol., **122**: 729, 1938.
‡ Sprague, R., and Ivy, A. C., Amer. J. Physiol., **115**: 389, 1936.
§ Chapman, S. W., and Fulton, J. F., Amer. J. Physiol., **123**: 35, 1938.

The reader is again referred to Chapter II for fuller details, but it is now well known in the case of anterior pituitary extracts that not only may a temporary diabetic state be produced but if the injections are long continued a permanently diabetic condition follows. The perpetuation of this is due to the secondary involvement and destruction of the islets of Langerhans. This observation by F. G. Young is certainly one of the most important that has been made in recent years since it indicates that a permanently diabetic state may follow a temporary period of hyperpituitarism. Since the anterior pituitary exhibits such temporary hyperactivity as a physiological event during the period of active growth and at the menopause the occurrence of peaks in the incidence of diabetes at these times may be and probably is related to the disturbed endocrine balance.

In the case of the adrenal cortex it is not so well known that intense but temporary glycosuria may also be produced in normal animals (rats) given sufficient quantities of certain of the steroids isolated from this gland. I am indebted to Dr. D. J. Ingle for permission to quote his unpublished work in this regard. Ingle has found that the daily administration to rats of 2 to 5 mg. of 11-dehydro 17-hydroxy corticosterone (compound E of Kendall) will produce glycosuria up to 7 gm. a day and also increase the nitrogen excretion and evoke acetonuria.

It is also well known that the administration of thyroxin will produce atypical glucose tolerance curves and may also cause glycosuria. These effects, however, are mild in comparison to those produced by anterior pituitary or adrenal cortical extract although in an animal or individual with deficient pancreatic function such a period of hyperthyroidism may also precipitate a permanently diabetic state.

The Nature of the Defect in Depancreatized Animals.—In the depancreatized animal the disordered metabolism is of course precipitated by the loss of insulin but why this should bring about the observed events is still a matter for controversy. While we do not yet know the exact manner in which insulin affects carbohydrate metabolism, three major activities have been attributed to this hormone: (a) that it is necessary for a normal rate of muscle glycogen deposition, (b) that it is essential for the oxidation of glucose by the muscles and other tissues, and (c) that it inhibits glucose formation from noncarbohydrate sources in the liver. The present evidence would indicate that the first two constitute its primary action while the third is an indirect consequence of the former. None of these suggestions have, however, escaped criticism. Those who regard the sequence of events in diabetic animals as being initiated by a failure of glucose oxidation in the tissues find themselves in disagreement with those who regard the uninhibited formation of glucose from both protein and fatty acids by the liver as the essential defect.

The problem is further complicated by the recognition of the hormones of the anterior pituitary gland and of the adrenal cortex as agents that inhibit carbohydrate oxidation and increase the rate of gluconeogenesis. Consequently, pancreatectomy not only deprives the organism of insulin but also leaves unchecked the activity of other endocrine glands whose secretions normally influence carbohydrate metabolism in a manner diametrically opposed to that of insulin. That this is so is shown by the amelioration of a pancreatic diabetes that follows hypophysectomy or adrenalectomy.

The Nature of the Defect in Human Diabetes Mellitus.—It may be readily realized that if there exists a difference of opinion regarding the exact mechanism of insulin action, then the nature of the defect in human diabetes is still more obscure. Superficially everything would seem to point to insulin deficiency as the cause of the majority of cases and correct as such a view may ultimately prove to be it should not be accepted as a completely established fact, particularly when it is appreciated how greatly the discoveries of recent years have forced a reorientation of many of our views of carbohydrate metabolism and the endocrine factors that control it.

While too much emphasis should not be placed on the failure to demonstrate the universal occurrence of lesions of the islets of Langerhans in human diabetics nor on the inconsistency of the type of lesions found, since histological methods are notoriously unreliable as a measure of function during life, it would seem that the bulk of present evidence indicates that diabetes in man is continued by reason of the failure of the pancreas to supply sufficient insulin for the bodily needs.

Such a view does not necessarily imply that the islets of Langerhans are destroyed but rather that their capacity to produce insulin is inadequate to meet the circumstances under which the metabolism is operating.

Consequently, *insulin deficiency may be of two types:* (*a*) that in which there is an actual decrease in the insulin output of the pancreas due to a reduction in the quantity of islet tissue and (*b*) that in which the insulin production may be normal or above normal but owing to alterations in the metabolism of the tissues is inadequate to supply the needs of the organism. Such a situation is encountered in animals injected with anterior pituitary extract and others of an unknown origin may occur. It should be remembered, however, that (*b*) is likely to pass into (*a*) since sooner or later the islets fail and undergo characteristic changes.[7]

Differentiation of Human Diabetics.—There have been several attempts to differentiate between human diabetic patients. Perhaps the best known is found in the recent studies of Himsworth.[8] This investigator has followed the suggestion of Falta that these patients may be grouped into: (*a*) the *insulin-sensitive type* that require only minimal amounts of insulin to prevent glycosuria and (*b*) the insulin-insensitive or *insulin-resistant type*. The latter require large quantities of insulin to control their glycosuria. Conversely, the former type of patient develops hypoglycemia if the insulin dosage is only slightly increased while the latter requires much greater amounts to produce a comparable degree of depression of the blood glucose. Furthermore, as Himsworth points out, a test can be used to distinguish between these groups (Fig. 135). This consists of giving an intravenous injection of 5 units of insulin that is immediately followed by 30 gm. of glucose given by mouth for each square meter of body surface. Blood glucose estimations are then made at intervals during the first hour. In the first group of diabetic patients insulin suppresses the alimentary hyperglycemia but fails to control that of the second group. If the blood-glucose curve after glucose ingestion without insulin is also determined in a separate test the area between the two curves represents the effect of the insulin injected. This is termed the insulin area (I) and the ratio between this and the area of the glucose tolerance curve is termed by Himsworth the I/G ratio. In the insulin-sensitive group this area had an average value of 1.34 and in the insensitive group of 0.51.

According to Himsworth, the former group contains those diabetic patients who react favorably to a diet high in carbohydrate while the latter comprises those who do not tolerate such a regimen.

As Himsworth points out there is an obvious parallelism between the behavior of the insensitive group towards insulin and glucose and animals injected with anterior pituitary extract. However, definite evidence to indicate that diabetes in patients of this type is a result of an anterior pituitary imbalance is lacking except possibly in those cases associated with tumors of the pituitary gland.

Newburgh and his colleagues[9] have recently reported on a group of diabetic patients whom they also regard as a distinct class. These come from the middle-aged, obese group of persons who exhibit glycosuria on an unrestricted diet. When fed a diet which resulted in a marked reduction in body weight the majority showed a striking improvement in carbohydrate tolerance, to such an extent that they could no longer be termed "diabetic" (Fig. 136). These investigators emphasize that the diabetes in this group is

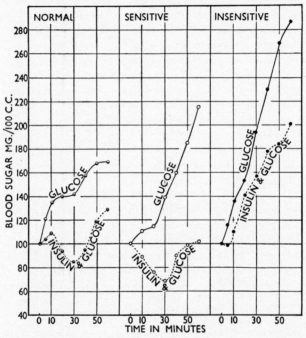

Fig. 135.—Glucose tolerance and insulin-glucose curves from a normal subject, from an insulin-sensitive diabetic and from an insulin-insensitive diabetic. The composition of the diet was approximately the same in each case. (From Himsworth and Kerr, Clin. Science, 4: 119, 1939.)

differentiated from "juvenile" diabetes by the normal ability of such patients to oxidize glucose, and that the disturbance in carbohydrate metabolism is consequently based not on an inability to utilize carbohydrate but on some factor or factors related to the excess weight. Since at least 50 per cent of diabetics between the ages of thirty and sixty years are obese this type of disturbance in carbohydrate tolerance accounts for a large proportion of those classed as "diabetics."

Factors Associated with the Appearance of Diabetes Mellitus in Man.— It has already been pointed out that a normal carbohydrate metabolism is a consequence of the integrated and correlated action between various organs and the hormones that influence their activity. Furthermore, insulin is only one member of this endocrine system and while an adequate supply is apparently decisive nevertheless alterations in carbohydrate metabolism may occur as a result of abnormalities either in the tissues or in other members of the glandular system. These at a later date may then involve the pancreas.

In human diabetes it has been known for some time that certain influences or conditions are associated with the appearance of diabetes although in many instances the "diabetes" may be expressed merely by hyperglycemia and glycosuria after food. Those most widely recognized are (*a*) heredity, (*b*) endocrine disturbances affecting particularly the pituitary gland and adrenal cortex, and to a less extent the thyroid gland, (*c*) obesity, and (*d*) a group of miscellaneous factors such as race, sex, infection and destructive lesions of the pancreas. Others of more doubtful relationship are trauma and arteriosclerosis.

The Hereditary Factor in Diabetes.—It is established that diabetes is an inheritable disease. There is a statistically significant increase in the prevalence of diabetes, among blood relatives of diabetic patients over that of a

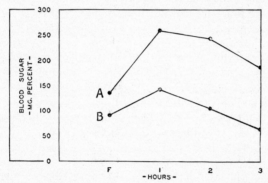

Fig. 136.—The composite glucose tolerance curves of twenty-one obese diabetic patients before and after reduction of weight. (From Newburgh, Conn, Johnson and Conn, Trans. Assoc. Amer. Phys., 53: 243, 1938.)

control group from the general population, the relative frequency being 6.7 and 1.23 per cent respectively; the onset of diabetes in *identical twins* has frequently been observed to be almost simultaneous; the occurrence of diabetes is believed to follow a mendelian recessive pattern and the prediction where diabetes will develop has become possible. It is predictable, based on the observations of White and Pincus,[10] that when both parents have diabetes, all their children eventually, if they live long enough, will develop diabetes; when one parent has diabetes and the other is a diabetic carrier, 40 per cent of their children may be expected to develop diabetes; whereas if a diabetic patient or carrier marries an individual who neither has diabetes nor is a diabetic carrier, none of their children will have diabetes. The last mentioned holds a possible solution to effective prevention of diabetes. Though a diabetic patient marries an individual who neither has diabetes nor is a diabetic carrier all their children, though they will not develop diabetes, are carriers. If these children marry nondiabetics of nondiabetic families the offspring have 1 chance in 2 of being carriers. Similarly in the next or third generation the chance would be 1 in 4, and in the fourth generation 1 in 8. Outbreeding of the disease by the consistent union of descendants of diabetic patients with those of nondiabetic families is therefore possible.

If a child of a diabetic patient develops diabetes it establishes (1) the nondiabetic parent as a carrier, and (2) a 50 per cent chance of the other children developing diabetes. It is obvious that the brother or sister of a diabetic patient may or may not be a carrier.

The predisposition to diabetes may be, and often is, transmitted through apparently normal individuals. This is in keeping with the fact that diabetes may skip one or more generations.

The onset of the diabetes, which we can agree has a hereditary basis, is influenced by several known factors, notably age, body weight, occupation, physical exercise, infections, and finally and of utmost importance, endocrine disturbances. Endocrine functions are known to be controlled by mendelian genes. From the fact that the onset of diabetes is most frequently delayed until middle life, it is obvious that the prediction regarding diabetes may not be fulfilled if the individual dies before reaching this age.

Endocrine Factors.—The perfection of the symbiotic function of the various endocrine glands under normal conditions is that their collective activities seem as one in the maintenance of normal metabolism. When this harmony is disturbed the discord may proclaim itself in many ways. A careful perusal of the scheme of endocrine control of metabolism on page 69 emphasizes the various possible disorders which may result. Among these may be the appearance of diabetes mellitus.

The Influence of the Previous Diet.—While there is a popular conception that an increased consumption of sugar is associated with the increasing incidence of diabetes, it can be said with considerable assurance that an excessive carbohydrate consumption in itself is not a direct cause of the disease. Nevertheless, the composition of the diet prior to the onset of the disease may be a factor of great significance particularly as the work of Himsworth and others has clearly indicated the alterations in the ability of normal individuals to utilize glucose that follow periods in which the composition of the diet is varied. These have been discussed elsewhere (Chapter II), and it will be recalled that Himsworth has found that both the shape and area of the glucose tolerance curve as well as the sensitivity to insulin is determined by the quantity of carbohydrate in the diet. Thus, as the carbohydrate intake is progressively restricted and the diet kept isocaloric by the substitution of fat, the response of the blood glucose to ingested glucose assumes a more and more "diabetic" character while at the same time the area of the insulin-depression curves also becomes less and less.

These very significant observations have naturally led Himsworth to speculate on the possible effects on carbohydrate tolerance of the exposure of individuals to regimens in which the diet is relatively rich in fat and correspondingly restricted in carbohydrate. From his analysis of the available data he has concluded[11] that diabetes is relatively common in those countries in which diets of this character are habitually ingested. Also of great interest is his suggestion that the hereditary predisposition to the disease is widespread and that it is in these individuals that long-continued ingestion of low carbohydrate diets may precipitate the disease. His views are perhaps best summarized in a quotation taken from the paper quoted above.

"Susceptibility and hereditary predisposition undoubtedly play a part in the etiology of the disease, but, in my opinion, their rôle is confined to that of diathesis. The great rise in the diabetic mortality rates of different countries, during the last thirty years, is difficult to explain on the ground that a sudden widespread dissemination of hereditary susceptibility has occurred. A more logical explanation is that the susceptibility to the disease is widespread and that the increasing pressure of some external factor, which provokes the development of diabetes, is disclosing the frequency of this susceptibility. It is suggested that this external determining factor is that of diet: the ingestion of a low-carbohydrate high-fat diet. In any population there will be an unknown number of susceptible individuals and the susceptibility of these individuals will vary considerably. When the diet of the country contains relatively large proportion of carbohydrate it will provoke diabetes only in those who are most susceptible and those who are less susceptible will not develop the disease. But if the diet changes so as to contain smaller proportions of carbohydrate, and correspondingly larger of fat, then the disease will be provoked in less susceptible subjects, and if the proportion of dietary carbohydrate becomes progressively smaller, individuals with slighter degrees of susceptibility will respond by developing diabetes. The incidence rate of diabetes mellitus in the population will thus rise in proportion as the diet changes. If this hypothesis is correct then it would be expected that the incidence of diabetes in different countries could be correlated with the proportion of carbohydrate in the national diet; that increase in the proportion of carbohydrate in the national diet would be associated with a fall in diabetic mortality; that variation in the proportion of dietary carbohydrate consequent upon change in environment would produce change in the incidence of the disease; and that variation in the proportion of carbohydrate in the diet of different classes and in different parts of one country would be reflected in changes in the diabetes incidence rate. The information presented in this paper fulfills these expectations." In further support of this view Himsworth and Kerr[12] have found in normal healthy individuals that insulin insensitivity is more common in the higher age groups and it is among these subjects that the authors believe the insulin-insensitive type of diabetics arises.

Obesity.—The above experiments and the analyses of the influence of the composition of the diet on the development of diabetes naturally lead to a discussion of the part played by obesity, for it is well known that overweight is a frequent precursor of the diabetic state and is most marked in those over forty-five years of age.

Obesity may contribute to the appearance of diabetes in the following ways: (*a*) Overweight is due to a disproportion between the energy ingested in the form of foodstuffs and the energy expenditure of the organism. While we do not know whether fat formation and deposition requires the activity of insulin it is known that an excess food intake either in human or experimental diabetes necessitates the administration of extra insulin; (*b*) Diets that produce obesity are those rich in fat with a high caloric value. As pointed out above Himsworth suggests that under these circumstances insulin insensitivity develops; (c) Newburgh and his colleagues incline to the belief that the diabetes associated with obesity is of a special character and that its etiological basis is different from that of the "juvenile" type; (d) Finally, if there is a group of individuals with a lessened pancreatic reserve, then the long-continued action of conditions that lead to obesity might well be expected to strain the islet function to a point at which insulin supply becomes inadequate.

Miscellaneous Factors in the Etiology of Diabetes.—*Age.*—The relative infrequency of diabetes in childhood and the increasing incidence in the fourth and fifth decades of life are dealt with in the section on the incidence of diabetes. The peak of the frequency curve occurring at puberty in the young diabetic and at the menopause in the adult suggests endocrine influences.

Race and Sex.—The high incidence of diabetes in the Jewish race may be explained by inbreeding, heredity, occupation, and the tendency to obesity in middle life, among other factors mentioned earlier in this chapter under Incidence.

The increasing incidence of diabetes in the females in the fourth and fifth decades of life coincide with an increasing prevalence of overweight and possibly to a decrease in the amount of physical exercise at this age. In addition, at this period the readjustments in the endocrine balance associated with the menopause undoubtedly plays an important part.

Infections.—Infection, generally speaking, plays a minor part in the etiology of diabetes. The far-reaching effects which infections have on a pre-existing diabetes are dealt with under the complications of diabetes.

An infection causing a pancreatitis may cause sufficient destruction of the islets to cause diabetes. Diabetes following a pancreatitis would probably be much more common if it were not for the high mortality caused by the latter condition. Infection of the gallbladder and biliary tract is found about three times as frequently at autopsy in diabetic as in non-diabetic subjects. There can be no doubt that biliary tract infection predisposes to diabetes in individuals with diabetic diathesis.

It is feasible that an acute infection may injure the pancreas, leaving it with a reserve weakened to such an extent that predisposing factors in later years, *i.e.*, obesity, etc., may lead to its failure.

Arteriosclerosis.—Arteriosclerosis cannot be considered a cause of diabetes. If it were, diabetes would be more prevalent in the sixth and seventh decades of life than in the fifth. As the patient ages the arteriosclerosis increases, but the diabetes tends to become milder, due probably to the reduction in the total metabolism after sixty years of age.

Trauma.—Trauma directly to the pancreas could conceivably cause extensive destruction of the pancreas and thus cause diabetes if the patient survives. Trauma to other parts of the body plays no apparent part in the etiology of diabetes. Diabetes appearing after injury is in all likelihood related to enforced inactivity, obesity, and hereditary diathesis.

Other Factors.—*Pancreatic tumors* occasionally cause diabetes by destruction of the islets of Langerhans. *Hemochromatosis* and *pancreatic calculi* cause diabetes in the same manner. The latter two are rare.

In *summary*, it may be said that diabetes mellitus is a disease affecting those processes of metabolism by which carbohydrate is both utilized and formed. As secondary consequences the metabolism of protein and fat are also disturbed as may be the electrolyte and water balance. Insulin deficiency, either relative or absolute, appears to play a central rôle in the continuation of the disease. The factors which initiate the disturbance in carbohydrate metabolism are of a varied character and the mechanism of their action is often obscure. Among them are hereditary influences, alterations in the endocrine balance and long-continued use of diets the composition and quantity of which appear to render the organism decreasingly sensitive to insulin. There is also satisfying evidence that any agent that imposes a long-continued strain on the insulin-producing mechanism of the pancreas will result in its final insufficiency. Consequently, while the disease may begin through the operation of extrapancreatic factors of a diverse character, it may ultimately be continued by the failure of the islet tissue.

Such a definition offers the possibility that if the factor precipitating the disturbance in carbohydrate metabolism is removed in time, a normal balance between insulin requirement and insulin supply may again be achieved. The amelioration of diabetes in certain obese individuals that results from weight reduction and a controlled dietary regime would appear to be an instance of this. Recently Lukens and Dohan[13] have shown that cats rendered severely diabetic by pituitary extract may be cured by a course of insulin treatment provided too long a time is not allowed to elapse before such treatment is begun. The success of such a procedure is graphically shown by the return of a normal histological appearance of the islets of Langerhans in such animals.

Note should be made of the recent papers by Haist, Campbell and Best,[14] who have shown that fasting or a diet high in fat leads to a reduction of the insulin content of the pancreas while a diet high in carbohydrate leads to an increased content. It is also noteworthy that the injection of anterior pituitary gland extract rapidly depletes the pancreas of insulin and as we know is ultimately followed by marked pathological changes in the islets of Langerhans. The authors suggest that the lowered insulin content after fat feeding indicates that the secreting cells are being rested and suggest that a diet high in fat might be useful as a prophylactic measure in children whose family history suggests that they might ultimately become diabetics.

BIBLIOGRAPHY

1. Barker, S. B., Chambers, W. H., and Dann, M., J. Biol. Chem., **118:** 177, 1937.
2. Lukens, F. D. W., Amer. J. Physiol., **122:** 729, 1938.
3. Collip, J. B., Selye, H., and Neufeld, A. H., Amer. J. Physiol., **119:** 289, 1937.
4. Chapman, S., and Fulton, J. F., Amer. J. Physiol., **123:** 35, 1938.
5. Dohan, F. C., and Lukens, F. D. W., Amer. J. Physiol., **122:** 307, 1938.
6. Houssay, B. A., Endocrinology, **18:** 409, 1934.
7. Richardson, K. C., and Young, F. G., Lancet, **1:** 1098, 1938.
8. Himsworth, H. F., Clin. Science, **4:** 119, 1939.
9. Newburgh, L. H., Conn, J. W., Johnson, M. W., and Conn, E. S., Trans. Assoc. Amer. Phys., **53:** 245, 1938.
10. Pincus, G., and White, P., Amer. J. Med. Sci., **186:** 1, 1933.
11. Himsworth, H. F., Clin. Science, **2:** 117, 1935.
12. Himsworth, H. F., and Kerr, R. B., Clin. Science, **4:** 153, 1939.
13. Lukens, F. D. W., and Dohan, F. C., Science, **92:** 222, 1940.
14. Haist, R. E., Campbell, J., and Best, C. H., New Eng. J. Med., **223:** 607, 1940.

SYMPTOMATOLOGY

By Garfield G. Duncan

Symptoms may suggest a diagnosis of diabetes but nothing more. Often I have suspected the presence of diabetes based on symptoms only to find the suspicion unsupported by the results of a more careful investigation. On the other hand the finding of glycosuria, the initial step toward a diagnosis, is not infrequent in the absence of classical symptoms.

The varied symptomatology of diabetes in a typical case is at once indicative of some systemic disorder. General weakness, loss of weight, excessive appetite and thirst, the frequent passing of large quantities of urine without discomfort, rising at night to void, itching of the skin (which in the female occurs particularly about the vulva), and backache are the most common symptoms of uncontrolled and uncomplicated diabetes. Impotence in the male is much less common than these but is more frequent than is generally supposed. Direct questioning of private patients may be required before this complaint is elicited. Impotence is more freely complained of in the free clinics and especially by colored patients.

It has been estimated that as high as 12 per cent of patients having diabetes have no symptoms of the disorder. This observation is based on the finding of glycosuria in applicants for insurance and those undergoing routine health examinations. There is no doubt that many persons who are genuinely free from symptoms have a mild diabetes of which they are ignorant. I am incredulous, however, of the value of figures based on applicants for life insurance who state that they have no symptoms.

General Weakness.—This may be the only symptom. It has been the most common complaint of my diabetic patients on the occasion of their first visit. This symptom common to so many debilitating diseases gives little indication of the nature of the underlying disorder. It is a symptom, however, that should always receive serious consideration and it is a good practice to investigate thoroughly each patient who complains of it.

Rapid Loss of Body Weight.—A rapid loss of body weight in the afebrile patient, especially in the young patient, should suggest the possibility that diabetes may be the cause. This symptom is readily accounted for. Sugar is lost in the urine in amounts varying from mere traces to as much as 15 per cent of sugar. One has but to recall that each gram of sugar lost represents a body deprivation of approximately 4 calories. Sugar in the urine means lost nourishment. It is an odd form of starvation but accounts for the seeming paradox which exists when with increased appetite the food intake greatly exceeds that of the normal and yet weight loss continues. There is excessive protein breakdown with abnormally large quantities of nitrogen excreted in the urine. Weight loss is due in part to the loss of body water by the diuresis resulting from the effect which the high concentration of sugar in the blood exerts on the renal epithelium. Further loss in weight is encountered in the presence of ketosis. In this instance dehydration and loss of nourishment in the form of acetone bodies are additional factors. This feature is dealt with in the section on Complications.

Great importance attaches to body weight and its changes in diabetes. A person with untreated and uncontrolled diabetes loses weight on an unrestricted diet. The diabetes at the same time becomes more severe. Loss of weight in this manner is injurious. This is true even in the obese patient because it leaves less weight to be reduced by a method which improves and controls the diabetes. This other method of weight reduction is brought about by reducing the patient's total food intake—exactly as one would reduce an obese nondiabetic patient. This restriction lessens the immediate demand on the islet function of the pancreas and at the same time consolidates this gain, since it reduces the total metabolism by virtue of the reduced body weight which ensues. Risking monotony in repetition concerning one of the most important aspects of clinical diabetes I will restate: A loss of weight, a decrease in total metabolism by restriction of the total diet, decreases the food loss, gives the pancreas functional rest, and affords the overweight patient with uncontrolled diabetes a remarkable improvement in carbohydrate and total food tolerance. A loss of weight due to the activity of the diabetes, whether due to ignorance or wilful neglect, destroys food tolerance, the diabetes becomes more severe, and the need for insulin increases. A previously obese patient who becomes emaciated because of the activity of the diabetes has lost all of the advantages of a reduction in weight by appropriate treatment, and the necessity of using insulin indefinitely is usually inescapable. I hope this is clear. It is of vital importance. It represents one of the fundamental considerations of diabetes the understanding of which we owe to Dr. Frederick M. Allen.

Excessive Appetite and Thirst.—These are in direct relation to the amount of glycosuria and the polyuria until ketosis intervenes. Anorexia then appears. Excessive appetite is a compensatory effort to replace lost nourishment; polydipsia, to replace lost fluids. The thirst and the frequent voiding of large amounts of urine are among the most common symptoms of diabetes occurring in about three-quarters of all cases. It is in this group of patients that backache is common. This symptom can be reproduced in normal persons by the intake of large quantities of water. Distention of the renal capsule by increased activity of the kidneys with greater than usual volumes of fluid passing through them is responsible. Fatigue in the debilitated patient accentuates the backache.

The physician who recognizes diabetes early does his patient a great service. No reliance is to be placed on the absence of symptoms. One has but to consider how much so many patients owe to chance examinations for other disorders, routine or insurance examinations to realize this. Diabetic patients who are free from symptoms are not immune to complications nor is the diabetes innocent in such cases. A routine urinalysis for every patient will reward one for the effort put forth. Diabetes will be found by this simple test more often than is supposed. Further it will be found earlier when the diabetes is mild, when it is easily controlled without exacting treatment, and insulin will usually not be needed.

Complications of diabetes very often prompt the patient to seek treatment. The discovery of diabetes, the presence of which the patient may be entirely ignorant, is often made on such consultations.

The symptoms of the various complications of diabetes will be dealt with later in this chapter, but for the sake of completeness the more common are recorded here. They are: pain, coldness and gangrene of the extremities, dimness of vision (cataract and retinitis), skin disorders (furuncles, carbuncles, intertrigo, epidermophytosis), and symptoms of peripheral neuritis, particularly pain. Loss of appetite should make one suspect the development of ketosis, especially if the thirst and polyuria are exaggerated and are accompanied by vomiting, intense fatigue, sleepiness, and pain in the abdomen.

PHYSICAL FINDINGS

Many diabetic patients have no physical evidence of the chronic disease from which they suffer. However, the more carefully the examination is made, the more often will the search be rewarded by the discovery of abnormalities which when correlated with the symptoms are found to be more or less characteristic. I refer especially to the appearance of *fatigue,* the *looseness* and *fine wrinkling of the skin* observed in patients who have lost in body weight, and to *dryness* of the skin in those patients who suffer from excessive thirst and polyuria. A mild degree of *pallor* characterizes the skin of many diabetic patients. This is particularly noticeable in those who are overweight and have advanced disease of the arteries. This may be in part attributable to the elevation of the blood lipids, but in most instances it is undoubtedly due to disease of the arteries and capillaries. It is especially common in patients suffering from disease of the coronary arteries. In the young patients, particularly females, taking large amounts of insulin, the skin has a *waxy transparency* with a smoothing out of wrinkles of the face. This has been referred to as an "insulin face." It is noticeable shortly after insulin therapy is begun and is due to water retention in the skin and subcutaneous tissues. This condition tends to disappear when the diabetes is controlled over a period of months. I can recall, however, several young women in whom this state remained unchanged for several years.

Other *skin disorders* may occur as a result of the diabetes, namely, *xanthelasma, xanthochromia,* and *rarely, xanthoma diabeticorum* and *necrobiosis lipoidica diabetica.*

Though all shades of health from the robust, normal-appearing diabetic patient to one critically ill with ketosis are observed, it is well to emphasize that most physical abnormalities observed in these patients are due to complications of the diabetes. The untreated diabetic patient is especially susceptible to *staphylococcal infections,* e.g., furuncles, carbuncles, and bacteremia. He is unusually prone also to develop pulmonary *tuberculosis.* This complication is most common among young patients who have had an attack of diabetic coma. Root and Bloor[1] found that 17.8 per cent of patients admitted in diabetic coma developed active tuberculosis within five years. The intelligent observation of a patient presenting himself with any of these disorders may bring to light a coexisting diabetes.

The physical examination frequently reveals *degenerative changes,* especially cataracts, diabetic retinitis, and generalized disease of the arteries (particularly the coronary arteries). Coldness of the extremities, cyanosis of feet in the dependent position, gangrene of the toes, heel, or foot occur as a result of extensive changes in the arteries. *Irritation of the skin,* either general or about the genitalia as a result of pruritus, is common as are *epidermophyton* infections; these infections involve the feet, between the toes most frequently, but may be found elsewhere on the body.

The physical signs of diabetic coma are considered in detail later but because signs of this complication should be looked for in every diabetic patient they are summarized here. They are: marked dehydration, an odor of acetone on the breath, "air hunger" (Kussmaul's respiration), reduced intraocular tension, dry skin and mucous membranes, low blood pressure, hypothermia, rapid pulse, abdominal tenderness with varying degrees of rigidity, and coldness of the extremities.

PATHOLOGY

There is a great diversity of pathologic changes associated with diabetes but those which arrest attention first are in the pancreas because of its etiologic relationship to this disease, and, in the arteries because of the prominent part they play in neglected diabetes. The immediate cause of death is much more likely to be due to some complication arising because of disease of the arteries than from alterations in the pancreas itself. Gangrene of an extremity and occlusion of a coronary artery with myocardial infarction—both on the basis of arteriosclerotic changes of the arteries—are illustrations of common occurrence. Important pathologic changes are found in the heart, liver, gallbladder, reticuloendothelial system, skin, eyes, and nervous system of diabetic patients. Involvement, primary or secondary, of the other endocrine glands is receiving more and more attention, and infections to which diabetic patients are especially prone (notably pulmonary tuberculosis and staphylococcal infection) are frequently encountered.

Pathologic Changes in the Pancreas.—In some cases of diabetes there is no evidence detectable by any laboratory methods, of the disease in the pancreas. This does not preclude functional changes in the islet cells. Extensive changes are not infrequently found in the acinar and insular tissues of nondiabetic persons. The following statement by Allen still holds: "Every anatomical hypothesis of diabetes still requires to be assisted by assuming the existence of a certain proportion of functional cases without known anatomical basis."

Disease of the pancreas did not receive serious consideration as a cause of diabetes until von Mering and Minkowski[2] discovered that they had caused diabetes by removing the pancreas from a dog. As a result of this observation the cause of diabetes in the first clinical case of diabetes with associated pancreatic disease became apparent. In this case Cawley[3] (1778) found, at autopsy, multiple pancreatic calculi and extensive secondary damage in the pancreas.

Von Mering and Minkowski established the relationship of the pancreas to diabetes produced experimentally. Laguesse, because of the relationship of the rich blood supply to the islets of Langerhans suggested that the islets produced an internal secretion. Opie's hypothesis that diabetes is due to alterations in the islets of Langerhans followed. Ssobolew failed to find any islets in three of thirteen cases of diabetes.

Evidence that disease of the islet tissue of the pancreas was at fault in diabetes was enhanced when Weichselbaum[4] observed hydropic degeneration of the islets in patients who died of diabetes. Allen[5] next produced hydropic degeneration of the islet cells by removing approximately nine-tenths of a dog's pancreas and producing functional overstrain of the remaining pancreatic remnant by overfeeding the animal. This degenerative change affected the beta cells of the islets, which are believed to be the site of insulin production.

Further evidence that the islet cells produced insulin was the actual recovery of insulin by Banting and Best from the islets after the acinar tissue had been allowed to atrophy by ligating the pancreatic duct. Hyperinsulinism due to tumors of the islets of Langerhans with complete cure following the removal of the tumor leaves no doubt of the part played by the islets of the pancreas as the producers of insulin. Insulin has been recovered in large quantities not only from the tumor of the islets but from the metastatic lesions in the liver as well.[6]

The part played by the islets of Langerhans in the production of insulin is established. Whether a decrease in this function is primary in the pancreas or secondary to disease of the pituitary or adrenal glands cannot at this time be determined clinically or even at autopsy. These features have been discussed in the section on Etiology.

Disease Processes Involving the Islets of Langerhans and the Pancreas as a Whole.—The islets may appear normal and yet the patient may have clinical diabetes. Is this because the insulin is neutralized, is it a poor product or is there a lack of insulin activation or transport? The answer probably rests in the interrelationship of the endocrine glands. This is a common refuge in our ignorance, but one which recent advances, particularly the work of Houssay, Long, Lukens, Young, and Best and their associates seem to justify. A progressive destruction of the islets of Langerhans will eventually cause diabetes. The processes by which this may occur are: invasion, destruction and replacement of the islets by hyaline material, fibrosis, abscess, tumors, and more rarely acute pancreatitis, pancreatic calculi, cysts, hemorrhage, amyloid changes, fat infiltration, and gummata, and finally, the cause which is receiving most consideration at the present time is the functional overstrain of the islets of Langerhans and their ultimate destruction by excessive secretion of the anterior pituitary gland.

Hyalinization.—Hyalinization of the islets is the most typical lesion of the pancreas in diabetes mellitus. Its cause is unknown and its origin and the process of selective localization in the islets are under dispute.

Warren[7] believes that hyalinization of the islets is a cause of and not a result of diabetes and may be considered as due to production of intercellular substance by fibroblasts and possibly by endothelial cells. He believes that the hyaline material thus produced "separates the cells from the blood supply and finally forces them out of existence, growth occurs at the periphery of the islet, particularly if adjacent to fat or fibrous tissue into which expansion can take place more readily than into acinar tissue."

Eventually large hyaline masses are formed exceeding the size of the original islet. This chronic process of destruction of epithelial cells and replacement with hyaline material sooner or later reduces the capacity of the islets to produce insulin below the level necessary for the maintenance of normal metabolism. Diabetes mellitus results.

Hyalinization is a slow process. A variety of stages between complete hyalinization of one islet to other islets scarcely affected is the rule. The hyaline material remains intercellular and in close approximation with the walls of the vessels of the islets giving the appearance of perivascular deposits. Calcification of hyalinized islets occurs occasionally. Hyalinization is unusual in the young, occurring most frequently in patients of the older age group having mild diabetes over a long period. Fifty per cent of Warren's cases who had diabetes over ten years had hyaline deposits in the pancreas. Of Warren's 200 cases of hyalinization of the islets, 97 per cent occurred in individuals over forty years of age. It occurs infrequently in nondiabetic persons in later life.

Opie,[8] who first described hyalinization, believes, because of staining characteristics of the islet cells, that the hyalin is epithelial in origin, hence of intra- and not intercellular manufacture, and that it is a product of degeneration of the islets.

Though the origin of the hyalin is still under dispute, and MacCallum states that in routine autopsies at the Johns Hopkins Hospital they have seldom found obvious disease of the islets of Langerhans, certain conclusions can, nevertheless, be drawn: 1. Hyalinization of the islets usually occurs in diabetes. 2. It is most common in patients over forty years of age. 3. It has been observed in nondiabetic persons in later life. 4. It is usually, but not always, absent in young persons having severe diabetes. 5. Coincident with the progress of hyalinization there is destruction of islet cells and a diminution in the total number of functionally active islets ensues.

To realize the extent of damage to the islets when hyalinization causes diabetes one has but to recall that, experimentally, nine-tenths of the pancreas must be removed to cause diabetes. The functional capacity of the islet tissue is tremendously reduced or a potent insulin antagonist is or has been at work when diabetes appears.

Great practical significance is attached to whether hyalinization is the cause or the effect of diabetes. If it is the cause we are in a relatively helpless state. If it is the effect of diabetes then its progressiveness should certainly be altered by satisfactory control of the diabetes. Clinical impressions, based on observations of function, admittedly less certain than laboratory observations with the microscope, lead one to believe that hyalinization in the islets is a penalty for neglect of the diabetes—a result of disturbed metabolism and not of inflammatory reaction.

The underlying cause of changes in the pancreas leading to diabetes is probably extrapancreatic. Experimental evidence shows the anterior lobe of the hypophysis to be at fault. Hyaline changes were observed to develop in Young's dogs who received crude extracts of this gland. They developed permanent diabetes.

Fibrosis.—Fibrosis is an index of the extent of a chronic pancreatitis. This may be on the basis of repeated mild attacks of acute pancreatitis predisposed to by chronic disease of the gallbladder. There may be little or no fibrosis present yet all stages are seen, varying from the commonly found small amount of fibroblastic tissue about an islet to the uncommon extensive penetration and destruction of islet and acinar tissue with replacement by scar tissue. The fibrous tissue formation is a chronic process and begins at the capsule and penetrates by extension along the course of the vessels. Cecil found fibrosis in 54 per cent and Warren in 27 per cent of his cases of diabetes. Like hyalinization, and at times occurring with it, fibrosis occurs most frequently in patients over forty years of age.

Hydropic Degeneration of the Islets.—In contrast to the foregoing chronic and common changes in the pancreas hydropic degeneration of the islets is an acute and rarely observed process. It was first observed by Weichselbaum and Stangl in 1901.[4] In the process of hydropic degeneration the islet cells become swollen, the granules of the beta cells—the pre-insulin state—decrease in number and finally disappear and are replaced by vacuoles. Failing appropriate treatment of the diabetes the vacuoles coalesce and nuclear degeneration and disappearance of the affected cells follow. Allen[5] produced these changes experimentally, by suddenly inducing diabetes, and showed them to be due to functional overstrain of the islets of Langerhans.

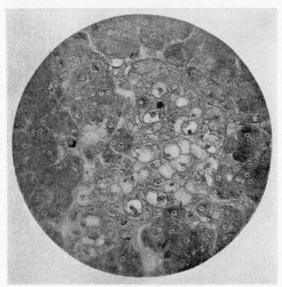

Fig. 137.—A photograph of a typical islet of Langerhans undergoing hydropic degeneration. The pancreatic tissue was taken from a diabetic dog before insulin treatment. (Copp and Barclay, J. Metab. Research.)

Though it is not to be expected that the human, suffering from diabetes, would show the same degree of changes, nevertheless typical hydropic degeneration has been observed in cases when death was due to diabetic coma. Allen[9] believed hydropic degeneration of the islets to be positive microscopic proof of the diagnosis of diabetes. He observed the progressiveness of the hydropic degeneration and an increasing severity of the diabetes when animals were overfed and that these effects were reversible in the early stages by restricting the diet. This reversibility was made more striking when insulin was used (Copp and Barclay[10]). New importance attaches to Allen's observations in the revealing work of Young and Best, and they have been recently confirmed by Lukens and Dohan. (See Etiology of Diabetes.)

Clinically how important is hydropic degeneration? It is an acute process and has been proved to be reversible. The prompt control of a rapidly progressive diabetes may restore islet cells in which the degree of degeneration has not proceeded to a point beyond which the cell and its function cannot be redeemed. It is fascinating to speculate that the remarkable reduction in the need for insulin, which all physicians who have treated many diabetic patients have observed, has been due in part at least to the rescue of these cells. This consideration is a stimulation to secure prompt control of the diabetes.

Lymphocytic Infiltration.—Infiltration of the islets of Langerhans by lymphocytes, occasionally accompanied by endothelial leukocytes, occurs in young patients with severe diabetes.[11] In one instance, a girl of twelve years, the diabetes progressed rapidly, ending fatally, in spite of intensive treatment, five days after the condition was discovered.

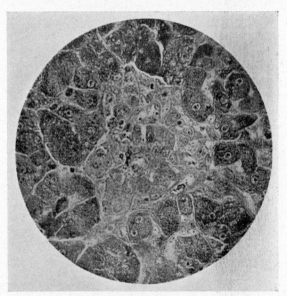

Fig. 138.—A typical islet of Langerhans after fifteen days of symptomatic control of the diabetes with insulin. Note the absence of hydropic degeneration and vacuolization. (Copp and Barclay, J. Metab. Research.)

The youthfulness of the patient, the rapidity of the progressiveness of the diabetes and the presence of numerous endothelial leukocytes and lymphocytes in the islets of the pancreas were considered to be related to each other.

Less Common Changes in the Islets of Langerhans.—Pyknosis or thickening of the nuclei in shrunken islet cells was observed in six cases of diabetes by Warren. Occasionally these were the only abnormal findings. Gibb and Logan encountered these changes in fifteen of 142 cases.

Hypertrophy of islet tissue occurring in the diabetic patient has been considered as evidence of regeneration from duct epithelium. Cecil observed thirty-four instances of hypertrophy in 100 diabetic necropsies.

Hemorrhage into the islets and islet cell *adenomata* have been recorded as complicating diabetes. They are admittedly rare and are in no way characteristic of the pathological changes seen in diabetes.

Fat infiltration of islet tissue is common but usually not extensive. Deposits of fat are more frequently found throughout the acinar tissue and its occurrence and extent is more or less directly related to the obesity of the patient. Most adult diabetic subjects are overweight and the fatty deposits in the pancreas are not surprising. It is not unusual to find extensive fatty infiltration and fibrosis in the same pancreas.

Acute pancreatitis preceded the onset of diabetes in five of Warren's cases. The high mortality in acute pancreatitis is an obvious reason for the relatively small number of cases of diabetes developing from this cause.

It is rare indeed for diabetes to follow *trauma*. Direct injury to, with extensive destruction of the tail of the pancreas might conceivably have the same effect as surgical removal of nine-tenths of the pancreas. The scarcity of such reports adequately emphasizes the extreme rarity of traumatic diabetes if indeed there is such a condition.

Syphilitic fibrosis and *gummata* may be found in the pancreas in the diabetic patient. Syphilis and diabetes are rarely associated with each other except in the Negro race and here there is no convincing evidence that diabetes has ever been caused by syphilitic changes in the pancreas.

Duct Obstruction and Islet Cell Loss from Obvious Causes.—The pancreatic duct may be obstructed by pressure from without, involvement of the duct wall by neoplasm, inflammatory reaction, metaplasia of the epithelium as occurs in vitamin A deficiency, and concretions in the lumen of the duct. All are potential causes of pancreatic diabetes.

A patient under the care of Dr. David L. Farley at the Pennsylvania Hospital illustrates the possible sequelae of obstruction to the pancreatic duct.

A Negress, aged forty-two years, was admitted for the treatment of an arsenical hepatitis in June 1936. In the study of her liver function a glucose tolerance test was conducted and with a normal response. This patient was readmitted in a semistuporous state on March 2, 1939. She had been well until February 27, 1939, when she first complained of weakness. This symptom progressed, anorexia developed, and she vomited once. The physical signs were those of marked dehydration. There was glycosuria, acetonuria and albuminuria. The CO_2 combining power of the blood plasma was 27 volumes per cent and the blood sugar was 424 mg. per 100 cc.

Large amounts of insulin (845 units in twenty-four hours), with the other measures for combating ketosis did not appreciably affect the blood sugar level or the CO_2 combining power of the blood, though there was a temporary clinical improvement. She gradually became comatose and died on the second day. She had fever during the last day of life.

The necropsy revealed no gross changes in the pancreas, but microscopically the islet tissue was scarred and necrotic, and purulent exudate was present throughout and about the ducts. The ducts showed a marked squamous metaplasia of the epithelium. No islet tissue was found.

It seemed probable that a vitamin A deficiency, epithelial metaplasia, duct obstruction, stasis, and secondary infection provided the sequence of events which caused the diminution in the number of islets, the diabetes, the resistance to insulin and the fatal complication.

Metastatic abscesses may also affect the pancreas. Warren has reported four such instances occurring as complications of a staphylococcus pyemia.

Pancreatic Calculi.—Calculus formation in the pancreas as a cause of diabetes is uncommon. Dillon[12] reported that of 2800 autopsies at the Pennsylvania Hospital, two cases of pancreatic calculi were found and in one of these there was evidence of diabetes. There were slightly over 100 cases of pancreatic calculi recorded in the literature prior to 1932 (Ackman and Ross). The condition is, nevertheless, of great historic interest. The first positive autopsy evidence of disease of the pancreas in a case of diabetes was a case of multiple pancreatic calculi reported by Cawley.[3] Furthermore Warren states that it was such a case reported by Barron[13] which "aroused Banting's interest and thus played a part in the development of insulin." Mason[14] observed marked resistance to insulin in a case of pancreatic calculi. Stasis and infection are the secondary factors which doubtless cause most of the destruction.

Neoplasms.—It is remarkable how infrequently neoplasms of the pancreas cause sufficient destruction of islet cells to precipitate the clinical manifestations of diabetes. Carcinoma is the most common neoplasm to occur in the pancreas and it usually involves the head, whereas the islet tissue, most abundant in the tail, has a good chance of escaping destruction. Adenoma, sarcoma, lymphoma, and cysts of the pancreas are rare. New growths of the islet tissue are dealt with in Chapter XIII.

Vascular Lesions—Lesions of the Circulatory System.—Lesions of the vascular system are responsible for the deaths in more than 50 per cent of patients who have had diabetes for more than fifteen years.

Arteriosclerosis can be rightly blamed for the heart disease so commonly observed in the diabetic patient, and for the gangrene of the extremities. It is the diabetic patient's greatest enemy. It progresses insidiously, consolidating its gains as it goes, and when attention is attracted to it by symptoms or examination one finds it permanently established and incurable. It is with difficulty that any impression is made on its relentless progress. The long start and the process of aging both favor the disease and tend to annul efforts to correct it. Sir Clifford Allbutt in writing of arteriosclerosis has said: "Marvellous as in the human frame are the symmetry of parts and the harmony of function, yet it cannot be supposed that the stealthy hours carry away no qualities of tissue, no quantities of energy."

One is struck by the frequency with which advanced arteriosclerosis accompanies diabetes. Even the young patients are not spared. The full-blown condition is readily identified. It is the process of the development of these changes that awaits solution. Is the high lipid content of the blood in these patients an important predisposing factor? Does this cause the fatty infiltration of the intercellular substance of the intima producing the atheromatous plaques of intimal thickening which is the outstanding arterial lesion in the diabetic patient?

Aschoff explains these changes in the intima on the basis of Virchow's "imbibition theory," according to which there is, as a result of wear and tear, a primary loosening of the intimal layer due to infiltration of blood plasma, which is accompanied or followed by a reparative proliferation of intimal cells and a more marked vascularization of the media. The intimal thickening progresses and eventually a stage is reached when lipid substances are precipitated in the depths of the thickened intima. A softening process follows with extension to the surface. Calcium deposits occur in these areas of softening.

Irreversible changes are represented by swelling and hyaline degeneration of the ground substance of the intima, the infiltration with lipids and mucin, and fibrous proliferation. The combination of these two phases, the atheromatous and the arteriosclerotic or atherosclerotic, is prevalent in diabetic patients and are seen most frequently in the aorta, but the coronary, cerebral vessels and smaller arteries are commonly affected. Some of the common results of these changes are discussed in the chapter on gangrene.

Winternitz[15] believes that the atheromatous plaques are the result of extravasation of blood within the wall affording a possible source of lipid deposits.

Pathologic Distribution of Glycogen in the Diabetic Patient.—*In the Kidney.*—Accumulation of glycogen in the renal epithelium—especially in the loops of Henle, but also in the convoluted tubules and glomeruli—has been erroneously regarded as being pathognomonic of diabetes. The condition was described by Armanni in 1875 but the glycogen was not identified until Ehrlich did so in 1883. It is now known that glycogen accumulations may occur in the renal epithelium in the presence of glycosuria from any cause. At first thought this might reduce to insignificance the observation of these changes. To appreciate evidence to the contrary one has but to realize that approximately four-fifths of all persons having glycosuria also have diabetes. Hence when these alterations are found it is likely that they are the result of diabetes.

In ordinary sections of kidney tissue for microscopic examination the glycogen stands out as clear areas in the epithelial cells. The glycogen is readily observed if thin slices of tissue are fixed in absolute alcohol within an hour or two after death and stained with Best's carmine stain according to the technic advised by Mallory.[16]

It is established (1) that glycosuria predisposes to glycogen infiltration in the renal epithelium, particularly in the loops of Henle, (2) that this is not a constant finding in diabetes, (3) that the amount of glycogen in the renal tubules is reduced and disappears with proper control of the diabetes, with or without the use of insulin, (4) that there is an indirect relationship between the amount of glycogen present in the liver and skin. Uncontrolled diabetes leads to depletion of liver and skin glycogen and to glycosuria with glycogen infiltration in the renal tubules. Control of the diabetes reverses conditions, *i.e.*, the glycogen in the liver and skin increases and the renal glycogen disappears.

In the Skin.—Severe and untreated diabetes interferes with the normal deposition and storage of glycogen in the epithelia of the stratum corneum, of the sweat glands and of the hair follicles. The glycogen content of the skin becomes greatly depleted. The normal state, however, is restored with correction of the glycosuria and the hyperglycemia by appropriate treatment of the diabetes.

The part, if any, which depleted skin glycogen plays in the susceptibility which diabetic patients have to pruritus and infections of the skin is not known. Excess sugar in the absence of glycogen may be one factor, but the mechanism by which it operates is by no means clear.

In the Liver.—Glycogen storage in the liver is also interfered with in untreated diabetes. As the disease progresses the liver glycogen is reduced and oddly enough as the glycogen disappears from the cytoplasm it accumulates to the degree of engorgement in the cell nuclei. Lacking treatment with insulin, cytoplasmic glycogen is reduced to mere traces or indeed it may be entirely absent. This is in contrast to the amount of glycogen (400 gm.) occurring in the liver of a robust man under normal conditions, and to that of the diabetic patient who has been properly treated. As the cytoplasmic glycogen is restored the intranuclear glycogen decreases. This return to normal is impeded and indeed may be prevented by acute infections, the effect of which has a definite clinical bearing. The sudden development of sensitiveness to insulin after abrupt relief from acute infections is undoubtedly exaggerated by this scarcity of glycogen. On the other hand large quantities of glycogen in the liver reduce remarkably the likelihood of hypoglycemic reactions because of the readiness with which it is converted to glucose.

Decreasing glycogen depots infer poor treatment or no treatment at all for the diabetes. The hazard of developing ketosis is thus increased and this risk is magnified by complicating infections.

Glycogen is a carbohydrate reserve. Insulin is essential for its storage and for the utilization of its end product, glucose. Insulin and glycogen are dependent one upon the other for their normal functioning.

In the Muscle.—The muscle glycogen is not greatly reduced in untreated diabetes as it is not directly convertible to glucose for use by the body tissues in general.

There is a glycogenic infiltration in excess of the normal in the heart muscle of untreated diabetes. Whether this (1) is due to an inability of the muscle to use the glycogen or (2) is a safety device to safeguard a muscle upon which the life of the individual depends is not known. This finding refutes the belief that the heart muscle of the diabetic patient is unable to take up sugar from the blood and should dampen the ardor of those who advocate maintaining a moderate hyperglycemia because of this erroneous belief.

Miscellaneous Distribution of Glycogen.—Glycogen occurs in small quantities in the pancreas, brain, hypophysis, placenta, and in leukocytes, but no outstanding importance or characteristics are attached to this distribution in the diabetic patient.

Objective Pathologic Changes in Fat Metabolism in Diabetes.—The common and striking abnormalities associated with fat metabolism in untreated diabetes are (1) excess cholesterol in the circulation, (2) increased blood fats, and (3) the accumulation of ketone bodies in the blood. The foregoing disturbances are directly related to the clinical complications, *e.g.*, xanthomata, atheromatosis and ketosis. Hepatomegaly and splenomegaly are also directly attributable to the disturbed fat metabolism as a result of which lipids are deposited in the phagocytic reticuloendothelial cells—*lipid histiocytosis.*

These deposits are most abundant in the spleen, which becomes enlarged. The rarity of lipid histiocytosis in an advanced stage is emphasized by the remarkable infrequency of a spleen sufficiently enlarged to be palpable.

Fat infiltration and moderate *enlargement of the liver* is a fairly common finding in diabetes, especially in diabetic children. Warren points out that increased water content of the liver has accounted for some of the increased weight of the liver formerly attributed to fat accumulations. An enlarged and tender liver is much more likely to be due to distention of the liver capsule by rapid accumulations of water than by the slower process of fat deposition.

The reader is referred to the review of lipid histiocytosis by Warren and Root.[17]

There is a great temptation to compare the human diabetic patient with the depancreatized dog. Realizing that there are definite limitations to this method of explaining alterations from the normal we are justified in noting that the depancreatized dog, even though treated with insulin, cannot survive for long periods and that at death the outstanding changes are fat infiltration and degeneration of the liver (Fisher, 1924). McLeod and his associates prevented these changes and permitted the dogs to survive for long periods by adding raw pancreas to their diet. A possible acinar as well as the insular deficiency was at once considered as the explanation of the enlarged and fatty livers found in some of the diabetic patients. The addition of either lecithin[18] or choline,[19] both ingredients of raw pancreas, to the diets of the depancreatized dog prolonged life in each instance, and the changes in the liver were prevented. Dragstedt (1936) attributed similar results to a hitherto undescribed internal secretion of the pancreas and suggested the name *lipocaic* for this new hormone. Dragstedt[20] has recently reviewed and extended this work. He points out that if there is an enlarged, fatty and poorly functioning liver with a subnormal blood lipid level, a decreased dextrose excretion and an unusually great sensitiveness to insulin in a diabetic patient or animal, that it is due to a lipocaic insufficiency. He notes that Grayzel and Radwin (1938) secured a striking decrease in the size of the liver in three young diabetic patients by giving lipocaic. Enlargement of the liver is reported as having returned within one or two months of the withdrawal of the lipocaic. Lipocaic is administered in doses of 1.0 to 1.5 gm. daily. Though the extension of the use of lipocaic in its clinical application deserves careful scrutiny, the satisfactory control of the diabetes, particularly with protamine zinc insulin, is a very effective means of dealing with enlargement of the liver in diabetic children.

DIAGNOSIS

General Considerations.—The diagnosis of diabetes mellitus is made by the appropriate consideration of the patient's symptoms, family and past history, physical findings and laboratory data. The clinical signs and symptoms are of utmost value as they arouse the suspicion of the presence of diabetes and of its complications. Quite as important and much more sensitive are the confirmatory laboratory data. Without them the diagnosis may be considered probable but without them a positive diagnosis can never be made. Of these data sugar in the urine and the elevation of the blood sugar level above normal values are the most significant. Other abnormalities, notably increased blood cholesterol and fat values, an accumulation of acetone bodies in the blood and their excretion in the urine, and a reduced carbon dioxide combining power of the blood plasma are found in studying the diabetic patient. They are actually of little value in the diagnosis of diabetes but they do indicate complications of this disease. Special tests may be necessary to detect or to exclude a very mild diabetes.

Any evidence of diabetes should instigate an investigation calculated to confirm or disprove the tentative diagnosis. The important considerations, with the diet unrestricted, are:

(a) Glycosuria—occurring concomitant with a hyperglycemia.

(b) Hyperglycemia—fasting blood (venous) sugar values above 120 mg. per 100 cc. and postprandial values in excess of 160 mg. per 100 cc., or if capillary blood is used the fasting value for sugar above 120 or a postprandial value above 190 mg. per 100 cc. The diagnosis should not be made on the basis of only one determination of the level of the blood sugar.

(c) Special tests for doubtful cases.

    1. Effect of a meal containing 100 gm. of carbohydrate, on the level of the blood sugar. Values above 160 mg. per 100 cc. at one or two hours after the meal are indicative of diabetes providing there is no complication present which might alter the carbohydrate tolerance.

    2. One-hour two-dose glucose tolerance test (Exton Rose procedure).

    3. Standard glucose tolerance test.

The Urine—Glycosuria.—This term is loosely used in general to mean sugar in the urine. It actually means glucose in the urine as distinct from the other forms of melituria (Chapter XV). A relatively innocent glycosuria occurs in nondiabetic subjects who have permanently low renal thresholds for glucose, and others who have temporary reduction in the renal threshold as occurs during pregnancy and in hyperthyroidism. It is obvious that glycosuria alone does not warrant the diagnosis of diabetes. No glycosuria should be passed by lightly, however. Glucose, a fermentable dextrorotatory copper-reducing sugar, appearing in the urine in amounts demonstrable by the Benedict test (p. 737), should be considered as being due to diabetes until proved otherwise. The glycosuria of diabetes is not innocent. The problem of diagnosis is an individual one for each patient: Is the glycosuria due to diabetes or is it not? This is a more important question and one which is more simply answered than the actual identification of the type of sugar. A search for hyperglycemia before and after the strain of a meal will usually give the answer. If not, the special tests referred to below are resorted to. Glycosuria is the most common, though not the most sensitive sign which leads ultimately to the diagnosis of diabetes mellitus. It ordinarily is the result of hyperglycemia, sugar being lost when the blood sugar level exceeds the renal threshold, usually between 150 and 180 mg. per 100 cc. Glycosuria is an important sign because it is tested for in the conduct of a routine urinalysis, hence the chance of its discovery is great and the detection of the diabetes more likely in contrast with the more delicate test for diabetes—an abnormal elevation of the blood sugar. Yet the determination of the blood sugar level is not a routine test for all patients in most hospitals. The value of a routine urinalysis for every patient, diabetic and nondiabetic, therefore cannot be overemphasized. Tragedies of neglect are too common. One must be continuously on the alert. Penalties will be exacted sooner or later if we relax in our standards. These penalties are incorrect diagnoses, and delayed treatment of uncomplicated diabetes and of acute and chronic complications of this chronic disease. Either or both may cause the patient great inconvenience or even jeopardize his life. Both constitute an unfavorable reflection on the physician.

There is a minute quantity of copper-reducing substance in normal urine but this is too small to be detected by the usual tests, notably Benedict's and Fehling's. Sugar occurring in the urine in concentrations below 0.1 per cent may be considered as normal.

Glucose when boiled with an alkaline copper solution (Benedict's test, p. 737) reduces the copper to cuprous oxide, thus changing the color of the solution from blue to green, greenish yellow, orange or brick red with increasing concentrations of sugar. Ordinarily glucose occurring in sufficient quantities in the urine to be detected by the Benedict test indicates a pathologic condition.

Glycosuria, it is generally believed, may occur in some normal persons for short periods after an unusually great carbohydrate intake. This is *alimentary glycosuria*. This represents either a low renal threshold for glucose or a hyperglycemia of short duration following "a carbohydrate debauch." It is questionable whether hyperglycemia of this degree, even if it does occur after an unusually great intake of carbohydrate, should be considered as normal.

The glycosuria which occurs as the result of diabetes varies from mere traces scarcely detectable to large amounts, 15 per cent or more. It is unusual to find a concentration of sugar in the urine of diabetic patients in excess of 10 per cent. The determination of the amount of sugar lost (see method, p. 737) in each twenty-four-hour excretion of urine is a valuable aid in assaying the effectiveness of treatment. For practical purposes qualitative tests (p. 737), which are crudely quantitative also, applied to fractional collections of urine serve admirably as guides in adjusting the insulin dosage. More will be said of this in the section on treatment.

In the patient suffering from a mild diabetes glycosuria is most apt to occur during the daytime and in the evening, that is, during the time of the day when three meals are taken in fairly close succession. Glycosuria is least apt to occur in this patient in the morning before breakfast—at the end of the longest period without food. An evening specimen and not the first one voided in the morning is the best one to examine if diabetes is suspected. In contrast, the severe grades of diabetes cause continuous glycosuria until corrected by appropriate treatment.

Sugar having been found in the urine, the level of the blood sugar should be determined. If the value is normal before and after meals and when the patient is subjected to one or both glucose tolerance tests the diagnosis of a nondiabetic melituria is justified. Identification of the sugar may then be proceeded with as outlined by Cantarow in Chapter XV.

False positive reactions to tests for glycosuria are common. The copper solution used in Fehling's and Benedict's qualitative tests for glycosuria is slightly reduced and may be mistaken for sugar when large quantities of the conjugate glycuronates occur in the urine. They appear in decomposing urine and may be avoided by examining freshly voided specimens. The glycuronates appear in the urine in considerable quantities and give a positive Benedict's test after the ingestion of salicylates, camphor, menthol, chloral hydrate, borneol, morphine, phenol, naphthol, pyramidon, and turpentine. As a group, the glycuronates reduce the copper in Benedict's and Fehling's solutions but unlike glucose are nonfermentable.

The homogentisic acid of alcaptonuria reduces the alkaline copper solutions, thus giving false positive tests for sugar. In this disorder if the urine is allowed to stand and become alkaline by ammoniacal putrefaction or if alkali is added, the urine assumes a black or gray color. I have seen only one case of alcaptonuria.

Benedict's Qualitative Test[21] *for Sugar in the Urine* (*Modified*):

EQUIPMENT.—

1. Qualitative Benedict's Solution (when purchasing testing solution, specify *Qualitative* Benedict's Solution, as Benedict's Quantitative Solution does not change color when boiled with glucose).
2. Test tubes marked at 5 cc. and at 2.5 cc. levels.
3. Dropper pipette.
4. Water-bath.

TECHNIC.—

1. Put 2½ cc. (approximately ½ teaspoonful) of Benedict's Solution in a test tube.
2. Add 4 drops of the urine to be tested. Hold pipette perpendicularly while adding drops.
3. Shake tube to mix urine and Benedict's solution thoroughly.
4. Put the tube in a water-bath of boiling water and boil for five minutes.
5. Let cool and read reaction.

INTERPRETATION.—

Clear blue solution: no sugar. Light greenish-yellow: faint trace of sugar. Yellow to orange: moderate amount of sugar, about 1 per cent. Chocolate-brown or brick-red: large quantities of sugar, over 2 per cent.

Millard Smith's Micro-modification of Benedict's Quantitative Test for Sugar in the Urine:[12]

EQUIPMENT.—

1. One small ring stand with test tube clamp, a micro Bunsen burner or small alcohol lamp.
2. A Pyrex test tube (18 by 160 mm.).
3. A Millard Smith pipette* No. 2 and a 1 cc. Ostwald pipette.

TECHNIC.—

1. Transfer 1 cc. of Benedict's quantitative solution to the test tube (held in ring stand clamp) and add 0.2 to 0.7 gm. of anhydrous sodium carbonate. Bumping is prevented by adding a thoroughly dried pebble, a piece of quartz or a pinch of talcum powder.
2. The mixture is raised to and kept at the boiling point.
3. The urine is added slowly from the Smith pipette until all of the blue color disappears. Care should be taken to allow time for complete reduction before adding

* Can be purchased from Emil Greiner Co., 55 Vandorn St., New York City.

more urine. The test is done slowly and care must be taken not to pass the end point. The percentage of sugar present is read directly from the pipette without calculation.

Urine containing less than 1 per cent of sugar is titrated directly. When larger amounts of sugar are present, the urine is diluted, 1 to 10 or 1 to 20 before titration.

Specific Gravity.—The specific gravity of the urine usually increases in direct proportion to the amount of sugar present. A specific gravity of 1.030 or above obtained on a pale urine is frequently due to sugar. The specific gravity is restored to normal when the glycosuria is corrected. However, a normal specific gravity, 1.008 to 1.025, is common even though glycosuria is present.

Urine Volume.—In untreated diabetes the twenty-four-hour urine volume characteristically exceeds the average normal of 1500 cc. In fact the quantities may reach several gallons. The great increase in the volume of urine gives but little index of the severity of the diabetes, but in general the greater the volume the greater is the amount of sugar present. Occasionally the polyuria is so great that amounts totalling more than 50 per cent of the body weight may be voided in twenty-four hours. Control of the diabetes restores the rate of urine excretion to normal.

Ketonuria.—Ketonuria is the first recognizable sign of ketosis though it is of little importance in the diagnosis of diabetes. It results when, from insulin lack and insufficient carbohydrate intake, the metabolism of fat is accentuated and ketones are produced in greater than normal quantities. Ketones are also derived from certain amino acids. Ketonuria occurs in a mild form in healthy nondiabetic patients whose food intake, especially the carbohydrate, is greatly curtailed. It is common in the diabetic patient without other evidence of ketosis. This was especially so in the pre-insulin era when diets high in fat and low in carbohydrate contents were popular. A considerable quantity of ketones may be excreted in the urine without their accumulation in the blood or without a reduction of the CO_2 combining power. Failing appropriate treatment, however, the rate of production of ketones eventually exceeds the rate at which they can be excreted. It is then that qualitative reactions for acetone and diacetic acid in the plasma (see footnote) or serum become positive and it is then that the acetone odor appears on the breath. Stadie[20] believes ketones accumulate because of a coincident breakdown of the fatty acid chains and not because of an interference in the process of fat metabolism at the acetone body stage.

The ketone bodies are *acetone, diacetic acid,* and *β-hydroxybutyric acid.* Acetone and diacetic acid appear under similar conditions and as the latter is, by far, the more injurious of the two it receives chief consideration. Both are identified by a modified Rothera test.*

An increasing loss of β-hydroxybutyric acid in the urine goes hand in hand with a deepening ketosis. In severe ketosis it is in this form that most of the ketones are lost, amounting to as much as 200 gm. in twenty-four

---

* Bedside test for plasma acetone and diacetic acid (Rothera-Wishart): Two drops of plasma, or serum, are placed in a Wassermann tube and supersaturated with ammonium sulfate crystals and shaken. Two drops of approximately 5 per cent sodium nitroprusside solution are added and shaken. Two drops of ammonia water are added and shaken. Allow to stand for three minutes.

Interpretation: Permanganate color   = trace of plasma acetone.
                Light blue   = moderate.
                Deep blue or almost black = heavy reaction for plasma acetone.

hours. The tests for acetone and diacetic acid in the urine are strongly positive before appreciable amounts of hydroxybutyric acid are excreted.

Ketonuria is a guide for further investigation. It is not the amount of ketones excreted that is of most importance, but their accumulation in the tissues and in the blood. It has been shown that mild degrees of ketonuria may persist for months and years without apparent harm.

Qualitative Test for (a) Acetone: (Rothera's Test):* To 5 or 10 cc. of urine add about 1 gm. of ammonium sulfate and two or three drops of fresh concentrated sodium nitroprusside solution and overlay with strong ammonia. A reddish purple ring shows the presence of acetone.

Qualitative Test for (b) Diacetic Acid in the Urine (Gerhardt's Test): To a few cc. of the urine add 10 per cent aqueous solution of ferric chloride, drop by drop, until the phosphates are precipitated; filter and add more of the ferric chloride. If diacetic acid is present, the urine assumes a Bordeaux red color.

The Blood.—*Sugar Content.*—Hyperglycemia is the most decisive sign of diabetes. Without it the diagnosis cannot be made. A concentration of sugar in a specimen of venous blood, taken after an eight- to fourteen-hour fast, in excess of 120 mg. per 100 cc. or a value exceeding 160 mg. after a hearty meal is usually due to diabetes. There is practically no difference in the sugar concentration in venous and arterial (capillary) blood in the postabsorptive (fasting) state. After a meal, however, and in the normal person the arterial blood sugar level (taken for micro method determinations) is from 20 to 50 mg. per 100 cc. higher than that in the venous blood. This difference represents utilization of sugar by the tissues and as might be expected the difference is reduced in untreated diabetes and the normal variation is restored by adequate treatment.

A diagnosis of diabetes should never be made on the basis of a single blood analysis unless the hyperglycemia is accompanied by glycosuria and characteristic symptoms. The most certain criteria are repeatedly elevated fasting blood sugar values and the appearance of glycosuria, especially after meals. It is significant that in the patient with an untreated but mild diabetes glycosuria tends to subside toward morning—at the end of the longest period without food. It is then that the blood sugar level is the lowest in the twenty-four hours.

Sugar is present in the blood of normal persons in concentrations varying (according to Benedict's test[†]) from 70 to 120 mg. per 100 cc. (fasting). There are slight differences in the values according to the method of determination employed, but clinically these differences are insignificant. The blood sugar levels in the average untreated diabetic patient without acute complications range between 200 and 280 mg. per 100 cc.

Patients with a mild diabetes frequently have normal fasting blood sugar values. On no account should this be a basis on which to exclude diabetes. An example in which this error was made is presented:

* Todd and Sanford Laboratory Methods, Seventh Edition, Saunders & Co., Philadelphia, pp. 153 and 154, 1934.

† The macro method of Benedict's test for the determination of the blood sugar value is employed at both the Pennsylvania and Jefferson hospitals. Micro methods in which capillary blood is withdrawn from the finger tip may be desirable, but I have found little need for them and unless the blood is taken by one who is an expert at doing so the results are not as dependable as those of the macro method.

P. B., a male, aged sixty years, was treated in January, 1929, for an acute pharyngitis and heart disease. A trace of sugar was found in the urine on one occasion. A normal fasting blood sugar value served, but falsely, to exclude diabetes. The patient was admitted in June of the same year in diabetic coma with a blood sugar concentration of 1280 mg. per 100 cc. (Folin-Wu method).[24]

The hyperglycemia and glycosuria of diabetes behave in a characteristic manner. Liberal additions to the carbohydrate and total caloric intake tend to increase their severity, while restricted carbohydrate and total food allowances have the opposite effect. The administration of insulin accentuates the reduction of the sugar level in both the blood and the urine.

Hyperglycemia may be present for only short periods, two to four hours after each meal, with normal fasting values in patients having mild diabetes. The likelihood of identifying these mild cases is enhanced by taking the blood specimen for determination of the sugar value two hours after the biggest meal of the day. Values in excess of 160 mg. per 100 cc. and sugar in the twenty-four-hour collection of urine make the diagnosis obvious.

The blood sugar alone is not an accurate index of the severity of the diabetes. An untreated obese patient may have a blood sugar level of 500 mg. or more per 100 cc. and yet the mildness of the diabetes is apparent when the hyperglycemia is promptly corrected by merely restricting the total food intake, in this manner securing a moderate reduction in weight. It is a good rule that "Every untreated overweight diabetic patient has a mild diabetes." In contrast the underweight patient with untreated diabetes has a severe diabetes even though the blood sugar level may not exceed 250 mg. per 100 cc. For the restoration of this patient to health a gain in weight is indicated. This end is achieved by a liberal food intake and insulin therapy. To repeat, the level of the blood sugar is not a reliable index of the severity of the diabetes. The degree of hyperglycemia in the light of the relationship of the patient's weight with that of the normal is a more reliable guide. The fat diabetic patient has a mild diabetes and the lean diabetic patient with a persistent fasting hyperglycemia has a severe diabetes. It is well in most instances to delay giving an opinion on the severity of the diabetes in underweight patients until repeated blood sugar values are known and their response to appropriate treatment is observed.

Other departures from the normal composition of the blood (p. 812) are not of special value in arriving at a diagnosis of diabetes. They are for the most part observed during complications of this disorder and will be dealt with under the respective complications. I refer to alterations in the hemoglobin, urea nitrogen, plasma acetone, CO_2 combining power, plasma or serum chloride and blood volume as seen in ketosis, and abnormal cholesterol and fatty acid values where disturbance of fat metabolism is evident but not necessarily to the degree of ketosis.

Potential diabetes is a term reserved for a small group of patients whose fasting blood sugar level does not exceed 120 mg. per 100 cc., whose glycosuria readily subsides after slight dietary restrictions, and whose blood sugar concentration does not exceed 170 mg. per 100 cc. even after meals.

Special Tests.—Special tests are indicated when there is doubt about the diagnosis of diabetes. They should be reserved for these cases and not carried out promiscuously. Too frequently we see patients with glycosuria and a fasting hyperglycemia needlessly exposed to the inconvenience and expense of these tests. Furthermore if the diagnosis is already clear by the presence of glycosuria and hyperglycemia grave doubts as to the physician's understanding of the subject are created if additional unwarranted and even possibly harmful tests are demanded. The object of these tests should be (a) to identify a latent diabetes at a time when slight restraint in diet will prevent the potential disorder from becoming active and (b) to remove the suspicion that diabetes is present when it does not exist.

An example of these cases so frequently seen, in which special tests are valuable is the individual who is refused life insurance because of a transient glycosuria and yet on the preliminary examination, thus prompted, no glycosuria or hyperglycemia is found. In other words, when the diagnosis of diabetes is considered but cannot be made because under usual conditions the blood and urine are normal, it becomes necessary to observe the ability of the individual to deal with carbohydrate.

Individuals from diabetic families may be contemplating marriage or for other reasons even without evidence of diabetes may want assurance that they do not have diabetes in a latent or potential form. For these persons the special tests are of value.

Patients having glycosuria without hyperglycemia may have the indictment of diabetes waived by such tests. One can recall seeing patients who have been needlessly and ineffectively dieting and even taking insulin when the disturbance actually was an innocent renal glycosuria.

Assuming that the fasting blood sugar value has not exceeded 120 mg. per 100 cc. and that the value obtained on a specimen of blood taken two hours after a meal is not in excess of 160 mg. per 100 cc., it is well to obtain a reading of the blood sugar level two hours after the patient has eaten a meal containing 100 gm. of carbohydrate, there having been no previous restriction in diet.

TABLE 4

TEST MEAL CONTAINING 100 GRAMS CARBOHYDRATE

		P.	F.	C.
Banana	155 grams (1 medium)	1.5		34.1
Shredded wheat	30 grams (1 biscuit)	3.3	0.3	22.5
Milk	240 grams (1 cup)	7.2	9.6	12.0
Bread (white)	60 grams (2 slices)	5.4	0.6	31.8
Butter	10 grams (2 teaspoonsful)		8.5	
Total calories 642		17.4	19.0	100.4

Should this value exceed 160 mg. per 100 cc. it is good evidence of an impaired carbohydrate tolerance and it may be that further tests are necessary to establish the diagnosis. If there is doubt or if the blood sugar value is below 140 mg. per 100 cc. and one wishes to exclude diabetes with certainty, a glucose tolerance test should be done. Greater reliance can be placed on such tests if the patient has received an adequate diet containing 300 gm. of carbohydrate daily for three days before the test is conducted.

The One-hour Two-dose Dextrose Tolerance Test introduced by Exton and Rose,[25] based on principles established by Hamman and Hirschmann (1919), is a valuable aid in the diagnosis of doubtful cases of diabetes. The test is simple to perform; it is completed in one hour and is thus available as an office procedure; the interpretation of the results is readily made, the verdict obtained is correct in nearly all cases, and fewer vein punctures and fewer chemical tests are necessary than when the standard glucose tolerance test is employed. With these advantages this test has gained widespread popularity. It is steadily replacing the so-called standard glucose tolerance test.

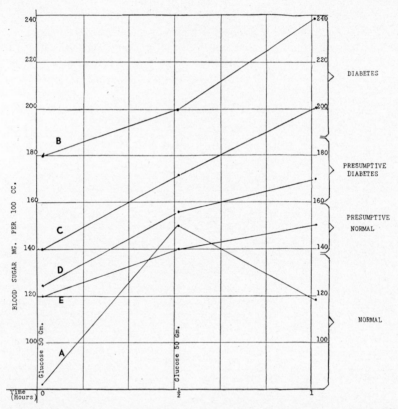

Fig. 139.—Results of the one-hour two-dose glucose tolerance test (Exton-Rose procedure). Note: *A*, the normal curve, the rapid rise and prompt fall of the blood sugar level; *B* and *C*, characteristic of diabetes with the continued increase in the sugar concentration with fasting values above normal. Curve *D* represents presumptive diabetes, and curve *E* presumptive normal; both are nondiagnostic.

In the normal individual one dose of glucose given by mouth will cause a reduction of the blood sugar concentration after a second dose.[26] The explanation of this phenomenon which is generally put forward is that the first dose of dextrose stimulates the pancreas to produce more insulin, in consequence of which, in the normal individual, the blood sugar falls instead of increasing after the second dose. This is also spoken of as the *Staub-Traugott effect*. In the diabetic patient whose pancreas is unable to respond in this normal manner the blood sugar level does not fall after the second dose of glucose. However, Ellis[27] demonstrated a temporarily reduced insulin requirement in diabetic patients by giving hourly doses of glucose and insulin. Soskin[28] and Himsworth believe that this is the result not of increased insulin production but of a progressively increasing sensitivity to insulin. Best and Taylor,[29] however, believe the effect is a direct stimulation of the islets of Langerhans increasing the production of insulin and they present convincing evidence to this effect.

The Exton-Rose Glucose Tolerance Test:

TECHNIC.—

The patient reports before breakfast having had a daily carbohydrate intake of at least 300 gm. for three days preceding the test.

One hundred grams of glucose are dissolved in 650 cc. of water. This is flavored with lemon and divided into two equal parts. The test is conducted after an overnight fast.

1. The bladder is emptied.

2. A sample of venous blood (5 cc.) is taken and immediately thereafter one of the portions of glucose in solution (50 gm. of glucose) is given by mouth.

3. After a thirty-minute interval a second sample of blood is taken, a urine specimen secured and the remaining glucose (50 gm.) solution is given.

4. After another thirty-minute interval specimens of blood and urine are obtained.

The sugar concentration in each specimen of blood and the amount of sugar, if any, in the urine are determined.

INTERPRETATION.—

The results of the test should be interpreted in the light of general clinical observations. For instance, a patient suffering from an acute infection might be labelled a diabetic if cognizance of the effect of infection on the carbohydrate tolerance is not considered. Such a patient should be given the benefit of a second test several weeks after the infection has been corrected. It is important that coexisting conditions, especially infections, disease of the liver and endocrines other than the pancreas, which might modify the results of the test one way or the other be given due consideration.

Various interpretations of this test have been reviewed by Matthews.[30] I have given little heed to what happens to the blood sugar level in the first half hour. The fasting blood sugar values in all of my cases have been normal, the test being used only in the doubtful cases. The important phase of the test is the second half hour and it is largely on the blood sugar value at the end of this period contrasted with the half-hour value that the interpretation is based.

Normal Tolerance Curve

1. The fasting blood sugar level is below 120 mg. per 100 cc.

2. The one-hour level does not exceed 160 mg. per 100 cc.

3. The blood sugar level is lower at the end of one hour than at the end of the first half hour.

Tolerance Curves Indicating Diabetes

1. The fasting blood sugar value may be normal or in excess of 120 mg. per 100 cc.

2. A continued increase of more than 25 mg. in the sugar level during the second half hour.

3. A one-hour blood sugar value in excess of 160 mg. per 100 cc.

This interpretation is almost identical with that of Matthews[30] who, using the normal fasting value of below 120 mg. and 158 mg. at the end of one hour as the critical value, reports that 95 per cent of the normal persons were designated in agreement with the clinical findings and all the patients with diabetes were so designated making for his entire series 98 per cent in agreement with the clinical diagnosis.

This test is an aid in making a diagnosis. It is not nearly so valuable as an indicator of the severity of the diabetes. This is determined with much greater precision by taking into consideration the persistence of a fasting hyperglycemia, the body weight and the response to treatment.

The Standard Glucose Tolerance Test.—The indications and clinical considerations are the same for this as for the preceding test. It is still widely used and gives valuable information but carries the disadvantage of five venipunctures and a time period of three hours to carry out.

TECHNIC.—The patient reports in the morning having had a daily intake of at least 300 gm. of carbohydrate for three days but having had no food since the previous evening.

The bladder is emptied, a sample of venous blood (5 cc.) for sugar determination is taken and 100 gm. of glucose dissolved in 300 cc. of water and flavored with the juice of a lemon are given by mouth.

Specimens of blood and urine for sugar determination are secured one-half hour later, and at one, two and three hours.

In interpreting the results of this test thought has to be given to factors which alter the results. I refer to (*a*) the temporary impairment of the carbohydrate tolerance during the course of acute infections. Staphylococcal infections are especially prone to produce this effect; (*b*) the diet which precedes the test is of importance. A normal person taking liberal amounts of fat and with a small carbohydrate intake[31, 32] or an undernutrition diet with a low carbohydrate allowance prior to the test is likely to give the same response as a patient with mild diabetes. Himsworth[33] states that, "with progressive restriction of dietary carbohydrate there is a progressive impairment of sugar tolerance, which is shown by a corresponding heightening of the blood sugar curve." It is remarkable on the other hand how constant the results of the test are under constant dietary conditions. In fairness to the patient and for precision of diagnosis a low carbohydrate *should be avoided* for at least three days before the tolerance test is made. The daily intake of 300 gm. of carbohydrate for three days preceding the test is now a routine on my service at the Pennsylvania Hospital. It is well to outline the diet to be taken during the three-day preparatory period.

The preparation for a glucose tolerance test by restricting the carbohydrate intake by individuals anxious to obtain life insurance defeats their unworthy purpose. This restriction is likely to give rise to a diabetic type of curve when in fact with a normal carbohydrate intake the curve might be normal. The importance of this aspect of studying the carbohydrate tolerance has been illustrated by Himsworth (Fig. 5, in Chapter II).

The glucose solution occasionally causes nausea. This delays absorption and distorts the character of the curve. The test should be repeated.

If the foregoing pitfalls are avoided diabetes can be excluded with reasonable certainty (1) if the fasting blood sugar level is below 120 mg. per 100 cc., and (2) if the sugar value returns to normal within two hours after the ingestion of 100 gm. of glucose. If these two qualifications are present the actual height reached by the blood sugar concentration is of little moment. The ability of the individual to provide an insulin response sufficient to bring about a rapid fall in the curve is the significant feature.

Contrast these results with the curve obtained when a diabetic patient is given this test. (1) The fasting blood sugar may be normal (70–100 mg. per 100 cc.) or it may exceed this level. (2) The values have exceeded 180 mg. per 100 cc. during the test and have not returned to normal in three hours.

Barring complicating circumstances of a nondiabetic nature which might give such evidence this curve is typical of diabetes, see figure 140.

The curves which fall between the two represented above are difficult of interpretation. If the evidence is not clearly defined the test should be

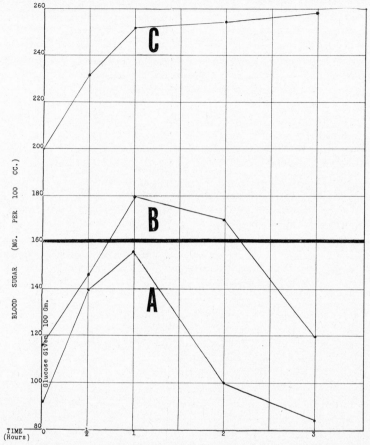

Fig. 140.—Three glucose tolerance curves. *A* depicts the normal glycemic response to the oral administration of 100 gm. of glucose. The rise in the blood sugar level is rapid, but a normal value is restored in two hours. In *B* the glycemic response is slower and normal values are not restored until the third hour as is found in mild diabetes. *C* depicts the fasting hyperglycemia and the continued increase in the blood sugar level even at the third hour as seen in severe diabetes. Glycosuria usually occurs when the blood sugar level is maintained (for several hours) above 160 mg. per 100 cc. as depicted by the heavy black line.

repeated after a lapse of a week or ten days. In instances of doubt it may be wise to study the response of such cases to the one-hour two-dose dextrose tolerance test (Exton-Rose procedure, p. 743).

DIFFERENTIAL DIAGNOSIS

Diabetes may be confused with other disorders which cause glycosuria and hyperglycemia. The wrong diagnosis incurs wrong treatment. The life of an unconscious patient who has glycosuria and a hyperglycemia as the result of an intracranial hemorrhage may be jeopardized if careful investigation fails to reveal the real illness. Should the condition be mistaken for diabetic ketosis and large amounts of insulin be given, the danger is obvious. This occurs too frequently.

Glycosuria.—The presence in the urine of substances which reduce copper in solution to cuprous oxide may be mistaken for glucose. These are pentose, lactose, levulose, maltose, and rarely galactose, conjugate glycuronates, homogentisic acid, vitamin C, and creatinine. The recognition of these various factors are dealt with in detail in Chapter XV. Glucose appearing in the urine of a nondiabetic patient is apt to be especially misleading. It occurs in *renal glycosuria* and following *intracranial injuries*.

Renal Glycosuria.—Glucose appearing in the urine in the presence of a normal blood sugar concentration is known as renal glycosuria, referred to also as "benign glycosuria" and "diabetes innocens." Renal glycosuria is a symptomless and innocent condition requiring no treatment. It has to do with alterations in the renal threshold for glucose and represents a reduction in the ability of the renal tubules to reabsorb sugar which has passed through the glomeruli. The blood sugar level above which glycosuria occurs is the so-called *renal threshold* for glucose. If the blood sugar level in a normal individual is increased artificially glycosuria occurs between 150 and 180 mg. per 100 cc. In long-standing diabetes the renal threshold is often higher, even as high as 250 mg. per 100 cc. On the other hand in renal glycosuria glucose appears in the urine without any elevation of the blood sugar above the normal concentration (70 to 100 mg. per 100 cc.). This innocent disorder occurs in two forms. The one in which there is a constant loss of glucose in the urine, the quantity of which is not altered by changes in the diet and only with great difficulty by giving insulin, and the other in which there is a temporary lowering of the renal threshold as observed during pregnancy, hyperthyroidism, and nephrosis, and in disease of the hypophysis. Renal glycosuria is not a forerunner of diabetes. Experimentally this condition is produced by giving phloridzin to animals.

Importance is attached to renal glycosuria because of the danger of mistaking it for diabetes. The safety of the patient lies in the correct diagnosis. The combination—diabetes and a low renal threshold for glucose—occurs occasionally, as in case M. K. (p. 870).

Renal glycosuria is probable if, when the diet is restricted, or when insulin is given there is no decline in the amount of glycosuria. Furthermore, from day to day there is little change in the amount of glycosuria. These inconclusive observations are suggestive but it is only by parallel examinations of the blood sugar level and the urine that the condition is clearly demonstrated.

A simple method of identifying a renal glycosuria is as follows: The patient's bladder is emptied and urine discarded; a sample of venous blood is taken; in thirty minutes a specimen of urine is obtained and at the end of another thirty minutes blood is again obtained. If both blood sugar values are normal (70 to 100 mg. per 100 cc.) and if there is a considerable amount of sugar in the urine collected at the midway period, the diagnosis of a low renal threshold is confirmed. One may carry the test further by securing a second urine specimen and a third blood sugar value as illustrated in table 5.

TABLE 5

The Relationship of the Blood Sugar Level and the Sugar in the Urine in a Case of Renal Glycosuria

1 P.M.	1:30 P.M.	2 P.M.	2:30 P.M.	3 P.M.
Blood Sugar	Urine Sugar	Blood Sugar	Urine Sugar	Blood Sugar
Per cent	Per cent	Per cent	Per cent	Per cent
0.100	1.5	0.108	1.4	0.098

The glucose tolerance tests are normal in the nondiabetic patient having renal glycosuria. Occasionally we see the tragic error of a mistaken diagnosis in these patients, resulting in needless dieting, anxiety, and frustration of efforts to rid the urine of sugar by giving insulin.

Pregnancy and the Renal Threshold.—In 10 to 15 per cent of normal pregnant women there is a lowering of the renal threshold for sugar, allowing glucose, not lactose as is generally supposed, to escape in the urine. Lactosuria is common during lactation but does not occur during gestation. Lactosuria and glycosuria may be observed simultaneously in the same patient. The renal threshold for glucose returns to normal after the lactation period has ended.

Hyperthyroidism.—In hyperthyroidism it is not unusual to find a lowering of the renal threshold for glucose. The problem is not as simple, however, as that which occurs during pregnancy. These patients are apt to have a hyperglycemia, and diabetes occurring in the same patient as hyperthyroidism is not uncommon. What appears to be a transitory diabetes may be observed. The tolerance for carbohydrate in these patients frequently is restored to normal by appropriate treatment of the hyperthyroidism. Unfortunately this is not always the case.

Nephrosis.—The renal threshold for glucose is lowered in nephrosis. It is assumed that degenerative changes in the tubular epithelium impair the absorption of glucose from the glomerular filtrate.

Alimentary Glycosuria.—Alimentary glycosuria is believed by some to represent a decreased threshold for sugar but that the threshold is sufficiently high to prevent continuous glycosuria, and that it occurs after extra "loads" of carbohydrate. This interpretation should be accepted with reserve and a careful study of the individual's carbohydrate tolerance should be made in each instance. So-called "alimentary glycosuria" may be due to a reduced renal threshold for sugar or to an increased permeability of the intestinal mucosa for sugar. Both causes are innocent. It should be suspected, however, until proven otherwise, that glycosuria, no matter what the ultimate cause proves to be, is due to impaired removal of sugar from the blood as seen in diabetes and rarely in extensive disease of the liver.

Diseases of the Hypophysis.—Hyperglycemia and glycosuria indistinguishable from that occurring in uncomplicated diabetes are common in *acromegaly*. The excessive elaboration of the growth hormone of the acidophilic cells of the anterior lobe of the pituitary gland in the adult is responsible for this disease. It is readily recognized by the overgrowth of the bones of the hands, feet, and face. The mandible protrudes and the teeth become separated from each other. The nasal bones and supraorbital ridges are involved in this excessive growth. Thickening of the skin with hirsutism is the rule and enlargement of the viscera—heart, liver, spleen, thymus, and tongue—occurs and there is increased secretion (hypertrophic or adenomatous changes) of the thyroid, parathyroid and adrenal glands.

The diabetes which occurs as the result of changes in the hypophysis in the acromegalic patient doubtless had its origin in the excessive activity of the pituitary gland. The fact that irreparable changes take place in the pancreas as a result of these changes has been conclusively shown by Young.[34]

The important consideration is that acromegalic patients who have hyperglycemia and glycosuria have two disorders, acromegaly and diabetes, and should be treated accordingly.

Pituitary basophilism (Cushing's disease) due to tumor growth of the basophilic cells of the anterior lobe of the pituitary gland also causes hyperglycemia and glycosuria. Here also at least two disorders—basophilism and diabetes—coexist. The diabetes is doubtless due indirectly to the changes in the hypophysis and should be reviewed in this light when a patient presents the characteristics of basophilism, *i.e.*, sudden onset of obesity involving the trunk, purplish cutaneous striae, the tense, tender, and pigmentated skin, demineralization of bones, arterial hypertension, suppression of sexual function, hyperglycemia, and glycosuria.

Pituitrin may account for a transitory glycosuria and hyperglycemia when administered subcutaneously.

Disease of the Adrenal Glands.—Hyperglycemia and glycosuria may occur as the result of a *tumor of the adrenal cortex*.[35] The diabetes is genuine, though it may be ameliorated by removal of the tumor. The clinical signs of tumor of the cortex of the adrenal gland are indistinguishable clinically from those of basophilism presented above.

The subcutaneous, intramuscular, or intravenous injection of epinephrine, an extract of the adrenal medulla, provokes hyperglycemia and may cause glycosuria. This is a transitory effect lasting only a matter of minutes. It neither causes nor predisposes to diabetes. The hyperglycemic response is due to a liberation of glucose from the liver. The same mechanism, under control of the sympathetic nervous system, operates in fear and anger and permits unusual effort to resist threatened danger.

Intracranial Injury.—Clinically glycosuria and hyperglycemia are common after intracranial trauma. This may result from violent accidents in which the base of the brain is injured and in event of intracranial hemorrhage as a result of injury or disease of the vascular system, or from injury caused by intracranial tumors and acute infectious processes. Of these, glycosuria and hyperglycemia have occurred in my experience most frequently following hemorrhage into the subarachnoid area.

It is understood that glycosuria of this type is in no way related to diabetes. It should be equally clear, however, that a patient having diabetes may suffer an intracranial injury and so glycosuria should not be dismissed lightly. I recall one patient, a young girl who was taken to a hospital in an unconscious condition with lacerations of the scalp sustained in an automobile accident. The glycosuria found was not considered unusual in this type of injury but fortunately a "diabetic identification card" with information regarding her diet and insulin was found on the patient. She required 75 units of insulin daily and hence the real danger of any delay in recognizing the diabetes in a young adult who had had diabetes since childhood is obvious.

The glycosuria and hyperglycemia occurring as a result of intracranial injury are attributable to injury in the pons, the floor of the fourth ventricle, and the hypothalamic area. Stimulation of the thoracic autonomic center and the parasympathetic system ensues and it is believed that such disturbances of centers or pathways carrying glycogenolytic impulses to the liver, or injury involving nerve communications with the adrenals, pancreas, or hypophysis may be held accountable for the hyperglycemia and glycosuria that follow.

PROGNOSIS

The prognosis is excellent for the intelligent and cooperative patient if the diabetes is identified early and treated diligently by a physician who has interest and training in this field of metabolism. The gain in duration of life has risen steadily with each succeeding advance in treatment.

Basing his statement on computations by the Statistical Department of the Metropolitan Life Insurance Company, Joslin[36] concludes, "At ten years of age the normal child has an expectancy of fifty-seven years, but the diabetic child has an expectancy of forty-seven years, in contrast to a scant two years a half generation ago."

The normal expectancy of life at sixty-five is twelve years but the expectancy for the corresponding diabetic patient is eight years. Forty per cent of Joslin's "physician diabetics" died of coma in the Naunyn era, 5.6 per cent in the Allen era, but of the physicians having diabetes there have been no deaths from coma since 1936.

The prognosis becomes progressively less favorable if the diabetes is not identified early, if the patient is unintelligent or uncooperative or both, if incurable complications are already present, and if the patient is deprived of good medical advice and treatment. Carelessness on the part of the patient and a laxity about the control of the diabetes shorten the lives of many patients. If a physician fails to do his part he must bear his part of the responsibility for a tragic outcome.

The standards set by various authors concerning the control of the diabetes vary from very rigid rules and strict measures to those representing very little in the way of treatment. The standards believed by the author to enhance a favorable prognosis are outlined in the section on Treatment.

PREVENTION

In view of the increasing incidence of diabetes, the prevention of this disease should concern everyone. The problem is especially vital to members of families in which diabetes is prevalent. It has to do with the side tracking of a hereditary predisposition of an organ of biological inferiority. *Diabetic patients should not intermarry.* As surely as they do, their offspring, if they live long enough, will develop diabetes. The observations of Pincus and White[37] leave no doubt about this. A diabetic patient may, without fear of such a catastrophe, marry into a family whose record is clear of diabetes. The mendelian recessive character of diabetes provides this guarantee. Looking further into the future, the children of this marriage should also marry into nondiabetic families. Wilder[38] suggests that members of diabetic families limit their families to one or two children. The advice presented will not always be heeded, but it is our duty as physicans to acquaint our diabetic patients with the hereditary nature of this disease.

Members of diabetic families are predisposed to diabetes by heredity and there can be no doubt that the appearance of this disorder will often be prevented if other precipitating factors are not added to the hereditary diathesis. I refer especially to obesity and to infections. The correction and prevention of obesity are the greatest practical means available for the prevention of diabetes. Every member of every diabetic family should be made aware of this. This is a form of public welfare that is grossly neglected.

Overeating should be avoided. Increasing weight should be checked by curtailing the diet, especially the fats. A mere restriction of the foods high in caloric value which may suffice—notably fat meat, butter, cream, cheese, salad oil, mayonnaise, salad dressing, ice cream and confectionery. The ultimate effect which can be accomplished by observing, inviolate, these simple restrictions is remarkable. The treatment of obesity, dealt with in Chapter X should be applied when necessary.

Physical exercise is an important preventive measure. It inhibits the development of obesity and it develops muscles which are carbohydrate-consuming; at the same time muscular exercise is an "insulin-sparer." Accumulations of fatty tissue, on the other hand, increase the total metabolism in quite a different way and in one that increases the need for insulin. Observe the diabetic patient who institutes and maintains a program of active daily exercise. His insulin requirement decreases. Observe the sedentary diabetic patient who gains considerably in weight. His need for insulin increases.

The importance of keeping the body weight at or a trifle below the normal standard (see Appendix) after the age of thirty-seven years cannot be overemphasized. Regulation of body weight in this manner and the limitation of the size of diabetic families are the most practical means of preventing diabetes.

It has been suggested that diabetic patients be sterilized, or that members of diabetic families remain childless via contraceptive means, as measures to stamp out the disease. This would not solve the problem unless extended to include those relatives of diabetic patients who pass on the hereditary predisposition. If it were possible to identify such persons (which it is not) we should realize, as Joslin has estimated, that the relatives of the 2,500,0000 people in the United States (who, it is believed, have or will have diabetes) number approximately 32,500,000 or, one in four of the entire population.

The part played by *infection* in the etiology of diabetes is under dispute. It is generally agreed, however, that chronic infections of the gallbladder, because of proximity and connection *via* biliary and pancreatic ducts and lymphatics to the pancreas, predispose to diabetes and that its correction is an important prophylactic action. When medical treatment fails surgical measures should be considered.

The prevention of infections by isolation and immunization, and the correction of infections and hyperthyroidism by medical or surgical means.

in any case, are advisable even though it is not known how effective these measures will be in preventing diabetes.

I seriously doubt if a change of climate has any value in preventing diabetes. The adoption of more physical exercise in the new environment is probably responsible for the advantages usually attributed to the climate. For example, patients from the northern United States and Canada who go south in the winter require less insulin while in the south. This improvement has been attributed to changes in temperature, a special variety of grapefruit, or a change of water. Compare the physical exercise of a comparatively "shut-in" patient in Canada during the winter season with that of the patient in Florida, where swimming, tennis, golf, and other sports are the order of the day. Exercise tends to reduce the weight of the body and to improve the total food tolerance, hence, commercial exploitation notwithstanding, a program of exercise dutifully carried out in the north will give the advantages of the south so far as the diabetes is concerned.

The well-informed diabetic patient has ample opportunity to do missionary work among his relatives and obese friends by influencing them to adopt the following precautionary *plan:*

(1) A careful examination for the primary purpose of excluding diabetes. This will include a *postcibal* blood analysis for sugar, as well as an analysis of the urine.

(2) An annual examination in order that any deviation from normal may be recognized and treated in its incipiency.

(3) Correction of obesity and avoid becoming overweight, particularly after thirty-five years of age.

(4) Attention to the advantages that are to be derived from at least one-half hour of active outdoor exercise each day.

Diabetes occasionally makes its appearance in the child before it develops in the parent who has transmitted the predisposition to the disease. Parents of a diabetic child should adopt the same preventive measures as descendants of a diabetic family.

Education of diabetic patients and their families along the lines outlined in this section, though sadly neglected, holds great promise in the satisfactory control of diabetes of posterity.

TREATMENT

Appropriate treatment promises life to the diabetic child; it rescues the adult from the prospect of irreparable organic changes and creates a justified hope for a life of usefulness and service where the abyss of despair once prevailed. The object of the treatment should be to restore and maintain physiological blood sugar and cholesterol values, to correct and prevent glycosuria and acetonuria, to secure normal nutrition, and by virtue of these accomplishments, to restore the patient to a normal sense of well being with courage, ambition and ability to carry on a useful existence. Diabetes should be considered an incurable disease and in consequence treatment is life-long.

Failure to secure treatment, no matter what the reason, be it through ignorance or neglect, promotes the development of incurable distressing complications and premature death.

The measures used in the treatment of uncomplicated diabetes are (a) special diet, (b) insulin, (c) exercise, (d) general care, (e) training of the patient, (f) miscellaneous measures.

It is desirable to have the patient spend the initial period of a few days to a fortnight in a hospital. Acquaintance with the characteristics of the individual patient is thus made possible. Furthermore treatment under controlled conditions inspires in the patient a proper respect for the disease with which he is afflicted. A short course of training in the preparation of the diet, the administration of insulin, testing the urine for sugar, and in special hygiene for the diabetic patient, *vide infra*, under suitable conditions and given by a nurse and dietitian is also permitted.

The initial treatment or so-called "standardization" conducted at the physician's office is time-consuming and is often doomed to failure. In the unusual instance, however, and where a properly trained office personnel is available the efforts may be rewarded with success. I know of nothing, however, that has such a lasting impression on these patients as the hospital routine and training, and I know of no patient who regretted having had this experience.

DIET

Every diabetic patient relies to some extent on restrictions in the diet for the uniform success of treatment. Flexibility of the diet to meet the individual needs is essential. It will be found that diabetic patients require neither more nor less food than the nondiabetic subject to execute the same work, providing the diabetes is under control.

TABLE 6

RELATIVE PROPORTIONS OF PROTEIN, FAT AND CARBOHYDRATE AND THE TOTAL CALORIES IN A, THE NORMAL DIET, AND B, THE DIET FOR PATIENTS WITH UNCOMPLICATED DIABETES

Food	*A* Quantity (gm.)	Total Calories
Carbohydrate	250–400	1000–1600
Protein	60–120	280– 480
Fat	60–120	540–1080
		1820–3160

	B	
Carbohydrate	120–250	480–1000
Protein	60–110	240– 440
Fat	60–100	540– 900
		1260–2340

In prescribing the diet cognizance is taken of the respective importance of protein, fat, and carbohydrate, and of the total caloric value of the diet. In view of the importance which attaches to carbohydrate in the treatment of this disease we must not lose sight of the possible sources of sugar in the diet. Approximately 58 per cent of the protein, 10 per cent of the fat, and 100 per cent of the carbohydrate are available as sugar. (Glucose equivalent of diet = .58 Protein + .10 Fat + Carbohydrate.) Regarding the effects of the respective foods in diabetes Allen's words remain valid, "The food which tends most strongly to produce glycosuria is carbohydrate. Protein comes second and its glycosuric action in average cases is not equal to its theoretical glucose value. Fat seems to be important chiefly through the calories furnished by it, rather than as a theoretical direct source of glucose. *The most important factor governing the insulin requirement with the ordinary diet is not the carbohydrate content, but the total caloric content."* Diets which will result in the reduction in weight of obese patients are still essential but we can rejoice that starvation programs and "fast days" as methods of treatment are no longer necessary. It must not be assumed that the caloric needs of an individual can be predicted in advance. A certain amount of juggling with diet values is necessary for most patients and even then the best that can be said is that the diet closely approximates the individual's needs and that changes in his or her needs are subject to many influences.

Vitamin Content.—Diabetic patients require as high vitamin intake as do normal persons, if not a higher. The reader is referred to the Chapter VIII on Vitamins for consideration of this vitally important feature of all diets. Fortunately foods which are rich in vitamin content may be selected for the diabetic patient.

Protein Content.—*One gram of protein per kilogram of the standard, not the actual body weight** satisfies the protein requirement of the active adult and maintains nitrogen equilibrium. Protein allowances as low as $\frac{2}{3}$ gm. per Kg. are permissible but not desirable unless protein restriction is indicated by some complicating disorder such as nephritis with nitrogen retention in the blood. Increases to 1.25 gm. per Kg. may be allowed. Children require a higher quota of protein. Diets for diabetic children are dealt with in the section on Diabetes in Childhood and Adolescence.

Carbohydrate Content.—The carbohydrate quota is varied with the severity of the diabetes. The patient who has mild diabetes and does not need insulin is allowed less carbohydrate than the patient who has a more severe diabetes and who requires insulin.

The initial dose—if it is probable that insulin will not be needed—may contain 100 to 120 gm. of carbohydrate. With control of the diabetes small additions are made from time to time until the total carbohydrate for each day reaches 150 and preferably 200 gm. if this amount can be tolerated without *postcibal* glycosuria or hyperglycemia. Greater restriction of the carbohydrate than that necessary to prevent glycosuria and hyperglycemia appears to be unwise. The tolerance for carbohydrate is actually reduced by unnecessary reduction of the intake of carbohydrate.

The initial carbohydrate allowance is greater for the child or for the undernourished adult diabetic patient who obviously needs insulin from the outset. One hundred and twenty-five to 150 gm. of carbohydrate are allowed at once and after the diabetes is controlled the amount is gradually increased over a period of weeks or months until the so-called permanent diet contains between 200 and 250 gm. Such liberal quotas are made possible by insulin. It must be borne in mind that considerable increases in the carbohydrate intake may be made with but relatively little effect on the insulin requirement, providing the total caloric value of the diet is not increased.

Total Calories.—I consider the total caloric value of the diet to be one of the most important considerations when dealing with the dietary needs

* Standard weights according to age and sex are presented in the Appendix.

of the diabetic patient. Restrictions of or additions to the total caloric value of the diet have a far-reaching effect which must be understood if the patient is to derive the most benefit (see tables 7 and 8).

Starvation and "fast days" are no longer necessary in the treatment of diabetes. Reducing diets are of great importance, however. Approximately 75 per cent of adult diabetic patients are overweight and it cannot be emphasized too strongly that the most powerful means of improving their carbohydrate tolerance is by a reduction in body weight. All authorities on diabetes are agreed that the obese diabetic patient should be reduced and yet it is incomprehensible why this efficient means of controlling the disease and avoiding the use of insulin is so often entirely neglected. The untreated obese diabetic patient has a mild diabetes and, barring complications, control of the diabetes can be maintained readily by reducing the total caloric intake sufficiently to accomplish a slow reduction in weight.

Eighteen calories per kilogram of the standard body weight are allowed for the *overweight diabetic patient*. A reduction in weight will ensue. Adjustments may be made if the reduction is too rapid or too slow, keeping in mind that patients may be losing flesh but retaining water sufficient to prevent any appreciable change in the actual weight for a period of several days.

The rate of the reduction of body weight may be slowed up to a pound or two per month as soon as the diabetes is controlled. Suitable increases in the total caloric allowance of the diet are made to secure this end and when the body weight reaches the standard level,* which may require several months, further increases are made to prevent little if any further decrease in weight. The return to overweight, of course, would restore the hazards which accompany it. Patients are warned of this.

Diets of a low caloric value are employed to reduce weight and to secure the benefits that follow but care should be taken that they do not harm. It is especially important that the intake of certain vital food factors should not be reduced beyond the minimal requirements. The daily diet for the average male adult should contain calcium, 0.8 gm.; phosphorus, 1.3 gm.; iron, 12 mg.; Vitamin A, a minimum of 5000 International Units; thiamine, 1.8 mg. (1 mg. thiamine equals 333 International Units); ascorbic acid, 75 mg. (1 mg. ascorbic acid equals 20 International Units); riboflavin, 2.7 mg.; nicotinic acid, 18 mg. and Vitamin D when not available from sunshine should be provided up to the minimal amounts recommended for infants.

The mineral and vitamin requirements according to the age and sex, physical activity and during pregnancy and lactation, as recommended by the Committee on Food and Nutrition, National Research Council, are tabulated on page 492. These food requisites are emphasized at this point because it is when diets aimed at reducing body weight are employed that they are most likely to be neglected. All diets should be supervised in these respects. The caloric values may be adequate but other essential food factors may be lacking.

The diabetic patient whose weight is about at the *standard level* is allowed a more liberal diet even in the early days of treatment. Twenty-five

* See Appendix.

calories per kilogram of body weight are given until the diabetes is controlled. Thereafter gradual additions are made to the total calories, in fat or carbohydrate or both, to prevent a loss in weight. In fact the restoration of the few pounds lost in the initial weeks of treatment may be warranted. Insulin may be necessary in addition to the dietetic measures to control the diabetes.

The initial diet for the *undernourished adult diabetic patient* approximates 35 calories per kilogram of the standard weight. As the weight increases to about 5 or 10 pounds (2 to 4 Kg.) below the standard, weight decreases in the total calories, sufficient to prevent further gain, should be made. The behavior of the weight level from month to month will dictate further changes in the caloric value of the diet. The ultimate aim for adult diabetic patients is to keep the body weight a trifle, 5 to 10 pounds, below the standard weight. On no account is overweight to be fostered.

Fat Content.—The fat quota is automatically accounted for when the protein, carbohydrate and total calories already are decided upon. The fat merely makes up the balance of calories not provided for by the protein and carbohydrate. With the knowledge that, for practical purposes, each gram of protein provides 4 calories, each gram of carbohydrate 4 calories and each gram of fat 9 calories, this calculation is quite simple.

Special attention to the restriction of the fat is given to patients with hyperlipemia and hypercholesterolemia and xanthoma diabeticorum. These will be considered under complications.

Distribution of Meals.—The division of the diet is adjusted to the individual patient's needs: (*a*) For the patient having a mild diabetes and not requiring insulin the diet is divided into three equal meals. (*b*) For the patient taking a single dose of protamine zinc insulin, one-fifth of the carbohydrate is given for breakfast, two-fifths for lunch and two-fifths for the evening meal with a small portion of the evening meal (10 to 20 gm. of carbohydrate) held over and taken on retiring. (*c*) For the patient taking a dose each of crystalline and protamine zinc insulin before breakfast, with or without a dose of crystalline insulin before the evening meal the diet is divided into three equal meals, but a part of the noon meal, usually the fruit, is taken at 11 A.M. and a part of the evening meal is held over and taken at bedtime. This practice reduces the peak loads at meal times, more evenly distributes the intake of carbohydrate and aids in preventing hypoglycemic reactions. Patients taking a daily dose of globin or histone zinc insulin have done best in my experience when the insulin was given at least one hour before breakfast and the diet was divided as follows: one-fifth for breakfast, two-fifths for the noon meal and two-fifths for the evening meal, with part of the evening meal, usually a banana, taken at 3 P.M.

The foregoing outline, intended to aid in the prescribing of the diet for the uncomplicated diabetic patient, is offered as a basis upon which further treatment is planned. It permits flexibility. This is essential as each patient must have individual consideration if the best results are to be secured. Furthermore readjustments of the diet may be indicated occasionally to meet new conditions.

The following diets are illustrative of the observation diets employed at the Pennsylvania and Jefferson Hospitals:

(*A*) Obese diabetic patient,* female, aged 45 years, height 5′3″ (157 cm.), weight 200 pounds (91 Kg.). Standard weight 63 Kg.

Diet:† Protein   65 gm.   (Approximately 1 gm. per Kg. of standard weight)

Carbohydrate   110 gm.
Fat   48 gm.
Total calories   1134   (18 calories per Kg. of standard weight)

(*B*' Diabetic patient,‡ male, aged 39 years, height 5′10″ (177 cm.), weight 167 pounds (76 Kg.). Standard weight 76 Kg.

Diet: Protein   75 gm.   (A trifle less than 1 gm. per Kg.)

Carbohydrate   150 gm.
Fat   111 gm.
Total calories   1900   (Approximately 25 per Kg.)

(*C*) Undernourished adult diabetic female,§ aged 21 years, height 5′6″ (165 cm.), weight 105 pounds (48 Kg.). Standard weight 133 pounds (60 Kg.)

Diet: Protein   60 gm.   (1 gm. per Kg. standard weight)
Carbohydrate   180 gm.
Fat   151 gm.
Total calories   2100   (35 calories per Kg. of standard weight)

The foregoing plan of the dietetic treatment of diabetes adheres in principle to that advised by Allen and Joslin, though the average allowance of carbohydrate is somewhat higher than that allowed by Joslin. The carbohydrate content is neither very low nor is it extremely high. The same is true of the fat, though by restricting the fat the advantages of a reduced caloric intake for the overweight diabetic patients are secured. Accuracy in planning the diet is considered of utmost importance. The trend is toward a more liberal allowance of carbohydrate with a restriction in the total caloric content of the diet.

Diets employed by Wilder[39] in the routine treatment of diabetes contain more fat and considerably less carbohydrate than those employed by us. The amounts of carbohydrate advised by Wilder vary from 121 to 167 gm., the protein from 57 to 84 gm. and sufficient fat to supply the remaining calories.

Other Diets.—It is proper and desirable that different diets should be tried in the treatment of diabetes by the various authorities. It is only in this way that the best general plan of diet will be obtained. There is danger, however, that one authority may become so interested in the good features of one form of treatment, especially if his name becomes attached to it, that the advantages of others may be overlooked. An open mind on this subject is essential. The diets which have already been discussed are those with which I am most familiar, but excellent clinical results are reported by the exponents of the various extremes of diet recorded below.

The *high carbohydrate diet liberal in calories* has been employed and

* Does not require insulin.
† Diet No. 2, page 762.
‡ May or may not require insulin.
§ Requires insulin from the beginning of treatment.

advocated by Sansum and his co-workers,[40] Geyelin,[41] and Porges and Adlersberg.[42] An illustrative diet prescription is as follows: protein, 70 gm.; carbohydrate, 425 gm.; fat, 125 gm.—(3000 calories).

TABLE 7

TYPICAL RESPONSE OF THE BLOOD SUGAR LEVEL AND GLYCOSURIA IN THE OBESE DIABETIC PATIENT, TO THE RESTRICTION OF THE TOTAL CALORIC CONTENT OF THE DIET WITHOUT THE AID OF INSULIN

A. Fe., Female, White, Aged 51, Height 61 Inches, Ideal Weight 135 Lbs., 39% Overweight

Date	Weight, Lbs.	Diet P.	Diet C.	Diet Calories	Glycosuria	Blood Sugar, mg. per 100 cc.
July 7, 1933	188	70	80	1100	2.1%	250
July 21	184	70	80	1100	0	177
July 28	181½	70	80	1100	0	144
August 11	179	70	80	1100	0	122
October 20	170	70	95	1300	0	115
January 26, 1934	167¼	70	85	1200	0	110
August 24	153	70	95	1300	v. ft. trace	113
March 8, 1935	148	70	105	1400	0	113
July 12	147	70	115	1600	0	110
October 9, 1936	157½	70	115	1600	0	110
December 10	156	70	140	1600	0	120
June 25, 1937	165	75	160	1800	0	113
August 13	161	75	160	1800	0	109

Summary. With a loss of weight of 9 pounds, the blood sugar level fell from 0.250% to normal. Subsequently, the carbohydrate tolerance was much improved. Even with an increase in weight of 14 pounds from the lowest level, the blood sugar remained normal.

High carbohydrate, low fat, and restricted calorie diets are advocated by Rabinowitch.[43] It has not been proved that the benefits secured by this dietetic regimen are due to the high carbohydrate allowance and not to the accompanying restriction in the total calories. The benefits to be gained by judicious restriction of the total calories are legion, as shown by Allen as early as 1914. Rabinowitch believes that tuberculosis and ketosis develop

TABLE 8

EFFECT OF RESTRICTED CALORIC INTAKE AND THE REDUCTION IN BODY WEIGHT ON THE BLOOD SUGAR CONCENTRATION AND ON THE GLYCOSURIA

D. d'G., Female, White, Aged 46, Height 59¼ Inches, Ideal Weight 126 Lbs., 49% Overweight

Date	Weight, Lbs.	Diet P.	Diet C.	Diet Calories	Glycosuria	Blood Sugar, mg. per 100 cc.
March 25, 1932	186	70	80	1100	1.3%	238
April 1	178½	70	80	1100	0	152
April 15	174	70	80	1100	0	130
April 29	173½	70	80	1100	v. ft. trace	99
May 13	167	70	80	1300	0	88
July 8	155¼	70	80	1300	0	93
December 16	153½	70	120	1700	0	77
April 7, 1933	151	70	150	1700	0	76

less frequently when patients are on his regimen and that the development of arteriosclerosis in the diabetic patient is impeded. Certainly the blood lipids which seem to play an important part in this respect are readily reduced to and maintained at a normal level on this dietetic program.

An illustrative diet prescription of the Rabinowitch plan of diet is: protein, 70 gm.; carbohydrate, 400 gm.; and fat, 50 gm.—(2330 calories).

Free diets, or food with practically no restriction have been used by Stolte.[44] He and other pediatricians report good results when the diet values are practically ignored and complete dependence is placed on substitution therapy, insulin. The important question is, What is the eventual outcome? Do these patients pay a penalty long after they are lost sight of by the pediatrician? I am convinced that this "free diet" plan carries many potential dangers and advise against its use.

Menu-making.—Accuracy is encouraged if all diabetic patients weigh their diets. This exacting detail need not be continued by all after a knowledge of approximate amounts of food is obtained. The overweight patient with very mild diabetes may need only moderate restriction of sweets and foods containing large amounts of fat. I refer to butter, cream, cheese, salad oil, fat meat, ice cream, sugar, syrups, and confectionery. Standard household measuring utensils and standard helpings (teaspoon, tablespoon, ounce measure, cup, slice of bread, shredded wheat biscuit, crackers, strips of bacon, egg, etc.) are sufficiently accurate for all but the patients with severe diabetes. This is a liberty formerly enjoyed only by patients not taking insulin but now made possible for most of the "insulin patients" also by the slowly acting protamine zinc insulin, the use of which permits greater leeway with the diet than was formerly advisable.

Adequate control of the more severe diabetes as seen in the child and the undernourished adult is much more likely to be maintained if the diet is weighed.

TABLE 9

CHIEF SOURCES OF PROTEIN, FAT AND CARBOHYDRATE IN THE DIETS OF DIABETIC PATIENTS

Protein	Fat	Carbohydrate
Meat (lean)	Butter	Fruits
Fish	Cream	Vegetables
Eggs	Cheese	Cereals
Milk	Meat (fat)	Breads
Cottage cheese	Salad oil	
Peas, soy beans	Lard	
Nuts	Nuts	
Gluten, gelatin	Egg yolks	
	Cheese (cream)	

Syrups, jams, molasses, candies, sugar, etc. are carbohydrate foods but are so concentrated and high in carbohydrate value that they have no place in the diet for these patients.

Diets are prescribed in grams, the menu specifies the number of grams of each food allowed and gram scales are used to weigh the specified amounts. The Hanson and the Chatillon scales* are well adapted for this purpose. Each has a revolving dial which allows the pointer to be placed at zero when the empty container is placed on the pan. The food may then be weighed off directly without any subsequent calculation for the weight of the container.

The selection of the suitable foods to fill the respective amounts of protein, fat and carbohydrate quotas prescribed may be aided by consulting table 10, in which are outlined the important sources of these food components.

* These scales can be obtained from Hanson Brothers Scale Company, 525 N. Ada Street, Chicago, Illinois, and John Chatillon and Sons, New York City, respectively.

The filling of the diet prescription is much simpler than it at first appears. Nevertheless it is remarkable how frequently medical students and physicians, otherwise well versed in the management of diabetes, have difficulty in interpreting the diet prescription into the correct quantities of suitable foods. A little practice in making out menus from the diet prescription convinces one of its simplicity. The calculation of a sample menu for one meal is presented. Assuming that a diet of 75 gm. protein, 75 gm. fat and 150 gm. carbohydrate (1575 calories) is prescribed, and that the

TABLE 10

APPROXIMATE COMPOSITION OF FOODS FOR DIABETIC PATIENTS

Food	Wt., Gm.	Approx. Meas.	P.	F.	C.	Cal.
Cereal:						
Cooked...................	120	½ c.	3	..	16	76
Dry.....................	20	½ c.	3	..	16	76
Shredd. wheat...............	28	1 biscuit	3	..	21	96
Bread......................	30	1 slice	3	..	16	76
Bread......................	20	1 thin slice	2	..	11	52
Crackers, soda..............	6	2 biscuits (2" x 2")	1	1	4	29
Milk, whole................	240	1 c.	7	10	12	166
Milk, skimmed..............	240	1 c.	7	..	12	76
20% cream.................	120	½ c.	4	24	4	248
40% cream.................	120	½ c.	2	48	2	448
3% vegetable...............	100	½ c. 1 serving	2	..	3	20
6% vegetable...............	100	½ c. 1 serving	2	..	6	32
9% vegetable...............	100	½ c. 1 serving	3	..	9	48
12% vegetable..............	100	½ c. 1 serving	4	..	12	64
15% vegetable..............	100	½ c. 1 serving	4	..	15	76
18% vegetable..............	100	½ c. 1 serving	5	1	18	101
3% fruit...................	100	½ c. 1 serving	..	..	3	12
6% fruit...................	100	½ c. 1 serving	..	..	6	24
9% fruit...................	100	½ c. 1 serving	..	..	9	36
12% fruit..................	100	½ c. 1 serving	..	..	12	48
15% fruit..................	100	½ c. 1 serving	..	..	15	60
18% fruit..................	100	½ c. 1 serving	..	..	18	72
Egg.......................	50	1	7	5	..	73
Meat and chicken...........	30	1 oz.	7	5	..	73
Fish, fresh.................	30	1 oz.	6	2	..	42
Cheese, American...........	30	1 oz.	9	11	..	135
Cheese, cream..............	30	1 oz.	8	10	1	126
Cheese, cottage, skim........	30	1 oz.	6	..	1	28
Gelatin....................	3	1 tsp.	3	..	..	12
Bacon, lean................	15	3 thin strips, crisp	3	8	..	84
Butter.....................	10	2 tsp.	..	8.5	..	77
Oil........................	10	2 tsp.	..	10	..	90
Mayonnaise................	14	1 tbsp.	..	12	..	108
Cocoa.....................	5	2 tsp.	1	1	2	21
Ice cream, plain.............	120	1 gill (¼ pint)	3	15	19	223

c: cup   tsp: teaspoon   tbsp: tablespoon

portion for each meal for practical purposes will be one-third of these amounts, *i.e.*, 25 gm. protein, 25 gm. fat and 50 gm. carbohydrate (525 calories for each meal). Sometimes unequal division of the diet is desirable. (A division of one-fifth, two-fifths and two-fifths is not infrequent, p. 755.) Assume that the foods selected for breakfast are fruit, cereal, milk, eggs, bread or toast, and butter.

Consider the *carbohydrate* foods first. The average helping of cereal (dry) is 20 gm. or ½ cup (cooked). This amount of cereal contains 3 gm.

of protein and 16 gm. carbohydrate. A cup of milk, 240 gm. contains 7 gm. protein, 10 gm. fat and 12 gm. carbohydrate. One slice of bread, 30 gm.,

TABLE 11

THE CARBOHYDRATE PERCENTAGE OF COMMON FRUITS AND VEGETABLES

3 per cent	6 per cent	9 per cent
Vegetables	*Vegetables*	*Vegetables*
Asparagus, fresh or canned	Beans, scarlet runner	Artichokes
Beans, green, wax, fresh or canned	Beans, snap	Beets
	Beets, canned	Brussels sprouts
Beet greens	Chives	Carrots
Broccoli	Collards	Onions
Cabbage	Dandelion greens	Peas, very young
Cauliflower	Eggplant	Peas, canned
Celery	Kohlrabi	Rutabagas
Chard	Okra	
Cucumbers	Peppers	*Fruits*
Endive	Squash, winter	Blackberries
Lettuce	Tomato, pureed, canned	Cranberries
Mustard greens	Turnips	Currants
Radishes		Grapefruit
Sauerkraut, fresh or canned	*Fruits*	Grapefruit juice
Spinach	Blackberry juice	Lemons
Squash, summer	Muskmelon, including canta-	Lemon juice
Tomatoes, fresh or canned	loups and honeydew	Loganberry juice
Turnip tops	Strawberries	Tangerines
Watercress	Watermelon	

Fruits
  Rhubarb

12 per cent	15 per cent	18 per cent
Vegetables	*Vegetables*	*Vegetables*
Beans, lima, canned	Corn, green, very young	Beans, baked
	Parsnips	Beans, kidney (red), cooked
Fruits	Peas, medium	Corn, canned
Apple juice	Salsify	Potatoes
Apricots		Succotash, canned
Cherries, sour	*Fruits*	
Oranges	Apples	*Fruits*
Orange juice	Blueberries	Cherries, sweet
Peaches	Grapes	Crabapples
Peach juice	Pears	Figs
Pineapple		Grapejuice, unsweetened
Pineapple juice (fresh)		Bananas
Plums (excluding prunes)		
Raspberries		

TABLE 12

INCOMPLETE BREAKFAST MENU IN WHICH THE CARBOHYDRATE QUOTA IS FILLED

	Wt., Gm.	Approx. Measure	P. 25	F. 25	C. 50	Cal. 525
Fruit, 6 per cent..............	100	½ cup	..	..	6	24
Cereal (dry)..................	20	½ cup	3	..	16	76
Egg...........................						
Milk.........................	240	1 cup	7	10	12	166
Bread........................	30	1 slice	3	..	16	76
Totals.....................	....	....	..	..	50	..

accounts for 3 gm. protein and 16 gm. carbohydrate. There are still 6 gm. of carbohydrate lacking. This is made up by including 100 gm. of a 6 per cent fruit. The carbohydrate quota is thus completed (see table 12).

The *protein* quota still lacks 12 gm. The addition of 2 eggs accounts for 14 gm. protein—the slight excess is permissible—and 10 gm. fat (see table 13).

TABLE 13

Incomplete Breakfast Menu with the Protein and Carbohydrate Quotas Filled

	Wt., Gm.	Approx. Measure	P. 25	F. 25	C. 50	Cal. 525
Fruit, 6 per cent...............	100	½ cup	..	..	6	24
Cereal (dry)...................	20	½ cup	3	..	16	76
Egg.........................		2	14	10	..	146
Milk.........................	240	1 cup	7	10	12	166
Bread.......................	30	1 slice	3	..	16	76
Butter.......................						
Totals......................	......	....	27	..	50	

The fat quota is lacking by 5 grams.

One teaspoonful of butter (5 gm.) provides 4 gm. of fat which brings the total sufficiently close to the quota. The completed breakfast menu is shown in table 14. That for the midday and evening meals are made in like manner.

The need of making menus for each patient is reduced by employing standard diets. Twelve such diets are presented in Table 15. They will answer the needs of most diabetic patients. Diets employed during acute complications are presented on p. 820. Suitable substitutions will prevent the diet from becoming monotonous.

TABLE 14

Completed Breakfast Menu with the Quotas of Carbohydrate, Protein, Fat and Total Calories Filled

	Wt., Gm.	Approx. Measure	P. 25	F. 25	C. 50	Cal. 525
Fruit, 6 per cent...............	100	½ cup	..	..	6	24
Cereal (dry)...................	20	½ cup	3	..	16	76
Eggs........................		2	14	10	..	146
Milk.........................	240	1 cup	7	10	12	166
Bread.......................	30	1 slice	3	..	16	76
Butter.......................	5	1 tsp.	..	4	..	36
Totals......................	......	....	27	24	50	524

For the sake of simplicity and practical purposes, the fruits and vegetables have been more or less roughly classified according to their carbohydrate content in to 3, 6, 9, 12, 15, and 18 per cent groups, in table 11. The protein content of these fruits may be ignored. The substitution of any fruits or vegetables of the same value or half the amount of those having twice the carbohydrate value is permissible and adds to the variety of the diet. For example, substitutions for 100 gm. of a 6 per cent vegetable may include any one of the following: 200 gm. 3 per cent vegetable; 50

TABLE 15

STANDARD DIETS

Each diet outlined in this table contains at least:

Calcium	0.8 gm.
Phosphorus	1.3 gm.
Iron	12 mg.
Vitamin A	5000 International Units
Thiamine (Vitamin B₁)	1.8 mg.
Ascorbic Acid (Vitamin C)	75 mg.
Riboflavin	2.7 mg.
Nicotinic Acid	18 mg.

	1* 900 Calories P, 60; F, 29; C, 100		2* 1100 Calories P, 65; F, 44; C, 110		3* 1300 Calories P, 70; F, 60; C, 120		4 1300 Calories P, 75; F, 48; C, 140		5 1500 Calories P, 75; F, 62; C, 160		6 1700 Calories P, 80; F, 73; C, 180	
	Wt., gm.	Household measure	Wt., gm.	Household measure	Wt., gm.	Household measure	Wt., gm.	Household measure	Wt., gm.	Household measure	Wt., gm.	Household measure
Breakfast												
Milk	240 skim	1 c.	180 skim	⅔ c.	240 skim	1 c.	240 skim	1 c.	240 skim	1 c.	240 skim	1 c.
12% fruit	100	1 serv.	100	1 serv.	100	1 serv.	100	1 serv.	100	1 serv.	100	1 serv.
Cereal, whole grain	10	¼ c.	20	½ c.	20	½ c.	30	¾ c.	20	½ c.	20	½ c.
Eggs	100	2	100	2	100	2	100	2	100	2	100	2
Butter			5	1 tsp.	10	2 tsp.	10	2 tsp.	15	1 tbsp.	15	1 tbsp.
Bread, whole grain									30	1 sl.	45	1½ sl.
Noon Meal												
Milk	240 skim	1 c.	240 skim	1 c.	240 skim	1 c.	240 skim	1 c.	240 skim	1 c.	240 skim	1 c.
Cheese	30	1 oz.	30	1 oz.								
Meat, fish, or fowl					45	1½ oz.	60	2 oz.	30	1 oz.	30	1 oz.
3% vegetable	300	3 serv.	200	2 serv.	100	1 serv.	100	1 serv.	100	1 serv.	100	1 serv.
6% vegetable			100	1 serv.	100	1 serv.	100	1 serv.				
9% vegetable					100	1 serv.	100	1 serv.	100	1 serv.	100	1 serv.
12% fruit	100	1 serv.	100	1 serv.					100	1 serv.	100	1 serv.
Bread, whole grain					15		15	½ sl.	30	1 sl.	45	1½ sl.
Butter	5	1 tsp.	10	2 tsp.	15	1 tbsp.	5	1 tsp.	15	1 tbsp.	10	2 tsp.

Evening Meal

Meat, fish, or fowl	45	1½ oz.	60	2 oz.	60	2 oz.	60	2 oz.	60	2 oz.	60	2 oz.
3% vegetable	100	1 serv.	200	2 serv.	200	2 serv.	100	1 serv.	200	2 serv.	100	1 serv.
9% vegetable	200	2 serv.	100	1 serv.	100	1 serv.	100	1 serv.	100	1 serv.	100	1 serv.
18% vegetable	....	......	....	......	....	......	....	......	....	......	100	1 serv.
12% fruit	100	1 serv.	100	1 serv.	100	1 serv.	100	1 serv.	100	1 serv.	100	1 serv.
Bread, whole grain	....	......	15	½ sl.	30	1 sl.	45	1½ sl.	45	1½ sl.	30	1 sl.
Butter	5	1 tsp.	5	1 tsp.	15	1 tbsp.	5	1 tsp.	15	1 tbsp.	15	1 tbsp.

c.—cup; tbsp.—tablespoon; tsp.—teaspoon; serv.—serving (approximately ½ cup).

The first diet (900 calories) is the skeleton diet. Each succeeding diet is equivalent to the preceding diet with certain additions to provide the specified increases in protein, fat, carbohydrates and calories.

* Diets 1, 2 and 3 must be supplemented with compressed brewer's yeast, grains 36 (6 tablets) daily.

TABLE 15—*Continued*

	7 — 1900 Calories P, 80; F, 87; C, 200		8 — 2100 Calories P, 80; F, 109; C, 200		9 — 2300 Calories P, 85; F, 120; C, 220		10 — 2500 Calories P, 90; F, 135; C, 230		11 — 2700 Calories P, 100; F, 145; C, 250		12 — 2900 Calories P, 100; F, 167; C, 250	
	Wt., gm.	Household measure	Wt., gm.	Household measure	Wt., gm.	Household measure	Wt., gm.	Household measure	Wt., gm.	Household measure	Wt., gm.	Household measure
Breakfast												
Milk	180 whole	⅔ c.	180 whole	⅔ c.	240 whole	1 c.	240 whole	1 c.	240 whole	1 c.	240 whole	1 c.
12% fruit	100	1 serv.	100	1 serv.	100	1 serv.	100	1 serv.	100	1 serv.	100	1 serv.
Cereal, whole grain	20	½ c.	20	½ c.	20	½ c.	20	½ c.	20	½ c.	20	½ c.
Eggs	100	2	100	2	100	2	100	2	100	2	100	2
Butter	15	1 tbsp.	20	4 tsp.	15	1 tbsp.	20	4 tsp.	20	4 tsp.	25	5 tsp.
Bread, whole grain	60	2 sl.	60	2 sl.	60	2 sl.	60	2 sl.	75	2½ sl.	75	2½ sl.
20% cream					30	2 tbsp.	30	2 tbsp.	60	¼ c.	60	¼ c.
Noon Meal												
Milk	240 whole	1 c.	240 whole	1 c.	240 whole	1 c.	240 whole	1 c.	180 whole	⅔ c.	180 whole	⅔ c.
Cheese												
Meat, fish, or fowl	30	1 oz.	30	1 oz.	30	1 oz.	30	1 oz.	45	1½ oz.	45	1½ oz.
3% vegetable	100	1 serv.	100	1 serv.	100	1 serv.	100	1 serv.	100	1 serv.	100	1 serv.
6% vegetable												
9% vegetable	100	1 serv.	100	1 serv.	100	1 serv.	100	1 serv.	100	1 serv.	100	1 serv.
18% vegetable					100	1 serv.	100	1 serv.	100	1 serv.	100	1 serv.
12% fruit	100	1 serv.	100	1 serv.	100	1 serv.	100	1 serv.	100	1 serv.	100	1 serv.
Bread, whole grain	60	2 sl.	60	2 sl.	30	1 sl.	45	1½ sl.	60	2 sl.	60	2 sl.
Butter	15	1 tbsp.	25	5 tsp.	25	5 tsp.	30	2 tbsp.	15	1 tbsp.	20	4 tsp.
20% cream							30	2 tbsp.	30	2 tbsp.	30	2 tbsp.
Oil									15	1 tbsp	15	1 tbsp

Evening Meal												
Meat, fish, or fowl	60	2 oz.	60	2 oz.	60	2 oz.	60	2 oz.	60	2 oz.	60	2 oz.
3% vegetable	100	1 serv.	100	1 serv.	100	1 serv.	100	1 serv.	100	1 serv.	100	1 serv.
9% vegetable	100	1 serv.	100	1 serv.	100	1 serv.	100	1 serv.	100	1 serv.	100	1 serv.
18% vegetable	100	1 serv.	100	1 serv.	100	1 serv.	100	1 serv.	100	1 serv.	100	1 serv.
12% fruit	100	1 serv.	100	1 serv.	100	1 serv.	100	1 serv.	100	1 serv.	100	1 serv.
Bread, whole grain	45	1½ sl.	45	1½ sl.	60	2 sl.	60	2 sl.	75	2½ sl.	75	2½ sl.
Butter	20	4 tsp.	30	2 tbsp.	30	2 tbsp.	25	5 tsp.	15	1 tbsp.	25	5 tsp.
20% cream	....		....		30	2 tbsp.	60	¼ c.	60	¼ c.	60	¼ c.
Oil	....		....		....		....		10	2 tsp.	15	1 tbsp.

c.—cup; tbsp.—tablespoon; tsp.—teaspoon; serv.—serving (approximately ½ cup).

The first diet (900 calories) is the skeleton diet. Each succeeding diet is equivalent to the preceding diet with certain additions to provide the specified increases in protein, fat, carbohydrates and calories.

gm. of a 12 per cent vegetable or fruit; 75 gm. of a 9 per cent vegetable or fruit. Similarly, 30 gm. of bread (one slice) may be substituted for 120 gm. of cooked cereal or 20 gm. of one of the dry cereals.

Fruits are weighed raw, cooked in individual containers and served complete with any juice that there may be. Dried fruits, because of the great variation in their carbohydrate values, are to be avoided.

All *dry cereals* have approximately the same food values and may be interchanged one for the other in like amounts. *Cooked cereals*, of which oatmeal is recommended because of its vitamin B content, take up varying amounts of water. The error which results may be considerable. The cereal may be weighed in the dry state, usually 20 gm., and cooked in an individual container. Ordinarily the food value of 120 gm. of the cooked cereal approximates that of 20 gm. of dry cereal.

Bacon may be weighed in the raw or cooked state. When it is weighed raw the fat which separates out in the cooking is used or substituted for by an equal amount of butter. If cooked before weighing this substitution is not necessary and the fat which escaped during the cooking is not used.

The other meats are weighed after cooking. Those referred to in the Standard Diets are lean meats—beef, mutton, lamb, veal and fowl. The various food recipes and substitution lists are beyond the scope of this book. The reader is referred elsewhere* for this information.

INSULIN

Insulin is an antidiabetic hormone, a protein, containing at least nine amino acids and is produced by the islets of Langerhans, presumably by the beta cells, of the pancreas. In the mammalian organism the pancreas appears to be the only organ which manufactures or stores insulin (Best and Taylor).

Insulin was obtained by Banting and Best[2] in a form which when injected intravenously or subcutaneously caused a reduction in the blood sugar level, a restored ability to utilize sugar and a disappearance of glycosuria, in dogs previously made diabetic by partial pancreatectomy. The insulin was secured by isolating the islets of Langerhans in an ingenious manner. The pancreatic duct was firmly ligated, whereupon degeneration of the acinar cells occurred, leaving the islet cells intact. Banting's greatest contribution was the realization of his idea that an active hypoglycemic factor might be secured from this remaining portion of the pancreas. Banting describes the first results with such an extract as follows, "On 27th of July, 1921, we had a depancreatized dog and we decided to begin treatment. A duct-tied dog was chloroformed and the degenerated residue of pancreas was removed. It was chopped into small pieces in a chilled mortar and frozen in brine. The mass was ground up and about 100 cc. of saline was added. Of this extract 5 cc. was administered intravenously into the depancreatized dog. Samples of blood were taken at half-hour intervals and showed that the blood sugar had fallen from 0.200 to 0.11 per cent in two hours. The clinical condition of the dog was remarkably improved."

The discovery made, it was not long before practical means of obtain-

* Pattee, A. F., Practical Dietetics with Reference to Diet in Health and Disease, 22nd Ed., published by the author, Mt. Vernon, N. Y., 1939, and Proudfit, F. T., Nutrition and Diet Therapy—A Textbook of Dietetics, 7th Ed., The Macmillan Co., New York, 1938.

ing insulin in large quantities from beef and pork pancreases was evolved. For this accomplishment we are indebted to Banting, Best, McLeod, Collip, the staff of the Connaught Laboratories in Toronto, and to Clowes of Indianapolis. Later (1927) insulin crystals were obtained by Abel.[45] They proved to be the most active form of insulin available.

Clinical Use of Insulin.—Insulin was standardized and is measured in units. A *unit* is the amount of the crystalline preparation required to reduce the blood sugar level of a normal fasting (twenty-four hours) rabbit weighing 2 Kg., from normal (120 mg.) to 45 mg. per 100 cc. In clinical use the amount and distribution of insulin necessary to control the diabetes must

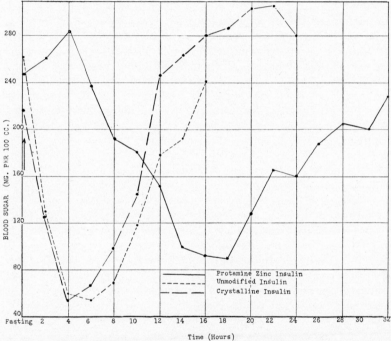

Time (Hours)

Fig. 141.—The comparative effects of 80 units of protamine zinc insulin, of crystalline and of unmodified insulin on the blood sugar level under strictly controlled conditions. Twenty grams of carbohydrate were given every two hours. Note the delayed but prolonged action of the protamine zinc insulin and the rapid action of short duration of both the unmodified and crystalline insulins. (Patient H. M., an adolescent male having a severe diabetes.) (After Duncan, G. G. and Barnes, C. E., Amer. Jour. Med. Sci., **202**: 553, 1941, Lea & Febiger, Publishers.)

be determined for each patient. No one can predict in advance the number of units which will accomplish a specified effect clinically.

The subcutaneous injections of insulin are followed by a reduction in the amount of sugar in the blood and in the urine, and carbohydrate storage and utilization are increased. This blood sugar lowering effect is more marked in juvenile than in middle-aged or elderly patients owing to a smaller glycogen reserve in the former. The apparent action of insulin is intensified by an undernutrition dietary regimen, by physical exercise, and by certain disease states when the glycogen reserve is low (*e.g.*, the eradication of infections and toxemia), and by disorders in which cachexia is out-

25

standing, notably malignant diseases. The apparent action of insulin is also intensified by certain endocrine disturbances in which antagonistic hormones are reduced, notably hypophyseal cachexia (Simmonds' disease), Addison's disease, and hypothyroidism. Extensive disease of the liver with reduced glycogen reserve, as seen in malignant disease and in some cases of cirrhosis of the liver, increases the apparent hypoglycemic effect of insulin.

The apparent intensity of insulin action is reduced especially by high caloric diets, by obesity, infections, and certain endocrine disorders, notably basophilic adenoma of the anterior lobe of the pituitary gland (Cushing's disease), acromegaly, hyperthyroidism and some cases of tumors of the cortex of the adrenal glands.[35]

Various Preparations of Insulin and Their Relative Effects.—From 1922 until 1936 insulin was available commercially in only one form, an aqueous solution, insulin hydrochloride. This preparation is now generally known as *unmodified* or *regular insulin,* a terminology used to prevent confusion with other insulin preparations, of which some are already available and others are under investigation.

A solution of crystalline insulin to which has been added minute amounts of zinc is available, commercially, as *zinc insulin crystals in solution.**

The effect of this product, given subcutaneously or intravenously, is, for practical purposes, indistinguishable clinically from unmodified insulin.[46, 47, 48] Because of its greater purity, lower protein content and the reduced likelihood of allergic reactions following its use this preparation is rapidly replacing unmodified insulin in clinical practice. Few references are made to unmodified insulin in this section, since it has been replaced at the Pennsylvania Hospital and for my patients at the Jefferson Hospital by zinc insulin crystals in solution, which for the sake of brevity is denoted hereafter as crystalline insulin.

Effect of Crystalline Insulin in Solution.—Crystalline insulin injected *intravenously* in a diabetic or normal person causes a reduction in the blood sugar level within a few minutes. The greatest hypoglycemic effect is noted between two and four hours, and, depending on the size of the dose, the effect wears off between four and six hours. A large dose has longer effect.

Injected *subcutaneously* as it is employed in the treatment of diabetes the hypoglycemic effect appears in about one-half hour with its greatest effect between three and five hours with the return of the blood sugar to the starting level between six and eight hours. Again, the size of the dose influences the degree of effect and the length of apparent action.

Crystalline insulin is especially valuable in emergencies because of its rapid action. It reduces the blood sugar from hyperglycemic levels to normal, or below normal if too much is given; it causes glycosuria to disappear and it restores the ability of the organism to utilize sugar. As a result of these effects it is invaluable in the treatment of the acute complications of diabetes. Through improved carbohydrate metabolism it makes possible the correction of ketosis—the CO_2 combining power of the blood is increased to normal, acetone bodies disappear from the blood and ketonuria is corrected. Furthermore, the insulin improves operative risks and en-

* Specified throughout this book as crystalline insulin.

hances tremendously the likelihood of a diabetic patient's recovery from acute infections.

Crystalline insulin is used widely in conjunction with protamine zinc insulin in the control of uncomplicated diabetes.

Protamine Zinc Insulin.—Protamine insulin (without zinc) was introduced by Hagedorn and his associates[49] in 1936. By adding to insulin a mono protamine, obtained from the sperm of the "salmine" species of fish, they produced a precipitate which when adjusted to the pH of the tissue fluids was absorbed more slowly than unmodified insulin when injected subcutaneously. The advantages of protamine insulin rested on two properties—slow absorption and a correspondingly retarded insulin effect. The Danish product was unstable and rapidly lost its potency at room temperature, but this was overcome by Scott and Fisher[50] who, by adding zinc in minute and harmless amounts, made the product stable for periods of many months.

This new preparation, *protamine zinc insulin*, is the one now in general use. Because of its slow action it cannot replace the crystalline insulin in the treatment of the acute complications of diabetes. In uncomplicated diabetes, however, either alone or combined with crystalline insulin, protamine zinc insulin, because of its prolonged effect (twenty-four to thirty-six hours), greatly reduces the extent of the oscillation of the blood sugar level; it allows more uniform control of the diabetes, with fewer injections; glycosuria is less and the danger of complications, notably ketosis, is reduced.

Most of our patients at the Pennsylvania and Jefferson Hospitals who require insulin are receiving protamine zinc insulin. The number in which good control of the diabetes is possible with this insulin alone is small, however. It is supplemented usually by one, and in patients with severe diabetes, by two doses of crystalline insulin.

Other Insulins.—Among several preparations now in the experimental stage two new ones, histone zinc insulin (Lilly) and globin insulin (Burroughs and Wellcome) have a more prompt but not so prolonged hypoglycemic action as protamine zinc insulin. They do not become effective as quickly, but their action is longer than that of crystalline insulin.

The diabetes is controlled by a single dose of either globin or histone zinc insulin in a greater percentage of patients than is possible with protamine zinc insulin alone. Globin insulin has the advantage of being a "clear insulin" and rarely indeed does it cause allergic reactions.

In using globin and histone zinc insulin, it has been my experience that the insulin should be administered at least one hour before breakfast if glycosuria during the forenoon is to be prevented, the diet is divided as follows: one-fifth for breakfast, two-fifths for lunch and two-fifths for supper with a part of the evening meal (usually a banana) at 3 P.M. to prevent the tendency to hypoglycemic reaction between 4 and 6 P.M. It is at this time that reactions are prone to occur when these insulins are employed and not during the night or early morning hours (as is the case with protamine zinc insulin). Globin and histone zinc insulin are not available commercially at this time (January, 1942).

Commercial Preparations of Insulin.—Three brands of insulin are commercially available. These are:

1. *Unmodified insulin* which, with several improvements, has been in use since 1922, is obtainable in rubber-capped vials in four different concentrations (*a*) "U. 20" in which there are 20 units in each cubic centimeter, (*b*) "U. 40" containing 40 units per cc., (*c*) "U. 80" containing 80 units per cc., and "U. 100" containing 100 units per cc.

2. *Zinc insulin crystals in solution* (crystalline insulin), which is marketed in "U. 40" and "U. 80" concentrations.

3. *Protamine zinc insulin*, which appears in trade vials of 10 cc. each and in two strengths, "U. 40" and "U. 80." Each cc. of "U. 40" contains 0.16 mg. of zinc.

The active material is the finely divided white precipitate which gives a milky opalescent appearance to the protamine zinc insulin solution. For accuracy in administration, uniform distribution of the precipitate in the solution is essential. One cannot place too great emphasis on the need of thorough mixing of the precipitate and solution. Successful treatment depends upon it. It must be done before each administration. Bubble formation is prevented by slowly inverting the bottle repeatedly in a tumbling fashion or placing it on a flat surface and describing circles with it. Violent agitation is to be avoided; it causes froth formation with unequal distribution of the precipitate.

With the mixing completed the protamine zinc insulin is withdrawn at once—before any settling of the precipitate occurs—into a cool and preferably dry syringe and immediately injected subcutaneously, *never intravenously*.

Patients should be cautioned not to use a hot syringe, since it causes the precipitate to adhere to the barrel and thus escape injection. Furthermore, they should be instructed to complete the injection immediately on withdrawal of the solution from the bottle, thus preventing the settling of the precipitate in the syringe. In other words, accuracy of dosage hinges on securing and maintaining an equal distribution of the suspension until it is deposited subcutaneously. Failure to do this will result in variations in the effect of protamine zinc insulin.

Technic of Insulin Administration.—The measuring of the insulin for administration may prove confusing in view of the various strengths employed. Patients find it difficult to realize that a unit of insulin is constant whether it be of "U. 20," "U. 40" or "U. 80" preparation. The measuring is simplified by employing a 1-cc. syringe graduated in tenths—$\frac{1}{10}$ cc. of "U. 20" insulin provides 2 units; $\frac{1}{10}$ cc. of "U. 40" 4 units; $\frac{1}{10}$ cc. of "U. 80" equals 8 units and $\frac{1}{10}$ cc. of "U. 100," 100 units. If finer graduations are indicated syringes which are calibrated in twentieths as well as tenths of a cubic centimeter are available. Also larger syringes which deliver $1\frac{1}{2}$ and 2 cc. are advisable when the 1-cc. syringe does not hold the entire single dose.

Sterilization of the syringe and needle is done by immersing the needle, already adjusted on the syringe, in grain alcohol (70 per cent) and filling the barrel of the syringe with the alcohol. (Ordinary 70 per cent rubbing alcohol is satisfactory but undenatured alcohol is preferable.) The alcohol is then expelled and the syringe is dried by pumping air in and out for a few minutes. It is important that no alcohol remain, in order to avoid the danger of injecting minute quantities of it into the bottle of insulin. Aseptic precautions are observed in the withdrawal of the insulin from the bottle and during its administration to the patient. Unmodified and crystalline insulin may be given intravenously in emergencies, but in their routine use they are given subcutaneously. Protamine zinc insulin is never given intravenously. The site of injection should be systematically varied. It is undesirable to use the same site twice within a fortnight.

Oral administration of insulin is useless. All forms of insulin are rendered inert by the digestive juices when given by mouth.

Unmodified insulin and crystalline insulin will remain potent indefinitely at room temperature. Refrigeration is not necessary. Freezing causes some loss of potency and, as Wilder has pointed out, this loss is reduced to a minimum if the thawing process is allowed to proceed slowly at room temperature. Clumping of the protamine zinc insulin is likely if it becomes frozen. Our practice has been to advise patients to discard insulin which has been frozen. This may be wasteful, but it eliminates uncertainty and teaches the patient to avoid such loss in the future.

Indications for Insulin Therapy in the Treatment of Uncomplicated Diabetes.—Insulin therapy is indicated in the treatment of diabetes when this disorder is not or obviously will not be controlled satisfactorily by suitable dietetic measures and exercise, and during acute complications for all diabetic patients, many of whom under usual circumstances may not need it. Some authorities give insulin in the initial days of treatment for all diabetic patients. In favor of this plan is the more rapid control of the diabetes and the training of the patient in the administration of insulin while he or she is under competent supervision. It also emphasizes that many patients can discontinue insulin. The majority of diabetic patients have a mild diabetes and ultimately do not need insulin. This information has a good effect in neutralizing a general and erroneous belief that once one uses insulin he must always use it. Unfortunately this is usually true for the thin patient having severe diabetes, but it is not true for those having mild diabetes.

All patients who have an acute onset of the diabetes which may be mild or severe, should be given insulin with the hope, in the light of recent work by the Toronto group, that some may be cured. These patients are practically always the young or the thin patients with severe diabetes who are ordinarily given insulin from the outset of treatment. The obese, untreated diabetic patient has a mild diabetes which develops insidiously when the body mass has increased to such an extent and has been maintained for a sufficient period to exhaust an already reduced pancreatic reserve. In these patients I believe the pancreas is a *locus minoris resistentiae* in which heredity has played a prominent part in which hypophyseal hyperactivity years before laid the groundwork but fell short of causing clinical diabetes. Obesity serves to bring the disorder to the surface.

The amounts of insulin needed in the individual case will vary, not only with the severity of the diabetes but with the total caloric value of the diet, the carbohydrate allowance, changes in total metabolism and in weight, exercise, and the presence or absence of complications. These factors will be considered in the following pages.

The amount of insulin needed is not relative to the degree of hyperglycemia with any constancy nor can it be calculated with any degree of exactness according to the amount of sugar in the urine. If glycosuria exists more insulin is needed, but what 5 units will do in ridding the urine of sugar in one patient may require 25 or more units in another.

The insulin needed cannot be computed according to the so-called glucose equivalent in the diet. Case No. U 5805 on the late Dr. Elmer Funk's service at the Jefferson Hospital illustrates this nicely: With a blood sugar of 0.205 per cent she received 50 units of insulin when the total glucose of the diet was 95 gm. Three days later on a new diet, with a total glucose of 146 gm., 46 units reduced the blood sugar to 0.165 per cent. The total calories remained constant.

How are we to decide which patients need and which patients do not need insulin?

It is a good working rule, barring acute complications which will be considered later, that all untreated diabetic patients who are considerably overweight will not need insulin notwithstanding the presence of a high fasting blood sugar level on the first examination. Every physician who sees many diabetic patients has seen fat patients with blood sugar levels above 300 mg. per 100 cc. and yet insulin was not necessary to control their diabetes.

It is a good working rule, too, that all children and underweight diabetic patients require insulin even if the initial level for fasting blood sugar should not be high. The certainty that insulin will be needed by the growing children and the underweight adult is based on the knowledge that to promote normal health and physical growth, a gain in weight and a liberal diet, each of which increase the need for insulin, are necessary. The combination of a persistently elevated fasting blood sugar level and undernutrition make insulin therapy imperative if good health is to be restored. It has been our practice at the Pennsylvania and Jefferson Hospitals never to give insulin to overweight diabetic patients unless during some acute complication. We are desirous that the merit for the control of the diabetes should go to the dietetic measures and not to a preliminary and temporary course of insulin treatment. In this manner the patient can be deeply impressed by the value of a restricted diet. Approximately 70 per cent of the patients attending my metabolic clinic at the Pennsylvania Hospital do not need insulin to maintain satisfactory control of their diabetes. We have observed the effect of insulin on obese diabetic patients at other clinics and, for purposes of study, we have given insulin to similar patients. Knowing that the diabetes is inherently mild and that the reduction of a few pounds in weight would control it, one might expect that a small dose of insulin would suffice to accomplish the same result. This is not so. These patients are relatively resistant to insulin due, I believe, to their obesity. Repeatedly over 100 units of insulin a day were necessary to accomplish, in reducing the blood sugar level, what was as readily obtained by a slight reduction in weight. These patients have three means to control their diabetes without insulin, e.g., a low caloric diet, a reduction in weight and physical exercise. All three are powerful agents in reducing the need for insulin. Various attempts have been made, especially by Himsworth,[51] to classify diabetic patients into insulin-resistant and insulin-sensitive groups. Most of the insulin-resistant patients were middle-aged and overweight. There seems to be a general lack of appreciation for the fact that the overweight insulin-resistant patient loses this resistance to insulin in direct proportion to the reduction of body weight. One is secure in stating that any factor which reduces the total metabolism, with one exception (*i.e.*, the cessation of physical exercise), aids in the control of the diabetes. Reduction in body mass seems to be the most effective of these factors. Newburgh[52] has confirmed our work and extended the proof of benefit secured by reduction in weight in the obese diabetic patient.

Selection, Dosage and Distribution of Insulin.—Protamine zinc insulin is employed for practically all uncomplicated diabetic patients who require insulin. It is supplemented with crystalline insulin when necessary. The protamine zinc insulin is given in one dose in the morning, fifteen to thirty minutes before breakfast. The initial dose may be 6 to 8 units for a child and 15 to 20 units for an adult. Additions of 4 to 12 units may be made every second or third day until the level of the fasting blood sugar is normal (70 to 100 mg. per 100 cc.). This accomplished, no further increases in the amount of protamine zinc insulin should be made. If this advice is not heeded hypoglycemic reactions will occur early in the morning. The maximum amount of protamine zinc insulin which can be given with safety is that amount which restores a normal fasting blood sugar level.

It is not necessary to have daily blood sugar determinations while early morning glycosuria persists. When the urine voided before breakfast is free from sugar a normal blood sugar value is to be expected.

The amount of protamine zinc insulin necessary to restore normal fasting blood sugar values varies greatly—from 10 to as much as 200 units a day. The average amount to achieve this end in our patients falls between 30 and 60 units a day.

In only a small number of patients, and these with relatively mild diabetes, will a single dose of protamine zinc insulin suffice to control the disorder throughout the twenty-four hours. Additional crystalline insulin is usually needed. Those who require supplementary assistance with the quickly acting insulin are identified in two ways.

First: As the protamine zinc insulin reaches its maximum dosage the 9 P.M. to 7 A.M. collection of urine* becomes aglycosuric. If large amounts of sugar are still lost in the 7 to 11 A.M., the 11 A.M. to 4 P.M., and the 4 to 9 P.M. urine collections, a supplementary dose of crystalline insulin is indicated. This is given within fifteen minutes before breakfast at the same time as the protamine zinc insulin but they are injected separately.†

* Fractional urine collections are made over specified periods; namely, 7 to 11 A.M., 11 A.M. to 4 P.M., 4 to 9 P.M. and 9 P.M. to 7 A.M.

† Lawrence and Archer[53] have reported satisfactory results following the simultaneous injection of the two insulins from the same syringe. Wilder[54] also has adopted this method. It has the advantage of one injection over two. My own experience with the simultaneous injection of both insulins covered approximately one year, after which I abandoned it, possibly without sufficient reason, because of irregularity of effect, difficulty of the technic for the patient and the fact that somewhat greater amounts of insulin were needed to control the diabetes with the mixed than with the separate injections. Watson[55] has shown that to gain the individual physiological effects of unmodified and protamine zinc insulin they must be injected separately. When the mixed insulins are injected it is important to avoid introducing even minute quantities of the alkaline protamine zinc insulin into the bottle of crystalline insulin. This is accomplished by the irrevocable practice of withdrawing the crystalline insulin into the syringe before withdrawing the protamine zinc insulin.

Second: A normal fasting blood sugar level having been accomplished with protamine zinc insulin, blood sugar determinations are done at 11 A.M., 4 P.M., and 10 P.M. Supplementary crystalline insulin should be given if the blood sugar exceeds 150 mg. per 100 cc. in any of these. The initial dose, 4 to 8 units, may be safely increased 2 to 8 units daily until the 7 to 11 A.M. urine collection is aglycosuric and the 11 A.M. blood sugar level is normal. During this process it may be necessary to make a modest reduction in the protamine zinc insulin because the former dose, now supported with a rapidly acting insulin, may prove excessive as indicated by hypoglycemic values and actual clinical insulin reactions before breakfast.

The average supplementary dose needed to restore a normal blood sugar level at 11 A.M. varies, with unusual exceptions from 8 to 80 units. The average dose is between 10 and 40 units.

This program, a single dose of protamine zinc insulin and a single daily dose of crystalline insulin, both given fifteen minutes before breakfast, controls all but the very severe diabetes. An additional or second dose of crystalline insulin in those patients, usually children or those who have been markedly undernourished because of the diabetes, is indicated when in spite of satisfactory blood sugar values at 7 and 11 A.M. there is a hyperglycemia in excess of 150 mg. per 100 cc. at 10 P.M. A small dose, 4 to 8 units, of crystalline insulin is given before the evening meal. Small increases, 2 or 3 units, are made daily until the 4 to 10 P.M. urine is aglycosuric and the 10 P.M. blood sugar level is at or below 150 mg. per 100 cc. If this program of three doses, one dose each of protamine zinc and crystalline insulin before breakfast and one dose of crystalline before supper, does not uniformly control the diabetes when the increases have reached a point where further additions would cause hypoglycemic reactions it is because of some complication and an insulin regime as outlined for acute complications on p. 828 should be adopted.

After the diabetes is controlled examinations for sugar in single urine specimens voided before breakfast, before lunch, and at bedtime (9 or 10 P.M.) provide reliable information regarding the state of control of the disorder, providing the renal threshold for sugar is normal.

Whether or not sugar appears in the early morning specimen determines whether or not to increase or decrease the protamine zinc insulin, whereas results of the examination of the specimen voided before lunch determines the action to be taken with the morning dose of crystalline insulin. For patients requiring an evening dose of crystalline insulin the examination of the late evening (9 or 10 P.M.) specimen, will guide the changes in the amount of insulin to be given.

Some patients (2 to 4 per cent of those needing insulin) because of allergic manifestations or unsatisfactory response with protamine zinc insulin or a desire to continue with unmodified or crystalline insulin may have to be treated with crystalline insulin alone. It is for the treatment of this small group that the following outline is presented.

The fractional collections of urine as indicated above are used as guides in increasing the insulin until the urine is free from or contains only a trace of sugar.

One dose, 8 to 12 units, of crystalline insulin given twenty minutes before breakfast may suffice to control a relatively mild diabetes. Usually more is necessary. While sugar continues to appear in the 7 to 11 A.M. specimens 2 to 6 units may be added daily. When the dose reaches 18 or 20 units or if the 7 to 11 A.M. urine becomes free from sugar while the other fractions contain sugar, it is well to give *two doses*. This may be given as follows: 12 units twenty minutes before breakfast and 8 units before supper. It is well to make no increase in the total dose at the time it is divided. The mere splitting of the dose has the same effect as an increase. The smaller the dose of crystalline insulin, the more effective is each unit.

Further increases, 2 to 4 units daily, are made to the morning dose while glycosuria persists in the 7 to 11 A.M. urine fraction, and to the evening dose while there is sugar in the 4 to 10 P.M. fraction.

Three doses are usually indicated when the amounts have reached the neighborhood of 20–0–16. The division might be as follows: 16 units before breakfast, 8 units before lunch and 12 units before supper, prescribed as 16–8–12. Small additions, 2 to 4 units, may be made daily as outlined above. Glycosuria in the 11 A.M. to 4 P.M. collection indicates an increase in the noon dose while freedom from glycosuria would suggest no change. This applies also to the other doses and specimens. An occasional patient does better with a small third dose given at bedtime instead of before lunch.

The foregoing plan of treatment serves the majority of patients who require insulin. There is, however, a group of more severe cases in which a point is reached when, if additions are made to any one of the three doses of insulin, a hypoglycemia results during the day and yet a hyperglycemia occurs in the early morning. This is due to three large doses fairly close together on one hand, and a long night period without insulin on the other. The diabetes is so severe that when the effect of the evening insulin is exhausted and the patient has not enough endogenous insulin to keep the blood sugar at a normal level during the remainder of the night, a progressive increase in the blood sugar concentration occurs. This accounts for the morning hyperglycemia despite the normal blood sugar values throughout the remainder of the day. Allen[56] has suggested lengthening the day periods between doses and shortening the night period without insulin by giving the morning insulin one hour earlier. The timing of the noon dose remains unchanged but the evening dose is given one or two hours after supper. When the severity of the diabetes calls for this plan, there need be no fear of a hypoglycemia during the night. A portion of the supper may be taken at bedtime if a safeguard seems necessary.

When a *fourth dose* is necessary as occasionally occurs in patients having severe diabetes, it is well to give it at midnight with a small amount of nourishment (5 to 10 gm. of carbohydrate). The other three doses, in event of the fourth dose being needed, should be given prior to the respective meals. The fourth dose is usually needed for a short period only.

Frequent doses, every four or six hours or more frequently, are needed during emergencies. This is true in dealing with ketosis, acute infections, and surgical conditions. They will be dealt with under their respective headings.

The value of examining fractional collections of urine for sugar is apparent. Ordinarily after discharge from the hospital, for the patient who takes only the quickly acting insulin, the examination of single specimens affords the required information. The patient taking one dose of insulin should examine an evening specimen preferably two hours after supper as this is the time glycosuria is most likely to occur. If two doses of insulin are taken the urine voided before breakfast and before supper are examined and if three or four doses are used a specimen voided before each meal and at bedtime should be examined for sugar.

TABLE 16

FACTORS WHICH ALTER THE NEED FOR INSULIN

Those Increasing Need for Insulin	*Those Decreasing Need for Insulin*
Gain in weight	Reduction in weight (therapeutic)
Increased diet	Reduced caloric intake
Cessation of exercise	Increased physical exercise
Pregnancy	Termination of pregnancy
Therapies:	Termination of the following therapies:
Thyroid	Thyroid
Epinephrine	Epinephrine
Dinitrophenol	Dinitrophenol
Pituitary gland preparations	Pituitary gland preparations
Deep roentgen ray	Deep roentgen ray
Toxemias	Correction of:
Hyperthyroidism	Hyperthyroidism
Sepsis	Acute infections
Acute infections	Burns
Fever	Ketosis
Ketosis	Fever
Ultraviolet ray burn	

COMPLICATIONS DIRECTLY ATTENDANT ON INSULIN THERAPY: INSULIN REACTIONS* (HYPOGLYCEMIA)

An insulin reaction is characterized by a depression of the blood sugar level below normal—usually below 60 mg. per 100 cc., though values down to zero have been recorded. The more or less characteristic symptoms which follow the depression of the blood sugar level generally, but by no means always, vary in intensity with the degree of hypoglycemia. Little attention is given in current medical writings on this subject to the frequent occurrence of abnormally low blood sugar values without symptoms. This is a frequent happening in patients treated with protamine zinc insulin.

Causes.—In general, too much insulin or too little food or both embrace the factors causing hypoglycemic reactions following insulin treatment.

The causes can be presented more specifically as follows:

1. Unusual exercise without reducing insulin or increasing the diet. Exercise, in all but very severe and untreated diabetes, has a blood-sugar lowering effect. As a result the routine dose of insulin becomes excessive and insulin reactions are likely.

2. Failure to eat all the food allowed, or delaying meals, particularly breakfast and lunch, too long after the insulin has been given.

3. Overdose of insulin because of error in measuring.

4. Vomiting.

* Insulin reactions are often loosely spoken of as "insulin shocks." This, of course, is an incorrect term. Clinical evidences of a hypoglycemia are not those of shock. If we are to encourage clear thinking we must use the least confusing terms possible. Wilder has suggested the term "insulin collapse." This is descriptive and at the same time not likely to be confused with local insulin reactions. However, "hypoglycemic reactions" seems to be the most suitable term.

5. Diarrhea.

6. Failure to anticipate gains in carbohydrate and total food tolerance, and a proportionate reduction in the need for insulin following (*a*) the control of the diabetes, (*b*) a reduction in weight, (*c*) eradication of infections and toxemia, and (*d*) a reduction in diet.

7. Erroneous distribution of the insulin and diet.

8. A too rapid increase in the amount of insulin given.

9. The development of cachexia with poor glycogen storage as in malignant disease and in certain instances of tuberculosis. Underweight persons are more sensitive to insulin than those who are well nourished.

10. A change of the site of insulin injection from an insulin tumefaction to other areas may precipitate a hypoglycemia (p. 786).

Symptoms.—A mild reaction may be manifested in the development of *trembling*, a feeling of *tenseness, cardiac palpitation, hunger, weakness, perspiration* and *difficulty in mental concentration*. A rapid reduction of the blood sugar concentration from hyperglycemic levels to normal may on some occasions give rise to these symptoms.

The symptoms of hypoglycemia due to protamine zinc insulin do not appear quickly as do those due to crystalline insulin. The protamine zinc insulin acts so much more slowly that a compensatory transformation of liver glycogen to dextrose defers the acute symptoms. It is apparent that if the overdose is great enough the blood sugar level will continue to fall and when the patient loses consciousness it is much lower and the liver is much more depleted of glycogen than when the hypoglycemia is due to a rapidly acting insulin. Hence a hypoglycemia of any degree due to protamine zinc insulin should be regarded as an emergency. These reactions are most severe when they occur in the early morning. This is because of (*a*) the fasting state of the patient and (*b*) because the reactions are rarely recognized in the early stages.

Headache is the most common symptom of a low blood sugar due to excessive amounts of protamine zinc insulin. Loss of memory, emotional instability, disorientation, malaise, and areas of numbness are common. Nausea in a mild form is not uncommon. These symptoms occur most frequently between midnight and breakfast time.

As the severity of the reaction increases, whether from slowly or rapidly acting insulin, vertigo, faintness, perspiration (not as common when due to protamine zinc insulin as when due to crystalline insulin), diplopia, blurring of vision, cardiac palpitation, and coldness of the extremities occur. Difficulty in walking, disturbance in emotions, varying from shouting and a hilarious behavior to one of depression and lapses into quietness, are common. The patient may stubbornly resist treatment. Paresthesias, particularly of the tongue, the buccal and circumoral areas, and of the extremities may be noted in fairly mild reactions. Paraplegias and, in unusual instances, transient hemiplegia, have resulted from hypoglycemia. Vomiting may occur but it is not a common symptom of hypoglycemia. It is more frequent in reactions due to protamine zinc insulin than to those caused by one of the quickly acting insulins.

Severe reactions lead to disorientation, retrograde amnesia, muscle twitching, convulsions (occurring more frequently in children than in adults), unconsciousness, and if the overdose of insulin has been great and the patient is a child or an undernourished adult death may occur. Residual effects of cerebral damage may be permanent but they are usually transitory. Protracted coma or stupor for hours and days even after the blood sugar is restored to normal occurs occasionally and is an ominous sign. Bowen and Beck[57] reported nineteen fatal cases of insulin reactions collected from the literature. The symptoms of hypoglycemia have been identified by Wilder[58] as occurring under disturbances of (a) the sympathetic nervous system, (b) the central nervous system, and (c) of psychical nature. A mixture of all three are common. They are dealt with according to their individual characteristics in Chapter XIII, on Hyperinsulinism.

The hazards to which a patient may be exposed during an insulin reaction are many. Three illustrations are presented.

ILLUSTRATIVE CASES

Patient S. H.* (Pennsylvania Hospital), who, while out walking, felt quite warm and experienced difficulty in controlling his legs. Knowing from past experiences that these were premonitory symptoms of a severe hypoglycemic reaction he entered a restaurant, purchased some food but before he was able to partake of it his legs gave away and he collapsed on the floor. He was unable to rise. He was thrown out of the restaurant by two attendants who believed him to be intoxicated. His anger was aroused at this treatment, to which he offered considerable resistance. It is interesting that at this point his symptoms began to subside; he presented a police officer with his diabetic identification card, he returned with the officer to the restaurant, had his money refunded and walked half a block, unaided, to another restaurant where he secured some orange juice.

The stimulating effect which anger has on the adrenal glands may be exemplified clinically in this instance.

The removal of a patient having an insulin reaction, but believed to be intoxicated, to a police station is readily understood. The hazard is increased if a diabetic patient has the odor of alcohol on his breath during an insulin reaction. The attending risks are obvious. The practice of carrying a diabetic identification card should be unfailing. Legal entanglements may further involve matters. Patient S. H. brought suit against the restaurant proprietor. Settlement out of court gave the patient thirty-five and the lawyer forty dollars!

Another patient, J. H., aged eight years, left her school room and proceeded to her home, crossing several main thoroughfares en route. It was not until her mother noticed her "wolfing" her food that an insulin reaction was suspected. Upon recovery the patient had no recollection of having left the school room or of finding her way home.

Patient E. M., an insurance salesman, had no recollection of what occurred in a two-hour period during which he secured an applicant's signature for insurance. He proceeded to his automobile, and drove, alone, through Camden, New Jersey, to Medford (18 miles) along an extremely busy highway, around traffic circles, to end by running into a post. He was found in a nearby field by state troopers who, on finding his diabetic identification card, fed him orange juice, a supply of which they found in the patient's automobile. The possibilities attending this adventure are many.

* Case record reported in greater detail elsewhere.[59]

This experience was the result of an attempt on the part of a careless patient to balance a break in diet restrictions with an overdose of insulin.

Diagnosis.—A history indicating that the patient has diabetes and is receiving insulin treatment is helpful. This information is not always obtainable and, even if it is, the possibility of unconsciousness resulting from other causes makes a careful differential diagnosis important.

The patient in an insulin reaction may exhibit signs ranging from slight transitory moments of confusion to complete unconsciousness. The mode and time of onset of symptoms are important. The patient may appear "queer"; a fixed expression is common and conversation may be without proper sequence. He may behave like an automaton. He appears confused and is emotionally upset over trivial matters or without apparent cause. He may become boisterous and resist examination and treatment. The onset of unconsciousness before meal time should make one suspect hypoglycemia while if it occurs between one and three hours after a hearty meal hypoglycemia is less likely to be the cause.

There is usually some pallor of the skin but, in general, the patient's appearance is not that of a person who has been ill, but that of one who has fainted. The skin is wet. Beads of perspiration are common on the forehead at the hair margin; the face, body, and extremities are cold and clammy, and the underclothes are wet with perspiration. The body temperature may be slightly below normal. The pupils are dilated; the intraocular tension is not disturbed; the pulse rate is advanced with normal or increased force and the blood pressure is either normal or, as frequently occurs, is elevated. It falls below normal only when the patient is *in extremis*. The breathing is undisturbed. Marks from the injection of insulin are usually apparent on legs, arms, or abdomen. The tendon reflexes are overactive and a Babinski sign may be elicited during but not immediately after recovery from the reaction.

The examination of the urine offers little of value in confirming the diagnosis. The absence of glycosuria is suggestive evidence, however, in the case of an unconscious patient known to have diabetes and known to take insulin. Furthermore the absence of glycosuria and ketonuria is definite evidence against diabetic ketosis. On the other hand the patient whose blood sugar goes quickly from a high to a low level may have sugar in the bladder from the hyperglycemic phase. Sugar in the first specimen obtained from the unconscious patient should not rule out the possibility of a hypoglycemia. After the bladder has been emptied, a second specimen should contain no sugar.

A low blood sugar level, below 60 mg. per 100 cc., is the most important single evidence of an insulin reaction. One must make a diagnosis on clinical evidence, however, and begin treatment. The patient's welfare should not be jeopardized by delaying therapy until the blood sugar concentration is known.

Differential Diagnosis.—The most frequent causes of unconsciousness to be confused with insulin reactions are alcoholism, diabetic coma (ketosis), and intracranial lesions. The other causes, however, should receive consideration. I refer especially to trauma, poisonings, epilepsy, uremia, syphilis of the central nervous system, and rarely, hyperinsulinism and Addison's disease. Night sweats attendant upon tuberculous infections complicating diabetes are occasionally suggestive of, and may be confused with an insulin reaction.

Diabetic Coma (Ketosis).—The chief characteristics of diabetic coma are presented on p. 811 and the characteristic clinical differences between diabetic coma and an insulin reaction are presented in table 17. In contrast to the patient having an insulin reaction, the patient in coma (ketosis) has received too little insulin; there is marked *dehydration* and *air hunger* (Kussmaul breathing) with the *odor of acetone on the breath;* the onset of symptoms is slow, at least eight to twelve hours; and is preceded by *anorexia, thirst, polyuria* and later *vomiting;* the *pulse* is weak and rapid

TABLE 17

A COMPARISON OF THE CLINICAL EVIDENCES OF HYPOGLYCEMIA AND DIABETIC COMA (KETOSIS)

	Hypoglycemia	Diabetic Coma (Ketosis)
Cause	Too much insulin or not enough food	Too much food or not enough insulin
General appearance	A well person who has fainted	Very ill (to the inexperienced appears hopelessly ill)
Breathing	Normal	Rapid and deep (air hunger)
Onset	Rapid (minutes)	Slow, at least twelve hours
Hunger	Great	Anorexia
Thirst	None	Great
Vomiting	Rare	Common
Eyes	Staring, and pupils dilated	Sunken
Disturbed vision	Diplopia and difficulty in focusing	Haziness
Headache	Common	Absent
Intraocular tension	Normal	Decreased
Skin	Wet (especially forehead)	Dry
Tissues	Normal	Dehydrated
Pulse	Full and rapid	Weak and rapid
Air hunger	Absent	Present
Blood pressure	Elevated or normal	Subnormal
Cardiac palpitation	Frequent	Absent
Constipation	None	Present
Muscular twitching	Common	Absent
Nervousness	Common	Absent
Babinski's sign	May be present	Absent
Complicating infections	Absent	Common
Abdominal pain	Absent	Common
Urine sugar	None (after residual urine is discarded)	Present
Blood sugar	Below normal	Above normal
Acetonuria	Absent	Present
Response to treatment	Rapid (minutes)	Slow (hours)

(After Duncan, G. G., Diabetes Mellitus and Obesity, 1935, Lea and Febiger, Philadelphia.)

and the blood pressure is subnormal; the *tendon reflexes* are diminished and the plantar reflexes are normal; there is usually no twitching of the muscles or convulsions; glycosuria and acetonuria are present; there is often a complicating infection in the ketotic patient, and finally the blood sugar level is above normal and the CO_2 combining power of the blood plasma is reduced.

If there is any doubt whether one is dealing with diabetic coma (ketosis) or an insulin reaction (hypoglycemia) the therapeutic test of giving glucose (dextrose), 20 cc. of a 50 per cent solution in distilled water, intravenously should be made. This will do the ketotic patient no harm and it will restore the hypoglycemic individual to consciousness in most cases.

Intracranial Lesions.—The more common intracranial lesions that are likely to confuse one in making the diagnosis are: hemorrhage, thrombosis and emboli in cerebral vessels, tumors, and trauma. A careful physical examination will reveal signs of arterial disease, localizing neurological signs, or evidence of trauma and there will be no marks of the insulin injection. The blood sugar level will be normal or moderately elevated and glycosuria is common when there is injury to the base of the brain. This response is presumably due to stimulation of the sympathetic centers.

Treatment of Hypoglycemia.—The hypoglycemia should be corrected without delay. Mild reactions are readily remedied by having the patient drink a glassful (240 cc.) of orange juice, or take four or six glucose lozenges (8 or 12 gm.). All patients taking insulin should carry these lozenges or lumps of sugar with them. Any sweets will serve the same purpose. Cane sugar must be reduced to a monosaccharide before it is absorbed, hence is somewhat slower than glucose in correcting a hypoglycemia. Honey, molasses, syrup, and hard candy are all effective, but if not available other carbohydrate foods may be given if the patient is able to take food by mouth. Fruits, cereals, bread, crackers will correct mild reactions. Often it is only necessary to take a meal a trifle earlier than usual and make suitable changes in the insulin dosage on the following day.

It is dangerous to attempt to feed an unconscious patient. I have seen pneumonia result from the inhalation of food into the lungs during this procedure. If there is no alternative the risk is reduced if the patient is held in a sitting posture and fed slowly with a spoon. Liquids should not be poured into the mouth of an unconscious patient. One or two glucose lozenges* or, lacking these, a lump of sugar placed between the cheeks and teeth will dissolve slowly and be swallowed with little risk.

Dextrose, 20 cc. of a 50 per cent solution in distilled water, is given intravenously without delay to the patient who is unconscious or having convulsions as a result of a hypoglycemia. The recovery from unconsciousness is prompt. Often consciousness is restored before the intravenous injection is completed. Should this measure fail to restore consciousness a continuous intravenous administration of a 10 per cent solution of glucose (dextrose) in distilled water is begun. This latter measure is rarely necessary but in two instances where enormous doses of insulin were taken by mistake, I believe it was life saving. Consciousness having been restored intravenous treatment is no longer necessary, but when the reaction is due to protamine zinc insulin it is a good plan to give 10 or 20 gm. of carbohydrate half-hourly or hourly until the next meal is taken, or until glycosuria is provoked. In this manner one can prevent hypoglycemic reactions due to protamine zinc insulin which are apt to recur because of the continued action of insulin after their temporary correction. A recurrence of the reaction is not likely when the hypoglycemia follows overdosage with crystalline insulin.

If sterile glucose is unobtainable and if feedings by mouth are not practical, carbohydrate in liquid form may be administered *via* a tube passed through one nasal passage and into the stomach. The withdrawal of fluid

* Glucose lozenges of different flavors, each weighing 2 gm., are available.

which turns blue litmus red is proof that the tube is in the stomach and not in a bronchus. This precautionary test should always be made. Retention of food in the stomach may prevent absorption of carbohydrate, hence too much reliance should not be placed on oral or tube feedings if there is not a prompt (within ten or fifteen minutes), satisfactory clinical response.

The hypoglycemic individual absorbs considerable glucose if it is administered by rectum. Twenty grams of glucose or corn syrup dissolved in eight ounces of warm water and given by the Murphy drip or intermittent methods have served well in emergencies on several occasions when instructions regarding treatment had to be given to the patient's relatives by long distance communication.

Epinephrine, 0.5 to 1.0 cc. of a 1 in 1000 solution, given subcutaneously may cause a return of consciousness and allow food to be taken by mouth. It operates by liberating glucose from liver glycogen. Little effect can be expected from epinephrine in the emaciated patient or in the patient who has a severe reaction from protamine zinc insulin in which the liver glycogen is heavily drawn upon before symptoms of a hypoglycemia appear. Epinephrine is most effective in the well-nourished patient and when the hypoglycemia is the result of an overdose of a rapidly acting insulin, unmodified or crystalline. The effect of the epinephrine in any case is only transitory. It should never be relied upon alone but should be supported by the administration of food.

DIABETIC IDENTIFICATION CARD.—Every diabetic patient taking insulin should carry an appropriate identification card. Such a card, I am convinced, saved the lives of at least two of my patients and saved S. H. (see p. 778) from a sojourn in a prison cell. The cards employed at the Pennsylvania Hospital clinic carry the following information.

I HAVE DIABETES AND TAKE INSULIN

If I am found ill, unconscious or behaving unnaturally:
Place a candy or lump of sugar between my cheeks and
teeth, or feed me orange juice slowly
If not improved in *15 minutes*
take or send me to a hospital or notify my physician.

My name is ....

Address ....Telephone ....

My physician is ....

Address ....Telephone ....

Prevention of Insulin Reactions (Hypoglycemia).—A recurrence of an insulin reaction may be prevented by reducing the insulin on the day following a reaction and on succeeding days. If the reaction occurs before breakfast the protamine zinc insulin should be reduced by 2 to 8 units; if it occurs before lunch the morning dose of crystalline insulin is responsible and should be reduced by 2 to 8 units thereafter; if the reaction occurs in the late evening the dose of crystalline insulin given before supper should be reduced by a similar amount.

It is not wise to reduce the insulin dosage without determining the cause of the reaction. Should the hypoglycemia have followed unusual exercise, an omitted meal or vomiting, no reduction is indicated on the following day if normal conditions are restored.

Insulin reactions may be prevented in the following ways:

1. A small reduction of the insulin dosage, of 2 to 8 units, is made when unusual and strenuous exercise is planned. When the usual amount of insulin has been injected and extra exercise is taken a moderate addition to the usual diet such as a banana, a glass of milk or a glass of orange juice is advisable. A regular daily plan of exercise, uniform in time and amount, will reduce the likelihood of reactions.

2. In event of vomiting the amount of insulin is reduced to one-half the usual requirement if there is no glycosuria, keeping in mind that even if food is not ingested metabolism of the body tissues continues. Rarely indeed should a dose be completely omitted, though this is a common (and dangerous) practice. Each specimen of urine is examined separately and if heavy glycosuria should occur more insulin is given. This plan is also adopted in case of diarrhea. Close supervision of the diabetic patient who is vomiting or has diarrhea is essential as in one patient they may cause hypoglycemic reactions and in another ketosis. In case of vomiting food by mouth should be stopped. Nourishment in the form of a 10 per cent solution of glucose (dextrose) in normal saline may be given by vein, one liter every six hours. Crystalline insulin is given at four- or six-hour intervals (p. 828). In case of diarrhea, bland foods and those which tend to cause constipation are allowed though intravenous therapy may be needed in severe cases.

3. Appropriate reductions are made in the insulin dosage after the diabetes is brought under control. A gain in carbohydrate and total food tolerance occurs at this time and the need for insulin decreases proportionately. A decrease of four to eight units a day until glycosuria occurs is a good practice. At this point a small increase in the amount of insulin given will usually suffice to adequately control the diabetes. Greater reductions should follow the reduction in body weight and eradication of ketosis, infections and toxemia.

4. Increasing the insulin too rapidly is a cause of reactions which is easily avoided. The increases in the amount of insulin given should be small —2 or 4 units daily—as control of the diabetes is approached.

5. The timing and distribution of the insulin is arranged according to the plan presented on page 773. It is especially important, when a rapidly-acting insulin and protamine zinc insulin are given before breakfast, that the meal be not delayed more than fifteen minutes after the insulins are administered. The same is true of the evening meal if a dose of crystalline insulin is given before the meal. This precaution is necessary because of the presence of a combined action of protamine zinc insulin and crystalline insulin at the end of a considerable period without food.

6. The likelihood that reactions will occur before lunch is reduced, in the patient susceptible to reactions, by taking part of the lunch—the fruit or milk—at 10:30 or 11 A.M. Similarly the likelihood of early morning hypoglycemic reactions is greatly reduced by saving a part of the evening meal and taking it at bedtime. When globin insulin is employed, a banana,

deducted from the evening meal, taken at 3 P.M., aids in preventing late afternoon reactions.

7. A small reduction—four to twelve units—of the insulin dosage when the patient is discharged from the hospital is a wise precaution to offset the effect which the increased exercise has in precipitating low blood sugar levels.

Allergic Reactions to Insulin.—Local reactions about the site of the insulin injection, believed to be allergic, are manifested by swelling, redness, discomfort, and itching. They are common when protamine zinc insulin is used and unusual when the rapidly-acting insulins are given. Swollen and indurated areas about an inch or an inch and a half in diameter appear and become hot and tender. These local reactions first appear from six to twelve hours after the injection is given. The reaction is at its height from eighteen to twenty-four hours, after which the inflammatory reaction and the swelling gradually subside until there is no trace of them in three or four days. In the sensitive patient, there may be three or four of these "areas" in the various stages of progression and regression at one time. Fortunately within three or four weeks desensitization usually occurs spontaneously. However, should reactions of this nature continue even with crystalline insulin it may suffice to merely use the same product but from a different pharmaceutical firm.

The severity of the local reactions or their continued appearance after a month of treatment may make a change to another brand of insulin imperative.* The change may be from protamine zinc insulin to unmodified insulin or to crystalline insulin. Should these measures be of no avail insulin prepared from beef pancreases may be secured. Allergic reactions to this brand are fewer than when insulin of pork origin is used, though occasionally a patient is sensitive to beef and not to pork insulin. Allergic reactions are least likely to occur following the injection of crystalline insulin.

Generalized urticaria or constitutional reactions, especially edema of the face and mucous membranes, dyspnea, prostration, gastro-intestinal symptoms and stiffness of joints following insulin administration are uncommon but present a genuine problem when they occur. These reactions as well as the persistence of severe local reactions are dealt with by the immediate subcutaneous injection of epinephrine, 0.5 cc. (8 minims) of 1 in 1000 solution, followed by the oral administration of ephedrine sulfate, 0.024 gm. (grains ⅜) and calcium lactate, 0.325 gm. (grains 5) three times daily, and systematic desensitization is undertaken. Rapid desensitization as done by Bayer[60] by injecting, intradermally, minute amounts of the insulin at ten- or fifteen-minute intervals has proved satisfactory in my experience. Increases are made from the initial dose of ⅟₁₀₀₀ of a unit to ⅟₅₀₀, to ⅟₂₅₀, and so on until the dose reaches one unit. If no wheal develops subcutaneous doses may be started.

Roth and Rynearson[61] have desensitized their patients by giving histamine acid phosphate in doses of 0.05 mg. twice daily for two days and 0.075 mg. twice daily on the third and 0.1 mg. twice daily for the succeeding ten days.

* Globin insulin (Burroughs and Wellcome), as yet in the experimental stage, has, in my experience with two allergic patients, replaced protamine zinc insulin satisfactorily with a resulting disappearance of the allergic phenomena.

R. G., male, aged sixty-five years, with onset of diabetes in October, 1939, took insulin from January until March, 1940. In August, 1940, insulin was resumed because of a small carbuncle. After nine days the patient developed urticaria, and his face began to swell, especially his lower lip and under his eyes. He was found, by intracutaneous tests, to be sensitive to all available (seven) brands of insulin. He was rapidly and successfully desensitized with crystalline insulin beginning with $\frac{1}{500}$ of a unit in distilled water and doubling the dose at ten-minute intervals, except when a definite wheal formed in which case no increase was made when the next injection was given. This program was continued until, within three hours, it was possible to give 1 unit subcutaneously. A dose of 5 units was then given subcutaneously without ill effect. Treatment with histamine acid phosphate was begun when subcutaneous injections of insulin were resumed. The dose of histamine acid phosphate was 0.025 mg. This amount was given subcutaneously twice daily for two days, then 0.05 mg. twice daily for two days, and 0.1 mg. twice daily for the succeeding ten days.

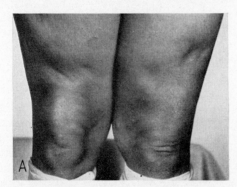 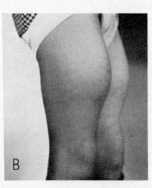

Fig. 142.—*A*, Pitting of the skin caused by atrophy of the subcutaneous fat following many injections of insulin in the same area. (Courtesy of Dr. J. West Mitchell.) *B*, Swelling of the anterior aspect of both thighs caused by hypertrophic changes in the subcutaneous adipose tissue following many injections of insulin in the same areas. (Courtesy of Dr. L. L. Pennock.)

There has been no return of the allergic response probably because he has had (September, 1941) no lapse in the insulin treatment since being desensitized.

A third method of treating allergy to insulin also recommended by Roth and Rynearson is the oral administration of histaminase—the potency of which varies—in doses of 6 to 8 tablets daily. Specialists in the field of allergy do not agree concerning the value of this remedy. I have had no experience with it.

Insulin Tumefactions.—Local painless, indurated areas of fat hypertrophy sometimes occur where insulin is injected in the same area over long periods. The swelling (see Fig. 142, *B*) is "rubbery" to palpation and the skin is adherent to the subcutaneous tissue. Not infrequently the overlying skin is peculiarly insensitive to pain. For this reason patients, especially children, wish to have the insulin injected into this area, but as the induration interferes with absorption of the insulin, this practice should be forbidden.

Treatment consists of changing the site of injection in such a manner that one site will not be used a second time in any fortnight. The swelling gradually subsides. Injections of insulin elsewhere with a more rapid absorption may precipitate hypoglycemic reactions until suitable adjustments in the dosage are made.

Fat Atrophy Due to Insulin.—Every large clinic for the treatment of diabetes has had one or more patients who have developed a pitting of the skin due to fat atrophy at the site of repeated injections of insulin (Fig. 142, *A*). The first case of this nature was reported by Barborka (1926).[62] In the few cases of this complication which I have seen this disfigurement occurred, presumably, because the patients disregarded the advice to vary the sites of injection. These depressions or concavities are due to the disappearance of subcutaneous fatty tissue. They develop slowly over a period of weeks and months. The cause is unknown beyond its direct relationship to injection of insulin too frequently in one area. The condition is not peculiar to the patient with diabetes mellitus, however, as it is occasionally seen after repeated injections of pituitrin in the treatment of diabetes insipidus. Several factors have been blamed, notably faulty technic of administration of insulin, impurities in the alcohol used for sterilizing purposes, the preservative present in insulin, and the low temperature of the insulin when injected.

The cases of fat atrophy complicating insulin therapy which I have seen were in females and all but one were young. The complication is met with in males.

This disfiguring condition is corrected by varying the sites of injection of insulin in such a manner that a site will not be used for injection twice in any fortnight. Furthermore, aseptic technic, the changing of methods of sterilization of syringe and needle from alcohol to boiling, the injection of insulin which has been allowed to reach room temperature, and the use of concentrated insulin, U. 80 or U. 100, may be adopted with benefit. The pitting disappears slowly requiring from two to four months and rarely one to two years to completely subside.

Insulin Edema.—A filling out of the face, giving it a waxy appearance, smooth and free from wrinkling with a reduction of facial expression is seen in some patients following the rapid control of a severe diabetes with insulin. An imbalance in the osmotic pressure between circulatory and tissue fluids caused by withdrawal of glucose from the blood is believed to be responsible. These patients are usually, but not always, young females. A patient seen recently had not only the "insulin facies" but extensive edema of his extremities and disturbance of vision as well, during the first few weeks he received insulin. This patient, M. C., had a complicating xanthoma diabeticorum with a blood cholesterol of 1666 mg. per 100 cc. and a severe diabetes. The water retention probably was exaggerated by the high carbohydrate diet which was allowed.

Ordinarily no special treatment is necessary for this "insulin edema," though in the case referred to above the edema was so extensive that the salt was withdrawn from his diet and for a few days he was given ammonium chloride 1.3 gm. (grains 20) three times daily. Wilder has found the intravenous administration of a solution of calcium lactate effective in these cases.

Presbyopia Due to Insulin.—A transient presbyopia occurs in a considerable number of patients when they receive insulin for the first time. This disturbance is attributed to a reduced elasticity of the lens and is probably the consequence of a disturbance of the adjusted osmotic pressure in the tissue of the lens and circulating fluids. The result is difficulty in focusing vision on nearby objects. The changes are bilateral. The degree of change usually amounts to about 2 diopters but in the young patients, in whom the condition is most troublesome, changes of 8 diopters are sometimes observed. This disturbing complication has occurred in my experience for the most part in young adult patients whereas Wilder[63] states, "This disturbance in vision is much more marked in individuals who are approaching the age of natural presbyopia and whose lenses, because of age, have already lost elasticity."

This disturbance is entirely apart from hypoglycemic reactions and fortunately after two to four weeks of treatment the presbyopia precipitated by insulin therapy disappears entirely.

The patient should be advised that the disturbance is temporary. Glasses purchased at such a time, though satisfactory during the period of presbyopia, would gradually become unsuitable with the restoration of the normal osmotic equilibrium between the lens and ocular fluids. Examinations preparatory to prescribing for glasses should be delayed until at least six weeks have elapsed subsequent to control of the diabetes. The temporary derangement will have disappeared by this time. In isolated instances it may be desirable to overcome this disturbance in vision from the beginning of treatment by securing suitable lenses for temporary use.

EXERCISE

Physical exercise judiciously employed by patients who have no contraindicating conditions is of inestimable value in the treatment of diabetes. It improves the total food and carbohydrate tolerance and reduces the need for insulin. Richardson[64] observed that the blood sugar level was raised by exercise if the fasting level exceeded 300 mg. per 100 cc. and that it was lowered if the fasting blood sugar concentration was below 175 mg. per 100 cc. In the overweight patient having a mild diabetes exercise has two beneficial effects. The first is its insulin-like action in reducing the blood sugar level and the second and more gradual effect is the reduction of body weight. The latter is especially valuable as a supplement to the restricted diet. Exercise speeds the control of the diabetes in the overweight person. This patient quickly learns that glycosuria tends to occur when he is physically inactive and that it subsides when he is active.

In untreated undernourished patients having severe diabetes exercise is not helpful but actually accentuates the wasting processes characteristic of this disease and the blood sugar level is increased instead of lowered. But exercise becomes a helpful instead of a harmful agent in these cases when the diabetes is adequately treated by diet and insulin. Its blood sugar lowering effect is restored and all the advantages that accrue as the result of a good physical condition are added. The decrease in the need for insulin following discharge from the hospital is largely due to the effect of exercise.

How should exercise be prescribed? Unless specific instructions as to time and amount of exercise are given the maximum benefit will not be secured. For the patients for whom exercise would be advantageous a half hour's walk daily is prescribed. The walk should include climbing of hills, grades, or steps; little energy is expended by walking on the level unless it is done briskly. Substitution of various forms of exercise is quite as important as substitutions in the diet. Golf, tennis, badminton, horseback riding, quoits, and gymnastic exercises are satisfactory. Irregularities in time and amount of exercise are permissible for the overweight diabetic person who does not require insulin. For the patient who has severe diabetes and is taking insulin approximately the same amount of exercise at about the same time each day is desirable. Irregularities in exercise call for a reduction in the insulin or an increase in the diet on the days of unusually great exercise and *vice versa*. In general, excessive exercise is contraindicated, since undue fatigue is undesirable.

Patients who use protamine zinc insulin only are free to exercise briskly in the forenoon, afternoon, or evening without risk of a hypoglycemic attack, but when the exercise is excessive it would be well for them to take extra nourishment such as a banana, a glass of orange juice, or a medium-sized apple at bedtime. If the exercise is a part of their daily routine this food may be saved from the evening meal, but if the exercise is "extra" the bedtime nourishment may be added to the usual diet.

Patients who take a dose of protamine zinc and crystalline insulin before breakfast should be cautioned about "extra" exercise in the forenoon because of the likelihood of a reaction occurring before lunch time. An "extra" mid forenoon nourishment is highly desirable if "extra" exercise is indulged in the morning.

Patients who are taking a third dose of insulin (crystalline) before supper may precipitate a severe hypoglycemic reaction during the night by unusually active late afternoon or evening exercise. This is prevented by taking additional nourishment at bedtime, such as a helping of cereal, a banana, a glass of milk, or an orange, or, in case the exercise is planned, a moderate reduction (2 to 6 units) in the evening dose of insulin is permissible.

GENERAL CARE

General care of the patient under treatment for diabetes mellitus embraces his mode and habits of living, diet customs, environment, occupation, vacations, social activities, and personal hygiene. The home conditions of the patients in the diabetic clinic are investigated by the social service workers of the hospital. These workers do a great deal to improve the home conditions of the patient. Instruction in the ordering and preparation of foods is carried out by the dietitians in the food clinic. Public funds may be necessary to secure the proper foods. This is arranged by the social service department through the departments of public assistance.

The habit of securing adequate rest and sleep is quite as important as that of obtaining sufficient exercise. Tobacco used in moderation has no apparent deleterious effect on the diabetic patient, though it is contraindicated if there is disease of the peripheral arteries or if there is a complicating disease of the coronary arteries. Alcohol may be injurious because of the added nourishment it provides. When used temperately and when the food value is allowed for by detracting a like amount from the regular diet it has no serious effect on the diabetes but neither can it be considered beneficial. Patients who require insulin may be exposed to special hazards if they use alcohol (p. 778).

Occupations requiring considerable physical exercise are to be desired over those which are sedentary. The part played by exercise in diabetes has been discussed in the foregoing pages. An occupation which allows the patient to live and eat at home is to be advised in preference to that which entails travelling. Patients with severe diabetes who require large doses of insulin should avoid occupations which necessitate their driving an automobile or working with power-driven machinery.

Social activities bring up innumerable problems. Irregularities in diet and in time of meals are common difficulties. Sensitive individuals may break diet rather than let their friends know they have diabetes. Diabetes is nothing to be ashamed of. Rarely, if ever, can the patient be blamed for having it. It is not infectious. It may be wise to point out to certain patients the illustrious persons who have had and who have diabetes, in order to make them realize that diabetes is no disgrace. It involves sacrifices, truly, but they are not great, and in fact they often prove to be excellent character builders. It is not wise to vary from the general principles of accurate treatment no matter how socially prominent the patient may be. They respect discipline who have little of it, even though they may resent it at first.

Though personal hygiene refers to habits, clothing, and cleanliness, we are particularly interested in the special hygiene made necessary by diabetes. I refer to the care of the feet. This aspect will be dealt with under the section on the prevention of gangrene (p. 801).

The Training of the Patient.—Patients should have a general knowledge of diabetes. Otherwise they give up treatment early and may think themselves cured. They should be instructed regarding the incurability of diabetes and the effect which infection has upon it. They should be taught how to test the urine for sugar, and in some cases acetone, how to prepare, weigh, or measure their food, how to administer insulin, and how to care for their feet. It is important that every diabetic patient be made to realize with what speed acute complications may overtake them. Any indisposition should be regarded by them as possible ketosis.

MISCELLANEOUS FACTORS IN THE TREATMENT OF DIABETES

The Vitamin B Complex.—This complex plays an important part in the intermediary metabolism of carbohydrate. The neuritis which results from vitamin B_1 (thiamine) deficiency is intensified by a high carbohydrate diet. Furthermore lactic acid and pyruvic acid, and methylglyoxal, intermediates in the metabolism of carbohydrate, accumulate in the nerve tissues and elsewhere as a result of this deficiency. Evidence is accumulating that in diabetic patients ample vitamin B complex has some effect on the carbohydrate tolerance and I have observed an apparent economy of insulin in several instances after its administration.

Some believe that diabetic patients need more vitamin B_1 (thiamine) and possibly more of the vitamin B complex than do normal persons.

Thiamine in large doses, 10,000 units once or twice daily, is an effective measure in the treatment of peripheral neuritis in conjunction with the treatment of the diabetes.

Sodium Chloride.—Some moderation of glycosuria, hyperglycemia, and ketonuria has followed the oral and intravenous administrations of large amounts of sodium chloride.[65] The insulin requirement has been reduced and MacClean[66] has observed a correction of a relative insensitiveness to insulin following the administration of sodium chloride. Wilder[67] states concerning the therapeutic use of sodium chloride in the treatment of diabetes, "We have treated successfully a number of patients having a relative insensitivity to insulin, with satisfying results."

The oral administration of innumerable preparations have failed to stand the tests of time and clinical trial. Of these the most recent are synthalin, neosynthalin (guanidine derivatives), plant extracts, of which myrtillin attracted considerable interest, extracts of the duodenal mucosa, dilute hydrochloric acid, and succinic acid.

There is no known remedy which when given orally will control diabetes. Yet there is probably no field more exploited than this one. Improvement which follows the oral administration of any one of the many useless preparations, presumably, is due not to the drug but to the restrictions in diet which are invariably adopted at the same time.

Estrogenic preparations given subcutaneously[68] have some effect in alleviating diabetes (Soskin quoted by Wilder), as has *parathyroid extract.*[69] An extract of the *anterior lobe of the hypophysis* was given by Woodyatt[70] in an attempt to stimulate an antihormone effect. An improvement followed the interruption of the treatment. These measures, while they have some effect and may even hold considerable promise, are strictly in the experimental phase.

Surgery.—There is no known surgical measure which has a specific curative action in the treatment of diabetes mellitus. Yet the condition is often moderated by the surgical correction of acute infections and toxemia. The surgical measures which have been attempted for their possible curative values are: Pancreatic transplants, celiac ganglionectomy, denervation of the adrenal glands, bilateral section of the splanchnic nerves, thyroidectomy, and hypophysectomy. None has proved of abiding clinical value and none is without serious risk.

Roentgen-ray irradiation over the hypophysis, adrenal glands, and thyroid has been tried with unimpressive results. None have proved to have sufficient merit to play a part in the routine treatment of diabetes.

COMPLICATIONS

There are few greater emergencies in the practice of medicine than the acute complications of diabetes mellitus. Three problems confront the physician: *first,* the change in the character of the diabetes as a result of the complications; *second,* the management of the complication, and *third,* the proper evaluation of and the institution of appropriate measures to combat the influence which the diabetes has upon the complication, and *vice versa.*

A fatalistic attitude still exists toward diabetic patients suffering from acute complications. This attitude must be destroyed before these patients will receive adequate treatment. Although it is difficult to instil optimism where pessimism has ruled for centuries, the younger physicians and surgeons have a more effective investigative and therapeutic equipment than their older colleagues had for the management of these patients, hence their therapy is on a more secure footing. This does not mean that conservative judgment is no longer necessary, but it does mean that diabetic patients now, more than ever before, are being given the same opportunities to recover from acute illnesses as nondiabetic patients. It cannot be emphasized too strongly that with the diabetes properly controlled there need be no fear to carry out any procedure which would be indicated if the patient did not suffer from diabetes. It is true that arteriosclerotic heart disease is prevalent in the older diabetic patients and that this complication increases the risk of surgical intervention.

DEGENERATIVE CHANGES

Approximately two-thirds of all cases of diabetes develop in persons over thirty-nine years of age and approximately nine-tenths of the total diabetic population is above this age. It is not surprising, then, that degenerative conditions of all types will be associated frequently with this disease. The lengthening of the life span of diabetic patients brings continually a greater number of these patients to an age which exposes them to causes of degenerative diseases other than diabetes.

The degenerative changes which attract chief attention in diabetic patients are: (1) arteriosclerosis, leading especially to extensive involvement, with occlusive tendencies, of the coronary arteries and of the arteries of the legs and feet, predisposing to gangrene; (2) diabetic retinitis; (3) diabetic cataract, and (4) peripheral neuritis.

ARTERIOSCLEROSIS

Of the four distinct **types** of arteriosclerosis it is the *atheromatosis* and *patchy thickening* of the intima of the larger arteries which predominates in diabetic patients. Lipid material accumulates in thickened intimal cells; the lumen of the vessel is encroached upon, calcification of the atheromatous plaques occurs and later degenerative changes involve the media. Distortion of the intima favors thrombosis. Atherosclerosis in a muscular artery alone or with calcification of the media is strongly suggestive of diabetes.

These atheromatous changes may occur alone or simultaneously with a second type of arteriosclerosis; namely, *Mönckeberg's sclerosis*. This type of sclerosis is less common than atherosclerosis in diabetic patients. The degenerative patchy process, necrosis, and calcification involve the media without lipid invasion, and there is a predilection to involve the muscular arteries of the legs though the characteristic beading of the radial arteries is not uncommon.

A third type of arteriosclerosis characterized by diffuse *arteriolar sclerosis* with hyperthrophy of the media and proliferation of the intima which involves the smaller arterioles may occur coincidentally as a complication of diabetes. An associated arterial hypertension and sclerosis of the retinal and renal vessels is the rule.

The fourth type is *senile arteriosclerosis*, in which there is a diffuse aging of progressive degeneration, a splitting of the internal elastic membrane which is replaced by new fibrous tissue. The degree of fibrosis may be extreme. The cause of arteriosclerosis is not known. Advanced arteriosclerotic changes with a great tendency to atherosclerosis and to occlusion of the lumina of the arteries are more prevalent among the diabetic than among the nondiabetic population of the same age groups. This is especially noticeable in women. It has been predicted that over one-half of the diabetic patients now living in the United States will die of some form of occlusive vascular disease.

Infections, hypercholesterolemia, hyperlipemia, obesity, arterial hypertension, hyperglycemia, differences in diet, individually or combined, have been considered as factors in the etiology and prevalence of arteriosclerosis in diabetic patients. The process in the diabetic patient does not differ pathologically from that seen in the nondiabetic subject, except in the matter of degree and the predilection to involve the coronary arteries and the arteries of the distal extremities. It is significant, however, that there is no direct relationship between the severity of the diabetes and the degree of arterial change. In fact, the greatest degrees of arterial changes are seen in patients having mild diabetes. Wilder[71] believes that obesity has received more emphasis than it deserves and states that "thin patients suffer from gangrene as frequently as do those who are overweight." My experience is in disagreement with this attitude toward obesity. I believe that obesity is of extreme importance in predisposing to degenerative changes in the arteries. Furthermore, though patients may be thin when gangrene develops, the vast majority give a history of having been overweight.

The etiology of arteriosclerosis in diabetic subjects is controversial. It is my impression that neglected mild diabetes in the overweight patient is the most important factor but that additional predisposing influences such as hyperlipemia, hypercholesterolemia, and arterial hypertension may or may not be present.

The following facts are significant: Advanced degrees of arteriosclerosis and the complications which result are becoming steadily more prevalent among the diabetic population. Deaths from these complications have steadily increased during the first four decades of this century, while deaths from diabetic coma have decreased. Arteriosclerosis in diabetic patients predilects to affect the arteries of the heart and of the legs in contrast to cerebral and renal vessels, involved in the nondiabetic patient. The discovery of insulin has contributed to the increasing frequency of arteriosclerosis among diabetic patients because it has permitted them to live longer. Diabetes in some manner hastens the development of arteriosclerosis.

Disease of the Coronary Arteries.—Disease of the heart has been the most common cause of death in adult diabetic patients in the past fourteen years at the Pennsylvania Hospital. Its incidence as a complication of diabetes is increasing. Nathanson[72] found extensive disease of the coronary arteries in forty-one of 100 autopsies on patients with diabetes mellitus. The incidence was 52.7 per cent in those over fifty years of age in contrast to 8 per cent in a large series of nondiabetic patients.

Disease of the coronary arteries occurs in diabetic women with almost the same frequency as it does in men. This is in contrast to the incidence in the general population in which disease of the coronary arteries is five times more common in men than in women.

Vander Veer[73] observed that in the last 100 consecutive cases of infarction of the myocardium resulting from coronary occlusion at the Pennsylvania Hospital, there were eighthy-one men and nineteen women, a ratio of 4 to 1. An analysis of these cases revealed that five of the nineteen women had diabetes. The youngest patient, a diabetic, had her first coronary artery occlusion at forty-four and a second and fatal attack at forty-six years of age. Of four patients fifty years of age or younger, three had suffered from diabetes and the other had a severe long standing hyperpiesia. The other two diabetic patients were aged sixty-five and sixty-nine years. The average age of the female patients was fifty-nine years. Excluding the diabetic patients the average age was sixty-five years.

In Warren's[74] large series of postmortem examinations on diabetic patients death was attributed to cardiac infarction in 16.4 per cent, and 41 per cent of these were in women! It is well established that the incidence of coronary thrombosis with infarction of the heart muscle is unusually frequent in diabetic patients. This is most pronounced in the group of older patients with diabetes, usually mild, who are already in the arteriosclerotic age group.

Wilder[75] emphasizes that it is the advanced arteriosclerotic lesions that are more frequent in the diabetic patient and that actually when all degrees of involvement are considered the incidence of arteriosclerosis is not greater in the diabetic than in the nondiabetic patients.

The essential type of cardiac lesion in the diabetic patient is an atherosclerosis of the coronary arteries. This disorder tends to be progressive and depending upon the degree of involvement there may be periods of temporary ischemia of the ventricular muscle causing attacks of *angina pectoris* or permanent occlusion of a coronary artery. The degree of atherosclerosis of the coronary arteries bears a more direct relationship to the duration than it does to the severity of the diabetes.

Prevention and Treatment of Arteriosclerosis Complicating Diabetes Mellitus.—Until a rational explanation of the increased frequency of arteriosclerosis of an advanced degree in diabetic patients is at hand, the prevention and treatment of this complication must be broad and general.

Careful and constant control of the diabetes is, in my opinion, the most logical and most important measure. In the great majority of patients it is quite a simple matter to prevent glycosuria and even transient and minor degrees of hyperglycemia. In most patients this exactness of treatment will not expose the patient to the danger of hypoglycemic reactions. In fact, the patients having a mild diabetes and who are prone to develop and have arteriosclerosis present less of a problem in maintaining strict control of the diabetes than the patient having a severe diabetes and a small margin of safety between a hyper- and a hypoglycemia. I am convinced, though I cannot prove it, that the restoration of a normal physiological status, inasmuch as hyperglycemia, hypercholesterolemia, and glycosuria are corrected and prevented, is the most powerful factor in preventing and treating arteriosclerosis in the diabetic patient. It is my firm belief that those who encourage glycosuria and a mild degree of hyperglycemia are encouraging the progressiveness of this incurable complication.

The maintenance of normal values for the blood lipid, especially that of cholesterol (155 to 200 mg. per 100 cc.) will do no harm and, as believed by many, it will prove effective in preventing or alleviating the progress of atheromatous degeneration. This end is gained by control of the diabetes and by adding to the carbohydrate and subtracting from the fat contents of the diet until normal values for the blood cholesterol are maintained.

The correction and prevention of obesity are of great value. The ease with which this can be done and the advantages thus gained have been stressed in the foregoing pages. There may be some difficulty in controlling the diabetes, even though mild, unless there is a reduction in weight. Insulin is remarkably ineffective when given to obese patients unless a low caloric diet is employed simultaneously. This aspect has been well supported by Durkin and Fetter[76] in my clinic. A reduction in body weight is valuable also in alleviating the hypertension which is common in the obese diabetic patient.

It is not known what effect *dietary deficiencies* have on the progress of atherosclerotic changes in diabetic patients, but in any event the preliminary and permanent diets should contain *sufficient amounts of vitamins and minerals* and as the body weight reaches the desired level the caloric intake should be increased to prevent undernutrition.

Insulin therapy in patients with known or suspected disease of the arteries should be conducted cautiously. If the diabetes can be controlled without insulin this is the better plan. Insulin is not contraindicated in these cases and it should be used when needed, but care should be exercised to avoid rapid lowering of the blood sugar level. Special care should be taken to prevent hypoglycemic reactions as there is no doubt that they increase the risk of occlusion of the coronary arteries. One physician had the experience of having, in a single fortnight, three patients develop coronary artery occlusions during insulin reactions.

The treatment of cardiac failure is conducted, in addition to measures outlined above, identically as for the nondiabetic patient. Diabetes presents no contraindication to the usual measures employed in the treatment of this complication.

Occlusion of the Coronary Arteries.—Occlusion of the coronary arteries is not a contraindication to insulin therapy. In diabetic patients who previously have needed insulin the requirement is usually temporarily increased. The signs and symptoms of coronary thrombosis in some cases may be masked by the development of ketosis and coma. Great care should be taken in the conduct of treatment to avoid even mild degrees of hypoglycemia. In fact, during the first few days a mild degree of hyperglycemia will do no harm and will increase the margin of safety.

For the patient who has a mild diabetes and occlusion of a coronary artery, a diet similar to that recommended by Master[77] for the treatment of nondiabetic patients is used. It contains approximately 250 gm. of carbohydrate, $\frac{2}{3}$ gm. of protein per Kg. of body weight, and sufficient fat to bring the total calories to 16 per Kg. For patients with a more severe diabetes where control of the diabetes may be difficult, the use of equally-divided and equally-spaced feedings with the same amount of rapidly-acting insulin given before each feeding is best employed (see p. 828). This regimen is a very effective and safe means of controlling severe diabetes in the presence of acute complications, whether surgical or medical in type.

Absolute rest and adequate sedation are important in the treatment of a patient suffering from a recent occlusion of a coronary artery. The period of absolute rest in bed depends upon the extent of the infarction but is usually six weeks or more. Morphia is employed early in dealing with this complication in doses of 0.016 gm. (¼ grain) or even 0.032 gm. (½ grain) or more to allay the initial pain. This is followed by phenobarbital in doses of 0.065 gm. (1 grain) or less four times a day. Aminophyllin (N. N. R.), a combination of theophylline and ethylenediamine, 0.2 gm. (3 grains) three times daily is widely used. Effort at defecation should be avoided. Mineral oil, 15 cc. (½ ounce) each evening before retiring will aid in this respect.

GANGRENE

Gangrene is a local death of tissue following obstruction of the circulation to the part. As seen in diabetes it occurs on the basis of arteriosclerosis and may affect any part of the body, though the lower extremities, especially the toes and heels, are most often affected. Intermittent claudication is a frequent precursor of gangrene.

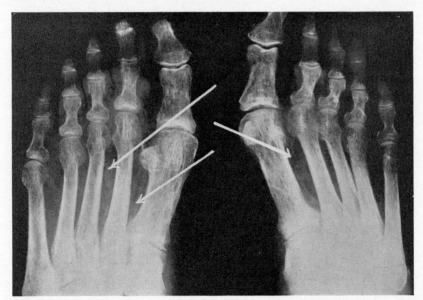

Fig. 143.—Roentgenogram depicting extensive calcification of the small arteries in the feet and the demineralization of the bones of a diabetic patient aged seventy-two years.

Gangrene is one of the most common and one of the most serious complications of diabetes mellitus. It occurs for the most part in patients with mild diabetes and in those who are over forty years of age.

Pathogenesis.—The progressive encroachment on the lumen of an artery by the atheromatous thickening of the intima reduces the circulation to the extremity. Deposits of calcium in the atheromatous areas follow and it is common to find extensive calcification which permits complete delineation of an artery by roentgen-ray photography (see Fig. 143). The development of a collateral circulation is stimulated and between the waning blood supply from the main artery and the function taken on by the collateral vessels the circulation is adequate for the ordinary needs of the limb. A sudden increase in the demands made upon the circulation may follow injury by trauma, burn, undue exercise, or infection, and make apparent the inadequacy of the makeshift circulation. There is an insufficient blood supply to maintain the life of the tissues and too much to allow mummification. A wet necrosis ensues. A secondary infection, which tends to spread rapidly usually follows, creating the danger of a general sepsis. An extensive lymphangitis is the rule. This is the most common type of gangrene, and most to be feared.

A "dry" type of gangrene occurs when the arterial occlusion develops rapidly and there is little or no time for the development of a collateral circulation. The gangrenous area becomes completely devoid of an arterial supply and as a result mummification with a sharp line of demarcation develops. This is spoken of as arteriosclerotic or senile gangrene.

Embolic or thrombotic gangrene is not related to diabetes, though the distortion of the intima by the atherosclerotic processes predisposes to thrombosis. The onset is sudden with severe pain, and gangrene appears quickly. There is no opportunity for the development of a collateral circulation, hence the gangrene is of the "dry" type. The extent of the involvement depends upon the size of the artery and the site of the occlusion.

Causes.—The part played by arteriosclerosis as a predisposing cause of gangrene has already been discussed. Its importance cannot be overemphasized. Without it diabetic gangrene would not occur.

Age is a factor. The incidence of gangrene in diabetic patients increases with each decade of life after forty years. Of Joslin's[78] patients in whom diabetes developed after seventy years of age one in seven also developed gangrene. The frequency of gangrene was just half as great when the onset of the diabetes was in the sixties. As to *sex*, gangrene affects the male slightly more often than the female. In Joslin's hospital series 215 males and 197 females suffered from gangrene. More cases of gangrene are seen during the winter than during the summer season. Feet with impaired circulation are more sensitive to injury from low temperatures. Actual frost-bite is especially dangerous. Concerning *uncleanliness*, there can be no doubt that infection and subsequent gangrene are more prone to develop in dirty than in clean feet.

Hyperglycemia and Hypercholesterolemia.—There is disagreement about the effect of hyperglycemia as a predisposing cause of gangrene. Allen insists on a normal blood sugar as the surest means of preventing diabetic gangrene. Rabinowitch believes that normal levels for blood cholesterol and blood fats are more important. It is my impression that both play a part and that a safe and simple means of prophylaxis at our disposal is the maintenance of both normal blood sugar and cholesterol values. I have no fear in reducing the blood sugar of arteriosclerotic patients to normal and keeping it there, provided the reduction is made gradually over a period of several weeks, and provided that there is ample carbohydrate (150 to 200 gm.) in the diet. I do not subscribe to the belief that mild or moderate degrees of hyperglycemia are beneficial to these patients. On the contrary, I believe they are distinctly harmful in contributing to the progressiveness of the degenerative changes. It is my impression (and admittedly one difficult to prove) that mild diabetes if neglected causes a

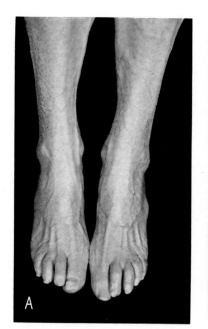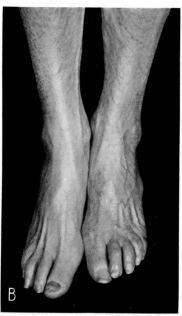

Fig. 144.—Photographs illustrating the blanching test in a diabetic patient with extensive disease of the arteries of the extremities. Both limbs, *A*, were allowed to become cyanotic in the dependent position. The patient's right leg was then elevated until it blanched, which required about one minute. The blanched limb was then lowered and a photograph, *B*, was taken immediately to depict the contrast between the cyanosed and blanched limb.

higher incidence of advanced degrees of arteriosclerosis than if normal blood sugar and cholesterol levels are maintained.

Exciting Causes of Gangrene.—Injury is the exciting cause of diabetic gangrene. This may be in the form of *trauma* from a direct blow, stubbing toe, ill fitting shoes, nail in shoe, carelessly treated corn or callus, or it may follow exposure to *extremes of temperature*, excessive heat or cold. Hot water bottles, electric pads, diathermy treatments, and the use of excessively hot water in bathing each contribute their quotas as causes of gangrene. Failure to wear warm hose in very cold weather is also a factor. The injury may be from *irritating local applications*, especially tincture of iodine, solutions of bichloride of mercury, carbolic acid, medicated ointments, and patent corn removers.

Finally, and among the most important, is *infection*. Infection tips the balance, making inadequate a circulation which hitherto had been adequate. The two great influences contributing to the admission of pyogenic organisms to the tissues are uncleanliness and the presence of an epidermophytosis of the feet. These features will be dealt with in greater detail under Prevention of Gangrene (p. 801).

Estimating the Circulation in the Feet.—In evaluating the circulation of a leg or foot, reliance cannot be made on any single test. Clinical evaluation by all the means at our disposal is desirable.

A history of fatigue and of cramps in the legs, pain, coldness, numbness, and tingling or burning sensations in the extremities singly or combined may suggest the presence of an inadequate blood supply to the extremity. The effect of exercise in provoking intermittent claudication or pain in the feet, caused by placing the legs in a dependent position and relieved by walking slowly or elevating the limbs, suggests extensive vascular damage.

The *physical examination* of the patient should be thorough. Evidence of vascular disease elsewhere, especially in the retinal vessels, heart, and kidneys, may influence the conduct of treatment. Examination of the affected limb should be no less thorough.

A foot has a good circulation if it has good color, does not become cyanotic when placed in a dependent position, has a good pulsation in the dorsalis pedis and in the posterior tibial arteries, and is warm to the touch.

A foot has a grossly impaired circulation if it becomes cyanotic when allowed to hang vertically over the edge of the bed; if it blanches promptly when elevated above the level of the patient's body, when the patient is in the recumbent posture, and if it is persistently cold to the touch with no palpable pulsation in the dorsalis pedis and posterior tibial arteries. The pulsation of the popliteal artery may have disappeared. The effect of the blanching test is presented in Fig. 144. Atrophy of the muscles of the leg is a common sequela of impaired circulation.

It is not unusual to find a foot which is warmed by a good collateral circulation yet in which the pulsations of the dorsalis pedis and posterior tibial arteries are absent. On the other hand the capillary circulation may be gravely impaired with coldness of the foot persisting in spite of good pulsations in these vessels.

Special Tests.—Special tests are usually unnecessary. Good clinical judgment is more reliable but for the sake of completeness and for the few cases in which they may exert a deciding influence, they are included.

Histamine Flare.—Histamine in dilute solution when inoculated into the skin causes, within two and one-half to ten minutes under normal conditions, (1) a dilatation of the capillaries at the site of injection, (2) a surrounding zone of erythema (flare), and, (3) an elevated and palpable wheal due to an exudation of plasma from the capillaries into the skin. This reaction was observed by Lewis,[79] who also found that the reaction was influenced by a reduced arterial blood supply. Starr[80] observed that in the occlusive vascular disease, of the type which may complicate diabetes, the reaction was impaired and in advanced cases the reaction failed to appear within ten minutes after the inoculation of the histamine.

The test for the level of impaired circulation in the recumbent diabetic patient is conducted as follows: After cleansing the selected areas with alcohol, and allowing to dry, one drop of histamine acid phosphate solution (1:1000 preserved by 0.5 per cent chloretone) is placed on the dorsum

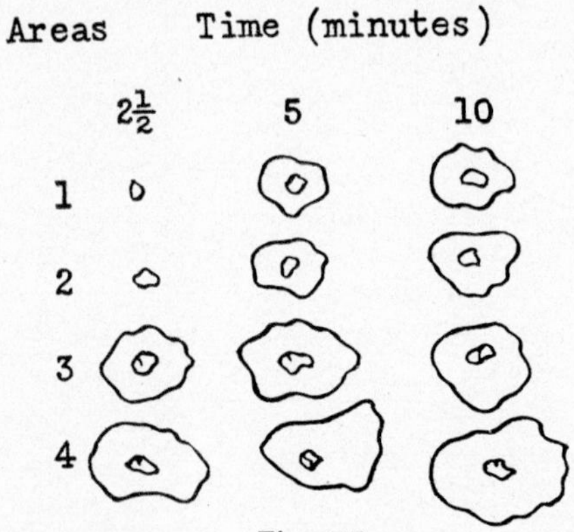

Fig. 145. 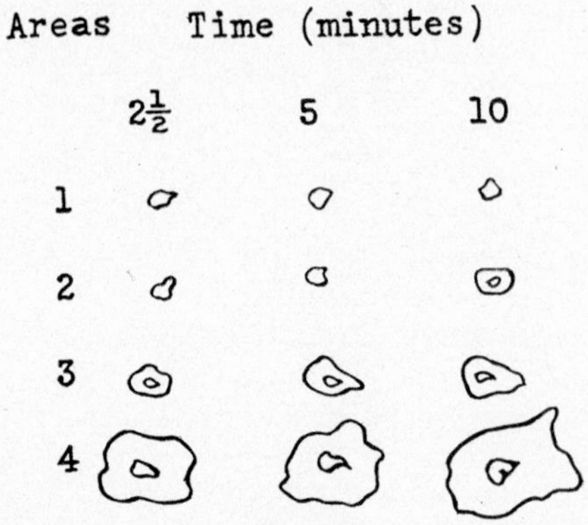   Fig. 146.

Fig. 145.—A normal response to intracutaneous inoculation with histamine acid phosphate.

Fig. 146.—An abnormal response to histamine flare tests. No flare or palpable wheal appeared in area 1, dorsum of foot, a flare delayed in appearance and abnormally small appeared in area 2, above the ankle. There is a moderate reaction below and a normal reaction above the knee. These results indicate a good circulation above and an impaired circulation below the knee with extreme degree of vascular occlusion below the ankle.

of the foot, area 1, another on the leg approximately three inches above the external malleolus, area 2, another about the same distance below the knee (lateral aspect), area 3, and one the same distince above the patella, area 4. Multiple pricks into the skin with a fine needle are made through each drop of solution without drawing blood.

Interpretation.—The results of the tests are read after ten minutes have elapsed. The development of a palpable wheal with a flare (zone of erythema) appearing in about two and one-half minutes with maximum development at ten minutes is a normal response, as illustrated in figure 145. The erythema or flare may be lacking in an otherwise reliable test, but an area of pallor without a palpable wheal should be considered abnormal.

A diminished wheal response (see Fig. 146) indicates an impaired supply of arterial blood to the part and when no wheal develops within ten minutes there is an extreme degree of vascular occlusion. The response may become normal with the establishment of a good collateral circulation.

This test is an aid in determining the degree and extent of vascular disease in the extremities of diabetic patients. As such, occasionally it may be of some assistance in determining the site of amputation.

Intradermal Saline Wheal Test.—Under normal conditions a wheal produced by injecting 0.2 cc. of 0.85 per cent salt solution intradermally remains for an hour or more.[81, 82] In advanced occlusive vascular disease the wheal becomes impalpable and disappears in five or ten minutes. This test has no advantages over the histamine flare test and carries more discomfort for the patient.

Dermatherm.—The dermatherm* permits the determination of the temperature of the skin at any point. This information is especially valuable in

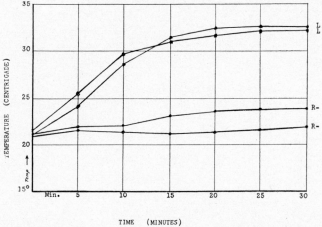

TIME (MINUTES)

Fig. 147.—Skin temperature vasodilation test. Immersion of upper extremities in water bath 44° C. (111.2° F.) caused no appreciable rise in skin temperature of toes of right foot as recorded by the dermotherm, whereas there was almost an immediate rise in skin temperature of the toes of the left foot. This would indicate that the symptoms in the right leg are due to organic occlusion of the peripheral arterioles and that symptoms in the left leg are due to spastic vasoconstriction. (Test performed on H. W., by Dr. M. Sackey.)

differentiating between organic and spastic arterial occlusion. The temperature of the skin over the tips of the toes, the dorsum of the affected foot and various other levels are taken, the patient having been in a room the temperature of which is approximately 20° C. (68° F.) for one-half hour. These readings are recorded and compared with those taken one hour after both arms and hands have been immersed in hot water, 43 to 45° C. This technic, as advocated by Gibbon and Landis,[83] causes a definite reflex vasodilatation and a rise in temperature in the distal extremities from a normal temperature of about 24.7° C. on the toe and 30.2° C. on the sole of the foot, to 33.5 or 34.5° C. if the vascular supply is normal or if occlusion has been due to vascular spasm (Fig. 147). There is little or no rise in the skin temperature of the feet in the event of an advanced occlusion of the arteries due to organic changes. This test is especially desirable if a

* Manufactured by the Taylor Instrument Company.

26

periarterial sympathectomy is considered. It identifies the vascular spastic type of occlusion in which the operation holds promise of success in contra-distinction to the organic occlusive vascular disease, in which sympath-ectomy would be not only valueless but dangerous. Satisfactory evaluation of the alterations in circulation is obtained without the more radical nerve-blocking procedures, notably spinal anesthesia or injection of the peroneal nerve with a solution of procaine hydrochloride. For more detailed infor-mation regarding this test the reader is referred to a recent publication by Kramer.[84]

Plantar Ischemia Test.—This simple test is an outgrowth from the ob-servations made by Parkes-Weber[85] in which he noted blanching of the feet following exercise in patients with circulatory disease of the extremi-ties. These observations were incorporated into a test (Samuels[86]) in which the patient in the reclining position elevates a foot or feet at an angle of 90 degrees. He is instructed to flex and extend his feet and toes rapidly for one minute. If the circulation of the extremities is normal, very little alteration in color occurs but in event of advanced occlusive vascular disease an alabaster-like pallor of the plantar surface of the foot results. The same principles are involved as in the blanching test outlined and illustrated in Fig. 144.

Roentgenography.—Roentgen-ray examinations of the extremities are of value in identifying the extent of calcification of the arteries (see Fig. 143). In one of my patients it was obvious by this examination that extensive calcification of the arteries ceased four inches above the knee. This infor-mation aided in deciding upon the site of amputation. This method of examination also gives valuable information concerning demineralization of the bones of the affected extremity.

Roentgen-ray examination may be misleading unless one is aware that it gives no information concerning the collateral circulation, inflammatory changes in the arteries or vascular occlusion when there is no calcification of the arterial walls.

Arteriography.—We have not employed this method of studying the circulation in the extremities of diabetic subjects. It seems to carry a need-less risk and I doubt very much if it adds to the information secured by simpler measures. The method, as employed by Pearse and Warren,[87] comprises the rapid injection of 15 or 20 cc. of a radiopaque material, such as a 20 to 24 per cent of colloidal thorium dioxide into the femoral artery and a roentgen-ray film is taken of the distal extremity after three seconds have elapsed.

Oscillometric Readings.—The oscillometer is an instrument which per-mits the recording of the magnitude of pulsation in the larger arteries at various levels in the extremities. The value of this instrument has been dis-cussed by Samuels.[88] Its usefulness in studying the diabetic patient is lim-ited. The progression or regression of arterial occlusion may be measured and recorded by a recording oscillometer or sphygmotonometer. The instrument is of no value in determining the efficiency of the collateral circulation and may therefore mislead. For instance, there may be no pul-sation recorded by the oscillometer, indicating extensive occlusive vascular disease, yet the limb may be warm and the circulation may be actually good by virtue of an efficient collateral circulation.

Symptoms and Diagnosis of Gangrene.—Premonitory symptoms are usually present before the development of gangrene. Coldness of the extremities, fatigue with cramps in the muscles of the legs following exercise (intermittent claudication), a sensation of numbness and burning in the foot, singly or combined, usually antedate the onset of gangree. Discrete reddish areas which later become pigmented, wine-colored cyanosis of the feet in the dependent position with cadaveric pallor when elevated and shiny reddish and somewhat swollen toes are common signs which precede actual gangrene.

Following some minor injury vesicles may appear as the first sign of gangrene. Blebs on the foot of an adult diabetic patient should be viewed with concern. They appear innocent at first but their true nature is apparent when the underlying tissues become discolored as necrosis progresses. Bluish-gray discoloration of the skin may be the first sign of gangrene. The gangrene extends until it is bounded by areas fertile in arterial blood. Relatively painless demarcation and mummification may ensue and the affected areas become hard, shrivelled and black. More often, however, a secondary infection causes local inflammatory changes with an extensive lymphangitis. Constant pain, frequently burning in character, is the rule. Lacking appropriate treatment generalized sepsis and ketosis with the associated signs and symptoms of toxemia may appear with remarkable rapidity.

Prevention of Diabetic Gangrene.—The prevention of gangrene is confined in a broad sense to control of the diabetes (p. 751) and special care of the extremities.

It is, I believe, largely attributable to the measures outlined here and to the training of our patients that between 1932 and 1941 only two patients from the diabetic clinic at the Pennsylvania Hospital have required major amputations.

Printed instructions, as follow, regarding the care of the feet should be given to each diabetic patient over thirty-five years of age.

CARE OF THE FEET IS EXTREMELY IMPORTANT

A. Cleanliness.

1. Wash feet with warm (not hot or cold) water and a bland soap each evening, rinse until free of soap, dry thoroughly but very gently between toes, then rub feet gently with "rubbing alcohol." If the skin is dry, toilet lanolin or cocoa butter should be applied two or three times weekly.
2. Clean under toe nails with an orangewood stick.
3. Wear clean hose, loosely fitting and without seams or wrinkling, every day.
4. Insert lamb's wool between overlapping toes.

B. Avoid Injuries to Feet.

Toe Nails.—Cut nails only with scissors or nail clipper, never with a knife, and only after a foot bath and an alcohol rub, and in a good light. The nails should be cut straight across and should not be shorter than the end of the toe. If the nail edges are injuring the flesh they may be raised by inserting a small wedge of cotton, soaked in alcohol, under the corners of the nail.

Shoes.—Shoes should be made preferably of soft leather, with a smooth lining, snugly fitting over the instep, and allowing plenty of play for the toes. Pointed shoes and a loose-fitting heel are dangerous and should be avoided. New shoes should be broken in gradually; they should be worn not more than two hours per day at first.

Put bedroom shoes on before stepping from the bed. Adult diabetic patients should never go barefoot, even in their bedrooms. Many injuries to the feet occur by neglecting this precautionary measure.

Corns are caused by ill-fitting shoes. They are corrected by relieving pressure over the affected area. Properly fitting shoes are most important and protective corn pads (nonmedicated) will bring comfort. Further treatment should be conducted by an accredited chiropodist. Cutting or filing of corns, or their treatment with medicated pads should never be carried out by the patient. Minute injuries, apparently innocent at the time, have cost patients limbs and lives.

Calluses may be corrected by corrective shoes and by soaking the feet in warm (not hot) soapy water for twenty minutes each evening.

Temperature Changes.—The feet should not be exposed to the extremes of temperature. Very hot or very cold water, hot water bottles, electric heating pads, foot cradles which are not thermoregulated, low temperatures, and actual frost-bite are among the more common dangers in this regard.

Feet with impaired circulation often lose the normal sensitiveness to heat and cold, hence far-reaching injury may follow thermal changes which at the time caused no discomfort. Relief of cold feet may be obtained by placing them in a thermoregulated heat cradle set at approximately 32° C. (89.6° F.) or by wearing loose-fitting woolen socks. Immersing the hands and arms in hot water may aid in warming the feet in cases of vascular spasm. Foot exercises are also effective in warming cold feet.

C. Eradication of Infections.

Antiseptics such as alcohol (75 per cent), hexylresorcinol (S.T. 37), and hydrogen peroxide may be applied to minor abrasions of the skin of the feet. All injuries or infections, even the minor ones, affecting the feet of diabetic patients over thirty-five years of age should be treated by a physician. Many local applications which may be suitable for a normal person may be hazardous for the diabetic patient. Among these are *tincture of iodine,* carbolic acid (phenol), medicated ointments, and bichloride of mercury. Iodine, phenol, and salicylic acid may be used as suggested below but only under the supervision of the physician.

Epidermophytosis is a fungus infection which occurs in approximately 80 per cent of the general population and with greater frequency among diabetic patients. It involves special hazards for the latter by invading impoverished tissues and opening portals of entry for other organisms, notably the Staphylococcus aureus. Epidermophytosis may occur in the form of vesicles or it may give the skin between the toes a parboiled or macerated appearance. It may appear as fissures between, under, or elsewhere on toes or as soft corns, or as a dermatitis which may occur on other parts of the body. A weeping of the affected area is not uncommon. The feet have a foul odor and there is considerable itching of the skin about the areas thus infected.

Identification of the *Epidermophytons* establishes the diagnosis. They are obtained for microscopic identification by placing a surface scraping from the lesion on a slide to which 20 per cent sodium hydroxide is added and allowed to stand for at least one-half hour. They may also be secured by culture. Positive intracutaneous tests may be obtained in susceptible persons.

Prevention and Treatment of Epidermophytosis.—The prevention of epidermophytosis entails avoiding contact of bare feet with floors where the *Epidermophyton* is known to be prevalent, notably in public swimming pools, gymnasiums, clubs, hotels, and in the home where other members of the family are infected with this fungus.

Once cured it is important to avoid reinfection from infected shoes and socks. Prophylaxis is accomplished by dusting the stockings and feet with an antiseptic powder. The following has been found useful:

℞	Thymol	1.0 gm.	gr. xv
	Pulv. alum	20.0 gm.	dr. v
	Pulv. kaolin ....q.s.	100.0 gm.	oz. iii

The *Trichophytons* grow best when there is a mildly alkaline medium, warmth, and moisture. Taking these requisites into consideration a recurrence of the disorder is usually corrected and is readily prevented by (*a*) rinsing the feet in a weak solution of vinegar (1 dram to a quart of warm water), after bathing, and (*b*) drying thoroughly but gently between the toes.

An alternate plan to reduce the danger of reinfection is to immerse the feet in a 0.5 per cent solution of sodium hyposulphite after bathing in public places.

The feet infected with this fungus may be soaked in a solution of 1:4000 potassium permanganate or 1 per cent aqueous solution of aluminum acetate for thirty minutes daily for moist or vesicular lesions. Castellani's paint* is daubed on the exfoliative soft corn or fissured lesions. Roentgen-ray therapy may be resorted to, the amount of exposure being determined by a competent dermatologist or roentgenologist. Overtreatment is to be avoided. This is the chief danger in using proprietary preparations. A vigil must be maintained for any evidence of skin injury by chemical parasiticides. For treatment of the mild form of the infection and for daubing affected areas between the toes after bathing and for several weeks after the infection has apparently subsided, the following prescription is recommended:†

* Castellani's Paint (modified):

    10 cc. Saturated alcoholic solution basic fuchsin
   100 cc. 2 per cent Aqueous solution carbolic acid
     1 gm. Boric acid
     5 cc. Acetone
    10 gm. Resorcin

Directions: To the 10 cc. of alcoholic solution of basic fuchsin, add 100 cc. of 2 per cent carbolic acid solution; filter, then add 1 gm. of boric acid; allow to stand for two hours. Add 5 cc. of acetone; allow to stand for two more hours. Finally add 10 gm. of resorcin. Filter.

† Recommended by Dr. John Ludy in a personal communication.

Potassium iodide	....	2.0 gm.	gr. xxx
Iodine crystals	....	1.0 gm.	gr. xv
Acid salicylic	....	3.0 gm.	gr. xlv
Acid benzoic	....	3.0 gm.	gr. xlv
Acid boric	....	2.5 cc.	gr. xl
Acetone	....	4.0 cc.	dr. i
Alcohol	.... q.s.	120.0 cc.	℥ iv

D. Avoid Constriction of the Lower Extremities.

Patients are instructed to avoid circular garters; stockings should not be "rolled," crossing of the knees should be avoided, and tightly fitting footwear or any form of clothing which might interfere with the circulation of the feet is forbidden.

E. Special Measures for Improving the Circulation of the Feet.

I. Foot Exercises. The patient, in the supine position, may extend the feet, flex and rotate them first laterally and then medially, and continue this sequence for five minutes and then reverse the sequence for another five minutes.

Buerger's[89] passive exercises are also of value in improving the circulation in the feet of the middle aged and elderly diabetic patients. The patient, lying on his back, raises one or both feet at an angle of 45 to 60 degrees, and allows them to rest on an adjustable boards,* until the feet are quite blanched or until the foot becomes painful. This usually requires about one minute if foot exercises are conducted in this position and somewhat longer, up to three minutes, if the feet are passive. The patient then assumes the sitting position with the legs hanging over the edge of the bed until a reactionary hyperemia develops or until pain is experienced in the legs or feet. After two to five minutes in this position a rest period for about three minutes is allowed in the horizontal position. This cycle may be repeated several times daily at first and increased gradually until the exercises last from one-half to one hour daily.

II. Alternate Positive and Negative Pressure to Extremities.[90, 91] The affected limb is placed in a chamber, a "glass boot," properly fitted with rubber cuffs and exposed to alternating positive pressure of 40 to 50 mm. Hg for fifteen seconds and a negative pressure of 80 to 100 mm. Hg for twenty-five seconds. This method of passive vascular exercise is carried on automatically by an electrically driven air pump for one-half to one hour or even longer and repeated daily, two or three times weekly, or once weekly, as indicated.

In my experience this treatment has been of some value for patients suffering from intermittent claudication. It has distinct limitations, however, and should not be used in the presence of extensive or moist gangrene, cellulitis, osteomyelitis or any inflammatory involvement of the arteries, veins or lymphatics. If treatment causes discomfort it should be discontinued.

* A Buerger board which is adjustable to different angles is made simply by having two boards, each ¾ inch thick, 30 inches long and 12 inches wide, hinged at one end, with a supporting prop between, which is adjustable to fit on various cleats according to the angle desired.

III. Intermittent Venous Occlusion. A cuff fitted above the knee is inflated to a pressure of 70 to 80 mm. of Hg obstructing the venous return for one, two or three minutes followed by a like period of release. This treatment, aimed to produce a reactive hyperemia, is continued for one or two hours or longer each day.

Favorable effects on the peripheral circulation of the feet of diabetic patients have been observed.[92] Intermittent claudication has been relieved and chronic ulcers have subsided following a course of these treatments. Intermittent venous occlusion has a broader scope of application than the treatment with intermittent positive and negative pressure, as it may be used in the presence of localized gangrene and open wounds, though its use should be carefully supervised and with any sign of progression of the complication the treatments should be stopped.

IV. Iontophoresis. The introduction of acetyl-β-methylcholine chloride (mecholyl) into the body by iontophoresis causes vasodilatation. Its use may be warranted in the diabetic patient if the impaired peripheral circulation is found to be of a functional or spastic rather than of an organic occlusive type.

The danger of burns makes the treatment a hazardous one unless it is carried out by a skilled personnel. Kramer[93] recommends the treatment as follows, "After extensive use of this form of therapy we feel this procedure is useful because of its vasodilator properties, by overcoming vasospasm and helping to improve the peripheral circulation."

V. Oscillating Bed (Sanders[94, 95]). Postural changes similar to those accomplished by the Buerger exercises are made possible without effort on the part of the patient by the oscillating bed, electrically driven, mechanically controlled, and adjustable to suit the needs of each patient. It has the advantage of allowing continuous passive exercises for days at a time. My experience with this bed is limited but I share the present optimism regarding its beneficial effect in selected patients.

VI. Sympathectomy and Ganglionectomy. Rarely indeed will a periarterial sympathectomy or ganglionectomy be indicated in a diabetic patient. However, should troublesome symptoms persist in spite of all conservative measures and the impaired circulation to the limb prove to be of a spastic nature and not organic in origin, this operation might be considered. It is useless in organic occlusive arterial disease.

Patients with vasospastic occlusions may be helped by the reflex hyperemia of the distal extremities which follows the immersion of hands and arms in hot water. This, on the basis of observations made by Gibbon and Landis,[96] has been recommended as a mode of treatment. Recently I have seen two patients who were helped by this immersion treatment carried out for ten to fifteen minutes night and morning. Electric heating pads wrapped around the arms are equally effective.

Treatment of Diabetic Gangrene.—Consultation with a surgeon who has an abiding interest in diabetic patients and who is skilled in the surgical treatment of these patients is among the first considerations in the treatment of diabetic gangrene.

Diet and insulin therapy for the patient having diabetic gangrene is the same as that for those having acute infections and other surgical complications. They will be dealt with in detail in the section on the management of acute infections and surgical conditions complicating diabetes mellitus.

NONOPERATIVE TREATMENT.—Conservative nonoperative treatment is justifiable when the gangrenous patch is demarcated and superficial, when the feet and toes are warm, when there is a good pulsation over the dorsalis pedis artery, when the extremity retains a normal color on elevation and when in a dependent position, and when there is no evidence of active extension of a complicating secondary infection.

The treatment for these patients comprises: (1) control of the diabetes by means of diet and insulin, (2) eradication of infection by adequate drainage, by slight elevation of the affected limb, and, when indicated, by irrigation with Dakin's solution or one of its substitutes, such as hychlorite or dichloramine-T (2 per cent), having first protected the skin areas as recommended by Farr,[97] by painting with ordinary rubber-tire cement diluted with ether in proportions of 1 to 3. Gangrenous slough is gently excised. Wet dressings should not be used unless a secondary cellulitis is also present.

Improvement of the circulation may be facilitated in patients in the pregangrenous state by foot exercises, passive exercises as in Sanders' oscillating bed or Buerger's exercises, and active foot exercises, alternate positive and negative pressure to the affected limb, intermittent venous occlusion, warmth in thermoregulated cradle 31° to 33° C. (87.8° to 91.4° F.), and possibly iontophoresis. Baking, diathermy, and "vibration treatment" to the extremities of elderly diabetic patients are dangerous and should not be used. All pressure from bed clothing should be taken off the feet by the use of a foot board.

Arteriosclerotic changes are not confined to the legs and feet in the diabetic patient with gangrene of a lower extremity. Thorough consideration should be given to the heart, and especially to the likelihood of disease of the coronary arteries. Retinoscopy will often give the physician a good estimate of the condition of the smaller arteries and veins.

OPERATIVE TREATMENT.—It is not within the realm of this book to go into the surgical technic for the treatment of gangrene of the extremity.* Nevertheless it is important for physicians to be familiar with the indications for surgical intervention.

The usual *indications for amputation* of a leg are: (1) gangrene which fails to localize, involving one or more toes or a toe and the heel in a foot which is cold to the touch and in which there is pain in the elevated or dependent positions, (2) in event of intractable pain the leg or foot with evidence of extensive vascular occlusion (although great care should be taken not to confuse a peripheral neuritis with the pain due to an inefficient vascularity), and (3) deep, extensive and extending infection and especially if osteomyelitis involving the metatarsal bones is present. (A phalanx may be safely and satisfactorily removed if the osteomyelitis is limited to the phalangeal bones.)

Site of Amputation. Individual toes may drop off or may be removed

* For details regarding the surgical aspect of these cases the reader is referred to: McKittrick, L. S., and Root, H. F., Diabetic Surgery, Lea and Febiger, Philadelphia, 1928; also McKittrick, L. S., Surg., Gynec. & Obstet., **68**: 508, 1939, and McKittrick, L. S., Arch. Surg., **40**: 352, 1940.

with a successful outcome. Less common and usually less successful are partial amputations of the foot. The most common site of amputation is in the region of the midthigh.

Careful evaluation of the circulatory deficiency as outlined on pages 797–800 will aid in deciding this important question. In general, midthigh amputations are safest. The operative field is within a well vascularized area and the risk of a second operation is minimal. When partial amputations of the foot are performed the results are less dependable, although they are justified if the patient is not suffering great pain and if the foot is warm, with a good pulsation in the dorsalis pedis artery, and if osteomyelitis does not extend beyond the phalanges and the gangrenous areas and the complicating infections are localized. Amputation of a foot leaves an unsatisfactory stump for weight-bearing. Before one consents to allow the surgeon to amputate the foot or part of the foot it is well to ponder Wilder's[98] statistics—an ultimate mortality of 20 per cent of fifteen cases in which primary amputation through the foot was done, against a mortality of 7 per cent of seventy-one cases in which early and high amputations were done.

The entire obliteration of the circulation of a gangrenous and secondarily infected limb by placing a tourniquet above the knee and the refrigeration of the limb by packing in ice had been recommended as a preoperative measure by Allen.[99] No anesthetic is necessary for the ensuing amputation.

OCULAR COMPLICATIONS

Diabetic Retinitis.—Ophthalmologists frequently make a diagnosis of diabetes on the basis of a characteristic type of retinitis appearing for the most part in the middle-aged and elderly patients with mild but neglected diabetes of long standing. The *pathogenesis* of diabetic retinitis is not clear. It is clear, however, that insulin therapy is in no way responsible for nor does it aggravate the condition. Minute oval punctate hemorrhages appear deep in the retina in the macular region. These hemorrhages have no correlation with arterial hypertension but the hemorrhages are more numerous with diabetes of long duration. Deep retinal hemorrhages are the most characteristic of the retinal abnormalities (see table 18[100]). These hemorrhages are infrequently seen in patients under forty years of age. Shiny or waxy punctate exudates as described by Waite and Beetham[100] are visible in a later stage of diabetic retinitis. Both processes tend to extend involving more and more of the retina. Later the exudates tend to coalesce to form large grayish-white plaques; these are especially prevalent in the macular region. Disturbance in vision ensues. It is not uncommon to find reduced caliber of the arteries and venous engorgement of hyperpiesia and the cotton wool patches of arteriolonephrosclerosis associated with diabetic retinitis.

It is of interest that Waite and Beetham found no greater degree of sclerosis in the retinal arteries of diabetic patients than in the nondiabetic control series. The most serious type of retinitis associated with diabetes is described by Wilder[101]: "Segments of a vein may be ensheathed in a layer of heavy grayish-yellow exudate and other segments may be obliterated. Usually large hemorrhages are also found with this marked disease of the veins and rather commonly hemorrhages occur into the vitreous. As a result of, or as a sequel to the latter, bands of scar tissue form and new vessels proliferate into the vitreous giving rise to a picture of retinitis proliferans, which resembles that described in tuberculosis and syphilis. Contraction of the bands of scar tissue may cause detachment of the retina."

Treatment.—Control of the diabetes aids in preventing the progressive tendency of diabetic retinitis. It is my impression that a liberal quota of carbohydrate, not less than 150 gm. per diem, is of additional value. Insulin is used if necessary. Wilder has had encouraging results following the use of moccasin venom as described by Watkins, which has been found helpful in treating other hemorrhagic states. Ascorbic acid, 200 mg. daily, has been recommended and ophthalmologists favor the use of potassium iodide. Hanum[102] believes vitamin P (citrin) is indicated in view of the lowered capillary resistance in cases of diabetic retinitis.

TABLE 18

RETINAL ABNORMALITIES (WAITE AND BEETHAM)[100]

	Of 3915 Visible Fundi in Diabetic Patients		Of 101 Visible Fundi in Nondiabetic Patients	
	Number	Per Cent	Number	Per Cent
Deep retinal hemorrhages..............	730	18.6	34	3.0
Waxy exudates......................	420	10.7	7	0.7
Nerve fiber layer hemorrhages.........	196	5.0	33	3.0
Cotton wool exudates.................	168	4.3		
Cholesterol crystals..................	28	0.7	35	3.0
Proliferation of capillaries in retina.....	26	0.7	4	0.4

Diabetic Cataract.—Cataracts occur in diabetic patients in two forms. First is the *senile cataract* which occurs in the older patients who have a mild diabetes of long standing. This cataract is identical, clinically, with those appearing in nondiabetic persons. However, Carey and Hunt[103] found on chemical examination three times as much calcium and a lower phosphorus content in cataractous lenses of diabetic than in those of nondiabetic patients. The senile type of cataract was present in approximately 6 per cent of diabetic patients observed by Waite and Beetham.[100] The incidence of senile cataracts increases with the duration of diabetes. The lens opacities are not reversible with control of the diabetes.

The second type, the *true diabetic cataract*, is rare, occurring in less than 0.5 per cent of diabetic patients. It occurs bilaterally and is a rapidly-forming cataract, maturing in a few days. It is seen only in diabetes, and occurs only in young patients (see Juvenile Cataract, p. 903). The subcapsular vacuolar degeneration of the lens characteristic of this type of cataract is often retrogressive with control of the diabetes. This form of cataract has been called the true diabetic cataract by Duke-Elder[104] and has been referred to as "flocculi cataract" by Waite and Beetham.[100]

The *treatment* of the senile cataract in the diabetic patient is identical with that in the nondiabetic subject. The results are equally good. It is believed that hypoglycemic reactions during the postoperative period may precipitate a hemorrhage in the operative field. No harm will come from a mild degree of hyperglycemia during this period and if this will guard against the hazards of hemorrhage it is worth while.

Other Ocular Complications of Diabetes.—Control of the diabetes is the most effective prophylactic measure as well as treatment for the "true diabetic cataract."

Other ocular complications which appear more frequently in the diabetic than in the nondiabetic subjects are: Wrinkling of Descemet's membrane, paresis of accommodation, depigmentation of the epithelial layer of the iris, transitory refractive errors, preretinal hemorrhages with proliferation of vessels and connective tissue, lipemia retinalis, and abnormalities involving the optic tracts. Of these there are: Tobacco amblyopia first stressed in this country by De Schweinitz and Fewell,[105] sector defects, and homonymous hemianopsia. Waite has stressed the susceptibility of older diabetic patients to tobacco and also that improvement following the withdrawal of tobacco was impeded in patients who were in the habit of using alcoholic drinks. That vitamin deficiency may have played a part is suggested by the improvement which followed the administration of thiamine chloride.

DIABETIC PERIPHERAL NEURITIS

Peripheral neuritis is a common complication of diabetes. The disorder affects patients who are over thirty-five years of age and who have uncontrolled, usually mild, and unfortunately, often unrecognized diabetes. It affects the undernourished more frequently than the well-nourished patient and it is notable that there is a greater frequency of disease of the vascular system in these patients. Many of them have associated hemorrhagic lesions in the retina. Neuritis is disabling and tends to become chronic if its true nature is not recognized and appropriately treated. These patients have pain, which may be intense, and tenderness along the course of the affected nerves. Cramps and paresthesia are prominent when the neuritis involves the legs in which the circulation is impaired. It may be difficult to determine to what degree the symptoms are due to neuritis *per se*, and to a deficient circulation. Involvement of the arms cannot be explained on a purely circulatory basis. Numbness and tingling of the hands and feet are complained of, and a burning sensation also may be experienced particularly when the nerves of the legs are involved. Shooting pains along the course of the nerve, weakness of the muscles with an exaggeration of the symptoms on exposure to cold are among the symptoms of which these patients complain.

On examination one notes that the affected limb is spared and protected by the patient, that in chronic cases there is some atrophy of the muscles supplied by the involved nerve, hyperesthesia over the affected area, and exquisite tenderness on deep pressure over the trunk of the affected nerve with a radiation of paresthesia throughout its distribution. Paralysis of groups of muscles, sometimes present, increases the disability. Involvement of the peroneal nerve may result in a "foot-drop." Any group of muscles may be involved—the muscles of the eye, the bladder and rectum may be affected. Paresis occurs much less frequently, however, than sensory disturbances. In case of sciatica the trouble may be bilateral. The tendon reflexes of the affected limb become reduced and often disappear. Trophic ulcers may occur.

Diabetic pseudotabes is a rare complication. It is characterized by the following signs and symptoms: Argyll Robertson pupillary response (absent light reflex but with normal accommodation to distance), urinary incontinence or retention, absence of the patellar reflexes, numbness of the feet, and epigastric pain. Only four such cases were observed in 2000 cases of diabetes reviewed by Waltman and Wilder.[106]

Abnormalities affecting the spinal cord in diabetes may be confused with other disorders. Of these the most important are: subacute combined degeneration of the spinal cord as seen in pernicious anemia, pressure on the cord by new growth, hypertrophy of the ligamenta flava, hernia of the nucleus pulposus and a displaced intervertebral disk.

Pathogenesis.—Diabetic patients suffering from neuritis frequently have extensive disease of the vascular system. Furthermore, the diabetes is usually uncontrolled. Evidences of a deficiency of vitamin B_1 are suggested not only by the neuritis but by the response to treatment with thiamine chloride.

Patchy degeneration occurs in the nerve trunks, especially of the afferent nerves near the periphery and there is a thickening of the nutrient vessels. Waltman and Wilder consider these as the significant lesions in diabetic neuritis. This view is receiving general adoption.

Prognosis.—The changes which occur in diabetic neuritis are not permanent though the symptoms varying from mild discomfort to intractable and severe pain may last for many months. The speed with which recovery is attained depends upon the identification of the disorder, the complete control of the diabetes and upon other measures as outlined below.

Treatment.—Control of the diabetes—fasting blood sugar level below 120 mg. and postcibal levels below 150 mg. per 100 cc.—is usually essential if the other measures employed in the treatment of this disorder are to be effective.

Diets aimed at undernutrition actually exaggerate the symptoms for a short time. The response to treatment has in my experience been facilitated by markedly restricting the allowance of carbohydrate but allowing adequate calories (30 to 35 per Kg. of the normal body weight) by providing a high vitamin content and at the same time employing large doses of thiamine chloride (25 mg. twice a day). Instead of a carbohydrate content of between 200 and 250 gm. in the diet, an allowance of between 100 and 150 gm. is prescribed until relief is secured. The carbohydrate quota is then gradually restored to its former level.

Insulin aids in controlling the diabetes and is employed during an attack of diabetic neuritis even if the diabetes is mild.

During the acute stages of the disorder the patient is kept at rest. Heat to the affected parts is soothing. Exposure to infra-red rays for one-half to one hour twice daily is helpful. The patient's room should be warm, approximately 24° C. (75.2° F.). Codeine sulfate, 0.03 gm. (½ grain), given simultaneously with acetylsalicylic acid, 0.325 gm. (5 grains), is especially valuable and may be used three or four times daily while the pain is severe. Morphine should not be used.

Thiamine chloride is given intramuscularly in large doses; usually 25 mg. twice daily, though in intractable and severe cases improvement seems to be more prompt when this amount is doubled.

The oral administration of sodium chloride, in doses of 30 gm. or more, is worthy of trial as recommended by Sanstead and Beams.[107] I have found it dramatically effective in a few cases in which the neuritis involved the distal extremities and in which there were extensive vascular changes.

Strict interdiction of alcohol is advisable and where there is disease of the vascular system tobacco should be avoided. Splints should be employed in case of footdrop or wristdrop to hold the limb in a normal position.

KETOSIS (DIABETIC COMA)

Coma due to ketosis is a preventable and curable outcome of uncontrolled diabetes. It is an intoxication by accumulated products of intermediary fat (and to a limited extent protein) metabolism in an organism unable to properly utilize carbohydrate. Under normal conditions fat is readily and completely oxidized and the end-products, CO_2 and water, are eliminated. Failing an adequate supply of insulin a corresponding reduction of carbohydrate utilization ensues, and as a result the metabolism of fat and of protein is accentuated to meet the energy requirements. With greater mobilization and catabolism of fat and of protein there is an increased production of ketone bodies by the liver. When the rate of ketogenesis exceeds the rate at which the ketones are oxidized in the tissues ketonemia and ketonuria ensue (see Chapter III). In ketosis the concentration of ketones in the blood exceeds normal and when they reach a relatively low renal threshold they are excreted in the urine as acetone and diacetic acid.

Acetone is the first of the ketone bodies to appear in the urine. These ketones may be lost in small quantities over long periods without apparent harm. The amount of ketones appearing in the urine increases as the ketosis deepens. The last of the ketone bodies to reach the urine is betahydroxybutyric acid. In severe ketosis it is in this form that most of the acids are eliminated, hence its appearance in increasing amounts is a crude index of the gravity of the intoxication. Diacetic acid and betahydroxybutyric acid as such are excreted only by way of the kidneys. The reaction of the urine is acid, but neither this nor the degree of ketonuria is a reliable indication of the severity of the ketosis.

As the oxidation and excretion of ketones fail to keep up with their production they accumulate in great quantities in the blood, and barring treatment, give rise to the characteristic symptoms and physical changes of ketosis leading to unconsciousness and death.

Diabetic ketosis may develop slowly, in which case it is compensated for a considerable time by increased oxidation of ketones up to a certain level, by an increased excretion of acids, by increased ammonia production and neutralization of acids, and by the buffer action of the blood by which the carbon dioxide is displaced from the bicarbonate of the plasma by the ketone bodies. Fixed base, particularly sodium, is lost to the body when the ketosis becomes severe, whether the onset is gradual or rapid. A dehydration and hemoconcentration occur. The onset of ketosis is usually rapid and severe in the young diabetic patient and during acute complicating infections. The compensatory mechanisms are overwhelmed, large quantities of acetone, diacetic acid and finally betahydroxybutyric acid are excreted in the urine, acetone bodies accumulate in the blood and an acetone odor is noted on the breath. The carbon dioxide combining power of the blood plasma is reduced in proportion to the severity of the ketosis. It decreases from the normal of 55 to 65 volumes per cent to 35 volumes per cent in a mild ketosis, to 20 volumes per cent and below in severe ketosis or coma. Joslin[108] has set an arbitrary figure of blood CO_2 at 20 volumes per cent below which the patient can be considered, for comparative statistical purposes, to be in coma. Wilder[109] considers the level of 25 volumes per cent a more suitable dividing point. Strictly speaking, a patient may be in coma—a state of unconsciousness—with a CO_2 combining power of the plasma between 20 and 30 volumes per cent and yet another patient may be mentally lucid with a level of 15 volumes per cent. One of Joslin's patients walked into the hospital and shortly thereafter the CO_2 combining power of his blood was found to be 4 volumes per cent. The fact that this patient died seven hours after admission emphasizes the danger these patients may be in, even though they have not lost consciousness.

TABLE 19

COMPOSITION OF HUMAN BLOOD*

Constituent	Normal Range, mg. per 100 cc.†	In Diabetes
Hemoglobin per cent (Haden)	15.6	Increased in ketosis
Urea N	10–15	Increased in ketosis
Glucose	70–100	Increased
Total fatty acids	290–420	Increased
Cholesterol	150–190	Increased
Lipid phosphorus (lecithin)	12–14	Increased
Total acetone bodies (as acetone)	1.3–2.6	Increased
Acetone aceto-acetic acid (as acetone)	0.3–2.0	Increased
β-hydroxybutyric acid (as acetone)	0.5–3.0	Increased
CO_2 capacity (plasma) vol. per cent	55–75‡	Decreased in ketosis
CO_2 content (arterial blood) vol. per cent	45–55‡	Decreased in ketosis
CO_2 content (venous blood) vol. per cent	50–60‡	Decreased in ketosis
Chlorides as NaCl	450–500	Decreased in ketosis
Sodium (serum)	330	Decreased in ketosis

* Extracted from Hawk and Bergeim's Practical Physiological Chemistry, by courtesy of P. Blakiston's Son and Co.

† Figures express concentration in milligrams per 100 cc. of whole blood unless otherwise indicated in first column.

‡ Figures represent weighted averages of the observations of several investigators.

As the ketosis develops the following outstanding alterations from normal become accentuated: (1) The carbon dioxide combining power of the blood plasma decreases. (2) The continued loss of fixed base which entails a reduction of the sodium chloride and electrolyte concentrations in the body fluids causes a reduction in the alkali reserve, a diuresis, and dehydration. These changes are accentuated by vomiting. (3) Ketonuria and ketonemia. (4) Concentration of the blood ensues and there is a (5) a shift of the hydrogen ion concentration of the blood toward the acid side, and (6) the patient becomes less sensitive to insulin.

It is to these changes that the clinical manifestations of diabetic coma can be attributed. Despite the rapid excretion of the ketone bodies, their production in the body exceeds the rate at which they can be oxidized or excreted. They accumulate in the blood and as the compensatory mechanisms fail Kussmaul breathing, "air hunger," ensues. As the store of fixed base is reduced the ensuing diuresis and dehydration account for the hemoconcentration, the fall in blood pressure, circulatory collapse, the depression of renal activity and the ensuing retention of nitrogen in the blood, and the subnormal temperature.

Incidence.—No better illustration of the beneficial effects of insulin can be had than the reduction in the deaths from ketosis following its discovery. The reduced mortality from ketosis is directly attributable to (1) the improvement in the treatment of diabetes during acute complications, (2) a decreased incidence of diabetic coma attributable to better treatment of the diabetes in general, and (3) to the training of the diabetic patients to recognize danger signs and secure treatment immediately. Joslin[110] has contrasted the death rates from coma in his series in the Naunyn, Allen and Banting eras:

> 1898 to 1914—60.8 per cent of all diabetic deaths were in coma
> 1914 to 1922—42.0 per cent of all diabetic deaths were in coma
> 1930 to 1936— 6.1 per cent of all diabetic deaths were in coma

It is tragic that this splendid improvement has not been nearly equaled throughout this country as a whole. It is tragic that many diabetic patients die of coma without receiving insulin. It is tragic that such a disparity exists between the available scientific knowledge of diabetic ketosis and the application of this knowledge in its treatment.

The unpleasant fact that 18 per cent of deaths of diabetic policyholders of the Metropolitan Life Insurance Company in 1935 were due to diabetic coma emphasizes that too frequently either the diagnosis is not made early enough, or that insulin and other appropriate treatment is not started soon enough or if started is not carried out vigorously enough.

Etiology.—Ketosis is precipitated by: (1) acute infections, (2) omission of insulin, (3) vomiting, (4) diarrhea, (5) prolonged neglect of the diabetes, (6) indiscretions in the diet, (7) surgical operations, (8) pregnancy, (9) thyrotoxicosis, and (10) insensitiveness to insulin.

One young patient omitted her insulin and was beyond aid within eighteen hours. Another on the advice of her physician, I am sorry to say, omitted her insulin because of vomiting. She recovered from a profound coma but for hours the outcome was uncertain.

The pathologic physiology of ketosis has been considered already in this section and also in Chapter III.

Symptoms.—Recognition of the onset of ketosis is not always easy. The onset is so variable that any indisposition in a known diabetic patient should at once suggest the possibility of ketosis.

Ordinarily if there is no complicating infection the patient experiences a gradually increasing fatigue and listlessness. The appetite for food disappears, dryness of the mouth and thirst increase as does the polyuria. Drowsiness with nausea and, later, vomiting with pain in the abdomen (due to dilatation of the stomach in some instances, but most frequently to chloride depletion, and rarely to an acute pancreatitis) occur. The stupor deepens, and the deep breathing of air hunger (Kussmaul's breathing) becomes marked. Complete loss of consciousness with fatal termination results if rescue by treatment is deferred.

This process in uncomplicated and uncontrolled diabetes is a gradual one requiring several days to develop fully. The onset is quite different if an acute infection is present. Recently I saw a girl, seventeen years of age, who had a blood sugar level of 156 mg. per 100 cc. and yet within twenty-four hours, because of multiple staphylococcal infections, she was in diabetic coma with a CO_2 combining power of the blood plasma of 8 volumes per cent and a blood sugar level of 850 mg. per 100 cc.

Large quantities of sugar, diacetic acid and acetone in the urine of a patient showing the progress of events outlined above give sufficient evidence to make a tentative diagnosis of diabetic coma. Treatment should be started at once and modified later as indicated by further chemical analyses. The blood sugar level is high, usually between 400 and 800 mg. per 100 cc., but what is of more importance is the fall in carbon dioxide combining power of the blood, which in coma is below 20 volumes per cent. Tests for acetone and diacetic acid in the blood plasma or serum are also positive. This test (the Rothera-Wishart test) is especially valuable because it remains positive even if the carbon dioxide combining power of the plasma is artificially increased by large doses of alkali. A decreasing plasma acetone content is an index of genuine improvement and its disappearance means that the patient is out of immediate danger from the ketosis *per se*.

Other concomitant findings in diabetic coma are: high specific gravity of the urine, albuminuria usually with showers of hyaline or granular casts, a high cholesterol content of the blood, a lipemia, a low sodium chloride value, and a leukocytosis. The values may vary from 12,000 to 60,000 leukocytes per cu. mm. The cause of the leukocytosis is frequently unexplained. The retention of nitrogen in the blood which is doubtless due to a low filtration pressure in the kidneys disappears with the treatment of the ketosis except when a coincidental true diffuse glomerular nephritis exists. Examination of the blood reveals a high red cell count, usually above 5,000,000 erythrocytes per cu. mm. which is attributable to hemoconcentration.

Physical Findings.—The patient in diabetic coma appears desperately ill. The cheeks are flushed. Air hunger, as evidenced by an increased rate and depth of respirations, is pronounced. Replacement of this Kussmaul breathing by feeble, rapid, and gasping respirations is an ominous sign. The sweetish odor of acetone is noted on the breath. It may in fact permeate the patient's room. General dehydration is pronounced. The skin is dry. *The skin of a patient in diabetic coma is always dry.* This is important in differentiating coma due to ketosis from unconsciousness due to an insulin reaction, in which the skin is characteristically moist. In ketosis the intraocular tension is reduced, the eyeballs are sunken, the mucous membranes of the nasal passages, lips and mouth are dry. The tongue is dry and has a dirty brownish coating. The pharynx is dry and beefy red, and stringy dried secretions may be seen in the mouth and dried deposits are observed on the teeth.

The blood pressure has been low in every patient I have seen in diabetic coma. The pulse rate is rapid and lacks normal force, and the heart sounds may be distant. The extremities are cold and the body temperature is usually subnormal, but rises above normal in the presence of infection shortly after treatment has been instituted. Patients in uncomplicated coma are afebrile. Fever in a ketotic patient should suggest a complicating infection. The abdomen may be tender, especially in the epigastrium and frequently there is considerable rigidity of the abdominal muscles. These findings with leukocytosis and vomiting may mislead one to the conclusion that an acute surgical condition exists in the abdomen. The colon may be distended by a collection of hard feces. The reflexes tend to be sluggish. In examining a patient in coma, one must always be on the alert for signs of complications. The history is usually incomplete and the unconscious patient can tell us no more than we are able to observe. It is so easy to overlook an otitis media, mastoiditis or an early pneumonia. Also furuncles, carbuncles, infections of the respiratory tract, surgical conditions in the abdomen or pelvis, infections of the urinary tract, gangrene, and septicemia are among the more common complications which precipitate ketosis and which tend to load the scales against recovery.

Differential Diagnosis.—The conditions likely to be confused with diabetic coma are intracranial hemorrhage and severe insulin reactions (hypoglycemia). Trauma to the head, uremia, drug poisoning and meningitis deserve special consideration as glycosuria is frequently encountered in these conditions.

Hypoglycemia.—The hazard of treating an insulin reaction as a diabetic ketosis is obvious. It is best to withhold insulin until the effect of intravenous dextrose (see page 780) is observed in any case in which the differential diagnosis between these two conditions is doubtful.

The chief differentiating points between unconsciousness due to hypoglycemia and to ketosis are presented in table 13. The most important of these are: the quickness of onset of unconsciousness in the insulin reaction as against the gradual onset in coma. Furthermore the hypoglycemic patient has a wet skin, no evidence of dehydration, normal breathing, usually no vomiting, no reduction of intraocular tension, a normal or elevated blood pressure, no abdominal tenderness or rigidity, no sugar* or acetone in the urine, and the blood sugar level is below normal in contrast to the hyperglycemia of the patient in diabetic coma.

Intracranial Hemorrhage.—Glycosuria is common following intracranial hemorrhage, especially if the hemorrhage occurs into the ventricles and if there is injury to the floor of the fourth ventricle. The onset is sudden. Asymmetries in contour, muscle tone, and reflexes, if present, are helpful in making a diagnosis. The patient in coma as a result of intracranial hemorrhage is not dehydrated. The skin is moist, the intraocular tension is not decreased, and the blood pressure is usually elevated. The spinal fluid may contain gross blood. Compared with diabetic coma the degree of unconsciousness is marked in contrast to the moderate elevation of the blood sugar; there is little or no acetonuria; no plasma acetone is demonstrable and the carbon dioxide combining power of the blood is not greatly depressed.

* The first specimen of urine from the hypoglycemic patient may contain sugar which has been secreted several hours previously but the bladder being emptied, a second specimen will be aglycosuric.

Uremia.—The patient in uremia is less dehydrated than the patient in diabetic coma. There is an ammoniacal odor on the breath, an enlarged heart, an elevated blood pressure, and usually no glycosuria. No acetone is demonstrable in the blood and the blood sugar is not elevated.

Findings common to both uremia and diabetic coma are: unconsciousness, reduced carbon dioxide combining power, elevated blood urea nitrogen values, and moderate dryness of the skin.

There should be no difficulty in differentiating between diabetic coma and other forms of unconsciousness if a history is carefully obtained and physical and laboratory examinations are conducted.

Prognosis.—The prognosis is good if the patient is young, if he is only drowsy or semiconscious, if the blood pressure is not greatly reduced, if there is no complicating infection, and if the carbon dioxide combining power of the blood plasma is not below 20 volumes per cent and the plasma acetone is detectable in only small amounts.

The prognosis is grave if the patient has been completely unconscious for more than twelve hours, if he is over forty years of age, if the systolic blood pressure is below 50 mm. of Hg, if a severe complicating infection is present, especially a septicemia, if the carbon dioxide combining power is below 12 volumes per cent, if there is anuria with a marked retention of nitrogen in the blood, if there is concomitant arteriosclerotic heart disease, and, in general, if the level of the blood sugar is extremely high—above 1000 mg. per 100 cc.

Age is one of the most important prognostic factors. The mortality of Wilder's patients in diabetic coma in the first four decades of life was 4 per cent, and in the next four decades it was 40 per cent.

The *degree and duration of unconsciousness* are also important. In Dillon's and Dyer's[111] series the mortality in the patients which could be aroused was 28 per cent, and in the completely unconscious it was 81 per cent. Of ten patients reported by Baker[112] who were completely unconscious for more than twelve hours only three survived.

The *degree of disturbance in kidney function* is also a prognostic index. Of 268 cases of coma reported by Dillon and Dyer[111] the mortality was 22 per cent in those in whom the blood urea nitrogen value was 20 mg. per 100 cc. or less, but in those in whom this value was exceeded the mortality was 62.4 per cent.

Infection, its nature and severity, influences greatly the outcome of a case of diabetic coma.

The degree of *hyperglycemia* and depression of the *carbon dioxide combining power* of the blood influence the prognosis but not to the same extent as the foregoing factors. These values are of greatest importance in measuring the objective progress of treatment.

Prevention.—Diabetic coma is preventable. In all but rare occasions it develops because of ignorance or neglect. *Diabetic coma will not develop while the diabetes is under control.*

The tragic effect of acute infections by rapidly producing ketosis should be made known to every diabetic patient. It is remarkable how often patients, even those who should know better, test the urine for sugar while they are in good health, but fail to do so when they are indisposed. Every patient should make arrangements to have the urine tested at least once a day at all times. The indisposition is too often a forerunner of ketosis or is actually due to ketosis. In either case large quantities of sugar are found in the urine. This is the danger signal; if it is heeded, coma can be prevented by administering larger doses of insulin.

A dose of insulin should never be omitted because of loss of appetite unless the urine at that time is free from sugar. It is much safer to take one-half the usual dose and in either case each subsequent specimen of urine should be tested for sugar and the insulin increased if need be until normal conditions are restored. Even though food is not ingested the metabolic needs of the body are being largely taken care of by the body tissues and the need for insulin persists.

The omission of insulin because of anorexia has become one of the most common causes of diabetic coma. Furthermore, physicians have not been blameless in advising such action.

Acute complications, notably surgical conditions, infections, and other predisposing causes of diabetic coma call for very definite changes in the diet and insulin treatment if ketosis is to be prevented. Diabetic patients should secure early treatment for any illness no matter how minor, if the urine tests (Benedict) are "orange" or "brick red." They are in imminent danger if in addition drowsiness, anorexia, nausea, abdominal pain with increasing thirst, and polyuria, singly or in combinations develop.

Treatment.—Each patient in coma is an individual problem. He should be in a hospital and have a capable nurse in constant attendance and should be seen hourly by a physician especially trained in this field of metabolism, until he is out of danger. Too much responsibility is often placed on the intern in the treatment of these cases. A qualified "team" will produce better results. The "team" at the Pennsylvania Hospital comprises: the consultant in metabolism, the resident in medicine, the senior intern, the intern on laboratory service, and a nurse.

Each patient responds differently to treatment, hence no routine treatment will be applicable to all. In general the treatment of diabetic coma is considered under the following heads:

(*a*) Insulin
(*b*) Carbohydrate
(*c*) Fluids
(*d*) Chlorides
(*e*) Alkali
(*f*) Correction of disturbances in the circulatory system
(*g*) Gastric and colonic lavage
(*h*) Warmth and rest.

Insulin.—The administration of insulin should not be delayed once the diagnosis of diabetic coma is made. It is the specific treatment. It restores normal carbohydrate metabolism and by doing so removes the abnormal accentuation of fat and protein metabolism. If the diagnosis is made with certainty before the patient leaves home for the hospital, the first dose of crystalline insulin should be given at once. Two plans of insulin treatment of diabetic coma are presented: (*a*) protamine zinc insulin and crystalline insulin, and (*b*) crystalline insulin.

Protamine Zinc and Crystalline Insulin.—For the adult 80 to 100 units of protamine zinc insulin and 60 units of crystalline insulin are injected subcutaneously at different sites and 40 units of crystalline insulin are given intravenously. Patients in circulatory collapse with the likelihood of poor absorption of insulin should be given a larger proportion of the insulin intravenously, even though much of it may be promptly excreted or neutralized in some manner not yet understood. One should not rely on insulin given intravenously but should give adequate amounts subcutaneously as well.

We have used this one dose of protamine zinc insulin, the initial dose, in conjunction with crystalline insulin in the treatment of coma, being mindful that the effect of protamine zinc insulin is carried over at least twenty-four hours and that with the correction of ketosis the effectiveness of insulin is greatly increased. Subsequent doses are of crystalline insulin, the amounts given being regulated according to the gravity of the clinical condition and the response to treatment. Usually 50 units are given four or six hours after the initial doses and again at eight or twelve hours. Thereafter small doses, 10 to 14 units, the amount depending upon the apparent need as indicated by the carbon dioxide combining power, the sugar concentration in the blood, and the presence or absence of glycosuria, are given at four-hour intervals until the patient is fully recovered from the ketosis and able to resume his diet. The diet for the first day or two following ketosis is divided into six equal feedings, one every four hours. In the presence of acute infections or other serious complications this equal division and distribution of the diet and insulin is continued until improvement warrants four feedings and four doses of insulin. Later with complete recovery the more permanent program may be renewed; three meals, each at the regular mealtime, with one dose of protamine zinc insulin with or without crystalline insulin before breakfast and for some patients a dose of crystalline insulin also before supper. This transition is illustrated in table 22 (p. 825).

Crystalline Insulin Alone.—Crystalline insulin may be used alone if for some reason one does not wish to use protamine zinc insulin. Small doses given frequently are more effective than large amounts given infrequently. An initial dose of 60 units, 20 units intravenously and 40 subcutaneously, is advised. Another dose, 10 to 50 units, the amount varying with the gravity of the patient's condition, is given after an interval of one-half hour.* Hourly, or if necessary half-hourly, administrations of insulin are continued on the same basis while large amounts of sugar are lost in the urine and until the carbon dioxide combining power of the plasma reaches a relatively innocent level (above 35 volumes per cent) or until plasma acetone is no longer detectable by the Rothera-Wishart test (p. 738). These analyses should be made every four hours while the patient's life is in danger. Failing expected improvement, the doses should be steadily increased. Occasionally enormous amounts of insulin are needed. Amounts exceeding 3000 units in twenty-four hours have been necessary to correct the ketosis.

* Fowler, Bensley and Rabinowitch[113] advocate giving 100 units of unmodified insulin intravenously, 100 units of unmodified insulin subcutaneously and 200 units of protamine zinc insulin subcutaneously to patients in coma. Large quantities of carbohydrate are given. The results with this program seem to be no better than with more conservative plans of treatment and I believe that in inexperienced hands it carries needless risk.

Carbohydrate,* Chlorides, and Liquids.—The continuous or intermittent intravenous administration of a 5 per cent solution of glucose (dextrose) in normal saline (warm) amounting to one liter every six hours until the patient can take food containing an adequate amount of carbohydrate and liquids by mouth is recommended. An additional liter or two of normal saline (warm) is given subcutaneously during the first twelve hours of treatment. Nothing should be given by mouth while there is vomiting, abdominal distention, or abdominal pain.

When fluids are taken by mouth and retained, parenteral therapy is discontinued and salty broths, ginger ale (noneffervescent), orange juice diluted with water, gruel, and weak tea are allowed *ad libitum* but are not forced.

When the plasma acetone has been reduced to barely detectable amounts and the carbon dioxide combining power has reached a relatively harmless level, above 35 volumes per cent, a liquid diet is allowed, *e.g.*, protein 50 gm., fat 33 gm., and carbohydrate 250 gm. (1500 calories). This diet, as illustrated in table 20, is divided into six equal feedings, at intervals of four hours. After twenty-four or thirty-six hours when the margin of safety has been increased, the diet is given in four equal feedings, one every six hours, and finally with complete recovery from the attack three meals are resumed. The liquid diet is replaced by "soft" and "solid" foods as the patient's appetite returns.

Sodium chloride and *water* depletions are corrected in the average adult patient in diabetic coma by (*a*) the normal saline intravenously†—one liter every six hours until the patient can take liquids by mouth or until evidences of dehydration are largely corrected, (*b*) normal saline subcutaneously—one or two liters in the first twelve hours of treatment, (*c*) normal saline, approximately 8 ounces, may be left in the patient's stomach before removing the tube after gastric lavage. Under no circumstances should fluid be "poured" into the mouth of a semiconscious or unconscious patient.

Alkalis.—It is with reluctance that one uses alkali in the face of advice to the contrary from an authority as great as Joslin, who believes alkalis are not needed and that they may, in some instances, be harmful.

---

* One may question why carbohydrate is given when the blood sugar level is abnormally high. One need only recollect that all of the available glycogen stores are depleted and at most there will be not more than 20 to 30 gm. of dextrose in circulation. This is a meager supply to balance against hundreds of units of insulin. Furthermore our object is to facilitate carbohydrate metabolism. This is best done by supplying glucose in liberal amounts and adequate insulin to assure its utilization. This is the quickest means of correcting the ketosis and it is the ketosis and not the hyperglycemia which threatens the patient's life.

† During the state of collapse of a severe ketosis or of a profound insulin reaction it is sometimes impossible to use the veins for injection of insulin or glucose precisely at a time when speed is essential. The arm and leg veins at such occasions contain little blood and in order to introduce the needle a phlebotomy is sometimes necessary. Since substances injected into the bone marrow are rapidly absorbed into the general circulation, blood, insulin, isotonic glucose or salt solution may be infused through the manubrium of the sternum, when veins are unavailable. To perform the injection the cavity of that bone is penetrated with a needle equipped with a bevelled obturator. The obturator is removed and suction is applied with a syringe. If marrow is obtained the material to be injected is, without delay, introduced through the needle or allowed to infuse by gravity. The rate of flow by gravity (1 meter height) into the manubrium of adults is between 5 and 20 cc. per minute.

TABLE 20

LIQUID DIET (SIX EQUAL FEEDINGS)

	Gm.	Protein	Fat	Carbohydrate
8 A.M.				
Skimmed milk..................	180	5.3	....	9
Cereal gruel (dry wt.)..........	20	3	....	16
Butter.......................	6	....	5	
Orange juice..................	140	....	....	17
	...	8.3	5	42
12 N.				
Grape juice...................	160	....	....	29
Skimmed milk..................	240	7	....	12.5
20 per cent cream.............	30	1	6	1
	...	8	6	42.5
4 P.M.				
Ginger ale....................	100	....	....	16
Pineapple juice................	100	....	....	12
Skimmed milk..................	240	7	....	12.5
20 per cent cream.............	30	1	6	1
	...	8	6	41.5
8 P.M.				
Skimmed milk..................	100	3	....	5
20 per cent cream.............	30	1	6	1
Orange juice..................	200	....	....	24
Egg white....................	35	4	....	
Glucose......................	12	....	....	12
	...	8	6	42
12 M.				
Soup { Skimmed milk..............	240	7	....	12.5
Carrot puree	50	1.5	....	4.5
Butter....................	6	....	5	
Grapefruit juice...........	270	....	....	24
	...	8.5	5	41.0
4 A.M.				
Soup { Broth....................	120	0	0	0
Egg......................	50	7	5	
Gelatin...................	3	2.5		
Grape juice...............	200	....	....	36
Lactose...................	5	....	....	5
	...	9.5	5	41
Total.........................	...	50.3	33.0	250.0

The division of a liquid diet containing 50 gm. of protein, 33 gm. of fat and 250 gm. of carbohydrate (1500 calories) into six equal feedings is illustrated. The timing of the feedings and the constituents of the diet are also shown. This is a typical diet arrangement for diabetic patients when the diabetes is complicated by acute medical or surgical conditions.

The use of alkali has not been a routine measure at the Pennsylvania and Jefferson Hospitals. Most patients in coma do not need alkali in addition to the treatment with insulin, glucose, and fluids, but for those in a profound ketosis with extreme hyperpnea, a carbon dioxide combining power of the blood below 15 volumes per cent, with or without anuria, 300 cc. of a 3 per cent solution of sodium bicarbonate* may replace a like amount of normal saline and be given intravenously. In extreme cases 500 cc. of a 5 per cent solution of bicarbonate of soda may be given instead. It is remarkable how rapidly extreme degrees of hyperpnea may be relieved by this measure.

Sodium r lactate solution has been recommended by Hartmann[113] as a substitute for bicarbonate of soda. It has the advantages of bicarbonate of soda and fewer disadvantages. It is obtainable commercially in sterile solution and needs only to be diluted and administered in appropriate amounts.

Sodium r lactate solution has certain advantages over sodium bicarbonate solution in the treatment of diabetic ketosis. It is readily sterilized by boiling or autoclaving and is stable. It may be injected intravenously or subcutaneously. The sodium lactate is slowly converted into sodium bicarbonate in the body and the lactate is converted into liver glycogen. Both processes are valuable in correcting ketosis. Furthermore, it is possible to predict with remarkable accuracy on the basis of the carbon dioxide combining power of the blood how much of the lactate solution is necessary to raise the carbon dioxide combining power to a desired level.

Molar sodium lactate solution (Lilly) is supplied in ampoules each containing 10 cc. of solution of which there is 1 cc. of lactic acid, 85 per cent as sodium lactate. The contents of one ampoule (10 cc.), when diluted with 50 cc. (five volumes) of sterile distilled water, make an isotonic solution (one-sixth molar) suitable for intravenous or subcutaneous injection. This amount (50 cc.) of the sixth molar is equivalent to 0.85 gm. (approximately 15 grains) of potential sodium bicarbonate. Hartmann[114] has devised a formula for determining the amount of sodium r lactate solution necessary to raise the carbon dioxide combining power to normal (60 volumes per cent). The amount in cubic centimeters of the *molar* sodium lactate = (60 − plasma CO_2 content) × (0.3 × body weight in kilograms).

In diabetic coma, with other powerful factors, especially insulin and carbohydrate, at work in correcting the ketosis, I do not believe it wise to give the full amount of sodium r lactate solution estimated to restore a normal plasma carbon dioxide combining power. It seems more logical and practical, and it has proved satisfactory, to give only that amount needed to restore the carbon dioxide combining power to a relatively harmless level—approximately 40 volumes per cent. *Example:* Patient's weight 60 Kg. Carbon dioxide combining power 12 volumes per cent. The amount (cc.) of *molar* sodium lactate necessary to restore the plasma CO_2 to 40 volumes per cent = (40 − 12 (plasma CO_2)) × (0.3 × 60 (body weight in kilograms)) = 504 cc. This *molar* solution is made isotonic (one-sixth molar) by diluting with 5 volumes (2520 cc.) of sterile distilled water.

Warmth and Rest.—The body temperature of a patient in diabetic coma is usually subnormal and the skin and extremities are cold. When it is known that a patient in diabetic coma is to be admitted to the hospital

---

* Sodium bicarbonate must not be sterilized by boiling, as this converts it into the caustic carbonate. The bicarbonate of soda is removed from a freshly opened package of a chemically pure brand with sterile apparatus into sterile distilled water. The solution is then ready for intravenous administration.

the bed clothes should be warmed in readiness to receive him. The provision of warmth is by no means the least important factor in the treatment of this condition. Blankets, hot water bottles and electric heating pads are used, special care being taken to prevent burns. The temperature of all fluids given by vein and subcutaneously should be about 38° C. (100° F.). Fluids by mouth should be hot but not hot enough to burn. The enema water should be warm, 38° to 43.4° C. (100.4° to 110° F.). Needless moving of the patient should be avoided.

Restoration of Normal Circulation.—The most effective means of improving the circulation is the correction of the dehydration and chloride depletion by the administration of insulin, glucose, chlorides and water. The blood volume is thus restored to normal, the blood pressure rises and the tendency to anuria is corrected.

Digitalis, caffeine sodium benzoate, pyridine betacarbonic acid diethylamide (coramine) and epinephrine are frequently given. Bopp[115] is especially enthusiastic about the effects of coramine given intravenously for circulatory collapse in diabetic coma. The dose is 1 cc. of a 10 per cent solution given intravenously or intramuscularly. In event of anuria from circulatory collapse and with a low blood sodium chloride level, 60 cc. (2 oz.) of a 10 per cent solution of sodium chloride given slowly by vein is recommended. In regard to blood transfusions there is no lack of cellular elements of the blood in diabetic coma. It would seem that if the blood volume is restored by administering water and sodium chloride without adding cells our object is achieved. The indications for blood transfusion rarely exist in these patients.

Gastric Lavage, Enema, and Catheterization of the Bladder.—In cases in which there is persistent vomiting, abdominal distention, or abdominal pain, gastric lavage with normal saline solution (warm) is especially valuable. It is remarkable the quantity of fluid, partially digested food, and changed blood ("coffee grounds") which may be recovered from the stomach. The evacuation of this material reduces the menace of cardiac and respiratory embarrassment, and the danger of inhalation of vomitus into the lungs. When the stomach is emptied 8 ounces (240 cc.) of normal saline or of a 5 per cent solution of bicarbonate of soda are left in the stomach as an aid in correcting the chloride depletion or replenishing with alkali respectively. The patient is frequently relieved in this manner of the nausea and vomiting, and the abdominal discomfort due to a distention of the stomach or chloride depletion is corrected, the way being prepared for giving liquids by mouth. Should the signs of an acute surgical condition in the abdomen not decrease after a gastric lavage the likelihood of some complicating infection such as appendicitis or cholecystitis should be considered.

A cleansing enema is necessary to evacuate the contents of the large bowel. Days of increasing dehydration have contributed to the dryness and hence delayed transportation of the intestinal contents. A quart of warm soapy water may be used and, if not effective, repeated after a few hours.

Catheterization of the bladder is usually unnecessary, but it may be necessary in order to secure specimens of urine. It should be done without fail if the bladder becomes distended. Evidence of such distention (obvious distention with a flat note on percussion over the suprapubic region) should be looked for at frequent intervals until consciousness is restored.

ILLUSTRATIVE CASES

Impending Coma.—Male, aged nineteen years. Weight 136 pounds (62 Kg.). Height 68 inches (170 cm.). This patient was known to have had diabetes four years when admitted to Dr. Hobart Reimann's Service at the Jefferson Hospital at 12:30 P.M. on April 28, 1939. He had been well until April 24 when he contracted an acute infection of the upper respiratory tract. There was no improvement and, on April 27, he began to vomit. He vomited twenty times and because of this omitted his insulin (60 units of protamine zinc and 12 units of unmodified insulin) on April 28.

When he was seen at 2 P.M. on this date the following observations were made: Marked air hunger with hiccoughs, flushed cheeks, dry skin, decreased intra-ocular pressure, tongue and pharynx red and dry, abdomen moderately distended with marked tenderness and moderate muscle rigidity, blood pressure 146 mm. Hg systolic and 75 mm. diastolic, pulse rate 98, and respirations 36 per minute. His body temperature was normal on admission, but shortly thereafter it rose to 102° F. and continued to be elevated for four days during the course of an acute tracheitis and bronchitis.

The urine contained 3 per cent of sugar and the reactions for acetone and diacetic acid were strongly positive.

The blood sugar level was 336 mg. per 100 cc. and the CO_2 combining power of the plasma was 24 volumes per cent. The leukocyte count was 14,500 per cu. mm.

The immediate treatment consisted of: (1) *Insulin,* 100 units of protamine zinc and 100 units of unmodified insulin given subcutaneously as soon as the diagnosis of diabetic ketosis was made. (2) *Carbohydrate.* One liter of a 10 per cent solution of dextrose in normal saline was given slowly by venoclysis. (3) *Chlorides.* An additional 1000 cc. of normal saline was given intravenously and, when tolerated, he was given salty broths by mouth. (4) *Additional fluids* were given freely by mouth after the vomiting and abdominal pain had subsided. (5) *Warmth* was provided by suitable coverings and hot-water bottles to the extremities. Hot liquids were given by mouth when the patient's condition warranted. (6) An enema was given early in the treatment. (7) A *gastric lavage* was *not* done. (8) *No alkalis* were given.

The CO_2 combining power of the blood plasma was determined at 1, 4 and 11 P.M. and was found to be 24, 24 and 40 volumes per cent and the level of the blood sugar was 336, 336 and 166 mg. per 100 cc., respectively. With satisfactory progress no additional insulin was given until midnight, when he was given the first nourishment by mouth. The diet contained 60 gm. of protein, 29 gm. of fat and 250 gm. of carbohydrate (1500 calories) and was divided into six equal meals at four-hour intervals. Twelve units of insulin were given before each meal. Each dose was increased to 16 units on April 30 because of a hyperglycemia (227 mg. of sugar per 100 cc.). As the infection subsided the nourishments were reduced to four daily, one every six hours, and finally on May 5 three meals were resumed. The multiple doses of insulin were then replaced by a dose each of protamine zinc and unmodified insulin, both given in the morning before breakfast.

The treatment of impending coma in this instance illustrates the use of both protamine zinc and unmodified insulin. One hundred units of each were given subcutaneously at the outset of treatment.

This plan avoided the frequent administrations of crystalline insulin during the first twelve hours of treatment. At the end of this period the patient was able to take liquid nourishment by mouth. A diet containing 60 gm. of protein, 250 gm. of carbohydrate and 29 gm. of fat (1500 calories) was prescribed. It was divided into six equal feedings with insulin accordingly.

Four-hour determinations of the CO_2 combining power of the blood plasma and the blood sugar level are advisable while the patient's life is in danger. In this manner the need for additional crystalline insulin to com-

TABLE 21

Showing the Method of Using a Large Single Dose of Protamine Zinc Insulin and Unmodified Insulin at the Outset of Treatment of Impending Diabetic Coma. The Alterations in Diet and Insulin Are Characteristic and Are in Keeping with the Decreasing Blood Sugar, and Alleviation of the Glycosuria and Acetonuria

Date, 1939	Diet				Insulin, Units		Blood		Urine		
	P., Gm.	F., Gm.	C., Gm.	Total Cal.	Distribution	Total	Sugar (Mg, per 100 cc.)	CO₂ (Vol. %)	Sugar	Acetone	
April 28	1000 cc. 10 per cent dextrose in normal saline.				200	200	226 (1 p.m.) 336 { 4 p.m.) 166 (11 p.m.)	24 24.2 40.2	4+ 1+ —	4+ 2+ —	100 units unmodified and 100 units protamine zinc insulin given stat. (1 p.m.). Insulin, 12 units every four hours, begun at midnight.
29	1000 cc. normal saline.				....	....	200	40.9	3+	—	Six meals.
30	60	29	250	1500	12—12—12—12—12—12	(72)	227	54	1++	0	
May 1	60	29	250	1500	12—12—12—12—12—12	(72)	81	48	1+	0	
2	60	29	250	1500	16—16—16—16—16—16	(96)	108	55	0	0	
3	60	84	250	1500	16—16—16—16	(64)	68	55	0	0	
4	60	84	250	2000	16—16—16—16	(64)					Four meals.

TABLE 22

THE TREATMENT OF A PATIENT IN DIABETIC COMA IS PRESENTED IN DETAIL, SHOWING THE AMOUNTS AND THE TIMING OF THE INSULIN ADMINISTRATION, THE CARBOHYDRATES, FLUIDS, CHLORIDES, AND THE DIET

Date, 1937	Time	Diet P., Gm.	F., Gm.	C., Gm.	Total Cal.	Insulin, Units per Injection.	Blood Sugar (Mg.) 100 Cc.	Blood Acetone, Rothera-Wishart Test	CO₂ (Vol. %)	Urine Sugar, Benedict's Test	Urine Acetone, Rothera Test	Remarks
Dec. 23	1 P.M.					40	426		8	4+	4+	1000 cc. 5% dextrose in normal saline. Gastric lavage. B. P. 90/44.
	1:30					40						
	2:00					40 (intravenously)					4+	
	2:30					40	422	3+	11	4+		Normal saline 240 cc. by stomach tube.
	3:00					40						500 cc. 2% sod. bicarb. intravenously.
	3:30					40						1000 cc. normal saline intravenously.
	4:00					40	423	3+	21			325 cc. 10% dextrose intravenously.
	4:30					40				4+	4+	B. P. 108/54.
	5:00					40						
	5:30					40						
	6:00					40	290	3+	29	4+		B. P. 110/60.
	6:30					40					3+	
	7:00					40						
	7:30					40						B. P. 100/60.
	8:00					40	416	2+	33	4+		
	8:30					40						1000 cc. normal saline subcutaneously.
	9:00					30						
	10:00					30						
	11:00					30	316	1+		2+		325 cc. 10% dextrose in normal saline intravenously.
	12:00					30						B. P. 90/40.
24	1 A.M.					30						
	2:30					30	374	0		3++		
	3:00					30						
	3:30					30						
	4:00											
	4:30											
	5:30						160			0		
	6:30											
	7:00											
	8:30								39			B. P. 90/44.
	9:00						133		53	0		
	12:00					30-30-30	149			0		6 equal feedings begun (liquid) at noon.
25		40	27	300	1600	30-30-30-20-20-20	80			-1+		4 equal feedings.
30		40	27	300	1600	10-10-10-10	140			-1+		3 equal feedings.
Jan. 7		40	27	300	1600	20-8-12	126			2+ -4+		
12		40	27	300	1600	24-10-14-10	294			0+ -4+		
28		40	102	200	2000	24-10-*(24)	266			0		
Feb. 11		70	102	200	2000	14-0-0	157					
						*(36)						

* Protamine zinc insulin.

bat ketosis and hyperglycemia, or for more carbohydrate to combat a tendency to hypoglycemia as the case may be, is recognized.

Coma.—Male, aged thirty-one years. Weight 125 pounds (56 Kg.). Height 66 inches (165 cm.). Admitted December 23, 1937, in diabetic coma.

This patient had been admitted to the Pennsylvania Hospital on two former occasions: in August, 1935, with diabetes and a furuncle of the cheek, and in January, 1936, because of "painful feet." He was taking 77 units of unmodified insulin a day when discharged from the hospital in 1936. In January, 1937, he was admitted to the Graduate Hospital in diabetic coma and he spent April, 1937, in the Chester Hospital, when he had pneumonia. In July, 1937, he was readmitted to the Graduate Hospital in impending coma and, in December, he entered St. Agnes Hospital where the same diagnosis was made. Following his discharge on December 19 he stated that because of financial difficulties he was unable to buy food and consequently he omitted his insulin. An intense thirst and polyuria developed, followed by anorexia and nausea. For twenty-four hours before admission he was stuporous, intensely weak, and vomited "black liquid."

He was admitted (December 23) in diabetic coma. He had marked air hunger and his tissues were generally dehydrated. The skin was dry and his eyes were soft and sunken; the tongue was dry and coated and the pharynx was dry and red. The precordial dullness was increased to the left and the cardiac sounds were obscured by loud rhonchi. There was diminished expansion over the left side of the chest (later there were evidences of pulmonary atelectasis on this side). The liver was palpable three finger breadths below the costal margin. The blood pressure was 90 mm. Hg systolic and 40 mm. diastolic. The body temperature was 97° F., the pulse rate 105 per minute, and there were 28 respirations per minute.

The CO_2 combining power of the blood plasma was 8 volumes per cent and there was a 3+ reaction for plasma acetone (Rothera-Wishart test). The blood sugar level was 426 mg. per 100 cc. There was 4+ glycosuria and the urine contained large amounts of acetone and diacetic acid. There was a moderate albuminuria. Occasional hyaline casts, an occasional red blood cell and a few leukocytes were found on microscopic examination of the urine. The blood count revealed: Hgb. 90 per cent, R.B.C. 5,000,000, and W.B.C. 28,000 (polynuclear leukocytes 85 per cent, lymphocytes 13 per cent, monocytes 2 per cent).

The foregoing findings confirmed the diagnosis of diabetic coma and there was a complicating partial pulmonary atelectasis. Within twelve hours of the institution of treatment the body temperature increased to 102° F. and remained elevated for two days.

Treatment.—*Insulin.*—Forty units of unmodified insulin were given subcutaneously at half-hour intervals (one dose, 40 units, was given intravenously). The level of the blood sugar, the CO_2 combining power of the blood plasma and the presence of plasma acetone were determined at frequent intervals (1 P.M., 3 P.M., 4:30 P.M., 7 P.M., 9 P.M., 12 midnight, 3:30 A.M. and 7 A.M.) until a satisfactory increase in the CO_2 combining power of the blood plasma and a disappearance of the plasma acetone were accomplished. It was necessary to give 40 units of insulin at half-hour intervals for sixteen doses, then 30 units hourly for six doses. In the first twelve hours of treatment 790 units of insulin were given, in the second twelve hours 150 units (a total of 940 units in twenty-four hours). The unusually large amount of insulin was indicated in view of the slowness of the response of the CO_2 combining power of the blood plasma and the plasma acetone (Table 22).

Carbohydrate, Liquids, Chlorides and Alkali.—One liter of 5 per cent glucose (dextrose) in normal saline was administered intravenously at the outset of treatment. Eight ounces (240 cc.) of normal saline were left in the stomach after the gastric lavage. Five hundred cubic centimeters of a 2 per cent solution of sodium bicarbonate were given intravenously three hours after treatment was started. This was followed by 1 liter of normal saline intravenously, which in turn was followed by 325 cc. of a 10 per cent solution of dextrose intravenously (5 P.M.) and five hours later (10 P.M.) 1 liter of normal saline was given subcutaneously. At 1 A.M., 325 cc. of a 10 per cent solution of glucose was given by venoclysis. A liter of water and salty broth was given by mouth in the first twenty-four hours of treatment.

A diet (liquid for three days) containing 40 gm. of protein, 300 gm. of carbohydrate and 27 gm. of fat (1600 calories) was begun at noon on December 25 (two days after admission). The diet was divided into six equal portions, a feeding every four hours. This was continued until December 30 when feedings at six-hour intervals were begun and finally, on January 7, the usual three-meal schedule was resumed.

The insulin was divided into the same number of doses as there were meals, and the amount given was steadily decreased as the blood sugar level became normal. When discharged, this patient was receiving 36 units of protamine zinc insulin and 14 units of unmodified insulin, both given before breakfast at separate injections.

Gastric Lavage.—The stomach was emptied of a large quantity of fluid containing minute black particles. This was done because of persistent vomiting and abdominal distention.

Enema.—A soapy water enema, which was effectual, was given early in the course of the treatment.

This illness and the past experiences of this unruly patient proved of no avail as he was readmitted on March 21, 1938, in diabetic coma of three days' duration. His blood sugar level was 380 mg. per 100 cc. and the CO_2 combining power of the blood plasma was 4 volumes per cent. In spite of 1040 units of insulin, 6500 cc. of fluids, including racemic sodium lactate solution, there was no improvement, from either the clinical or chemical point of view, and he died twelve hours after admission.

ACUTE INFECTIONS

Patients with uncontrolled diabetes have a subnormal resistance to infections, especially to the tubercle bacillus and Staphylococcus aureus. The cause of this well-known phenomenon is still obscure but there can be no doubt that it is closely related to poorly controlled diabetes, reduced liver glycogen and ketosis. It is well known also that an acute infection in a diabetic subject precipitates a hyperglycemia and ketosis, which may progress rapidly to coma. The action of insulin becomes impaired and often under these conditions very large doses are required to control the diabetes. The behavior of the diabetes is frequently a reliable index of the progress of an infection, favorable or unfavorable. The duration of insulin action is reduced as is its degree of action by acute infections, whereas artificially induced fever shortens the duration of insulin action but does not reduce the degree of its hypoglycemic action.[116]

Why infection makes the diabetes more severe is not, as yet, clearly understood. Probably a number of factors are involved. Weiland (1913) and Geiger (1925) observed that fasting nondiabetic subjects developed hyperglycemia during the period of rising temperature in febrile conditions. This hyperglycemia disappeared when the temperature returned to normal. Williams and Dick (1932) found that glycosuria occurred in 41 per cent of normal individuals during the course of acute infections, and Schmidt, Eastland and Burns (1934) have demonstrated a temporarily impaired glucose tolerance in nondiabetic patients suffering from pyogenic infections. The effect of infection on the level of the blood sugar is not, therefore, a peculiarity confined to diabetic subjects but tends to occur in normal individuals to a milder degree. A hitherto "latent diabetes" will often become manifest as a moderately severe diabetes during the course of an acute or chronic infection. The enormous doses of insulin which may be required by a diabetic patient with a severe infection seem to deprecate the suggestion of a mere suppression of endogenous insulin production, particularly since it can be shown that the action of this injected insulin is less effective in controlling the blood sugar level than would usually be the case. For this reason it is believed by some workers that insulin antagonists are produced which counteract the normal action of insulin. Karelitz, (1930), for example, showed that the action of insulin injected into rabbits was inhibited if it was previously mixed with the blood of diabetic patients. Control experiments in which the insulin was mixed with the blood of non-diabetic patients also showed some inhibition of the insulin action, but to a lesser degree. Some consider that hormones antagonistic to insulin, probably elaborated from the thyroid, anterior pituitary, or suprarenal glands, are produced in excess. Others consider that a coenzyme of insulin fails to be produced, or that some new enzyme is produced in the serum of patients with infections and that this "antihormone" actively opposes the action of insulin. It has been suggested that trypsin elaborated by degenerating leukocytes destroys insulin in the blood. The increase in the total metabolism of the patient is a factor and alterations in the acid-base equilibrium may play a part in some cases. Whatever the theoretical basis of the phenomenon may be the practical issue is plain and of extreme importance. Hyperglycemia and glycosuria develop as a result of the infection and the additional insulin given is less effective than it otherwise would be. Hence, it is essential to continue increasing the amount of insulin until it is adequate to control the hyperglycemia and glycosuria and to prevent the risk of ketosis and coma.

Treatment of Diabetes During Acute Infections.—The elderly and obese patient suffering from mild diabetes, which under ordinary conditions is satisfactorily controlled by a diet without insulin, will almost always require insulin if an infection is contracted.

These patients should be given insulin during the course of acute infections and febrile illnesses if the fasting blood sugar level exceeds 120 mg. per 100 cc., or if the *postcibal* value exceeds 160 mg. per 100 cc. If the infection is a mild one and the patient is already taking insulin, a simple addition to the usual doses of insulin over the course of a few days may be all that is required to control the glycosuria and the level of the blood sugar. In more severe infections, however, other measures are indicated.

Crystalline insulin is the preparation of choice in the presence of an acute infection. Its action is more prompt and shorter in duration than that of protamine zinc insulin. This makes it a simpler weapon to manipulate when both the blood sugar level and insulin requirement may be subject to rapid alterations.

The following *method of distributing the insulin* has been employed at the Pennsylvania Hospital for the past nine years with favorable results: During the course of moderately severe infections the insulin is given in four equal doses, at evenly spaced intervals. Thus a patient receiving 60 units of crystalline insulin would receive 15 units every six hours. The diet is similarly divided so that the patient receives the same amount of carbohydrate, fat, and protein after each injection of insulin. It is convenient to give meals and insulin at 6 A.M., 12 noon, 6 P.M. and 12 midnight. In more severe infections the day is divided into six periods, for example, the patient would receive at the outset 10 units of insulin with a sixth of the total diet every four hours. This program permits the uniform control of the blood sugar level during the most severe complications. Changes in the dosage of insulin are regulated according to the amount of sugar found in the urine, which is collected before each nourishment, and/or by the level of the blood sugar.

When meals and insulin are given at four-hour intervals, urine collections are made for the same period, and likewise when meals and insulin are given every six hours, the urine is collected each six-hour period. The bladder is emptied before each feeding and the quantity of reducing substance in the urine is determined. An estimation of the blood sugar level at the same time is helpful and often necessary. During critical periods determinations of the blood sugar level are made at 8 A.M. and 4 P.M. daily. While the urine contains sugar and the blood sugar level is unduly high, the amount of insulin given is steadily increased at each administration. The diabetic patient, when recovering from the more severe infections, changes from six feedings at four-hour intervals with six injections of insulin to four at six-hour intervals. As the infection subsides, guided by the freedom from glycosuria and the tendency of the blood sugar level to remain low, the insulin is reduced. An added advantage of the equal division of the diet and insulin is that one determination of the blood sugar level during the day is, theoretically speaking, as good as four or six. In practice there are naturally some variations, but on the whole these are small.

Though I prefer using a quickly acting insulin alone during acute infections, the amount of protamine zinc insulin formerly used may be continued unchanged with small doses of crystalline insulin every four or six hours, suitable increases being made until the diabetes is controlled.

Great reductions in the dosage of insulin are likely to be needed after the termination of an infection. This is especially true if the termination is rapid as in the crisis of pneumonia, the drainage of an abscess, or the amputation of a secondarily infected, gangrenous extremity. It is dangerous, however, to omit a dose of insulin during the course of an infection just because a low blood sugar value is obtained. It is remarkable with what speed hyperglycemia returns and ketosis supervenes. A reduction in the amount of insulin given rather than the omission of a dose is advisable. It is a good rule to anticipate a rapid return of the carbohydrate tolerance and hence a decrease in the need for insulin by reducing the amount of insulin by 4 to 20 units when the urine fraction becomes free from sugar. Further changes, decreases or increases, may be guided by the presence or absence of glycosuria. Dramatic reductions in the need for insulin and the danger of precipitating hypoglycemic reactions occur when the factor which in the first place increases the need for insulin suddenly disappears. At this time the glycogen reserve in the liver is low further increasing the risk of insulin reactions.

When the infection has subsided and the blood sugar remains at a more or less constant level it is possible to revert to the usual three meals a day with two or three doses of insulin. Finally, if insulin is necessary in health, a single morning dose of protamine zinc insulin, with or without crystalline insulin, may replace the more frequent injections of insulin.

Infections involving the urinary tract may invalidate glycosuria as a guide to the degree of hyperglycemia. The urinary infection may of itself lead to a disappearance or diminution of the sugar in the urine, although the blood sugar remains high. Thus a diabetic patient under our care in the Pennsylvania Hospital was found to have no sugar in her urine, although the blood sugar level at the same time was 480 mg. per 100 cc. and she had not received insulin. This patient's urine was thick with pus and on culture *B. coli* and streptococci were found.

When the diabetes is complicated by an infection the *diet* requires some modification from the usual form. The protein content of the diet must be reduced in most instances of acute infection because it becomes unpalatable. Liquid nourishment may be all that the acutely ill patient can take and this should consist largely of fruit juices, skimmed milk, cream, gruels and ginger ale with glucose (Table 20). In prolonged infections, however, adequate *protein*, 1 gm. per Kg. of the normal body weight, in an easily digestible form must be given. The daily *carbohydrate* intake is increased by 20 to 100 gm. or more, and the *fat* is reduced to 40 or 50 gm. a day. By this means the caloric requirements of the body are satisfied and the danger of ketosis is minimized.

A diet for a patient weighing 70 Kg. and having an acute infection of short duration, might contain protein 50 gm. (approximately ⅔ gm. per Kg. of body weight), carbohydrate 280 gm. (4 gm. per Kg.) and sufficient fat, 50 gm., to make a total of 1750 calories (25 calories per Kg.).

Additional Measures.—Beyond the treatment of the diabetes, infections should receive the same treatment as in the nondiabetic patients. On no account should these patients be deprived of specific methods of treatment such as serum therapy or chemotherapy. Sulfanilamide, sulfathiazole, sulfapyridine, sulfadiazine and mandelic acid, which are among the newer agents with which to cope with infections, are equally valuable in the diabetic and nondiabetic patients. Sulfathiazole and sulfadiazine, because they are less likely to cause vomiting, are preferable to sulfapyridine, though in cases of pneumococcal meningitis sulfapyridine is more effective and in such cases should be used.

ILLUSTRATIVE CASES

Female, aged forty-seven years. Weight 166 pounds (75 Kg.). Height 58 inches (145 cm.). This patient was obese but was not known to have diabetes. Admitted on December 7, 1938, with a history and physical findings typical of lobar pneumonia. A

TABLE 23

SHOWING PROMPT CONTROL OF THE HYPERGLYCEMIA FOLLOWING EQUAL DIVISION AND DISTRIBUTION OF THE DIET AND INSULIN. THE INCREASING NEED FOR INSULIN AS THE INFECTION PROGRESSED AND THE REDUCED NEED WITH RECOVERY ARE EXEMPLIFIED

	Blood Sugar (Mg.)	Urine Sugar	Insulin (Units)						Meals per 24 Hours
Dec. 8........	217	Traces	10	15	10				6
9........	197	"	10	10	10	10	15	15	6
10........	189	"	15	15	15	15	15	15	6
11........	126	Nil	15	15	15	15	15	15	6
12........	142	"	15	15	15	15	15	15	6
13........	121	"	15	15	15	15	15		5
16........	131	"	15	15	15	15			4
19........	...	"	15	15	15				3
21........	93	"	12	12	12				3
23........	...	"	8	8	8				3
26........	...	"	5	5	5				3
28........	...	"	Nil						3
30........	98	"	"						3

"head cold" was followed by pain in the left side of her chest which kept her in bed for some days. Her temperature was 104° F.; herpes labialis was present; there were signs of consolidation of the lower lobe of the left lung and a friction rub was audible. The blood count revealed 18,800 leukocytes per cu. mm. Pneumococci, type IV, were cultured from her sputum. Examination of the urine revealed sugar and acetone bodies and the blood sugar level was 217 mg. per 100 cc.

A liquid diet containing 250 gm. of carbohydrate, 50 gm. of protein and 60 gm. of fat (1740 calories) was prescribed. This diet was divided into equal meals which were given at four-hour intervals day and night (4 A.M., 8 A.M., 12 N., 4 P.M., 8 P.M. and 12 M.). As the fever subsided the feedings were reduced to five, then to four, and finally to three a day. Insulin was given in equal doses, one dose before each meal, and the urine collected before each meal was tested for sugar. The blood sugar was estimated daily for the first seven days (Table 23).

The patient made a satisfactory recovery. A dextrose tolerance test on January 6 showed a prolonged hyperglycemia, but there was no glycosuria.

Rumanian, male, forty-eight years old, was admitted to Jefferson Hospital on September 10, 1938, because of a large carbuncle in the suboccipital region and diabetes (blood sugar value 476 mg. per 100 cc. on September 9th). The patient first noticed "a lump" on his neck on August 29, 1938, but gave a history of having had a series of furuncles four to five months before entering the ward. He was being actively treated for tertiary syphilis at the Out-Patient Clinic.

On admission to the hospital the patient was moderately obese. The teeth were carious and the gums were infected. The neck was short and thick and there was a large carbuncle with extensive induration in the suboccipital region. There was moderate cardiac enlargement with a systolic murmur at the cardiac apex. The blood count September 12th: R. B. C. 3,900,000 and W. B. C. 18,500 per cu. mm., September 15th: W. B. C. 27,500 per cu. mm., September 30th: R. B. C. 4,800,000 per cu. mm. with W. B. C. 9400 per cu. mm. The Wassermann and Kahn reactions were positive.

The *treatment* was conservative. Several roentgen-ray treatments were given and the diabetes was controlled. Surgical measures were delayed until a localized collection of pus had formed. A small incision gave adequate drainage.

A diet liberal in carbohydrate content (200 gm.), though restricted in total calories (1400) was given. There was a prompt effect when unmodified insulin was given at four-hour intervals. Large amounts of insulin were given during the febrile course (September 10th to 15th) to maintain the blood sugar at normal levels. As the infection subsided, the need for insulin decreased and the regime was reduced to four meals and four doses of insulin a day as convalescence was established (September 23rd). There was a gradual transfer to protamine zinc insulin (October 9th to 17th) and the resumption of three meals a day on October 9th.

This case well illustrates the ease with which diabetes may be controlled in spite of a serious infection. The blood sugar was promptly reduced to normal and at no time were there signs or symptoms of a hypoglycemia. It should be emphasized that during the acute disturbance satisfactory blood and urine findings were obtained and that improvement in the local condition followed.

The treatment and relevant laboratory data are presented in table 24.

TUBERCULOSIS

The untreated diabetic patient, especially if young, is predisposed to tuberculosis. This is true now as it was in the preinsulin era. This predisposition is neutralized by proper control of the diabetes by measures now available. Undernutrition and emaciation are no longer necessary.

Insulin in appropriate amounts with adequate nutrition to keep the body weight at a normal level has done much to correct the predisposition

27

TABLE 24

The Diet and Insulin as Used in the Treatment of a Patient Having Diabetes Complicated by a Large Carbuncle Are Recorded. The Plasma Sugar Values, White Blood Cell Count and the Results of Examinations of the Urine for Sugar and Acetone Are Tabulated

Date, 1935	Diet				Insulin		Blood Sugar (Mg.)	Urine		Wt. Kg.	
	P.	F.	C.	Cal.	Distribution	Total Units		Sugar (Gm.)	Acetone		
Sept. 10	75	33	200	1400	12—12—12—12—12	72	476 (9/9/38)	3.7%–6%	0	..	6 equal meals and 6 equal doses of insulin.
12	75	33	200	1400	15—15—15—15—15	90	187	1.2%–8%	0		W. B. C. 18,500.
13	75	33	200	1400	20—20—20—20—20	120	238	.6%–5%	0		
14	75	33	200	1400	22—22—22—22—22	132	161	.3%—0	0	..	W. B. C. 27,500.
15	75	33	200	1400	22—22—22—22—22	132	86	.3%—0	0		
16	75	33	200	1400	18—18—18—18—18	108	111	0	0		
21	75	33	200	1400	14—14—14—14—14	84	75	0	0		
23	75	33	200	1400	14—14—14—14	56	90	0	0		4 meals and 4 doses of insulin.
29	75	33	200	1400	10—10—10—10	40	102	0	0	..	W. B. C. 9400
Oct. 8	75	33	200	1400	10—10—10—10	40	115	0	0		
9	75	33	200	1400	20 (A.M.)—10 (P. M.) / (8)*	38	...	0	0		3 meals resumed.
10	75	33	200	1400	16—6 / (16)*	38	114	0	0		
11	75	33	200	1400	12—4 / (24)*	40	104	0	0		
12	75	33	200	1400	8 / (24)*	32	102	0	0		
13	75	33	200	1400	8 / (24)*	32	99	0	0		
17	75	33	200	1400	(30)*	30	93	0	0	97	Discharged.

* Protamine zinc insulin.

to tuberculosis. Nevertheless tuberculosis is still between two and three times more frequent at autopsy in diabetic than in nondiabetic patients. Between 3 and 4 per cent of the deaths of diabetic patients are from tuberculosis (Root). Himsworth found that fifteen (6.5 per cent) of 230 consecutive diabetic patients had tuberculosis.

The development of tuberculosis in diabetic patients who are faithful with their diet and insulin is becoming rare. I have no doubt that the incidence of this disease will remain high in patients who are wantonly careless and whose physicians largely ignore hyperglycemia and the loss of large amounts of sugar in the urine. It is true as Tolstoi[117] has stated that patients may lose as much as 150 gm. of sugar in the urine some days and yet be apparently free from symptoms. It is equally true, in my estimation, that these patients are the leading candidates for tuberculosis, true diabetic cataracts, chronic degenerative disorders, and a gradual increase in the severity of their diabetes. These are complications the likelihood of which cannot be excluded in a few weeks or even a few months of observation. Root[118] states, "The less well controlled the diabetic, the greater the susceptibility to infection becomes." With this I agree.

Diabetes usually precedes the development of clinical tuberculosis and when it does the prognosis is less favorable than when the tuberculosis is first to appear. Root is less pessimistic in 1940 than he was in 1937 about the continued frequency of tuberculosis among diabetic patients. He finds that, "The incidence of pulmonary tuberculosis in adult diabetics is diminishing. The development of tuberculosis in the juvenile diabetics occurred more than twelve times as often as among nondiabetic Massachusetts grade and high school children. Pulmonary tuberculosis developed in 8 per cent of diabetic patients within three years after recovery from coma between 1923 and 1929. In 83 per cent of these cases the development of progressive tuberculosis appeared to follow the onset of diabetes." Eighty per cent of Bertram's[119] asthenic diabetic patients developed clinical tuberculosis after attacks of ketosis.

Diagnosis.—Tuberculosis has unusual and misleading signs in the diabetic patient. Loss of weight, common in untreated tuberculosis patients, may be attributed to the diabetes. Eleven of Himsworth's[120] thirteen patients with tuberculosis and diabetes denied having a cough; sputum was usually absent and physical signs of tuberculosis were present in only two of the thirteen cases.

Early diagnosis of tuberculosis in diabetic subjects depends upon the detection of (1) increased pulse rate, (2) mild degree of fever, (3) prolonged sedimentation rate, (4) the absence of clinical improvement with control of the diabetes, and—by far the most important—(5) the roentgen-ray evidence of the disease. *Roentgenography* will reveal early tuberculous lesions which fail to give detectable physical signs. Every diabetic patient should have a roentgen-ray examination of the lungs and every young diabetic patient, especially if the diabetes is not controlled, should have such an examination annually. Every patient with the rapidly-forming "true diabetic cataract" should be carefully examined for tuberculosis. Four of ten patients reported by Himsworth[120] had pulmonary tuberculosis. Both conditions are prone to occur in young patients with uncontrolled and severe diabetes. Root found that a number of diabetic patients dying of tuberculosis had low phospholipid content in the lung tissue. The low phosphorus content in true diabetic cataracts suggests a correlation.

Pathology.—The extension of the tuberculous process in the untreated diabetic patient is rapid. It is usually far advanced before it is recognized clinically. The fulminating course of the disease is attributable to the extension of the characteristically deep seated lesions, pneumonic in type, spreading toward the hilum of the lung with little tendency to fibrosis or pleural involvement. The freedom from pleural involvement and pleural adhesions explains why the induction of successful artificial pneumothoraces is possible in a high percentage of diabetic patients. Caseation proceeds promptly and rapidly with early cavitation but minimal amounts of sputum and, as might well be expected, if the disease is not recognized and energetically treated the prognosis is grave. Incipient tuberculosis is practically unknown in diabetic patients. The virulence of the tuberculous process in these patients may well be related to the disturbance of protein and fat metabolism in diabetes.

The effect of the tuberculous infection on the diabetes is variable. Usually the insulin requirement is increased but this increase is not so rapid nor so great as is observed with acute pyogenic infections. This may be due to the absence of leukocytosis and to the mildness of the degree of change in the metabolic rate caused by this infection. The increased insulin need is most striking in cases in which there is a predominating secondary infection with a leukocytic reaction.

In unusual cases the opposite effect is observed. The insulin need steadily decreases. This goes hand in hand with the declining weight and the progressiveness of the disease, hence it is a bad omen. It was the improvement of the diabetes which occurred with the progressive emaciation of these patients that led Allen to consider the effects of undernutrition on diabetic patients in general—and the greatest advance in the therapy of this disease prior to the discovery of insulin resulted.

Prevention and Treatment.—The prevention of tuberculosis is readily summarized as follows: (1) The avoidance of exposure to tuberculous infection, (2) the control of the diabetes, and (3) the provision of adequate nutrition to maintain a normal body weight.

Control of the diabetes is imperative as a prophylactic measure and as a method of arresting the infection once it is started. This is accomplished, in the more advanced febrile cases by frequent feedings and the frequent administration of crystalline insulin, as outlined on page 828. All diabetic patients suffering from tuberculosis should be given insulin. The amount needed is not so great as during pyogenic infections, and indeed, these patients are often particularly insulin sensitive and liable to hypoglycemic reactions from the slightest overdosage. In the less severe cases and as improvement in the more serious cases occurs, the three-meal-a-day regimen is sufficient with nourishments between meals and at bedtime. A transfer is made to protamine zinc insulin alone or if necessary supplemented by crystalline insulin. The diet should be liberal from the start, 35 to 45 calories per Kg. of body weight, and regulated, as necessary, to secure and maintain the body weight at a normal level. It should contain liberal amounts of carbohydrate, 200 to 300 gm. a day.

Successful treatment of these patients will depend upon the special interest in and the equipment for the treatment of diabetes as well as the conduct of the treatment of the tuberculous process.

Diabetic patients should be given the advantages of (1) prolonged rest in good hygienic surroundings, preferably in a sanatorium equipped to treat both diabetes and tuberculosis. If such conditions are not available these patients do better in a general hospital where the diabetes can be well treated. (2) Artificial pneumothorax, phrenic avulsion, and (3) thoracoplasty when the indications for such treatments are present.

It can be positively stated that the outlook for diabetic patients suffering from tuberculosis is quite as good as that for the nondiabetic having this disease, providing the diagnosis is made early, providing the diabetes is properly controlled, and providing proper treatment for the tuberculosis is conducted.

CANCER

Cancer appears more frequently in the diabetic population than in the population at large and this trend is becoming increasingly apparent as more diabetic patients live longer in "the cancer age." In the majority the onset of malignant disease occurs after the diabetes is established. Of 243 fatal cases Joslin[120] records carcinoma of the breast in 35, of the pancreas 33, of the uterus 27, of the stomach 17, of the urinary bladder 15, and of the liver 14. Carcinoma of the pancreas comprised 12 per cent of the total in contrast to 2.5 per cent in 5300 cases of cancer reported by Hoffman. Diabetic subjects are, therefore, more likely to develop cancer of the pancreas than are nondiabetic patients.

Some cases of carcinoma of the pancreas cause diabetes. This is not common, however, probably because of the independent blood supply to the islets of Langerhans and because cancer usually involves the head of the pancreas—that portion containing the fewest islets.

SYPHILIS

Syphilis in the diabetic patient is coincidental. There is no apparent etiologic relationship between the two in spite of past belief to the contrary.

SKIN DISORDERS COMPLICATING DIABETES MELLITUS

Carbuncles.—Carbuncles are among the most serious and yet are among the preventable complications of diabetes. Fortunately they are not common. The mortality rate is high in cases of large carbuncles, approximately 20 per cent. This is contributed to by disregard for the diabetes, obesity, neglect of the lesion or even meddlesome interferences in its early stages. Septicemia with or without metastatic abscesses results too frequently.

It has not been determined why diabetic patients are prone to develop staphylococcal infections. It is not due directly to the hyperglycemia but it is suggested by Urbach's work that the sugar content of the skin is the important factor. He found that the sugar content of normal skin averaged 59 per cent (61 mg.) of the average normal blood sugar of 103 mg. per 100 cc., whereas in diabetic patients with skin diseases the sugar content was higher than in diabetic patients without skin disorders, being on the average 69 per cent of the blood sugar level. Also in contrast with the large

quantity of glycogen in normal skin, Warren found almost none in the
skin of patients with untreated diabetes. Appropriate treatment of the diabetes reduces the glucose and increases the glycogen content of the skin.

Overweight patients who have a mild but neglected diabetes and who
are uncleanly in their habits and personal hygiene are especially likely to
contract furuncles and carbuncles. Carbuncles may occur anywhere on the
surface of the body, but are especially apt to affect the vulva in the female
and the neck in the male.

Some patients, though having an apparently severe diabetes during the
course of the infection, have no demonstrable sign of the diabetes a few
months after the infection has subsided.

Prevention.—Control of the diabetes, correction of obesity, cleanliness
of the skin and clothing, avoiding shaving the back of the neck, and early
and appropriate treatment for minor infections of the skin comprise the
outstanding prophylactic measures. The instruction of diabetic patients
in the treatment of "pimples" and "boils" will aid in reducing the incidence
of carbuncles. Suction treatment of these infections by means of a vacuum
bottle is to be condemned as are squeezing, pricking, and cutting of the
lesion. Patients should be instructed to daub the area gently with alcohol
(70 per cent) several times daily, to apply hot compresses of a saturated
solution of boric acid, to wash their hands thoroughly with soap and water
several times daily finishing off with an alcohol rinse, and to use freshly
laundered underclothes and bed linens each day. Clean hands, clean skin,
clean collar bands, clean razors, and clean towels are important aids in preventing furuncles and carbuncles.

Treatment.—Conservative treatment without incision in the early stages
promotes localization and reduces greatly the likelihood of a septicemia.
Carbuncles are serious. The patient should be treated in a hospital, kept in
bed, and emergency measures should be adopted to bring the diabetes
under control rapidly. Feedings and insulin injections at four-hour intervals, as outlined on page 828 are especially valuable measures in attaining
this end. Enormous amounts of insulin may be necessary. As the carbuncle
localizes and with free evacuation of pus a prompt decrease in the insulin
need ensues. Roentgen-ray therapy over the lesion is especially effective in
the early stages—before there is a local collection of pus. Indeed, it may
abort the carbuncle in the early stages. It facilitates localization and reduces
the likelihood of a septicemia. Treatments with ultraviolet light are also
of value. The constant application of compresses of thick gauze dressings
soaked with a saturated solution of warm boric acid are of value. Wilder[121]
recommends the daily intravenous injection of 10 cc. of 40 per cent solution of methenamine for one week. I have had no experience with this
measure.

Sulfathiazole, 2 gm. in the initial dose repeated in four hours and 1 gm.
every four hours thereafter, offers promise of being effective in preventing
a septicemia and of correcting it if present. This drug is admittedly not so
effective against the *Staphylococcus aureus,* the usual organism in carbuncles, as it is against the Pneumococcus. It may be continued for a week
or ten days and is discontinued when obvious localization of the infection
is well developed. *Sulfadiazine* bids fair to replace sulfathiazole in the

treatment of staphylococcal infections. It is used in the same amounts. No incision should be made in a "diabetic carbuncle" except that necessary to evacuate pus and afford good drainage. Extensive surgical interference is contraindicated.

Furuncles.—Furuncles, also staphylococcal infections, occurring in diabetic patients should be looked upon as potential carbuncles and treated as such. They may occur singly but more frequently, they are multiple and widespread. They tend to recur in crops from time to time.

The patient is instructed to keep "Hands Off" pimples and boils and to observe good hygiene as outlined above in the prevention of carbuncles.

Freshly laundered underclothes and bed linen daily aid in preventing the spread of the infection. Furthermore, the infected area should be protected from the rubbing of underclothes by a dressing held in place by a bandage or liquid adhesive. Adhesive tape should never be used in these cases.

Eradication of foci of infection occasionally gives dramatic results in preventing recurring furuncles. Correction of disturbances of the digestive tract, vaccine (autogenous) therapy, and active immunization with staphylococcal toxoid deserve a trial. The most important measure, however, and one which is frequently overlooked, is the strict control of the diabetes. Roentgen-ray therapy in the early stage is often effective in aborting furuncles. In my experience it has been of little help unless given early.

CASE ILLUSTRATING CARBUNCLE COMPLICATING DIABETES

An American male, sixty-five years old, was admitted to the Jefferson Hospital July 26, 1935, because of a large carbuncle on his neck (Fig. 148). The carbuncle was incised on July 31 and a roentgen-ray treatment was given on August 2. By August 8

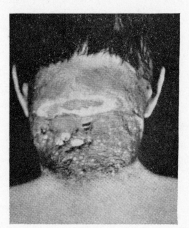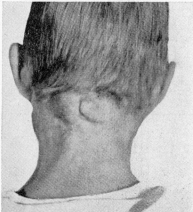

Fig. 148.—Photographs of a diabetic carbuncle taken when the infection was at its worst and when recovery was practically complete.

the area involved was considerably larger. The diabetes was not controlled. Crucial incisions were made on August 9. The patient was seen by the author for the first time on August 12. At that time the patient was irrational. There were evidences of arteriosclerotic heart disease with auricular fibrillation with a pulse deficit of twenty-four a minute. There was moderate albuminuria, 4 plus glycosuria (20.9 gm. in twenty-four hours), blood urea nitrogen 58 mg. and the plasma sugar 366 mg. per 100 cc. There were 18,650 leukocytes per cu. mm.

The carbohydrate intake was increased and the diet and insulin were equally divided and equally distributed. (If such a case presented itself now a higher carbohydrate quota, probably 250 gm., six equal nourishments and six equal doses of insulin to be given at four-hour intervals would be prescribed.)

The insulin was rapidly increased while glycosuria continued. The diabetes was readily controlled despite the fluctuating febrile course and with but two or three exceptions (August 16, 19 and September 3) the blood sugar values were satisfactory (See table 25). The extent of the carbuncle and the result are depicted in figure 148.

This patient died following an acute occlusion of a coronary artery in November, 1940.

Pruritus.—Pruritus is the most common symptom affecting the skin of the diabetic patient. It is especially common in females affecting the pudenda, the intense itching of which makes many patients seek treatment. To omit examination of the urine of a patient suffering from pruritus, generalized or local, especially if the genitalia are affected, is to miss the diagnosis and in many instances to deny the patient appropriate treatment.

The itching is caused (1) by the irritation of the skin set up by dried urine, which contains sugar, and (2) by fungi which find in the sugar-laden urine an ideal medium in which to multiply. Of the fungi the *Trichophyton* is the common offender. Minute injuries resulting from rubbing or scratching may be portals of entry for infecting organisms, notably the staphylococcus. Furuncles, carbuncles and erysipelas are contracted in this manner.

Treatment.—The treatment consists of local and general measures.

Local.—Cleanliness of the genitalia is essential. Gentle bathing of the parts with a cold solution of boric acid (saturated) after each voiding of urine is helpful. This is followed by daubing the affected areas with toilet lanolin or a bland ointment (such as α-butyloxycinchoninic acid-γ-diethylethylene-diamide [nupercaine]) having mild anesthetic properties. If, as not infrequently occurs, there is an associated vaginitis a douche, composed of a saturated solution of boric acid twice daily, is indicated. Failing prompt improvement some pelvic complication especially prolapsus uteri, cystocele, rectocele, or urethrocele should be considered.

General.—Control of the diabetes deprives the fungi of the glucose medium and by correcting the glycosuria the cause of the local irritation is corrected in most cases.

The nervousness and fatigue, due largely to disturbed rest, tending to intensify the symptoms and sometimes responsible for a generalized pruritus, are usually alleviated by sedation and analgesics though some patients are refractory to all forms of treatment. Phenobarbital gm. 0.0325 (½ grain) before each meal and gm. 0.097 (1½ grains) at bedtime, or sodium amytal, gm. 0.097 (1½ grains), two or three times daily alone or with acetylsalicylic acid, gm. 0.26 (5 grains), is of distinct value.

Xanthochromia.—Xanthochromia, or xanthosis as described by Salmon, is a yellowish tinting of the skin especially noticeable in the palms of the hands, the soles of the feet and the nasolabial folds. Associated with rubeosis —a rosy coloration of the skin of the face occurring in young patients with neglected diabetes—xanthochromia gives a "peaches and cream" complexion. It is due to an impaired destruction or impaired excretion of cer-

TABLE 25

The Diet and Insulin Regime Used and the Laboratory Results Obtained in the Management of a Patient Having Diabetes Complicated by a Large Carbuncle on the Neck Are Outlined

Date, 1935	Diet				Insulin (Unmodified)		Blood Sugar* (Mg.)	Urine		Wt. Kg.	
	P.	F.	C.	Cal.	Distribution	Total Units		Sugar (Gm.)	Acetone		
July 27	100	111	100	1800	None	..	268	62.5	+++	77	
Aug. 1	90	110	90	1710	None	..	263	29.6	+++		
3	90	110	90	1710	5— 5— 5	15	..	15.7			
7	90	110	90	1710	15—10—10	35	286	20.9			
13	60	51	175	1400	10—10—10—10	40	366	..	0	..	Equal division of diet and insulin begun.
15	60	51	175	1400	30—30—15—15	90	68	?	0		
16	60	51	175	1400	18—18—18—18	72	198	Trace	0		
17	60	51	175	1400	18—18—18—18	72	125	+ and 0	0		
19	60	51	175	1400	18—18—25—25	86	263	+	0		
22	60	51	175	1400	22—20—20—22	88	123	Neg.	0		
26	60	51	175	1400	20—20—20—20	80	125	Neg.	0		
28	70	80	175	1700	22—12—18	52	..	Neg.	..	..	3 meals and 3 doses of insulin resumed.
31	70	80	175	1700	22—12—18	52	98	Neg.	0		
Sept. 3	70	80	175	1700	22—12—18	62	232	Neg.	0		
5	70	80	175	1700	22—12—18	72	187	Neg.	0		
10	70	80	175	1700	22—12—18	80	112	Neg.	0		

tain lipochromes, the most conspicuous of which is carotin, derived from pigment-containing foods, notably carrots, sweet potatoes, corn, and butter and egg yolk. The nature of the disturbance and its relationship to diabetes has been discussed by Heymann.[128] An accumulation of the lipochrome in the blood, xanthemia, is a prerequisite to the xanthochromic discoloration of the skin. Fruits and vegetables rich in lipochrome have been extensively employed in diets for diabetic patients. Hence an increased supply superimposed on a faulty utilization, destruction, or excretion of the pigment makes the diabetic patient a susceptible subject to this disorder. The recent trend toward normal diets for diabetic patients and better facilities to control the diabetes has reduced the frequency of xanthochromia.

It appears that xanthosis occurring in diabetes does so as the result of the disturbance of carbohydrate metabolism. Contrasted with normal subjects diabetic children showed a marked delay in reducing an artificially increased blood carotin content to normal.

Xanthochromia may be confused with jaundice. The sclerae are not icteroid, however, the bilirubin content of the blood is normal, and there is no bile in the urine.

Treatment.—Beyond its cosmetic effect, which is not marked, xanthochromia is an innocent condition. It causes no symptoms but occasional embarrassment. The condition is corrected by continued control of the diabetes. In this manner normal utilization of the carbohydrate and of the lipochrome is restored. The xanthochromia subsides slowly. Its disappearance may be hastened by temporarily reducing foods rich in lipochromes, notably eggs, sweet potatoes, corn, butter, and carrots. Care should be taken not to interfere with the vitamin and mineral intake. Yeast concentrates and vitamins A and D may be administered. Skimmed milk will provide calcium. Iron and ammonium citrate, 2 to 4 gm. (30 to 60 grains) daily, may be given during the period of rigid dietary restriction.

Xanthelasma.—Xanthelasma occurs in nondiabetic as well as in diabetic patients though it occurs much more frequently in the latter. It should not be confused with xanthoma diabeticorum. It consists of a collection of slightly raised yellow, fatty, flattened tumors, and occurs about the inner canthus of the eyelids. It is usually bilateral. The condition is more prevalent in females than in males. No treatment beyond that of controlling the diabetes and maintaining a normal blood cholesterol is indicated. The tumors do not disappear unless excised or otherwise removed. This may be indicated for cosmetic reasons. If excised they tend to recur. Otherwise the condition is innocent.

Xanthoma Diabeticorum.—This rare complication of diabetes is manifested by discrete cutaneous nodules (Fig. 149), 1 to 3 mm. in diameter, appearing symmetrically for the most part about the elbows, knees, and buttocks though the forearms, dorsum of the hands, the toes, neck, and back are affected but to a much less degree. The eruption does not occur on the face. The nodules have a yellowish center with a reddish periphery, are hard, like kernels of wheat, and are not tender. Xanthomatous nodules may also occur on the tongue (see Fig. 150). Xanthoma diabeticorum is a manifestation of uncontrolled diabetes with hyperlipidemia. The patient (M. C.) of whom the photographs in figures 149 and 150 were taken, had an initial blood cholesterol level of 1666 mg. per 100 cc. (cholesterol ester

340 mg.), a blood sugar concentration of 488 mg. per 100 cc. and a carbon dioxide combining power of 33 volumes per cent. This patient also exhibited a classic example of lipemia retinalis, and his blood plasma had the appearance of cream. Further consideration of xanthoma diabeticorum is presented in Chapter XI.

Treatment.—Control of the diabetes is essential. The diet, until the disorder is corrected, should contain but little fat (30 to 40 gm.) and a liberal

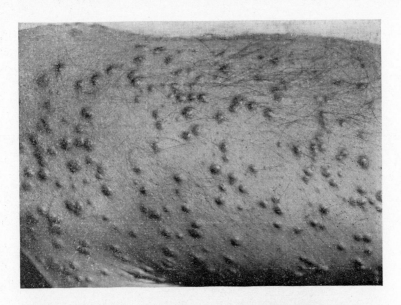

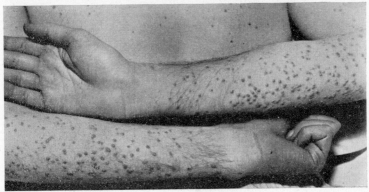

Fig. 149.—Nodular cutaneous eruption in a case of xanthoma diabeticorum (Patient M. C.).

carbohydrate quota (300 to 340 gm.). Patient M. C., aged twenty-five years, being 181 cm. (6 feet and ¾ inch) in height and weighing 72 Kg. (158 lb.) was given a diet of: protein 110 gm., carbohydrate 350 gm. and fat 40 gm. (2200 calories). M. C. required 44 units of protamine zinc and 24 units of crystalline insulin each morning. On the foregoing regimen the diabetes was controlled, the lipemia retinalis disappeared promptly, and the cutaneous nodules lost their firmness, the affected areas became flattened, and within two months all evidences of the disorder, including the xanthomatous nodules on the tongue, had disappeared.

Though the lesions disappear under treatment, they tend to recur if the diabetes is neglected. Subsequent to the control of the diabetes it is permissible to increase the fat and reduce the carbohydrate contents of the diet to amounts employed in the treatment of uncomplicated diabetes.

Necrobiosis Lipoidica Diabeticorum.—These discrete, clearly defined, reddish cutaneous papules, from 1 to 3 mm. in diameter, occur four times as frequently in the female with neglected diabetes as in the male. The condition is rarely seen in nondiabetic individuals. The lesion does not fade on pressure. It increases in size and progresses slowly from the reddish papule with a smooth glistening and firm surface. Eventually atrophic changes with ulceration in the center take place. At this stage the lesion

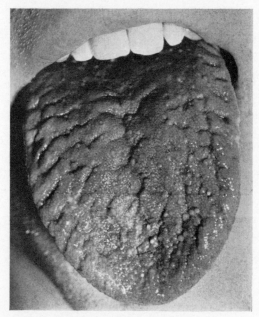

Fig. 150.—Xanthomatous nodules occurring on the tongue of a patient having xanthoma diabeticorum (Patient M. C.).

may be several centimetes in diameter surrounded by a reddish or violaceous region of infiltration.

A single lesion of necrobiosis lipoidica diabeticorum may appear but more frequently there are multiple lesions in various stages of development and located for the most part on the legs below the knees.

The etiology of this disorder is unknown. Local injury (*e.g.*, from scratching) may play a part. In most cases it occurs in patients with neglected diabetes and the majority of patients in whom this disorder appears are between ten and forty years of age.

Prevention as well as treatment lies in the control of the diabetes. Diets low in fat and containing liberal carbohydrate quotas (200 to 300 gm.) are indicated. No effective local treatment for this disorder has been found.

The reader is referred to comprehensive reviews of this subject by

Hildebrand, Montgomery and Rynearson,[124] and by Michelson and Leymon.[125]

Hirsutism.—Hirsutism appears in diabetes in two forms:

1. It occurs as a fine lanugo hair on the back and arms of the young patient who is undernourished and whose diabetes is not controlled. It occurs especially in individuals with a fair complexion. This type of hirsutism is corrected by control of the diabetes and by improved nutrition.

2. Achard and Thier (1921) attracted attention to the *diabète des femmes barbes*. They described the syndrome of hirsutism, amenorrhea, and obesity. This syndrome is due to hyperplasia or tumor growth of the adrenal cortex. The prevalence of hirsutism in diabetic women suggests that an increased functional activity of the adrenal cortex, either primary or secondary to hypophyseal dysfunction, is a common occurrence in diabetes. Adrenal cortical tumors on the other hand are uncommon and infrequently cause diabetes. The literature on this subject was reviewed by Duncan and Fetter,[126] who found only eleven cases recorded in which adrenal cortical tumors apparently accounted for the hirsutism and diabetes. They added a case of their own and five more have been recorded since their review.

Control of the diabetes is indicated. Removal of the adrenal tumors is advisable but only after careful preparation is made for the management of an acute adrenal insufficiency which may follow the operation.

Hirsutism similar to that seen in cases of adrenal cortical tumors occurs in pituitary basophilism. The treatment is directed toward reducing the functional effect of the tumor either by irradiation or removal.

Areas of Local Necrosis Following the Injection of Contaminated Insulin.—One patient was admitted to the Pennsylvania Hospital because of large (3 to 5 cm.) areas of necrosis appearing at the site of each "insulin injection." These reactions occurred immediately after the injection and after using insulin for eight years without any untoward reactions. On investigation it was discovered that the insulin in the bottle had been partially replaced by concentrated ammonium hydroxide apparently with homicidal intent.

Dermatitis Gangrenosa.—A rare condition of gangrene involving the skin of the trunk or extremities has been described by Riven.[127] Large vesicles occurred on the back, thighs, and legs with subsequent gangrene of the underlying areas. The patient had fever and staphylococci were recovered from the vesicle fluid.

Other Skin Disorders.—Epidermophytosis, lipodystrophies, and local allergic cutaneous reactions to insulin are dealt with elsewhere in the book. Diabetic patients may be subject to all skin disorders that are seen in nondiabetic persons. The treatment is the same as in the nondiabetic subject, but in general improvement will be facilitated if the diabetes is adequately controlled.

DISTURBANCES IN SEXUAL CHARACTERISTICS COMPLICATING DIABETES

Female.—Delayed development of secondary sexual characteristics, disturbance or absence of menstruation and an early menopause are frequent in women with untreated diabetes. Fertility is reduced, though the incidence of conception has increased during the insulin era. Libido is frequently reduced. It is rarely increased. Abortions are more prevalent in the diabetic than in the nondiabetic women. This is attributable, to a large extent, to faulty management or total neglect of the diabetes.

With control of the diabetes catamenia commences at a normal age. Catamenia is restored within a few months if amenorrhea has occurred as a result of the diabetes. A restoration of sexual desire is usual and the likelihood of conception is greatly increased.

Male.—The chief sexual disturbance in the male resulting from diabetes is impotence. There is apparently no disturbance in fertility. Impotence is rarely corrected by control of the diabetes. In fact, in several instances, I have observed that loss of libido was added to impotence after insulin therapy was begun. Loss of libido is more common in diabetic than in nondiabetic men.

DISEASES OF THE LIVER

Despite the important part played by the liver in carbohydrate metabolism, disease of this organ is an uncommon complication of diabetes. In uncontrolled diabetes enlargement of the liver is not infrequent, however. This is noted especially in children and is due to infiltration of fat, and in some cases to accumulation of water in the intercellular spaces. Rapid changes in the size of the liver are attributed largely to changes in the water content. Distention of the liver capsule in this manner causes discomfort and tenderness in the hepatic area. Tests of liver function usually show normal responses.

The hepatomegaly of diabetes is corrected by controlling this metabolic disorder. Protamine zinc insulin has made uniform control of diabetes, even in young patients, a simple matter. As a consequence it has aided in correcting and preventing hepatomegaly. Experimentally the feeding of raw pancreas, and the administration of lecithin, choline or betaine, and lipocaic have prevented and corrected hepatomegaly in depancreatized animals. Resort to these measures is not necessary clinically. Uniform control of the diabetes suffices.

CHOLECYSTITIS AND CHOLELITHIASIS IN DIABETES

Cholecystitis and cholelithiasis are so frequent in obese, but otherwise normal patients, that it is not surprising to find them to be common in the middle-aged diabetic population, the majority of whom are overweight. Warren[128] found that 31 per cent of 453 diabetic patients who were over thirty years of age and who came to autopsy had gallstones. In contrast he found gallstones in 21 per cent in the same age group of 500 nondiabetic patients.

Extension of infection from the gallbladder via the biliary passages, lymphatics, contiguity and blood stream to the pancreas has been considered as a cause of diabetes. An associated hepatitis, as described by Conn and his associates,[129] may cause hyperglycemia and glycosuria after the ingestion of carbohydrate and yet very low blood sugar values occur during fasting periods. More will be said of these cases in the discussion of chronic hypoglycemia in Chapter XIII.

Treatment.—A chronic cholecystitis occurring in the diabetic patient should be treated medically. Regularity of the hours of work and rest, avoidance of overeating, frequent vacations, a diet consisting of frequent meals of easily digested foods comprise the treatment. Fried foods are avoided, as are pork, pies, pastries, and excessive sweets. Biliary drainage is worth a trial as a therapeutic as well as a diagnostic measure. Acute fulminating cholecystitis in the person with diabetes does not subside as it may in the nondiabetic person, with bed rest and nursing care. Instead, the inflammatory process tends to become progressively worse. Surgical intervention is indicated and the operation should be performed without needless delay.

Cholelithiasis associated with colic is an indication for surgical intervention. Furthermore, since the diabetic patient withstands a chronic infection poorly, surgical drainage or removal of the gallbladder should be seriously considered when gallstones are observed roentgenologically, in the symptom-free patient. The risk, in biliary tract disease, as well as in surgery of the biliary tract, is somewhat greater in the diabetic than in the nondiabbetic person, but one must accept a slightly higher mortality in the diabetic patient with gallstones than in the nondiabetic of comparable age and pathological processes.

Surgery and Diabetes Mellitus

The majority of diabetic patients at one time or another acquire or develop conditions which require surgical treatment. It should be stressed, in dealing with diabetic patients, that each is a candidate for ketosis, no matter how mild the diabetes. Notwithstanding, wound healing is normal if the diabetes is controlled, and as I have previously stated, "Reparative, prophylactic, and emergency surgery are conducted successfully in the presence of diabetes. Insulin, although it has increased tremendously the margin of safety, has not simplified the management of the diabetes in these cases. No other complications call for more experience and skill with insulin. Simultaneous medical and surgical attention is essential. A surgeon might better ignore Lister's contributions to surgery than to be oblivious to the need of cooperation with the internist." Best results are secured when both surgeon and internist have an abiding interest in and are qualified by long experience to deal with diabetic patients suffering from surgical complications.

The internist is responsible for the treatment of any complicating medical condition, for prescribing the diet and the insulin, and for securing the laboratory analyses. Intravenous glucose (dextrose) and saline prior to and following the operation is prescribed by the internist after determining the surgeon's wishes for any modification from the routine. The internist is present at the operation and he sees the patient twice daily, at least, until the emergency has passed.

The surgeon is responsible for the surgical aspect of the case. This comprises (1) sharing the responsibility of diagnosing the surgical condition, (2) the decision regarding the time to operate, (3) the conduct of the operation, and (4) postoperative surgical care.

Rarely is it necessary for the internist to delay operation, because of the diabetes. The circumstances which make surgical measures necessary are among the common causes of the disturbances in metabolism which imperil the lives of these patients. Eradication of the provocative condition simplifies the correction of these secondary disturbances.

Surgical intervention is delayed if the carbon dioxide combining power of the blood plasma is below 35 volumes per cent or if the plasma gives a strongly positive reaction for acetone. Under these conditions, despite the urgency or gravity of the surgical condition, a short delay in operation is essential to allow correction, partial or complete, of the ketosis. Active treatment as for impending coma will reduce remarkably, within a few hours, the risk of operation by correcting the ketosis and adding to the glycogen reserve. Barring ketosis, a hyperglycemia need not deter surgical intervention. It is the ketosis and the accompanying deprivation of glycogen reserve and not the hyperglycemia which adds to the risk. In fact it is desirable that a diabetic patient be presented for operation with a sufficient degree of hyperglycemia, 150 to 220 mg. per 100 cc., to guard against any likelihood of a hypoglycemia, due to continued insulin action, during the operation.

Diet.—If immediate operation is not imperative two or three days are well spent in reducing the hyperglycemia and glycosuria, and in eradicating any ketosis. In this manner the risk of the operation is decreased, the glycogen reserve is increased and knowledge of the patient's general reaction to treatment can be obtained.

The diet contains: *Protein* ⅔ to 1 gm. per Kg. of the estimated normal weight; a liberal *carbohydrate* quota, approximately 3 gm. per Kg. of the normal weight. Under no conditions should the allowance of carbohydrate be curtailed during the preoperative period; *total calories*, 25 calories per Kg. of the normal weight; *fat* makes up the calories not provided by protein and carbohydrate. A liberal intake of fluid is encouraged. If there is dehydration it may be necessary to give normal saline subcutaneously or by vein in addition to broths, tea, and coffee by mouth. If there is a high fever or if the patient is seriously ill the diet is divided into six equal meals, one given every four hours. If the fever is moderate or of a mild degree four equal nourishments, one every six hours, usually suffices; if the patient is not apparently ill and is afebrile the usual three meals daily may be continued until the day of operation.

The diet may be made up of liquid, soft, or solid foods as conditions warrant.

Insulin.—Afebrile patients who are allowed the regular three meals daily until the day of operation continue also on their usual program of protamine zinc insulin alone or with crystalline insulin until the day of operation. The protamine zinc insulin is then replaced by an equal amount of crystalline insulin and the total is divided into four or six doses as the need demands (*vide infra*). In the presence of infection, fever, and toxemia the amount of insulin given is steadily increased until it is adequate to control the hyperglycemia and glycosuria, and to prevent ketosis.

The elderly and obese patient suffering from mild diabetes, which under ordinary conditions is satisfactorily controlled by a diet without insulin, almost always requires insulin if an infection or acute surgical condition is contracted.

These patients are given insulin during the course of acute complications if the fasting blood sugar level exceeds 120 mg. per 100 cc., or if the *postcibal* value exceeds 160 mg. per 100 cc. If the disturbance is mild and the patient is already taking insulin, a simple addition to the usual doses of insulin may be all that is required to control the glycosuria and the level of the blood sugar prior to operation. In more severe conditions, however, other measures (presented in the following pages) are indicated.

Crystalline insulin is the insulin of choice in the management of diabetes during the course of an acute surgical complication. Its action is more prompt and shorter in duration than that of protamine zinc insulin. These properties make it a simpler weapon to manipulate when both the blood sugar level and insulin requirement may be subject to rapid alterations. The amounts given and the distribution of the insulin are determined for the surgical patient as for the patient with an acute infection (see p. 828).

Day of Operation.—On the day of operation one-sixth of the preoperative diet is given, in liquid form, at 6 A.M. and is preceded by one-sixth of the previous day's total dosage of insulin. Only crystalline insulin is employed throughout the emergency period.

One hour before operation (preferably four hours after the 6 A.M. nourishment) 250 cc. (approximately 8 oz.) of a 10 per cent solution of glucose (dextrose) in normal saline is given by venoclysis without insulin. This measure guards against any hypoglycemic hazard during the operation and presumably adds to the glycogen stores. No insulin is given immediately before or during the operation, but immediately after operation a sixth of the former day's total is given subcutaneously.

Two to four hours after operation a liter (approximately 1 qt.) of a 5 per cent solution of glucose (dextrose) in normal saline is given slowly and continuously by venoclysis and is repeated at six-hour intervals until four-hour liquid nourishment can be taken by mouth—usually within twenty-four hours. Should the intravenous glucose therapy be indicated for several days, as in the illustrative case (Table 26), every third liter is given as glucose (dextrose) in saline and the remainder as glucose in distilled water unless more or less chlorides are indicated.

During postoperative convalescence the crystalline insulin is given at four- or six-hour intervals, as the case may demand. The insulin need may decrease abruptly after drainage of an abscess, after the removal of a secondarily infected gangrenous foot, or after the removal of a pyonephrotic kidney. On the other hand, in reparative and prophylactic surgery the postoperative insulin need is elevated during the healing process. The amount of insulin given is regulated in a crude way by the amount of glycosuria. If there is a marked glycosuria the insulin is steadily increased and as glycosuria disappears a modest reduction in the dosage is made. This flux one way or the other is continued until a normal status is restored. As convalescence proceeds, usually within three days, four nourishments at six-hour intervals are given in the twenty-four hours and when recovery is practically complete three meals with a bedtime nourishment are resumed. Insulin administrations are reduced accordingly. When recovery is complete a gradual return is made to protamine zinc insulin alone or combined with crystalline insulin.

Appendicitis is one of the most frequent reasons for emergency surgery and merits special mention. As in children, acute appendicitis in the diabetic patient is frequently atypical. It may give rise to few characteristic symptoms and the first signs of it may be the ketosis which it readily precipitates. Surgeons may predict the stage of this disorder in the nondiabetic patient, but almost invariably in the diabetic patient, as ascertained by a laparotomy, the process has extended beyond the limits predicted.

Choice of Anesthetic for the Surgical Diabetic.—Local, regional, and spinal anesthetics are best suited for diabetic patients undergoing surgery. The nature of the operation may necessitate a general anesthetic, in which case nitrous oxide, ethylene, or cyclopropane may be used. The degree of anoxia and the poor muscle relaxation count against the use of nitrous oxide in long operations. In view of the anoxia during ether anesthesia and the reduction in the glycogen of the heart muscle and in the liver, the period of anesthesia should be as short as possible. If sedatives are indicated preoperatively a small dose of morphia is suitable.

Intermittent spinal anesthesia as introduced by Lemmon[130] is the anesthesia of choice when it is applicable. Avertin anesthesia has been satisfactory in our experience.

Chloroform or ethyl chloride should not be given to a diabetic patient.

The detailed management of diabetic patients needing major surgery is presented below. Another case record illustrating the treatment of diabetes complicated by a large carbuncle is presented on page 837.

Female, aged forty-three years. Admitted to the Jefferson Hospital under the care of Dr. T. Shallow on February 19, 1938. She complained of abdominal pain which was generalized at first (February 17th); later the same day the pain became localized in the right lower quadrant. She had no desire for food.

This patient had been attending the diabetic clinic since January, 1938. She had a mild diabetes and did not require insulin.

Abdominal pain had been complained of "off and on" since April, 1937, but this was attributed to a "cyst." On February 17, 1938, the pain was sudden, sharp, and caused her to "double up." In an attempt to obtain relief a dose of magnesium sulfate was taken. This was effective but the pain did not abate. The patient attended the diabetic clinic on February 19th and was admitted to the hospital. She was extremely ill. Her temperature was 100° F., pulse rate 142 and respirations 36 per minute. The blood pressure was 190 mm. Hg systolic and 128 mm. diastolic. There was considerable sclerosis of the peripheral arteries. The skin was dry and hot, the tongue and pharynx dry and red, the heart sounds distant, and the abdomen was obese. The muscles of the right side of the abdomen were spastic with marked tenderness over the entire right lower quadrant.

The urine contained 1.4 per cent of sugar and acetone was present. The CO_2 combining power of the blood plasma was 37.5 volumes per cent and the blood sugar (fasting) level was 220 mg. per 100 cc.

The diagnoses were: acute suppurative appendicitis with localized peritonitis; diabetes mellitus; ketosis; generalized arteriosclerosis with arterial hypertension, and obesity.

An immediate operation was advised. One liter of 5 per cent dextrose solution in normal saline was given intravenously and 25 units of unmodified insulin were injected subcutaneously. The patient was given morphine sulfate, gm. 0.016 (grain ¼), and atropine sulfate, gm. 0.0004 (grain 1/150), at 3:15 P.M. and spinal anesthesia was given at 4:30 P.M.

A perforated appendix and a localized accumulation of pus was found in the appendiceal region. The appendix was removed and two drains were left in place.

Immediately after the operation 1000 cc. of 10 per cent dextrose in normal saline were given slowly by venoclysis and 20 units of unmodified insulin were given subcutaneously (Table 26).

The plasma sugar content at 8:30 P.M. was 200 mg., and the CO_2 combining power of the blood plasma was 37.5 volumes per cent. A 10 per cent solution of dextrose was given slowly but continuously. Every third liter of dextrose solution was given in normal saline. The insulin was increased until, on February 21st, a satisfactory blood sugar

TABLE 26

SHOWING THE DETAILS OF TREATMENT AND THE LABORATORY DATA IN A CASE OF DIABETES COMPLICATED BY ARTERIOSCLEROSIS AND A LOCALIZED PERITONITIS FOLLOWING A RUPTURED APPENDIX

Date, 1938	Diet				Insulin		Blood		Urine		Fluids		Remarks
	P., Gm.	F., Gm.	C., Gm.	Total Cal.	Units per Injection	Total Number of Units	Sugar in Mg. per 100 cc.	CO₂ (Vol. %)	Sugar, %	Acetone	Intake in cc. 24 Hours	Output in cc. 24 Hours	
Feb. 19	Preoperative. 1000 cc. 5% glucose. Postoperative.				25 35—35	... 95	220*	....	1.4	...	4000	1175	Fasting blood sugar before admission. Operation 4.30 P.M.
20	2000 cc. 10% glucose. 3000 cc. 10% glucose. 1000 cc. 10% glucose intravenously.				35—35—35—35—........—45 35—35—35—45—45	230	210 200 (8:30 P.M.) 222 (A.M.)	37.3 34.7	2.9	+	4000	1000	Glucose alone and with saline given slowly and continuously via indwelling venous cannula.
21	4000 cc. 10% glucose. 1000 cc. 10% glucose in normal saline.				45—45—40—40—40—40	250	236 (P.M.) 194 (A.M.)	51.9 51.9		+	5000	950	
22	3000 cc. 10% glucose. 2000 cc. 10% glucose in normal saline.				40—40—40—45—45	250	139 (P.M.) 215 (A.M.)	67.2 55.8	2.5	0	5000	1025	
23	3000 cc. 10% glucose. 2000 cc. 10% glucose in normal saline.				45—45—45—45	225	182 (A.M.) 126 (4 P.M.)	62.3	1.6	0	5000	1350	45 units given before each liter of glucose solution.
24	3000 cc. 10% glucose. 2000 cc. 10% glucose in normal saline.				45—45—45—40	175	98 (A.M.) 114 (4 P.M.)	....	1.0	0	4000	1300	
25	60	51	200	1500	40—40—40—40	160	141 (A.M.)	....	0	0	5000	900	Diet (liquid) in 4 equal feedings 1 every 6 hours.
26	60	51	200	1500	30—30—30—30	120	69 (P.M.)	....	0	0	2000	1000	
27	60	51	200	1500	16—16—16—16	64	....	....	0	0	2100	1000	
28	60	51	200	1500	16—16—16—16	64	....	....	0	0	3000	1000	Solid food permitted.
Mar. 3	60	51	200	1500	16—16—16—16	64	109	....	0	0	2100	800	
6	60	51	200	1500	14—14—14—14	56	....	....	0	0	3800	800	
8	70	44	180	1400	14—14—14—14	56	....	....	0	0	3600	1075	
13					*(50)—0—0 14	...	....	....	0	0	4000	1700	
20	70	44	180	1400	14 (46)—0—0 14	...	98	....	0	0	3000	800	
23	70	44	180	1400	(46)—0—0 14	...	....	....	0	0	2900	900	Discharged.

* Protamine zinc insulin in parentheses.

level was obtained (139 mg. per 100 cc.) and the CO_2 combining power of the blood plasma was 67.2 volumes per cent.

The abdomen had become soft by February 22nd, though there was continuous fever. Neither food nor liquids had been allowed by mouth. Nutrition was maintained by the slow, continuous, intravenous administration of 10 per cent dextrose. On February 25th, fluids were allowed by mouth and a diet (liquid) containing 60 gm. of protein, 200 gm. of carbohydrate and 51 gm. of fat (1500 calories) was begun.

There was a gradually diminishing purulent discharge from the incision until March 18th. The infecting organism was the *Staphylococcus aureus*.

Comment.—There were several important considerations in the management of this patient:

1. An overweight patient having a mild diabetes acquired an acute infection. The effect of acute infections with fever is always unfavorable in diabetic patients. The anorexia with the resulting reduction in the carbohydrate intake occurring at a time when the total metabolism is increased by fever predisposes to ketosis. The increased metabolism is carried on at the expense of the body fats. A vicious circle is thus established: infection and fever, loss of appetite, low carbohydrate intake, increased total metabolism, increased fat breakdown, and ketosis.

The vicious circle is broken by four measures: (1) an adequate carbohydrate intake; (2) sufficient insulin (these measures correct the disproportionately high fat metabolism); (3) the eradication of the infection (this reduces the total metabolism, dissipates the fever and restores the appetite); and (4) adequate liquids are of value in correcting and preventing dehydration. The need for insulin decreases as convalescence is established. Shortly after her discharge from the hospital this patient no longer required insulin.

I wish to emphasize again that although the diabetes was mild in this overweight patient, nevertheless the demands created by an acute infection aggravated the diabetes and emergency measures were necessary. *It is remarkable how frequently the changing status of the diabetes during acute infections is disregarded.*

2. This patient, though only forty-three years of age, had an arterial hypertension with extensive arteriosclerosis. The latter is common, especially when the diabetes is mild and has been untreated for long periods. It can be assumed that any diabetic patient at or beyond middle life presents, because of these changes, a greater surgical risk than nondiabetic subjects.

3. A point of interest was the activity of the patient in spite of the seriousness of her illness. Widespread abdominal infections in diabetic patients often cause fewer symptoms than is ordinarily found in patients not having diabetes.

4. The *preoperative treatment* of the diabetes. Was it wise to operate so early, or should the surgeon have waited for a lower blood sugar level and a higher CO_2 combining power of the blood plasma? Major surgical procedures should be delayed if the blood sugar exceeds 300 mg. per 100 cc. with a CO_2 combining power of the plasma below 35 volumes per cent, with strong reactions for acetone bodies in the blood plasma and urine. During this delay the ketosis may be corrected by giving fluids, glucose, chlorides and insulin.

For the patient under consideration no delay was necessary. In fact, as in most cases, the most important step in the treatment was to eradicate the infection as early as possible. Hence a safe dose, 25 units, of unmodified insulin was given and partial correction of the dehydration was accomplished by the intravenous administration of 1 liter of a 5 per cent solution of dextrose in normal saline.

DISEASE OF THE THYROID GLAND COMPLICATING DIABETES

General Considerations.—Hyperthyroidism (exophthalmic goiter) occurred as a complication of diabetes in 180 of Joslin's[131] 15,601 patients (1.15 per cent). Diabetes complicates toxic nodular goiter more frequently than it does toxic diffuse goiter. This is probably because the former is a disease of longer duration. The disease of the thyroid gland precedes the development of diabetes in a slight majority of cases. It occurs for the most part in relatively young patients and is more frequent in female than in male patients.

Hyperthyroidism activates a borderline or potential diabetes. It intensifies a preexisting diabetes as noted by the increase in the concentration of sugar in the blood and the amount of sugar in the urine, and it reduces the apparent efficiency of insulin. Besides having a neutralizing effect on insulin it, by virtue of its effect upon the adrenal glands, depletes the storage of glycogen in the liver. An unusual sensitiveness to the *overdosage* of insulin ensues. The normal endogenous means of combating a hypoglycemia is reduced, hence insulin reactions in these patients are likely to be severe. Furthermore, hyperthyroidism reduces the renal threshold for glucose. (Under normal conditions glucose—dextrose—may be given continuously without causing glycosuria, but in the subject suffering from hyperthyroidism, 0.6 gm. per Kg. is sufficient to provoke glycosuria.) A normal threshold is restored after correction of the hyperthyroidism. In hyperthyroidism there is a reduction in the ability of the liver to store glucose as glycogen and in diabetes there is an impairment in the utilization of glucose in general. A greater tendency for glucose to accumulate in the blood ensues and with the reduction in the level of the renal threshold it is readily understood why large quantities of sugar are lost in the urine, why a rapid reduction in body weight ensues and why ketosis develops with remarkable rapidity in the untreated diabetic subject suffering from hyperthyroidism. Occasionally a diabetic patient may, with the onset of hyperthyroidism, develop anorexia and lose body weight rapidly. In such a case the diabetes may be alleviated to a considerable degree.

Diagnostic Considerations.—Glycosuria occurring in the patient suffering from hyperthyroidism requires special consideration. It occurs in between 30 and 40 per cent of cases of hyperthyroidism without diabetes, being slightly more frequent in toxic diffuse goiter than in toxic nodular goiter. Furthermore the blood sugar level tends to be higher than normal in patients suffering from hyperthyroidism. Not infrequently what appears to be a mild diabetes disappears after thyroidectomy.

The hyperglycemia occurring in hyperthyroidism *per se* is under more control than that occurring in the diabetic patient with hyperthyroidism. In the former there is a rather persistent ceiling, at a moderate level, 150 to to 200 mg. per 100 cc., which the blood sugar level rarely exceeds in the absence of diabetes. In the latter insulin therapy is essential if severe degrees of hyperglycemia are to be prevented.

A tentative diagnosis of diabetes in a patient also suffering from hyperthyroidism may be safely made if the fasting blood sugar exceeds 150 mg. per 100 cc. This is in contrast with 120 mg. as the upper border of normal in those who have not hyperthyroidism. Glucose tolerance tests are affected by both disorders, yet they are of value in detecting a diabetes coexisting with hyperthyroidism. In diabetes the hyperglycemia develops gradually after the ingestion of 100 gm. of glucose and the blood sugar value does not return to normal within two hours, and indeed rarely within three hours. When this test is applied in uncomplicated hyperthyroidism the hyperglycemia develops abruptly with an ensuing prompt reduction of the blood sugar level, reaching normal within two hours. The glucose tolerance test applied in the presence of diabetes and hyperthyroidism may or may not reveal a fasting hyperglycemia, but there is a prompt elevation of the blood sugar usually exceeding 200 mg. per 100 cc. one hour after the administration of glucose, and the two-hour level exceeds 170 mg. per 100 cc.

Hyperthyroidism may be overlooked in a patient in coma even though it may have been the precipitating cause of this complication. If the clinical history is suggestive, if there is a continued tachycardia, tremor, or other manifestation of hyperthyroidism, treatment should include the administration of iodides, as outlined in Chapter V.

Treatment of the Diabetic Patient Suffering from Hyperthyroidism.— The margin of safety for the diabetic patient is reduced by hyperthyroidism, a cure of which should not be needlessly delayed. Control of the diabetes preliminary to operation is readily secured and a storage of glycogen in the liver is encouraged by giving a diet liberal in carbohydrate content (300–400 gm.) and divided into six equal feedings, one every four hours. A liberal protein content of the diet (1 to 1.25 gm. per Kg. of body weight) is desirable. This is a greater allowance than was permitted before iodine was used. Iodine has reduced the risk of exaggerating the hyperthyroidism by the liberal intake of protein. Protection of the liver is further enhanced by giving thiamine (vitamin B_1), 3 to 10 mg. a day. The vitamin B complex supplemented by vitamin A is also recommended. The insulin (crystalline) is divided into equal doses, one given before each nourishment. Additions are made to the insulin as indicated by the persistence of glycosuria in the fractional urine collections. Great quantities of insulin may be necessary. The insulin may appear ineffective but if sufficient amounts are given this apparent insulin resistance is overcome.

Treatment of the hyperthyroidism is conducted as in the nondiabetic patient. Complete rest in bed and oral administration of compound solution of iodine (Lugol's solution), 0.6 cc. (minims 10) or saturated solution of potassium iodide three times daily is advisable for about ten days in preparation for a subtotal thyroidectomy. Potassium iodide is preferred to Lugol's solution by some and is given in doses of 0.3 cc. (5 minims) of the saturated solution three times daily. Sedation is provided by phenobarbital 0.03 to 0.09 gm. (½ to 1½ grains) three times daily. Iodine therapy is continued for about two weeks after operation. The effect of iodides is less in degree and in uniformity in cases of toxic nodular goiter than it is with cases of toxic diffuse goiter. A reduction of the basal metabolic rate, an alleviation of the symptoms of hyperthyroidism and a decrease in the insulin requirement ensue. The ideal time for surgery is when these evidences of improvement, as judged clinically and by the reduced metabolic rate, have reached their maximum. The conduct of treatment on the day of operation and postoperatively is the same as for other surgical conditions (see page 847).

Experience with these patients emphasizes that the prognosis is bad if they are not operated upon. Operative measures are desirable for the toxic diffuse goiters, the toxic and nontoxic nodular goiters.

The results following a subtotal thyroidectomy are usually gratifying. The diabetes is made milder, but is not cured, insulin is more effective, the metabolism rate is restored to normal, and a restoration of normal nutrition is readily secured.

Irradiation of the thyroid is resorted to when operation is refused or when some cardiovascular or other complication contraindicates surgical intervention. Repeated treatments are necessary. They should be conducted by a competent radiologist.

The treatment during a thyroid storm or crisis which may occur before thyroidectomy or a few hours or several days after thyroidectomy is outlined in Chapter V, on page 246.

Myxedema.—Myxedema (hypothyroidism) is an uncommon complication of diabetes. The subnormal metabolism characterizing hypothyroidism alleviates rather than intensifies a tendency to diabetes.

Hypothyroidism has been intentionally produced by Wilder (1934) and by Rudy, Blumgart and Berlin (1935) in cases of severe diabetes. A decrease in the severity of the diabetes with a proportionate reduction in the need for insulin ensued.

Correction of hypothyroidism in a diabetic patient by giving thyroid intensifies the diabetes, reduces the carbohydrate tolerance, and raises the need for insulin. These changes parallel increases in the metabolic rate.

INSULIN-REFRACTORY AND INSULIN-RESISTANT CASES

Insulin-refractory are separated from insulin-resistant patients for practical purposes. This division is desirable for contrast and clarity. Patients who are *insulin-refractory* may be defined as those patients who show no response whatever to injections of large amounts of insulin. In contradistinction is the *insulin-resistant* diabetic patient who may require large amounts of insulin, even several hundred units a day, but who is definitely benefited by it.

Insulin-refractory Group.—Diabetic patients who are unaffected by insulin fortunately are exceedingly rare. Refractoriness to insulin is due to some complication, recognition of which indicates the plan of therapy. It is unknown why patients become refractory to insulin. It is conjectural whether the condition is due to insulin destruction, as appears to be the case in some instances, to insulin neutralization, to the excretion of insulin, to some unexplained influence exerted by disturbed function of the liver, or to a combination of these influences. Patients completely refractory to insulin so far as can be determined by the usual chemical data have been found to have (*a*) progressive destruction of the pancreas, (*b*) extensive disease of the liver, (*c*) overwhelming sepsis, or (*d*) profound and prolonged ketosis. Progressive destruction of the pancreas occurred in one of Dr. David Farley's patients recently observed at the Pennsylvania Hospital. The lesion was an extensive *abscess* permeating the full length of the pancreas. Enormous doses of insulin were ineffective in preventing deepening coma and death. A deficiency in vitamin A with metaplasia of the cells of the pancreatic ducts may have predisposed to the secondary infection. The combined effect of destruction of the insulin-producing mechanism and sepsis accounts in some way for insulin refractoriness.

Hemochromatosis with its relentless destruction of the functional integrity of the islets of Langerhans and its effect upon the function of the liver also in some patients causes complete ineffectiveness of insulin as interpreted by its failure to reduce the level of the blood sugar. To such a patient Root gave 1680 units of insulin in twenty-four hours without preventing death in coma. That there is some factor at work other than the destruction of the insulin-producing mechanism is obvious as the amounts of insulin given to these patients surely exceeds the normal production of insulin.

TABLE 27

CONDITIONS DETRACTING FROM THE EFFECTIVENESS OF INSULIN

Insulin-refractory Group	Insulin-resistant Group
1. Progressive destruction of the pancreas	1. Ketosis
(a) Abscess of pancreas	2. Increased total metabolism
(b) Hemochromatosis	(a) Obesity
(c) Invasion of pancreas by neoplasms	(b) High caloric diet
(d) Multiple pancreatic calculi	(c) Fever, infections and toxemias
(e) Acute pancreatitis	(d) Pregnancy
2. Certain diseases of the liver	3. Skin disorders
(a) Cirrhosis	(a) "Sunburn"
(b) Unexplained	(b) Reaction to deep roentgen ray therapy
3. Overwhelming sepsis	(c) Eczema and pruritus
4. Profound and prolonged ketosis	(d) Aseptic skin wounds
	4. Allergy
	5. Cardiovascular disease
	(a) Atheromatous changes in arteries (?)
	(b) Myocardial insufficiency with edema and enlarged liver
	6. Hepatic disease
	7. Disturbance of other endocrine glands
	8. Polycythemia (?)

A patient of Mason's[132] was given 2075 units of insulin in twenty-four hours. At autopsy *calcareous degeneration of the pancreas*, also a cyst in the midbrain were found.

Invasion of the pancreas by *new growths, multiple pancreatic calculi, acute pancreatitis* and extensive epithelial proliferation in the ducts of the pancreas with secondary infections also cause progressive destruction of the pancreas and in so doing may make the patient refractory to insulin. This does not always occur, however. An amazingly small amount of functioning islet tissue may be found without apparent lack of insulin function.

Disease of the Liver.—Occasionally extensive disease of the liver causes a refractoriness to insulin though more frequently it has the opposite effect. The *modus operandi* is not understood. A patient having cirrhosis of the liver was unaffected by 1100 units of insulin in one day as reported by Mohler and Goldburgh (1932).

Overwhelming Sepsis.—The manner by which the patient suffering from overwhelming sepsis becomes refractory to insulin is unknown. Destruction of insulin by a trypsin-like ferment elaborated by the leukocytes has been offered as a possibility. Secondary damage to the liver may play a prominent part in this group. Neutralization of insulin by antagonistic hormones increased during infections or the excretion of insulin in the urine are probably unimportant factors.

The treatment of "insulin-refractory" patients is considered at the end of this section, see below.

Insulin-resistant Group.—Increased resistance to insulin is common. It is caused by many conditions and at one time or another is observed in varying degrees in every diabetic patient taking insulin. One factor alone may be at work as is observed when the total calories increase, or a combination of influences such as infection, fever, leukocytosis, increased total metabolism, and ketosis may be responsible. Occasionally no apparent cause is detectable.

Simple increases in the total metabolism accomplished by artificially induced fever and by single doses of dinitrophenol were shown, by Hayward and Duncan,[116] to reduce the effectiveness of insulin. An insulin resistance of a much greater degree occurs as the result of ketosis or infection, especially if there is a concomitant leukocytosis. That this insensitiveness to insulin occurs as a result of a secondary hepatic disturbance seems likely. Changes in insulin sensitivity may be considered under the following: (1) the increasing severity of the diabetes which occurs as the result of neglect, overstrain of pancreatic function by a continuous and abnormal demand; (2) disturbances of hepatic function due to cardiac decompensation and of infection with associated toxemia, fever, and ketosis; (3) the effect of hormonal antagonists to insulin, pituitary, adrenal, and thyroid; (4) toxemias due to ultraviolet-ray burns and to deep roentgen-ray therapy; (5) increases in total metabolism which occur with increasing body weight, increased caloric intake, pregnancy, artificially induced fever, thyrotoxicosis, administration of thyroideum, and the administration of dinitrophenol.

It is obvious that these groups of disturbances may overlap and intensify the insulin resistance by occurring simultaneously in the same patient.

Overweight patients tend to be resistant to insulin. A dose of insulin given to a thin, young patient having a severe diabetes usually will have a greater blood sugar lowering effect than will an identical dose given to an obese adult subject with mild diabetes. Attempts have been made to explain this on a hypophyseal basis. This may be the explanation but the difference in the total metabolism in the two patients whether due to endogenous or exogenous differences seems to explain the disparity in the effectiveness of the insulin. Differences in the sensitivity of diabetic patients to insulin have been especially well shown by MacBryde[133] and Himsworth.[134]

Considerable resistance to insulin may occur following "sunburns," deep roentgen-ray therapy, allergic disturbances, eczema, pruritus of old age, deficiency in the vitamin B complex, and aseptic wounds. A search for a broken needle in the subcutaneous tissues of a young diabetic patient resulted temporarily in nearly doubling the insulin need, yet there was no infection. Fear, anxiety, and pain may cause a transitory increase in the resistance to insulin.

Treatment of Insulin-refractory and Insulin-resistant Patients.—The factors in this treatment include: (1) Identification and correction, if possible, of the complicating disease is the first consideration. (2) The control of the diabetes. (3) The sparing and reenforcing of the function of the liver.

Diet.—In insulin-refractory and insulin-resistant cases the diet therapy is the same. Sufficient *protein* is given to maintain nitrogen balance, two-thirds to 1 gm. per kilogram of body weight. A liberal *carbohydrate* quota is important, 250 to 400 gm. being allowed while the *fat* quota is kept low, 40 to 50 gm. The diet is divided into six equal nourishments, one being given every four hours. In milder cases four meals, one every six hours, is satisfactory. The meals may comprise liquid, soft or solid foods as indicated by fever, acuteness of the complicating infection and the ability of the patient to take the different foods. The intake of carbohydrate is important. It may be necessary to pass a tube into the stomach or into the duodenum and give liquid feedings by this route.

Insulin.—The insulin (crystalline) is given as frequently as are the meals and the amount is steadily increased even if many hundreds of units are necessary to overcome the peak of the insulin resistance. A precipitous decline in the insulin need may follow the eradication of a complication and the control of the diabetes. Prompt and great reduction in the amount of insulin given may be necessary if hypoglycemic reactions are to be avoided.

The increasing resistance to insulin which occurs in uncomplicated diabetes is often an index of neglect. Adequate control of the disorder will accomplish a reduced rather than an increased need for insulin.

PERNICIOUS ANEMIA

Pernicious anemia and diabetes occasionally occur in the one patient. Heredity plays an important part in each. These two diseases, both of which may cause degenerative changes in the spinal cord, are readily controlled. These changes are more likely to occur and be more severe in the diabetic patient who has a primary anemia than in a nondiabetic subject. No effort should be spared to keep the erythrocyte count at 5,000,000 per cu. mm. or more by means of the intramuscular injection of liver extract or by the oral administration of desiccated hog's stomach (ventriculin) (see Chap. VII). Adequate control of the diabetes is likewise important. Pernicious or primary anemia and diabetes have in common (1) the influence of heredity, (2) incurability, (3) ready controllability, and (4) tendency to become progressively more severe if neglected. The reader is referred to Root's[135] articles in which he reports seventy-nine cases of pernicious anemia occurring in diabetic patients.

INFECTIONS OF THE URINARY TRACT

Infections of the urinary tract are frequent and serious complications of diabetes. They may present few symptoms and their presence should be carefully sought for in every case of diabetic coma. They occur much more frequently in patients whose diabetes is neglected than in those in whom this metabolic disorder is under control.

The infection may be hematogenous, as occurred in a patient observed recently at the Pennsylvania Hospital. A male adult admitted because of metastatic abscesses resulting from a minor injury and infection of the hand, and diabetes. During his final illness the duration of which was eight months, he had, at different times, subcutaneous abscesses, purulent adenitis, pyelonephritis, and finally, a cerebellar abscess. In each instance the *Staphylococcus aureus* was the causative organism and it was also recovered in numerous blood cultures.

Another patient, an adult male, had pyelonephritis caused by a nonhemolytic *Staphylococcus aureus* and prior to to its correction with ammonium mandelate, he required 690 units of insulin a day. As the infection subsided the resistance to insulin disappeared and the patient when discharged a short time later did not require insulin.

Seiple[136] reported a case of diabetes complicated by staphylococcal septicemia with multiple abscesses and a pyelonephritis in which recovery from the infection took place following the removal of the original focus of infection by amputation of a leg. Chemotherapy (sulfapyridine) was used and also ammonium mandelate. Multiple transfusions were given and the original focus was exposed to roentgen-ray therapy.

Bertram[137] cites an instance of an ascending pyelonephritis following catheterization of a patient in diabetic coma. Catheterization of any diabetic patient should be avoided if possible. If catheterization is essential it should be done with great care, and urinary antiseptics should be employed as a prophylaxis against infection.

The treatment of infections of the urinary tract are the same in the diabetic as in the nondiabetic patients. This applies to surgical as well as medical measures. The management of diabetic patients requiring surgery and during acute infections has been dealt with earlier in this chapter.

HEMOCHROMATOSIS (BRONZE DIABETES)

Hemochromatosis is a cause, not a result of diabetes mellitus. It is a rare, chronic, and progressive disorder of metabolism, the first case of which was decribed by Trousseau in 1865. The outstanding characteristics of hemochromatosis are (*a*) an abnormal deposition of pigments, especially hemosiderin, an iron-containing pigment, in the skin and viscera. Pigmentation of the skin is absent in approximately 20 per cent of cases. (*b*) A cirrhosis of the liver and pancreas. Progressive cirrhotic changes take place in the various organs. The liver and pancreas are the first organs affected and are the sites of the more extensive cirrhotic changes. (*c*) Diabetes mellitus is present in most, but not all cases. Diabetes mellitus occurs as a complication of hemochromatosis and is an index of the damage done to the islet cells of the pancreas. Diabetes is usually a late manifestation of the disease.

Hemochromatosis occurs in the great majority of instances in patients between the ages of forty-five and fifty-five years. The condition is unknown before the age of twenty years but from this age to forty-five years there is a consistent increase in its incidence. A decline in the incidence occurs between the ages of fifty-five and seventy years. Females are rarely affected before the fifth decade of life. The disorder affects males from twenty to twenty-five times as frequently as females (see table 28). The disease is rare. Sheldon was able to collect only 311 authentic cases of hemochromatosis in the entire medical writings on this subject. Only thirty-four cases of hemochromatosis were observed at the Mayo Clinic in seventeen years (1923–1940).

Etiology.—The cause of hemochromatosis is obscure. Von Reckling-hausen, in 1889, identified two pigments derived from hemoglobin, (*a*) hemosiderin, an iron-containing compound, loosely bound with fat and protein, which turns black when brought in contact with ammonium sulfide, and (*b*) hemofuscin, which contains no iron but stains readily with basic aniline dyes and is believed to be related to the melanins. It is the iron-containing hemosiderin which plays the more prominent part in hemochromatosis. It is retained and deposited chiefly in the connective tissue of the glandular organs, the lymph nodes, striated muscles, reticulo-endothelial system, alveolar epithelium, cartilage, and the synovia. Why these deposits occur is not known. It is known, however, that the cirrhotic changes progress in direct proportion to the amount of hemosiderin deposited in the organs. Necrosis of the pigment-containing cells is followed by the cirrhotic process. Mallory[139] produced hemochromatosis experimentally by the administration of copper, and he believes that the disease as seen clinically is a manifestation of poisoning with copper. This hypothesis has not gained general acceptance. Neither has poisoning with bacterial toxins, alcohol, lead or zinc proved to be a likely cause of hemochromatosis.

TABLE 28

THE AGE AND SEX INCIDENCE IN 290 CASES OF HEMOCHROMATOSIS*

Age Group	20 to 25	26 to 30	31 to 35	36 to 40	41 to 45	46 to 50	51 to 55	56 to 60	61 to 65	66 to 70	71 to 75
No. of cases (male).......	2	7	13	37	48	59	56	34	9	8	4
No. of cases (female).....	..	1	1	..	..	2	5	1	3	1	
	2	8	14	37	48	61	61	35	12	9	4

* After Sheldon.[138]

Dry[140] and Sheldon[138] believe that the disease is an inborn constitutional abnormality of iron metabolism. Sheldon states, "This hypothesis of an inborn error of metabolism appears to be the only one which will encompass the enormous array of facts provided by the clinical, pathological, and chemical aspects of the disease." Hemochromatosis has been observed to occur as the result of a familial and hereditary predisposition. Whatever the cause, there is an abnormal retention of iron. The total iron content of the body reaches 25 to 50 gm. in hemochromatosis in contrast to approximately 3 gm. in the normal person.

Hemochromatosis is distinct from hemosiderosis in which iron pigments, resulting from the excessive destruction of erythrocytes, are deposited in the tissues. In the latter condition there is irrefutable evidence to indicate that such iron pigments are used again in the formation of blood, whereas in hemochromatosis the hemosiderin is not used again, and, furthermore, there is no apparent abnormal destruction of red blood cells in hemochromatosis.

There is convincing evidence that minute quantities of iron in excess of body needs, are retained and accumulate over a period of many years.

Eventually this retention of iron brings about the clinical characteristics of hemochromatosis. This retention may be due to an inherited abnormal avidity of the tissues for iron with an inability of the cells to rid themselves of the ferrous compounds.

Pathology.—Hemosiderin and to a less extent hemofuscin are found in excess of normal throughout the organs and tissues of the body with the exception of the brain and nervous system.

Hemosiderin is deposited in the propria of the sweat glands and in the deeper strata of the malpighian layer of the skin. The liver is reddish, rusty, or of an ochre tint. It is enlarged and the capsule is thickened. The surface is firm and nodular (hob-nail appearance) and there are massive accumulations of hemosiderin and lesser amounts of hemofuscin. The hemosiderin predominates in the extracellular areas but is present also in large amounts in the cells of the liver, in the fibrous tissue, in the Kupffer cells, in the liver capsule, and in the walls of the blood vessels.

The *pancreas* is also heavily pigmented with hemosiderin and some hemofuscin, giving it a reddish or rusty color. It is enlarged, firm and cirrhotic. The normal architecture of the pancreas is largely replaced by fibrous tissue, and there is degeneration and actual loss of acinar and islet tissues. Acute necrosis of the pancreas is, in rare instances, the cause of death.

Melanin, normally present in the deeper layers of the epidermis, is present in excessive quantities. Deposits of hemosiderin are found also in the spleen, lymph nodes, the pituitary, thyroid, and salivary glands, and in the myocardium. Hemofuscin is found in the cells of glandular organs, in connective tissue, in smooth muscle, and particularly in the walls of the medium-sized and small arteries.

On *physical examination* the pigmentation of the skin and mucous membranes and the enlargement of the liver (the most constant findings in this disease) may be noted. The liver is quite firm, not tender, and is usually smooth but may be rough (hob-nail) if the disorder is well advanced. In late states of the disease the liver is small and cannot be palpated. The spleen is palpable in about 60 per cent of cases. Ascites appears frequently as a late manifestation.

Laboratory Investigations.—A moderate hypochromic anemia, hyperglycemia, glycosuria, and reduced serum albumin with a reversal of the albumin-globulin ratio are common findings. Icterus, though an unusual complication of this disorder, may be present and cause an elevation of the serum bilirubin. Hypercholesterolemia with xanthomatous eruptions is sometimes present. Moderate elevations of the basal metabolic rate are not uncommon.

Dry[140] found no significant departure from normal in the iron balance studies in cases of hemochromatosis, indicating that the average daily retention is exceedingly small but must be greatly prolonged to account for the large quantities of iron in the tissues.

A summary of an unusual case of hemochromatosis reported by Cantarow and Bucher[141] is as follows:

Hemochromatosis was observed in a patient who did not have glycosuria or iron-containing pigment in the skin. The skin, however, was blue-

bronze in color due to excessive deposits of melanin. The absence of glycosuria and of iron-containing pigment in the skin with the presence of
cutaneous xanthomatosis and with hypercholesterolemia and hyperbilirubinemia, caused considerable difficulty in making a correct diagnosis. The
true nature of the condition was established by examination of a section
of liver removed during a peritoneoscopic examination. Evidences of
adrenal cortical hormone and male sex hormone deficiencies were obtained
during life. The possibility was suggested that a reduced carbohydrate
tolerance or actual diabetes which might otherwise have been present might
have been mitigated by the hypocorticoadrenalism.

Chemical examination of the tissues revealed enormous quantities of iron
in the liver, pancreas, and retroperitoneal lymph nodes, but relatively little
iron was found in the heart and skeletal musculature. Death was due to the
unusual complication of acute necrosis of the pancreas.

Diagnosis and Symptomatology.—The diagnosis is easily made when
the outstanding characteristics—*pigmentation of the skin, diabetes mellitus,*
and *cirrhosis of the liver*—are present. The urinary sediment may contain
hemosiderin but the identification of the pigment in a section of skin taken
at biopsy remains the most conclusive of the diagnostic criteria. A specimen of liver secured during a peritoneoscopic examination will serve to
establish the diagnosis in a puzzling case of hemochromatosis.

The disorders which are likely to be confused with hemochromatosis
are argyria and Addison's disease. Pigmentation is the only characteristic
which these three conditions have in common. An adequate history and
careful physical examination should establish the correct diagnosis. Hemochromatosis and Addison's disease occasionally occur in the same patient.
The clinical and chemical characteristics of the latter are discussed in
Chapters V and VI.

The *pigmentation* of the skin is visible in approximately 80 per cent of
patients suffering from hemochromatosis. It occurs as the first sign of the
disease in about a quarter of the cases and gives the skin a bronzed, bluish-
metallic, leaden, or slate color. This color involves the entire body but is
more obvious in parts normally pigmented, about the genitalia and perineum, and in the folds of the skin, scars and on exposed portions—the face,
the extensor surfaces of the forearms, and the dorsum of the hands. Pronounced pigmentation may be due to increased melanin in the malpighian
layer of the skin without any iron-containing pigment being present. Pigmentation of the buccal mucosa occurs in about 16 per cent of cases. The
conjunctiva may also be pigmented. Pigmentation has been observed to
decrease during insulin therapy. Some patients have intense itching of the
skin.

Diabetes mellitus, with its characteristic symptoms, notably excessive
thirst, polyuria, excessive appetite, loss of weight, and lassitude, may result
from hemochromatosis. Though the symptoms of diabetes were the first
noted in 25.7 per cent of Sheldon's[138] collected cases, diabetes is usually a
late manifestation of the disease and before insulin was available the diabetes became progressively worse. Death within twelve months usually followed the onset of diabetes. The diabetes may now be controlled but it may
in rare instances become exceedingly severe and the patient may pass

through a state of increasing insulin resistance to one in which insulin is completely ineffective.

Twenty-six of the thirty cases of hemochromatosis observed by Butt and Wilder[142] had diabetes as demonstrated by laboratory methods, and diabetes was present in 78 per cent of Sheldon's cases.

Asthenia is a common symptom of hemochromatosis. It may be secondary to disturbances in the function of the adrenal glands, to the cirrhosis of the liver, or to the diabetes if this complication is not controlled.

Cirrhosis of the liver and the symptoms which it causes, notably lassitude, discomfort in the epigastrium, the sensation of heaviness in the abdomen, distention of the abdomen due to ascites, and enlargement of the liver are usually present. In the final stages of the disease the liver is usually small. Hematemesis, purpura, icterus, diarrhea, dyspepsia, vomiting, lanugo-like hair appearing on the scalp and loss of normal hair are among the infrequent manifestations of this disease.

Tuberculosis, hypogonadism, hypocorticoadrenalism, and carcinoma of the liver are not infrequent complications of hemochromatosis. When present they influence the symptomatology.

Prognosis and Treatment.—Hemochromatosis is a chronic disease, the clinical manifestations of which appear gradually, over periods of months and years. We can anticipate with considerable justification that the cause of death will change, if it has not done so already, from diabetic coma to hepatic failure or to complications arising as a result of cirrhosis of the liver. If it were not for insulin therapy, diabetic coma would still be the most common cause of death in these patients. Control of the diabetes has prolonged life and indeed in some cases insulin treatment seems to have interrupted the progressiveness of the hemochromatosis. The more common causes of death in patients suffering from hemochromatosis are recorded as: diabetic coma, 50 per cent; cirrhosis of the liver, 11 per cent; pneumonia, 10 per cent; tuberculosis, 9 per cent; and carcinoma of the liver, 7 per cent.

The outlook for patients suffering from hemochromatosis is undergoing a change, the outcome of which is not predictable. In the cases collected by Sheldon, the average interval between the first medical consultation and death was a trifle over eighteen months. Most of these patients were seen before the discovery of insulin. The survival now depends upon the ability of the patient's liver to regenerate more rapidly or at least as rapidly as it is destroyed.

The **treatment** of hemochromatosis comprises (*a*) treatment of cirrhosis of the liver; (*b*) control of the diabetes.

The diabetes is controlled as outlined elsewhere in this chapter. The diet should contain large amounts of carbohydrate (300 to 400 gm. a day) and adequate protein (at least 1 gm. per Kg. of the normal body weight). Insulin therapy is usually necessary. The amount given is increased until the diabetes is controlled. Usually moderate amounts suffice but occasionally the insulin may be remarkably ineffective. Huge doses may then be necessary.

Wilder[143] advocates the use of concentrated vitamin preparations, especially those of A and B_1 (thiamine). In treatment for the cirrhosis of the liver, abstinence from alcohol is advisable, as are the curtailment of activities, restriction of the sodium chloride intake (if ascites is present), the administration of diuretics, and, when necessary, abdominal paracentesis.

Restriction of the iron intake is futile as it would require many years to make any impression on the quantities of stored ferrous compounds.

DIABETES MELLITUS AND PREGNANCY

By Garfield G. Duncan and Ferdinand Fetter

The problem of pregnancy complicating diabetes has assumed increasing importance for both obstetrician and internist since the introduction of insulin. Before the advent of insulin, pregnancy rarely occurred in diabetic women. This was fortunate since the pregnant woman with severe uncontrolled diabetes was in grave danger of losing her life with no likelihood of producing a living child.

Today, with improved methods of management, diabetes, even if severe, is not incompatible with pregnancy; diabetes is not a contraindication to pregnancy, and rarely, if ever, does it justify a therapeutic abortion. Although fertility in diabetic women is still less than in nondiabetics, the pregnancy rate has risen to between 10 and 15 per cent in contrast to 2 to 6 per cent in the pre-insulin era. The maternal mortality rate has been greatly reduced, and the few deaths that do occur are rarely attributable to the diabetes *per se*. Pregnancy carries but little risk for the intelligent and cooperative diabetic woman who understands the problems of diabetes. She is instructed in the necessity of strict control of the diabetes, frequent analyses of the urine and blood for sugar, and in addition, determinations of the blood prolan level and the estrin and progestin excretion at two- or three-week intervals after the twenty-fourth week of pregnancy. The hormonal determinations offer the possibility of an early prediction and the appropriate management of the toxemia of pregnancy in these patients. While the outlook for the diabetic mother has progressed favorably, that for the fetus has not shown the same degree of improvement. Stillbirths are yet frequent, occurring about six times as often as in nondiabetic women. If we have a means (the estimation of the serum prolan) of predicting accidents in diabetic pregnancies, a great reduction in fetal mortality is to be expected. White[144] has already observed this in her series.

Consideration of the Diabetic Mother

Ketosis.—Pregnant diabetic women are prone to develop ketosis—one of the most dangerous complications of pregnancy. Unless carefully guarded against, it develops rapidly, facilitated by a reduced supply of glycogen associated with an increasing total metabolism. The likelihood of developing ketosis is increased further by the changing need for insulin, hyperemesis, and nutritional deficiencies, notably to a deficiency in the vitamin B complex.

Sterility.—The cause of the relative sterility in diabetic women is not known. Disturbed hormonal relationships are probably responsible. A decrease in the amount of gonadotropic hormone of the anterior pituitary (follicle and luteinizing principles) is especially likely. Nutritional deficiencies in uncontrolled diabetes may also be a cause of sterility.

Abortion and Miscarriage.—In Joslin and White's series[145] of 130 pregnancies in eighty diabetic women in the pre-insulin period, 22 per cent of the patients aborted. The incidence of abortion has been reduced to 10 per cent in 176 pregnancies occurring in 132 women since the introduction of insulin. Abortion and miscarriage are directly proportional to the lack of control of the diabetes. Abortion or miscarriage occurred in 33 per cent of a series of uncontrolled diabetic patients, as compared with an incidence of only 2 per cent in patients whose diabetes was well controlled. Adequate control of the diabetes makes abortions or miscarriages fifteen times less likely to occur.

Stillbirths and Toxemia.—Stillbirths, despite insulin therapy, are six times as common in diabetic women as they are in nondiabetic women. There are several factors that operate to produce this. One is the well-known propensity of the babies of diabetic women to be overdeveloped. The tendency to polyhydramnios, attributed to fetal diuresis caused by hyperglycemia, in diabetic mothers also increases the number of stillbirths. The abnormalities in the chemistry of the blood (sugar and CO_2) of the diabetic mother has been considered a factor; however, with exact control of the diabetes, abnormal chemical changes in the blood should not be present. Probably most important is the undoubted high incidence of toxemia (usually mild) in the pregnant diabetic patient who is thus predisposed by (1) a high incidence of arteriosclerosis, and (2) hormonal abnormalities. These factors are associated with an increased incidence of toxemia in pregnant women in general. In Joslin and White's series of 306 pregnancies, toxemia occurred in 12 per cent of the cases; in Mengert and Laughlin's[146] series of thirty-three pregnancies, it occurred in 24 per cent, and in Potter and Adair's[147] series of sixteen pregnancies, it occurred in 50 per cent.

That the preeclamptic toxemia is predictable in most of these patients on the basis of an excess serum prolan (chorionic gonadotropin) after the sixth month of pregnancy is apparent from the investigations of Smith and Smith[148, 149] and the clinical observation of White.[144] Of fifty-one pregnant diabetic women, White reports: (1) that the pregnancy was uneventful in twenty whose serum prolan values were repeatedly normal (less than 200 rat units per 100 cc. of blood) during the last trimester of pregnancy; (2) that of eleven patients having excessive serum prolan values which rose steadily to term and who received no hormonal therapy (estrin and progestin) all developed complications. Eight developed toxemia, five (62 per cent) of whom required emergency deliveries, and three delivered prematurely; (3) that in two successive pregnancies in the same patient there was in each instance a temporary excess of serum prolan which subsided spontaneously. The reduction in the serum prolan was preceded by a rise in the estrin excretion. Following these two events the signs of toxemia were ameliorated; (4) that of seventeen patients who had excess serum prolan and who received continuous substitution treatment (estrin and progestin) there were no emergency deliveries.

The high frequency of excess serum prolan in pregnant diabetic women is in contrast to its occurrence in one of fifty pregnancies in normal women.

Maternal Mortality.—In the pre-insulin era the maternal mortality was

28

between 25 and 30 per cent. Joslin has reduced the rate in his patients to 3.8 per cent since the introduction of insulin. This is an appreciable reduction, but it is still more than six times the maternal mortality of 0.6 per cent for nondiabetic women. Mengert and Laughlin had no maternal deaths in thirty-three pregnancies in twenty-eight diabetic women. We had one maternal death (3.2 per cent) resulting from a ruptured uterus in the last twenty-eight pregnancies* in diabetic women. The trend is toward a lower maternal mortality in diabetic women. Prior to the general use of insulin the maternal deaths were largely the result of the diabetes. Now, theoretically at least, there is no excuse for diabetes itself being responsible for a maternal death.

Fetal Mortality.—Abortions, miscarriages, and stillbirths occur more often in the diabetic than in the nondiabetic woman. Stillbirths are still six times as common in diabetic as it is in nondiabetic women. White has reported a fetal mortality of 22 per cent (including neonatal deaths) in diabetic women in the insulin era who were delivered at term. This contrasts unfavorably with the 3.8 per cent of stillbirths reported for the general registration area. The means by which the frequency of stillbirths can be reduced are now at our disposal. These are: (1) strict control of the diabetes; (2) the prediction of toxemia by high serum prolan values; (3) treatment of such cases by the substitution of estrin and progestin, and (4) emergency deliveries in the cases in which toxemia develops.

THE DIAGNOSIS OF DIABETES IN THE PREGNANT WOMAN

The woman known to have diabetes who becomes pregnant offers no diagnostic problem. However, when a pregnant woman develops diabetes, the second diagnosis, because of the great frequency with which sugar is found in the urine of pregnant women, is not always easy to make. Aside from lactosuria, which may be considered physiological during the period of lactation, glycosuria has been reported to occur at times during the course of pregnancy in from 35 to 60 per cent of nondiabetic pregnant women. In these cases the glycosuria is due to the lowering of the renal threshold for sugar, which is common in pregnancy. Hence the finding of considerable amounts of reducing substance in the urine of a pregnant woman is not sufficient evidence upon which to base a diagnosis of diabetes. A method of establishing the diagnosis of a low renal threshold is presented on p. 747. The same criteria for making a diagnosis of diabetes in the pregnant as in the nonpregnant diabetic patient are used (p. 734). To be on the safe side, pregnant women showing glycosuria, even with normal glucose tolerance curves during and three months after the termination of pregnancy, should be watched for the development of diabetes for several years.

THE EFFECT OF PREGNANCY ON THE DIABETES

There is a loss of carbohydrate tolerance and an increase in the insulin requirement during the first trimester of pregnancy, the period of greatest metabolic readjustment. During the second trimester, the period of greatest qualitative fetal development, the carbohydrate tolerance usually remains fairly stationary. The behavior of the carbohydrate and total food toler-

* Not published.

ance, and in consequence, the changes in the insulin requirement vary greatly in the final trimester of pregnancy. It has been our experience that if the diabetes is kept under strict control, the insulin requirement increases steadily in every case in the final three months. This is as one might expect with the increase in body weight and in the total metabolism. In patients with uncontrolled diabetes the glycosuria and hyperglycemia may subside in the final trimester due, we believe, to assistance rendered the mother by overactivity of the islets of the fetal pancreas. Some patients may show no apparent change in their carbohydrate or total food tolerance during pregnancy. Diabetes, if adequately controlled, is rarely, if ever, made permanently worse by pregnancy.

In view of these experiences we cannot agree with those who permit constant glycosuria and a mild degree of hyperglycemia in pregnant diabetic women. The danger of causing hypoglycemic reactions by strict control of the diabetes is grossly exaggerated. Actually, hypoglycemic reactions are difficult to produce in these patients and when they do occur there is no evidence that they appreciably harm either the mother or the fetus.

MANAGEMENT OF THE PREGNANT DIABETIC PATIENT

General Measures.—With certain limitations the regimen is the same as for a diabetic woman who is not pregnant. Good general hygiene and outdoor exercise are encouraged, but exercise should not be carried to the point of fatigue. The patient is closely observed by the obstetrician and the internist throughout the pregnancy. She should be seen at least every two weeks during the first two, and weekly during the final trimester.

Diet.—The diet should contain adequate amounts of calcium and the accessory food factors (see Chapters V and VIII respectively). Diets for diabetic patients tend to be low in vitamin B. The diet should be supplemented by the vitamin B complex, preferably in the form of eight to twelve compressed brewer's yeast tablets daily. Calcium is provided in adequate amounts by 1 quart of milk a day and in the form of tablets of calcium gluconate or lactate. The pregnant woman requires a liberal allowance of *protein*—not less than 1.5 gm. and preferably 2 gm. per Kg. of the standard weight.* An adequate supply of glycogen to meet the demands of pregnancy are provided by 3 to 4 gm. of *carbohydrate* per Kg. of the standard body weight. The *total calories* are regulated to prevent undernutrition during gestation—between 30 and 40 calories per Kg. of the standard body weight. During the last four or six weeks of pregnancy it may be well to lower the caloric intake sufficiently to prevent an undue gain in weight. This measure and the provision of adequate allowance of protein and vitamins may aid in preventing oversized babies. The difference between the total calories and those provided by the protein and carbohydrate is made up by *fat*.

Insulin.—We give insulin to every pregnant diabetic patient. The initial dosage may be estimated as for uncomplicated diabetes (p. 771). Adequate increases are made to maintain normal fasting and *postcibal* blood sugar values. The amount required to do this may treble or quadruple that required before gestation.

The importance of controlling the diabetes during pregnancy is shown

* See Appendix, page 938.

by White's[143] figures: Diabetes controlled, the percentage of living babies was 80; diabetes poorly controlled, the percentage was reduced to 52. Of our twenty-eight cases the only two fetal deaths were in cases in which the mother's diabetes was neglected. One of these women was not seen by us until she was in labor, and the other patient's diabetes was not controlled during pregnancy.

Management of the Pregnant Diabetic Woman during the First Trimester.—Nausea and vomiting are the chief complications of the first trimester. Feedings at intervals of from two to four hours supplemented by intravenous glucose, may be necessary to maintain an adequate intake of carbohydrate (3 to 4 gm. per Kg. of standard weight). If frequent small feedings are necessary, crystalline insulin should be given every three or four hours, the amounts being increased to correct glycosuria and hyperglycemia, or decreased to prevent insulin reactions. If the vomiting is not severe and frequent feedings are not needed, protamine zinc insulin may be used, supplemented by crystalline insulin before breakfast and before the evening meal if needed. The insulin requirement usually increases during the first trimester.

The Second Trimester.—This period is usually freest of complications. Ordinarily, the insulin requirement and carbohydrate tolerance do not change appreciably.

The Third Trimester.—In our experience,[150] when the diabetes has been successfully controlled in the first two trimesters, there is a steady increase in the insulin requirement during the final trimester. Exact control of the mother's diabetes spares the fetal pancreas and helps to prevent hypoglycemia in the new-born from excessive activity of the islet cells. It seems that if adequate exogenous insulin is supplied to the mother, the fetal pancreas does not react by compensating for the lack of endogenous insulin in the maternal pancreas. The increasing insulin need in the third trimester is a natural result of the rapid increase in total metabolism.

Since the observation which Carlson and Drennan[151] made on dogs, an increase in carbohydrate tolerance during the last trimester has been attributed to insulin supplied by the fetal pancreas. Gray and Feemster[152] observed a gain in the carbohydrate tolerance in a diabetic mother during the third trimester of pregnancy. The new-born infant developed a spontaneous and fatal hypoglycemia. The postmortem examination revealed hypertrophy and hyperplasia of the islet cells in the infant's pancreas.

TERMINATION OF PREGNANCY

There is some disagreement about the method of delivery of the pregnant diabetic woman. The question is whether cesarean section or spontaneous delivery is the method of choice.

Cesarean Section vs. Spontaneous Delivery.—Wilder[153] at the Mayo Clinic and White and Titus, associated with Joslin, have elected premature delivery by cesarean section, though White[144] states, "By this procedure alone there was no favorable effect upon the outcome of the pregnancy as shown by the almost constant rate of fetal deaths up to the year 1938." It is true that cesarean section spares the diabetic woman the effort of a normal labor, but, on the other hand, it substitutes in its place a major surgical procedure.

We advocate normal spontaneous delivery in all women whose diabetes is adequately controlled and who are normal from the obstetrical point of view. Cesarean section should not be undertaken because of the diabetes alone. Other indications for cesarean section, of course, may be present in a diabetic woman. In only two of our twenty-eight patients was this method of delivery resorted to. Mengert and Laughlin have reported thirty-three pregnancies in twenty-eight diabetic women. Of these, twenty-eight terminated in spontaneous delivery, two were breech extractions, two by outlet forceps, and one by cesarean section. There were no maternal deaths. The fetal mortality was six, or 18.2 per cent. This is but little higher than the fetal mortality of 17 per cent (which, however, includes neonatal deaths) reported by White in seventy-nine pregnant patients. The number of these patients delivered by cesarean section is not stated, but it was higher than the incidence of 3 per cent reported by Mengert and Laughlin. Considering that the fetal mortality from cesarean section alone ranges from 8 to 16 per cent a study of the comparative fetal mortality in these two series reveals that conservative management of these patients produces as many live births as does cesarean section, and is therefore to be preferred to the more radical methods, unless there are obstetrical or hormonal indications for a cesarean section.

A new era for the offspring of diabetic mothers is promised[143, 147, 148, 153] by the methods of predicting and controlling the preeclamptic toxemia of pregnancy. I refer first to the excess serum prolan (chorionic gonadotropin) and the reduced excretion of estrin and progestin, which precede the other signs of toxemia, i.e., increasing blood pressure, albuminuria, and edema; and second, to the substitution therapy with estrin and progestin. White states, "Substitution estrin and progestin therapy has controlled the rise of the serum gonadotropin, brought about the rise of estrin and progestin, and as a result late fetal mortality has fallen from 32 to 6 per cent, or nearly to the level of nondiabetic pregnancies; namely, 3.4 per cent." *

These encouraging results were secured by giving estrin (progynon B) 150,000 to 300,000 international units daily when the serum prolan was found to exceed normal after the sixth month of pregnancy. Also progestin (proluton) was given in doses of 10 to 20 mg. a day during the same period with the object of preventing excessive destruction of estrin. Substitutions of testosterone, stilbestrol, and pranon for estradiol and progestin are being observed.

These observations and those recorded on page 866 strongly recommend that (1) pregnant diabetic mothers who have normal serum prolan values be allowed to deliver spontaneously, barring obstetrical indications for a cesarean section; (2) that spontaneous delivery be permitted in those cases in which the serum prolan is reduced from excessive to normal values and estrin and progestin excretion increased to normal either spontaneously or by means of estrin and progestin therapy; (3) that in event of a failure to control the hormonal imbalance cesarean section be done without delay with the onset of signs of toxemia, i.e., a rising blood pressure, albuminuria and edema. If substitutional therapy fails to reduce the serum prolan to normal and if the baby is overdeveloped cesarean section is justified early in the ninth month of pregnancy.

* Based on 600 cases delivered at Faulkner Hospital, 1939.

Cesarean sections in diabetic women should not be resorted to, however, as a routine procedure. Diabetes *per se* does not constitute an indication for this procedure.

TREATMENT OF THE DIABETIC PATIENT DURING LABOR AND DELIVERY

The patient should receive the equivalent of 10 to 15 gm. of carbohydrate per hour during labor, which amounts to 150 to 200 gm. if the labor is long. The carbohydrate may be given by mouth or, barring this, by the intravenous route as a 10 per cent solution of glucose (dextrose) in distilled water or normal saline.

Crystalline insulin should be given in small doses at four-hour intervals, the amount given being increased or decreased according to whether sugar is present or absent, respectively, in each specimen of urine. The administration of carbohydrate and insulin reduces greatly the danger of ketosis during a long labor.

A prompt reduction in the insulin need after delivery is most marked in the patient whose insulin requirement had increased in the final three months of pregnancy. Obese patients who required large amounts of insulin during pregnancy can usually do without it within a few days after delivery. An increased need for insulin may develop following delivery, however, in those patients whose diabetes was ameliorated during the course of pregnancy. In these patients the withdrawal of the hyperactive fetal pancreas increases the mother's dependence upon exogenous insulin.

Lactation.—Diabetic women lactate poorly, even though they are allowed an ample diet. Diabetic animals also fail to lactate normally. The deficiency in the supply of milk may be due to a decrease in the lactogenic hormone of the anterior lobe of the pituitary gland. If the mother is anxious to nurse her baby, she should be allowed to do so, but supplementary feedings are almost certain to be needed. Patients, almost without exception, need less insulin while nursing their babies than they did before they became pregnant. In fact the lactating woman may be exceedingly sensitive to insulin. Lactose in the urine may be mistaken for glucose, and lochia renders the urine useless for examination during the early postpartum period, hence the amount of insulin given should be guided by frequent determinations of the blood sugar level.

CARE OF THE FETUS AND NEONATAL INFANT OF THE DIABETIC MOTHER

The infant born to a diabetic mother needs special care. The fetal mortality is too high. The challenge is presented in (1) death of the fetus followed by abortion in the early months of pregnancy, (2) stillbirths, and (3) the maceration of overdeveloped babies.

Fetal Anomalies.*—Congenital defects are more frequent in babies born of diabetic mothers than in the babies of nondiabetic women. Of 208 babies in Joslin and White's series,[143] an incidence of congenital anomalies of 3.4 per cent occurred, which is almost twice the incidence for the general population (1.8 per cent). The congenital defects noted were microcephaly, mongolian idiocy, congenital heart disease, atresia of the gastro-intestinal

---

* Experimental injections of prolan into pregnant rats and rabbits produced maceration and death of oversized fetuses, such as occurs in the toxemic diabetic patient.

tract, and achondroplasia. The congenital defects occurring in White's fifty-one cases all occurred in the abnormal hormone group—excessive serum prolan.

Large Babies.—Babies born to diabetic mothers are often unusually large. The exact cause for the overgrowth of these babies is not known. Wilder[152] states, "A large, flabby (edematous) fetus is an effect of nutritional deficiency of the mother." Maternal hyperglycemia or overnutrition may be factors. Exact control of the diabetes throughout the pregnancy and especially in the third trimester, usually prevents overgrowth of the fetus and results in the birth of a baby of normal size. With control of the mother's diabetes, and the prevention or correction of hormonal imbalance, the outlook for the infant born to a diabetic mother is good.

The special dangers of the neonatal period are hypoglycemia and asphyxia. We believe that inadequate control of the mother's diabetes during gestation may result in compensatory overactivity of the fetal pancreas, and thus predispose to the development of hypoglycemia in the infant after birth. Of our two fatalities, one infant apparently normal at birth was found dead at feeding time, and within a few minutes of being examined, on the second day of life. An intracardiac specimen of blood secured immediately contained 24 mg. of sugar per 100 cc. (Blood sugar values as low as 50 mg. per 100 cc. during the first day or two after delivery are physiological.) The fetal pancreas showed some hypertrophy and hyperplasia of the islets of Langerhans. The mother's diabetes had not been controlled during gestation. The other fetal death was a macerated fetus delivered of a diabetic mother who had had no prenatal care.

Randall and Rynearson[155] have advocated the intramuscular injection of 5 cc. of 10 per cent glucose (dextrose) solution* into each of the infant's buttocks shortly after birth. Further injection, of 10 cc. of 10 per cent dextrose solution by mouth, at four-hour intervals, are continued during the first forty-eight hours. These precautions are especially indicated if the infant shows clinical signs of hypoglycemia, or if the infant's blood sugar is low (less than 50 mg. per 100 cc.).

Feedings every two hours from birth through the first three days of life are important in preventing a hypoglycemia. Lactose water (5 per cent of lactose in water) is fed by means of a medicine dropper. Since the adoption of this plan we have not found intramuscular or subcutaneous infusions of glucose to be necessary.

Asphyxia.—Respiratory difficulties occur more often in infants born of diabetic than of normal mothers. Ketosis, hypoglycemia, or trauma to the cerebral cortex from a long labor associated with a large baby may contribute to the production of asphyxia. In White's series, 60 per cent of the infants showed some degree of respiratory difficulty. The usual care in removing the mucus from the infant's mouth and throat, and the use of an incubator in which the temperature is 29° C. (84.2° F.) and the atmosphere contains a large amount of oxygen will reduce the danger of asphyxia.

Outcome to the Infant.—If the infant of a diabetic mother is born alive its chances of survival are good. White found the neonatal mortality of

---

* This treatment is not devoid of the danger of causing a slough of the subcutaneous tissues.

these babies to be only 4 per cent, which is but 1 per cent higher than the 3 per cent neonatal mortality of other babies. The mortality during the first year of life of babies born to diabetic women was the same, 5 per cent, as that for babies born of nondiabetic subjects.

As to the probability that the infant will develop diabetes, if, as we believe, diabetes is carried as a recessive Mendelian trait, the child cannot inherit the disease from the mother alone. Unless the father has diabetes also, or carries a recessive factor for diabetes, the child will not develop this disease.

ILLUSTRATIVE CASES

M. K., aged twenty-seven years. Weight 155 pounds (70 Kg.). Height 59 inches (147 cm.). Admitted to Dr. Clifford Lull's service at the Philadelphia Lying-In Hospital on April 4, 1939, for the termination of a full-term pregnancy by a cesarean section. The patient was known to have had diabetes for fifteen years. Just prior to becoming pregnant she required 40 units of crystalline insulin daily (two doses). Her insulin requirement increased particularly during the first and third trimesters, until she was taking 130 units daily in three doses. Two weeks before term the diet was reduced gradually from 1800 to 1100 calories because of a rapid gain in weight. A reduction in the insulin given, from 130 to 88 units, ensued.

On admission her diet contained protein 60 gm., carbohydrate 150 gm. and fat 29 gm. (1100 calories). She received 88 units of crystalline insulin *per diem*.

The blood sugar (fasting) level was 155 mg. per 100 cc. There was constant glycosuria due to a proved low renal threshold for dextrose.

A roentgen examination of the pelvis revealed some contraction of the transverse diameter. The patient had developed puffiness of the face and ankles. Her blood pressure had increased over a period of one week from 150 mm. of Hg systolic and 90 mm. diastolic to 190 mm. systolic and 110 mm. diastolic and showers of granular casts were found in the urine. These evidences of toxemia and not the diabetes *per se* were the indications for the cesarean section.

On the day of operation, April 6th, this patient was given a liquid breakfast containing protein 15 gm., carbohydrate 62 gm. and fat 5 gm. (350 calories) at 6 A.M. preceded by 22 units of insulin (unmodified), one quarter of her usual daily requirement.

At 11 A.M., 250 cc. of a 10 per cent solution of dextrose were given intravenously and the operation was performed at 11:30 A.M., under nitrous oxide, oxygen and ether anesthesia. Unmodified insulin, 22 units, was given immediately after operation.

At 2 and 8 P.M., and at 2 A.M., 1000 cc. of a 10 per cent solution of dextrose in normal saline were given by venoclysis, each preceded by 22 units of insulin. At 8 A.M. on April 7th a diet containing protein 60 gm., carbohydrate 250 gm. and fat 18 gm. (1400 calories) was prescribed. This food was given in liquid form and was divided into six equal feedings, one every four hours. Beginning on April 11th it was given in four feedings.

The insulin requirement fell rapidly after delivery to 6 units before each meal on April 11th.

The mother had inadequate breast milk and, with the cessation of nursing, a gradual increase in the insulin requirement followed. At the time of discharge, on April 21st, she required 28 units of crystalline insulin before breakfast and 20 units before supper and her diet after April 18 contained 60 gm. of protein, 175 gm. of carbohydrate and 84 gm. of fat (1600 calories).

On this regimen the sugar content in her blood was 112 mg. per 100 cc. on April 25th.

The baby was a normal male and weighed, at birth, 6 pounds and 6 ounces. Lactose solution was given to the baby every two hours for the first three days of life.

F. V., white, aged twenty-nine years when seen in November, 1934. This patient had had five pregnancies; two ended in miscarriages; one in a full-term stillbirth; two were living children, of whom one died fourteen hours after birth and the other was living and well. Symptoms suggestive of diabetes had been present for about one month when she was seen in November, 1934. A diet aimed at undernutrition containing protein 80 gm., carbohydrate 90 gm. and fat 69 gm. (1300 calories), prescribed because she was overweight, served to control the diabetes without insulin. She became pregnant in December, 1934. Insulin therapy was begun at once and at the end of the first trimester 30 units a day were required. The diet had been increased to protein 80 gm., carbohydrate 150 gm., fat 87 gm. (1600 calories). At the end of the second trimester, she required 36 units and at the end of the third trimester 52 units of insulin a day. The diet was not changed. The diabetes was satisfactorily controlled throughout the period of gestation. The highest blood sugar value (fasting) was 144 mg. per 100 cc. This patient had a spontaneous precipitate delivery of a living, full-term normal female infant weighing 6 pounds 13 ounces.

The mother was given small doses of insulin for two days after delivery. Insulin was then discontinued and the diabetes was satisfactorily controlled. The diet contained 80 gm. of protein, 150 gm. of carbohydrate and 65 gm. of fat (1500 calories).

This patient became pregnant again in January, 1938. At the end of the first trimester, she required 22 units of insulin, and at the end of the second trimester, 42 units. The diet contained: protein 80 gm., carbohydrate 200 gm. and fat 87 gm. (1800 calories). At the end of the third trimester, the insulin need had risen to 98 units of protamine zinc insulin and 30 units of unmodified insulin a day. The diet was constant. In spite of the diet, which contained only 1800 calories a day, her weight increased from 79 Kg. (175 pounds) during pregnancy to 89 Kg. (197 pounds) at term. She was delivered on September 10, 1938, of a baby weighing 8 pounds 11 ounces. The baby gave evidence of moderate respiratory difficulty and cyanosis for the first forty-eight hours. Two ounces of a 5 per cent lactose solution were given to the baby every two hours. The infant's blood sugar level forty-four hours after birth was 55 mg. per 100 cc. Subsequently the infant developed bronchitis, but after recovery progressed normally. The diabetes was not so well controlled during the second pregnancy because of poor cooperation on the part of the patient. The blood sugar values varied for the most part from 140 to 210 mg. per 100 cc. We believe that the undue gain in weight on the part of the mother, the large baby and consequently a difficult delivery with asphyxia are related to lack of cooperation and to the failure to control adequately the diabetes. After delivery the mother did not require insulin.

BIBLIOGRAPHY

1. Root, H. F., and Bloor, W. R., Am. Rev. Tuberc., **39:** 714, 1939.
2. Von Mering, J., and Minkowski, O., Arch. of Exper. Path. in Pharmakol., **26:** 371, 1899.
3. Cawley, R., London Med. Jour., **9:** 286, 1788.
4. Weichselbaum, A., and Stangl, E., Wien. klin. Wchnschr., **14:** 968, 1901.
5. Allen, F. M., J. Metabolic Research, **1:** 1, 1922.
6. Wilder, R. M., Allan, F. N., Power, N. H., Robertson, H. E., J.A.M.A., **89:** 348, 1927.
7. Warren, S., Pathology of Diabetes, 2d ed., Lea & Febiger, Philadelphia, 1938, p. 39.
8. Opie, E. L., Jour. Exper. Med., **5:** 397, 1901; also in Special Cytology edited by E. V. Cowdry, New York, 1928.
9. Allen, F. M., Jour. Metabolic Res., **1:** 5, 1922.
10. Copp, E. P., Barclay, A. J., Jour. Metabolic Res., **4:** 445, 1923.
11. Warren, S., J.A.M.A., **88:** 99, 1927.
12. Dillon, E., Bull. Ayer Clin. Lab. Pennsylvania Hospital, **8:** 35, 1924.
13. Barron, M., Surg., Gynec. and Obstet., **31:** 437, 1920.
14. Mason, E., Jour. Clin. Invest., **9:** 31, 1930.
15. Winternitz, M. C., Thomas, R. M., and Le Compte, P. M., The Biology of Arteriosclerosis, Charles C. Thomas, Springfield, 1938.
16. Mallory, F. B., Pathological Technique, p. 126, 1938.
17. Warren, S., and Root, H. F., Amer. Jour. Path., **2:** 69, 1926.
18. Hershey, J. M., and Soskin, S., Am. Jour. Physiol., **98:** 74, 1931.
19. Best, C., Am. Int. Med., **7:** 145, 1933.
20. Dragstedt, L. R., J.A.M.A., **114:** 29, 1939.
21. Benedict, S. R., J.A.M.A., **57:** 1193, 1911.
22. Smith, M., J. Lab. Clin. Med., **7:** 364, 1922.
23. Stadie, W. C., Lukens, F. D. W., and Zapp, J. A., Jr., J. Biol. Chem., **132:** 423, 1940.
24. Folin, O., and Wu, H., J. Biol. Chem., **41:** 367, 1920.
25. Exton, W. G., and Rose, A. R., Proc. Assn. Life Ins. Med. Dir. Am., **18:** 252, 1931.

26. Hamman, L., and Hirschman, J. J., Bull. Johns Hopkins Hosp., **30:** 306, 1919.
27. Ellis, A., Quart. J. Med., **3:** 137, 1934.
28. Soskin, S., Allweiss, M. D., and Cohn, D. J., J. Physiol., **109:** 155, also **110:** 142, 1934.
29. Best, C. H., and Taylor, N. B., The Physiological Basis of Medical Practice, Williams and Wilkins Co., Baltimore, 1939, p. 938.
30. Matthews, M. W., Magath, T. B., and Berkson, J., J.A.M.A., **113:** 1531, 1939.
31. Adlersberg, D., and Porges, O., Klin. Wchnschr., p. 32, 1926; also Die Behandlung der Zuckerkrankheit mit fettarmer Kost, Vienna, 1929.
32. Sweeney, J. S., Arch. Intern. Med., **40:** 818, 1927.
33. Himsworth, H. P., Lancet, **22:** 1, 1939.
34. Young, F. G., Brit. Med. J., **2:** 393, 1939.
35. Duncan, G. G. and Fetter, F., Med. Clin. N. Amer., **18:** 261, 1934.
36. Joslin, E. P., Ibid., p. 277.
37. Pincus, G., White, P., Am. J. M. Sc., **186:** 1, 1933.
38. Wilder, R. M., Clinical Diabetes and Hyperinsulinism, W. B. Saunders Company, Philadelphia, 1940, p. 54.
39. Wilder, R. M., Ibid., p. 122.
40. Sansum, W. D., Blatherwick, N. R., Bowden, Ruth, J.A.M.A., **86:** 178, 1926.
41. Geyelin, H. R., Atlantic M. J., **29:** 825, 1926; also J.A.M.A., **104:** 1203, 1935.
42. Porges, O., and Adlersberg, D., Med. Klin., No. 40, 1932.
43. Rabinowitch, I. M., Canad. M. A. J., **23:** 489, 1930; Ibid., **33:** 136, 1935.
44. Stolte, K., Med. Klin., **27:** 831, 1931.
45. Abel, J. J., Geiling, E. M. K., Rouiller, C. A., Bell, F. K., and Wintersteiner, O., J. Pharm. Exper. Therap., **31:** 65, 1927.
46. Marbel, A., and Virtiainen, I., J.A.M.A., **113:** 1303, 1939.
47. Ricketts, H. T., and Wilder, R. M., J.A.M.A., **113:** 1310, 1939.
48. Duncan, G. G., Cuttle, T. D., and Jewesbury, E. C. O., Bull. Ayer Clin. Lab., **3:** 293, 1939.
49. Hagedorn, H. C., Jensen, B. N., Krarup, N. B., and Wodstrup, I., J.A.M.A., **106:** 177, 1936.
50. Scott, D. A., and Fisher, A. M., Proc. Am. Soc. Biol. Chem., **8:** 88, 1936.
51. Himsworth, H. P., Lancet, **1:** 127, 1936.
52. Newburgh, L. H., and Conn, J. W., J.A.M.A., **112:** 7, 1939.
53. Lawrence, R. D., and Archer, N., Brit. M. J., **1:** 487, 1937.
54. Wilder, R. M., Ibid., p. 92.
55. Watson, E. M., Canad. M. A. J., **43:** 444, 1940.
56. Allen, F. M., J.A.M.A., **82:** 1937, 1924.
57. Bowen, B. D., and Beck, G. M., Ann. Int. Med., **6:** 1412, 1933.
58. Wilder, J., Deutsch. Ztschr. f. Nervenh., **112:** 192, 1930.
59. Duncan, G. G., Canad. M. A. J., **33:** 71, 1935.
60. Bayer, L. M., J.A.M.A., **102:** 1934, 1934.
61. Roth, G. M., and Rynearson, E. H., Proc. Staff Meet. Mayo Clinic, **14:** 353, 1939.
62. Barborka, C. J., J.A.M.A., **87:** 1646, 1926.
63. Wilder, R. M., Ibid., p. 98.
64. Richardson, R., Jour. Clin. Invest., **13:** 699, 1934.
65. McQuarrie, I., Proc. Staff Meet. Mayo Clin., **10:** 239, 1935.
66. MacLean, A. R., Proc. Staff Meet. Mayo Clin., **10:** 321, 1935.
67. Wilder, R. M., Ibid., p. 162.
68. Wilder, R. M., Ibid., p. 167.
69. Zunz, E., and Labarre, J., Compt. rend. Soc. de biol., **112:** 1544, 1933.
70. Woodyatt, R. T., Tr. Assoc. Am. Physicians, **51:** 127, 1936.
71. Wilder, R. M., Ibid., p. 335.
72. Nathanson, M. H., Amer. J. Med. Sci., **183:** 495, 1932.
73. Vander Veer, J. B., M. Clin. N. Amer., **23:** 1569, 1939.
74. Warren, S., The Pathology of Diabetes Mellitus, 2d ed., Lea & Febiger, Philadelphia, 1938.
75. Wilder, R. M., Ibid., p. 332.
76. Durkin, J. K., and Fetter, F., M. Clin. N. Amer., **23:** 1499, 1939.
77. Master, A. M., Amer. Heart J., **12:** 549, 1936; also J.A.M.A., **105:** 377, 1935.
78. Joslin, E. P., Treatment of Diabetes Mellitus, Lea & Febiger, Philadelphia, 1937, p. 539.

79. Lewis, T., Heart Journal, **11**: 119, 1924.
80. Starr, I., Amer. J. Med. Sci., **188**: 4, 1934; J.A.M.A., **90**: 2092, 1928.
81. Cohen, M. B., J.A.M.A., **86**: 1677, 1926.
82. Stern, W. G., Annals of Int. Med., **1**: 5, 1927.
83. Gibbon, J. H., and Landis, E. M., Jour. Clin. Invest., **11**: 5, 1932.
84. Kramer, D. W., Manual of Peripheral Vascular Disorders, The Blakiston Company, Philadelphia, 1940, p. 57.
85. Parkes-Weber, D., Proc. Royal Soc. Med., **1**: 44, 1907.
86. Samuels, S., Diagnosis and Treatment of Disease of the Peripheral Arteries, Oxford publication, 1936.
87. Pearse, H. E., Jr., and Warren, S. L., Ann. Surg., **94**: 1094, 1931.
88. Samuels, S., J.A.M.A., **88**: 1780, 1927.
89. Buerger, L., Circulatory Disturbances of the Extremities, W. B. Saunders Company, Philadelphia, 1924, p. 436.
90. Herrmann, L. G., and Reid, M. R., Arch. of Surg., **29**: 697, 1934.
91. Landis, E. M., and Gibbon, J. H., Jr., J. Clin. Invest., **12**: 925, 1933; also Arch. Int. Med., **52**: 785, 1933.
92. Collens, W. S., and Wilensky, N. D., J.A.M.A., **109**: 2125, 1936.
93. Kramer, D. W., Ibid., p. 226.
94. Saunders, C. E., J.A.M.A., **106**: 916, 1936.
95. Barker, N. W., Proc. Staff Meet. Mayo Clin., **14**: 618, 1939.
96. Gibbon, J. H., Jr., and Landis, E. M., Jour. Clin. Invest., **11**: 1019, 1932.
97. Farr, R. E., Surg. Clin. N. A., **3**: 1175, 1923.
98. Wilder, R. M., Ibid., p. 217.
99. Allen, F. M., Trans. Assn. Am. Phys., **52**: 189, 1937.
100. Waite, J. H., and Beetham, W. P., New Eng. J. Med., **212**: 367, 1935.
101. Wilder, R. M., Ibid., p. 224.
102. Hanum, S., Acta. ophth. Scand., supp., **16**: 3, 1939.
103. Carey, H. W., and Hunt, H. M., New Eng. J. Med., **212**: 463, 1935.
104. Duke-Elder, S., Recent Advances in Ophthalmology, ed. 2, P. Blakiston's Son & Co., 1929, p. 283.
105. de Schweinitz, G. E., and Fewell, A. G., Therap. Gaz., **42**: 623, 1926.
106. Waltman, H. W., and Wilder, R. M., Arch. Int. Med., **44**: 576, 1929.
107. Sanstead, H. R., and Beams, A. J., Arch. Int. Med., **61**: 371, 1938.
108. Joslin, E. P., Ibid., p. 210.
109. Wilder, R. M., Ibid., p. 174.
110. Joslin, E. P., Treatment of Diabetes Mellitus, Lea & Febiger, Philadelphia, 1937, p. 351.
111. Dillon, E. S., and Dyer, W. W., Ann. Int. Med., **11**: 602, 1937.
112. Baker, T. W., Arch. Int. Med., **58**: 373, 1936.
113. Fowler, A. F., Bensley, E. H., and Rabinowitch, I. M., Canad. M. A. J., **42**: 336, 1940.
114. Hartmann, A. F., Arch. Int. Med., **56**: 413, 1935.
115. Bopp, W., Deutsch. med. Wchnschr., **61**: 218, 1935.
116. Hayward, G. H., and Duncan, G. G., Amer. Jour. Med. Sci., **198**: 396, 1939.
117. Tolstoi, E., J.A.M.A., **115**: 454, 1940.
118. Root, H. F., Treatment of Diabetes Mellitus (E. P. Joslin), Lea & Febiger, Philadelphia, 1940, p. 563.
119. Bertram, F., Die Zuckerkrankheit, 2d ed., Leipzig, Georg Thieme, 1939, p. 114.
120. Himsworth, H. P., Quart. J. Med., **7**: 373, 1938.
121. Joslin, E. P., Ibid., p. 582.
122. Wilder, R. M., Ibid., p. 221.
123. Heymann, W., J.A.M.A., **106**: 2050, 1936.
124. Hildebrand, A. G., Montgomery, H., and Rynearson, E. H., Arch. Int. Med., **66**: 851, 1940.
125. Michelson, H. E., and Leymon, C. W., J.A.M.A., **103**: 163, 1934.
126. Duncan, G. G., and Fetter, F., Med. Clin. N. Amer., **18**: 261, 1934.
127. Riven, S. S., Amer. J. Med. Sci., **189**: 550, 1935.
128. Warren, S., Ibid., p. 246.
129. Conn, J. W., Newburgh, L. H., Johnston, M. W., and Sheldon, J. M., Arch. Int. Med., **62**: 765, 1938.

130. Lemmon, W. T., Annals of Surgery, **3**: 141, 1940.
131. Joslin, E. P., Ibid., p. 656.
132. Mason, E. H., Jour. Clin. Invest., **9**: 31, 1931.
133. McBryde, C. M., Arch. Int. Med., **52**: 932, 1933.
134. Himsworth, H. P., Lancet, **1**: 127, 1936.
135. Root, H. F., New Eng. Jour. Med., **208**: 819, 1933; also J.A.M.A., **96**: 928, 1931.
136. Seiple, H. H., Penna. Med. Jour., **44**: 50, 1940.
137. Bertram, F., Ibid., p. 38.
138. Sheldon, J. H., Haemochromatosis, London, Oxford University Press, 1935, p. 11.
139. Mallory, R. B., Amer. J. Path., **1**: 117, 1925.
140. Dry, T. J., Proc. Staff Meet. Mayo Clin., **8**: 56, 1933.
141. Cantarow, A., and Bucher, C. J., Arch. Int. Med., **67**: 333, 1941.
142. Butt, H. R., and Welder, R. M., Arch. Path., **26**: 262, 1938.
143. Wilder, R. M., Clinical Diabetes Mellitus, W. B. Saunders Company, Philadelphia, 1940, p. 325.
144. White, P., in Joslin, E. P., The Treatment of Diabetes Mellitus, Lea & Febiger, ed. 8, Philadelphia, 1940, p. 693.
145. White, P., in Joslin, E. P., The Treatment of Diabetes Mellitus, Lea & Febiger, ed. 7, 1937, p. 618.
146. Mengert, W. F., and Laughlin, K. A., Surg., Gynec. and Obstet., **69**: 615, 1939.
147. Potter, E. L., and Adair, F. L., Amer. Jour. Obstet. and Gynec., **35**: 256, 1938.
148. Smith, G. V., and Smith, O. W., Amer. Jour. Physiol., **107**: 128, 1934.
149. Smith, O. W., and Smith, G. V., Amer. Jour. Obstet. and Gynec., **33**: 365, 1937.
150. Duncan, G. G., and Fetter, F., Amer. Jour. Med. Sci., **187**: 347, 1934.
151. Carlson, A. J., and Drennan, F. M., Amer. Jour. Physiol., **28**: 391, 1911.
152. Gray, S. H., and Feemster, L. C., Arch. Path. and Lab. Med., **1**: 348, 1926.
153. Wilder, R. M., Ibid., p. 223.
154. Murphy, D. P., Surg., Gynec. and Obstet., **56**: 914, 1933.
155. Randall, L. M., and Rynearson, E. H., J.A.M.A., **107**: 919, 1936.

DIABETES IN CHILDHOOD AND ADOLESCENCE

By Tracy D. Cuttle

Diabetes in children presents problems distinct from those encountered in adults. In childhood, diabetes is a more severe disease and with growth and development there is a progressive increase in the requirements for food and insulin. The complications and the speed with which they may prove fatal differ from the complications of diabetes in later life. These differences and the need for closer supervision of the treatment in the diabetic child warrant the consideration of diabetes in childhood and adolescence apart from the problems presented by diabetes in the adult.

Although diabetes is not now curable, present-day physiologic research indicates that there is hope for the cure particularly of the acute form seen in childhood. Closely simulating this acute form of childhood is experimental diabetes, produced by a disturbance of endocrine regulation. Clinical evidence of endocrine imbalance has likewise been noted in a high percentage of children suffering from diabetes mellitus.[1] Diabetes mellitus, experimentally produced in cats by the administration of a diabetogenic hormone following partial removal of the pancreas, has been cured[2]; perhaps in the near future corresponding results may be obtained with children suffering from diabetes. Until this favorable outcome is achieved our aim should be to make the diabetic child as nearly normal as possible, to permit full physical development and function, to offer a minimum of physical and social handicaps, and in all other ways to promote a normal expectancy of life and health. Such plans are directed toward the restoration and maintenance of physiologic conditions in the patient insofar as the nature of the disease and necessary limitations of therapy will permit. It is possible in the majority of children to fulfill these aims and to prevent or correct such complications as failure of growth, coma and hepatomegaly, but degenerative complications, such as premature arteriosclerosis and juvenile cataract, may still develop in the generation of diabetic children whose present existence was made possible by the introduction of insulin. Modern management with the use of the slowly and rapidly acting insulins, liberal diets, and the prevention of hypercholesterolemia, should give rise to a generation of diabetic children free from degenerative complications.

INCIDENCE

Diabetes in childhood is not a common disease. Children make up about 5 per cent of the diabetic population of this country. In our clinics at the Pennsylvania and Jefferson Hospitals 5.5 per cent of the diabetic patients had the onset of the disease before the age of fifteen.

Priscilla White estimates that 1000 new cases of diabetes in childhood occur each year, that one child in 8000 contracts diabetes under the age of fifteen years and that there are between 19,000 and 25,000 people with diabetes in the United States who are now alive and who developed diabetes in childhood. Her own series, which is admittedly not a representative group because of her special interest in children, comprises 10 per cent of the patients treated by Joslin and his associates.[3] The survey by the National Institute of Health in 1935 and 1936 of 2,500,000 persons showed an incidence of one diabetic child in 2500.[4]

Sex.—The sex incidence in the large series reported is almost equally divided. Grishaw, West, and Smith[5] in a series of 341 children, all of whom had developed diabetes before their sixteenth birthday, found 184 girls and 157 boys. White's[3a] large series of 1430 diabetic children consisted of 725 boys and 705 girls. The National Health Survey found a ratio of 35 males to 41 females in the group in which the onset of diabetes was noted before the fifteenth year.[4] Brown and Thompson[6] in a small but thoroughly studied group of diabetic children found 62 per cent girls and 38 per cent boys. These findings correspond with our own in which the sex incidence is 60 per cent boys and 40 per cent girls.

TABLE 1

SEX INCIDENCE OF DIABETES—COMPOSITE SERIES

Age of Onest	Male	Female	Total
0– 1	4	7	11
1– 2	29	29	58
2– 3	51	38	89
3– 4	50	55	105
4– 5	57	45	102
5– 6	63	51	114
6– 7	57	64	121
7– 8	71	60	131
8– 9	60	67	127
9–10	51	78	129
10–11	53	84	137
11–12	76	99	175
12–13	79	85	164
13–14	86	57	143
14–15	70	65	135
15–16	22	9	31
	879	893	1772

Age.–The age at onset of diabetes is of interest as the peaks of increased incidence follow the most rapid periods of growth. The age at onset for 1772 diabetic children has been graphically shown in figure 151. It may be seen that the greatest incidence for both boys and girls occurs at the time of puberty. There is a sharp drop in the incidence of onset during the fifteenth year.

Race.–The incidence of childhood diabetes according to race is difficult to determine as there are no figures available which are statistically significant. All authorities agree that the disease is more common in Jewish

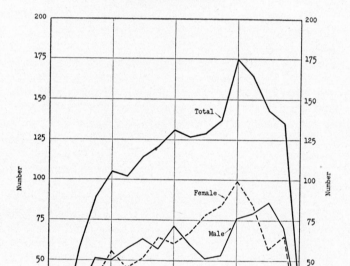

A COMPOSITE GRAPH SHOWING THE
INCIDENCE ACCORDING TO AGE AT ONSET
OF DIABETES IN 1772 CHILDREN

Fig. 151.–The 1772 juvenile patients used in compiling this graph have been collected from our own and published case reports which included the age at onset in juvenile diabetic patients. (See table 1.)

than in Gentile children, that is to say, the percentage of Jewish children who develop diabetes is greater than that of Gentiles. Approximately 8 per cent of White's living juvenile patients were Jews (1932).[7] In her latest report[3a] (1940) she referred to 87 Jewish children in 1211 consecutive cases (7 per cent). Grishaw[5] found 37 Jewish children in 341 juvenile diabetic patients, an incidence of 10.6 per cent. The expected incidence would be between 3 and 4 per cent if the disease were no more frequent in Jewish children, since Jews comprise 3.7 per cent of the population in this country.

ETIOLOGY

Heredity.—The predisposition to diabetes is inherited. Ample proof of this statement has accumulated in the thirteen centuries since its hereditary nature was suggested. The evidence in favor of this theory is as follows:

1. Diabetes occurs in both members of pairs of identical twins.

2. The incidence of diabetes is greater in the blood relatives of diabetic patients than in those of a control population.

3. In a large series of cases selected at random it is possible to demonstrate that the incidence of diabetes follows the ratios for a mendelian trait of the recessive type.

4. Hyperglycemia occurs in the relatives of diabetic patients in approximately the incidence which would be expected for a simple mendelian recessive factor.

White has reviewed the medical writings on this subject and from her series of diabetic children has concluded that diabetes mellitus is inherited as a mendelian recessive characteristic.[3b]

Grishaw[5] reports 110 cases with a positive family history in a series of 341 diabetic children. In fifteen cases it was not known whether diabetes had existed in the antecedents. Brown and Thompson[6] found that 56.7 per cent of their juvenile diabetic patients had at least one diabetic relative. Only 10 per cent of the children had a sibling or parent in whom the disease was manifest. The mean number of diabetic relatives of the subjects who reported any instance of diabetes in the family was two. Chiari[8] reports a familial incidence of 25 to 30 per cent. About 5 per cent of the children had a diabetic brother or sister.

White[3b] states that "the evidence of an hereditary predisposition to diabetes can be demonstrated in proportion to the number of years of diabetes observed." At the onset of diabetes only one child in five had a relative with the disease. After fifteen years, one-half of the children had one or more diabetic relatives, and after twenty years the incidence had increased to nearly three out of five.

If we agree that the predisposition to diabetes is hereditary, we must explain why the disease manifests itself at varying ages and during particular phases of development. In children the onset of diabetes occurs most frequently during adolescence (see figure 151). Many etiologic factors have been suggested and we shall consider the most important ones.

Infection.—Acute illness, especially infections, have been considered of etiologic importance. It is generally agreed that infections lower the carbohydrate tolerance and make established diabetes more severe, but there is no convincing evidence to show that infections cause diabetes. Grishaw[5] found in 24 per cent of his entire group a history of an acute illness sufficiently near to the onset of recognizable symptoms of diabetes to be considered a possible causative factor or precipitating event. The records of preceding illness varied little from those obtained in the cases of other non-diabetic children of a similar age. White[3c] reported that infections occurred with less frequency in the past histories of diabetic children than was noted in the average American school child. Only 10 per cent of the children had an acute infection in the year of onset of diabetes. Brown and Thompson[6] obtained a history of some acute infection other than "colds" in 33 per cent of their patients within the six months preceding the onset of diabetes. Measles, tonsillitis and scarlet fever were the most common infections.

Obesity.—In adults obesity is the most common predisposing factor to bring out the inherited disposition to diabetes. This is not true for children, in whom obesity is uncommon at the onset of diabetes. Brown and Thompson[6] found that a majority of their group of children were 4.1 Kg. (10 pounds) or more below the average weight at the onset of diabetes and before the disease was controlled.

Endocrine Imbalance.—The production of permanent diabetes in the dog by the injection of extracts from the anterior lobe of the pituitary gland suggests that a hyperactivity of this gland may be a precipitating factor in some or all cases of diabetes mellitus in humans. There is more evidence to substantiate this hypothesis in juvenile than in adult diabetic patients. White[1] reviewed the data concerning 1250 patients with juvenile diabetes and found that 177 showed evidence of prolonged pituitary involvement. She states[3d] "Clinical evidence of excessive hormonal production is suggested by the advanced growth, development, and pubescence of the diabetic child, examined at the recognition of the disease." Eighty-six per cent of 417 children were taller than normal when measured within three months of the onset of symptoms of diabetes. These 417 children were, on the average, 2.5 inches above the standard average heights.* The diabetic child exceeded the normal in stature by all standards. Of the 114 juvenile patients observed, forty-six boys exceeded the standard average height by 3.2 inches and forty-three girls by 2.8 inches. When this group was compared with a control group of privileged children, it was found that more of the diabetic children exceeded the Meredith height standards than did those of the control group.

Brown and Thompson,[6] however, did not find that the height in their series of children varied significantly from normal (Burgess standards). A greater number of children were below than above the average height for every age group when compared with the local standards for Minneapolis school children. Few measurements, it must be noted, were taken prior to or at the time of the onset of symptoms. Two patients had an enormous spurt in growth during the year preceding the onset of diabetes. The same writers believe that derangement of the pituitary gland may be the precipitating factor in some cases, infection in others, but some unknown factor in the majority.

Young[9, 10] believes that the results of his work on the production of diabetes in dogs by the administration of large doses of diabetogenic hormone from the anterior lobe of the pituitary gland may be the answer to the question regarding the onset of diabetes in human beings. He believes that short periods of overactivity of the pituitary gland may liberate excessive amounts of diabetogenic hormone. This excessive amount of hormone, by producing irreversible changes in the islets of Langerhans, may thus cause diabetes mellitus.

The theory of overactivity of the anterior lobe of the pituitary gland is in accord with the clinical findings in diabetic children. These are: (1) evidence of precocity, which is presumptive evidence of hyperactivity of

* See Appendix.

the pituitary gland at the onset of diabetes, (2) bone and dental development twelve to eighteen months in advance of their chronological age,[11] (3) an elevated basal metabolic rate (average + 12 per cent[3]), and (4) precocious development and precocious puberty.

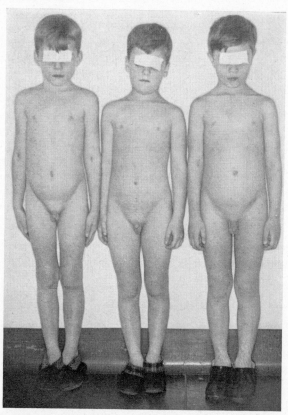

Fig. 152.—These three boys aged six years are within two months of the same age. The boy in the middle is a normal boy of over average height for his age (117 cm.; 46 inches). The boy to the left and the boy to the right are diabetic children. This photograph was taken within three months of the onset of diabetes in both boys. The boy to the left measures 119.5 cm. (47 inches); the boy to the right measures 120.5 cm. (47½ inches) in height. The average height for boys of this age is 106.5 cm. (42 inches). It may be seen that these boys are 5 and 5½ inches respectively above the average height for their age (see Appendix) and 1 and 1½ inches respectively above the upper limit of normal height for six years of age.

The usual absence of pathologic changes in the pituitary gland and in the pancreas in no way refutes the theory, since functional changes may occur without anatomical changes.

The theory that the tendency or potentiality for diabetes is an hereditary mendelian recessive factor and that the disease appears as the result of hyperactivity of the pituitary gland producing secondary changes in the pancreas is most plausible (see section on etiology, p. 711).

SYMPTOMS

The onset of symptoms is abrupt and violent in contrast to the onset in adults, in whom it is usually insidious. Joslin[12] has been able to date the onset of the disease in 44 per cent of the children in his clinic within a period of two months. Grishaw[5] classified the onset as acute if the symptoms developed on a given day or within about two weeks. If the symptoms were noted later the onset was classified as gradual. In 329 records, eighty-nine were of patients who developed diabetes before the age of five years. Of this group 88.5 per cent had an acute onset of symptoms. In 122 patients the onset of symptoms occurred between six and ten years of age. Of these, 82.8 per cent had an acute onset. In the remaining group with an onset between the ages of eleven and fifteen years, 78.8 per cent had an acute onset of symptoms.

In younger children the first recognition of diabetes is often made in acidosis or coma. In this respect the onset resembles that of diabetes produced experimentally in dogs by the injection of large amounts of diabetogenic hormone.[9, 10] Grishaw found that of 274 patients approximately four of every ten had more or less severe ketosis, and one of every five was in coma at the time the diagnosis of diabetes was made.

TABLE 2

INCIDENCE OF KETOSIS AND COMA AT THE TIME THE DIAGNOSIS OF DIABETES WAS MADE[5]

Age at Onset	Total Number of Patients	Ketosis, Per Cent	Coma, Per Cent	No Acidosis, Per Cent
0– 5	76	47.4	21.1	31.5
6–10	99	35.4	18.2	46.4
11–15	99	32.4	25.2	42.4

In older children the symptoms of untreated diabetes are, in most cases, classical: *polyuria, polydipsia, polyphagia,* and *loss of weight* and *strength.* Pruritus is a frequent symptom, and infections of the skin, visual changes, personality changes, mental confusion, and failure in school are common complaints.

In a series of 329 cases, polyuria occurred in 91.4 per cent, polydipsia in 89 per cent, loss of weight and strength in 79 per cent and polyphagia in 73.2 per cent. There was little difference when the patients were divided as to the age of onset.[5]

DIAGNOSIS

The difficulty of making a diagnosis of diabetes mellitus in childhood has often been stressed.[13, 14, 15, 16] Grishaw[5] found in calculating the number of days elapsing between the onset of symptoms and the discovery of sugar in the urine that, in spite of the typical nature of the symptoms and acuteness of their onset, the diagnosis was delayed for an average of 54.5 days in 265 cases. The younger children fared better than the older ones, owing, it is suggested, to closer observation of their bathroom habits and the general condition of the younger children.

History.—The history, in the great majority of cases, is that of an acute onset of the classical symptoms of diabetes. A history of infections of the skin, furunculosis, visual changes, pains in the muscles of the extremities, personality changes, and lack of capacity for school work are also frequent complaints. In these children the history of loss of appetite, nausea, vomiting, shortness of breath, and loss of consciousness usually follows the classical symptoms of diabetes, but in some cases the first sign of diabetes may be acidosis or coma. Although diabetes is rare in infants, the possibility of this disease should be considered in any thirsty and marasmic baby.

A careful family history is more important in juvenile diabetes since the hereditary factor is more frequently demonstrable in young than in adult patients.

Physical Examination.—At the onset of symptoms, the diabetic child is overheight but underweight for his age.

If a group of children with inadequately controlled diabetes is examined several years after the disease is established, the children are found to be shorter and stouter than the children of a similar age group in the general population. The precocious development of the child at the onset of diabetes has therefore been followed by retarded development in the succeeding years.

Some authors have reported a high incidence of *congenital anomalies* such as, syndactylism (webbed fingers and toes), clubbed fingers, and curved fingers, in diabetic children; this has not been our experience.

Diabetic children who have had the disease for several years may develop *skin complications* such as, xanthosis, xanthoma diabeticorum, and necrobiosis lipoidica diabeticorum. Premature arteriosclerosis and juvenile cataracts are also much more common in this group than in nondiabetic children.

Dentition is precocious, but *dental caries* and pyorrhea are so commonly associated with juvenile diabetes that their presence in young children should lead the dentist to suspect the possibility of unrecognized diabetes.

Hepatomegaly and splenomegaly are not uncommon in diabetic children. This is particularly true if the diabetes has not been properly controlled.

Precocious puberty and the early development of secondary sex characteristics is the rule for both male and female diabetic children.

Urinalysis.—The presence in the urine of substances which reduce Benedict's solution is unfortunately common in childhood. Examination of a large number of specimens from any healthy child will reveal an occasional specimen which contains enough reducing substance to produce a green color when boiled in Benedict's solution, p. 737. Although this degree of glycosuria is common, its presence should not be lightly dismissed. Joslin[12] found that of a group of children showing sugar in the urine, 80 per cent had true diabetes and only 0.9 per cent had renal glycosuria.

The diagnosis of diabetes is made on the basis of a persistent glycosuria and hyperglycemia. No child should be placed on a diabetic regimen until the diagnosis of diabetes is clearly established.

Examinations of the Blood.—Some authors believe that a level for the fasting blood sugar above 130 mg. per 100 cc. indicates diabetes. The disease in childhood is usually so severe, however, that no artificial yardstick is necessary to make a diagnosis. (If the fasting level is not above 150 mg. per 100 cc., and in all doubtful cases, a glucose tolerance test should be performed.) *Glucose tolerance tests* are rarely necessary, but they are indicated if the urine contains sugar and if random determinations of the blood are within the limits of normal. The quantity of glucose used for the test dose depends upon the weight of the child since the utilization of glucose is governed by body size. White[3] found that the normal child could tolerate 1.8 gm. of glucose per Kg. of body weight and we have adopted this amount for our test. The single dose or the one-hour two-dose tolerance test (Exton-Rose procedure)[17] may be used. In the single dose test 1.8 gm. of glucose is given for each Kg. of body weight. The technique and interpretation of the test are the same for the child as for the adult, see p. 744.

In the *one-hour two-dose* tolerance test the dose is calculated according to the child's weight in the same manner as for the one-dose test (1.8 gm. of glucose per Kg. of body weight is given) but the calculated amount is divided and given in two equal doses, exactly as for adults (see p. 741).

TREATMENT

Diabetes in childhood differs in several important aspects from the disease in adults, hence the treatment must be varied to take account of these differences.

The essentials of correct treatment are *diet, insulin, exercise,* and *education* and *protection* of the patient. The treatment should be so conducted that the following standards for controlled diabetes are fulfilled.

1. Adequate nourishment.
2. A fasting blood sugar level below 150 mg. per 100 cc. and a *postcibal* level below 200 mg. per 100 cc.
3. Glycosuria of less than 10 gm. of glucose in twenty-four hours.
4. Cholesterol content of the blood below 230 mg. per 100 cc.
5. A normal physiologic adjustment and development.

The first four criteria are generally agreed upon, but the last, equally important, is frequently neglected.

To attain these desired results, two phases of treatment must be considered: (1) initial adjustment and (2) periodic readjustment to allow for growth and development. The latter is important and merits special emphasis. Furthermore, in contrast with the adult, one must contend with the greater physiologic and emotional instability of the child.

The initial treatment for diabetes in children should be carried out in the hospital. This period of institutional care is important, for it not only supplies the facilities for adequate investigation, but it allows for a period of supervised instruction.

Diet.—The diet must allow for adequate nutrition and must supply the needs for normal growth and development. Numerous methods have been suggested by which the caloric requirements may be calculated. Some are based on statistics, some on laboratory investigation, and some are empirical. Three satisfactory methods of calculating the caloric requirements for the child are:

1. An accurate and simple method of determining the basal energy requirements (p. 940) is based upon the surface area of the body, which may be determined by consulting the DuBois Body Surface chart (p. 9). The surface area is expressed in square meters. The surface area of the patient multiplied by the normal caloric requirement per square meter as modified by age and sex (p. 940) yields the basal energy requirement, expressed in calories for the average person of this height, weight, age and sex. The energetic child requires at least a 100 per cent increase over the basal requirements. The basal energy requirements should, therefore, be increased in accord with the child's activities.

2. A second method for the determination of the caloric requirements of the diet for a child is based on the energy requirements according to age and body weight. This method is in my opinion the most satisfactory for general use. There are differences in the energy requirements for boys and for girls after puberty but before the thirteenth year the requirements are the same for both sexes. The energy requirements for children are listed in table 3, which follows.

TABLE 3

ENERGY REQUIREMENTS OF CHILDREN—TOTAL CALORIES FOR CHILDREN IN TERMS OF BODY WEIGHT*

Age in Years	Calories per Kilogram		Calories per Pound	
1– 2............	100–90		50–45	
3– 5............	90–80		40–36	
6– 9............	80–70		36–32	
10–13............	70–60		32–27	
	Boys	Girls	Boys	Girls
14–15............	60–55	50–45	27–25	23–20
16–17............	60–55	45–40	27–25	20–18
18–19............	55–50	40–35	25–23	18–16

* Rose, Foundation of Nutrition, The Macmillan Co., 1933.

The calculations are based on the ideal rather than on the actual weight of the child. This ideal weight may be determined from the Height-Weight-Age Tables for boys and girls of school age.† The ideal weight is expressed in pounds in the Height-Weight-Age Tables. This should be converted to kilograms by dividing by 2.2 (the number of pounds in a kilogram).

After the caloric requirements have been determined (by Method 1 or Method 2) the calories are apportioned in the basic food constituents, namely: carbohydrate, protein, and fat. These nutritional requirements for children are presented in table 4 (p. 884). Finally, the respective protein, fat, and carbohydrate values are converted into terms of actual daily menus for the patient. The following diets will illustrate how this is done (see tables 5, 6, 7, 8).

3. A simple and practical method of calculating the diet based on the child's age is advocated by White.[3f] One thousand calories are allowed

† See Appendix, pp. 936, 937.

TABLE 4

APPROXIMATE AMOUNTS OF THE FOOD CONSTITUENTS NEEDED A DAY FOR BODY BUILDING AND
FUNCTIONING IN TERMS OF THE STANDARD OR OPTIMAL REQUIREMENTS FOR CHILDREN*

Carbohydrate:
  6–10 gm. per Kg. of body weight per day, or 50 per cent of the total calories per day.

Fat:
  2–3 gm. per Kg. of body weight per day, or 35 per cent of the total calories per day.

Protein:
  2–3 gm. per Kg. of body weight per day, or 15 per cent of the total calories per day.

Iron:
  6 mg. under 1 year; 8 mg. 4–6 years; 15 mg. 12–20 years.

Calcium:
  1 gm. (15 grains) per day.

Phosphorus:
  1–1.5 gm. (15–23 grains) per day.

Vitamins:
  Vitamin requirements supplied by liberal amounts of foods containing the various vitamins.
    See table 4, p. 492.

Fluid:
  3 to 4 glasses in addition to milk.

CALORIES

  To estimate the total calories, multiply the number of grams of carbohydrate and the
grams of protein by 4 and the number of grams of fat by 9. The sum of these figures represents
the total calories.
  To secure the number of calories needed for light activity use the median figures for carbohydrate, protein and fat.
  For moderate or greater activity increase either the carbohydrate or the fat or both.
  * Modified from Stern[18] and table 4, p. 492.

TABLE 5

DIET† FOR 6-YEAR-OLD BOY—1750 CALORIES

Food		Protein 50 Gm., Fat 83 Gm., Carbohydrate 200 Gm.			
	Gm., Wt.	Household Measure	P.	F.	C.
Breakfast:					
Milk....................	240	1 cup	7	10	12
Fruit, 12 per cent.............	100	1 serving	..	..	12
Cereal....................	20	½ cup	3	..	16
Cream, 20 per cent.............	30	2 tablespoons	1	6	1
			11	16	41
Noon meal:					
Vegetable, 9 per cent............	100	1 serving	3	..	9
Vegetable, 18 per cent...........	100	½ cup	5	1	18
Fruit, 12 per cent.............	200	2 servings	..	..	24
Milk....................	240	1 cup	7	10	12
Bread....................	30	1 slice	3	..	16
Butter....................	25	5 teaspoons	..	21	
			18	32	79
Evening meal:					
Vegetable, 6 per cent...........	100	1 serving	2	..	6
Vegetable, 18 per cent...........	100	½ cup	5	1	18
Milk....................	240	1 cup	7	10	12
Fruit, 12 per cent.............	100	1 serving	..	..	12
Bread....................	60	2 slices	6	..	32
Butter....................	30	2 tablespoons	..	25	
			20	36	80
			49	84	200

† Divided as follows: one-fifth for breakfast; two-fifths each for the noon and evening meals.

for a child one year old and 100 calories are added for each year of age until the completion of growth. The calories for girls are limited to 2200 as epiphyseal closure in girls occurs at the menarche. After maturity adolescent female obesity is avoided by restricting the diet to between 30 and 40 calories per Kg. of the ideal weight for height and age. For boys a maximum of 2800 calories is reached at nineteen years of age.

The diets advocated by White contain carbohydrate, protein, and fat in the following respective gram ratios: 2.0 : 0.9 : 1.0. In other words, for

TABLE 6

DIET* FOR 6-YEAR-OLD BOY—1750 CALORIES

Food	Protein 50 Gm., Fat 83 Gm., Carbohydrate 200 Gm.				
	Gm., Wt.	Household Measure	P.	F.	C.
Breakfast:					
Milk.........................	240	1 cup	7	10	12
Cereal.......................	20	½ cup	3	..	16
Fruit, 12 per cent...............	100	1 serving	..	..	12
Bread........................	45	1½ slices	4.5	..	24
Butter.......................	20	4 teaspoons	..	17	
			14.5	27	64
Noon meal:					
Vegetable, 9 per cent............	100	1 serving	3	..	9
Vegetable, 18 per cent...........	100	½ cup	5	1	18
Fruit, 12 per cent...............	100	1 serving	..	..	12
Milk.........................	240	1 cup	7	10	12
Bread........................	30	1 slice	3	..	16
Butter.......................	20	4 teaspoons	..	17	
			18	28	67
Evening meal:					
Vegetable, 3 per cent............	100	1 serving	2	..	3
Vegetable, 6 per cent............	100	1 serving	2	..	6
Milk.........................	240	1 cup	7	10	12
Bread........................	45	1½ slices	4.5	..	24
Butter.......................	20	4 teaspoons	..	17	
Fruit, 12 per cent...............	200	2 servings	..	..	24
			15.5	27	69
			48	82	200

* Divided into three equal meals.

every 2 gm. of carbohydrate, 0.9 gm. of protein and 1 gm. of fat is prescribed. This makes for the utmost simplicity in the actual construction of the diets as the prescribed figure for carbohydrate is 10 per cent of the figure for the total calories. For example, in prescribing a diet for a boy or girl aged nine years, 1800 calories are allowed comprising carbohydrate 180 gm., fat 90 gm., and protein approximately 80 gm.

The calculation of the diet prescription is aimed at providing adequate nutrition and a diet relatively high in carbohydrate content. This is in accord with the changes in diet prescriptions which have taken place during the past fifteen years. The plea for more liberal diets was initiated by Sansum and others in 1926.[19] Physicians were reluctant to change from the diets high in fat and low in carbohydrate which were aimed at undernutrition, and which formed the basis of the treatment of diabetes before the advent of insulin. In the last ten years carbohydrate allowances have been

TABLE 7

Diet* for 15-Year-Old Girl—2500 Calories

Food	Protein 95 Gm., Fat 124 Gm., Carbohydrate 250 Gm.				
	Gm., Wt.	Household Measure	P.	F.	C.
Breakfast:					
Milk	240	1 cup	7	10	12
Cereal	20	½ cup	3	..	16
Fruit, 12 per cent	100	1 serving	..	..	12
Bread	15	½ slice	1.5	..	8
Egg	50	1	7	5	
Butter	10	2 teaspoons	..	8.5	
			18.5	23.5	48
Noon meal:					
Meat	45	1½ oz.	10.5	7.5	
Vegetable, 3 per cent	100	1 serving	2	..	3
Vegetable, 9 per cent	100	1 serving	3	..	9
Vegetable, 18 per cent	100	½ cup	5	1	18
Fruit, 12 per cent	100	1 serving	..	..	12
Milk	240	1 cup	7	10	12
Bread	90	3 slices	9	..	48
Butter or other fat	35	2 tablespoons and 1 teaspoon	..	31	
			36.5	49.5	102
Evening meal:					
Meat	30	1 oz.	7	5	
Vegetable, 3 per cent	200	2 servings	4	..	6
Vegetable, 6 per cent	100	1 serving	2	..	6
Vegetable, 18 per cent	200	1 cup	10	2	36
Milk	480	2 cups	14	20	24
Fruit, 12 per cent	100	1 serving	..	..	12
Bread	30	1 slice	3	..	16
Butter	30	2 tablespoons	..	25	
			40	52	100
			95	125	250

* Divided as follows: one-fifth for breakfast and two-fifths each for noon and evening meals.

gradually increased until the pendulum has swung in the other direction and some authors now recommend the so-called "free diet."[20] We do not subscribe to the use of the "free diet," since it introduces another variable into an already difficult problem. We also deprecate the use of diets aimed at undernutrition, or undue restriction of the carbohydrate allowance in the treatment of juvenile diabetic patients.

TABLE 8

DIET* FOR 15-YEAR-OLD GIRL—2500 CALORIES

Food	Protein 95 Gm., Fat 124 Gm., Carbohydrate 250 Gm.				
	Gm., Wt.	Household Measure	P.	F.	C.
Breakfast:					
Milk	240	1 cup	7	10	12
Cereal	40	1 cup	6	..	32
Fruit, 15 per cent	100	1 serving	..	..	15
Bread	45	1½ slices	4.5	..	24
Eggs	100	2	14	10	
Butter	25	5 teaspoons	..	21	
			31.5	41	83
Noon meal:					
Meat	45	1½ oz.	10.5	7.5	
Vegetable, 9 per cent	100	1 serving	3	..	9
Vegetable, 18 per cent	100	½ cup	5	1	18
Fruit, 12 per cent	100	1 serving	..	..	12
Milk	240	1 cup	7	10	12
Bread	60	2 slices	6	..	32
Butter	25	5 teaspoons	..	21	
			31.5	39.5	83
Evening meal:					
Meat	30	1 oz.	7	5	
Vegetable, 3 per cent	200	2 servings	4	..	6
Vegetable, 6 per cent	100	1 serving	2	..	6
Vegetable, 18 per cent	100	½ cup	5	1	18
Milk	480	2 cups	14	20	24
Fruit, 12 per cent	100	1 serving	..	..	12
Bread	30	1 slice	3	..	16
Butter	20	4 teaspoons	..	17	
			35	43	82
			98	124	248

* Divided into three equal meals.

The "high carbohydrate diet," which may arbitrarily be defined as a diet containing more than 200 gm. of carbohydrate *per diem* has the following advantages:

1. It is less expensive.
2. It is more palatable.
3. It approximates the average American diet, so that all the members of the family may partake of it.
4. There is less temptation for the child to indulge in forbidden food. "Diabetic children cannot be expected to adhere to inadequate diets."[21]
5. The more nearly normal diet has a beneficial psychologic effect on the child.
6. Hypoglycemia is less frequent.
7. The liberal allowance of carbohydrate with the high antiketogenic factors decreases the incidence of ketosis.
8. There is a greater efficiency in the utilization of insulin.[21, 22]
9. Hypercholesterolemia occurs less frequently.[23]

Menus, calculated from the diet prescription, contain foods which are easily available and palatable. This calculation is usually done by the dietitian, but with the help of the standard tables for food values and a little simple arithmetic, the menu may be constructed by the physician. Many patients are taught to do this for themselves before they leave the hospital.

Mineral, Inorganic, and Vitamin Requirements.—In addition to the nutritional elements mentioned, namely, carbohydrate, protein, and fat, consideration must be given to the mineral and inorganic elements which are necessary in the diet and to the accessory food factors, the vitamins. The sample diets given in the text contain an adequate amount of these essential substances for ordinary circumstances. The present diets are adequate in all respects and contain at least one gram of calcium a day. Iodine, phosphorus, sodium, and iron are present in adequate amounts. It is possible that a deficiency may arise because of abnormal absorption of vitamins from the gastro-intestinal tract and, under certain conditions of disease, supplementary vitamin therapy is recommended. This is particularly true of vitamin B_1 (thiamine), which has been shown to be intimately related with carbohydrate metabolism. It appears to act as a catalyst in pyruvic acid oxidation and without it carbohydrates may not be metabolized beyond the pyruvic acid stage. Faulty utilization of *vitamin A* has been frequently reported in children suffering from diabetes. This may be associated with a carotinemia and in some cases hepatomegaly. This disturbance is due to two factors: first, the diabetic diet is usually high in carotene and second, there seems to be a faulty metabolism of this vitamin associated with the disease. Vitamin A is formed in the liver by the splitting of carotene hence the disturbance of liver function associated with diabetes may account for the disturbance in vitamin A metabolism. *Vitamin B_1 (thiamine) deficiency* is more common in adult patients with diabetes than it is in children. In children whom we have observed, the only cases of peripheral neuritis due to a lack of vitamin B were caused by poor absorption of the vitamin because of disturbance in the gastro-intestinal tract. The failure of growth of certain diabetic children may be associated with a deficiency in vitamin B_2 an assumption which is still theoretical. A deficiency in *vitamin C* is even more uncommon, chiefly because the diets for diabetic patients contain an abundant supply of this vitamin. It has been suggested that pyorrhea and retinal hemorrhages may be due to a vitamin C deficiency, but quantitative determinations of the vitamin C content of the blood and urine have failed to show any significant deficiency of this factor. It is true, however, that the retinal hemorrhages associated with diabetes may show striking improvement following treatment with large doses of ascorbic acid.[24] Disturbances in the calcium and phosphorus metabolism associated with vitamin D deficiency are also rare. Cod liver oil is prescribed in the diets of diabetic children. Deficiencies in vitamin E and vitamin K, associated with juvenile diabetes, have not been reported, though a vitamin K deficiency is as likely to develop in a diabetic child in the presence of obstructive or hepatic jaundice as in any other child.

The number of meals and the proportion of the daily diet allowed at each meal are specified in each diet prescription. This last aspect of the dietary is important. In the absence of complications the meals should correspond with the family's meal hours. The diet is divided so that one-fifth of the total is allowed for breakfast, two-fifths for lunch, and two-fifths for dinner. If *"buffer* meals" are required, 30 gm. of carbohydrate are taken from the total diet and given 10 gm. in the middle of the morning, 10 gm. in the middle of the afternoon, and 10 gm. at bedtime. If a large breakfast is preferred, three equal meals are prescribed and similar "buffer meals" may be used. During the course of an intercurrent acute or chronic infection, or complications requiring surgical treatment, the diet is divided into equal feedings which are equally spaced throughout the twenty-four hours at 4- or 6-hour intervals. This method, the equal division and distribution of diet and insulin, suggested by Duncan, Fetter, and Durkin,[25, 26] for the treatment of these complications in adult diabetic patients, has proved to be of value in the treatment of those of children. (Example—case J. J., Case 2, p. 894.)

Insulin.—All authorities agree that children having diabetes require insulin, and preferably continuously from the day the diagnosis is made.[13, 14, 27, 28, 29, 30] The question, therefore, is not whether insulin should be used, but what *type* of insulin should be used. The answer to this question will depend upon the individual case, but in the great majority of cases a combination of protamine zinc insulin and unmodified insulin gives the best results. In the presence of acute complications, we employ the quickly acting unmodified insulin or zinc insulin crystals in solution* in conjunction with the equal division and distribution of the diet. When the complication is corrected and the diabetes is controlled, the diet is changed to regular meals and the slowly-acting protamine zinc insulin is used to replace the crystalline insulin in whole or in part. The transfer from four injections of crystalline insulin, with four equal meals, to one injection of the protamine zinc insulin or to the combination of the protamine zinc insulin and the crystalline insulin is carried out in the following manner:

The total dose of insulin needed to control the diabetes is divided by five. Three-fifths† is given as protamine zinc insulin in the morning before breakfast. The remaining two-fifths is now divided into thirds, of which two-thirds is given as crystalline insulin with the morning dose of protamine zinc insulin and the remaining third is given as crystalline insulin before the evening meal. This is a very rough guide and further adjustments are almost always necessary. The evening dose of crystalline insulin is omitted after a few days by gradually reducing the dose and adding it to the morning injection in the form of protamine zinc insulin. Most children require both crystalline and protamine zinc insulin, which are given daily as separate injections before breakfast.[31, 33]

It should be reemphasized that the initial adjustment of the diabetes and the establishment of proper control with insulin should be carried out in the hospital, the time spent there depending largely upon the individual patient.

* The action of zinc insulin crystals in solution (crystalline insulin) corresponds so closely to the action of unmodified insulin that they may be used interchangeably.[31] For the sake of brevity *crystalline insulin* is referred to in the text.

† If three-fifths of the total dose of crystalline insulin is *more than 40 units*, it is safer to employ two-fifths instead, with one-third of the remainder as crystalline insulin in the morning and one-third at night. The dosage is then modified depending on the result of the tests for sugar in the urine.

The initial prescription of protamine zinc insulin for the newly developed uncomplicated diabetes in the juvenile is based upon the age of the patient—under five years of age, 8 or 10 units; between five and ten years, 15 or 20 units; between ten and fifteen years, 20 or 30 units given in each instance twenty minutes before breakfast. Protamine zinc insulin is increased by 2 or 4 units on alternate days until the fasting urine specimen is free of sugar or until the blood sugar level is normal. Then, to avoid a cumulative action, the dose is decreased by 2 or 4 units daily until traces of sugar reappear in the urine or until the blood sugar has reached the upper limits of normal. Most diabetic children require supplementary doses of crystalline insulin. The ultimate regulation of the insulin dosage and distribution is accomplished for the child as for the adult, p. 773.

The patient should be free of glycosuria and free of symptoms before being discharged from the hospital. Unless this initial stabilization has been completed, the management of the child as an ambulatory patient will be difficult and an unsatisfactory state of control fluctuating between hypoglycemic reactions and hyperglycemia is likely to ensue. Such a state predisposes to progression of the diabetes and to complications, sequelae, and fatalities which characterize uncontrolled diabetes.

The insulin requirement after reaching a peak is usually considerably reduced during the succeeding weeks, often to half of the amount needed to overcome the glycosuria and hyperglycemia in the earlier stages of treatment. Furthermore, with increased glycogen storage the patients become somewhat fortified against insulin reactions. The insulin needs are governed by the severity of the diabetes, the diet, body weight, and exercise. The dose of insulin cannot be satisfactorily based upon the age of the patient. Appropriate insulin treatment requires close supervision of the patient throughout the period of regulation, with the observance of a regimen which is constant. If it is established that the patient's renal threshold is normal (160–180 mg. per 100 cc.), much can be accomplished by examining the urine for sugar alone, without other laboratory studies. The determination of the level of the blood sugar is more accurate and the final determination of the oscillation of this level throughout the twenty-four hours should be determined before the patient is discharged from the hospital, as described on page 774. Several new insulins which have an action which is delayed between that of the crystalline insulin and protamine zinc insulin have been developed in the last few years. We have used two of these, globin insulin (Burroughs and Wellcome) and histone zinc insulin[*] (Lilly) with definite advantages in the treatment of juvenile diabetic patients. Their chief characteristics are presented on page 769.

The following case report is typical of uncomplicated juvenile diabetes. Crystalline, protamine zinc, histone zinc, and globin insulins were used at various times in the treatment of this child. The improvement obtained from adequate treatment over a period of two months may be seen by comparing the photographs taken before with the one taken after this period of treatment.

[*] These insulins are not available commercially at the present time (December, 1941). For a more complete study see Barnes, C. A., Cuttle, T. D., and Duncan, G. G., Histone Zinc Insulin, J. Pharmacol. & Exper. Therap., **72:** 331, 1941; also Duncan, G. G., and Barnes, C. A., Globin Insulin, Amer. Jour. Med. Sci., **202:** 553, 1941.

CASE ILLUSTRATING USE OF VARIOUS TYPES OF INSULIN FOR UNCOMPLICATED DIABETES
IN CHILDHOOD

Case 1.–M. G., a white female, aged fourteen years, weight 43 Kg. (95 pounds); height 155 cm. (61 inches).

This patient was first admitted to the Pennsylvania Hospital on November 13, 1940, because of the loss of 15 pounds in weight in a period of four months. She had always been healthy and well nourished until June, 1940. At that time she weighed 88 pounds. She noted an increasing appetite but a loss in weight, until at the time she was admitted to the hospital, she weighed 73 pounds. She became weak and apathetic, and in

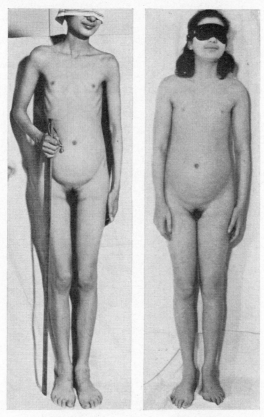

Fig. 153   Fig. 154

Fig. 153.–Case 1, M. G., aged fourteen years, height 153.7 cm. (60.5 in.), weight 33 Kg. (73 pounds). Photograph taken November 13, 1940, at the time of her first admission to hospital. She is over height and under weight for her age.

Fig. 154.–Case 1, M. G., aged fourteen years, height 155 cm. (61 in.), weight 43 Kg. (95 pounds). Photograph taken January 18, 1941, approximately two months after her first admission to the hospital. It may be seen that a definite improvement in her nutrition and general condition has resulted during this short period of treatment.

August, 1940, developed cramping pains in her legs following exertion, which were alleviated with rest. She began to drink increasing amounts of water and she was forced to get up three or four times nightly to urinate. She finally was sent to the hospital by the family physician because he suspected the presence of tuberculosis. The child was tall and thin, height 60.5 inches, weight 73 pounds. She was apathetic and listless. Her skin was dry and scaling, the mucous membranes were of good color, the teeth were poor, the tongue was dry and coated. There was no odor of acetone on the breath. No further significant abnormalities were noted on physical examination.

Her urine was concentrated (specific gravity 1.033) and completely reduced Benedict's solution. Neither acetone nor diacetic acid was present in the urine. The blood sugar level was 468 mg. per 100 cc. and the carbon dioxide combining power of the blood plasma was 61 volumes per cent (27.5 milliequivalents per liter). The blood cholesterol level was 524 mg. per 100 cc. Roentgenograms of the chest and sella turcica showed no abnormalities. Roentgenograms of the long bones showed an osseous development compatible with an age of nineteen years. The photograph (Fig. 153) was taken at this time. The following diet was prescribed: carbohydrate 250 gm., protein 100 gm., fat 110 gm. (2400 calories). This was divided into four equal feedings given at six-hour intervals and 40 units of crystalline insulin were given before each feeding. After one week the blood sugar was within the limits of normal and the urine was free of sugar. The meals were then changed to three equal portions at the regular meal hours and 50 units of protamine zinc and 15 units of crystalline insulin were given each morning before breakfast, and 8 units of crystalline insulin were given before the evening meal. The diabetes remained well controlled. Fifty-eight units of histone zinc insulin, in one injection in the morning, were required at a later date to control her diabetes, and satisfactory blood sugar levels for a twenty-four-hour period were obtained when 58 units of globin insulin were substituted for the histone zinc insulin. The patient gained in weight, the level of the blood sugar remained below 150 mg. per 100 cc. (fasting level), and below 200 mg. per 100 cc. (post cibum level). The cholesterol value for the blood was reduced to 258 mg. per 100 cc. She was discharged from the hospital on December 29, 1940, and when last seen she weighed 95 pounds (Fig. 154, taken January 18, 1941). This photograph was taken two months after the original photograph. The improvement in her nutrition is obvious.

Exercise.—Juvenile diabetic patients are encouraged to take normal exercise and enter into all the usual activities of childhood. This not only improves their general health and psychologic adjustment to their disease, but tends to lower their requirements for insulin. Hypoglycemia is the only danger associated with exercise if the patient's diabetes is controlled. The risk is proportional to the severity and duration of the exercise. Hypoglycemia can be avoided by decreasing the dose of insulin by several (4 to 12) units before unusual exercise or by adding extra carbohydrate. This slight inconvenience to the patient is far outweighed by the benefits derived from allowing the child to indulge in the normal activities of childhood. Every effort is made to prevent the diabetic child from developing a feeling of inferiority.

Education.—The treatment of the diabetes is relatively simple but the treatment of the child may be exceedingly difficult. If this difficulty is to be surmounted, the child must be taught to overcome the handicap and to realize that some of the finest accomplishments have been achieved by diabetic patients. During the period in the hospital the child receives a basic education concerning diabetes and, at subsequent visits, the instruction is continued. The child and the parents are instructed in the preparation of the diet, weighing, substitutions, and the changes necessary for increased exercise or periods of mild illness when the child is confined to bed. Children over ten years of age are taught to give their own insulin under the supervision of the parent or nurse. They are taught how to make the simple tests of the urine—the tests for glucose, acetone, and diacetic acid. They are also taught to recognize and to correct the early symptoms of hypoglycemia so that severe reactions may be avoided.

COMPLICATIONS OF INSULIN TREATMENT IN CHILDREN AND ADOLESCENTS

The complications of insulin treatment may be discussed under the following headings:

A. General reactions
    1. Hypoglycemia
    2. Insulin resistance
B. Local reactions
    1. Localized lipodystrophy
    2. Local allergic reactions
    3. Induration at the site of insulin injections
C. Transitory refractive changes.

Hypoglycemia.—Hypoglycemia is more frequently seen in diabetic children than it is in adults. This is probably due to the greater variation in physical activity in the presence of a smaller storage capacity for glycogen. Gastro-intestinal upsets and variations in the diet are also more common in children and the child is less likely to observe the warning symptoms of hypoglycemia.

Hypoglycemic reactions occur when the blood sugar level falls too low, usually below 60 mg. per 100 cc., or when the fall is too rapid. Protamine zinc insulin causes a slow reduction in the blood sugar level and a lower level is reached before symptoms appear than when crystalline insulin is employed. The most common time for "protamine reactions" is in the early hours of the morning. The severity of the reactions at this time is due to the fact that the patient during sleep has failed to recognize the warning symptoms and also that this is the longest period without food.

The symptoms of hypoglycemia vary greatly but are usually fairly constant for the individual patient. Some of the symptoms which have been noted are:

1. Listlessness
2. Difficulty of speech
3. Pallor
4. Sweating
5. Dull intractable headache
6. Gnawing epigastric pain
7. Excitability or unruliness
8. Personality changes ("The quiet child or the child in tantrums")[34]

If these warning symptoms are not heeded, the more severe hypoglycemic reactions progress to unconsciousness and convulsions.

Hypoglycemic reactions are promptly corrected by giving carbohydrate by mouth if the patient is conscious and by vein if unconscious. A 50 per cent solution of glucose (dextrose) is the solution of choice for intravenous administration, and 20 cc. of the solution is usually adequate. This provides the needed carbohydrate quickly and tends to combat the cerebral edema which may occur in severe hypoglycemic reactions. Epinephrine, pituitrin or pitressin may be used, as noted on page 782, in an emergency; namely, when the patient is unconscious and sterile solutions of glucose (dextrose) are not available. These hormones act by the liberation of liver glycogen and may result in the temporary improvement of the patient; *i.e.*, the unconscious child may regain consciousness. They should be followed, however, by the administration of glucose.

Insulin Resistance.—Relative resistance to insulin may result from ketosis, infections, or the administration of a diet which is low in carbohydrates. Some children, however, require extremely large doses of insulin over a long period of time and have been termed "insulin resistant." DeWesselow and Griffiths[22] were unable to demonstrate this condition in their investigations and concluded that insulin resistance could be changed to insulin sensitivity by the administration of large amounts of carbohydrate. Their conclusions are applicable to the majority of children, but occasionally a patient is encountered in whom true insulin resistance seems to be present. White reports two such cases[3g] and the following case will serve as an example:

CASE ILLUSTRATING INSULIN RESISTANCE—PROGRESSIVE LIPODYSTROPHY COMPLICATED BY DIABETES MELLITUS

Case 2.—J. J., male, white, aged four years, height 41 inches (104 cm.), weight 42 pounds (19 Kg.).

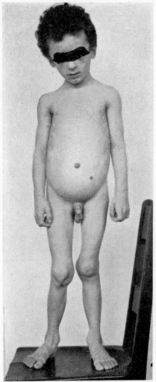

Fig. 155.—J. J. Progressive lipodystrophy associated with diabetes, hepatomegaly, splenomegaly, and dysfunction of the adrenal glands. Note the complete loss of subcutaneous fat, the protuberant abdomen, the pigmentation of the skin in the axillae and groin, and the precocious development of the genitalia.

This boy was admitted to Jefferson Hospital under the care of Dr. E. L. Bauer on October 21, 1938. He was referred to the hospital by the family physician because of swelling of the abdomen and failure to gain in weight. His mother stated that he had developed normally following an uneventful spontaneous delivery until he was one year old. She then noticed that his legs became thin, and "lumps" appeared on his legs and face. The face became thin and the abdomen prominent. His appetite was voracious; he was exceedingly thirsty and he passed large quantities of urine.

There was no history of diabetes in the family.

At the time of admission he was extremely emaciated and had the facial expression of an old man. The skin was very dry and smooth and there were atrophic changes over the face. There was a loss of subcutaneous fat and a wasting of the muscles of the face, hands, feet, and arms. He was tall for his age and the emaciation accentuated his height. The hair was thick, abundant, coarse, and brittle, and lanugo was present over the chest and back. There were areas of hyperpigmentation about the axillae and groin. The tongue was dry and coated, and the pharynx was injected. The heart was not enlarged but a blowing systolic murmur was audible at the apex. The abdomen was protuberant and the edge of the liver was palpable 5 cm. below the costal margin in the right midclavicular line. The spleen extended 10 cm. below the costal margin in the left midclavicular line. Both organs were smooth, firm and movable. There were no signs of free fluid in the peritoneal cavity. The tendon reflexes were absent. There was no apparent loss of muscular power.

Shortly after admission the following investigations were reported:

Urine: Specific gravity 1.035, sugar 1.25 per cent, albumin moderate amount present, acetone negative. Microscopic: occasional hyaline and granular casts.

The *blood count* was within normal limits and the Wassermann and Kahn tests on the blood were negative. The blood sugar was 135 mg. per 100 cc. Shortly after admission the following investigations of the blood were reported: calcium 11.9 mg. per 100 cc., phosphorus 5.6 mg. per 100 cc., CO_2 combining power 60 volumes per cent, chlorides 601 mg. per 100 cc., N. P. N. 25.0 mg. per 100 cc., total cholesterol 175 mg. per 100 cc., free cholesterol 121 mg. per 100 cc.

Examination of the stools: No starch or undigested meat fibers; moderate amount of neutral fat.

Roentgen-ray examination of the skull and the entire bony skeleton showed no evidence of any abnormalities suggestive of endocrine dysfunction or nutritional disease. A barium enema showed the colon to be capacious but there was no evidence of Hirschsprung's disease.

A diagnosis of progressive lipodystrophy was made, and it was noted that there was evidence of the endocrine imbalance which frequently accompanies this disorder.

On November 5, 1938, a glucose tolerance test was performed and a typical diabetic tolerance curve was obtained:

Blood sugar, mg. per 100 cc.	Fasting	30 minutes	60 minutes	2 hours
	117	198	206	235

The child, when seen by us in December, 1939, showed evidences of uncontrolled diabetes mellitus. The fasting blood sugar was 282 mg. per 100 cc., the urine contained 5 per cent of sugar and the alkali reserve, as indicated by the carbon dioxide combining power of the blood plasma, had fallen to 39 volumes per cent.

Because of the rapid increase in the severity of the diabetes and the development of ketosis, the following *treatment* was instituted:

Diet: Carbohydrate 125 gm., protein 45 gm., fat 30 gm. This prescription was divided into six equal feedings, which were given at four-hour intervals (8 A.M., 12 noon, 4 P.M., 8 P.M., 12 midnight, and 4 A.M.).

Insulin: Unmodified insulin, 14 units, administered with each feeding.

Within twenty-four hours the urine was free of sugar and acetone, and the blood sugar taken immediately before the 8 A.M. feeding was 84 mg. per 100 cc. This regimen was continued with minor changes in the diet and a progressive increase in the insulin dosage for an unusually long time because of the increasing severity of the diabetes and the presence of a chronic and recurring acute tracheobronchitis with a fever at times as high as 105° F. The details of the treatment, the method employed for the transfer to regular meals, and the use of a combination of unmodified and protamine zinc insulin are summarized in table 9, p. 896.

Comment.—Several estimations of the gonadotrophic and estrogenic hormone levels in the serum and urine were made by Dr. A. E. Rakoff. There was a definite excess of estrogenic hormone in the serum and urine. This result, in conjunction with the areas

29

of hyperpigmentation about the axillae and groin, was highly suggestive of dysfunction of the adrenal glands.

This patient was found to have an intelligence quotient of 102 by the revised Stanford-Binet scale.

TABLE 9

SUMMARY OF DATA OBTAINED FROM THE RECORD OF J. J. (CASE 2) FOR A PERIOD OF SEVEN MONTHS

1. *The period of febrile illness during which time the equal division and distribution of the diet and insulin regimen was followed.*

Date	Diet (gm.)*				Insulin (Unmodified)		B. Sug. (mg. per cent)	Urine Sug.	Wt. (Kg.)	Ht. (cm.)
	P.	F.	C.	Cal.	Distribution	Total				
1938										
Dec. 14	45	30	125	950	14—14—14—14—14—14	84	84	Neg.	18.0	104
15	45	55	150	1300	14—14—10—10—10—10	68	41	Neg.		
23	50	60	165	1500	16—16—16—16—16—16	96	161	1.0	18.5	
1939										
Jan. 18	60	85	200	1800	34—34—34—34—34—34	204	154	1.2	20.5	
Mar. 6	60	70	230	1800	62—62—62—62—62—62	372	102	Neg.	21.0	
19	60	70	230	1800	68—68—68—68—68—68	408	115	Neg.	21.5	
May 14	60	70	230	1800	68—68—68—68—68—68	408	114	1.1	22.0	112

2. *The transfer from six equal feedings and six equal doses of insulin to three regular meals and the administration of protamine zinc insulin and unmodified insulin.*

Date, 1939	Diet (gm.)				Insulin		Blood Sugar (mg./100 cc.)		Urine Sugar (gm.)
	P.	F.	C.	Cal.	7 A.M.	5 P.M.	11 A.M.	4 P.M.	
May 15	60	70	230	1800	160† 70	80	108	258	22
18	..	..	...	....	160† 70	80	103	251	29
20	..	..	...	....	160† 70	80	195	251	32
22	..	..	...	....	172† 80	80	43	180	18
24	..	..	...	....	180† 74	80	110	264	22
26	..	..	...	....	192† 70	84	116	218	18
28	..	..	...	....	200† 74	84	180	208	6
June 2	..	..	...	....	212† 80	84	60	171	4

3. *The adjustment with three regular meals, breakfast at 7:30 A.M., lunch at 11:30 A.M. and dinner at 5 P.M. and two buffer meals containing 10 gm. of carbohydrate at 10 A.M. and 8 P.M.*

Date, 1939	Diet (gm.)				Insulin		Blood Sugar (mg./100 cc.)					Urine Sugar (gm.)	Wt. (Kg.)	Ht. (cm.)
	P.	F.	C.	Cal.	7 A.M.	5 P.M.	9 A.M.	11 A.M.	1 P.M.	4 P.M.	9 P.M.			
June 12	60	70	230	1800	212† 86	84	103	...	86	70	112	1.4	22.5	115
16	..	..	...	....	200† 80	80	...	125	..	138	...	2.5		

* During this period the diet was divided into six equal feedings given at 8 A.M., 12 N., 4 P.M., 8 P.M., 12 M., and 4 A.M.
† Protamine zinc insulin.

When the patient was discharged from the hospital on June 17, 1939, his liver was no longer palpable. The spleen, however, had not decreased in size. Tests of liver function (bromsulfalein test, hippuric acid synthesis, van den Bergh) gave results which were within normal limits both during the stage of hepatomegaly and after the liver was no longer palpable.

He was admitted to the Wilkes-Barre General Hospital in January, 1940, at which time he was receiving 450 units of insulin a day. In spite of this his urine contained large quantities of sugar, although the level of the fasting blood sugar was usually within the limits of normal. Dr. J. M. Klein has kindly advised me that the child has had recurring eruptions of multiple xanthomata, which subsided after a decrease in the fat content of his diet. It was decided to reduce the quantity of insulin given. This was done gradually with a careful watch for evidence of ketosis. Over a period of three months the insulin was reduced to 15 units of protamine zinc insulin a day without the development of ketosis. The liver and spleen have remained enormously enlarged and the muscular dystrophy has become increasingly prominent. The patient is bright and cheerful and his general condition is satisfactory. Roentgenograms of the skeleton and skull have been within the limits of normal. The blood cholesterol level on July 9, 1940, was 480 mg., and on December 14, 1940, 280 mg. per 100 cc. The fasting level for the blood sugar was 81 mg. per 100 cc. The tolerance which this child has for insulin is remarkable, as has been the lack of change in the level of the blood sugar with the withdrawal of insulin.

Localized Lipodystrophy.—Localized lipodystrophy is frequently seen in diabetic children. This may result from the repeated administration of insulin in the same site, but even when insulin is administered properly this condition is occasionally seen. It is more common following the administration of protamine zinc insulin than following crystalline insulin. The patients are advised to use "insulin maps," *i.e.*, an imaginary checker board is drawn on the anterior aspect of both thighs. Each daily dose is given in a different square so that several weeks intervene between injections in the same square. Should lipodystrophy result the prognosis is good since spontaneous recovery usually occurs in from six months to two years. It is well to advise the patient to administer insulin in areas which will not be disfiguring should lipodystrophy develop.

Local Allergic Reactions.—Local allergic reactions are commonly seen in diabetic children. Sometimes merely changing the brand of insulin will correct this disturbance. General allergic reactions have not been reported and the local reactions are less frequent when crystalline insulin is substituted for unmodified insulin and are less frequent with histone insulin than with protamine zinc insulin. Desensitization results spontaneously in a few weeks if the administration is continued.

Induration at the Site of Insulin Injections. ("Insulin pads, lipomatosis").—This condition is seen less frequently with protamine zinc insulin than with unmodified insulin. It may follow repeated injections at the same site or the injection of large doses of insulin at one site. It may be prevented by the use of "insulin maps" and by the spreading of the sites of injection if large daily doses are necessary.

Transitory Refractive Changes.—These refractive changes are not a complication of insulin therapy but are most commonly noted at the onset of treatment and may last from a few days to a few weeks. This change, though transitory, may be very troublesome. The magnitude of the change usually amounts to two diopters or less, but in diabetic children the shift in refraction may amount to eight diopters.[35]

The cause of these transitory refractive changes is not completely understood. Granström[36] believes that the changes are due to altered curvature and refractive index of the lens rather than to changes in the aqueous humor.

Suffice it to say that the child and his parents should be advised of the possibility of this change in vision before treatment is instituted and they should be warned of the transient nature of this change so that they will not be put to needless expense by consulting an ophthalmologist until at least four weeks after the child's diabetes has been properly controlled.

COMPLICATIONS OF DIABETES IN CHILDHOOD AND THEIR TREATMENT

The complications of juvenile diabetes are conveniently divided into:
1. The acute or direct complications
    (*a*) Ketosis and coma
    (*b*) Acute infections
    (*c*) Surgical complications
2. The chronic or indirect complications
    (*a*) Lowered resistance to infections
    (*b*) Pseudodwarfism, retarded growth and development
    (*c*) Premature arteriosclerosis
    (*d*) Juvenile cataracts
    (*e*) Metabolic disturbances of the skin
        (1) Xanthosis
        (2) Xanthoma diabeticorum
        (3) Necrobiosis lipoidica diabeticorum
    (*f*) Hepatomegaly
    (*g*) Deficiency diseases

Ketosis and Coma.—This dreaded complication is still the most common cause of death in children suffering from diabetes. The reasons for the higher incidence of coma in juvenile as compared with adult diabetic patients are obvious. Children are less likely to keep to a strict diet and are more likely to omit their insulin. They are also more prone to infections and in the presence of infection have less carbohydrate reserve. Then, too, the disease is more severe in childhood. Fortunately, the incidence of coma has decreased since the advent of the slower-acting insulins and the introduction of more liberal diets. The *signs and symptoms* of diabetic coma are the same in the child as they are in the adult. The onset is often abrupt. Coma may develop within twelve hours of the onset of hypoglycemia. Coma usually follows dietary indiscretions or the failure to take insulin. In spite of careful instruction, parents often fail to give the child insulin when he is ill and has refused food, or when the child has vomited. If the child does not take nourishment, does not receive insulin, and vomits, he becomes dehydrated and ketotic, and if treatment is not instituted, coma may develop with amazing rapidity. The signs, symptoms, and methods of recognizing impending and established coma are the same in the child as in the adult. For consideration of these aspects, the reader is referred to pp. 813–815.

Treatment.—The treatment of coma in the child, as in the adult, is aimed at the correction of the ketosis in as speedy a manner as possible. Insulin is given early and in repeated doses. The amount depends upon the size and age of the child, the severity and duration of the coma, and the duration of the diabetes. Protamine zinc insulin has been used successfully in the treatment of coma, but at the present time, particularly in the treatment of coma in children, it is safer to rely upon the quickly-acting crystalline insulin.

It is a good rule in the treatment of coma, to keep the blood sugar level above 200 mg. per 100 cc. and the urine containing considerable amounts of sugar until the carbon dioxide combining power of the blood plasma is above 40 volumes per cent, or the urine and plasma are free of ketone bodies. If the insulin is given too rapidly without sufficient glucose (dextrose), the child may become hypoglycemic before the ketosis is corrected. I have seen this occur recently. The administration of fluid is next in importance to insulin therapy. If the child is unconscious the intravenous administration of a 5 per cent solution of glucose (dextrose) in normal saline and the parenteral administration of normal saline by hypodermoclysis are essential. The intravenous administration of fluids to children may present difficulties. Several methods of administration have been devised.[37, 38, 39, 40]

Most children respond promptly to treatment with insulin, fluids, salt and glucose, but in the presence of a suppressed renal function administration of buffered sodium lactate solution (Hartmann's solution) may be a valuable adjunct,[41] page 821.

Gastric lavage should not be done routinely but should be reserved for those patients who are vomiting persistently or who have abdominal pain with distention.

The other measures in dealing with diabetic coma, *i.e.*, warmth, transfusions, circulatory support and enemata are dealt with on pp. 817–823.

Acute Infections.—For some reason not yet understood there is a lowered resistance to infection in diabetes mellitus. Many attempts have been made to determine the nature of this lowered resistance but no satisfactory explanation has been found.[42] Suffice it to say that a lowered resistance to infection exists in these patients and even the most trivial infection has a profound effect on the severity of the diabetes. Almost any degree of abnormal health in the juvenile patient must be considered an emergency because slight deviations from the normal may precipitate acidosis and coma even in a patient whose diabetes has been well controlled prior to the infection. In the presence of a mild infection this change may take place in from twelve to twenty-four hours. For this reason the children and their parents are instructed to notify their family doctor or to report to the clinic immediately in the case of illness.

Intercurrent infectious diseases are practically always associated with an increase in the severity of the diabetes. Sometimes an increase in the insulin requirements will be noted before the infection manifests itself. Under no circumstances must the insulin treatment be interrupted or reduced during a febrile illness. *At least half of the customary dose of insulin must be administered, no matter how little food is absorbed, and even if it is vomited.* Only if the urine is free from sugar at the time is it safe to reduce the insulin. Each subsequent voiding of urine is tested for sugar and the insulin dosage is adjusted according to the presence or absence of sugar until the acute disorder subsides.

If the illness is of a mild nature, injections of crystalline insulin may be given in addition to the usual injection of protamine zinc insulin. Fruit juices, gruels, cereals, and ginger ale may be substituted for lack of other food. If the infection is severe the child should be admitted to a hospital. If the child has a fever, the equal division and distribution of the diet and insulin is employed to control the diabetes until the temperature returns to normal. After convalescence, protamine zinc insulin may be used again but the previous doses may not suffice. The former equilibrium is seldom exactly reestablished, hence a readjustment is necessary. This is accomplished before the patient leaves the hospital.

Surgical Complications.—Diseases which require surgical intervention occur as frequently in the diabetic as in the nondiabetic child. Severe infections of the skin, osteomyelitis, and infections of the urinary tract are slightly more common in diabetic children but with the introduction of roentgen-ray and chemotherapy the prognosis for these conditions has greatly improved. For the pre- and postoperative treatment of children requiring operations we have found the equal division and distribution of food and insulin to be a great help. The diet is usually divided into six equal feedings, and given at four-hour intervals. The total daily dose of insulin is divided into six doses of crystalline insulin, one of which is given before each feeding. If it is necessary to substitute parenteral fluid for oral feedings immediately before and after the operation, the calculated amount of carbohydrate in the feeding is replaced by an equal amount in the form of 5 per cent glucose (dextrose) in normal saline or distilled water. This plan greatly simplifies the diabetic treatment during this crucial period and allows for satisfactory control of the diabetes at a time when it is extremely important.

Greene, Swanson, and Jacobs[43] question the generally accepted opinion that wound healing is delayed and wound infection is more common in the presence of hyperglycemia. They believe that there is no relationship between the height of the blood sugar level and degree of glycosuria, and the incidence of delayed healing of wounds or of infection in originally clean wounds in cases of diabetes mellitus. We are not in agreement with these authors. Our results have corresponded with those of McKittrick,[44] who has found a steady improvement in the results of treatment in diabetic patients who had undergone surgical operations. This improvement is closely correlated with the improvement in the control of the diabetes during the pre- and postoperative periods. We strive to maintain the level of the blood sugar within normal limits during these periods save for the day of operation. On that day it is advisable to allow the blood sugar level to reach 180 or 200 mg. per 100 cc. in order to be certain that there is no danger of hypoglycemia during the operative procedure.

Lowered Resistance to Infections.—With the introduction of the slowly-acting insulin a striking improvement in the control of juvenile diabetes has been made possible. Coincident with this improvement there appears to be an increased resistance to infections on the part of these well-treated children. Children in whom the diabetes is poorly controlled have a decreased resistance to infections. No diabetic child can cope with an established infection as well as can a normal child.

The incidence of tuberculosis is higher in children suffering from diabetes than it is in the general population and it is frequently seen in patients who have been in diabetic coma.[12, 14, 45] Himsworth[46] concluded, however, that if the diabetes is properly controlled, these patients are no more prone to develop *pulmonary tuberculosis* than nondiabetic subjects. White reports an incidence of pulmonary tuberculosis of the adult type in 1.4 per cent of her diabetic children.[3h] This figure compares favorably with the incidence of tuberculosis in the general population, which is estimated at between 1 and 2 per cent. Of the diabetic children who contracted the disease, 66 per cent died. Tuberculosis is second only to coma as a cause of death in diabetic children. Diabetic children who develop tuberculosis present a difficult problem. It is essential that their diabetes be kept under control in order that the tuberculous process may be arrested. If the tuberculous process advances, the diabetes becomes more difficult to control and a vicious circle may develop. These children do better if they are treated in a general hospital, where physicians specially trained in the treatment of both diabetes and tuberculosis are available. The chances of a tuberculous patient receiving satisfactory care in a general hospital are greater than that the diabetes will be properly controlled at a sanatorium. It is a routine procedure at the Pennsylvania and Jefferson Hospitals to obtain a roentgenogram of the chest at least once a year in our diabetic children. The results of tuberculin tests in diabetic children may be of some value. White[3h] found that 13 per cent of the children tested between the ages of five and nine gave positive reactions, 39 per cent between ten and fourteen years, and 22 per cent between sixteen and nineteen years. From these data she concluded that there was no increased susceptibility to tuberculosis as indicated by this test.

Pseudodwarfism.—This complication of juvenile diabetes is fairly common and its onset is insidious. White reports the occurrence of retarded growth and development in 121 diabetic children.[31] This complication was first thought to be due to undernutrition, and it was thought that the only treatment necessary was an adequate diet.[27] Since the work of Houssay,[47] Long,[48, 49] Lukens,[48, 2] Young,[50] and others, the relationship between juvenile diabetes and abnormalities of the anterior lobe of the hypophysis has been more closely investigated (see section on Etiology, p. 711). It is now believed that dwarfism associated with diabetes mellitus results from diminished secretion of the growth hormone by the anterior lobe of the hypophysis and does not result from undernutrition.

Dwarfism does not precede the onset of diabetes. Data obtained within the first year of the onset of diabetes in thirty-six cases indicate that the patients were typical tall diabetic children. "Dwarfism was not recognized as a rule until the fifth year of diabetes" (White[1]). At the onset of diabetes the child is on the average 2 inches above the standard height for the age. Since these children grow a little, retarded growth is not evident before the fifth year. This will serve to emphasize the importance of checking the annual rates of growth as well as the deviations from the standard for height.

The children with pseudodwarfism resemble the hypopituitary dwarf in physical appearance. They are short in stature with infantile proportions. There is a delay in the development of the teeth and the epiphyses close later than normal. The psyche is childlike although the intelligence quotient is frequently above the average. The texture of the skin is fine and the skin is usually covered with fine hair (lanugo). Puberty is often delayed. These children are overweight for their height and age. In contradistinction to the true pituitary dwarfs, hepatomegaly and an elevation of the basal metabolic rate frequently accompany pseudodwarfism. The incidence of pseudodwarfism predominates in males over that of females in a ratio of 75 to 44.[3j]

Treatment.—Treatment comprises an abundant diet and careful control of the diabetes. One of the extraction products of the anterior pituitary gland which contains large amounts of growth hormone should be given. The administration of "growth hormone" (Antuitrin G) has been followed by increased growth in those patients treated before the closure of the epiphyses was completed.[1, 14] The administration of thyroid substance is followed in some cases by an increase in the rate of growth, due possibly to the stimulating effect which thyroid exerts on the acidophilic cells of the anterior lobe of the pituitary gland. Thyroid may be administered in conjunction with pituitary extract. Roentgenograms of the joints should be taken before therapy is started, as improvement should not be looked for after the epiphyses have closed. The prognosis is poor if treatment is not instituted before the fifteenth year. After seventeen years of age results are usually unsatisfactory.

White observed no untoward effects from the administration of anterior pituitary extract and she states that there was no evidence of the production of antihormones. There was, however, an increase in the insulin requirements in the group which was treated with growth hormone. In fact this group required more insulin per kilogram of body weight than any other group studied.[3j]

The following case will illustrate this complication of juvenile diabetes.

CASE ILLUSTRATIVE OF DIABETIC PSEUDODWARFISM

Case 3.—C. J., a white male, aged twenty-seven years, was first seen by us in 1937 when he was admitted to the hospital in impending coma. He had developed diabetes in 1923 when he was nine years of age. At the time of onset he was a well developed child and for the first two years his diabetes remained well controlled. A restricted diet was prescribed and he received a small dose of insulin daily. In 1925 he was admitted to another hospital in diabetic acidosis. Two years later (1927) he was admitted to the same hospital in a profound insulin reaction (hypoglycemia). He continued under the care of his family physician until 1932. During this period he suffered frequent hypoglycemic reactions. He was treated in the diabetic clinic of a second hospital from 1932 to 1937 and on one occasion was admitted for readjustment of the diet and insulin. He was subject to frequent hypoglycemic reactions, and his blood sugar level fluctuated widely from 30 to 500 mg. per 100 cc. His diet was restricted to less than 1200 calories a day during this period and he failed to gain in height after he reached the age of fourteen years.

When admitted to the hospital in 1937, he weighed 104 pounds and was 58 inches tall (see Fig. 156). He was well nourished but had the appearance of a fifteen-year-old boy. His face was full and rounded; his hair was fine and silky; the eyes were normal, and there was no evidence of peripheral arteriosclerosis. A roentgenogram of the skull and sella turcica showed no abnormalities. Similar studies of the skeleton showed the epiphyses of the long bones to be closed. The basal metabolic rate was + 13 per cent. Desiccated thyroid gland and whole pituitary substance had been administered before that time, but in view of the roentgenographic evidence of closed epiphyses this form of therapy was discontinued.

At present (1941) this patient weighs 50 Kg. (110 pounds) and measures 147.5 cm. (58 inches) in height. His diabetes is well controlled. The diet contains 175 gm. of carbohydrate, 80 gm. of protein, and 86 gm. of fat (1800 calories). He is taking 14 units of protamine zinc insulin every morning and 16 units of crystalline insulin every evening before dinner. He has an occasional hypoglycemic reaction but is able to earn his living as a clerk in a clothing store.

The history of this boy's illness and the physical characteristics he portrays are typical of the type of dwarfism associated with diabetes. It may also be observed that this type of dwarfism resembles pituitary infantilism.

Premature Arteriosclerosis.—Arteriosclerosis does not antedate the onset of diabetes in children but it does develop rapidly in certain patients. This complication is fortunately becoming more infrequent with the better control of diabetes resulting from the use of protamine zinc insulin and diets containing adequate amounts of carbohydrate and limited amounts of fat. It is now believed that hypercholesterolemia is a contributory factor in the development of premature arteriosclerosis and for this reason a blood cholesterol level below 230 mg. per 100 cc. is included in the standards for the control of diabetes. The arteries of the eyes, kidneys, and extremities, particularly the legs, are frequently involved, and the coronary arteries are also the site of atheromatous and calciferous deposits. The symptoms depend

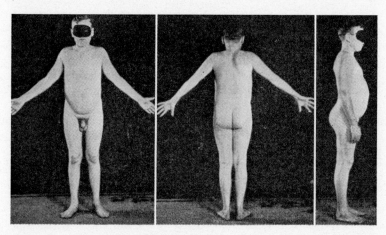

Fig. 156.—C. J. Photographs taken in 1937, fourteen years after the onset of diabetes; age twenty-four years, weight 104 pounds (46 Kg.), and height 58 inches (147 cm.). The stature and bodily contour are illustrative of the type of dwarfism associated with diabetes mellitus.

upon the degree of involvement; in fact, premature arteriosclerosis often causes no symptoms. An associated diabetic retinitis with retinal hemorrhages is the most frequent manifestation of the arterial changes. With adequate treatment and satisfactory control of the diabetes the development of this complication may be arrested and, indeed, the retinal changes are often reversible. We have found the administration of large amounts of ascorbic acid (50 mg. a day) has been followed by improvement in the retinal changes.[24]

Juvenile Cataract.—This, one of the most distressing complications of juvenile diabetes, is fortunately a very infrequent one. Like the other degenerative complications, it is more frequently seen in children in whom the diabetes has been inadequately controlled. This complication may also be associated with hypercholesterolemia and tuberculosis. With the control of the diabetes, immature cataracts and cataractous lesions may be arrested with no further loss of visual acuity.

Juvenile cataracts present the development of a distinctive type of opacity, distinctive in the sense that it does not occur in normal individuals although it is indistinguishable from the cataracts induced by various metabolic disorders and by dinitrophenol therapy. These opacities occur in the anterior and posterior cortical portions of the lens and resemble a chemical flocculent precipitate.[51] The lens is always soft and is sometimes fluid and milky. Treatment consists of the proper control of the diabetes. In some cases restoration of vision may depend on surgical removal of the lens. Discission has proved satisfactory in some cases but occasionally there are remains of the lens which do not become absorbed and must subsequently be removed by linear extraction. Semifluid cataracts are removed by linear extraction.

Metabolic Disturbances of the Skin.—*Xanthosis.*—Xanthosis or xanthochromia is the term applied to a yellow discoloration of the skin which is frequently seen in diabetic children. The pigmentation is particularly noticeable on the palms of the hands and the soles of the feet. It may also be present about the face, especially in the nasolabial fold, but this distribution is less common and involvement of the entire body is rare.

The discoloration of the skin is due to the presence of an excess of lipochrome pigment in the blood and tissue fluids. Lipochrome is a pigment which is found in green vegetables, fruit, carrots, corn, butter, and egg yolk, and is closely related to carotene.

Xanthosis results from the faulty utilization of lipochrome and carotene by diabetic children. Furthermore the usual diet prescribed for the diabetic child contains large quantities of foods rich in lipochrome.

Heyman[52] performed carotene tolerance tests upon normal and diabetic children and demonstrated its faulty utilization in the diabetic children. Xanthosis occurs in association with severe diabetes in children in whom the evidence of disordered fat metabolism is present.

Xanthochromia is not confined to diabetic children. It is often seen in adult diabetic patients and in other diseases in which there is a disorder of fat metabolism. It has also been reported in otherwise normal people who have been maintained on a vegetable diet containing large amounts of lipochrome.

The condition may be corrected by:

1. Adequate control of the diabetes.
2. Temporary exclusion from the diet of fruit and vegetables of high carotene content, notably carrots and spinach, and the restriction of butter and eggs.
3. The replacement of the vitamins contained in the foods restricted by concentrated vitamin products.

Xanthoma Diabeticorum.—This is an unusual complication of diabetes in children and it is becoming more infrequent with the better control of diabetes. Xanthoma diabeticorum should not be confused with xanthoma or xanthosis. Xanthoma diabeticorum is distinguished by tumor-like lesions of a brilliant yellow color with a reddish periphery. The lesions may appear within a few days and may extend over the entire body. They are more numerous on the extensor surface of the forearm and about the elbows and knees, where the lesions may be confluent. The palms, soles, and flexor surfaces of the large joints are seldom involved. The lesions vary in size from 1 to 6 mm. in diameter.

Joslin reports twelve cases, three males and nine females. Four of the twelve were children under fifteen years of age.[3k]

The level of the blood fat and cholesterol is usually elevated in xanthoma diabeticorum.

The lesions usually involute coincident with the adequate control of the diabetes and the fall in the level of the blood cholesterol. A diet high in carbohydrate and low in fat content is advisable.

Necrobiosis Lipoidica Diabeticorum.—The lesions of this unusual complication of diabetes appear as sharply demarcated, elevated, red papules capped by a slight scale and they do not disappear under pressure. The lesions measure from 1 mm. to several cm. in diameter. They may be single or multiple and the legs and ankles are the most common sites involved. The original papules may progress to form arcuate, oval, or irregular plaques of firm consistency with well-defined borders and a glistening surface which has been likened to the appearance of slightly stretched cellophane. The lesion may go on to atrophy and ulceration.

This condition more commonly involves females than males[53] and is most common in juvenile patients. The treatment, since the cause is unknown, is limited to the care of the local lesions and to the adequate control of the diabetic condition. A diet liberal in carbohydrate but limited in fat content should be prescribed.

Hepatomegaly.—This complication is not an infrequent finding in diabetic children in whom the diabetes has not been properly controlled. Hepatomegaly is diagnosed if the liver extends at least four fingerbreadths below the costal margin. The enlarged liver may extend into the pelvis.

Hepatomegaly frequently accompanies pseudodwarfism, progressive lipodystrophy, splenomegaly, and other complications of juvenile diabetes. The abdomen is usually protuberant and these children frequently complain of a dragging sensation in the abdomen or of bouts of abdominal pain.

The exact cause of hepatomegaly in these children is not known as biopsy and autopsy material has not been available. Biopsy material from the liver of a boy, aged twelve years, with diabetes, hepatomegaly, splenomegaly, ascites, jaundice, and hyperpyrexia revealed tremendous amounts of intracellular glycogen on microscopic examination.[54]

Biopsy of the liver in a similar case,[31] a woman, aged twenty-five years, with diabetes of eleven years' duration, revealed a large amount of fat (10.15 per cent) and a high glycogen content (12.1 per cent). The latter finding was considered to be due to a temporary hypoglycemia (blood sugar 0.03 per cent on the morning of operation).

The hepatomegaly may be due to gross fatty infiltration, glycogen deposition or hydropic degeneration, but further work is required to determine the pathogenesis of the enlargement of the liver. Tests of liver function and estimations of the cholesterol level and fat content of the blood usually reveal values within the limits of normal.

The prognosis is good. With adequate control of the diabetes, made possible by protamine zinc insulin, a decrease in the size of the liver occurs in the great majority of cases.

Deficiency Diseases.—*Vitamin Deficiency.*—Diabetic children are as likely to develop vitamin deficiencies as other children, but with modern treatment the prescribed diets contain sufficient amounts of the accessory food factors to prevent these complications, provided normal absorption takes place. None of our diabetic children has developed a recognizable vitamin deficiency.

PATHOLOGY

Introduction.—Diabetes is a disease in which disturbances in function are far greater than disturbances in structure. The paucity of pathologic changes in the diabetic child is indeed disappointing to the pathologist but encouraging to the clinician, for in the absence of irreversible changes in structure we may hope to obtain reversible changes in function.

Cause of Death.—Prior to the advent of insulin, coma was almost invariably the cause of death. Of twenty-two fatal cases reported by Warren[51a] prior to 1930, all died in coma and in five cases coma was uncomplicated by infection. Of 126 deaths in diabetic children between the years 1923 and 1938, White[3m] reported sixty-three that died in coma, eleven of sepsis, eleven of tuberculosis, six of pneumonia, and the remainder of miscellaneous causes. Grishaw[5] reported forty-one deaths in 301 children who were treated since the introduction of insulin. Of the forty-one who died, twenty-one died in coma and, of these, twelve were uncomplicated, nine were complicated by severe infection, seven died of acute infections, and one of tuberculosis. Before insulin was in general use, coma was almost invariably the cause of death. Although it is still the most common cause of death, coma now is almost always complicated by an infection. Diabetic children when properly treated do not ordinarily die of diabetes itself but of one of its complications.

Pathology of the Pancreas.—In children having died of diabetes one would expect to find diabetic lesions uncomplicated by the degenerative processes which occur in the aged. The pancreas of the diabetic child, however, seldom shows any striking or diagnostic changes. The pancreas may be small but there is a great individual variation in its size. Minkowski's extirpation experiments showed that diabetes did not develop in animals if one-tenth of the gland was allowed to remain. Since in animals almost all of the pancreas must be removed to produce diabetes, slight variations in the size of the human pancreas would not appear significant if the amount of insular tissue was in normal proportion to the acinar tissue. However, the pancreas may be relatively poor in islet tissue. In many diabetic children a definite decrease in the number of islets has been observed and in some cases only a few small cell groups could be found. In these cases there would seem to be a congenital deficiency in the amount of islet tissue which might become an actual insufficiency if the slight factor of safety were reduced by infection or by any increase in the insulin requirements. The islet tissue may be morphologically and quantitatively normal and yet be functionally abnormal. Estimations of the insulin content of the pancreas in fourteen normal and eighteen diabetic patients revealed that the normal pancreas contained on the average 1.7 units of insulin per gm., whereas the diabetic pancreas contained less than 0.4 of a unit per gm.[55]

There is no lesion of the pancreas which is pathognomonic of diabetes. In twenty-nine autopsies of diabetic children, Warren[51b] encountered hyaline changes in two cases, whereas lymphocytic infiltration, the most characteristic lesion of the islets in diabetic children, was noted in five cases. It is rarely seen in older individuals. It has been suggested that this lymphocytic infiltration may result from the action of some toxic substance or from necrosis of the islet cells.[51b] Such lesions are not found in dogs made diabetic by the parenteral administration of crude extracts from the anterior pituitary gland or its globin fraction. In these dogs, the characteristic lesions are degranulation and hydropic degeneration of the beta cells of the islets of Langerhans.[56]

Hydropic degeneration was diagnosed in four cases and suspected in one by Warren[51b] but the islets appeared normal in fifteen and were normal both in number and in appearance in ten of the twenty-nine cases. The absence of irreversible changes in the pancreas in diabetic children cannot be overemphasized, for where there is no irreparable damage there is hope of cure.

Copp and Barclay[57] working with Allen in 1923 and recently Lukens and Dohan[2] have shown that animals made diabetic by partial extirpation of the pancreas and by partial extirpation plus the injection of crude extracts of the anterior pituitary gland can be cured by the administration of insulin during the period characterized by hydropic degeneration of the islets of Langerhans. In children one can expect the regenerative powers of the pancreas to be at their height and such regeneration has been reported.[58]

Arrested cases of juvenile diabetes are infrequent. Joslin and White have followed sixteen children in whom a diagnosis of diabetes was established, but with one exception these children have shown no evidence of diabetes since 1934.[3p]

Acute pancreatitis should always be suspected in a child dying in coma.[51b]

Central Nervous System.—There have been only a few scattered reports of histologic studies of the brain in diabetic children. Dillon, Riggs, and Dyer[59] found that in eight patients, the youngest of whom was aged fourteen years, who died from uncomplicated diabetic acidosis, brain lesions similar to those seen in acute asphyxia were present. The primary pathologic changes occurred in the cerebral capillary bed.

CASE ILLUSTRATIVE OF DEATH FROM DIABETIC COMA WITH PATHOLOGIC CHANGES IN
THE CEREBRAL CORTEX

Case 4.—J. B., a white male, aged twenty-two years, was admitted to Jefferson Hospital under the care of Dr. Hobart Reimann on October 19, 1940, in diabetic coma. He had developed diabetes in the summer of 1933, at the age of fourteen years, and his diabetes had remained satisfactorily controlled through most of the intervening years.

When this patient had last been seen at the clinic, October 5, 1940, his blood sugar level was 102 mg. per 100 cc. and there was no sugar in the urine. He consulted his family doctor because of a "cold" three days before his last admission to the hospital and on the following day was confined to bed with a fever and a severe cough. He gradually lost consciousness and his family doctor finally had him admitted to the hospital fourteen hours after the onset of coma. At that time his blood sugar was 544 mg. per 100 cc. and the CO_2 combining power was 15.7 volumes per cent. He was comatose, the pupils did not react to light, and there was a reduction in his intraocular tension.

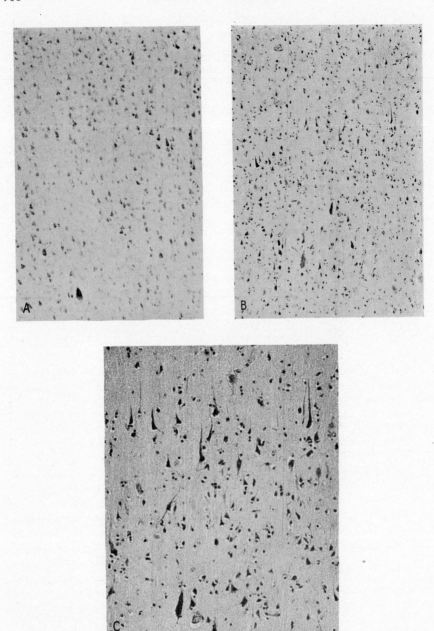

Fig. 157.—*A*, A portion of the motor cortex from a normal brain. *B*, An equivalent area from a case of diabetes (Case 4), showing the pyknotic cells and the prolonged and somewhat tortuous apical dendrites as well as the shrunken appearance of the cells. *C*, A photomicrograph from the same section showing these features in a higher power of magnification. (Photomicrographs by the courtesy of Drs. Bernard J. Alpers and Calvin S. Drayer.)

There were fine crepitant râles audible over the base of each lung, the heart sounds were distant and of poor quality, the abdomen was distended, and the urinary bladder was palpable 3 cm. below the umbilicus. The tendon reflexes were absent, skin and mucous membranes were cold and dry, and there was an odor of acetone on the breath. Treatment was instituted in the form of intravenous 5 per cent dextrose in normal saline and crystalline insulin was given subcutaneously. At 4 P.M., twenty-four hours after admission, the blood sugar was 110, the CO_2 combining power had risen to 48 volumes per cent. In spite of this improvement in the constituents of the blood the patient failed to regain consciousness and died at 1 P.M. on October 21. At autopsy the only remarkable findings were the changes noted in the brain, illustrated in the photomicrographs (Fig. 157).

Abnormalities of the Carbohydrate and Fat Metabolism.—Histochemical studies on autopsy material obtained from diabetic children have shown that glycogen is deposited in the tissues normally free of glycogen and that glycogen is absent from the tissues in which it is normally present. Normal glycogen stores are displaced by fat and *vice versa*. Glucose is found in the skin in place of glycogen, and the glycogen in the liver cells is found in the nuclei instead of in the cytoplasm. Glycogen is also found in tissues such as the renal tubules, which do not normally contain glycogen. Abnormally large amounts of glycogen may be found in the muscle of the heart.

Disturbances in fat metabolism are more evident in children than they are in adults. Atheroma and abnormal deposits of lipids in the reticuloendothelial system (lipid histiocytosis) and fatty infiltration of the liver are the characteristic changes. Lipid histiocytosis is the most striking of these lesions.

Arteriosclerosis is infrequent but is the most common complication after infections in diabetic children. The skin, lungs, and kidneys are the organs most frequently involved by infection.

PROGRESS OF THE DIABETIC CHILD

At present the diabetic child may be expected to live to late middle age and may become a useful member of society if he is willing to abide by the rules of conduct essential not only for his well being but for life itself.

Fortunately most diabetic children are intelligent enough to respond to instruction, but constant kind supervision is necessary to prevent a maladjustment on the part of the child to his disease.

Intelligence.—Cone[30] tested the intelligence of 169 diabetic children. The intelligence quotient (I.Q.) was found to be higher, by an average of 10 points, than the control group in which the median age was the same. Fifty-seven per cent of the diabetic children had an intelligence quotient between 90 and 109; 31 per cent between 110 and 150, and only 12 per cent were classified as inferior.

McGavin, Schultz, Peden and Bowen[60] tested the intelligence of forty-nine diabetic children under the age of eighteen years. The mean intelligence of the whole group was 103 and the standard deviation 16–8; they were in fact neither significantly brighter nor duller than the nondiabetic children.

Brown and Thompson[6] found in a group of sixty children tested for intelligence as determined by the Stanford-Binet test, that there was a normal distribution in regard to intelligence.

Grishaw[5] reports an average I.Q. of 105.4 (standard deviation 11.7–0.89) for sixty-two unselected diabetic children. The intelligence quotients for the children in this group were well in advance of the normal distribution for unselected children as indicated by intelligence quotients above 110 (42.1 per cent), between 90 and 110 inclusive (47.4 per cent), and below 90 (10.5 per cent). The normal or expected distribution according to Terman for unselected children is as follows: above 110, 20.6 per cent; 90–110, 60 per cent; and below 90, 19.4 per cent.

Psychological Problems of the Diabetic Child.—The diabetic child may be said to have an average or slightly superior intelligence, but when these same children are studied psychologically many are found to harbor a resentment to their diabetes which usually manifests itself a year or more after the initial adjustment of the diabetes.

A psychiatric investigation of forty-five juvenile diabetic patients by McGavin[60] brought out the striking fact that thirty-two of them were maladjusted.

Some children respond by aggressiveness and others by retiring and seclusive behavior. Maladjustment is more common among diabetic children who are undersize for their age. They are usually more concerned about their stature than about their illness.

The parents are often more affected by the diabetes than is the child. Oversolicitude on their part is to be discouraged as is a tendency to err too far in the other direction, *i.e.*, indifference and neglect.

Growth.—Since underdevelopment in stature has such a detrimental effect on the morale and the future happiness of diabetic children, everything possible should be done to promote normal physical development. For this reason it is important to check the annual rate of growth for each child as well as to compare his height with the standards for his age. If growth is retarded treatment should be instituted as outlined on p. 902.

Sexual Development of Diabetic Children.—Approximately 90 per cent of all diabetic children show normal or slightly precocious sexual development. In girls, if we use rounding of the hips, breast development, growth of pubic and axillary hair, and the menarche respectively as progressive evidence of the development of secondary sexual characteristics, it has been found that the first two characteristics appear earlier than in normal girls and the menarche may be slightly delayed. The normal cycle for boys may be taken as the development of pubic and axillary hair, voice changes, development of body hair and maturity. Here, too, the early signs of puberty come earlier. The development of body hair and maturity may be delayed.

Pseudodwarfism has been found in approximately 10 per cent of diabetic children up to the present time. In these children puberty is delayed. In girls the menarche may not be established until the age of seventeen or later, and in some the onset of catamenia is noted after the age of twenty. Male pseudodwarfs remain childish in their appearance, and changes of voice and maturity are greatly delayed (see p. 901).

Parenthood.—Diabetic children are now living to reach maturity and the question as to the advisability of marriage and parenthood will be frequently asked.

Diabetes is a hereditary disease of the mendelian recessive type. Diabetic patients who marry into families which are free from diabetes will not transmit diabetes to the children in the first generation but some of the children will carry a recessive gene for diabetes.

The German attitude is exemplified by Chiari[8] who states, "Since diabetes is not included in the law for the prevention of inferior offspring, there are only indirect possibilities for reducing diabetic offspring, but, as a rule, thorough enlightenment suffices, if not, the marriage certificate may be withheld."

Grishaw and others[5] report eighteen pregnancies in twelve diabetic children who had reached maturity. Seven Caesarean sections were performed on six women. There were five abortions, one of which was induced because of intractable ketosis and vomiting before the patient came under their care. In another case hysterectomy was done at the time of the abortion. The other abortions were spontaneous. One child died at birth. There was no maternal mortality.

White[3p] reported fifty-three marriages in patients including both sexes who had had diabetes since childhood. There were sixty-one subsequent pregnancies, thirty-six of which resulted in living children of whom one developed diabetes at the age of thirty-four. She was also a deaf mute.

From these and our own experiences, we can say that if the diabetic child who has reached maturity has chosen a nondiabetic mate whose antecedents have not had diabetes, there can be no legitimate objection to the marriage. If pregnancy results the problem is further complicated, but with proper care the maternal mortality should be almost zero, and normal children should result from the majority of such pregnancies.

Diabetes in Children as Contrasted with that in Adults.—Diabetes mellitus in childhood and adolescence differs in several important aspects from the disease as seen in adults:

1. The onset is abrupt and violent. In the majority of diabetic children (79 to 85 per cent)[5] the symptoms develop so dramatically that the onset may be dated to within a period of two weeks. This is in contrast to the usual gradual onset in adults.

2. It is a more severe disease in the child than it is in the adult. All children suffering from diabetes require insulin but of our adult patients, only 25 to 35 per cent require insulin.

3. Coma is ten times more frequent in children than it is in adult diabetic patients. Fortunately in spite of the higher incidence of coma in children, less vigorous treatment is necessary and the mortality rate of the diabetic juvenile patients treated in the hospital is almost zero. The mortality from coma is far higher for adults.

4. The disease is more labile in children than it is in adults. There is frequently a "facile replacement of controlled diabetes by acidosis or hypoglycemia."[61] This lability may be due to the greater activity of the child and the relatively small glycogen reserve which the child possesses.

5. The disease is usually progressive. With growth, development and increased total metabolism, larger doses of insulin are required and frequent readjustments of the diet are necessary to allow for proper development. These requirements increase more markedly during puberty.

6. There is a more definite relationship between juvenile diabetes and hyperfunction of the anterior lobe of the hypophysis than is the case in adults (see p. 878).

7. The hereditary factor is demonstrable in a larger proportion of juvenile diabetic patients than in adults who have this disease.

8. The increased susceptibility to infection is present for both juvenile and adult patients, but the site of infection is different. Children are more likely to develop tuberculosis and infections of the urinary tract; adults more commonly develop cutaneous infections.

9. Diabetes in children is rarely preceded by the obesity or degenerative changes which often foreshadow the onset of this disease in adults.

10. Degenerative complications are less frequently seen in diabetic children; arteriosclerosis, retinitis and retinal hemorrhages occur less frequently (but in many more times than the expected incidence in nondiabetic children) in the child than in the adult.

11. Deficiency-like diseases common in the adult are rare in the child.

12. The lesions of the skin characteristic of diabetes, namely: xanthosis, necrobiosis lipoidica diabeticorum and xanthoma diabeticorum are more specific for children.

13. Hepatomegaly is observed frequently as a complication in the juvenile but not in the adult diabetic patient.

14. There is more difficulty in sustaining a strict dietary regulation in children than in adults.

CASE ILLUSTRATING CLINICAL DIFFERENCES BETWEEN DIABETES IN CHILDREN AND IN ADULTS

Case 5.—G. D., a white female, aged fourteen years. Weight 126 pounds (57 Kg.), height 66 inches (167.6 cm.).

The patient was first admitted to the Pennsylvania Hospital on February 19, 1934, when she was eight years of age. She had enjoyed good health until three weeks before admission when there was such a marked increase in the frequency of urination that within two weeks she was voiding every twenty minutes, day and night. She also developed a ravenous appetite and a great thirst. "The urine was syrupy and, when it dried on her clothing, left a crisp area." She lost 8 pounds in two weeks and at the time of admission weighed 60 pounds (27.2 Kg.) and measured 54 inches (137 cm.) in height. None of her relatives had diabetes.

The child was tall and thin and lay comfortably in bed in no apparent discomfort. Her face was flushed and her skin and mucous membranes were dry. There was a slight odor of acetone on her breath. Respirations were not increased either in rate or depth. Her tonsils were enlarged and inflamed. No further significant abnormalities were noted on physical examination.

Her urine was concentrated (specific gravity 1.045) and completely reduced Benedict's solution. Acetone and diacetic acid were present in the urine. The blood sugar level was 230 mg. per 100 cc. and the carbon dioxide combining power of the blood plasma was 38 volumes per cent.

The following diet was prescribed: carbohydrate 110 gm., protein 45 gm., and fat 53 gm. (1100 calories). This was divided into three equal meals. Four injections of unmodified insulin a day (16 units before breakfast, 14 units at 11:30 A.M., 16 units before dinner, and 10 units at midnight) were required to control the glycosuria, ketonuria, and hyperglycemia.

Before the patient left the hospital the diet was increased to 1500 calories because of her failure to gain weight. It has been altered frequently during the seven years she has been under our care in the clinic and the hospital (table 10). One admission was necessitated by a dietary indiscretion, which resulted in ketosis, and three were for readjustment to new forms of insulin and for further investigation. She has attended the clinic at intervals of from one to three weeks during the entire period.

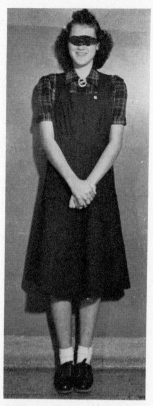

Fig. 158.—Photograph of G. D. taken November 8, 1940, approximately seven years after the onset of diabetes. It may be seen that she is a well-developed and well-nourished girl of fifteen years although she requires 150 units of insulin a day to control her diabetes.

PROGNOSIS

The prognosis of diabetes in childhood is more difficult to predict. With modern treatment the prognosis as to life expectancy has increased from 1.3 years in 1914 to 40.2 in 1940.[3q] If he will abide by the timed and measured regimen which is essential to his well-being, the diabetic child should live to be a healthy and useful citizen.

Occupation for these children is a serious problem. The civil services exclude diabetic patients from employment. These patients are not eligible for life insurance or for positions with companies which insure their employees. Since they are usually above the average intellectually, it is advisable that they receive an education which will enable them to earn a livelihood either in a profession or in independent business. Farming has been suggested as an ideal occupation for diabetic boys who are preparing for a future livelihood.

They should choose a husband or wife who does not have diabetes, in fact one who cames from a family which is free of diabetes

TABLE 10

FIGURES OBTAINED FROM THE RECORD IN CASE 5 AT INTERVALS OF THREE MONTHS FOR A PERIOD OF SEVEN YEARS

Date	Age, yrs.	Ht., in.	Wt., lbs.	Diet				Insulin, Units	Urine. Per Cent Sugar	Blood	
				P.*	C.*	F.*	Cal.			Sugar†	Chol.†
1934											
Mar. 27	8	54	61	60	120	86	1500	0‡	neg.	112	200
Jun. 22	9	55	65	65	130	100	1700	0‡	neg.	129	
Sep. 21	..	..	67	70	140	115	1900	12–0–8	neg.	239¶	
Dec. 21	..	..	75	70	140	115	1900	14–4–12–10	neg.	250¶	
1935											
Mar. 22	..	..	77	70	140	85	1700	27–10–23–8	neg.	100	
Jun. 7	10	56	81	70	140	85	1700	26–10–22–11	neg.	163	
Sep. 27	..	..	82	70	140	85	1700	22–13–0–23	neg.	247¶	
Dec. 20	..	..	86	70	140	85	1700	21–13–19–8	neg.	226¶	
1936											
Mar. 9	..	..	87	70	140	85	1700	19–11–19–6	neg.	126	
Jun. 26	11	60	90	70	140	85	1700	16–11–8 (8)	1	234¶	
Sep. 25	..	..	91	70	140	85	1700	(32) (24)	neg.	286¶	
Dec. 18	..	..	88	70	200	102	2000	((45)) ((40))	0.7	240¶	190
1937											
Mar. 26	..	..	92	70	200	102	2000	[72] 20–0–8	1.6	107	
Jun. 25	12	63	89	80	250	131	2500	[72] 3–0–12	3.0	183	
Sep. 17	..	..	89	80	250	131	2500	[72] 8–0– [16]	neg.	132	
Dec. 24	..	..	94	95	250	180	3000	[76] 10–0– [24]	3.0	231	
1938											
Mar. 25	..	..	103	95	250	180	3000	[80] 10–0– ((16))	2.0	324¶	
Jun. 17	13	65	111	95	250	180	3000	[84] 50–0– [24]	neg.	74	
Sep. 23	..	..	115	95	250	180	3000	[88] 46–0– [32]	1.4	120	
Dec. 16	..	..	117	95	250	180	3000	[90] 46–0– [30	1.5	282	
1939											
Mar. 10	..	..	121	95	250	147	2700	[106] 46—— [30]	2.5	105¶	
Jun. 2	14	66	123	95	250	113	2400	[120] 40——10	neg.	167	173
Sep. 22	..	..	119	95	250	130	2550	[120] –0–10 40	1.4	73	
Dec. 1	..	..	124	95	250	130	2550	[118] –0–0–8 34	neg.	60	
1940											
Mar. 8	..	..	124	95	250	130	2550	[118] –0–0–8 34	neg.	70	
Jun. 14	15	66	126	95	250	130	2550	[108] –0–0– ((12)) ((34))	0.9	67	167
Sep. 27	..	..	125	95	250	130	2550	[108] –0–0– ((12)) ((34))	1.1	105	
1941											
Jan. 24	..	..	126	95	250	130	2550	[108] –0–0– ((10)) ((34))	1.4	80	

* Gm.
† mg./100 cc.
‡ Reference 62 (Case 6).
¶ Blood taken ½ hour after breakfast and insulin.
( ) Protamine insulin.
(( )) Crystalline insulin.
[ ] Protamine zinc insulin.

BIBLIOGRAPHY

1. White, P., Arch. Int. Med., **63:** 39, 1939.
2. Lukens, F. D. W., and Dohan, C., Science, **92:** 222, 1940.
3. Joslin, E. P., Root, H. F., White, P., Marble, A., The Treatment of Diabetes Mellitus, 7th ed., Lea & Febiger, Philadelphia, 1940, p. 672.
3a. Ibid., p. 673.
3b. Ibid., pp. 47–60.
3c. Ibid., p. 670.
3d. Ibid., p. 671.
3e. Ibid., p. 674.
3f. Ibid., pp. 674–675.
3g. Ibid., p. 678.
3h. Ibid., p. 682.
3i. Ibid., p. 684.
3j. Ibid., p. 685.
3k. Ibid., p. 524.
3l. Ibid., p. 473.
3m. Ibid., p. 693.
3n. Ibid., p. 691.
3o. Ibid., p. 679.
3p. Ibid., p. 690.
3q. Ibid., p. 692.
4. National Institute of Health, 1935–1936: United States Public Health Service, Washington, D. C., 1938.
5. Grishaw, W. H., West, H. F., and Smith, B., Arch. Int. Med., **64:** 787, 1939.
6. Brown, G. D., and Thompson, W. H., Am. Dis. Child., **59:** 238, 1940.
7. White, P., Diabetes in Childhood and Adolescence, Lea & Febiger, Philadelphia, 1932.
8. Chiari, O., Wien. klin. Wchnschr., **52:** 1058, 1939.
9. Young, F. G., New England J. Med., **221:** 635, 1939.
10. Young, F. G., Brit. M. J., **2:** 393, 1939.
11. Bogan, L. K., and Morrison, A. B., Am. J. Med. Sci., **174:** 313, 1927.
12. Joslin, E. P., South. M. J., **26:** 1, 1933.
13. Payne, W. W., Brit. M. J., **2:** 960, 1936.
14. White, P., Section in Joslin, E. P., Treatment of Diabetes Mellitus, 6th ed., Lea & Febiger, Philadelphia, 1937, pp. 587–617.
15. O'Donnell, J. A., Pennsylvania M. J., **38:** 610, 1935.
16. Oakley, W., Diabetes Mellitus, The British Encyclopaedia of Medical Practice, **3:** 662, Butterworth & Co., Ltd., London, 1937.
17. Exton, W. G., and Rose, A. R., Am. J. Clin. Path., **4:** 381, 1934.
18. Stern, F., Applied Dietetics, Williams & Wilkins, Baltimore, 1937, p. 99.
19. Sansum, W. D., Blatherwick, N. R., and Bowden, R., J.A.M.A., **86:** 178, 1926.
20. Lichtenstein, A., J. Pediat., **12:** 183, 1938.
21. Nelson, W. E., and Ward, D., Am. J. Dis. Child., **55:** 487, 1938.
22. deWesselow, O. L. V., and Griffith, W. J., Quart. J. Med., **7:** 17, 1938.
23. Butler, A. M., New England J. Med., **212:** 760, 1935.
24. Stockwell, H., and Cuttle, T. D., yet unpublished work.
25. Duncan, G. G., Fetter, F., and Durkin, J., Surgery, **1:** 939, 1937.
26. Duncan, G. G., Internat. Clin., **2:** 31, 1939.
27. White, P., Bull. New York Acad. Med., **10:** 347, 1934.
28. Beattie, B., New England J. Med., **212:** 473, 1935.
29. Payne, W. W., Brit. M. J., **2:** 960, 1936.
30. White, P., Practitioner, **142:** 576, 1939.
31. Duncan, G. G., Cuttle, T. D., and Jewesbury, E. C. O., Bull. Ayer Clin. Lab., Pennsylvania Hosp., **3:** 293, 1939.
32. Nelson, W. E., and Dummer, C. M., J. Pediat., **10:** 446, 1937.
33. White, P., and Winterbottom, L., J.A.M.A., **112:** 1440, 1939.
34. Bader, G. B., J. Pediat., **4:** 77, 1934.
35. Root, H. F., Section in Joslin, E. P., The Treatment of Diabetes Mellitus, 7th ed., Lea & Febiger, Philadelphia, 1940, p. 546.
36. Granström, K. O., Acta Ophth., **11:** 1, 1933.

37. Aldrich, C. A., Stokes, J., Jr., Killingsworth, W. P., and McGuiness, A. C., J.A.M.A., **111**: 129, 1938.
38. Ormiston, G., Lancet, **1**: 82, 1938.
39. Hogg, P., Virginia M. Monthly, **65**: 46, 1938.
40. Cuttle, T. D., St. Barth. Hosp. J., **45**: 293, 1938.
41. Hartmann, A. F., Arch. Int. Med., **56**: 413, 1935.
42. Marble, A., White, H. J., and Fernald, A. T., J. Clin. Invest., **17**: 423, 1938.
43. Greene, J. A., Swanson, L. W., and Jacobs, C. A., J.A.M.A., **115**: 1518, 1940.
44. McKittrick, L. S., Arch. of Surg., **40**: 352, 1940.
45. Root, H. F., Tuberculosis Complicating Diabetes, Joslin, E. P., Treatment of Diabetes Mellitus, Lea & Febiger, Philadelphia, 1937, p. 499.
46. Himsworth, H. P., Quart. J. Med., **7**: 373, 1938.
47. Houssay, B. A., and Biasotti, A., Endocrinology, **15**: 511, 1931.
48. Long, C. N. H., and Lukens, F. D. W., Proc. Soc. Exper. Biol. and Med., **32**: 743, 1935.
49. Long, C. N. H., Medicine, **16**: 215, 1937.
50. Young, F. G., Lancet, **2**: 372, 1937.
51. Warren, S., Pathology of Diabetes, 2nd ed., Lea & Febiger, Philadelphia, 1938, p. 191.
51a. Ibid., pp. 167–168.
51b. Ibid., pp. 169–170.
52. Heymann, W., J.A.M.A., **106**: 2050, 1936.
53. Wilder, R. M., Clinical Diabetes and Hyperinsulinism, W. B. Saunders Company, Philadelphia, 1940, pp. 296–297.
54. Stetson, R. P., and Ohler, W. R., New England J. Med., **217**: 627, 1937.
55. Scott, D. A., and Fisher, A. M., J. Clin. Invest., **17**: 725, 1938.
56. Richardson, K. C., Proc. Roy. Soc. London, **128**: 153, 1940.
57. Copp, E. F. F., and Barclay, A. J., J. Met. Res., **4**: 445, 1923.
58. Boyd, G. L., and Robinson, W. L., Am. Jour. Path., **1**: 135, 1925.
59. Dillon, E. S., Riggs, H. E., and Dyer, W. W., Am. J. Med. Sci., **192**: 360, 1936.
60. McGavin, A. P., Schultz, E., Peden, G. W., and Bowen, B. D., New England J. Med., **223**: 119, 1940.
61. Bennett, T. I., and Gill, A. M., Lancet, **2**: 415, 1936.
62. Duncan, G. G., Shumway, N. P., Williams, T. L., and Fetter, F., Am. J. Med. Sci., **189**: 403, 1935.

APPENDIX*

By Garfield G. Duncan

COMPOSITION OF FOODS

The protein, fat, carbohydrate and caloric values of foods in common use are presented. The respective amounts occurring in 100 gm. (percentage) are presented as are the food values, weights and household measures of portions commonly served. The source of the data, unless otherwise indicated,† is the recently published Proximate Composition of American Food Materials, Chatfield and Adams, Circular No. 549, United States Department of Agriculture, published in June, 1940. All values are for edible portions of fresh foods unless otherwise indicated.

ABBREVIATIONS

A. P.–as purchased
av.–average
C.–8-ounce measuring cup
ckd.–cooked
diam.–diameter
lb.–pound
lg.–large
med.–medium

oz.–ounce
pkg.–package
sc.–scant
sl.–slice
sm.–small
sq.–square
T.–tablespoon
t.–teaspoon
"–inch

FOOD EQUIVALENTS

3 teaspoons   = 1 tablespoon
16 tablespoons = 1 cup
2 cups   = 1 pint

1 teaspoon   =   5 cc.
1 tablespoon = 15 cc.
1 cup   = 236 cc.
1 ounce   = 28.35 gm.

The top row of figures for each food listed indicates the percentage composition of that food. The second row indicates the composition of an average serving.

---

* The author is grateful to Miss Martha Tarbox, formerly Director of the Food Clinic at the Pennsylvania Hospital, for assistance in compiling the Appendix.

† The key to other sources is as follows:
  A. Food and Beverage Analyses, Milton A. Bridges, Lea & Febiger, Philadelphia.
  B. Campbell Soup Company, Camden, New Jersey.
  C. Nutritive Value of Foods, Dorothy S. Waller. Revised by George Wahr, Department of Dietetics, University of Michigan Hospital, Ann Arbor, Michigan.

Food	Grams	Household Measure	P.	F.	C.	Cal.	Source
Ale*..			.5	....	3.5	45	A
	230	1 c.	1.1		8.0	100	
Almonds.....................................			18.6	54.1	19.6	640	
	30	20	5.6	16.2	5.9	192	
Apple, fresh.............................			.3	.4	14.9	64	
	130	1, 2½" diam.	.4	.5	19.4	84	
Apple, dried.............................			1.4	1.0	73.2	307	
	60	2 oz.	.8	.6	43.9	184	
Apple butter...........................			.4	1.1	48.9	207	A
	40	1 heaping T.	.2	.4	19.6	83	
Apple juice.............................			.1		12.5	50	
	120	½ c.	.1	....	15.0	60	
Applesauce, unsweetened................			.2	.2	10.9	46	
	135	½ c.	.3	.3	14.7	63	
Apricots, fresh.........................			1.0	.1	12.9	53	
	50	2, 2½" diam.	.5		6.5	28	
Apricots, dried........................			5.2	.4	66.9	292	
	25	6 halves	1.3	.1	16.7	73	
Artichokes, globe......................			2.9	.4	11.9	63	
	200	1, 3" diam.	5.8	.8	23.8	126	
Asparagus..............................			2.2	.2	3.9	26	
	100	8, 6" stalks	2.2	.2	3.9	26	
Asparagus soup A. P., Campbell..........			1.3	1.2	7.0	44	B
	140	½ c.	1.8	1.7	9.8	62	
Avocados, Guatemalan type..............			2.0	17.2	5.4	184	
	85	½, 3½" long	1.7	14.6	4.6	157	
Bacon, raw, medium fat.................			9.1	65.0		621	
	40	3 strips	3.6	26.0	....	248	
Bacon, cooked, crisp...................			25.0	55.0	1.0	599	
	15	3 strips	3.8	8.2		89	
Bacon, Canadian, raw...................			22.0	15.0		223	
	30	1 oz.	6.6	4.5	....	67	
Bamboo shoots.........................			2.5	.3	5.1	33	
	100	¾ c.	2.5	.3	5.1	33	
Banana................................			1.2	.2	23.0	99	
	125	1 med.	1.5	.3	28.8	124	
Barley, flour..........................			10.2	1.7	76.9	364	
	130	1 c.	13.3	2.2	100.0	473	
Barley, pearl..........................			8.7	1.0	78.3	357	
	30	3 T.	2.6	.3	23.5	107	
Barracuda..............................			21.2	3.1		113	
	120	¼ lb.	25.4	3.7	....	135	

* Alcoholic content of ale usually 4–6 per cent by weight.
 The percentage composition figures are *underlined*.

Food	Grams	Household Measure	P.	F.	C.	Cal.	Source
Bass................................			20.6	1.8	....	99	
	230	½ lb.	47.4	4.1		227	
Bean soup A. P., Campbell...............			6.1	1.8	14.0	97	B
	140	½ c.	8.5	2.5	19.6	135	
Beans, baked with pork.................			5.7	2.0	19.0	117	
	250	1 c.	14.3	5.0	47.5	292	
Beans, dried navy, kidney, pea, pinto, red, etc....................................			22.0	1.5	62.1	350	
	75	½ c.	16.5	1.1	46.6	262	
Beans, lima, fresh.....................			7.5	.8	23.5	131	
	75	½ c.	5.6	.6	17.6	98	
Beans, Mung bean sprouts...............			2.9	.3	4.0	30	
	125	1 c.	3.6	.4	5.0	38	
Beans, string, green or wax.............			2.4	.2	7.7	42	
	100	⅔ c.	2.4	.2	7.7	42	
Beef, chuck, medium fat................			18.6	16.0		218	
	120	¼ lb.	22.3	19.2	....	262	
Beef, flank, medium fat................			14.6	40.0		418	
	120	¼ lb.	17.5	48.0	....	502	
Beef, loin, medium fat.................			16.9	25.0		293	
	120	¼ lb.	20.3	30.0	....	351	
Beef, neck, medium fat.................			18.2	19.0		244	
	120	¼ lb.	21.8	22.8	....	292	
Beef, plate and brisket, medium fat........			15.8	30.0		333	
	120	¼ lb.	19.0	36.0	....	400	
Beef, rib, medium fat..................			17.4	23.0		277	
	120	¼ lb.	20.9	27.6	....	332	
Beef, round, medium fat................			19.3	13.0		194	
	120	¼ lb.	23.2	15.6	....	233	
Beef, rump, medium fat................			15.5	31.0		341	
	120	¼ lb.	18.6	37.2	....	410	
Beef, corned, medium fat................			15.8	25.0		288	
	120	¼ lb.	19.0	30.0	....	346	
Beef, dried...........................			34.3	6.3		194	
	60	2 oz.	20.6	3.8	....	117	
Beef soup A. P., Campbell..............			5.6	1.3	8.2	67	B
	120	½ c.	6.7	1.6	9.8	80	
Beer*................................			.6			48	
	230	8 oz.	1.3	....	....	110	
Beets................................			1.6	.1	9.6	46	
	100	⅔ c. diced	1.6	.1	9.6	46	
Beets, canned, sieved...................			1.3	.1	8.5	40	
	15	1 T.	.2		1.3	6	

* Alcoholic content of beer 3–5 per cent by weight.

Food	Grams	Household Measure	P.	F.	C.	Cal.	Source
Beet greens			2.0	.3	5.6	33	
	100	1 c.	2.0	.3	5.6	33	
Biscuits, baking powder			7.3	13.0	46.2	331	
	30	1, 2¼″ diam.	2.2	3.9	13.9	100	
Blackberries			1.2	1.1	11.9	62	
	75	⅔ c.	.9	.8	8.9	46	
Blueberries			.6	.6	15.1	68	
	100	⅔ c.	.6	.6	15.1	68	
Bluefish			20.5	4.0		118	
	230	½ lb.	47.2	9.0	....	271	
Bologna			14.4	17.8		218	
	75	6 sl.	10.8	13.4	....	164	
Bonito			24.0	7.3		162	
	230	½ lb.	55.2	16.8	....	372	
Bran, wheat			15.9	4.2	66.2	366	
	5	2 T.	.8	.2	3.1	17	
Bran flakes			13.0	1.9	74.9	369	
	15	½ c.	2.0	.3	11.2	56	
Brazil nuts			14.4	65.9	11.0	695	
	30	4	4.3	19.8	3.3	209	
Bread Boston			4.9	2.5	41.2	207	
	30	1 sm. sl.	1.5	.8	12.4	63	
Graham			9.5	3.5	48.0	262	
	30	1 sl.	2.9	1.1	14.4	79	
Rolls			8.2	6.1	54.1	304	
	50	1 med.	4.1	3.1	27.1	153	
Rye			8.9	2.0	49.7	252	
	30	1 sl.	2.7	.7	14.9	76	
White			8.5	2.0	52.3	261	
	30	1 sl.	2.6	.6	15.7	79	
Broccoli			3.3	.2	5.5	37	
	100	2, 5″ stalks	3.3	.2	5.5	37	
Brussels sprouts			4.4	.5	8.9	58	
	100	1 c.	4.4	.5	8.9	58	
Butter			.6	81.0	.4	733	
	10	2 t.		8.1		73	
Buttermilk			3.5	.5	4.6	37	
	240	1 c.	8.4	1.2	11.0	88	
Cabbage			1.4	.2	5.3	29	
	100	½ c.	1.4	.2	5.3	29	
Cabbage, Chinese			1.4	.1	2.4	16	
	100	1 c.	1.4	.1	2.4	16	
Cantaloupe			.6	.2	5.9	28	
	100	¼, 5″ diam.	.6	.2	5.9	28	

Food	Grams	Household Measure	P.	F.	C.	Cal.	Source
Carrots................................			1.2	.3	9.3	45	
	100	½ c. diced	1.2	.3	9.3	45	
Carrots, canned, sieved..................			.7	.1	6.7	30	
	15	1 T.	.1		1.0	4	
Cashew nuts...........................			19.6	47.2	26.4	609	
	15	8	2.9	7.1	4.0	92	
Cauliflower...........................			2.4	.2	4.9	31	
	100	1 c.	2.4	.2	4.9	31	
Caviar................................			26.9	15.0	....	243	
	15	2 t.	4.0	2.3		37	
Celery................................			1.3	.2	3.7	22	
	40	3, 5″ stalks	.5	.1	1.5	9	
Chard................................			2.6	.4	4.8	33	
	100	½ c.	2.6	.4	4.8	33	
Cheese Camembert........................			19.7	25.2	....	306	
	40	1 triangle	7.9	10.1		123	
Cheddar, American..................			23.9	32.3	1.7	393	
	30	1 oz.	7.2	9.7	.5	118	
Cottage...........................			19.2	.8	4.3	101	
	55	¼ c.	10.6	.4	2.4	56	
Edam.............................			27.0	20.1	4.0	305	
	30	1″ cube	8.1	6.0	1.2	91	
Philadelphia cream....................			10.0	38.0	.2	382	B
	30	½ pkg.	3.0	11.4		115	
Cherries Sour.............................			1.3	.5	13.3	63	
	75	½ c.	1.0	.4	10.0	48	
Sweet............................			1.1	.5	17.8	80	
	75	½ c.	.8	.4	13.4	60	
Chestnuts, fresh........................			2.8	1.5	41.5	191	
	50	8	1.4	.8	20.8	96	
Chicken...............................			21.1	4.5	....	125	
	30	1 oz.	6.3	1.4		38	
Chicken soup A. P., Campbell............			3.6	1.2	2.6	36	B
	120	½ c.	4.3	1.4	3.1	42	
Chicken noodle soup A. P., Campbell			3.9	1.5	6.7	56	B
	120	½ c.	4.7	1.8	8.0	67	
Chicory...............................			1.6	.3	2.9	21	
	20	½ c.	.3	.1	.6	5	
Chocolate Bitter.............................			5.5	52.9	18.0	570	
	30	1 oz. (1 sq.)	1.7	15.9	5.4	172	
Sweetened...........................			2.0	29.8	60.0	516	
	30	1 oz.	.6	8.9	18.0	155	

Food	Grams	Household Measure	P.	F.	C.	Cal.	Source
Chocolate			6.0	33.5	54.0	542	
Milk...........................	30	1 oz.	1.8	10.1	16.2	163	
Cider, sweet..........................			.1	....	12.5	50	
	240	8 oz.	.2		30.0	121	
Clams, long and round................			12.8	1.4	3.4	77	
	60	6 med.	7.7	.8	2.0	46	
Clam chowder A. P., Campbell..........			3.0	4.1	9.7	88	B
	140	½ c.	4.2	5.7	13.6	123	
Coca-Cola............................			....	....	8.0	32	A
	180	1 bottle			14.4	58	
Cocoa...............................			9.0	18.8	31.0	329	
	5	2 t.	.5	.9	1.6	17	
Cocoanut, prepared, sweetened, dried, shred-			3.6	39.1	53.2	579	
ded.................................	100	1½ c.	3.6	39.1	53.2	579	
Cod, fresh...........................			16.5	.4		70	
	120	¼ lb.	19.8	.5	....	84	
Cod, salted..........................			29.0	.7		122	
	60	2 oz.	17.4	.4	....	73	
Collards.............................			3.9	.6	7.2	50	
	100	1 c.	3.9	.6	7.2	50	
Corn							
Popcorn, popped.....................			11.4	5.2	77.8	404	
	15	¾ c.	1.7	.8	11.7	61	
Sweet corn, fresh.....................			3.7	1.2	20.5	108	
	100	1 ear, 8″	3.7	1.2	20.5	108	
Canned........................			2.5	.9	19.6	96	
	100	½ c.	2.5	.9	19.6	96	
Cornflakes...........................			7.9	.7	80.3	359	
	30	1 c.	2.4	.2	24.1	108	
Cornmeal............................			9.1	3.7	73.9	365	
	100	⅖ c.	9.1	3.7	73.9	365	
Corn syrup..........................			....	....	74.0	296	
	15	1 T.			11.1	44	
Cowpeas, dry........................			22.9	1.4	61.6	351	
	100	½ c.	22.9	1.4	61.6	351	
Crabmeat............................			16.1	1.6	.6	81	
	85	½ c.	13.7	1.4	.5	69	
Crackers							
Butter.............................			9.8	12.4	70.8	434	
	12	3, 2″ diam.	1.2	1.5	8.5	52	
Graham............................			8.0	10.0	74.3	419	
	15	2	1.2	1.5	11.1	63	
Saltines............................			9.2	11.8	71.1	427	
	20	6	1.8	2.4	14.2	86	
Soda..............................			9.6	9.6	72.7	416	
	15	2	1.4	1.4	10.9	62	

Food	Grams	Household Measure	P.	F.	C.	Cal.	Source
Cranberry sauce.....................			.1	.3	51.4	209	
	20	1 T.		.1	10.3	42	
Cream							
Light or coffee......................			2.9	20.0	4.0	208	
	60	¼ c.	1.7	12.0	2.4	125	
Heavy or whipping..................			2.3	35.0	3.2	337	
	60	¼ c.	1.4	21.0	1.9	202	
Cucumber...........................			.7	.1	2.7	14	
	75	⅓ med.	.5	.1	2.0	11	
Dandelion greens.....................			2.7	.7	8.8	52	
	50	½ c.	1.4	.4	4.4	27	
Dates..............................			2.2	.6	75.4	316	
	15	2 lg.	.3	.1	11.3	47	
Doughnuts..........................			6.6	21.0	52.7	426	
	45	1, 3″ diam.	3.0	9.5	23.7	192	
Duck..............................			21.4	8.2		159	
	120	¼ lb.	25.7	9.8	....	191	
Eggplant...........................			1.1	.2	5.5	28	
	100	2 sm. sl.	1.1	.2	5.5	28	
Eggs							
Whole..............................			12.8	11.5	.7	158	
	50	1	6.4	5.8	.4	79	
White..............................			10.8		.8	46	
	35	White of 1 egg	3.8	....	.3	16	
Yolk..............................			16.3	31.9	.7	355	
	15	Yolk of 1 egg	2.4	4.8	.1	53	
Endive.............................			1.6	.2	4.0	24	
	15	¼ sm. head	.2		.6	3	
Farina.............................			11.5	1.0	76.1	359	
	20	{2 T. dry					
		{½ c. ckd.	2.3	.2	15.1	71	
Fennel.............................			1.9		3.6	22	
	50	⅓ med.	1.0	....	1.8	11	
Figs							
Fresh..............................			1.4	.4	19.6	88	
	75	3 med.	1.1	.3	14.7	66	
Dried..............................			4.0	1.2	68.4	300	
	45	3 med.	1.8	.5	30.8	135	
Finnan haddie.......................			23.2	.4		96	
	120	¼ lb.	27.8	.5	....	116	
Flounder...........................			14.9	.5		64	
	120	¼ lb.	17.9	.6	....	77	
Flour							
Graham............................			13.0	2.0	72.4	360	
	100	¾ c.	13.0	2.0	72.4	360	
Pancake, self-rising..................			10.3	1.5	72.3	344	
	100	¾ c.	10.3	1.5	72.3	344	

Food	Grams	Household Measure	P.	F.	C.	Cal.	Source
Flour							
Wheat, patent..........................			10.8	.9	75.9	355	
	8	1 T.	.9	.1	6.1	29	
Frankfurters.............................			14.1	20.8	....	244	
	60	1 med.	8.5	12.5		147	
French salad dressing...................			60.0	....	....	540	A
	10	2 t.	6.0			54	
Frog's legs..............................			16.4	.3	....	68	
	120	¼ lb.	19.7	.4		82	
Gelatin, plain...........................			85.6	.1	....	343	
	3	1 t.	2.6			10	
Gin*....................................			....	....	....	250	A
	30	1 oz.				75	
Ginger ale..............................					9.0	36	
	225	1 c.	....	....	20.0	80	
Gingersnaps.............................			6.4	8.9	76.7	412	
	30	4 med.	1.9	2.7	23.0	124	
Goose...................................			22.3	7.1	....	153	
	120	¼ lb.	26.8	8.5		184	
Grapefruit...............................			.5	....	10.1	42	
	120	½ med.	.6		12.1	51	
Grapefruit juice.........................			.4	.1	11.1	47	
	120	½ c.	.5	.1	13.2	56	
"Grapenuts".............................			10.6	.6	83.2	380	A
	30	¼ c.	3.2	.2	24.9	114	
Grapes							
American type (Concord, Delaware, etc.)..			1.4	1.4	14.9	78	
	100	24	1.4	1.4	14.9	78	
European (Malaga, Thompson, etc.).....			.8	.4	16.7	74	
	100	15	.8	.4	16.7	74	
Grape juice.............................			.4	....	18.5	76	
	120	½ c.	.5		22.2	91	
Guinea hen..............................			23.1	6.4	....	150	
	120	¼ lb.	27.7	7.8		181	
Haddock.................................			17.2	.3	....	72	
	120	¼ lb.	20.6	.4		86	
Halibut.................................			18.6	5.2	....	121	
	120	¼ lb.	22.3	6.2		145	
Ham, lean..............................			19.5	25.0	....	303	
	120	¼ lb.	23.4	30.0		364	
Hazelnuts...............................			12.7	60.9	17.7	670	
	35	30	4.4	21.3	6.2	234	
Heart							
Beef.................................			16.9	3.7	.7	104	
	120	¼ lb.	20.3	4.4	.8	124	

* Alcoholic content of gin 35.0 per cent.

Food	Grams	Household Measure	P.	F.	C.	Cal.	Source
Heart							
Veal................................			15.4	7.1	.8	129	
	120	¼ lb.	18.5	8.5	1.0	154	
Herring............................			19.0	6.7		136	
	120	¼ lb.	22.8	8.0	....	163	
Hickory nuts.......................			13.9	67.4	13.2	715	
	35	¼ c.	4.9	23.6	4.6	235	
Hominy............................			8.5	.8	78.9	357	
	20	{2 T. dry {1½ c. ckd.	1.7	.2	15.8	72	
Honey, strained....................			.3		79.5	319	
	25	1 T.	.1	....	19.9	80	
Honeydew melon....................			.6	.2	6.0	28	
	200	⅛ med.	1.2	.4	12.0	56	
Ice cream							
Plain............................			3.9	13.0	20.3	214	
	100	⅝ c.	3.9	13.0	20.3	214	
Rich.............................			3.5	23.0	18.0	293	
	100	⅝ c.	3.5	23.0	18.0	293	
Jams and Preserves.................			.5	.3	70.8	288	
	12	1 T.			8.5	34	
Jellies............................			.2	....	65.0	261	
	12	1 t.			7.8	31	
Kale..............................			3.9	.6	7.2	50	
	100	½ c.	3.9	.6	7.2	50	
Kidney							
Beef.............................			15.0	8.1	.9	136	
	120	¼ lb.	18.0	9.7	1.1	164	
Veal.............................			16.8	5.2	.2	115	
	120	¼ lb.	20.2	6.2	.2	137	
Kohlrabi..........................			2.1	.1	6.7	36	
	100	½ c.	2.1	.1	6.7	36	
Kumquats.........................			.9	.1	17.1	73	
	50	3 med.	.5		8.6	36	
Lamb							
Leg..............................			18.0	17.5		230	
	120	¼ lb.	21.6	21.0	....	275	
Rib..............................			14.9	32.4		351	
	60	1 med. chop	8.9	19.4	....	210	
Shoulder.........................			15.6	25.3		290	
	120	¼ lb.	18.7	30.4	....	348	
Lambsquarters.....................			3.8	.7	8.3	55	
	25	½ c.	1.0	.2	2.1	14	
Lard..............................				100.0		900	
	10	2 t.	....	10.0	....	90	
Leeks, raw........................			2.5	.4	7.9	45	
	55	½ c.	1.4	.2	4.3	24	

Food	Grams	Household Measure	P.	F.	C.	Cal.	Source
Lemons..............................			.9	.6	8.7	44	
	100	1 med.	.9	.6	8.7	44	
Lemon juice..........................					8.3	33	
	15	1 T.	....	....	1.2	5	
Lentils, dry.........................			24.7	1.0	59 9	347	
	60	¼ c.	14.8	.6	35.9	208	
Lettuce.............................			1.2	.2	2.9	18	
	100	¼ head	1.2	.2	2.9	18	
Limes...............................			.8	.1	12.3	53	
	40	1 med.	.3		4.9	21	
Lime juice...........................					8.3	33	
	15	1 T.	....	....	1.2	5	
Lichi fruits..........................			3.6	.5	70.0	299	
	25	10	.9	.1	17.5	75	
Liver Beef...........................			19.7	3.2	6.0	132	
	120	¼ lb.	23.6	3.8	7.2	157	
Calf............................			19.0	4.9	4.0	136	
	120	¼ lb.	22.8	5.9	4.8	163	
Chicken........................			22.1	4.0	2.6	135	
	60	⅛ lb.	13.3	2.4	1.6	81	
Hog............................			19.7	4.8	1.7	129	
	120	¼ lb.	23.6	5.8	2.0	155	
Lobster.............................			16.2	1.9	.5	84	
	100	1 av.	16.2	1.9	.5	84	
Loganberries........................			1.0	.6	15.0	69	
	100	1 c.	1.0	.6	15.0	69	
Macaroni Dry........................			13.0	1.4	73.9	360	
	75	⅝ c.	9.8	1.1	55.4	270	
Cooked.......................			3.7	.4	19.4	96	
	100	½ c.	3.7	.4	19.4	96	
Mackerel............................			18.7	12.0		183	
	120	¼ lb.	22.4	14.0	....	216	
Mangos.............................			.7	.2	17.2	73	
	100	1 sm.	.7	.2	17.2	73	
Matzos.............................			15.0		70.0	340	A
	20	1, 6″ diam.	3.0	....	14.0	68	
Mayonnaise.........................			1.5	78.0	3.0	720	
	10	2 t.	.2	7.8	.3	72	
Meat and poultry—cooked Lean, medium done..................			30.0	6.0		174	
	120	¼ lb.	36.0	7.2	....	209	
Medium fat, medium done.............			27.0	18.0		270	
	120	¼ lb.	32.0	21.6	....	322	

Food	Grams	Household Measure	P.	F.	C.	Cal.	Source
Meat and poultry—cooked							
Fat, medium done...................			22.0	30.0		358	
	120	¼ lb.	26.4	36.0	....	430	
Milk							
Cow							
Fresh—whole......................			3.5	3.9	4.9	69	
	240	1 c.	8.4	9.4	11.8	165	
Fresh—skim.....................			3.5	.2	5.0	36	
	240	1 c.	8.4	.5	12.0	86	
Dry—whole.....................			25.8	26.7	38.0	496	
	8	1 T.	2.1	2.1	3.0	39	
Evaporated, unsweetened............			7.0	7.9	9.9	139	
	120	½ c.	8.4	9.5	11.9	167	
Malted powder.....................			14.6	8.5	70.7	418	
	8	1 T.	1.2	.7	5.7	34	
Goat.............................			3.3	4.2	4.8	70	
	240	1 c.	7.9	10.1	11.5	169	
Molasses...........................					60.0	240	
	190	½ c.	....	....	114.0	456	
Mulberries.........................			1.2	.6	14.6	69	
	75	⅔ c.	.9	.5	11.0	52	
Mushrooms...........................			....	....	....	...	
Muskmelons.........................			.6	.2	5.9	28	
	100	¼ med.	.6	.2	5.9	28	
Mustard greens.....................			2.3	.3	4.0	28	
	100	1 c.	2.3	.3	4.0	28	
Nectarines.........................			.5	.1	16.0	67	
	100	1 sm.	.5	.1	16.0	67	
Noodles, dry.......................			14.3	5.0	70.6	385	
	60	½ c.	8.6	3.0	42.4	231	
Cooked............................			2.6	.2	16.8	79	C
	100	½ c.	2.6	.2	16.8	79	
Oatmeal							
Dry............................			14.2	7.4	68.2	396	
	20	¼ c.	2.8	1.5	13.6	79	
Cooked............................			2.3	1.2	11.0	64	
	120	½ c.	2.8	1.4	13.2	77	
Oils, salad or olive.................				100.0		900	
	10	2 t.	....	10.0	....	90	
Okra.............................			1.8	.2	7.4	39	
	100	½ c.	1.8	.2	7.4	39	
Oleomargarine.......................			.6	81.0		733	
	10	2 t.		8.1	....	73	
Olives							
Green, pickled.....................			1.5	13.5	4.0	144	
	15	5 med.	.2	2.0	.6	21	
Ripe, pickled.....................			1.6	19.0	1.9	185	
	20	5 sm.	.3	3.8	.4	37	

Food	Grams	Household Measure	P.	F.	C.	Cal.	Source
Onions.............................			1.4	.2	10.3	49	
	100	2 med.	1.4	.2	10.3	49	
Young, green........................			1.0	.2	10.6	48	
	25	5 sm.	.3	.1	2.7	13	
Opossum.............................			13.0	40.0		412	
	90	3 oz.	11.7	36.0	....	371	
Oranges.............................			.9	.2	11.2	50	
	100	1 med.	.9	.2	11.2	50	
Orange juice........................					10.1	40	
	120	½ c.	....	....	12.1	48	
Oysters.............................			9.8	2.0	5.9	81	
	100	6 med.	9.8	2.0	5.9	81	
Papaws			5.2	.9	16.8	96	
	50	1, 4″ long	2.6	.5	8.4	48	
Papayas.............................			.6	.1	10.0	43	
	100	¼, 5″ diam.	.6	.1	10.0	43	
Parsnips.............................			1.5	.5	18.2	83	
	100	½ c.	1.5	.5	18.2	83	
Peaches.............................			.5	.1	12.0	51	
	100	1 med.	.5	.1	12.0	51	
Peanuts, roasted.....................			26.9	44.2	23.6	600	
	30	15 med.	8.1	13.3	7.1	181	
Peanut butter.......................			26.1	47.8	21.0	619	
	15	1 T.	3.9	7.2	3.2	93	
Pears...............................			.7	.4	15.8	70	
	100	1 med.	.7	.4	15.8	70	
Peas fresh..........................			6.7	.4	17.7	101	
	80	½ c.	5.4	.3	14.2	81	
Canned, sieved......................			4.0	.4	9.3	57	
	25	4 t.	1.0	.1	2.4	15	
Pea soup A. P., Campbell.............			4.8	1.6	12.4	83	B
	140	½ c.	6.7	2.2	17.4	116	
Peas, dry—split.....................			24.5	1.0	61.7	354	
	50	¼ c.	12.3	.5	30.9	177	
Pecans.............................			9.4	73.0	13.0	747	
	25	6 lg.	2.4	18.3	3.3	188	
Peppers, green or red................			1.4	.4	6.2	34	
	25	1 pepper	.4	.1	1.6	9	
Perch...............................			19.3	4.0		113	
	120	¼ lb.	23.2	4.8	....	136	
Persimmons..........................			.8	.4	33.5	141	
	50	1 sm.	.4	.2	16.8	71	
Pheasant............................			24.3	5.2		144	
	120	¼ lb.	29.2	6.2	....	173	

Food	Grams	Household Measure	P.	F.	C.	Cal.	Source
Pickles							
Cucumber							
Sweet............................			.4	.1	20.7	85	
	25	2 sm.	.1		5.2	21	
Sour and dill.....................			.5	.2	1.9	11	
	50	1 lg.	.3	.1	1.0	6	
Pineapple, fresh.......................			.4	.2	13.7	58	
	75	½ c. diced	.3	.2	10.3	44	
Pineapple juice, unsweetened..............			.3	.1	13.0	54	
	100	½ c.	.3	.1	13.0	54	
Pine nuts, pignolias....................			31.2	48.4	11.2	605	
	10	1 T.	3.1	4.8	1.1	60	
Pistachio nuts.........................			19.6	53.2	18.6	632	
	20	¼ c.	3.9	10.6	3.7	126	
Plantains............................			1.3	.4	32.8	140	
	100	1 med.	1.3	.4	32.8	140	
Plums, fresh (excluding prunes)...........			.7	.2	12.9	56	
	50	2 med.	.4	.1	6.5	29	
Pompano............................			18.8	9.5		161	
	120	¼ lb.	22.6	11.4	....	193	
Porgy...............................			21.4	.9		94	
	120	¼ lb.	25.7	1.1	....	113	
Pork							
Ham, medium fat.....................			15.2	31.0		340	
	120	¼ lb.	18.2	37.2	....	408	
Shoulder, medium fat.................			13.5	37.0		387	
	120	¼ lb.	16.2	44.4	....	464	
Spare ribs A. P......................			8.6	26.0		266	
	240	½ lb.	20.6	62.4	....	644	
Salt................................			6.2	76.0		709	
	120	¼ lb.	7.4	91.2	....	850	
Potatoes, white.......................			2.0	.1	19.1	85	
	100	1 med.	2.0	.1	19.1	85	
Potato chips..........................			6.7	37.1	49.1	557	
	25	1 c.	1.7	9.3	12.3	140	
Pretzels.............................			8.8	3.2	74.5	362	
	25	6 med.	2.2	.8	18.6	90	
Prickly pear..........................			.5	.1	10.4	45	
	100	1 med.	.5	.1	10.4	45	
Prunes							
Fresh..............................			.9	.2	21.8	93	
	50	2 med.	.5	.1	10.9	47	
Dried..............................			2.3	.6	71.0	299	
	25	3 med.	.6	.2	17.8	75	
Pumpernickel.........................			6.7	1.2	49.7	236	
	30	1 sl.	2.0	.4	14.9	71	

Food	Grams	Household Measure	P.	F.	C.	Cal.	Source
Pumpkin			1.2	.2	7.3	36	
	100	½ c.	1.2	.2	7.3	36	
Quail			25.0	6.8		161	
	100	1	25.0	6.8	....	161	
Rabbit			20.8	10.2		175	
	100	¼ med.	20.8	10.2	....	175	
Radishes			1.2	.1	4.2	23	
	50	8 med.	.6	.1	2.1	12	
Raisins			2.3	.5	71.2	299	
	60	⅓ c.	1.4	.3	42.7	179	
Raspberries Fresh 　Black			1.5	1.6	15.6	83	
	50	½ c.	.8	.8	7.8	42	
Red			1.1	.6	14.4	67	
	50	½ c.	.6	.3	7.2	34	
Reindeer, lean			20.0	6.0		134	
	120	¼ lb.	24.0	7.2	....	161	
Rhubarb			.5	.1	3.8	18	
	50	½ c. diced	.3	.1	1.9	10	
Rice 　Brown, uncooked			7.5	1.7	77.7	356	
	20	1 heaping T.	1.5	.3	15.5	71	
White, uncooked			7.6	.3	79.4	350	
	20	1 heaping T.	1.5	.1	15.9	71	
Boiled			2.2	.1	23.2	103	
	100	½ c.	2.2	.1	23.2	103	
"Rice Krispies"			6.0	.3	88.4	380	A
	20	½ c.	1.2	.1	17.7	77	
Rice .puffed			6.7	.3	83.3	363	
	15	1 c.	1.0		12.5	54	
Rice flakes			7.7	.5	82.0	363	
	15	½ c.	1.2	.1	12.3	55	
Rice flour			7.4	.5	79.5	352	
	50	⅓ c.	3.7	.3	39.8	177	
Roe, fish			26.2	3.1		133	
	120	¼ lb.	31.4	3.7	....	159	
Rum, Bacardi*						250	A
	30	1 oz.	....	....	....	75	
Rutabagas			1.1	.1	8.9	41	
	60	½ c.	.7	.1	5.3	25	
Rye flour, medium			11.0	1.2	75.8	358	
	50	½ c.	5.5	.6	37.9	179	
"Ry-Krisp," Ralston			13.1	2.0	61.9	308	A
	12	2	1.6	.2	7.4	38	

* Alcoholic content of rum, bacardi, 35.0 per cent.

Food	Grams	Household Measure	P.	F.	C.	Cal.	Source
Salmon, raw..........................			17.4	·16.5	....	218	
	120	¼ lb.	20.9	19.8		262	
Canned.............................			20.6	9.6	....	169	
	100	½ c.	20.6	9.6		169	
Salsify, vegetable oyster.................			3.5	1.0	15.5	85	
	100	½ c.	3.5	1.0	15.5	85	
Sardines, canned, in oil.................			25.7	11.0	1.2	207	
	50	4, 2½″ long	12.9	5.5	.6	104	
Sauerkraut............................			1.3	.2	4.9	27	
	80	½ c.	1.0	.2	3.9	21	
Sausage, pork........................			10.8	44.8		446	
	115	¼ lb.	12.4	51.5	....	513	
Scallops..............................			14.8	.1	3.4	74	
	100	½ c.	14.8	.1	3.4	74	
Shad.................................			18.7	9.8		163	
	120	¼ lb.	22.4	11.8	....	196	
Shad roe.......			20.9	3.8		118	
	140	½ lg.	29.3	5.3	....	165	
Shredded wheat.......................			10.4	1.4	78.7	369	
	30	1 biscuit	3.1	.4	23.6	110	
Shrimp...............................			17.8	.8	.8	82	
	65	8 med.	11.6	.5	.5	53	
Smelt................................			20.6	1.4		95	
	120	¼ lb.	24.7	1.7	....	114	
Soybeans Dried............................			34.9	18.1	12.0	350	
	100	½ c.	34.9	18.1	12.0	350	
Fresh.............................			12.5	6.5	6.0	133	
	75	½ c.	9.4	4.9	4.5	100	
Soybean flour........................			37.3	20.2	12.0	379	
	100	1¼ c.	37.3	20.2	12.0	379	
Soybean milk.........................			3.4	1.5	2.0	35	
	120	½ c.	4.1	1.8	2.4	42	
Spinach..............................			2.3	.3	3.2	25	
	100	½ c.	2.3	.3	3.2	25	
Squab................................			18.6	22.1		273	
	50	1 whole	9.3	11.1	....	137	
Squash Summer...........................			.6	.1	3.9	19	
	100	½ c.	.6	.1	3.9	19	
Winter............................			1.5	.3	8.8	44	
	100	½ c.	1.5	.3	8.8	44	
Starch (including corn, arrowroot, etc.).....			.5	.2	87.0	352	
	30	¼ c.	.2	.1	26.1	105	

Food	Grams	Household Measure	P.	F.	C.	Cal.	Source
Strawberries..........................			.8	.6	8.1	41	
	100	¾ c.	.8	.6	8.1	41	
Sugars							
Granulated........................					99.5	398	
	10	2 t.	....	....	10.0	40	
Powdered........................					99.5	398	
	10	1 T.	....	....	10.0	40	
Brown............................					95.5	382	
	10	1 T.	....	....	9.6	38	
Sweetbreads..........................			11.8	33.0		344	
	120	¼ lb.	14.2	39.6	....	413	
Sweet potatoes........................			1.8	.7	27.9	125	
	100	1 med.	1.8	.7	27.9	125	
Sword fish...........................			18.8	4.4		115	
	120	¼ lb.	22.6	5.3	....	138	
Tangerines...........................			.8	.3	10.9	50	
	100	1 lg.	.8	.3	10.9	50	
Tapioca..............................			.6	.2	86.4	350	
	20	2 T.	.1		17.3	70	
Terrapin.............................			21.2	3.5		117	
	120	¼ lb.	25.4	4.2	....	139	
Tomatoes, raw........................			1.0	.3	4.0	23	
	100	1 med.	1.0	.3	4.0	23	
Tomato juice.........................			1.0	.2	4.3	23	
	120	½ c.	1.2	.2	5.2	27	
Tomato puree........................			1.8	.5	7.2	40	
	100	½ c.	1.8	.5	7.2	40	
Tomato soup A. P., Campbell..........			1.6	1.4	8.9	55	B
	140	½ c.	2.2	2.0	12.5	76	
Tongue, medium fat...................			16.4	15.0		202	
	60	2 oz.	9.8	9.0	....	120	
Trout, brook.........................			19.2	2.1		96	
	120	¼ lb.	23.0	2.5	....	115	
Tuna fish, canned.....................			24.2	10.8		194	
	120	¼ lb.	29.0	13.0	....	233	
Turkey...............................			24.0	6.7		156	
	120	¼ lb.	28.8	8.0	....	187	
Turnips..............................			1.1	.2	7.1	35	
	100	½ c.	1.1	.2	7.1	35	
Turnip tops..........................			2.9	.4	5.4	37	
	100	½ c.	2.9	.4	5.4	37	
Veal							
Loin, medium fat....................			19.2	11.0		176	
	120	¼ lb.	23.0	13.2	....	211	

Food	Grams	Household Measure	P.	F.	C.	Cal.	Source
Veal							
Round................................			19.5	9.0		159	
	120	¼ lb.	23.4	10.8	....	191	
Shank................................			19.7	8.0		151	
	120	¼ lb.	23.6	9.6	....	181	
Vegetable soup A. P., Campbell..........			3.7	1.4	12.4	77	B
	140	½ c.	5.2	2.0	17.4	108	
Vegetable beef soup A. P., Campbell.......			7.9	2.1	5.6	73	B
	140	½ c.	11.1	2.9	7.8	102	
Venison..............................			20.0	6.0		134	
	120	¼ lb.	24.0	7.2	....	161	
Walnuts							
Black..............................			18.3	58.2	18.7	672	
	35	6	6.4	20.4	6.5	235	
English.............................			15.0	64.4	15.6	702	
	35	6	5.3	22.5	5.5	246	
Water chestnuts.......................			1.5	.1	15.6	69	A
	100	½ c.	1.5	.1	15.6	69	
Watercress...........................			1.7	.3	3.3	23	
	20	½ c.	.3	.1	.7	5	
Watermelon..........................			.5	.2	6.9	31	
	200	½ sl. 2″ thick	1.0	.4	13.8	63	
Wheat flakes.........................			10.4	1.3	79.9	373	
	20	½ c.	2.1	.3	16.0	75	
Whiskies							
Bourbon*...........................			....	....	....	283	A
	30	1 oz.				85	
Rye*................................			....	....	....	283	A
	30	1 oz.				85	
Scotch*.............................			....	....	....	250	A
	30	1 oz.				75	
Whitefish............................			22.9	6.5		150	
	120	¼ lb.	27.5	7.8	....	180	
Wines							
Champagne							
Dry*..............................			....	....	1.2	85	A
	100	1 wine glass			1.2	85	
Sweet*.............................			.2	....	10.0	120	A
	100	1 wine glass	.2		10.0	120	
Claret*.............................			.2	....	.5	60	A
	100	1 wine glass	.2		.5	60	
Sauterne*...........................			.2	....	2.0	80	A
	100	1 wine glass	.2		2.0	80	
Port*...............................			.3	....	6.0	130	A
	100	1 wine glass	.3		6.0	130	

* Alcoholic content of Bourbon whiskey 40.0 per cent., rye 40.0 per cent., scotch 35.0 per cent., champagne, dry 11.5 per cent., sweet 11.0 per cent., claret 8.0 per cent., sauterne 10.5 per cent, and port 15.0 per cent.

Food	Grams	Household Measure	P.	F.	C.	Cal.	Source
Wines							
Sherry*.............................			.3	....	3.0	120	A
	100	1 wine glass	.3		3.0	120	
Vermouth—French*..................				....	1.0	110	A
	100	1 wine glass	....		1.0	110	
Vermouth—Italian*..................				....	12.0	175	A
	100	1 wine glass	....		12.0	175	
Yams.................................			2.1	.2	24.1	107	
	125	1 med.	2.6	.2	30.1	133	
Zwieback.............................			10.9	8.6	74.3	418	
	7	1 piece	.8	.6	5.1	29	

* Alcoholic content of sherry 15.0 per cent., vermouth—French 15.0 per cent. and Italian 18.0 per cent.

HEIGHTS AND WEIGHTS OF CHILDREN BETWEEN ONE AND FOUR YEARS OF AGE (WITHOUT CLOTHES)[1]

5602 Boys		Age, Months	4821 Girls	
Height, Inches	Weight, Pounds		Height, Inches	Weight, Pounds
26.5	18.0	6	25.9	16.8
27.3	19.1	7	26.5	17.4
27.6	19.8	8	27.0	18.3
28.1	20.4	9	27.6	19.1
28.5	20.9	10	27.9	19.5
29.0	21.4	11	28.4	20.1
29.4	21.9	12	28.9	20.8
29.9	22.9	13	29.4	21.0
30.3	23.0	14	29.5	21.6
30.8	23.6	15	30.1	21.9
31.1	24.1	16	30.5	22.6
31.4	24.5	17	30.8	22.9
31.8	24.6	18	31.1	23.4
32.3	25.5	19	31.5	23.8
32.6	25.8	20	32.0	24.1
32.9	25.8	21	32.3	24.8
33.3	26.9	22	32.6	25.3
33.6	27.0	23	32.9	25.6
33.8	27.1	24	33.4	26.4
34.0	27.9	25	33.8	26.9
34.1	28.3	26	33.9	27.3
34.8	29.0	27	33.9	27.3
35.1	29.1	28	34.6	27.8
35.4	29.3	29	34.8	27.8
35.4	29.5	30	34.9	28.3
35.5	30.5	31	35.1	28.8
36.0	30.6	32	35.4	29.0
36.1	30.6	33	35.6	29.1
36.5	31.1	34	36.5	30.1
36.8	31.9	35	36.5	30.3
37.1	32.3	36	36.8	30.5
37.4	32.3	37	36.8	30.8
37.5	32.4	38	37.0	31.0
37.9	33.1	39	37.3	31.6
38.4	33.5	40	37.5	32.0
38.6	33.6	41	37.8	32.3
38.6	33.8	42	38.0	32.5
38.8	33.8	43	38.3	32.8
38.9	34.3	44	38.5	33.0
39.0	34.5	45	38.5	33.5
39.0	34.8	46	38.8	33.5
39.3	35.8	47	38.9	33.5
39.5	35.9	48	39.0	33.8

[1] Crum, F. S.: Quarterly Publication of the American Statistical Association, Boston, September, 1916, N.S., No. 115, 15, 332.

HEIGHT—WEIGHT—AGE TABLE (BOYS)

Height, Inches	5 Yrs.	6 Yrs.	7 Yrs.	8 Yrs.	9 Yrs.	10 Yrs.	11 Yrs.	12 Yrs.	13 Yrs.	14 Yrs.	15 Yrs.	16 Yrs.	17 Yrs.	18 Yrs.	19 Yrs.
38	34	34													
39	35	35													
40	36	36													
41	38	38	38												
42	39	39	39	39											
43	41	41	41	41											
44	44	44	44	44											
45	46	46	46	46	46										
46	47	48	48	48	48										
47	49	50	50	50	50	50									
48		52	53	53	53	53									
49		55	55	55	55	55	55								
50		57	58	58	58	58	58	58							
51			61	61	61	61	61	61							
52			63	64	64	64	64	64	64						
53			66	67	67	67	67	68	68						
54				70	70	70	70	71	71	72					
55				72	72	73	73	74	74	74					
56				75	76	77	77	77	78	78	80				
57					79	80	81	81	82	83	83				
58					83	84	84	85	85	86	87				
59						87	88	89	89	90	90	90			
60						91	92	92	93	94	95	96			
61							95	96	97	99	100	103	106		
62							100	101	102	103	104	107	111	116	
63							105	106	107	108	110	113	118	123	127
64								109	111	113	115	117	121	126	130
65								114	117	118	120	122	127	131	134
66									119	122	125	128	132	136	139
67									124	128	130	134	136	139	142
68										134	134	137	141	143	147
69										137	139	143	146	149	152
70										143	144	145	148	151	155
71										148	150	151	152	154	159
72											153	155	156	158	163
73											157	160	162	164	167
74											160	164	168	170	171

Prepared by Bird T. Baldwin, Ph.D., and Thomas D. Wood, M. D.

HEIGHT—WEIGHT—AGE TABLE (GIRLS)

Height, Inches	5 Yrs.	6 Yrs.	7 Yrs.	8 Yrs.	9 Yrs.	10 Yrs.	11 Yrs.	12 Yrs.	13 Yrs.	14 Yrs.	15 Yrs.	16 Yrs.	17 Yrs.	18 Yrs.
38	33	33												
39	34	34												
40	36	36	36											
41	37	37	37											
42	39	39	39											
43	41	41	41	41										
44	42	42	42	42										
45	45	45	45	45	45									
46	47	47	47	48	48									
47	49	50	50	50	50	50								
48		52	52	52	52	53	53							
49		54	54	55	55	56	56							
50		56	56	57	58	59	61	62						
51			59	60	61	61	63	65						
52			63	64	64	64	65	67						
53			66	67	67	68	68	69	71					
54				69	70	70	71	71	73					
55				72	74	74	74	75	77	78				
56					76	78	78	79	81	83				
57					80	82	82	82	84	88	92			
58						84	86	86	88	93	96	101		
59						87	90	90	92	96	100	103	104	
60					91		95	95	97	101	105	108	109	111
61							99	100	101	105	108	112	113	116
62							104	105	106	109	113	115	117	118
63								110	110	112	116	117	119	120
64								114	115	117	119	120	122	123
65								118	120	121	122	123	125	126
66									124	124	125	128	129	130
67									128	130	131	133	133	135
68									131	133	135	136	138	138
69										135	137	138	140	142
70										136	138	140	142	144
71										138	140	142	144	145

Prepared by Bird T. Baldwin, Ph.D., and Thomas D. Wood, M. D.

HEIGHTS AND WEIGHTS OF 136,504 WOMEN FIFTEEN OR MORE YEARS OF AGE (WITH CLOTHES)[1]

Age	Graded average Weight in Pounds with Clothes — Feet and Inches with Shoes																
	4–8	4–9	4–10	4–11	5–0	5–1	5–2	5–3	5–4	5–5	5–6	5–7	5–8	5–9	5–10	5–11	6–0
15	101	103	105	106	107	109	112	115	118	122	126	130	134	138	142	147	152
16	102	104	106	108	109	111	114	117	120	124	128	132	136	139	143	148	153
17	103	105	107	109	111	113	116	119	122	125	129	133	137	140	144	149	154
18	104	106	108	110	112	114	117	120	123	126	130	134	138	141	145	150	155
19	105	107	109	111	113	115	118	121	124	127	131	135	139	142	146	151	155
20	106	108	110	112	114	116	119	122	125	128	132	136	140	143	147	151	156
21	107	109	111	113	115	117	120	123	126	129	133	137	141	144	148	152	156
22	107	109	111	113	115	117	120	123	126	129	133	137	141	145	149	153	157
23	108	110	112	114	116	118	121	124	127	130	134	138	142	146	150	153	157
24	109	111	113	115	117	119	121	124	127	130	134	138	142	146	150	154	158
25	109	111	113	115	117	119	121	124	128	131	135	139	143	147	151	154	158
26	110	112	114	116	118	120	122	125	128	131	135	139	143	147	151	155	159
27	110	112	114	116	118	120	122	125	129	132	136	140	144	148	152	155	159
28	111	113	115	117	119	121	123	126	130	133	137	141	145	149	153	156	160
29	111	113	115	117	119	121	123	126	130	133	137	141	145	149	153	156	160
30	112	114	116	118	120	122	124	127	131	134	138	142	146	150	154	157	161
31	113	115	117	119	121	123	125	128	132	135	139	143	147	151	154	157	161
32	113	115	117	119	121	123	125	128	132	136	140	144	148	152	155	158	162
33	114	116	118	120	122	124	126	129	133	137	141	145	149	153	156	159	162
34	115	117	119	121	123	125	127	130	134	138	142	146	150	154	157	160	163
35	115	117	119	121	123	125	127	130	134	138	142	146	150	154	157	160	163
36	116	118	120	122	124	126	128	131	135	139	143	147	151	155	158	161	164
37	116	118	120	122	124	126	129	132	136	140	144	148	152	156	159	162	165
38	117	119	121	123	125	127	130	133	137	141	145	149	153	157	160	163	166
39	118	120	122	124	126	128	131	134	138	142	146	150	154	158	161	164	167
40	119	121	123	125	127	129	132	135	138	142	146	150	154	158	161	164	167
41	120	122	124	126	128	130	133	136	139	143	147	151	155	159	162	165	168
42	120	122	124	126	128	130	133	136	139	143	147	151	155	159	162	166	169
43	121	122	125	127	129	131	134	137	140	144	148	152	156	160	163	167	170
44	122	124	126	128	130	132	135	138	141	145	149	153	157	161	164	168	171
45	122	124	126	128	130	132	135	138	141	145	149	153	157	161	164	168	171
46	123	125	127	129	131	133	136	139	142	146	150	154	158	162	165	169	172
47	123	125	127	129	131	133	136	139	142	146	151	155	159	163	166	170	173
48	124	126	128	130	132	134	137	140	143	147	152	156	160	164	167	171	174
49	124	126	128	130	132	134	137	140	143	147	152	156	161	165	168	172	175
50	125	127	129	131	133	135	138	141	144	148	152	156	161	165	169	173	176
51	125	127	129	131	133	135	138	141	144	148	152	157	162	166	170	174	177
52	125	127	129	131	133	135	138	141	144	148	152	157	162	166	170	174	177
53	125	127	129	131	133	135	138	141	144	148	152	157	162	166	170	174	177
54	125	127	129	131	133	135	138	141	144	148	153	158	163	167	172	174	177
55	125	127	129	131	133	135	138	141	144	148	153	158	163	167	171	174	177

[1] Association of Life Insurance Directors and Actuarial Society of America, New York, 1912 p. 67. Published by a committee. Allow 1½ inches for shoes and 6 pounds for clothes.

HEIGHTS AND WEIGHTS OF 224,819 MEN FIFTEEN OR MORE YEARS OF AGE (WITH CLOTHES)[1]

Age	Graded Average Weight in Pounds with Clothes — Feet and Inches with Shoes																	
	5–0	5–1	5–2	5–3	5–4	5–5	5–6	5–7	5–8	5–9	5–10	5–11	6–0	6–1	6–2	6–3	6–4	6–5
15	107	109	112	115	118	122	126	130	134	138	142	147	152	157	162	167	172	177
16	109	111	114	117	120	124	128	132	136	140	144	149	154	159	164	169	174	179
17	111	113	116	119	122	126	130	134	138	142	146	151	156	161	166	171	176	181
18	113	115	118	121	124	128	132	136	140	144	148	153	158	163	168	173	178	183
19	115	117	120	123	126	130	134	138	142	146	150	15ʳ	160	165	170	175	180	185
20	117	119	122	125	128	132	136	140	144	148	152	156	161	166	171	176	181	186
21	118	120	123	126	130	134	138	141	145	149	153	157	162	167	172	177	182	187
22	119	121	124	127	131	135	139	142	146	150	154	158	163	168	173	178	183	188
23	120	122	125	128	132	136	140	143	147	151	155	159	164	169	175	180	185	190
24	121	123	126	129	133	137	141	144	148	152	156	160	165	171	177	182	187	192
25	122	124	126	129	133	137	141	145	149	153	157	162	167	173	179	184	189	194
26	123	125	127	130	134	138	142	146	150	154	158	163	168	174	180	186	191	196
27	124	126	128	131	134	138	142	146	150	154	158	163	169	175	181	187	192	197
28	125	127	129	132	135	139	143	147	151	155	159	164	170	176	182	188	193	198
29	126	128	130	133	136	140	144	148	152	156	160	165	171	177	183	189	194	199
30	126	128	130	133	136	140	144	148	152	156	161	166	172	178	184	190	196	201
31	127	129	131	134	137	141	145	149	153	157	162	167	173	179	185	191	197	202
32	12⁷	129	131	134	137	141	145	149	154	158	163	168	174	180	186	192	198	203
33	127	129	131	134	137	141	145	149	154	159	164	169	175	181	187	193	199	204
34	128	130	132	135	138	142	146	150	155	160	165	170	176	182	188	194	200	206
35	128	130	132	135	138	142	146	150	155	160	165	170	176	182	189	195	201	207
36	129	131	133	136	139	143	147	151	156	161	166	171	177	183	190	196	202	208
37	129	131	133	136	140	144	148	152	157	162	167	172	178	184	191	197	203	209
38	130	132	134	137	140	144	148	152	157	162	167	173	179	185	192	198	204	210
39	130	132	134	137	140	144	148	152	157	162	167	1⁷3	179	185	192	199	205	211
40	131	133	135	138	141	145	149	153	158	163	168	174	180	186	193	200	206	212
41	131	133	135	138	141	145	149	153	158	163	168	174	180	186	193	200	207	213
42	132	134	136	139	142	146	150	154	159	164	169	175	181	187	194	201	208	214
43	132	134	136	139	142	146	150	154	159	164	169	175	181	187	194	201	208	214
44	133	135	137	140	143	147	151	155	160	165	170	176	182	188	195	202	209	215
45	133	135	137	140	143	147	151	155	160	165	170	176	182	188	195	202	209	215
46	134	136	138	141	144	148	152	156	161	166	171	177	183	189	196	203	210	216
47	134	136	138	141	144	148	152	156	161	167	171	177	183	190	197	204	211	217
48	134	136	138	141	144	148	152	156	161	166	171	177	183	190	197	204	211	217
49	134	136	138	141	144	148	152	156	161	166	171	177	183	190	197	204	211	217
50	134	136	138	141	144	148	152	156	161	166	171	177	183	190	197	204	211	217
51	135	137	139	142	145	149	153	157	162	167	172	178	184	191	198	205	212	218
52	135	137	139	142	145	149	153	157	162	167	172	178	184	191	198	205	212	218
53	135	137	139	142	145	149	153	157	162	167	172	178	184	191	198	205	212	218
54	125	137	139	142	145	149	153	158	163	168	173	178	184	191	198	205	212	219
55	135	137	139	142	145	149	153	158	163	168	173	178	184	191	198	205	212	219

[1] Association of Life Insurance Directors and Actuarial Society of America, New York, 1912, p. 38. Published by a committee. Allow 1 inch for shoes and 10 pounds for clothes.

DETERMINATION OF BASAL ENERGY REQUIREMENTS*

THE DuBOIS NORMAL STANDARDS† AS MODIFIED BY BOOTHBY AND SANDIFORD (FROM THE MAYO CLINIC), PRELIM. REPORT, AM. J. PHYSIOL., **90**: 291, 1929

Calories per Square Meter per Day

Age	Males	Females	Age	Males	Females
5..........	1272	1238	20–24	984	886
6..........	1265	1217	25–29	967	878
7..........	1248	1162	30–34	955	869
8..........	1229	1154	35–39	931	859
9..........	1210	1126	40–44	919	847
10..........	1188	1099	45–49	907	840
11..........	1166	1070	50–54	893	828
12..........	1147	1042	55–59	878	818
13..........	1130	1028	60–64	864	811
14..........	1109	984	65–69	847	802
15..........	1087	950	70–74	(835)	(787)
16..........	1073	924	75–79	(820)	(775)
17..........	1049	898			
18..........	1030	895			
19..........	1010	892			

* From Frances Stern: Applied Dietetics, Williams and Wilkins, Baltimore, 1936, p. 105.

† For convenience the calories for the day have been used, rather than calories per hour, as in the original table.

To determine the basal requirements, use the Body Surface Chart (Table 2 in Chapter I of this book). Refer to table above, using the age (nearest birthday) and sex; read the calories needed per square meter per day; multiply the surface area by this figure. (To determine the surface area of children use the Hannon Nomogram, Fig. 3, p. 9.) The result is the Basal Energy Requirement in calories per day for the average person of this height, weight, age, and sex.

INDEX

Edema in pneumonia, 317
in pregnancy, treatment, 342
in pregnant diabetics, 867
in tetany, 204
inflammatory, in gout, 631
malnutrition, 311
minerals in, 249
of pituitary origin, 313
of portal obstruction, 310
protein as affecting, 84
pulmonary, in beriberi, 427
subcutaneous, effect on urine
volume, 291
treatment, 307
wasting and, 505
Edestin, cystine and methionine
contents, 107
effect on fatty livers, 151
Education in diabetes, juvenile,
892
Effort, effect on blood glucose, 66
mental, effect on metabolism,
2
physical, effect on metabolism,
2
Effusions in avitaminosis C, 462
joint, in gout, 631
synovial, in gout, 639
Egg albumin, cystine and methionine contents, 107
effect on rickets, 409
extrinsic factor in, 355
vitamin A in, 396
D in, 406
white, flavin in, 452
in mercury poisoning, 339
injury factor, 478
syndrome, 474
yolk, biotin in, 474
Eicosapentenoic acid, 138
Elaidic acid in fat studies, 143
in lipid disposition, 165
Electrocardiogram, effect of vitamin D, 411
in beriberi, 429
in hyperparathyroidism, 194
in myxedema, 236
in nephritis, 332
in tetany, 204
Electroencephalogram, effect of
thiamin, 432
Electrolyte balance, effect of adrenalectomy, 66
in diabetes, 721
in diuresis, 306
kidney in, 285
diffusibility, 272
equilibrium, disturbances, 298
water in, 270
exchange, measurement, 300
excretion, 289, 292
in dehydration, 264
in diabetes insipidus, 290
inactivation by proteins, 277
patterns of gastro-intestinal secretions, 284
of ingested substances, 284
Electroneutrality in kidney function, 292
Embden ester in carbohydrate
decomposition, 43
Emboli, intracranial, hypoglycemia and, 781
Emotion, disturbances, in beriberi, 428
effect in toxic goiter, 241
on basal metabolism, 4, 11
on blood glucose, 66
on liver glycogen formation,
31

Emotion, effect on simple goiter,
233
glycosuria in, 29, 696
gout and, 637
instability in hyperinsulinism,
657
upset in insulin reaction, 777
Emphysema, hypercalcemia in,
185
Emulsification of fat, 142
Enamel, effect of avitaminosis A,
394
hypoplasia in hypoparathyroidism, 217
mottled, 218
Encephalitis, diabetes insipidus
and, 680
hyperinsulinism and, 660
Encephalography, effect on diabetes insipidus, 687
Enchondromata, multiple, hyperparathyroidism and, 200
Endocrine glands, 56
ablation, effect on carbohydrate metabolism, 70
amino acid requirement, 92
control of carbohydrate metabolism, 55
of metabolism, scheme, 69
diabetes in childhood and,
874
disease, from overeating, 529
effect on acid-base balance,
313
on carbohydrate metabo-
lism, 23, 655
on glucose tolerance, 26
on insulin action, 768
on water metabolism, 313
glycosuria in, 29
obesity and, 586
weight gain in, 513
in diabetes, 700, 717, 718, 725
in glucose tolerance test, 743
in glycogen disease, 598
in metabolism, 1
insulin and, 854, 855
imbalance in diabetes in childhood, 878
system, integration by anterior
pituitary, 57
interdependence, 57
iodine in, 229
obesity from, 513, 576
vitamin E and, 369
Enema, glucose, absorbability, 21
in ketosis, 822
Energy balance in obesity, 514,
523. See also Basal
metabolism.
treatment, 561
exchange in obesity, 536
expenditure for physical work
2
for work, 1
in toxic goiter, 241
from ketolysis, 163
from ketone oxidation, 162
lactic acid and, 44
metabolism, control, 1
needs, individual, 523
of children, 883
of heart action, 50
output in obesity, 561
production of muscle, 41
requirements, 504
computation, 505
fat deposition and, 164
in obesity, 528
reserve, fat as, 139

Energy source, 56
supply of muscle, 49
Enterokinase, 89
Environment in diabetes, 788
internal, constancy, 55
water and, 271
Enzymes, amino acid catabolism,
96
diastatic, 20
function, 478
hexokinase, yeast, 41
in body fluids, 275
in deamination of amino acids,
99
in fat hydrolysis, 141
in oxidation of purine nucleotides, 613
intestinal, 21
nucleolytic, 615
oxidizing, 45
pancreatic, 21
phosphatase, 38
function, 174
phosphorylase, 38
protein nature, 92
proteolytic, gastric, 87
intracellular, 93
pancreas, intestine, 87
respiratory, riboflavin and, 450
Warburg's, 46
synthesis, 90
thiamine as, 422
transaminating, 101, 103
yellow, 452
Ephedrine, effect on serum potassium, 266
in insulin allergy, 784
Epidermophytosis in diabetes,
724, 802, 843
in diabetic gangrene, 797
in obesity, 585
Epiglottis, tophi in, 626
Epilepsy, hyperinsulinism and,
660, 673
hypomagnesemia in, 222
insulin reaction and, 779
Epinephrine, amino acid relationship, 114
effect on basal metabolism, 11,
13
on blood phosphorus, 187
on carbohydrate metabolism,
64
on glycogen, 598
on insulin need, 776
on liver glycogen formation, 31
on potassium, 251
on serum potassium, 266
on uric acid excretion, 617
from tyrosine, 115
glycosuria from, 29, 748
in adrenal crisis, 262
in diuresis, 313. See also Adrenal glands.
in hyperinsulinism, 673, 675
in hypoglycemia, 782, 893
in insulin allergy, 784
in ketosis, 822
test in glycogen disease, 599
Epiphysis, separation, in avitaminosis C, 463
Episcleritis in gout, 646
Epistaxis in avitaminosis C, 464
Epithelium, effect of vitamin A,
393, 394
Epulis in hyperparathyroidism,
193
Equilibria, osmotic, 272
Erb's phenomenon in latent tetany, 414